WITHDRAWN

Safety with Lasers and Other Optical Sources

A Comprehensive Handbook

Safety with Lasers and Other Optical Sources

A Comprehensive Handbook

DAVID SLINEY
U.S. Army Environmental Hygiene Agency
Aberdeen Proving Ground, Maryland

and

MYRON WOLBARSHT
Duke University Medical Center
Durham, North Carolina

PLENUM PRESS · NEW YORK AND LONDON

Library of Congress Cataloging in Publication Data

Sliney, David.
  Safety with lasers and other optical sources.

  Includes bibliographical references and indexes.
  1. Lasers—Safety measures. 2. Lasers—Physiological effect. 3. Light—Physiological effect. 4. Electric lamps—Safety measures. 5. Electric welding—Safety measures. I. Wolbarsht, Myron, joint author. II. Title. [DNLM: 1. Lasers—Adverse effects—handbooks. 2. Ultraviolet rays—Adverse effects—Handbooks. 3. Infrared rays—Adverse effects—Handbooks. 5. Radiation protection—Handbooks. WN650 S633s]
TA1677.S44   621.36′6   80-16591
ISBN 0-306-40434-6

First Printing — July 1980
Second Printing — August 1981
Third Printing — March 1982

© 1980 Plenum Press, New York
A Division of Plenum Publishing Corporation
233 Spring Street, New York, N.Y. 10013

All rights reserved

No part of this book may be reproduced, stored in a retrieval system, or transmitted, in any form or by any means, electronic, mechanical, photocopying, microfilming, recording, or otherwise, without written permission from the Publisher

Printed in the United States of America

Dedication

To the Memory of

Walter J. Geeraets, M.D.
27 September 1922 - 14 September 1977

H. Christian Zweng, M.D.
27 August 1922 - 26 August 1977

They both were pioneers in the field of laser effects on the retina. Although often at odds with each other, their combined influence transformed an art into a science. Their loss within a single month is deeply felt by all.

Preface

Nearly a decade ago a general review article on the evaluation of optical radiation hazards was published in *Applied Optics* (Sliney and Freasier, 1973). This article received many favorable comments but also prompted many inquiries regarding specific optical hazard problems. From this it became evident that a monograph rather than a supplemental and expanded article was needed to fill this literature gap relating to laser and optical radiation hazards. The present work is designed to fill that gap, and is structured to permit either classroom or self-study use. Much of the material in this book was developed in connection with short courses on laser safety and radiometry in which we have participated, as well as from our previous articles. In particular, the sequence of chapters is based upon the experiences which we have had in lecturing in courses with different schedules. One of the great difficulties in developing a text of this nature is that a broad, multidisciplinary background must be included in order that the reader can comprehend all of the subject matter readily. For this reason, the material presented on anatomy and physiology is oriented toward the engineer or physical scientist, while the review material on basic optical physics is intended more for the physician or life scientist.

The 1973 article by Sliney and Freasier in *Applied Optics* began with an excerpt from a much earlier work by Verhoeff, Bell, and Walker (1916) on the subject of optical radiation hazards. The earlier authors were concerned at that time with unwarranted fears of lamps. It seems appropriate to repeat that passage here also:

> "These relations have generally been left quite out of reckoning in discussing the subject, with the result of leading to vague and quite unwarranted conclusions as irrelevant as if one should condemn steam heating as dangerous because one can burn his finger upon a radiator."

Nevertheless, there are hazards to the eye and skin from lasers and certain modern lamps. These hazards should be known and understood by users and equipment designers. Our book is an attempt to place all of these hazards in perspective. It is divided into several sections. Chapter 1 is a broad sketch of laser safety. Chapters 2 and 3 provide background material in optics and biology which may be skipped by the more advanced reader. Chapters 4 through 6 present the biological effects of optical radiation. Chapters 7 through 10 discuss various aspects of safety standards. Chapters 11 through 14 cover radiometric measurements. Chapters 15 through 20 are concerned with laser safety, while Chapters 22 through 24 follow the same approach for non-coherent optical sources. Chapters 25 through 28 cover other general subjects of interest relating to safety with lasers and other optical sources. In this connection we owe a special note of thanks to J. Smith for contributing Chapter 25 on Safety Programs.

The collection of information, examples, and technical data for a work of this size would have been impossible without the aid and suggestions of many other past and present colleagues, in particular the permanent staff at the US Army Environmental Hygiene Agency: James K. Franks, Terry L. Lyon, Wesley J. Marshall, Darius L. Crews, and Nicholas P. Krial; and two associates of Dr. Wolbarsht, M. B. Landers, III and Henry G. Wagner. Many others have aided in providing insight into the problems discussed in this text: William T. Ham, Jr., H. A. Mueller, R. T. Wangemann, R. H. Duguid, W. H. Parr, B. Tengroth, F. Harlan, F. Hillenkamp, T. J. White, D. Berger, J. A. Parrish, E. A. Beatrice, B. Stuck, D. J. Lund, R. Allen, J. Marshall, R. C. Honey, A. Vassiliadis, R. McCutchen, J. Hinrichs, F. Urbach, R. Watson, J. A. Hathaway, R. J. Rockwell, J. Smith, D. Edmunds, E. Sutter, R. Landry, I. Matelsky, F. A. Anderson, D. L. McCarthey, M. J. Suess, W. Gibbons, C. E. Moss, and W. Murray. Two former associates of Mr. Sliney's deserve particular note: Benjamin C. Freasier of Lyon, Australia, and Frank C. Bason, of Silkeborg, Denmark. We are especially grateful to those who typed the drafts and the final copy of the text: Carol Sliney, Nancy Miller, Linda Westwick, Ida L. Sliney, and Karen Huntley.

We have borrowed liberally from Governmental reports for the text. We have endeavored to cite the sources in most cases. Many of the drawings were from the US Army's TB MED 279, a technical bulletin on "The Control of Hazards to Health from Laser Radiation."

In preparing this text we have been constantly concerned with accuracy, since a misinterpretation by the reader, or the use of incorrect data, could result in a serious problem or even a hazard. We have endeavored to produce an accurate text; nevertheless, the reader is cautioned to apply the safety data and exposure limits with great care. We would greatly welcome information about errors or suggestions for improvement of a possible future edition.

Fallston, Maryland; Durham, North Carolina
15 December 1979

REFERENCES

Sliney, D. H. and Freasier, B. C., 1973, Evaluation of optical radiation hazards, *Appl. Opt.* **12**: 1-23.
Verhoeff, F., Bell, L., and Walker, C. B., 1916, The pathological effects of radiant energy on the eye: an experimental investigation with a systematic review of the literature, *Proc. Am. Acad. Arts Sci.* **51**:630-818.

The opinions or assertions contained herein are the private views of the authors and are not to be construed as reflecting the views of the Department of the Army or the Department of Defense.

Contents

Chapter 1   **INTRODUCTION TO LASER SAFETY**
- 1.1   Introduction 1
- 1.2   Laser Hazards 3
  - 1.2.1   Skin Hazards 4
  - 1.2.2   Electrical Hazards 5
  - 1.2.3   Chemical and Associated Hazards 5
  - 1.2.4   Miscellaneous Ancillary Hazards 6
- 1.3   Laser Hazard Analysis and Control 6
- 1.4   Laser Classification 7
- 1.5   Safety Precautions 8
  - 1.5.1   Class I Controls 8
  - 1.5.2   Class II Controls 8
  - 1.5.3   Class III Controls 8
  - 1.5.4   Class IV Controls 9
  - 1.5.5   Applying the Safety Procedures 10
- 1.6   Laser Eye Protection 10
- 1.7   Non-Laser Sources 10
- 1.8   Review Questions 11
- 1.9   References 11

Chapter 2   **REVIEW OF OPTICAL PHYSICS**
- 2.1   Introduction 13
- 2.2   Wave Motion 13
- 2.3   The Electromagnetic Spectrum 14
- 2.4   Wave-Particle Duality 15
- 2.5   The Wave Picture of Radiation 16
- 2.6   The Particle Picture of Radiation 17
- 2.7   Interaction of Electromagnetic Radiation with Matter 19

	2.8	Interaction at an Interface. 21
		2.8.1 Specular and Diffuse Reflection 21
		2.8.2 Specular Reflection Formulas. 23
		2.8.3 Refraction. 23
	2.9	Interaction with a Medium 25
		2.9.1 Transmission. 25
		2.9.2 Absorption 26
	2.10	Interference and Diffraction Effects 29
		2.10.1 Interference. 29
		2.10.2 Diffraction 30
		2.10.3 Scattering 32
	2.11	Sources of Radiation. 33
	2.12	Molecular and Atomic Transitions. 34
	2.13	Incandescent Sources 38
	2.14	The Laser 39
		2.14.1 Lasing Medium 39
		2.14.2 Pumping System 40
		2.14.3 Optical Cavity 41
		2.14.4 Laser Operation. 41
		2.14.5 Types of Lasers 42
		2.14.6 Temporal Modes of Operation. 42
		2.14.7 Spatial (TEM) Modes. 46
		2.14.8 Longitudinal Modes. 47
		2.14.9 Beam Diameter 47
		2.14.10 Beam Divergence. 50
		2.14.11 Hot Spots 51
	2.15	Characteristics of Light Sources, Coherent and Incoherent. . 51
		2.15.1 Properties of Coherent and Incoherent Light Sources 51
		2.15.2 Spatial Coherence 53
		2.15.3 Temporal Coherence of Monochromaticity. 54
		2.15.4 Speckle 54
	2.16	Radiometric and Photometric Terms and Units. 54
		2.16.1 Radiometric Terms 55
		2.16.2 Describing Source Output 55
		2.16.2.1 Irradiation of a Surface 55
		2.16.3 Photometric Analogues of Radiometric Terms . . . 58
		2.16.3.1 Brightness 60
		2.16.3.2 Intensity 60
	2.17	Review Questions 60
	2.18	References. 62
Chapter 3	**REVIEW OF ANATOMY AND PHYSIOLOGY OF THE EYE AND SKIN**	
	3.1	Introduction 65
	3.2	The Eye. 65

Contents xi

	3.2.1	The Structure of the Eye.	65
		3.2.1.1 General	65
		3.2.1.2 The Cornea	67
		3.2.1.3 The Aqueous	67
		3.2.1.4 The Iris	69
		3.2.1.5 The Lens	70
		3.2.1.6 The Vitreous Body	71
		3.2.1.7 The Retina	71
		3.2.1.8 The Choroid	76
		3.2.1.9 The Sclera	76
	3.2.2	Refractive Power of the Eye	76
	3.2.3	The Standard Eye	77
	3.2.4	Image Formation and Accommodation	77
		3.2.4.1 Defects in Image Formation	78
		3.2.4.2 Chromatic Aberration	78
	3.2.5	Ocular Performance and Minimal Image Size	81
	3.2.6	Retinal Function and Organization	84
		3.2.6.1 Lateral Organization of the Retina	84
		3.2.6.2 Spectral Sensitivity to Light	86
		3.2.6.3 Visual Sensitivity in the UV and Near Infrared	87
		3.2.6.4 Spectral Characteristics of the Ocular Media	87
		3.2.6.5 Retinal Processing	89
		3.2.6.6 Eye Movements	91
		3.2.6.7 Dark Adaptation	92
		3.2.6.8 The Visual Field	92
3.3	The Skin		93
	3.3.1	Anatomy	93
	3.3.2	Optical Properties	96
	3.3.3	Body Heat Regulation	97
3.4	Review Questions		97
3.5	References		98
	3.5.1	General References: Eye	98
	3.5.2	General References: Skin	99
	3.5.3	Specific References	99

Chapter 4 **EFFECTS OF OPTICAL RADIATION ON THE EYE**
4.1	Introduction		101
4.2	Determining Thresholds		102
4.3	The Effects of Different Optical Spectral Bands		103
	4.3.1	Retinal Injury	103
	4.3.2	Injury to the Anterior Portion of the Eye	104
4.4	Ultraviolet Radiation Effects		108
	4.4.1	Photochemical Injury	108
	4.4.2	Effects Upon the Retina	108

	4.4.3	Effects Upon the Cornea	109
	4.4.4	Lenticular Effects	112
	4.4.5	Effects on the Iris	116
4.5	The Retinal Hazard Region (400-1400 nm)		116
	4.5.1	Background	116
	4.5.2	Determining the Retinal Exposure	117
		4.5.2.1 Pupil Size	117
		4.5.2.2 Spectral Transmission of the Ocular Medium	119
		4.5.2.3 Spectral Absorption by the Retina and Choroid	120
		4.5.2.4 Optical Image Quality	121
	4.5.3	Small Images	124
	4.5.4	Retinal Pigment Epithelium Absorption	126
	4.5.5	Chorioretinal Thermal Injury	128
	4.5.6	The Effect of Retinal Image Size	130
	4.5.7	The Effect of Pulse Duration	130
	4.5.8	Location of Retinal Burns	133
	4.5.9	Very Long Exposure Durations	134
	4.5.10	Large Temporary Changes in Visual Sensitivity; Flashblindness	138
	4.5.11	Discomfort Glare	141
	4.5.12	Veiling Glare	141
	4.5.13	Flashing Lights	142
	4.5.14	Injuries to the Iris at Retinal Hazard Power Levels	143
4.6	Infrared Radiation and the Eye		144
	4.6.1	Infrared Spectral Bands	144
	4.6.2	Infrared Cataract	144
	4.6.3	Infrared Radiation and the Cornea	147
4.7	Uncertainties		149
4.8	Review Questions		149
4.9	References		151

Chapter 5   **OPTICAL RADIATION HAZARDS TO THE SKIN**

5.1	Introduction		161
5.2	Thermal Injury		162
	5.2.1	Critical Temperatures	162
	5.2.2	Dependence Upon Exposure Duration	162
	5.2.3	Penetration Depth	163
	5.2.4	Reflection	164
	5.2.5	The Warmth Sensation and Heat Flow	166
5.3	Laser Injury Thresholds for the Skin		167
	5.3.1	Thermal Injury	167
	5.3.2	Delayed Effects	169
5.4	Ambient Environment and Heat Stress		169
5.5	Ultraviolet Radiation Effects on the Skin		170

Contents   xiii

		5.5.1 Ultraviolet Erythema.........................170

            5.5.1   Ultraviolet Erythema.........................170
            5.5.2   Delayed Effects............................175
    5.6   Photosensitivity and Photoallergy......................176
    5.7   Phototherapy...176
    5.8   Review Questions....................................180
    5.9   References...181

Chapter 6   OPTICAL HAZARDS FROM THE AMBIENT ENVIRONMENT
    6.1   Introduction...187
    6.2   Sunburn..188
    6.3   Skin Effects from Chronic Exposure....................189
    6.4   Corneal Effects......................................199
    6.5   Snow Blindness......................................200
    6.6   Solar Retinitis.......................................201
            6.6.1   A New Understanding......................201
            6.6.2   Retinal Irradiance.........................201
            6.6.3   Clinical Reports...........................202
            6.6.4   Damage Mechanisms......................203
            6.6.5   Optically Aided Viewing...................206
            6.6.6   Safety in Viewing the Sun..................207
    6.7   Reflected Sunlight and the Eye.........................207
    6.8   Sunlight and Cataract................................210
    6.9   Sunlight and Heat Stress..............................211
    6.10   Conclusions...211
    6.11   Review Questions....................................212
    6.12   References..212

Chapter 7   LASER SAFETY STANDARDS: EVOLUTION AND RATIONALE
    7.1   Introduction...217
    7.2   Historical Development...............................218
            7.2.1   Early History of Exposure Limits............218
            7.2.2   The ANSI Z-136 Development..............220
            7.2.3   Historical Development of Hazard Classification..221
                      7.2.3.1   High-Power Lasers—Class IV Limits....221
                      7.2.3.2   Medium-Power Lasers—Class III Limits.222
                      7.2.3.3   Low-Power Lasers—Class II Limits....222
                      7.2.3.4   Class I Limits......................223
                      7.2.3.5   Class III Limits for CW Lasers........224
                      7.2.3.6   Class V.........................225
                      7.2.3.7   ANSI Changes in 1976..............226
    7.3   Exposure Limits.....................................226
            7.3.1   The Concept of Threshold..................227
            7.3.2   The Safety Factor and Probit Plots...........229
            7.3.3   Means of Determining Thresholds of Injury.....235
                      7.3.3.1   Direct Observation.................235
                      7.3.3.2   Histological Studies................236

		7.3.3.3	Histochemical Studies of Laser Injury..236
		7.3.3.4	Electrophysiological Studies .... .237
		7.3.3.5	Behavioral Studies................237
	7.3.4	Limiting Apertures 241
		7.3.4.1	The 1-mm Aperture...............241
		7.3.4.2	The 11-mm Aperture..............241
		7.3.4.3	The 7-mm Aperture...............241
	7.3.5	Spectral Dependence of Exposure Limits 242
	7.3.6	Repetitively Pulsed Laser Exposure............244
	7.3.7	Special Use Restrictions 244
7.4	Present Standards 244
	7.4.1	Local and State Regulations 246
	7.4.2	Present Federal Standards...................246
	7.4.3	Foreign National Standards..................248
	7.4.4	International Standards.....................248
7.5	Future Trends...................................248
	7.5.1	Delayed Effects...........................251
	7.5.2	Injury Mechanisms 252
7.6	References......................................255
7.7	Review Questions 259

Chapter 8 **CURRENT LASER EXPOSURE LIMITS**

8.1	Introduction 261	
8.2	Present Exposure Limits 263	
	8.2.1	Commonality of Limits.....................263
	8.2.2	Limiting Apertures 268
	8.2.3	Correction Factors A and B (C_A and C_B) for Eye Exposure................................268
	8.2.4	Repetitively Pulsed Lasers...................269
8.3	Point Source or Extended Source? 271	
	8.3.1	Dual Limits in the Retinal Hazard Region.......271
	8.3.2	Alpha Min (α_{min}) 272
8.4	Spectral Correction Factors (C_A and C_B) 273	
8.5	Restrictions on EL's 273	
8.6	Repetitively Pulsed Lasers..........................273	
8.7	Using the Tables and Figures.........................274	
	8.7.1	Step 1 274
	8.7.2	Step 2 276
	8.7.3	Step 3 276
	8.7.4	Step 4 277
8.8	Examples.......................................277	
	8.8.1	Calculate or Determine the Exposure Limits for the Skin and the Eye for a 20-ns Pulsed Ruby Laser (Wavelength of 694.3 nm) 277
	8.8.2	Determine the Exposure Limits for a TEA Laser Which Has a Pulse Duration of 1 μs (10^{-6} s) and a Wavelength of 10.6 μm....................278

Contents   xv

		8.8.3	Determine the EL's for an Erbium Q-Switched Laser Operating at 1.54 μm with a 20-ns Pulse ..278

        8.8.4   Determine the EL for a Gallium-Arsenide Laser Operating at a PRF of 100 Hz at a Wavelength Varying Between 905 and 910 nm with 100-ns Pulses 278

        8.8.5   Determine the Exposure Limit for a Helium-Neon Laser (632.8 nm) which is Chopped to Produce 1-ms Pulses at a Frequency of 50 Hz..........281

8.9   Future Developments 282
8.10 Review Questions 282
8.11 References..283

Chapter 9 LASER HAZARD CLASSIFICATION

9.1 Introduction 285
9.2 Differences Between ANSI and BRH Laser Classification Schemes 286
9.3 The BRH Performance Standard for Laser Products 287
    9.3.1   General Concepts 287
    9.3.2   The Importance of the BRH Regulation 287
    9.3.3   Accessible Emission Limits 288
    9.3.4   Laser Products Versus Laser Systems 294
    9.3.5   Tests for Compliance......................294
    9.3.6   Performance Standards 296
    9.3.7   User Information.........................304
    9.3.8   Servicing and Maintenance 305
    9.3.9   Applicability of the BRH Standard 305
    9.3.10 Reporting and Record Keeping Requirements....307
    9.3.11 Specific Purpose Laser Products 308
    9.3.12 The Definition of Accessibility 309
9.4 Practical Examples 311
    9.4.1   Example 1...............................312
    9.4.2   Example 2...............................313
    9.4.3   Example 3...............................313
    9.4.4   Example 4...............................314
    9.4.5   Example 5...............................315
    9.4.6   Example 6...............................316
    9.4.7   Example 7...............................318
    9.4.8   Example 8...............................319
9.5 Conclusions......................................322
9.6 Review Questions 323
9.7 References.......................................323

Chapter 10 PROTECTION STANDARDS FOR NON-LASER SOURCES

10.1 Introduction 325
10.2 Criteria for Broad-Band Sources 326

10.3		Ultraviolet Radiation Criteria 327
	10.3.1	General 327
	10.3.2	The AMA Standard 328
	10.3.3	The Development of the Envelope UV Hazard Criteria 328
	10.3.4	Applying the Ultraviolet Standard. 332
	10.3.5	UV-A Exposure Limits .333
10.4		Visible Radiation Criteria 335
10.5		Applying the Tentative Guidelines of USAEHA and ACGIH. 336
	10.5.1	The Retinal Hazard Functions. 336
	10.5.2	Retinal Thermal Hazard Evaluation. 339
	10.5.3	Retinal Blue Light Hazard Evaluation 340
	10.5.4	IR-A Hazard Analysis 341
10.6		ANSI Efforts. 341
10.7		BRH Standards 341
10.8		Infrared Standards. 342
10.9		Conclusion 342
10.10		Review Questions 343
10.11		References. 343

Chapter 11 **LASER OUTPUT MEASUREMENTS: RADIOMETRY AND CALORIMETRY**

11.1		Introduction 347
11.2		Rationale for Measurement. 347
11.3		Laser Parameters to Measure 349
11.4		Measuring Output Beam Radiant Exposure or Irradiance . .349
11.5		Types of Radiometric Instruments 352
11.6		Detectors. 353
	11.6.1	Thermal Detectors. 353
	11.6.2	Quantum Detectors. 359
	11.6.3	Specifying Detectors 361
	11.6.4	Detectors to Resolve Short Pulses 366
11.7		Safety Meters 368
11.8		Calibration: The Standard Source or the Standard Detector 368
	11.8.1	Spectroradiometric Standards 369
	11.8.2	Electrical Substitution Method 370
	11.8.3	Broad-Band Calibration. 370
	11.8.4	Acceptance Angle and Surface Uniformity 371
	11.8.5	Calibration Techniques .372
11.9		Background Filtering. 372
11.10		Measurement Technique Pitfalls 374
	11.10.1	Sources of Difficulty. 374
	11.10.2	A Checklist for Good Measurements 375

Contents   xvii

	11.11	The Meaning of Accuracy and Precision 378
	11.12	Conclusions......................................379
	11.13	Review Questions 379
	11.14	References.......................................380

Chapter 12 LASER BEAM DIAGNOSTICS
- 12.1 Introduction 385
- 12.2 The Simplified Laser Beam 386
- 12.3 Beam Irradiance Versus Range 387
  - 12.3.1 Circular Beam 387
  - 12.3.2 Non-circular Beams........................388
  - 12.3.3 Irregular Beam Profiles 389
- 12.4 Hazard Distance 389
- 12.5 The Gaussian Beam Profile 392
- 12.6 Measuring the Beam Diameter....................392
  - 12.6.1 By Eye 393
  - 12.6.2 The Aperture Method 394
  - 12.6.3 The Ribbon Method 395
  - 12.6.4 The Knife Edge Method 396
  - 12.6.5 The Ronchi Ruling Method...............397
  - 12.6.6 The Photographic Methods 400
  - 12.6.7 Using Damage Profiles....................404
- 12.7 Calculating the Transmitted Power Through an Aperture Stop 404
- 12.8 Gaussian Beam Wavefronts 406
  - 12.8.1 Beam Divergence and Diameter............407
  - 12.8.2 Gaussian Beam Front Radius of Curvature 409
  - 12.8.3 Focused Gaussian Beam 409
- 12.9 Laser Beam Collimators.........................411
- 12.10 Plane Wavefronts...............................411
- 12.11 Review Questions 412
- 12.12 References....................................413

Chapter 13 ATMOSPHERIC PROPAGATION OF LASER BEAMS
- 13.1 General 415
- 13.2 Atmospheric Attenuation 415
  - 13.2.1 Scattering 415
  - 13.2.2 Absorption 421
  - 13.2.3 Measuring Atmospheric Attenuation.........421
- 13.3 Atmospheric Turbulence........................422
  - 13.3.1 Irradiance Fluctuations...................422
  - 13.3.2 Projected Laser Radiance 427
  - 13.3.3 Radiance Profiles........................428
  - 13.3.4 The Influence of Collection Aperture Size 429
  - 13.3.5 The Influence of Beam Path Height Above Ground 429

		13.3.6	Conceptual Arguments 430

- 13.4 Probabilities of Retinal Injury. 430
- 13.5 Atmospheric Turbulence and IR-C Laser Beams 431
- 13.6 The Propagation of Very High Power Laser Beams 431
- 13.7 Conclusions. 431
- 13.8 Review Questions 433
- 13.9 Demonstration 434
- 13.10 References. 435

Chapter 14 RADIOMETRIC MEASUREMENTS REQUIRED FOR BROAD-BAND OPTICAL SOURCES

- 14.1 Introduction 439
- 14.2 Required Radiometric Data. 439
  - 14.2.1 Spectral Irradiance 440
  - 14.2.2 Spectral Radiance 440
  - 14.2.3 Source Size 440
  - 14.2.4 Range Data 440
- 14.3 Evaluation of Line Spectral Emission 441
- 14.4 Spectral Histograms. 443
- 14.5 Biological Weighting of Spectroradiometric Data 444
- 14.6 The Monochromator Slit Function, and Stray Light 445
- 14.7 Radiance Distribution 450
- 14.8 Direct Reading Instruments. 451
  - 14.8.1 The NIOSH UV Meters .452
  - 14.8.2 Earlier Direct Reading Instruments 456
  - 14.8.3 The Outlook 456
- 14.9 Problems Associated with Measurements 456
  - 14.9.1 Stray Light 457
  - 14.9.2 Source Size 462
  - 14.9.3 Wavelength Measurements. 464
  - 14.9.4 Infrared Measurement Problems 464
  - 14.9.5 Spectroradiometric Standards. 464
- 14.10 Calculation of Blackbody and Tungsten Sources. 466
- 14.11 Computer Program Data Base 466
- 14.12 Review Questions 466
- 14.13 References. 467

Chapter 15 GENERAL HAZARD ANALYSIS AND CONTROLS

- 15.1 Introduction 471
- 15.2 The Laser's Hazard Potentials-System Safety 473
  - 15.2.1 Hazard Classification. 473
  - 15.2.2 General Concepts of System Safety. 473
- 15.3 Laser System Design 475
  - 15.3.1 Interlocks 476
  - 15.3.2 Manual Switches 476
  - 15.3.3 The Enclosure 477

	15.3.4	Accidental Laser Firing......477
	15.3.5	Safe Laser Projectors......477
	15.3.6	Multiple Wavelengths......480
	15.3.7	Mode Locking......481
	15.3.8	Beam Hotspots......482
15.4	The Population Potentially at Risk......483
	15.4.1	Age, Experience, and Frequency of Exposure...483
	15.4.2	Exposure Duration-Intentional vs. Non-Intentional Exposure......485
	15.4.3	Photo-Sensitive Individuals......486
15.5	Environmental Considerations-Reflections and the Probability of Exposure......486
	15.5.1	Reflections......487
	15.5.2	Probability of Exposure......488
	15.5.3	Diffuse Reflection Hazards......489
	15.5.4	Specular vs. Diffuse Reflections......491
	15.5.5	Retroreflection......493
	15.5.6	Calculations of Specular Reflection......495
	15.5.7	Diffuse Reflection......498
	15.5.8	Reflectance......500
15.6	Optically Aided Viewing......501
15.7	Scanning Laser Beam......506
	15.7.1	Linear Scans......506
	15.7.2	Lissajous Scans......507
15.8	Laser Accidents......508
15.9	General Control Measures......510
	15.9.1	Engineering Controls, Personnel Protection and Administrative Control......510
	15.9.2	Control Measures for Very High Power Lasers...511
	15.9.3	The Choice of Control Measures......513
	15.9.4	Class 4 Laser Controls......513
	15.9.5	Precautions for Class 3 Medium Risk Laser Systems......514
		15.9.5.1 Indoor Operations......514
		15.9.5.2 Authorized Operators......514
		15.9.5.3 Outdoor Operations......515
		15.9.5.4 Ancillary Hazard Controls......516
15.10	Conclusions......516
15.11	Review Questions......517
15.12	General References......518
15.13	Some Laser Accident References......519

Chapter 16 **EYE AND SKIN PROTECTION**

16.1	Introduction......521	
16.2	Applications......521	
16.3	Laser Viewing Enhancement Goggles......523	

	16.4	Parameters of Laser Eye Protection. 523
		16.4.1 Wavelength 523
		16.4.2 Optical Density 524
		16.4.3 Visual Transmittance of Eyewear 525
		16.4.4 Laser Filter Damage Threshold (Maximum Irradiance). 525
		16.4.5 Filter Curvature. 528
	16.5	Methods of Construction. 528
	16.6	Selecting Appropriate Eyewear Step-By-Step 531
		16.6.1 Step 1 531
		16.6.2 Step 2 531
		16.6.3 Selecting the Most Suitable Eye Protector. 533
	16.7	Commercial Sources of Laser Eye Protection 536
	16.8	Eye Protection for Infrared Lasers .536
	16.9	Testing Laser Eye Protection. 538
		16.9.1 Routine User Tests 538
		16.9.2 Testing Optical Density. .538
		16.9.3 Environmental Tests 540
		16.9.4 Tests of Translucent Side Shields or Frames 540
	16.10	Marking of Eye Protectors. 541
	16.11	Eye Protection For Pump Lamps and Tunable Wavelength Lasers 542
	16.12	Polarizing Filters 542
	16.13	Dynamic Eye Protection Devices. .543
	16.14	Image Converter Tubes 543
	16.15	Eye Protection Filters for Solar Radiation 548
	16.16	Proper Fit 552
	16.17	Skin Protective Agents for Ultraviolet Radiation (Sunscreens) 552
	16.18	Design Specifications for Laser Protective Eyewear. 554
	16.19	Protective Shields and Protective Garments. 555
		16.19.1 Window Ports 555
		16.19.2 Area Shields and Large Windows. 556
		16.19.3 Protective Garments 557
	16.20	Future Developments 558
	16.21	Review Questions 559
	16.22	References. 560

Chapter 17 **LASER SAFETY IN RESEARCH LABORATORIES AND MEDICAL FACILITIES**

	17.1	Introduction 563
	17.2	Hazard Evaluation of New Lasers .564
	17.3	Pump Lamps and Gas Discharge Tubes 564
	17.4	Beam Paths 566
	17.5	Diffuse Reflections and Beam Traps 568
	17.6	Control Measures for Open Beam Paths. 571

Contents

17.7	Controlled Entry	572
17.8	Standard Operating Procedures	573
17.9	Temporary Beam Enclosures	574
17.10	Very High Power CW Lasers	575
17.11	Associated Hazards	575
17.12	Safety Aspects of Lasers in Medicine	576
	17.12.1 Laser Surgical Facilities	577
	17.12.2 Laser Retinal Photocoagulators	581
17.13	Laser Diagnostic Equipment in Medicine	583
17.14	Laser Surveys	585
17.15	Review Questions	588
17.16	References	589

Chapter 18 SAFETY WITH LASERS USED IN CONSTRUCTION

18.1	Introduction	591
18.2	Protection Standards for Construction Lasers	593
18.3	Hazard Classification	596
	18.3.1 Class 1 Systems	596
	18.3.2 Class 2 Systems	596
	18.3.3 Class 3 Systems	596
18.4	Distance Measurement Laser Systems	598
18.5	Control Measures for Visible Class 3 CW Lasers Used for Surveying Alignment and Leveling	600
18.6	Weighing the Risks	604
18.7	Typical Laser Products	604
18.8	Review Questions	604
18.9	References	607

Chapter 19 SAFETY WITH LASERS USED IN MANUFACTURING

19.1	Introduction	609
19.2	Neodymium:YAG Laser Material Processing	610
	19.2.1 Viewing Optics	611
	19.2.2 Enclosures	612
	19.2.3 Reflections	613
19.3	High-Power CO_2 Laser Cutting and Welding Equipment (1 kW to 20 kW)	614
19.4	Lasers in the Printing Industry	617
19.5	Ancillary Hazards	618
	19.5.1 Noise Hazards	618
	19.5.2 Airborne Contaminants	618
19.6	Nondestructive Testing	620
19.7	Review Questions	621
19.8	References	623

Chapter 20 LASER SAFETY WITH CONSUMER AND OFFICE PRODUCTS

20.1	Introduction	625

	20.2	Laser Displays and Laser Art...........................625
		20.2.1 Lasers in Science Exhibits...................626
		20.2.2 Holographic Displays........................627
		20.2.3 Sound and Light Shows......................627
		20.2.4 Regulations and Standards for Laser Light Shows...................................631
		20.2.5 Laser Beams in the Airspace.................634
		20.2.6 The Speckle Pattern and Laser Displays.......635
		20.2.7 Raster Scanned Laser Displays...............635
		20.2.8 Demonstration Lasers in the Classroom.......641
	20.3	Laser Point-of-Sale Terminals.........................641
	20.4	Lasers in Office Machines............................644
	20.5	Laser Optical Fiber Transmission Systems..............645
	20.6	Laser Cane for the Blind.............................648
		20.6.1 General Characteristics......................648
		20.6.2 Beam Divergence...........................649
		20.6.3 Beam Irradiance............................650
		20.6.4 Projected Radiance.........................651
		20.6.5 Hazard Analysis............................652
	20.7	Review Questions....................................652
	20.8	References..653

Chapter 21 **LASER HAZARDS IN OUTDOOR APPLICATIONS: MILITARY AND LIDAR**

	21.1	Introduction..655
	21.2	Ocular Exposure Conditions..........................655
	21.3	Laser Hazard Analysis and Controls...................657
	21.4	Direct Beam Exposure................................659
	21.5	Reflected Beam Exposure.............................659
		21.5.1 Diffuse Reflections.........................661
		21.5.2 Specular Reflections........................661
		21.5.2.1 Standing Water.................662
		21.5.2.2 Snow..........................663
		21.5.2.3 Ice............................663
		21.5.2.4 Water-Covered Ice...............663
		21.5.2.5 Glass Windows and View Blocks....663
	21.6	Scanning Lasers.....................................664
	21.7	Extended Sources...................................668
	21.8	Optical Viewing Instruments..........................669
	21.9	Laser Range Controls................................670
		21.9.1 Hazardous Range (NOHD)...................670
		21.9.1.1 Caution Range....................671
		21.9.2 Backstops.................................672
		21.9.3 Buffer Zones...............................673
		21.9.4 Laser Range Safety Fan (LRSF).............673

| | | 21.9.4.1 | Hazardous Diffuse Reflection Area...674 |
| | | 21.9.4.2 | Hazardous Area....................674 |

- 21.9.5 Airborne Laser Controls 674
- 21.9.6 Eye Protection 677
- 21.9.7 Limitations on Targets 677
- 21.9.8 Laser Maintenance Tests 677
- 21.9.9 Medical Surveillance 679
- 21.10 Operational Use of Laser Systems......................679
- 21.11 Viewing Probability..................................679
- 21.12 Training Mode.......................................680
- 21.13 Conclusions About Military Laser Safety 681
- 21.14 Laser Aiming Devices 681
- 21.15 Open-Air Communications Links 682
- 21.16 LIDAR 682
- 21.17 Environmental Impact.................................684
- 21.18 Examples...685
- 21.19 Review Questions 689
- 21.20 References...690

Chapter 22 LAMPS AND LIGHTING SYSTEMS

- 22.1 Introduction 693
- 22.2 Lighting Terminology 694
- 22.3 Types of Lamps and Light Sources 695
  - 22.3.1 Incandescent Sources 695
  - 22.3.2 Low-Pressure Gaseous Discharge Lamps 703
  - 22.3.3 Fluorescent Lamps 703
  - 22.3.4 High Intensity Discharge (HID) Lamps 705
    - 22.3.4.1 Mercury Lamps....................705
    - 22.3.4.2 High-Pressure Sodium Lamps 707
    - 22.3.4.3 Metal Halide Lamps...............708
  - 22.3.5 Short-Arc Lamps............................709
  - 22.3.6 Carbon-Arc Sources.........................711
  - 22.3.7 Electroluminescent Lamps, Radioactive Sources, and Light-Emitting Diodes 714
  - 22.3.8 Flashlamps and Flashbulbs 715
- 22.4 Hazard Evaluation of a Lamp Source 716
  - 22.4.1 Preliminary Evaluation 716
  - 22.4.2 Required Data.............................721
  - 22.4.3 Hazard Evaluation Using the Proposed Army/ACGIH Criteria........................723
  - 22.4.4 The Sliney-Freasier Method for Retinal Hazard Evaluation.................................724
  - 22.4.5 Evaluating Blackbody Sources..............728
- 22.5 Protection and Control Measures for Broad-Band Optical Sources 733

22.5.1 Control Measures for Ultraviolet Sources-
Germicidal Lamps....................734
22.5.2 Phototherapy Lamps and Sunlamps..........736
22.5.3 "Black Light" Lamps.....................739
22.5.4 Ultraviolet Curing Equipment...............742
22.5.5 Office Copying Machines and Graphic Arts
Lighting.............................744
22.5.6 CRT Displays and Control Measures for Glare
from Visible Sources......................746
22.5.7 Hospital Light Sources...................747
22.5.8 Photographic Flashbulbs..................749
22.5.9 HID Lamps..........................752
22.5.10 Infrared and Light-Emitting Diodes..........753
22.5.11 Industrial and Home Baking Applications......755
22.5.12 Infrared Sources in Hospitals...............756
22.6 Concept of a Lamp Safety Standard for High-Intensity
Sources.....................................756
22.7 Review Questions..............................757
22.8 References...................................758

Chapter 23 PROJECTION SYSTEMS
23.1 Introduction..................................763
23.2 Projection Optics...............................763
23.3 Projected Radiance.............................767
23.4 Evaluating a Projection System.......................770
23.5 Examples of Specific Projectors.....................773
23.5.1 Example 1: Tungsten-Halogen Lamp
Spotlight............................773
23.5.2 Example 2: Xenon-Short-Arc Searchlight.....775
23.5.3 Example 3: Emergency-Vehicle Lights.......779
23.5.4 Example 4: Slide Projector................780
23.5.5 Example 5: Infrared Heat Gun.............781
23.5.6 Example 6: Eye Movement Recorder........784
23.6 Searchlight Safety Measures.......................786
23.7 Opthalmic Instruments...........................786
23.7.1 Diagnostic Instruments...................786
23.7.2 Operating Room Instruments...............787
23.8 Solar Simulators...............................789
23.8.1 Solar Simulator in Dermatology.............789
23.8.2 Aerospace Solar Simulators................790
23.9 Hazards from Solar Furnaces and Solar Power Facilities...791
23.10 Review Questions..............................797
23.11 References...................................799

Chapter 24 WELDING ARCS
24.1 Introduction..................................801

24.2	Welding Arc Characteristics................................802	
	24.2.1 Types of Welding Arcs Processes.............802	
	24.2.1.1 The Carbon-Arc....................804	
	24.2.1.2 The Shielded Metal Arc............804	
	24.2.1.3 The Gas Tungsten Arc.............806	
	24.2.1.4 Gas Metal Arc Welding 806	
	24.2.1.5 Flux Cored Arc Welding 808	
	24.2.1.6 The Plasma Arc...................808	
	24.2.2 Arc Size and Temperature Profile 809	
	24.2.3 Optical Radiation Emitted from Welding Arcs ..811	
24.3	Hazards to the Skin..827	
24.4	Eye Hazards 828	
	24.4.1 Corneal Injuries............................828	
	24.4.2 Retinal Injuries from Welding Arcs 830	
	24.4.3 A Case Report............................830	
24.5	Epidemiological Studies 832	
24.6	First Aid 833	
24.7	Evaluating Welding Operations 834	
24.8	Welding Hazard Index.....................................834	
24.9	Engineering Protective Measures 836	
24.10	Welding Eye and Face Protection 841	
24.11	Protective Clothing for Welders..............................847	
24.12	Recommendations for Future Protective Filter/Curtain Requirements 847	
	24.12.1 Welding Filter Plates 847	
	24.12.2 Welding Filter Curtains 849	
24.13	Flames and Molten Metal 850	
	24.13.1 Potential Hazards 850	
	24.13.2 Infrared Protection Measures for Heavy Industry 852	
24.14	Review Questions...855	
24.15	References..855	

Chapter 25 **SAFETY PROGRAMS AND FORMAL TRAINING
by JAMES SMITH, IBM**

25.1	Introduction 861
25.2	Laser Safety Program 861
25.3	Training Objectives/Considerations 862
25.4	Training..863
	25.4.1 Area Workers Training.....................863
	25.4.2 Laser Workers Training....................864
	25.4.3 Management Training 864
	25.4.4 Laser Safety Officer Training 865
25.5	Example Programs..866
	25.5.1 Comprehensive Expandable Classroom Program .867
	25.5.2 Movie-Tape/Slide Program..................870

		25.5.3	Computer-Assisted Instruction (CAI) 872
	25.6	Audio/Visual Sources 876
	25.7	Summary. 876
	25.8	References. 877

Chapter 26 MEDICAL SURVEILLANCE

- 26.1 Introduction 879
  - 26.1.1 Monitoring Related to Occupation 879
  - 26.1.2 Personnel Evaluation. 880
  - 26.1.3 Health Evaluation 880
  - 26.1.4 Medical-Legal 880
- 26.2 Rationale of Medical Examinations for Laser Workers 881
- 26.3 Types of Routine Eye Examination Protocols. 881
  - 26.3.1 Fundus 881
  - 26.3.2 Functional Examinations and Documentation . .883
  - 26.3.3 Anterior Portion of the Eye 886
- 26.4 Guidelines for the Examination of Laser Accident Victims 886
  - 26.4.1 External Examination-Lids, Brows, Cheek and Nose 886
  - 26.4.2 Corneal Involvement (only following either an ultraviolet or infrared C laser exposure) 886
  - 26.4.3 Lens 887
  - 26.4.4 Iris. 887
  - 26.4.5 Vitreous 887
  - 26.4.6 Retina. 887
- 26.5 Changes in Standards for Medical Surveillance 888
- 26.6 Case Histories 893
- 26.7 Conclusions. 895
- 26.8 Review Questions 895
- 26.9 References. 897

Chapter 27 ANCILLARY HAZARDS

- 27.1 Introduction 899
- 27.2 Common High Power Lasers and Their Applications. 900
- 27.3 Airborne Contaminants. 900
  - 27.3.1 Contaminant Concentrations. 900
  - 27.3.2 Removal by Ventilation 902
  - 27.3.3 Contaminant Detection. 903
  - 27.3.4 Respiratory Protective Devices 904
  - 27.3.5 Skin Hazards. 904
  - 27.3.6 Asbestos 907
- 27.4 Fire Hazards 907
- 27.5 Radiation Hazards. 908
- 27.6 Cryogenic Hazards. 909
- 27.7 Noise Hazards 909

	27.8	Review Questions 910
	27.9	References......................................912

Chapter 28 ELECTRICAL HAZARDS
- 28.1 Introduction 913
- 28.2 Electrical Accidents...............................913
  - 28.2.1 A Near Accident 914
  - 28.2.2 Severe Accidental Shocks 914
  - 28.2.3 Electrocutions............................915
- 28.3 Physiological Effects of Electric Shock................916
  - 28.3.1 Current Magnitude 916
  - 28.3.2 Frequency Effect 918
  - 28.3.3 Ventricular Fibrillation....................919
- 28.4 The Dangerous Electrical Supplies....................919
- 28.5 Regulations, Standards and Standard Operating Procedures (SOPs)................................920
- 28.6 Safety Guidelines to Prevent Electrical Shock..........920
- 28.7 First Aid for Severe Shock Victims...................924
- 28.8 Review Questions 925
- 28.9 References......................................925

Appendix A TERMS AND UNITS OF MEASURE—THE INTERNATIONAL SYSTEM OF UNITS (SI)
- A.1 The Three Classes of Units in the SI 929
- A.2 Base Units of the SI..............................930
- A.3 Supplementary Units..............................930
- A.4 Conversion Factors and Constants....................935
  - A.4.1 Useful Physical Constants 935
  - A.4.2 Useful Mathematical Constants..............935
  - A.4.3 Useful Conversion Factors..................935
  - A.4.4 Speed 941
  - A.4.5 Temperature Conversion Formulas 941
  - A.4.6 Optical Units............................941
- A.5 Mathematical Symbols 944
- A.6 Nomenclature for Radiation Dosimetry 945

Appendix B THE HUMAN EYE
- B.1 The Standard Eye 947
- B.2 Spectral Weighting Program for Eye Hazard Computations.947
- B.3 Transmission Through the Eye 959

Appendix C LASER WAVELENGTHS AND CHARACTERISTICS..........961

Appendix D LIST OF CAPITAL LETTER ABBREVIATIONS..............967

Appendix E	HAZARD CLASSIFICATION OF SOME REPRESENTATIVE PRE - 1976 LASERS	973
Appendix F	COPY MACHINE CHARACTERISTICS	983
Appendix G	GLOSSARY OF TERMS USED IN WELDING AND BIOLOGY	987
Appendix H	SOURCES OF US GOVERNMENT PUBLICATIONS	997
Appendix I	HAMMER SAFETY	999
	AUTHOR INDEX	1003
	SUBJECT INDEX	1025

Chapter 1
Introduction to Laser Safety

1.1 INTRODUCTION

Despite the fact that the laser was only first developed in 1960, it has found many uses in industry and other aspects of human endeavor. During this period the hazards, particularly to the eye, were revealed, and subsequently much biological research was performed to delineate these hazards. By 1968 some national safety guides, written mostly for voluntary compliance rather than governmental regulations, were being used in the field of laser safety. By 1973 a national consensus standard written by the American National Standards Institute (ANSI Z-136) had evolved which became the basis of the present Federal regulations of the Bureau of Radiological Health (BRH) and draft Occupational Safety and Health Administration (OSHA) standards for control of health hazards from laser radiation.

As the eye is often far more vulnerable to injury than the skin from visible and near-infrared laser radiation, it is considered the organ most important to protect from all wavelengths of laser radiation. The increased hazard to the eye from visible and near-infrared lasers is a consequence of the eye's imaging process. As shown in Fig. 1-1, parallel rays of visible light from a distant object, or from a laser at any distance, can be imaged on the retina in a very small area. This focusing effect of the cornea and lens of the eye will concentrate these rays by an enormous factor— 100,000 times. Such a concentration of radiant power can cause the retina to be burned in much the same way that a piece of paper can be set ablaze when a magnifying glass focuses the rays of the sun.

Although the sun is very distant and its rays are nearly collimated by the time they reach the earth the image of the sun upon the retina of the human eye is 160 μm in diameter. This is still ten times the diameter of an image upon the retina produced by the nearly parallel rays from a laser source. The brightness of a laser source exceeds all known natural and man-made light sources. For instance, the brightness

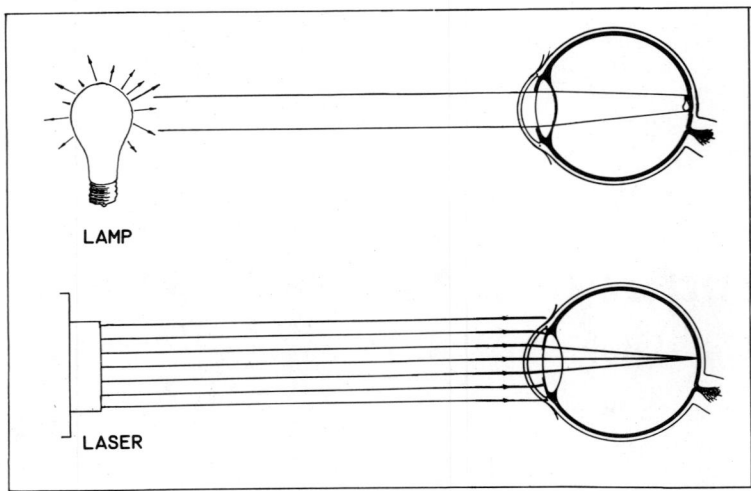

Figure 1-1. A 1-W visible laser beam represents a far greater hazard to the retina than a 100-W light bulb. The brightness of the collimated beam is more than one billion times greater than the light bulb.

of the sun or a xenon-arc lamp. The concentration of light falling upon the retina is dependent upon the brightness of the object being viewed.

Almost all types of lasers operating in the visible and near-infrared regions of the spectrum are so bright as to be hazardous to the eye. The exceptions are some very small, lower power semiconductor lasers which emit only a few microwatts of optical power. For this reason the safety measures necessary for controlling laser hazards normally concentrate upon making the beam path inaccessible, such as enclosing the laser in a box or controlled room to prevent access.

Until 1965 the only commonly available commercial lasers were helium-neon and ruby lasers. This resulted in simplified early guidelines for safe use of these lasers, which tended to place all lasers into only one, or at most, two safety categories. As more varieties of lasers evolved and the numbers of applications increased, it became necessary to make distinctions in the preparation of safety rules. It is now generally commonly accepted practice to consider all laser equipment under at least four classes. Hazard classes serve several purposes. Simplified and well-differentiated hazard control procedures can be listed for each class. Hazard classification of a laser product by the manufacturer enables the user to apply the proper set of safety rules. Product safety regulations use the same classification to specify the safety features required of the manufacturer depending upon the relative hazard of the laser product. Also, any medical surveillance or requirements for licensing operators can be easily indicated and based on the degree of hazard presented by the laser type.

Introduction to Laser Safety

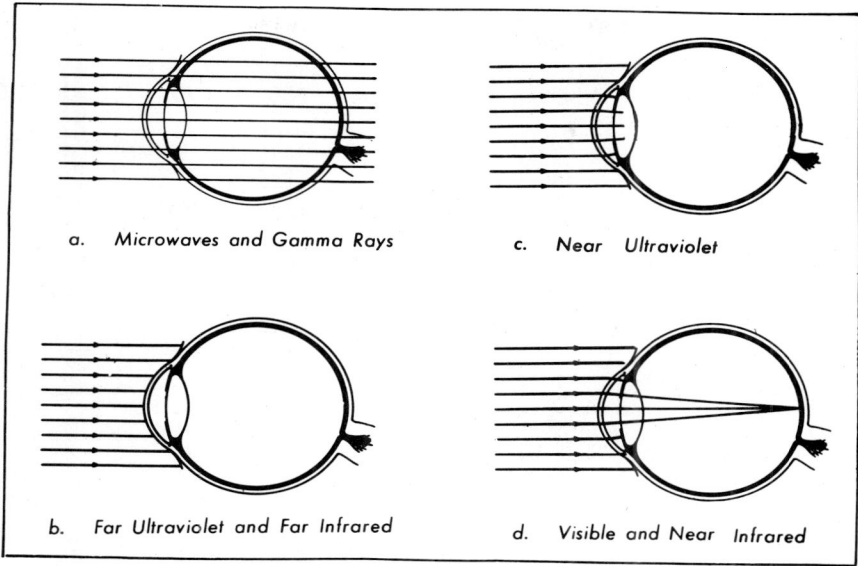

Figure 1-2. Schematic diagram of the absorption of electromagnetic radiation in the eye.

1.2 LASER HAZARDS

The hazards from laser equipment may best be grouped into four hazard categories: optical radiation hazards to the eye and skin; chemical hazards; electrical hazards; and casualty hazards. The type of potential injury depends upon the hazard.

Eye hazards are by far the most important. Different structures of the eye may be injured depending upon which structure absorbs the greatest radiant energy per volume of tissue. For instance, even though the greatest fraction of neodymium laser radiation is absorbed in the anterior optical structures of the eye, such as the cornea, lens and vitreous, the site of injury from a pulsed neodymium laser is the retina because the radiant energy absorbed per volume of tissue is much higher in that tissue. Retinal effects can be expected to occur when the laser wavelength is within the visible and near-infrared (IR-A) spectral regions (roughly between 400 and 1400 nm). The minimum image size on the retina of a highly-collimated laser beam depends upon the wavelength within this retinal hazard region only to a minor extent. The major factor, of course, is whether the eye is relaxed, i.e., imaged at infinity, or accommodated, i.e., imaged at a near object. Non-collimated beams or those that have been spread by reflection from a diffusing surface are of less importance.

As shown in Fig. 1-2, the retina is not very vulnerable if the laser radiation is

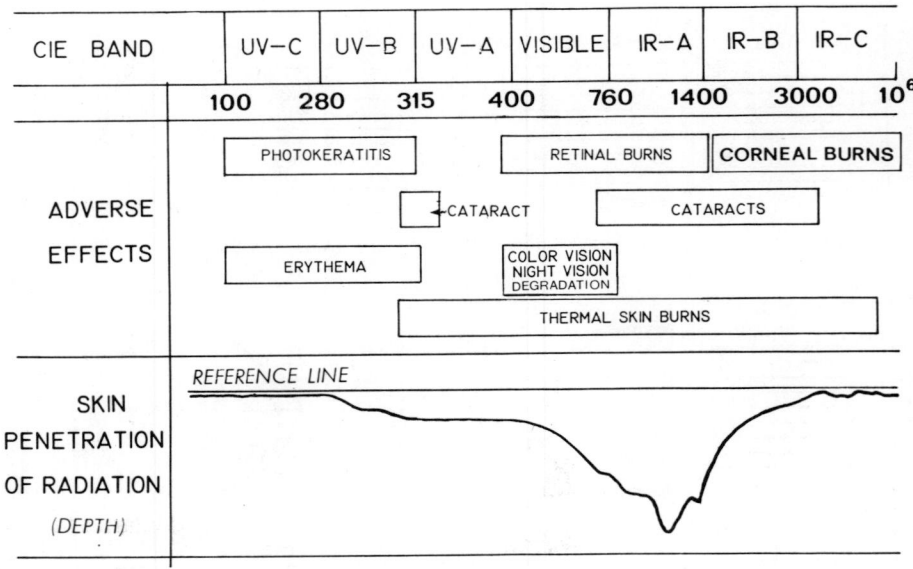

Figure 1-3. The International Commission on Illumination (CIE) divides the optical spectrum into seven spectral bands. Most biologic effects are limited to two or three spectral bands.

in the ultraviolet or far-infrared portions of the spectrum. This type of radiation is absorbed in the anterior portion of the eye, normally in the cornea or the lens. High exposure levels may permanently damage the cornea or lens. Intermediate levels in the UV cause greater injury of the cornea, which is severe but temporary. Even though it only lasts for one to two days, this type of injury to the cornea is an extremely painful experience, as can be attested to by anyone who has experienced snow blindness or its industrial counterpart, welder's flash. Both of these effects are known to the physician as ultraviolet photokeratitis and result from excessive exposure to the so-called "actinic" ultraviolet radiation (200-320 nm). In describing the biologic effects of optical radiation, the optical spectrum is often divided into spectral bands, as shown in Fig. 1-3. Chapter 4 will discuss laser effects upon the eye in greater detail.

1.2.1 Skin Hazards

Injury to the skin is far less likely than injury to the eye unless one is working with very high-powered lasers and protects only the eye. Skin injury is normally not possible with low power and medium power lasers. The levels of visible and infrared radiation required to cause injury to the skin are quite high, at least several watts-per-square-centimeter (W/cm^2) and depend not only upon the area of the skin absorbing the laser radiation but also upon the wavelength, the absorption depth (Fig. 1-3) and exposure duration.

The skin shares with the cornea a particular susceptibility to injury in the actinic ultraviolet spectral region (200-320 nm). This type of radiation causes sunburn and has also been indicted as the cause of many types of skin cancer. Instead of exposure levels of several watts-per-square-centimeter required to cause thermal injury, exposure levels of only microwatts-per-square-centimeter delivered over several hours are required to cause ultraviolet erythema (sunburn). Except for the ultraviolet spectral region laser radiation exposure is believed to cause only a thermal injury to the skin.

One other effect should be noted before leaving the subject of skin hazards. The sensitivity of the skin is greatly increased by certain photosensitizing chemicals and by previous exposure to specific wavelength bands (generally in the near-ultraviolet and visible portion of the spectrum). The light-sensitizing substances can occur in the skin as a result of disease states such as xeroderma pigmentosum, lupus erythematosus and herpes simplex. Other photosensitizing chemicals which reach the skin either directly from contact, or indirectly through oral administration include certain fungicides, plants and plant extracts, and the pitch and bacteriostatic agents, such as hexachlorophene, used in soaps. Some orally administered drugs such as tetracyclines are also known to cause photosensitization. Chapter 5 will discuss the effects of optical radiation upon the skin in greater detail.

1.2.2 Electrical Hazards

At least four individuals in the United States have been electrocuted from carelessness while working around high-voltage laser power supplies. Almost all laser power supplies have the potential of causing severe electrical shock and possibly resulting in electrocution. The safety standards for electrical safety should be followed when using any electrical or electronic equipment. Usually serious electrical hazards exist with the higher powered lasers used in material processing applications or with "breadboard" lasers in research laboratories. Chapter 28 of this book is devoted to electrical hazards.

1.2.3 Chemical and Associated Hazards

Many highly explosive and highly toxic materials have been used in laser research laboratories. Often potentially hazardous airborne contaminants are released into the atmosphere during laser material processing, as a very high laser beam irradiance incident upon a target can cause vaporization of this material. Laser welding or cutting of metals will form many of the same metal oxides and other fumes which are encountered in the environment of conventional welding activities. Good practice in industrial hygiene is to ensure that the general ventilation is adequate or to specify local exhaust ventilation. These and other environmental health subjects are discussed in Chapter 27.

Liquid nitrogen and other cryogenic fluids are utilized in cooling systems of certain lasers. Two examples are high-powered gallium-arsenide laser arrays and solid state ruby lasers operating in the continuous wave (CW) mode which are pumped continuously by a high intensity lamp. When cryogenic fluids evaporate they displace breatheable oxygen. As a result, cryogenic fluids should be used only in areas of good general ventilation. Other safety hazards associated with cryogenic fluids include explosions when ice collects in valves or connectors. This is most usual when the hardware is not specifically designed to operate with cryogenic materials. The more hazardous cryogenic fluids, liquid oxygen and liquid hydrogen, are less commonly used. Nevertheless, liquid oxygen, which is a serious fire or explosion hazard, often collects in open dewar flasks of liquid nitrogen, since the condensation temperature of liquid oxygen is some 13° higher than the boiling point of liquid nitrogen.

Both protective clothing and face shields are normally used when working with large quantities of liquid nitrogen. However, the quantities of liquid nitrogen used in cooling the infrared-sensitive detectors commonly used with infrared laser radiation are so small that they are not serious health hazards. There are a number of safety procedures that are required in using gas cannisters and in using cryogenic dewar flasks that must be followed to prevent serious accidents.

1.2.4 Miscellaneous Ancillary Hazards

The wide variety of equipment used in conjunction with lasers often have associated safety problems. Occasionally, special types of lasers pose some special health hazards. For example, X rays may be produced from high-voltage vacuum tubes used in laser power supplies or from electric-discharge lasers. Normally sufficient radiation shielding is installed around these high voltage (> 15 kV) components in commercial power supplies to prevent the leakage of potentially hazardous levels of x radiation.

Fire hazards may exist in and around some laser operations, but are normally limited to combustion of flammable materials such as paper by CW lasers which operate with an output power above one-half watt (0.5 W). Fire extinguishers should be kept around such lasers, and flammable materials should be kept out of the beam path.

Occasionally there is a noise hazard resulting from gas dynamic laser exhausts or from high-power pulsed laser discharges. The noise hazard may originate from electrical components such as high capacitance condensers producing impulse noises which exceed 140 dBA (the exposure limit for impulse noise). Impulse noises may also be associated with the very high energy pulsed discharges in TEA lasers. Hearing protection should be required for all individuals who may be exposed to these very high level noise levels.

1.3 LASER HAZARD ANALYSIS AND CONTROL

The safety procedures necessary for any laser operation vary with three aspects: (1) the *laser hazard classification;* (2) the *environment* where the laser is used and (3) the *people* operating or within the vicinity of the laser beam. The safety procedures are best presented by relating them to the laser hazard classification. The detailed safety procedures and laser hazard classifications will be presented in subsequent chapters. However, for the purpose of an introduction some general procedures can be presented along with a brief explanation of the commonly used hazard classification system. Hazard classification schemes differ only slightly depending upon which standard is being followed. All laser safety standards have a common overall concept.

1.4 LASER CLASSIFICATION

The lowest powered lasers are usually called "Class I" or "Exempt" lasers. This group is normally limited to gallium-arsenide lasers or certain enclosed lasers. These lasers are not considered hazardous even if the output laser beam can be collected by 80-mm collecting optics and concentrated into the pupil of the eye, or as in the case of an infrared or ultraviolet laser, if the radiation at its maximum possible concentration on the skin or eye will not cause injury at the maximum exposure duration possible during one day of laser operation. It is not surprising that most lasers by themselves do not fall into the Class I category. However, when lasers are incorporated into consumer or office machine equipment the resulting system often is Class I. If a Class I system contains a more dangerous laser, the access panel to it must contain a warning to alert the user of the hazardous laser radiation that will be encountered if the panel is removed. An outside panel covering the warning sign (which must be removed before the primary access panel is removed) is often permitted to give the illusion that nothing dangerous is inside the system to avoid unwarrented concern by the occasional user.

Class II lasers, often termed "Low-Power" or "Low-Risk" laser systems, are those lasers which are only hazardous if the viewer overcomes his or her natural aversion response to bright light and continuously stares into the source. Needless to say, such an event is considered remote. It could just as readily occur as blinding oneself by forcing oneself to stare at the sun for more than 10 to 20 seconds. Nevertheless, since this hazard, although rare, is as real as eclipse blindness, Class II lasers should have a caution label affixed to indicate that the individual should not purposefully stare into the laser.

Class III "Moderate Risk" or "Medium-Power" laser systems are those which can cause injury within the natural aversion response time, i.e., faster than the blink reflex (0.25 s). However, they are not capable of causing serious skin injury or hazardous diffuse reflections under normal use. These must have danger labels and the safety precautions required are often considerable.

Laser systems which are "High Power" and present a "High Risk" of injury and can cause combustion of flammable materials are in Class IV. They may also cause diffuse reflections that are eye hazards and may also cause serious skin injury from direct exposure. A more restrictive warning label is required and even more restrictive control measures are necessary for these lasers.

1.5 SAFETY PRECAUTIONS

The safety rules accompanying the above classifications can be summarized as follows.

1.5.1 Class I Controls

No user safety rules are necessary.

1.5.2 Class II Controls

a. Never permit a person to continuously stare into the laser source if exposure levels exceed the applicable permissible exposure level for the duration of intended staring.
b. Never point the laser at an individual's eye unless a useful purpose exists and the exposure level and duration will not exceed the permissible limit.

1.5.3 Class III Controls

a. Do not aim the laser at an individual's eye.
b. Permit only experienced personnel to operate the laser.
c. Enclose as much of the beam path as possible. Even a transparent enclosure will prevent individuals from placing their head or reflecting objects within the beam path. Terminations should be used at the end of the useful paths of the direct and any secondary beams.
d. Shutters, polarizers and optical filters should be placed at the laser exit port to reduce the beam power to the minimal useful level.
e. Control spectators.
f. A warning light or buzzer should indicate laser operation. This is especially needed if the beam is not visible, i.e., for infrared lasers.
g. Do not permit laser tracking of nontarget vehicles or aircraft.
h. Operate the laser only in a restricted area—for example, in a closed room without windows, and place a warning sign on the door.

Introduction to Laser Safety

i. Place the laser beam path well above or well below the eye level of any sitting or standing observers whenever possible. The laser should be mounted firmly to assure that the beam travels only along its intended path.
j. Always use proper laser eye protection if a potential eye hazard exists for the direct beam or a specular reflection.
k. A key switch should be installed to minimize tampering by unauthorized individuals.
l. The beam or its specular reflection should never be directly viewed with optical instruments such as binoculars or telescopes with sufficient protective filters.
m. Remove all unnecessary mirror-like surfaces from within the vicinity of the laser beam path.

1.5.4 Class IV Controls

a. Fortunately, these high-power lasers are seldom used outside of research laboratories and restricted industrial environments where personnel access is carefully controlled.
b. These lasers should only be operated within a localized enclosure, or in a controlled workplace, or where the beam is directed into outer space. If a complete local enclosure is not possible, laser operation indoors should be in a light-tight room with interlocked entrances to assure that the laser cannot emit while a door is open.
c. Eye protection is needed for all individuals working within the controlled area. If the laser beam irradiance is sufficient to be a serious skin or fire hazard, a suitable shielding should be used between the laser beam and any personnel.
d. Remote firing with video monitoring or other remote (safe) viewing techniques should be chosen when feasible.
e. Outdoor high-power laser devices such as satellite laser transmission systems and laser radar (LIDAR) should have positive stops on the azimuth and elevation traverse to assure that the beam cannot intercept occupied areas or non-target aircraft.
f. Beam shutters, beam polarizers, and beam filters should always be used to limit use to authorized personnel only. The flashlamps in optical pump systems should be shielded to eliminate any direct viewing.
g. Backstops should be diffusely reflecting-fire resistant target materials where feasible. Safety enclosures should be used around microwelding and microdrilling work pieces to contain hazardous reflections from the work area. Microscopic viewing systems used to study the work piece should ensure against hazardous levels of reflection of laser irradiation back through the optics.

1.5.5 Applying the Safety Procedures

All of the aforementioned safety rules would not necessarily be followed for any given laser operation as some are mutually exclusive. For instance, if the laser beam path is completely enclosed and the individual cannot observe any hazardous beam reflections, then there is no need for laser eye protection. For this reason, to aid the reader in formulating specific safety guidelines for his particular applications and specific laser system, detailed discussions of hazard control measures as applied to a variety of laser uses are given in Chapters 17-21.

To use these rules the laser must first be classified. This is given in the manufacturer's label for lasers made for sale in the U.S.A. since August 2, 1976. Standard labels are shown in Fig. 9-4 through Fig. 9-8. If the laser classification cannot be determined from the label or from the manufacturer's literature one must resort to calculations and measurements. The detailed information required to classify lasers is given in Chapter 9. Table I in Appendix E gives a listing of the most common lasers manufactured prior to August 1976 with a classification based upon the manufacturer's specifications. Some classification procedures are quite simple. For instance, all helium-neon lasers with an output power below 1 mW are classified as Class II, or below 0.4 μW as Class I. All continuous wave lasers with an output above 0.5 W are classified as Class IV.

1.6 LASER EYE PROTECTION

Filter goggles and spectacles are used for laser eye protection in many industrial laser operations and laser research laboratories, although such engineering controls such as closed beam paths and enclosures are far more preferable. However, safety goggles or spectacles are often an effective safety measure when engineering controls are not possible. It should be noted that the user must be careful that the filter material and side shields can withstand the maximum irradiance encountered in the environment for at least 3 seconds and the filter is of the required optical density. Any eye protection used in the outdoor environment should have curved surface lenses to assure that reflections are not collimated. Chapter 16 provides detailed information on laser eye protection.

1.7 NON-LASER SOURCES

Although most of the material in this book concerns laser safety, several chapters are related to hazards and controls of hazards from lamps, arcs, light projection systems and other non-laser optical sources (Chapters 6, 10, 14, 22, 23, and 24). The interest in optical radiation hazards from lasers has stimulated a greatly increased awareness of potential hazards from conventional light sources. An understanding of hazards from welding arcs and arc lamps will assist the reader in obtaining a better perspective of laser hazards. Hence if the reader is only responsible for the control of laser hazards he or she may also find reading these other chapters beneficial.

Introduction to Laser Safety

1.8 REVIEW QUESTIONS

1. The eye is generally more vulnerable than the skin to laser radiation. T or F

2. In which spectral bands may radiation cause photokeratitis?

3. The spectral range of 300 to 1400 nm is termed the "retinal hazard region." T or F

4. Laser standards have been well established since 1963. T or F

5. Laser hazard classification is useful for:
   (a) simple labeling
   (b) simplifying laser hazard analysis
   (c) is required of laser manufacturers marketing lasers in the U.S.A. since 1976
   (d) all of the above

6. There have been at least four electrocutions in the U.S.A. among laser users since 1960. T or F

7. What are some examples of environmental hazards associated with the use of high-power lasers?

8. What is the eye's aversion response?

1.9 REFERENCES

American Conference of Governmental Industrial Hygienists, 1973, "Guide for Control of Laser Hazards," ACGIH, P. O. Box 1937, Cincinnati, OH 45201 ($2.75).
American National Standards Institute, 1976, "Safe Use of Lasers," ANSI Standard Z-136.1, 1430 Broadway, New York, NY 10018 ($9.00).
Department of the Air Force, 1973, Laser Hazards Control AFM 161-8, Washington, DC (under revision).
Department of the Army, 1975, Control of Hazards to Health from Laser Radiation TB MED 279, Washington,DC, May 1975.
Laser Institute of America, 1977, "Laser Safety Guide 1977," LIA, 4100 Executive Park Drive, Cincinnati, OH 45241 ($2.50).
Occupational Safety and Health Administration, 1972, Title 29, Code of Federal Regulations 1910, OSHA Standards (under revision).
U.S. Department of Health, Education and Welfare, Bureau of Radiological Health, 1976, Laser Products, Performance Standard, (Part 1040, Code of Federal Regulations), *in* "Regulations for the Enforcement of the Radiation Control for Health and Safety Act of 1968," pp 44–58, BRH, Rockville, MD, January 1976 (free).

Chapter 2
Review of Optical Physics

2.1 INTRODUCTION

The material in this chapter is provided as an introduction to those aspects of optics which play an important role in the subject of optical radiation safety. It is not intended as a comprehensive discourse but is simplified for those individuals who have responsibilities for safety of laser equipment and high intensity light sources, yet have not had rigorous training in optical physics. It may be conveniently bypassed by those familiar with optics, although it may serve as a useful introductory or refresher presentation of the subject for the individual who has not recently worked in optics or optical engineering.

2.2 WAVE MOTION

Radiation is often referred to as an energy in transit. It is relatively simple to visualize energy in transit as high velocity particles. This is often the way gamma rays are visualized. It is decidedly more difficult to visualize electromagnetic radiation as wave motion, but some attempt must be made. In a discussion of wave motion there are three defining properties which are characteristic to all wave motion, including ocean waves or vibrations in a string. They are: *frequency, wave velocity,* and *wavelength*. The frequency is the number of vibrations per second and this is usually denoted by the Roman letter f or the Greek letter nu (ν). The velocity of a wave as it travels through space is normally represented in mathematical expressions as v. The wavelength is the distance occupied by one wave and is generally denoted by the Greek letter lambda (λ). For a wave velocity v and a frequency ν at at the end of one period of vibration t, there will be vt waves spread over a distance vt in space.

The three parameters of frequency, velocity, and wavelength are related by a very simple expression:

$$v = \lambda \nu \qquad (2\text{-}1)$$

All wave motions, regardless of the medium through which they propagate will exhibit certain phenomena. These include reflection, refraction and diffraction.

2.3 THE ELECTROMAGNETIC SPECTRUM

Electromagnetic radiation consists of oscillating electric and magnetic fields. Radio frequency, microwave, infrared, visible (light*), ultraviolet, x and gamma radiation are all electromagnetic radiation and are propagated both in free space and in matter. Other wave motion most commonly encountered as mechanical vibrations, or sound, can be propagated only in matter. Collectively these electromagnetic radiations form the electromagnetic spectrum when arranged according to frequency or wavelength. A chart of the spectrum is shown in Fig. 2-1. Equation (2-1) can be modified for electromagnetic radiation by giving the velocity of the radiation the value of the velocity of light, usually written as c. In a vacuum, this value c_o is:

$$\begin{aligned} c_o &= \lambda \nu \\ &= 3 \times 10^{10} \text{ cm/s} \\ &= 3 \times 10^{8} \text{ m/s} \end{aligned}$$

The ratio of the velocity of light c_o in a vacuum to the velocity c in a medium is termed the *refractive index* n of that medium ($n = c_o/c$). Equation (2-1) can also be expressed as

$$\lambda = c/\nu, \quad \text{or} \quad \nu = c/\lambda \qquad (2\text{-}2)$$

The inverse relationship between frequency and wavelength is clearly evident in Fig. 2-1. As the frequency increases from microwave radiation through the optical radiations to gamma radiation the wavelength becomes shorter and shorter. The electromagnetic radiations have a characteristic energy associated with each photon and the photon energy increases with an increase in frequency.

The electromagnetic spectrum is normally illustrated with at least 20 decades in frequency or wavelength as shown in Figure 2.1, but this should not suggest that there are actually ends of the spectrum. Quite often the spectrum is shown to at least 10^{22} Hz or 3×10^{-14} meter which is in the region of gamma radiation. Frequencies less than one Hz are likewise known. The references to one region or another as the "gamma-radiation region" or the "microwave region" are likewise arbitrary. and no internationally accepted set of terms exist for specifying each of the spectral regions. The spectral designations of the optical region will be further discussed in Section 2.6 (page 19).

---

*Light by definition is visible radiation; hence it is incorrect (but common) to speak of "ultraviolet light" or "infrared light."

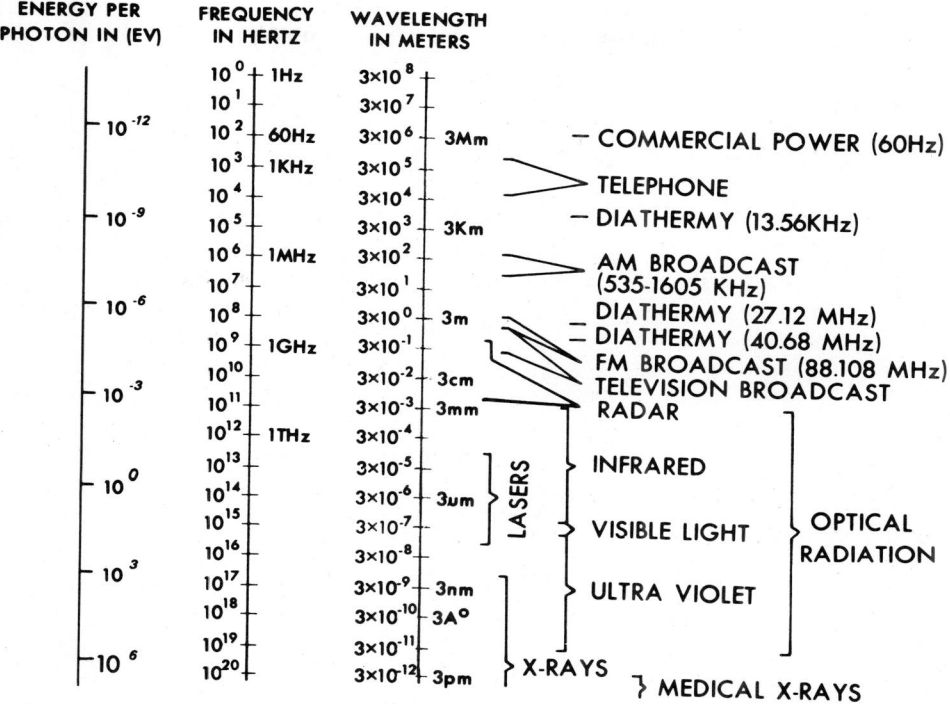

Figure 2-1. The electromagnetic spectrum.

2.4 WAVE-PARTICLE DUALITY

Certain phenomena such as the reflection and refraction of fast-moving particles are best explained by considering their wave properties, i.e. by a *wave description* of radiation. In fact even the electron is sometimes expressed as a wave motion. On the other hand, certain properties of electromagnetic radiation are more readily understood when they are considered to act as a series of discrete bundles or particles of energy which are called *photons* or *quanta*.

Perhaps the most helpful means to resolve this apparent confusion is the *principle of complementarity* suggested by Niels Bohr. In our study of the forms of matter and energy in the world, we are obliged to construct experiments in which we, as observers, and our tools must interact with the systems under examination. Thus the concepts of wave-like and particle-like behavior of radiation depend not only upon the radiation itself, but also upon the experimental arrangements used to observe it. The best description which we can achieve will depend upon many-fold observations and experiments, and the sum of this experience may enhance our understanding of what radiation "really is." The contradictions must be accepted

2.5 THE WAVE PICTURE OF RADIATION

Four fundamental laws of electricity and magnetism were mathematically expressed by James Clerk Maxwell in 1864 to derive equations governing the propagation of electromagnetic wave motion. Propagation equations for the electric and magnetic fields were shown to be a consequence of the fundamental laws describing earlier experiments with magnets and electric currents. The kind of wave propagation predicted by Maxwell's equations is shown in Fig. 2-2. The variation in the electric and magnetic field vectors (E and H) for monochromatic, plane-polarized waves propagating along the x-axis of a Cartesian coordinate system as a function of time t, position x, and angular frequency ω may be written:

$$E(x,t) = E_o \cos(kx - \omega t)$$
$$H(x,t) = H_o \cos(kx - \omega t)$$

(2-3)

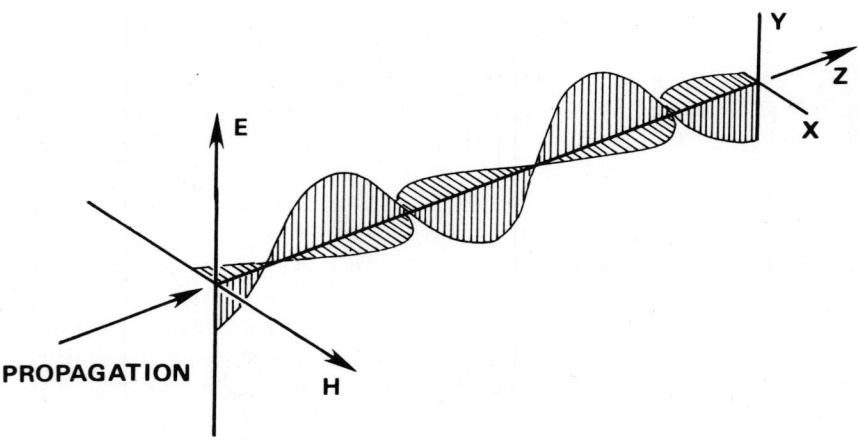

Figure 2-2. Propagation of an electromagnetic wave consisting of a sinusoidally oscillating electric field E and a magnetic field H with time in the Z direction.

These equations describe a particular solution to the wave equation. If the boundary conditions imposed on the wave equation are altered, other solutions are of course possible (for example, spherical waves in a spherical coordinate system). In this case:

$$k = 2\pi/\lambda$$
$$\omega = 2\pi\nu \quad (2\text{-}4)$$

where λ is the wavelength of the monochromatic waves and ν is the frequency of the radiation.

Polarization of radiation refers to the planes of oscillation of the electric and magnetic field vectors. Figure 2-2 shows a plane polarized wave for which the electric and magnetic vectors oscillate *normal* (perpendicular) to one another and *in phase* (in step). Radiation which has been scattered often exhibits random polarization with field vectors oscillating in all possible planes through the propagation axis. Light may be polarized by reflection from an interface or by passing through a medium which allows only one polarization direction to pass.

Using the wave description of radiation, many familiar phenomena can be described. The law of reflection and the law of refraction (*Snell's Law*) follow from the wave equation. The Fresnel equations, which can be derived from the wave equation, combine both of these laws and, in addition, provide reflection and transmission coefficients for optical power. The wave equation predicts absorption of electromagnetic radiation by conducting media. Cavity resonance, propagation in waveguides, and dipole radiation can all be described based upon the wave picture of electromagnetic waves.

2.6 THE PARTICLE PICTURE OF RADIATION

In spite of the many phenomena easily described by the wave approach, the *particle description* is particularly useful for gamma and X rays where the effects of individual particles are recorded. All types of radiation can be described either in terms of wave travel (a continuous electromagnetic field propagating in a medium or in a free space), or in terms of particle motion (rays of photons). This is termed *wave-particle duality*. Particle motion is used to describe the energy available in any given electromagnetic radiation in terms of photon energies. The energy in each photon (quantum) is directly related to the frequency as first proposed by the physicist Max Planck in 1900. The energy of a single photon Q_q is equal to

$$Q_q = h\nu \quad (2\text{-}5)$$

where Q_q is the photon energy in joules (J), ν is the frequency in hertz (Hz; wave cycles per second) and h (Planck's constant) is 6.6×10^{-34} joule-seconds (J·s).

As an example, a photon from a ruby laser which has a wavelength of approximately 0.7 μm, and hence from Eq. (2-2) a frequency of 4.3×10^{14} Hz, would have an energy Q_q (Eq. 2-5) of 2.9×10^{-19} J·s. This also means that a ruby laser which emits a pulse of energy of 0.29 J actually has 10^{18} photons in that one burst of radiant energy. A single photon is obviously a very small quantity of energy, yet several studies have shown that the human eye is capable of detecting a few photons of light.

Max Planck was forced to assume that radiation was quantized only after several years of fruitless efforts to explain the experimentally observed spectral emission from *blackbody radiators*. Such a radiator is created in a cavity of any shape in which electromagnetic radiation is in equilibrium at some absolute temperature T. The failure of Maxwell's wave theory of radiation to explain blackbody emission was serious in view of the impressive previous successes of that theory. By assuming that the radiation within the cavity could not exist with a continuous distribution of energies but only with certain energies $h\nu$, with particular frequencies determined by the boundary conditions within the cavity, Planck derived a radiation law which closely described blackbody emission spectra for radiators of different temperatures. Typical blackbody spectra for radiators at several absolute temperatures T are shown in Fig. 2-3.

Supporting evidence from Planck's quantization hypothesis was forthcoming in 1905 with Einstein's theoretical explanation of the *photoelectric effect*. The energy distribution of electrons emitted from a surface on which radiation was incident would only be understood if the incident radiation was assumed to arrive in energy packets or quanta of energy $h\nu$. Bohr's quantum theory of the hydrogen

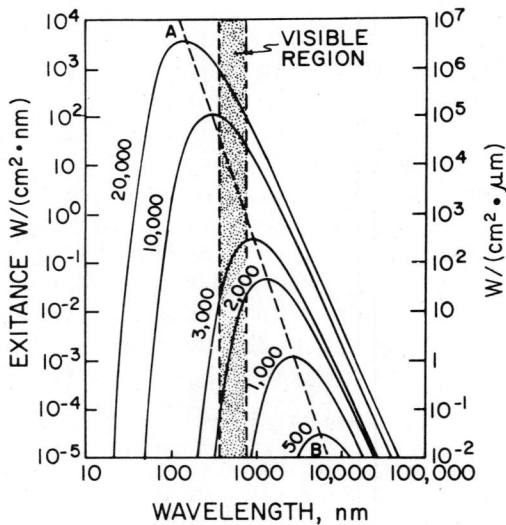

Figure 2-3. Blackbody spectra. Line AB shows Wien's Displacement Law for the shift of the peak wavelength with change in temperature.

atom developed in 1912 also rested on the assumption that radiation was emitted or absorbed only in discrete quanta.

Although quantum field theory has unified those conflicting pictures of the nature of radiation to some degree, the elementary level still presents the complementary wave-particle picture. Our choice of an appropriate mode of description will depend upon the particular experimental situation. In general, the wave picture is most useful for low energy, long wavelength phenomena, such as radiofrequency (RF) and microwave radiation. Both quantum and wave concepts are used in the optical region of the spectrum. High energy radiation such as X rays and gamma rays are most conveniently viewed as particle-like quanta. These customary divisions of the electromagnetic spectrum were illustrated in Fig. 2-1.

In a discussion of divisions of the electromagnetic spectrum caution is needed; any definition of a particular region has an overlap with adjacent regions. The spectral bands represent wavelength intervals within which a common state of the art and technology exists in sources, detectors, or in modes of interaction with matter. Indeed, neither the upper nor the lower limit to the entire spectrum are defined at present. The units used to describe energy, wavelength and frequency often differ from region to region as a matter of convention. Gamma and X radiation are generally described in terms of photon energy. Ultraviolet, visible (light) and infrared radiations, collectively known as optical radiation, are described in terms of wavelength; radiofrequency (including microwave) radiations are specified in terms of frequency. Sometimes the spectral region above approximately 100 nm is termed *ionizing radiation*, and wavelengths longer than 100 nm are placed in the *nonionizing radiation* spectrum. These terms are useful to biologists and certain health specialists who wish to distinguish between the biological effects of different radiations. Different disciplines make different divisions between adjacent spectral bands. For the physicist the optical spectrum generally consists of eight decades of wavelengths between 10 nm and 1 mm. On the other hand, photobiologists and health specialists who are not concerned about vacuum ultraviolet radiation begin at approximately 200 nm (which is the approximate long-wavelength edge of the vacuum ultraviolet) and go to far-infrared radiation at 1 mm. The International Commission on Illumination (the CIE, i.e. Commission International d'Eclairage) Committee on Photobiology has provided spectral band designations which are quite convenient in discussing biological facts. These customary divisions of the optical spectrum are given in Table 2-1.

2.7 INTERACTION OF ELECTROMAGNETIC RADIATION WITH MATTER

From a macroscopic point of view, the interaction of electromagnetic radiation with matter takes the form of absorption, transmission, reflection, refraction, and diffraction. In most instances one of these effects dominates almost to the exclusion of others. However, all effects are always present to some degree. For instance, if a beam of light passes through a sheet of transparent glass, at least 4% of the incident light is reflected from each surface. On the other hand, only a very small percentage

TABLE 2-1. Several Schemes for Dividing the Optical Spectrum

Physical #1	Physical #2	Photobiologic (CIE) *
Extreme UV (1-10 nm to 100 nm)	Vacuum or extreme UV (1-10 nm to 180 nm)	UV-C (100 nm to 280 nm)
Far UV (200 nm to 300 nm)		UV-B (280 nm to 315-320 nm)
Near UV (300 nm to 400 nm)	Near UV (300 nm to 400 nm)	UV-A (315 nm to 380-400 nm)
Light (380 nm to 760 nm)	Light (400 nm to 700 nm)	Light (380-400 nm to 760-780 nm)
Near IR (760 nm to 4000 nm)	Near IR (700 nm to 1200 nm)	IR-A (760-780 nm to 1400 nm)
Middle IR (4 μm to 14 μm)	Middle IR (1.2 μm to 7 μm)	IR-B (1.4 μm to 3 μm)
Far IR (14 μm to 100 μm)	Far IR (7 μm to 1 mm)	IR-C (3 μm to 1 mm)
Submillimeter (100 μm to 1 mm)		

* *Based on the recommendation of the Committee on Photobiology of the CIE (Commission International de l'Eclairage—the International Commission on Illumination) as published in the "International Lighting Vocabulary," published by the CIE in 1970. The scheme was originally proposed by W. W. Coblentz of the U. S. National Bureau of Standards in the 1930's. Today these divisions are almost universal except that the dividing line between UV-B and UV-A is often taken as 320 nm. It should also be noted that the photobiologic band UV-C need not extend very far into the vacuum ultraviolet region since biologic studies in a vacuum would have little practical meaning.*

(less than 1%) is usually absorbed within the clear glass even when marked refraction or bending of the light takes place. Similar effects occur in all spectral regions including radiofrequency and gamma-radiation bands.

2.8 INTERACTION AT AN INTERFACE

2.8.1 Specular and Diffuse Reflection

Reflection takes place at an interface. There are two basic types of reflections that are of interest to us—*specular* (mirror-like) and *diffuse*. Specular reflection is sometimes referred to as *regular reflection*. When light is specularly reflected from a mirror or other very smooth surface it obeys the law of reflection which states that the angle of reflection equals the angle of incidence. This is shown in Fig. 2-4. Specular reflection can occur when the size of surface irregularities or roughness is less than the wavelength of the incident radiation. This latter description of specular

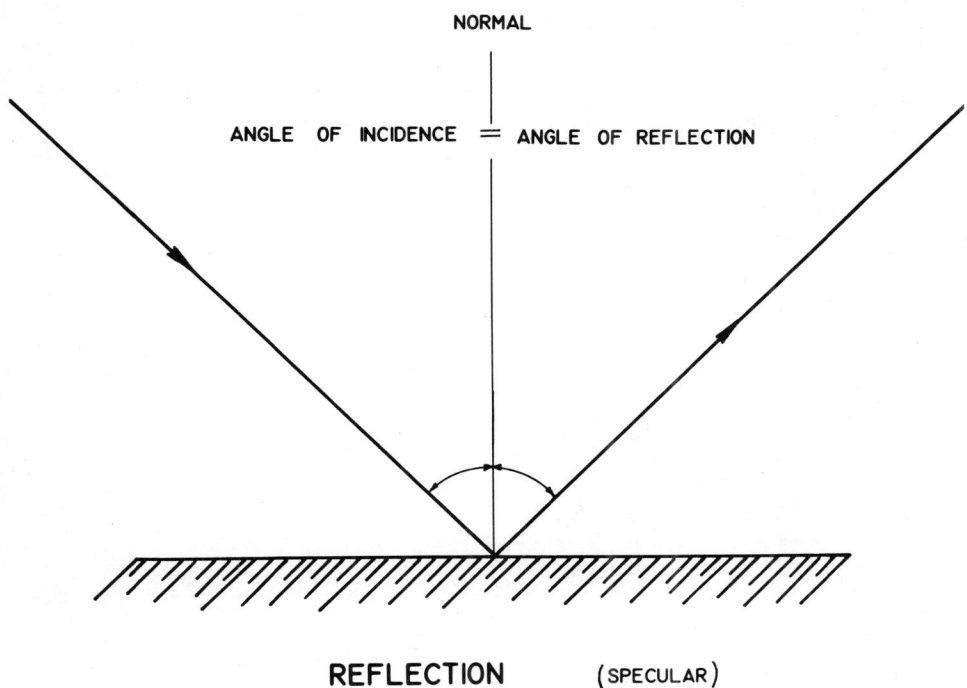

Figure 2-4. Regular reflection. Reflection from a specular surface behaves the Law of Reflection where the angle of reflectance equals the angle of incidence.

(mirror-like) reflection is important to keep in mind. Diffuse reflection occurs when the surface irregularities are randomly oriented and are much greater than the wavelength of the incident radiation; for example, when light is reflected from chalk, a black iron skillet, or a rough granite surface. Most naturally-occurring surfaces are diffusely reflecting in the visible light region of the spectrum. Diffuse reflection is shown in Fig. 2-5. Perfect diffuse reflection follows *Lambert's Law* which is also known as the *Cosine Law of Reflection*. A useful formula in radiometry is:

$$E = \Phi \rho \cdot \cos \theta / \pi r_1^2 \tag{2-6}$$

Here E is the irradiance reflected from the surface, Φ (phi) the laser beam power upon the surface, θ (theta) the angle that the incident beam makes relative to the surface's normal, ρ (rho) the diffuse reflection coefficient of the surface for the laser wavelength, r_1 equal to the distance from the beam spot on the diffuse target to the detector, and π (pi) the usual 3.14159... In radiometry two-place accuracy is usually sufficient to specify constants, e.g., 3.14.

It is important to remember that diffuse and specular reflections are highly wavelength dependent. A given surface may produce a reflection which is specular at one wavelength but it may or may not be specular at a greatly different wavelength. As an example, microwave radiation is reflected from a black cast iron skillet as a mirror-like reflection but light is completely diffused by such a surface. Obviously the size of the irregularities in the reflecting surface must be considerably greater than the wavelength of the incident radiation. If the size of the reflecting surface irregularities is of the order of the wavelength then the phenomena of diffraction and scattering take place.

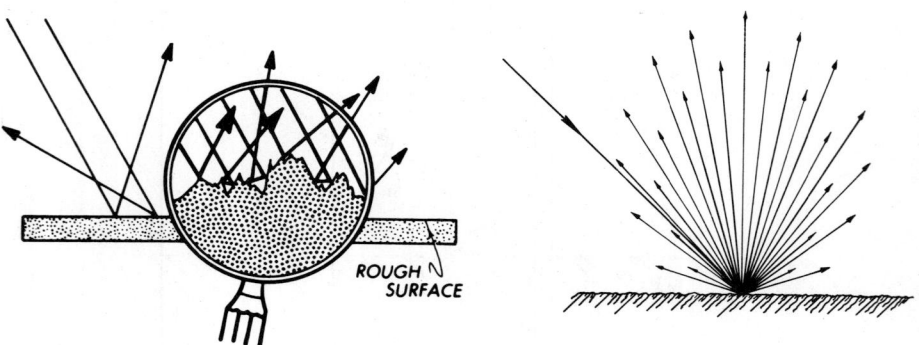

Figure 2-5. Diffuse reflection. Light reflected from a diffuse surface is redirected in a random fashion as a result of surface roughness (A); Totally diffused reflected light follows Lambert's Cosine Law of Reflection (B); the lengths of each reflected ray correspond to the radiant intensity in the direction of the ray.

2.8.2 Specular Reflection Formulas

The reflection and transmission coefficients for oblique incidence of plane-polarized light (the *Fresnel formulas*) follow directly from the wave equation. For light with the electric vector E vibrating in the plane of incidence (the plane formed by the propagation axis of an incident wave and a normal to the interface) the reflection coefficient is:

$$R_\| = \tan^2(\theta - \theta') / \tan^2(\theta + \theta') \qquad (2\text{-}7)$$

with $T_\| = 1 - R_\|$. For plane waves with the electric vector perpendicular to the plane of incidence, where $\theta' = \text{Arcsin}(\theta/n)$.

$$R_\perp = \sin^2(\theta - \theta') / \sin^2(\theta + \theta') \qquad (2\text{-}8)$$

and $T_\perp$ and $R_\perp$ are equal to 1. For unpolarized light, an averaging of these results leads to:

$$R = \tfrac{1}{2}R_\perp + \tfrac{1}{2}R_\| \qquad (2\text{-}9)$$

while T is $(1 - R)$. We shall see the usefulness of the Fresnel formulas many times in the analysis of specular reflection hazards.

At Brewster's angle

$$\theta_B = \tan^{-1}(n/n_o) \qquad (2\text{-}10)$$

No light which is plane-polarized in the plane of incidence can be reflected. This effect is shown in Fig. 2-6, where it is seen that the specular reflectance of glass vanishes at approximately 56° when n is 1.5. For water, with an index of refraction n of 1.33, θ_B is 53°.

2.8.3 Refraction

Refraction also takes place at an interface. Refraction occurs whenever a beam of light passes from one transmitting media to another having a different *refractive index* n. It is responsible for a bending of light near air-water and air-glass interfaces (Fig. 2-7). The law of refraction, which is also known as *Snell's Law* states that the angle of incidence (θ_1) and the angle of refraction (θ_2) are related by the equation

$$\sin\theta_1 / \sin\theta_2 = n_2/n_1 \qquad (2\text{-}11)$$

where n_1 and n_2 are the indices of refraction of the first medium and second medium respectively. Microwaves as well as optical radiation undergo refraction when passing from warm to cold air or vice versa, although the index of refraction of air is very nearly 1 (1.00006).

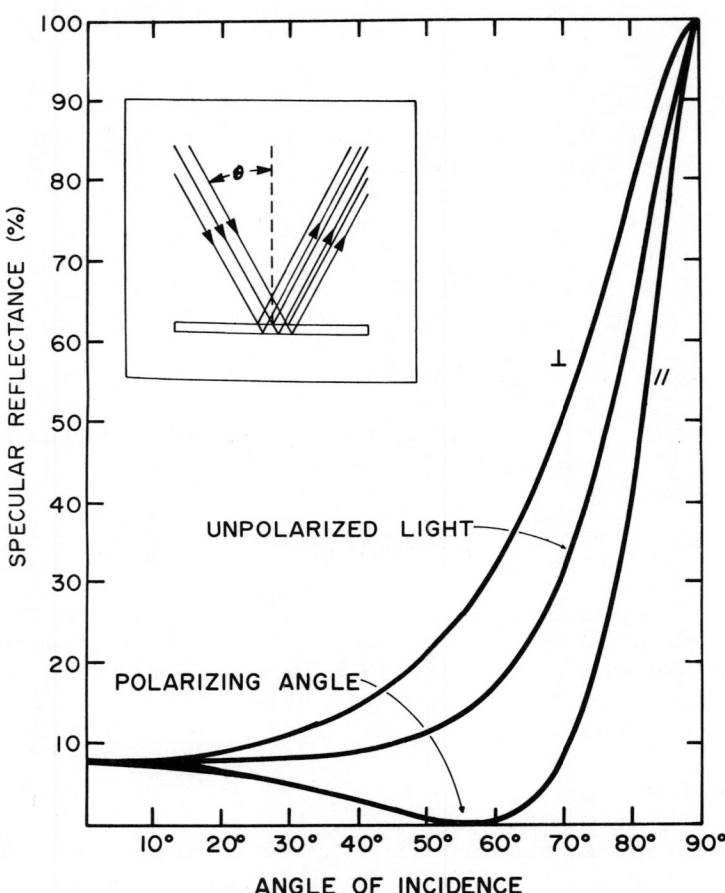

Figure 2-6. The specular reflectance for plate glass depends upon the polarization of the incident light and the angle of incidence. Light with the electric vector polarized perpendicular (⊥) to the plane of incidence is reflected more than light polarized parallel (‖) to the plane of incidence. The curves are for both surfaces of clear glass with an index of refraction of 1.5.

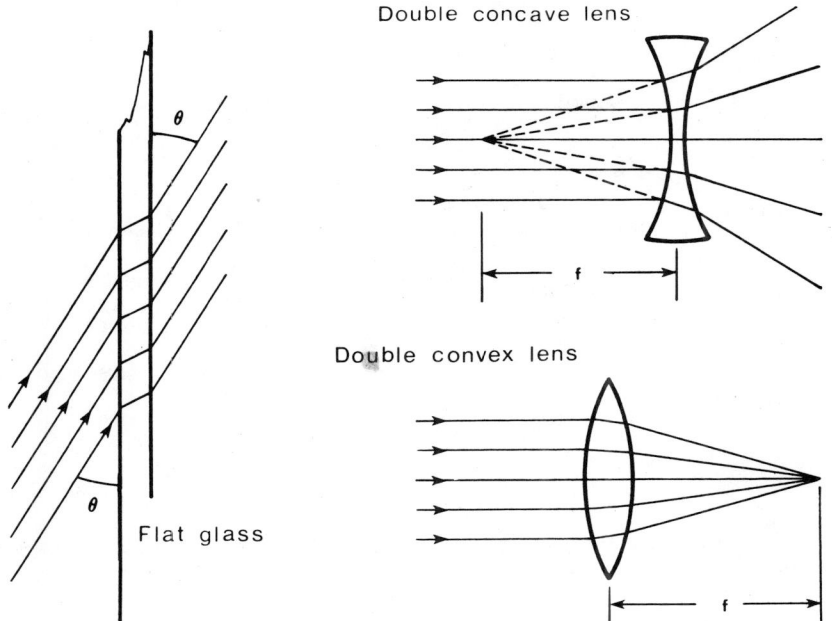

Figure 2-7. Refraction. A ray of light is displaced according to Snell's Law of Refraction by a transparent plate with parallel surfaces. The refraction by concave and convex lenses is also shown with f as the focal length.

Lenses and prisms are optical components which depend principally upon the phenomena of refraction. A prism bends blue light and red light differently since the index of refraction of glass is different for different wavelengths; hence for the same angle of incidence the two angles of refraction differ (Fig. 2-8) and blue light can be separated from red light). This effect (chromatic aberration) can be reduced by choosing a glass with very little *dispersion* or by glueing two lenses together which have complementary dispersion characteristics. Coatings are also used to further reduce dispersion to produce an achromatic optical system. On the other hand, the glass for a prism should have a great deal of dispersion to separate the different wavelengths. Often an optical system for a laser or other nearly monochromatic source is not required to be achromatic. Simple formulas of geometrical optics for lenses will be briefly presented later (Chapter 14).

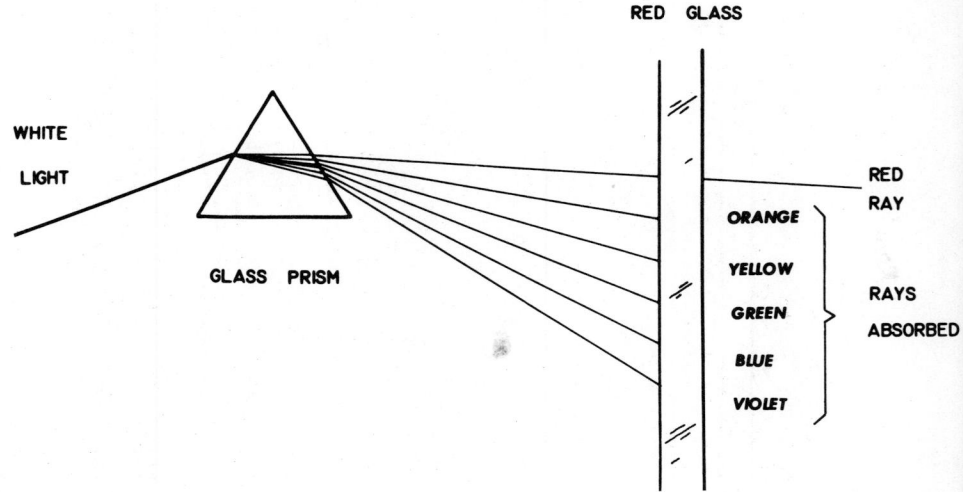

Figure 2-8. A prism is a dispersive refracting element which can be used to separate a beam of light into its spectral components. Also shown is selective spectral absorption by a colored glass filter.

2.9 INTERACTION WITH A MEDIUM

2.9.1 Transmission

The transmitted light which emerges from a medium is dependent upon the phenomena of absorption and scattering and also upon the reflection of some of the light at the interfaces between media. The transmittance of a medium is usually represented by τ (tau) and is for a certain wavelength and for a certain path length. The transmittance of most materials varies markedly across the optical spectrum. By the Law of Conservation of Energy the transmitted beam energy Q_τ is the incident beam energy Q_I less that lost due to absorption Q_A and reflection Q_R:

$$Q_\tau = Q_I - Q_R - Q_A \qquad (2\text{-}12)$$

2.9.2 Absorption

The absorption and transmission of optical radiation in any homogeneous, isotropic media is expressed in terms of the following formula.

$$\Phi = \Phi_0 e^{-\mu x} \qquad (2\text{-}13)$$

where Φ is the radiant power (radiant flux) leaving the medium, Φ_0 the initial radiant power in the laser beam entering the absorbing medium, x the thickness of the medium or path length of the beam and μ (Greek "mu") the attenuation coefficient of the absorbing medium.

When radiation is transmitted through a medium, it may lose power to the medium by a variety of processes. In a homogeneous and isotropic material, the proportion of radiant power lost per unit length is constant. For example, during its passage through absorbing glass, light of a certain wavelength may lose 10% of its optical power per centimeter. After 1 cm 10% of the initial beam power Φ_0 will be lost, and the power remaining will be 0.9 Φ_0. After one more centimeter, 10% of this transmitted power will be lost and 0.81 Φ_0 will remain, after the next cm it will be [(0.9) (0.9)(0.9) = 0.73]^S, and so on. (The absorption coefficient in this case is 0.1 cm^{-1}.) Under these conditions it is possible to derive the very useful *absorption law* (Eq. 2-13) giving the power Φ at any distance x from the starting point in the medium. Because the mathematical demonstration is quite straightforward, and because the resulting absorption equation can be applied in many other situations, the equation will be developed below. The reader may skip this next paragraph (in smaller print) and move directly to Eq. (2-14) without loss of continuity.

The differential change in flux dΦ during passage of radiation through a segment of homogeneous material of thickness dx is proportional to the radiant flux Φ of the radiation as it enters the segment and to the thickness dx.

$$d\Phi = -\alpha \Phi dx \qquad (2\text{-}13a)$$

where α is the constant of proportionality with units of inverse length and the minus sign represents a loss in radiant flux, or power. Rearranging,

$$d\Phi/\Phi = -\alpha\, dx \qquad (2\text{-}13b)$$

Integrating both sides from the initial radiant flux Φ_0 when x is 0 (for example, at an interface) to the flux $\Phi(x)$ at some depth x in the material,

$$\int_{\Phi_0}^{\Phi} \frac{d\Phi}{I} = -\alpha \int_0^x dx \qquad (2\text{-}13c)$$

$$\ln \Phi - \ln \Phi_0 = -\alpha x \qquad (2\text{-}13d)$$

$$\ln (\Phi/\Phi_0) = -\alpha x \qquad (2\text{-}13e)$$

Expressing both sides of the equation as powers of e:

$$e^{\ln(\Phi/\Phi_0)} = e^{-\alpha x} \qquad (2\text{-}13f)$$

and as $e^{\ln x}$ is x,

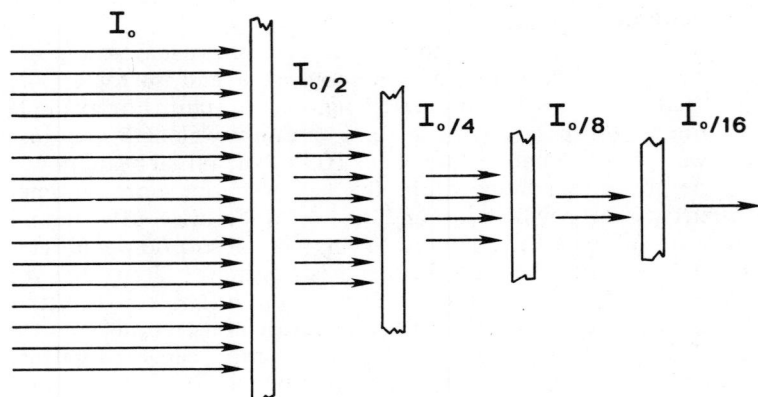

Figure 2-9. Exponential attenuation. Most attenuating media follow Beer's Law, that is, the initial beam intensity is reduced by an equal proportion for equal thickness of the medium.

$$\Phi/\Phi_0 = e^{-\alpha x} \qquad (2\text{-}13g)$$

which becomes Equation (2-13):

$$\Phi(x) = \Phi_0 e^{-\alpha x} \qquad (2\text{-}13h)$$

This is shown in a simple fashion in Figure 2-9.

The *Exponential Law of Absorption or Beer's Law* is the most important; the constant α is the *absorption coefficient*. It shows that the radiant power diminishes exponentially with distance during transmission through a uniformly absorbing medium. Likewise, for a scattering medium the same approach may be applied and absorption coefficient α is replaced by a *scattering coefficient* σ. The general equation for *attenuation* is:

$$\begin{aligned}\Phi &= \Phi_0 e^{-(\sigma x + \alpha x)} \\ &= \Phi_0 e^{-\mu x}\end{aligned} \qquad (2\text{-}13)$$

which was presented previously, where μ is the *attenuation coefficient*. The attenuation coefficient varies with wavelength as do α and σ, (see Fig. 2-9).

Similar arguments lead to similar laws for many natural phenomena with only the meaning of the variables and the value (and sign) of the proportionality constant changed. For example:

$$N(t) = N_0 e^{-xt} \qquad (2\text{-}14)$$

describes the process of spontaneous emission of a fixed quantity N_o of excited atoms in a fluorescent material.

Absorption in all substances is highly dependent on the wavelength of the incident radiation. Atoms or molecules become excited when they absorb a quantum of radiant energy. Following absorption this energy can be released as one or more photons of radiant energy. This is known as *fluorescence*. The energy may also be released as one or more quanta of mechanical energy (sometimes termed phonons). One cannot predict the exact time that will elapse between absorption and the emission of a photon but the physicist can predict an average time for a particular transition to occur and this is called the *fluorescent lifetime*. The fluorescent lifetime is an important parameter of any material used for an optically pumped laser.

2.10 INTERFERENCE AND DIFFRACTION EFFECTS

2.10.1 Interference

The bending or spreading of waves after passing an edge or passing through a small aperture is a wave phenomenon termed *diffraction*. The diffraction effects result from the constructive and destructive interference of adjacent waves. When the size of the barrier is small compared to the incident wavelength, the wave is bent around the barrier considerably. Thus, particles diffract light most dramatically when they are approximately the size of the wavelength of the incident radiation. The sum of the diffraction effects in this case is known as *scattering*.

Thomas Young demonstrated the phenomena of *interference* of light in 1801, firmly establishing the wave nature of light. Young's experiments and their interpretation were based on an earlier result due to the Dutch physicist Christian Huygens in 1678. Huygens proposed a geometrical construction which might be used to predict the evolution of wavefronts. He suggested that all points on a wavefront can be regarded as point sources from which secondary spherical wavelets are emitted. The new position of the wavefront will be a surface tangent to these wavelets after some time t. *Huygens' principle* leads to both the laws of reflection and to *Snell's Law*, discussed earlier. Young used Huygens' principle to explain the series of light and dark regions produced when the image of the sun passing through two pinhole apertures close together on a card was viewed on a screen some distance away. Each aperture was imagined to be the source of a spherical wave which spread out until it struck the screen. Where wavefronts intersected at the screen, constructive interference produced a bright spot, while dark spots would result where wavefronts were out of phase. Analogous interference effects may be seen in ripple tanks or bodies of water in which waves may overlap and add together. Figure 2-10 is reproduced from Thomas Young's original drawing illustrating interference maxima.

One of the simplest experiments illustrating interference involves the use of two parallel slits with widths on the order of a few wavelengths of light at a distance $\underline{a}$ apart. If radiation of wavelength λ is used, and if θ_d is the angular distance on the screen measured in a plane normal to the slit axes, it is easy to show that:

$$\underline{a} \sin \theta_d = m\lambda \qquad (2\text{-}15)$$

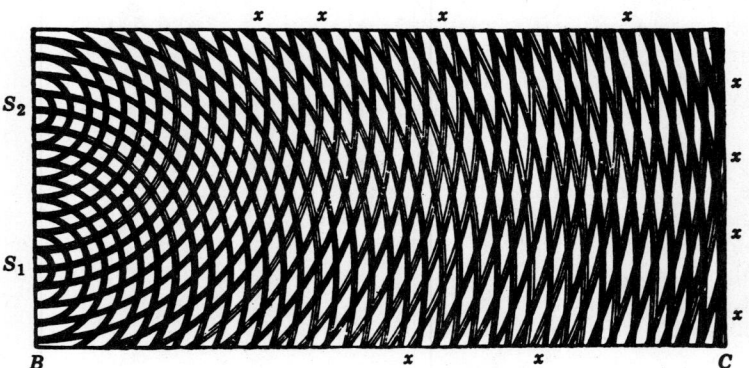

Figure 2-10. Young's original illustration showing interference of light waves from two sources S_1 and S_2.

where m being a discrete integer (i.e., m = 0, 1, 2, 3 . . .) describes the location of interference maxima. A detailed analysis will yield the exact irradiance distribution.

2.10.2 Diffraction

In the treatment of plane waves impinging upon an aperture, such as a circular aperture of diameter D, Huygens' principle may be employed again. Each point within the area of the aperture is regarded as a source of wavelets to explain the interference effects which produce a *diffraction pattern* at a screen some distance away.

Two types of diffraction situations are specified: *Fresnel* and *Fraunhofer diffraction*. Fresnel diffraction refers to effects produced when light from a point source at a finite distance from an aperture is intersected by a screen at a finite distance from the aperture, while the Fraunhofer case is a perfect plane wave diffracted onto a screen infinitely far away.

In the laboratory Fraunhofer diffraction may be realized by placing converging lenses before and after the aperture, or by the use of a collimated laser beam. Figure 2-11 illustrates Fresnel diffraction. A classical problem in the study of diffraction is diffraction by a circular aperture of diameter D. A British astronomer, Sir George Airy, solves the problem in 1835 to explain the characteristic rings observed around telescopic images of stars. The problem could be solved by assuming Fraunhofer conditions with the first minimum occurring at:

$$\sin \theta_d = 1.22 \ \lambda/D \qquad (2\text{-}16)$$

An exact solution yields a diffraction pattern as shown in Fig. 2-12. The pattern is

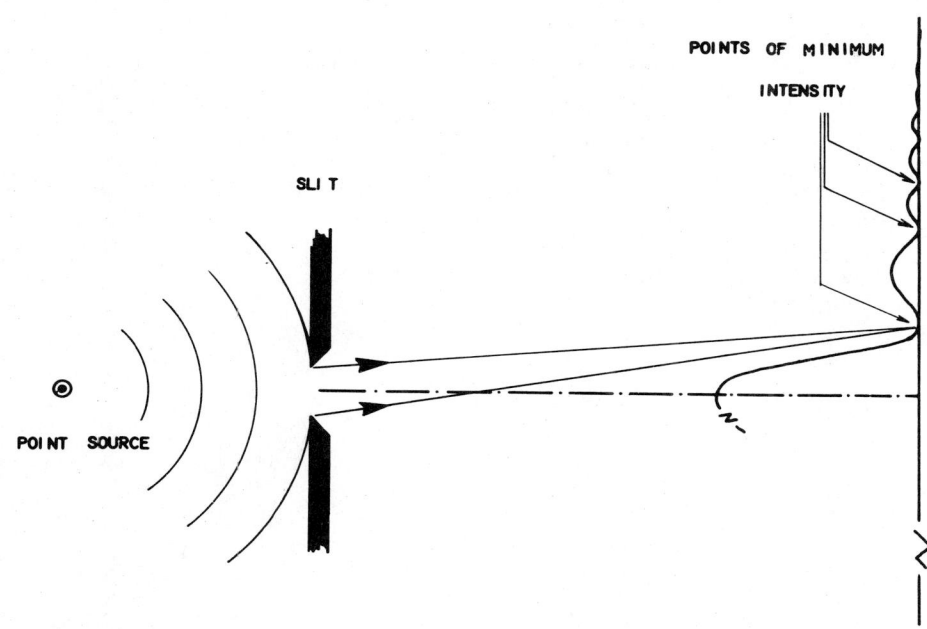

Figure 2-11. Relative intensity of light in a diffraction pattern produced by the passage of light through a narrow slit. The first minimum occurs where the path lengths from the slit edges differ by $\lambda/2$.

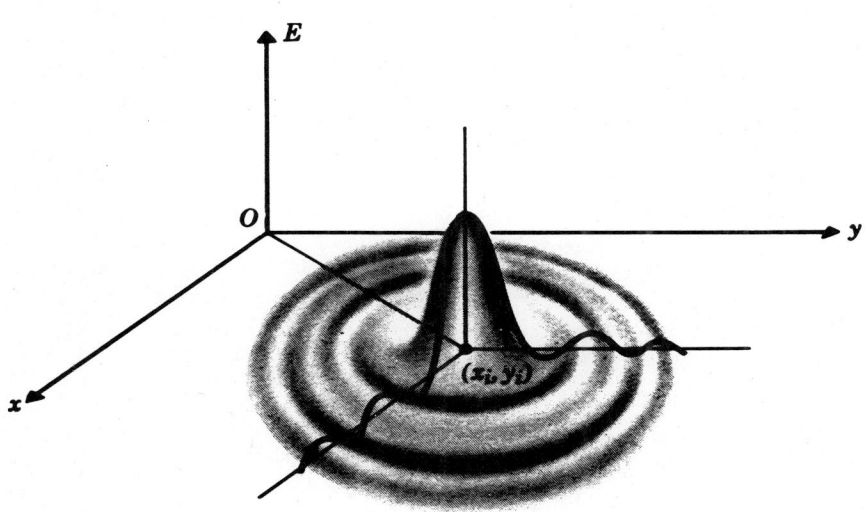

Figure 2-12. Airy intensity distribution for Fraunhofer diffraction from a circular aperture (from Klein, M. V., 1970, "Optics," John Wiley and Sons, New York, with permission).

often called the *Airy disc*. This formula will be used again in the discussion of minimal laser images on the retina in Chapter 3.

The foregoing sections have described very briefly the kinds of interactions which radiation exhibits with matter, with emphasis on the optical region of the electromagnetic spectrum. Many results, such as the laws of reflection, *Snell's Law,* the laws of absorption, and diffraction effects may be extended to radiation of longer or shorter wavelength. Applications to long wavelength radiation are limited only by practical considerations of size. These extensions break down significantly for higher energy photons (shorter wavelengths) due to the photoelectric effect, Compton scattering, and pair production, which occur at successively higher photon energies (i.e., at shorter wavelengths). These effects first become significant in the vacuum ultraviolet and x-radiation region when photon energies are in excess of a few electron volts which are sufficient to alter atomic structure.

2.10.3 Scattering

Small particles whose size approaches that of a wavelength of light scatter light as well as atoms and molecules. If the particles are much smaller than the wavelength of light (e.g., gas molecules) *Rayleigh scattering* takes place. Lord Rayleigh first demonstrated that the fraction of scattered radiation from a beam was inversely proportional to the fourth power of the wavelength of the radiation:

$$\Phi_{(scattered)} = k_1 \mu \Phi_0 / \lambda^4 \qquad (2\text{-}17)$$

where μ is an absorption coefficient and k_1 follows a function of $(1 + \cos^2 \theta_s)$ where θ_s is the angle from the beam axis. That is to say that this type of scattering increases dramatically for shorter wavelengths. For this reason the sky is blue and the sun at sunset is red. The atmospheric molecules strongly scatter the shorter wavelengths (blue) as the sunlight passes through the atmosphere. At sunrise and sunset this atmospheric path is much greater (see Chapter 6, section 6), and the direct sunlight is yellow-to-reddish since the shorter wavelengths have been scattered out of the beam. The Rayleigh scattered light goes in all directions with the intensity indicated by k_1. Rayleigh scattered light is also polarized to some extent. Looking at the blue sky through a polarizing filter will clearly demonstrate this.

If light goes through clouds of dust or condensed water vapor where the particle or droplet size is of the order of the wavelength of light or greater this strong wavelength preference is not seen in the scattered light. Clouds usually appear white or grey. This type of large-particle scattering is termed Mie scattering. Unlike Rayleigh scattering, Mie scattering is strongly directional. Normally, the forward component of Mie scattered radiation is much greater than backscatter.

The phenomena of scattering must be considered not only in terms of the atmospheric propagation of laser beams (Chapter 13), but also in reference to the light scattered in the ocular media of the human eye (Chapter 4). The scattering of light in a homogeneous medium from a light beam can also be expressed in terms of an exponential function:

$$\Phi = \Phi_0 e^{-\sigma x} \qquad (2\text{-}18)$$

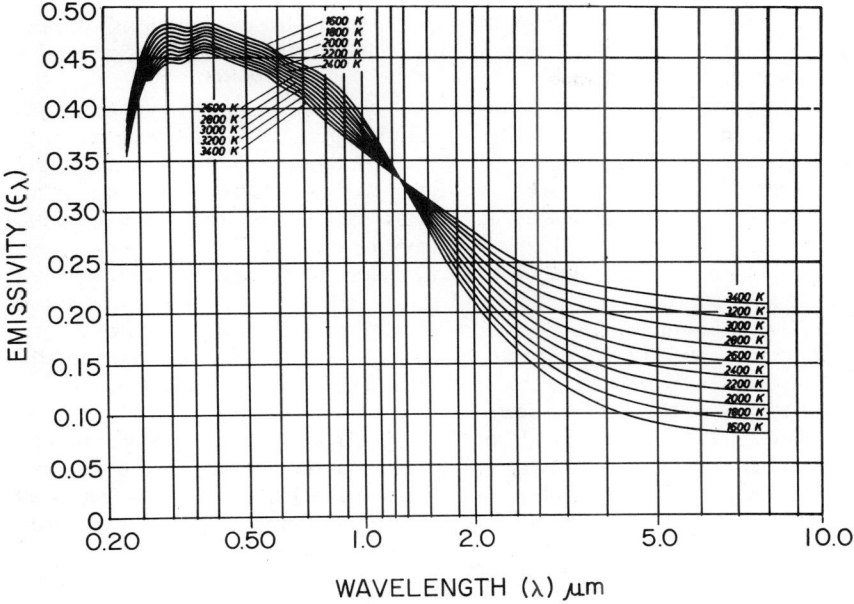

Figure 2-13. Spectral emissivity of tungsten (adapted from Ellenbass, 1972).

where σ is the scattering coefficient ($\sigma_M + \sigma_R$) and is the sum of the Mie scattering coefficient σ_M and the Rayleight scattering coefficient σ_R. When the absorption coefficient is added there is an attenuation coefficient μ, which once again gives as a result Eq. (2-13):

$$\Phi = \Phi_o e^{-(\sigma_R + \sigma_M + \alpha)} \qquad (2\text{-}19)$$
$$= \Phi_o e^{-\mu x}$$

2.11 SOURCES OF RADIATION

The sources of electromagnetic radiation can be categorized by several different methods. Sources can be grouped according to the type of material or the type of equipment which produces the radiation. The manner in which the radiation originated can be described in terms of nuclear, electronic, or molecular transitions between energy states. On an atomic scale it is useful to note that the very high energy photons which originate from transitions from one energy state to another in the nucleus of individual atoms have energies characteristic of the type of atoms. Likewise, the energy level transitions of electrons result in moderate energy photons within the soft X ray, ultraviolet, and visible portions of the spectrum. Slight modifications of vibrational, rotational, or translational energy states in molecular bonds can give rise to infrared or microwave photons. Physical chemists make use of these characteristics—photon absorptions and photon emissions—to identify the prescence of certain species of atoms or molecules by absorption and emission spectroscopy.

When the temperature of a body is elevated, a variety of energy transitions take place and photons are emitted. If the temperature of the body is approximately near that of the human body (37°C or 310 K) most of the emitted photons have wavelengths in the far infrared in the vicinity of 10 μm wavelength. If a material body is heated to incandescence, such as to 2000 K, the material could be described as red hot. The higher the temperature the greater percentage of high energy photons are released. But in all cases a wide range of photon energies are associated with the emitted incandescent radiation. A theoretical incandescent source has a characteristic "blackbody" spectrum. Figure 2-3 shows the blackbody spectrum for several different temperatures. In practice no material actually emits a perfect blackbody spectrum, but some materials such as solid tungsten or molten metals approach this distribution.

The ratio of the theoretically possible spectral emittance to the actual emittance of a gray body is the emissivity ϵ. For instance the emissivity of tungsten throughout the visible is approximately 0.4 (Fig. 2-13). Other sources of light such as carbon arcs, gas filled arc lamps, or gas discharge lamps, depart greatly from blackbody characteristics, i.e., ϵ varies greatly with the wavelength in the visible region. In these cases a stream of electrons flowing through a gas creates a release of photons characteristic of that particular gas. If gas has a low pressure and the current is not great, a line spectrum is emitted as shown in Fig. 2-14. As the gas pressure and the current density are increased, a continuous spectrum due to the temperature of the gas begins to appear. At very high current densities and gas pressures, this portion of the emission predominates as is shown in the bottom panel of Fig. 2-14.

2.12. MOLECULAR AND ATOMIC TRANSITIONS

For wavelengths shorter than 1 mm ($\nu > 30$ GHz) yet not shorter than typical atomic diameters, i.e., 1 to 10 nm (10 to 100 Å), molecular and atomic transitions are the most common sources of electromagnetic radiation. It is in this region that the "particle-like" character of radiation becomes increasingly apparent. To make matters more confusing the picture of an accelerated charge is no longer adequate to describe the generation of this radiation. Indeed, accelerated charges, namely electrons, moving in "orbits" around nuclei, quite specifically must *not* radiate an electromagnetic field. If they did, the electrons of all atoms would lose energy to the field, collapse to the positively-charged nuclei and lose all chemical identity. This is the kind of paradox which led Niels Bohr to the original quantum theory in 1911.

According to Bohr's theory, atoms emit radiation (photons) only when electrons move from a higher energy "orbit" (higher energy state) to a lower one. Within a stationary orbit they do not lose energy. When energy Q_q in the form of a photon is emitted due to such a transition (Fig. 2-15) the frequency of the emitted radiation is determined by the condition:

$$Q_q = \mathcal{E}_1 - \mathcal{E}_2 = h\nu \tag{2-20}$$

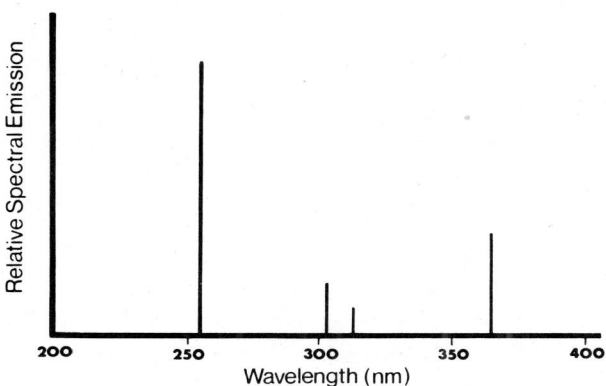

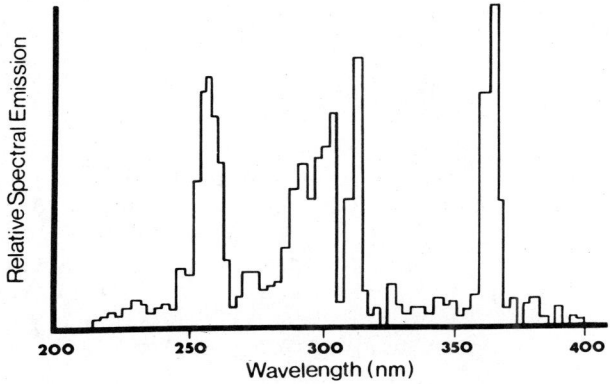

Figure 2-14. Spectra of Gas Discharge Lamps. The spectrum of a low-pressure gas discharge consists almost exclusively of the atomic emission spectral lines characteristic of the gas. The continuum is virtually non-existent. As the gas pressure in the lamp is increased, the continuum increases and the relative strengths of the lines change. This effect is clearly seen in the spectra plotted above. The solid bars are the lines of the spectrum of a very low-pressure 100-W mercury lamp; no continuum is seen even on this semilogarithmic plot. The solid line histogram is the spectrum of a high-pressure 250-W mercury lamp. The continuum now contains the majority of the energy. Note that the 254-nm line is predominant in the low-pressure gas discharge but is relatively weaker in the high-pressure discharge.

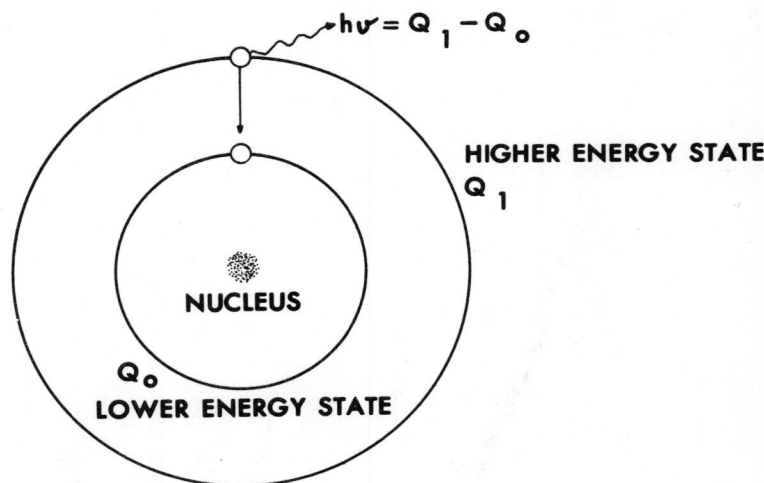

Figure 2-15. The fluorescent emission of light results from a transition of an electron from a higher energy state to a lower energy state in an atom.

where $\mathscr{E}_1$ and $\mathscr{E}_2$ are energies corresponding to the initial and final energy states. Finally, by quantization of the angular momentum of electrons in "orbit" the permissible values of the energies $\mathscr{E}_1$ and $\mathscr{E}_2$ are fixed. Emission or absorption of radiation (photons) by atoms will occur only for quanta with these discrete energies. Transitions in the wavelength region 400 to 760 nm are a common source of visible radiation. The photon energies expressed in joules are so small that many scientists have used electron volts (eV) for units where 1 eV is 1.6×10^{-19} J. A photon with an energy of 1 eV has a wavelength of 1,242 nm (see Appendix B).

It is important to note that several rules have been introduced in quantum theory which are in direct contradiction to classical nineteenth-century concepts. Nevertheless after over half a century of thought and experiment quantum mechanics remains firmly established as a description of many phenomena. However, for many applications Maxwell's wave theory is sufficient.

Energy transitions in molecular systems can cause radiation emission according to rules similar to those which apply to atomic systems. The energies (0.001 to 0.1 eV) of molecular transitions are typically less than those characteristic of atomic systems (1 eV to 100 eV). Instead of electron "orbital" potential and kinetic energies, the energy of molecular systems is associated with rotational and vibrational modes. Quantum theory predicts that the energy states of any harmonic system will be quantized, and this turns out to be true for many molecular structures. Emissions of this type occur in the infrared and microwave regions of the electromagnetic spectrum. The phenomena associated with heat arise from the vibrational energy of molecular systems.

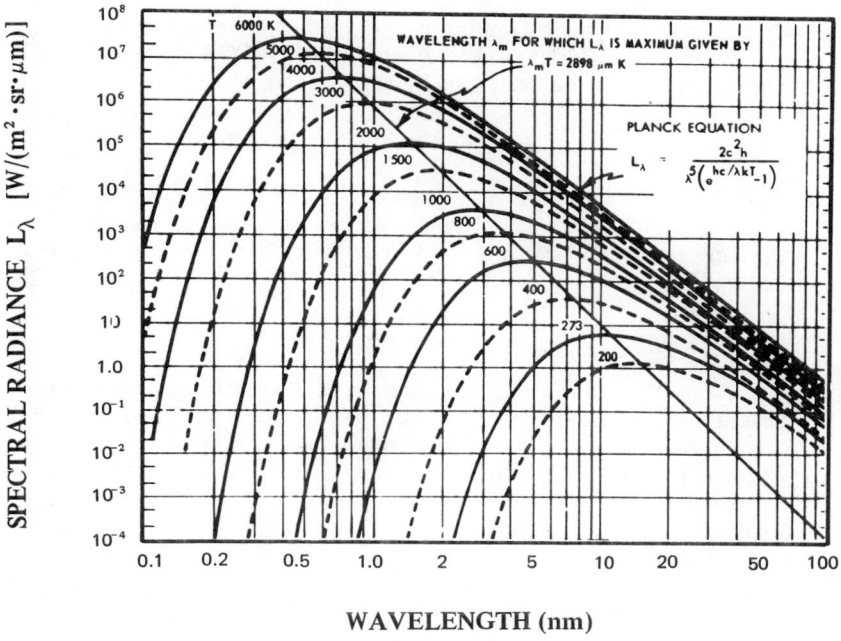

Figure 2-16. Spectral radiance L_λ of blackbodies at absolute temperature T in °K. Ordinate subdivisions are at 2 and 5 (adapted from RCA, 1974).

An important class of infrared sources for which radiation results from molecular vibrations is the *blackbody radiator*. As we noted earlier, it was the study of such emission by Planck which led initially to the quantum hypothesis. The derivations of Planck's formula for the *spectral radiant exitance* W_λ, i.e., the radiant power in watts-per-square-centimeter exiting from source area, as a function of wavelength, is given in many textbooks and need not be reproduced here. A useful form of Planck's radiation law is:

$$W_\lambda = \frac{2\pi c_1}{\lambda^5 (e^{c_2/\lambda T} - 1)} \qquad (2\text{-}21)$$

where c_1 is $c_o^2 h$ or 5.953×10^{-13} W/cm²; c_2 is $c_o h/k$ or 1.438 cm/°K; c_o is speed of light in free space; h is *Planck's constant* or 6.626×10^{-34} J·s; and k is *Boltzmann's constant* or 1.38×10^{-23} J/°K. If this formula is graphed for various values of the absolute temperature T, curves similar to those shown in Fig. 2-16 are obtained. The figure shows the absolute values of spectral radiance, the power per unit area of the source per unit solid angle into which radiation is emitted. For the blackbody radiator, and for a large number of other sources which appear equally bright viewed from all directions (i.e., *Lambertian*), the spectral radiance L_λ is related to the radiant emittance W_λ by the formula:

$$L_\lambda = W_\lambda/\pi \qquad (2\text{-}22)$$

Planck's radiation law leads directly to two other well known laws describing blackbody radiation, even though these laws had been established earlier. The *Stefan-Boltzmann Law* for radiant exitance describes the total radiant exitance of a blackbody. It states that:

$$W = \sigma T^4 \qquad (2\text{-}23)$$

That is, the radiant exitance W of a blackbody is proportional to the fourth power of the absolute temperature of the body. The Stefan-Boltzmann constant σ is $(2\pi^5/15)(c_1/c_2^4)$. This law follows from Planck's result by adding up the spectral radiant exitance for all wavelengths (integrating over all wavelengths).

Wien's Displacement Law is:

$$\lambda_m T = 0.288 \text{ cm}°\text{K}$$
or
$$\lambda_m = 0.228 \text{ cm}°\text{K}/T \qquad (2\text{-}23)$$

This expresses the familiar fact that the spectral distribution of a blackbody radiator and the wavelength λ_m of maximal spectral radiance shifts to shorter wavelengths with increasing temperature. As the substance surrounding a cavity is heated up, the cavity appears deep red, red hot, yellow, then "white hot," and finally blue or violet. Wien's displacement law follows at once from Planck's formula (2-21) by simple calculus to find the maximum value of a function. The first derivative is set equal to zero, and Wien's displacement law appears as the result.

2.13 INCANDESCENT SOURCES

Incandescent sources, such as filaments or heated wires, often emit light with spectral radiant exitance similar to, though not as intense as blackbody radiators. The ratio of any real source's emission to a blackbody's emission is termed the real source's emissivity, ϵ, which is a function of wavelength (as shown in Fig. 2-13) and of absolute temperature. The total emissivity over any spectral band may be defined as the average value of emissivity at each wavelength and is always less than 1. The theory for blackbody radiators may thus be applied to a variety of other sources with similar spectral distributions. For example, the radiance L of a source with emissivity ϵ may be written down at once using Eq. (2-22) and (2-23).

$$L = \epsilon \sigma T^4/\pi \qquad (2\text{-}25)$$

assuming that the source is equally bright when viewed from all directions.

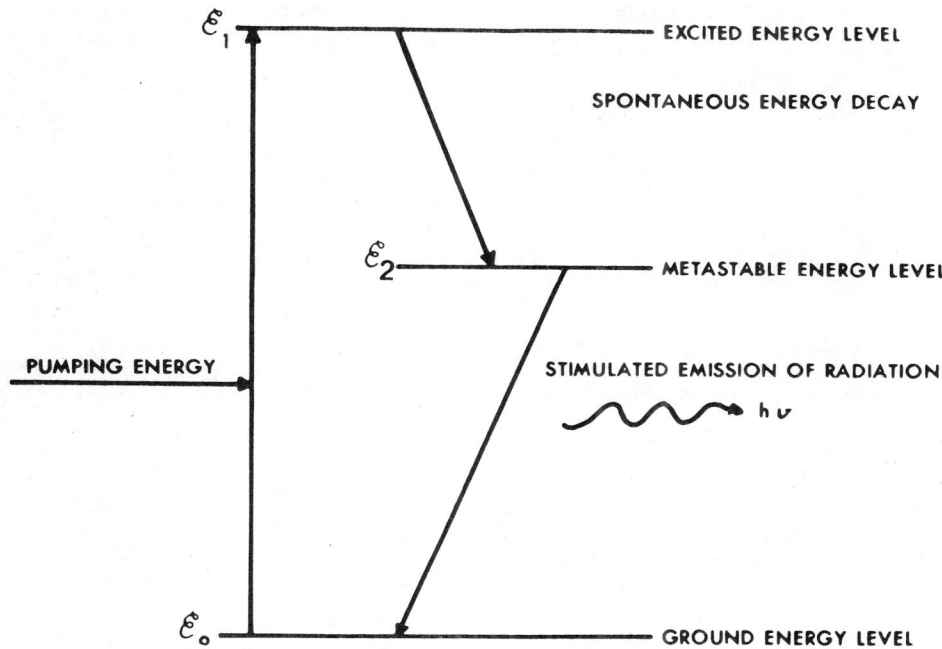

Figure 2-17. Three level energy diagram—one of the many possible sets of energy level transitions that can result in laser action. An absorbed photon (pumping energy) results first in an electron in an excited state at $\mathcal{E}_1$. However, the emitted laser photon energy corresponds to $\mathcal{E}_2 - \mathcal{E}_0$ since $\mathcal{E}_2$ is the longer-lived (metastable) level.

2.14 THE LASER

The laser has three basic components: (a) a lasing medium; (b) a pumping system (energy source); and (c) a resonant optical cavity. Lenses, mirrors, shutters, saturable absorbers, and other accessories may be added to the system to obtain more power, shorter pulses, or special beam shapes but only these three basic components are necessary for laser action.

2.14.1 Lasing Medium

A lasing medium, to have suitable energy levels, must have at least one metastable state long enough for a *population inversion* to occur, i.e., there are more electrons in the excited state than in the lower state to which these electrons decay when stimulated emission occurs. Figure 2-17 shows a simplified three-level energy diagram for a laser material. This is just one of the many possible systems of energy

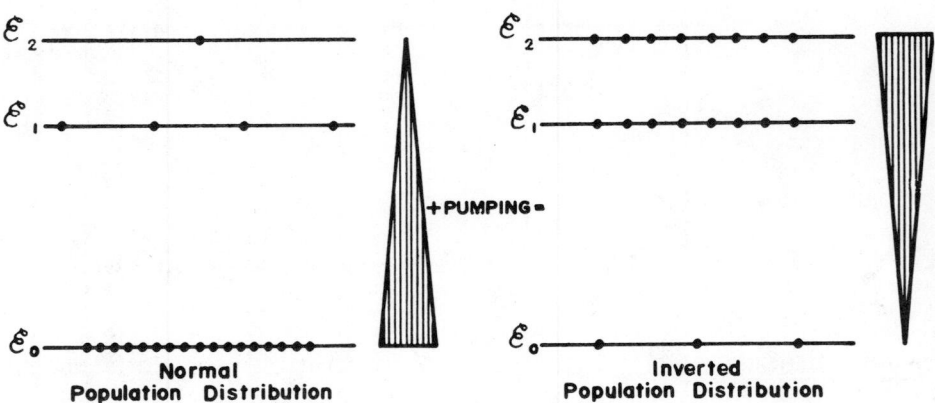

Figure 2-18. Population inversion is produced by pumping electrons from a lower energy state to a higher energy state so that the higher state has more electrons (larger population) than the lower state.

levels. Although laser action is possible with only two energy levels, most such actions involve four or more levels. The normal population of N_1 atoms in an excited state whose energy level is $\mathcal{E}_1$ (in joules) in comparison with the ground state energy level $\mathcal{E}_0$ compared to the total N_0 atoms is described by the Boltzmann equation:

$$N_1 = N_0 \, e^{-(\mathcal{E}_1 - \mathcal{E}_0)kT} \qquad (2\text{-}26)$$

k is the Boltzmann Constant (k = 1.38 × 10^{-23} J/°K). To obtain population inversion by temperature rise rather than photon excitation would require incredible temperatures.

2.14.2 Pumping System

To raise electrons to a higher energy level, lasers employ pumping systems. These systems pump energy into the laser material, increasing the number of electrons trapped in the metastable energy level until a population inversion exists sufficient to enable laser action (Fig. 2-18). Several different pumping systems are available—optical, electron collision, and chemical reaction.

Optical pumping uses a strong source of light, such as a xenon flashtube or another laser (e.g., an argon or nitrogen laser), generally of a shorter wavelength.

Electron collision pumping is accomplished by passing an electric current through the laser material, usually a gas (e.g., helium-neon) laser or a semiconductor junction (e.g., gallium-arsenide) laser, or by accelerating electrons in an electron gun to impact on the laser material, as in some semiconductor or gas lasers.

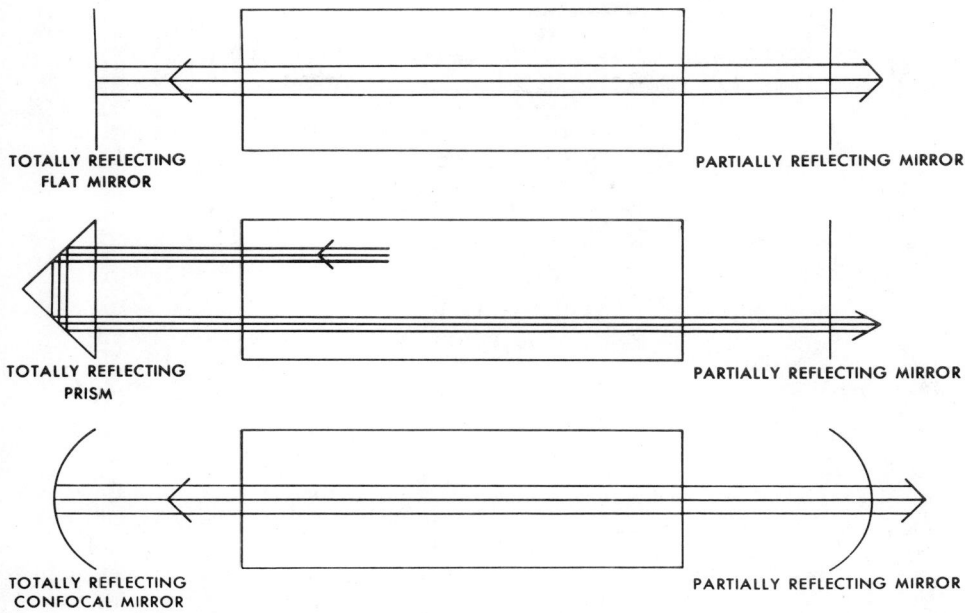

Figure 2-19. Three typical optical cavities: simple flat mirror system (top); rotating prism Q-switched system (middle); confocal mirror system (bottom).

Chemical pumping is based on energy released in the making and breaking of chemical bonds (e.g., some hydrogen-fluoride lasers).

2.14.3 Optical Cavity

A resonant optical cavity (such as a Fabry-Perot resonator) is formed by placing a mirror at each end of the laser material so that a beam of light may be reflected from one mirror to the other (Fig. 2-19). Lasers are constructed in this way so that the beam passes through the laser material many times and the number of emitted photons is amplified at each passage. One of the mirrors is only partially reflecting and permits part of the beam to be transmitted out of the cavity at each reflection.

2.14.4 Laser Operation

Energy is supplied to the laser material by the pumping system. This energy is stored in the form of electron trapped in the metastable energy levels. Pumping must produce a population inversion before laser action can take place.

When population inversion is achieved, the spontaneous decay of a few elec-

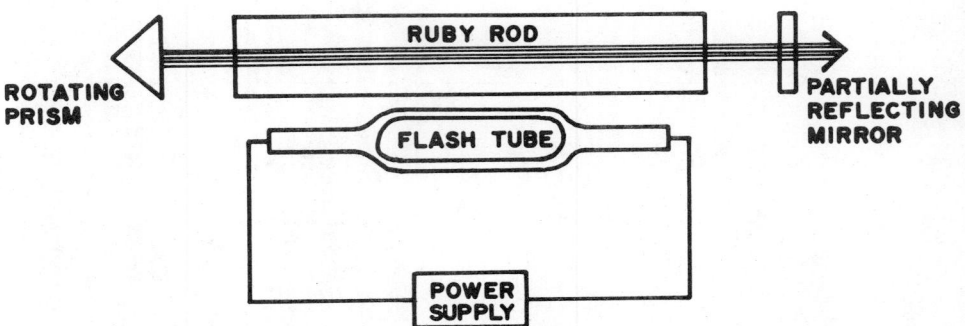

Figure 2-20. Schematic of "solid-state" ruby laser with xenon flash tube as the optical pump. The rotating prism permits "Q-switching" of the cavity.

When population inversion is achieved, the spontaneous decay of a few electrons from the metastable energy level to a lower energy level starts a chain reaction. The photons emitted spontaneously will hit (without being absorbed) other atoms and stimulate their electrons to make the transition from the metastable energy level to lower energy levels, emitting photons of precisely the same wavelength, phase, and direction.

To produce a laser this reaction must take place in an optical cavity. When the photons reach the end of the laser material they are reflected by the end-mirror back into the material where the chain reaction continues and the number of photons is increased. When the photons arrive at a partially-reflecting mirror, only a portion will be reflected back into the cavity and the rest will emerge as a laser beam.

2.14.5 Types of Lasers

Lasers are often designated by the type of laser material in the optical cavity. *Solid-state lasers* employ a glass or crystalline host material (Fig. 2-20); *gas lasers* employ a pure gas or a mixture of gases (Figs. 2-21 and 2-22); *semiconductor lasers* employ n-type and p-type semiconducting elements materials (Fig. 2-23); *liquid lasers* employ active material such as an organic dye in a liquid solution or suspension (Fig. 2-24). Solid-state and liquid lasers commonly employ optical pumping (both coherent and incoherent) while gas lasers usually employ electron-collision pumping, although some types of liquid and gas lasers have employed chemical-reaction pumping. Semiconductor lasers may be optically pumped by an electric current, another laser beam, or electron-collision from an electron beam. Table 2-2 provides an abbreviated list of commercially available laser wavelengths, while a more extensive list of most common laser wavelengths is given in Appendix C.

2.14.6 Temporal Modes of Operation

The different temporal modes of operation of a laser are distinguished by the

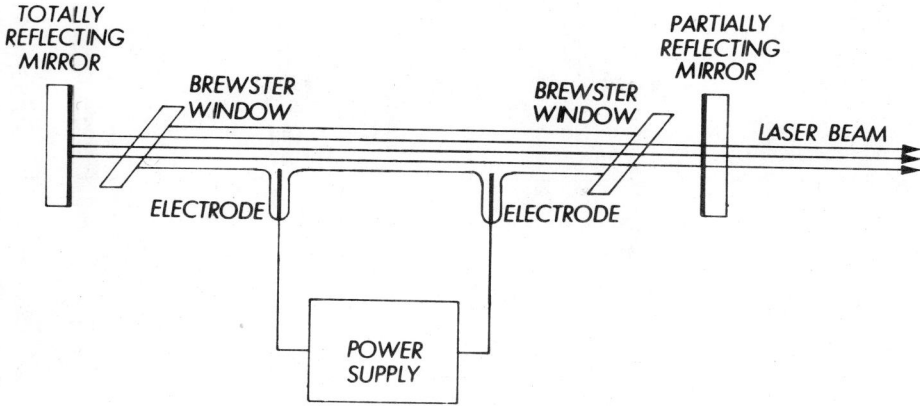

Figure 2-21. Schematic of helium-neon laser with electron collision pumping, representative of small gas lasers. The Brewster windows predominantly pass one polarization.

rate at which energy is delivered. In general, lasers operating in the *normal pulse* temporal mode have pulse durations of a few tens of microseconds to a few milliseconds, often referred to as *"long pulsed"* or just *"pulsed."*

Some lasers are able to operate continuously, termed *continuous wave* or CW. In this type of operation the peak power is equal to the average power output; that is, the beam irradiance is constant with time. Many lasers that appear to be CW may actually have a temporal structure that can only be resolved with very sophisticated measurement systems.

Pulsed lasers can be operated to produce repetitive pulses. The *pulse repetitions frequency* of a laser is the number of pulses which that laser produces in a given duration. Lasers are now available with pulse repetition frequencies as high as several hundreds of thousands of pulses per second. There is an enormous variation in the pulse widths and pulse repetition frequencies which can be generated and the specification of such pulse characteristics is extremely important in any evaluation of the interaction of laser radiation with biological systems.

The resonant quality of the optical cavity of a laser can be changed by rotating an end mirror or placing a shutter within the cavity. This enables the beam to be turned on and off rapidly and normally creates pulses with a duration of a few nanoseconds to a few microseconds. This operation is normally called Q-switching although it is sometimes referred to as *Q-spoiling* or *giant pulsing*. (The "Q" refers to the resonant quality of the optical cavity.) A Q-switched laser usually delivers *less* energy than the same laser operating to give normal pulses, but the energy is delivered in a much shorter time period. Thus, Q-switched lasers are capable of delivering very high peak powers of several megawatts or even gigawatts. Figure 2-25 shows oscilloscope traces of both a normal pulse and a Q-switched pulse.

When the phases of different temporal frequencies are intermixed, at the synchronization peaks the different oscillations will interfere with one another to

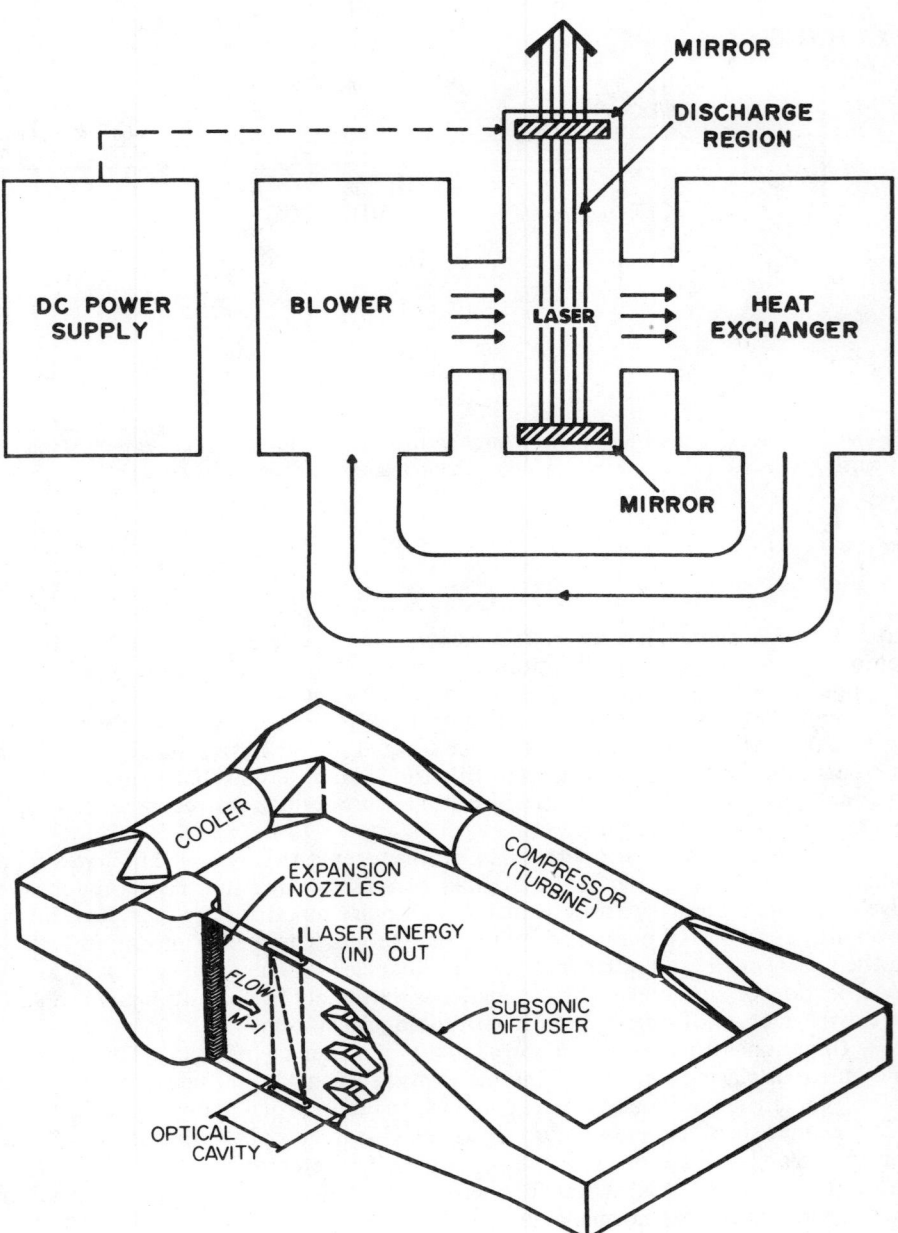

Figure 2-22. A gas laser schematic of CO_2 gas transport laser (GTL) (top panel) has rapid gas flow as indicated by the arrows. A gas-dynamic laser (GDL) (bottom panel) can produce far greater output power due to supersonic jet flow (from Dudley, 1976, with permission).

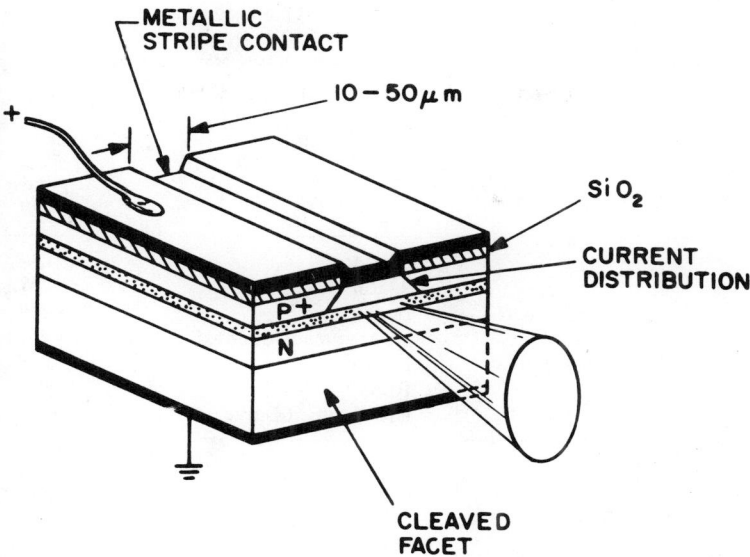

Figure 2-23. Schematic of gallium-arsenide laser with direct-current (electron collision) pumping, representative of semiconductor or injection lasers (from Gorog et al., 1976, with permission).

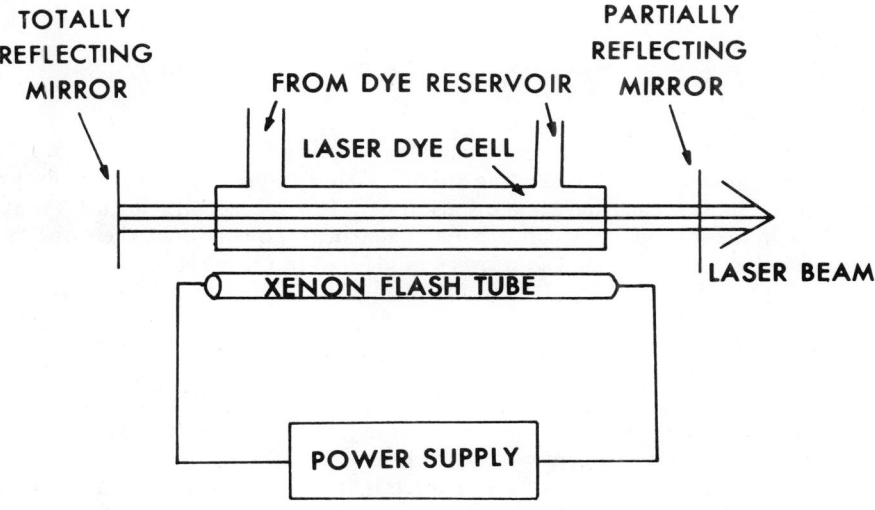

Figure 2-24. Schematic of liquid dye laser with flashtube optical pumping. A CW (e.g., argon) laser is also commonly used to pump a dye laser to provide a tunable CW laser output.

TABLE 2-2. Principal Wavelengths of Common Lasers*

CIE band	Wavelength (nm)	Medium	Typical operation
UV-A	325	He-Cd	CW
UV-A	337	Nitrogen	Pulse train
UV-A	350	Argon	CW
Light	441.6	He-Cd	CW
Light	458, 488, 514.5	Argon	CW
Light	458, 568, 647	Krypton	CW
Light	530	Nd frequency-doubled	Pulsed
Light	632.8	He-Ne	CW
Light	694.3	Ruby	Pulsed
Light	560–640	Rhodamine 6G dye	CW/pulsed
IR-A	850	GaAlAs	Pulse train
IR-A	905	GaAs	Pulse train
IR-A	1060	Nd:glass	Pulsed
IR-A	1064	Nd:YAG	Pulsed
IR-C	5000	CO	CW
IR-C	10,600	CO_2	CW

*These are only representative. See Appendix C for a far more complete listing.

generate a beat effect. The result will be a laser output which is observed as regularly spaced pulsations. Lasers operating in this fashion *(mode-locked)* usually produce trains of pulses, each having a duration of a few picoseconds to a few nanoseconds. A mode-locked laser can deliver higher peak powers than the same laser when Q-switched. Figure 2-25 also shows a mode-locked pulse train.

2.14.7 Spatial (TEM) Modes

Because lasers developed after masers (which were pumped by microwaves), it is only natural that some microwave terminology carried over into laser technology. Indeed, at one time lasers were known as "optical masers." A wave pattern across the direction of propagation is characteristic of all beam geometries (transverse electromagnetic wave or TEM). These wave patterns across the beam are identified with TEM mode notation. Figure 2-26 illustrates how some of the more common modes would look in cross section. Notice that the TEM_{01} mode looks like the TEM_{10} mode rotated 90°. A laser operating in the TEM_{10} mode can be considered as two lasers side-by-side, each with one-half the total power.

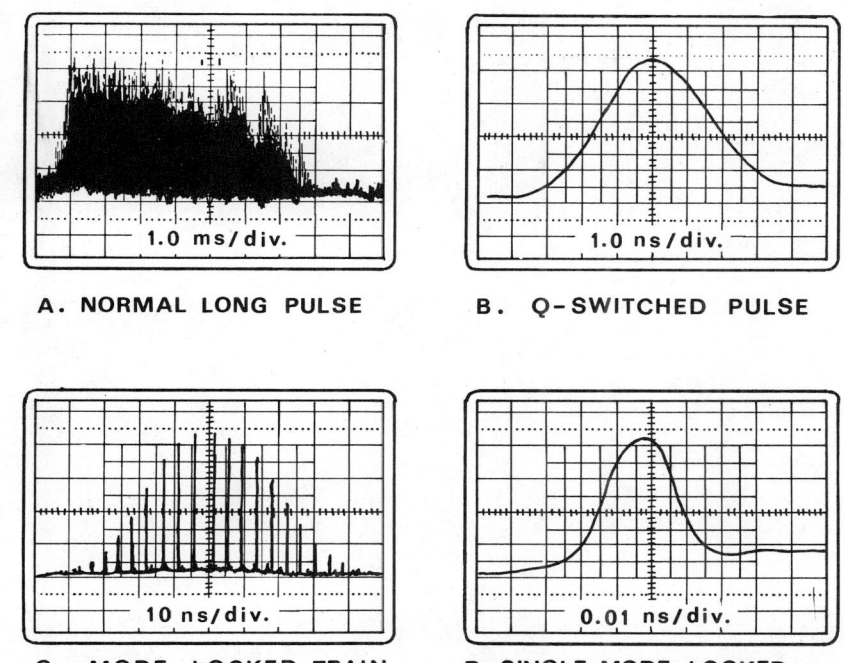

Figure 2-25. Oscilloscope traces of a long pulse laser (A), a Q-switched pulse (B), and mode-locked laser outputs (C and D).

2.14.8 Longitudinal Modes

Longitudinal (or axial) modes do not influence the emergent beam profile but influence the degree of coherency of the spatial and the frequency spectrum. Figure 2-27 illustrates the wavelength spectrum of a gas laser due to its longitudinal modes which are separated by wavelength intervals $\Delta\lambda$ depending upon cavity length b (mirror spacing):

$$\Delta\lambda = \lambda^2/2b \qquad (2\text{-}28)$$

2.14.9 Beam Diameter

The laser beam diameter is measured at the exit aperture of the cavity. For a laser operating in the TEM_{00} mode, the edge of the beam has been variously defined as the circle where the irradiance or radiant exposure is $1/2$, $1/e$, $1/e^2$, or

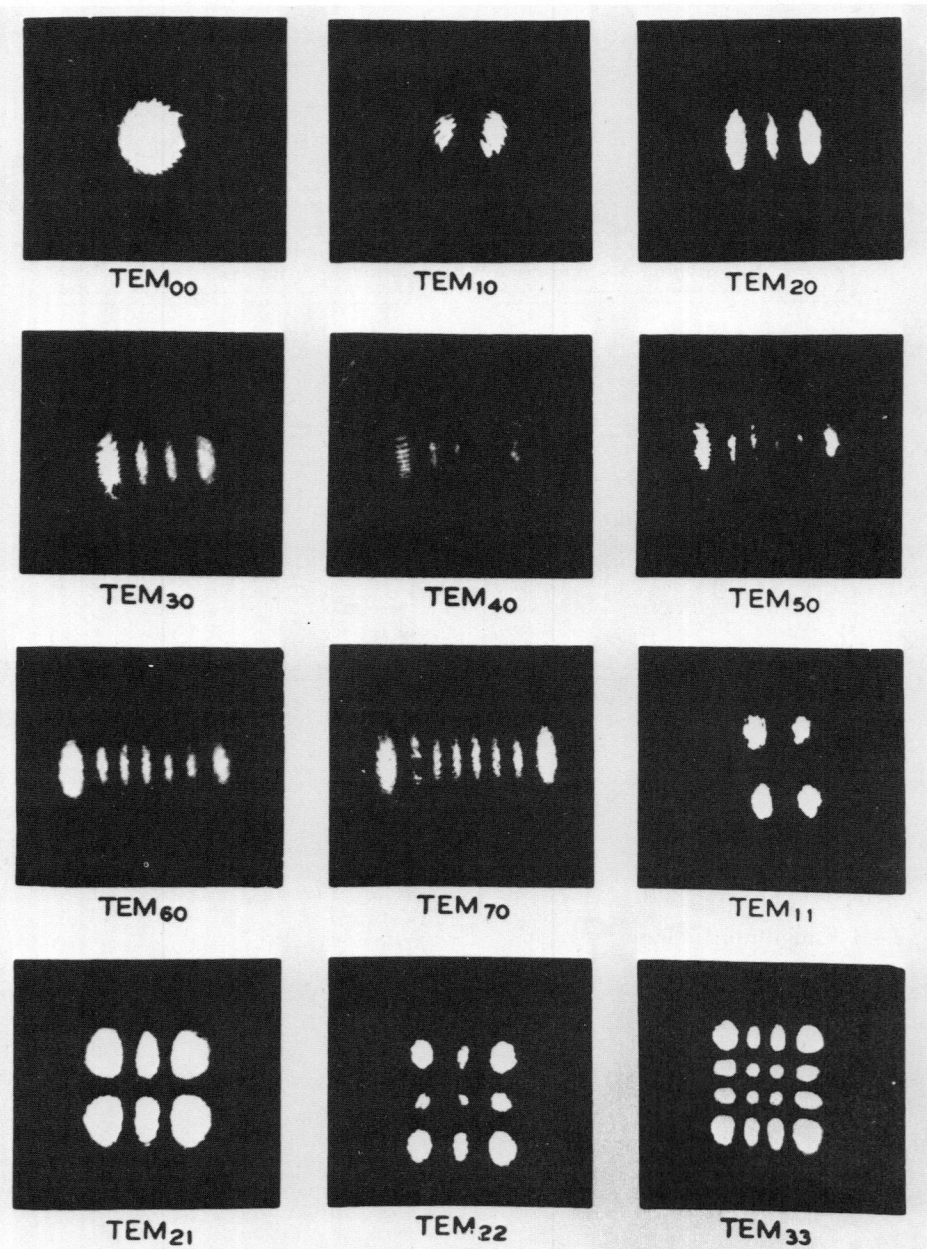

Figure 2-26. Typical transverse electromagnetic (TEM) modes as reflected in the emergent beam cross-sectional patterns of a He-Ne laser. From Kogelnik and Li, 1966, with permission.

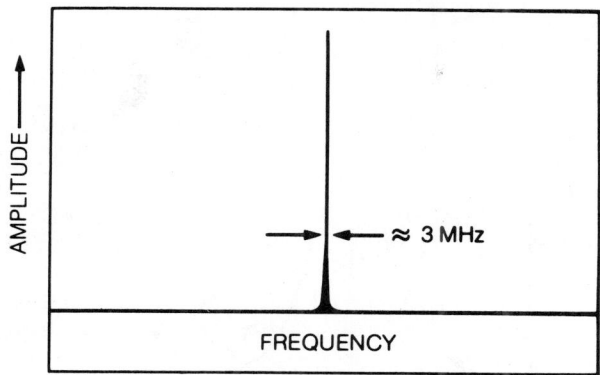

Frequency Stabilized Laser

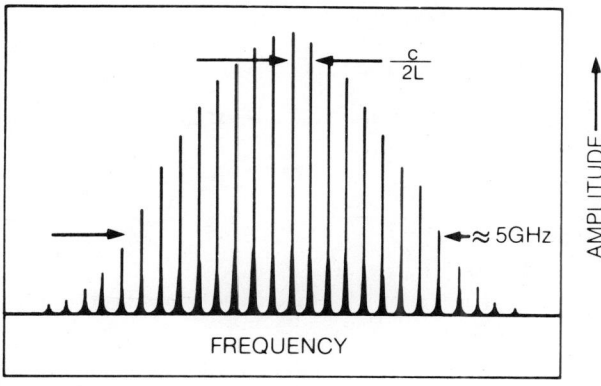

Typical Gas Laser

Figure 2-27. Longitudinal modes in a gas laser as expressed on a frequency or wavelength scale. The separation of modes is dependent upon cavity length L and the velocity of light c.

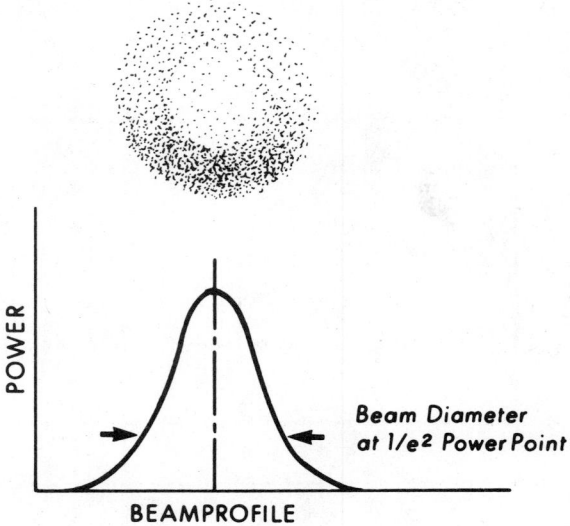

Figure 2-28. Gaussian profile of a single-mode laser beam is graphed by scanning across center of the beam pattern above.

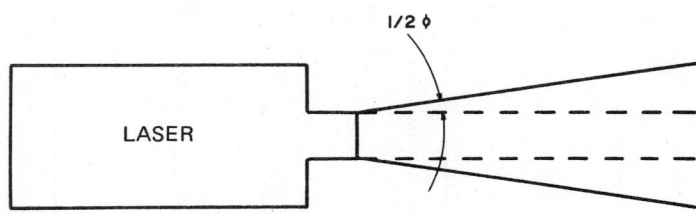

Figure 2-29. The beam divergence of a laser should be expressed at the full angle and not at the half-angle.

1/10 of the maximum (Fig. 2-28). All discussion and examples in this book define the edge of the beam as 1/e or 0.37 of the maximum unless otherwise noted. This subject is discussed at length in Chapter 12.

2.14.10 Beam Divergence

Lasers are unable to produce perfectly collimated beams due to the wave nature of light. However, the divergence, that is, the increase in beam diameter with increase in distance, can be made much smaller than with any conventional source of optical radiation now available, although synchotron radiation is comparable. The divergence angle at one time was expressed as the half-angle $\Phi/2$, as in Fig. 2-29, but is now almost always expressed as the full angle ϕ.

The beam divergence is determined with the laser operating (assumed) in the simplest spatial mode, TEM_{00}, and other modes negligibly small. The beam width is measured between the 1/e-peak-irradiance points. The radiant intensity distribution in the TEM_{00} mode is:

$$I = I_0 e^{-2\phi} \qquad (2\text{-}29)$$

2.14.11 Hot Spots

Hot spots are defined as localized areas of the beam where the beam irradiance is much greater than the average across the beam. They are of considerable concern for under some conditions a hot spot may be 100 times higher than the average beam irradiance. There are several sources of "hot spots": inhomogeneities in the laser cavity or areas where more energy is emitted than in other areas; imperfections in the mirrors and lenses of the laser system; and changes caused by atmospheric conditions.

Atmospheric inhomogeneities along the beam path produce lenticular effects (scintillation) which are responsible for atmospheric hot spots. Fog, rain, snow, dust, smoke, or other obscuring haze absorb and/or scatter the laser beam but do not cause "hot spots"; in fact, such scattering reduces the effect of hot spots. In Chapter 13, section 13.3 (atmospheric propagation) these effects are discussed in detail.

2.15 CHARACTERISTICS OF LIGHT SOURCES, COHERENT AND INCOHERENT

2.15.1 Properties of Coherent and Incoherent Light Sources

Now that laser sources have been discussed it is appropriate to go back and describe more fully the characteristics of two general categories of light sources—the point source and the extended source. Without an adequate appreciation of the distinction between extended sources and point sources it is difficult to understand either the properties of coherence or the problems in evaluating hazards peculiar to one or the other type of source.

If light were to originate from a single geometrical point it would be an ideal point source. Obviously there are no ideal point sources in nature since light has finite dimensions of wavelength, and even such minute sources of optical radiation as individual atoms have finite dimensions. Common sense would tell us that a source of no dimensions could radiate no optical power. However, in optical engineering one often speaks of a point source when the relative dimensions of the

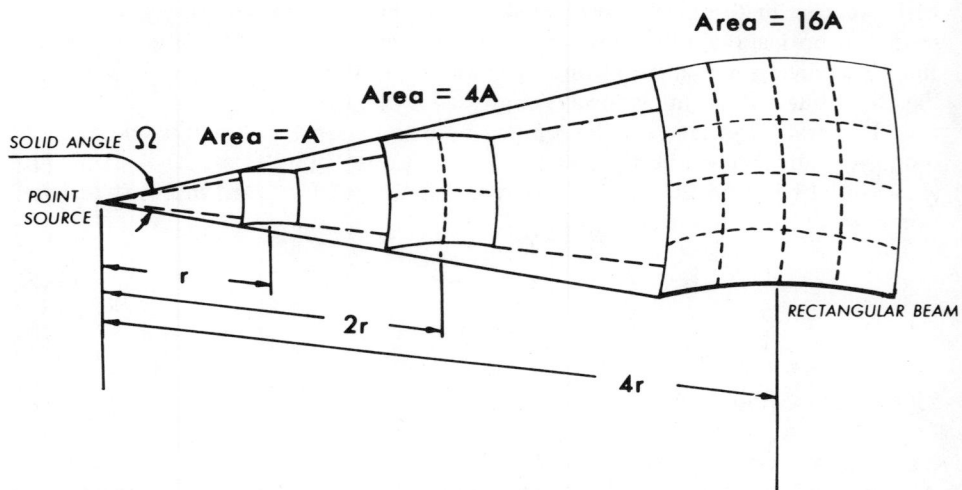

Figure 2-30. The inverse square law can be visualized best by imagining a square beam spreading out from a point source.

practical point sources as a star, which because of its distance subtends an angle so small that even the most powerful telescopes cannot enlarge it. In reality the stars are not point sources and the nearest star, our sun, certainly appears as an extended source.

The light from the sun emanates from an area whose linear angular subtense is approximately one-half of a degree. One could say that any extended source is made up of a large number of point sources and indeed many derivations in optics make use of this approach. To some people the light from the sun appears to be not too far different from that from a point source in that the direct rays from the sun are almost parallel. Nevertheless, if the direct rays of the sun are focused with a magnifying glass there is a finite geometrical image formed. This is especially noticeable during a partial eclipse when a non-circular image is formed. Such would not be the case if the light were from a star which more nearly approximates a point source. By comparing the sun with other stars, one obvious fact emerges, namely that any source behaves as a point source if the source is sufficiently far away so that it cannot be resolved. Very close to a point source all of the rays diverge very rapidly, but from an extended source the irradiance drops slowly. Figure 2-30 shows that a bundle of rays from a point source constantly diverge with a beam cross-sectional area which increases as the square of the distance. Also shown in Figure 2-30 is the decrease of the beam as irradiance (watts-per-square-centimeter) decreases inversely as the square of the distance. Obviously a bundle of light rays from an extended source would behave in a similar manner sufficiently far from the source. In fact, in radiometry the inverse square law is commonly used as a very close approximation for distance greater than 10 source diameters away from any uncollimated extended source. Distances less than ten source diameters

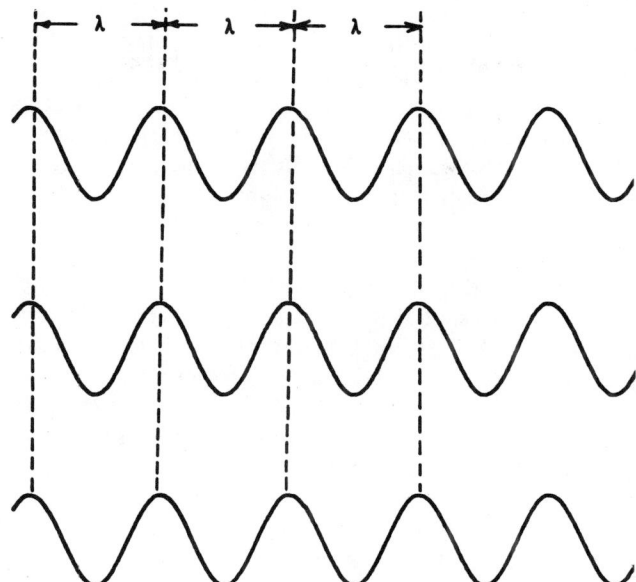

Figure 2-31. Phase relation for temporal coherence. In a laser beam, not only are the waves in step (spatial coherence), but the wavelengths of all the waves are the same and in phase (temporal coherence).

from the source are the "near field" while longer distances are the "far field." However, a well-collimated searchlight beam or a laser beam only obeys the inverse-square law at much greater distances (Chapter 12).

2.15.2 Spatial Coherence

Light emanating from a point source has a characteristic known as *spatial coherence;* that is, light waves all along the sphere of raidus from the point source have the same phase and are more or less in step. Light from an extended source close by is, for this reason, incoherent, since the rays are not all in step at a given radius from the source. Before the advent of the laser, the coherent light required to demonstrate diffraction and interference phenomena was obtained with a pinhole aperture and a reasonably monochromatic (such as a sodium lamp) bright light source. However, such a pinhole obviously limits the optical power output while the laser certainly suffers from no such restriction.

2.15.3 Temporal Coherence of Monochromaticity

A further degree of coherence is present when a light source emits only one wavelength. Again, to show interference and diffraction phenomena in the optical laboratory before the advent of the laser, a pinhole aperture was used in front of a sodium lamp, which emits most of its light in a nearly monochromatic doublet (589.0 and 589.6 nm). Monochromatic light is thought of as temporally coherent because all of the waves can retain their same phase relationships (e.g., to be in step) only if the wavelengths of all the rays in the bundle are the same as shown in Figure 2-31. Another way to look at this coherence is to say that the property of spatial coherence implies that if the properties of a beam of light at one point in space are known then its spatial properties at another point in space can be predicted; that is, the rays all travel in a fixed direction with one another and not in a random disarray as from an extended source. Furthermore, temporal coherence implies that if it is known that all of the waves are going through a maximum at a certain point, then it is also known that a given instant later (the period of the wave) the same maximum will occur; the waves are in phase with one another.

The distinction between coherent and incoherent light is analogous to a group of well-drilled marching soldiers compared with an unruly mob. The soldiers walk a given distance abreast in parallel rows (spatial coherence); they also march in step with the same stride (temporal coherence). The photons from an incandescent bulb is quite incoherent in both respects, more or less like an unruly mob, because the lamp emits different wavelengths, therefore lacks temporal coherence, and emits in different directions in a random fashion, and thereby lacks spatial coherence until a sample is taken at a great distance from the light bulb.

2.15.4 Speckle

A consequence of first-order coherence theory is the phenomenon of *speckle*. Speckle is the shimmering granular appearance of laser light reflected from a diffuse surface. Such speckle patterns may be observed using light from a carefully filtered arc lamp source and on some occasions at night when viewing distant colored light sources. When describing the degree of coherence of a source the parameter of *coherence length* is often used. The coherence length of some high quality gas lasers used in holography often exceed 100 m. The coherence length L_c is determined by the bandwidth (or linewidth) $\Delta \lambda$ of the laser:

$$L_c \simeq \lambda^2/2\pi \Delta\lambda \qquad (2\text{-}30)$$

2.16 RADIOMETRIC AND PHOTOMETRIC TERMS AND UNITS

Two systems of terms and units are used to describe optical radiation. One is a physical system called the radiometric system. Another one, the photometric system, attempts to describe the optical radiation in terms of its ability to elicit the

Review of Optical Radiation Physics

sensation of light by the eye. Table 2-3 gives the most commonly used terms and the "preferred" units for each system. There are generally analogous units in each of the two systems, and the table is arranged to show these similarities. Although the radiometric system of units can be used across the entire spectrum, the photometric system is limited to describing *light* (i.e., electromagnetic radiation that is visible) from approximately 300-400 nm to 760-780 nm.

2.16.1 Radiometric Terms

Of all the terms given in Table 2-3 the following will be encountered most often: *optical energy* (Q), *optical power* (Φ), or sometimes P) and the optical energy or power per unit area of absorbing source, which are known as *irradiance* (E), and *radiant exposure* (H) respectively. Most of these units have an area contribution. The preferred unit of area in the System International (SI) is the meter (m^2) or some 3-decade multiple or submultiple thereof (e.g., mm^2, μm^2, nm^2). However, since the cm is very nearly the size of some laser beams and only slightly larger than the dilated pupil of the eye, as well as a reasonable detector aperture size, cm^2 will be used freely in this text.

2.16.2 Describing Source Output

In classifying lasers, peak power or total energy emitted per pulse are often used for laser classification. On the other hand maximum permissible exposure (MPE) limits (or "exposure limits") are most often described in terms of *irradiance* and *radiant exposure*. The biological effect of radiant energy incident upon tissue is clearly not dependent upon the total energy but upon the energy absorbed per unit area of the absorbing tissue surface. The biological effect is usually also a function of duration.

2.16.2.1 Irradiation of a Surface

To describe effects of radiant energy (Q in joules) upon tissue, most investigators have used power or energy per unit area (e.g., W/cm^2 or J/cm^2) and in early years termed these "power density" or "energy density," as is standard in describing microwave biological effects. By standard CIE nomenclature *power density* and *energy density* refer to power or energy per unit volume and not per unit area and therefore their erroneous use should be discouraged. Rather than use *radiant energy* as a general term, the term "radiation" is preferable. Unfortunately, the term "radiation" has often meant only ionizing radiation to many. One other term once widely used to connote both irradiance and radiant exposure is "beam intensity." By CIE standard terminology, "radiant intensity," I, is power per unit solid angle (watts per steradian) from a point source. Figure 2-32 shows terms for a "solid angle," whose value in steradians is the area of the sphere's surface cut by

TABLE 2-3.

Photometric

Term	Symbol	Defining Equation	SI Units and Abbreviation
Quantity of light	Q_ν	$Q_\nu = \int \Phi_\nu dt$	Lumen-second (lm · s) (talbot)
Luminous energy density	W_ν	$W_\nu = \dfrac{dQ_\nu}{dV}$	Talbot per cubic meter (lm · s · m^{-3})
Luminous flux	Φ_ν	$\Phi_\nu = 680 \int \dfrac{d\Phi_e}{d\lambda} V(\lambda) d\lambda$	Lumen (lm)
Luminous exitance	M_ν	$M_\nu = \dfrac{d\Phi_\nu}{dA} = \int L_\nu \cdot \cos\theta \cdot d\Omega$	Lumen per square meter (lm · m^{-2})
Illuminance (luminous density)	E_ν	$E_\nu = \dfrac{d\Phi_\nu}{dA}$	Lumen per square meter (lm · m^{-2})
Luminous intensity (candlepower)	I_ν	$I_\nu = \dfrac{d\Phi_\nu}{dr}$	Lumen per steradian (lm·sr) or candela (cd)
Luminance[c]	L_ν	$L_\nu = \dfrac{d^2\Phi_e}{dr \cdot dA \cdot \cos\theta}$	Candela per square meter (cd·m^{-1})
Light exposure	H_ν	$H_\nu = \dfrac{dQ_\nu}{dA} = \int E_\nu dt$	Lux-second (lx·s)
Luminous efficacy (of radiation)	K	$K = \dfrac{\Phi_\nu}{\Phi_e}$	Lumen per watt (lm·W^{-1})
Luminous efficiency (of a broad band radiation)	V(*)	$V(*) = \dfrac{K}{K_m} = \dfrac{K}{680}$	Unitless
Luminous efficacy[d] (of a source)	η_ν	$\eta_\nu = \dfrac{\Phi_\nu}{P_i}$	Lumen per watt (lm·W^{-1})
Optical density[e]	D_ν	$D_\nu = -\log_{10} \tau_\nu$	Unitless
Retinal illuminance in trolands	E_t	$E_t = L_\nu \cdot S_p$	Troland (td) = luminance of 1 cd · m^{-2} times pupil area in mm^2

[a]The units may be altered to refer to narrow spectral bands in which case the term is preceded by the word spectral, and the unit is then per wavelength and the symbol has a subscript λ. For example, spectral irradiance H_λ has units of W·m^{-2}·m^{-1} or more often, W·cm^{-2}·nm^{-1}.

[b]While the meter is the preferred unit of length, the centimeter is still the most commonly used unit of length for many of the above terms and the nm or μm are most commonly used to express wavelength.

Useful CIE Radiometric and Photometric Terms and Units [a,b]

Radiometric

Term	Symbol	Defining Equation	SI Units & Abbreviation
Radiant energy	Q_e		Joule (J)
Radiant energy density	W_e	$W_e = \dfrac{dQ_e}{dV}$	Joule per cubic meter (J·m^{-3})
Radiant power (radiant flux)	Φ_e, P	$\Phi_e = \dfrac{dQ_e}{dt}$	Watt (W)
Radiant exitance	M_e	$M_e = \dfrac{d\Phi_e}{dA} = \int L_e \cdot \cos\theta \cdot d\Omega$	Watt per square meter (W·m^{-2})
Irradiance or radiant flux density (dose rate in photobiology)	E_e	$E_e = \dfrac{d\Phi_e}{dA}$	Watt per square meter (W·m^{-2})
Radiant intensity	I_e	$I_e = \dfrac{d\Phi_e}{d\Omega}$	Watt per steradian (W·sr^{-1})
Radiance[c]	L_e	$L_e = \dfrac{d^2\Phi_e}{d\Omega \cdot dA \cdot \cos\theta}$	Watt per steradian and per square meter (W·sr^{-1}·m^{-2})
Radiant exposure (dose, in photobiology)	H_e	$H_e = \dfrac{dQ_e}{dA}$	Joule per square meter (J·m^{-2})
—	—	—	—
—	—	—	—
Radiant efficiency[d] (of a source)	η_e	$\eta_e = \dfrac{P}{P_i}$	Unitless
Optical density[e]	D_e	$D_e = -\log_{10}\tau_e$	Unitless
—	—	—	—

[c] At the source, $L = \dfrac{dM}{d\Omega \cdot \cos\theta}$; at a receptor, $L = \dfrac{dE}{d\Omega \cdot \cos\theta}$

[d] P_i is electrical input power in watts.

[e] τ is the transmission.

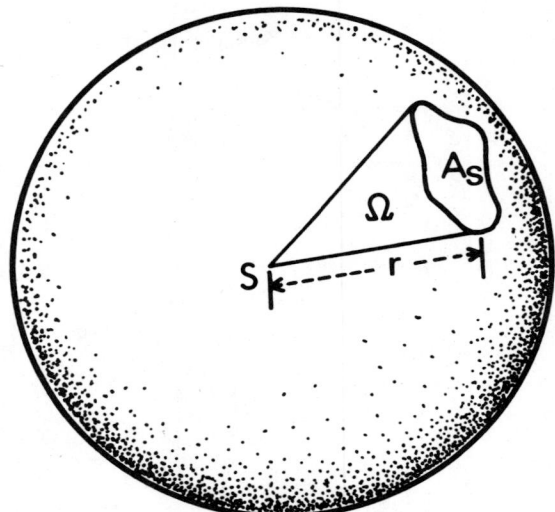

Figure 2-32. Solid angle. A solid angle Ω is defined by an area A_s on a sphere of radius r, e.g., $\Omega = A_s/r^2$. The solid angle is an important geometrical concept in considering luminance, luminous intensity, radiance and radiant intensity.

the angle divided by the square of the radius of the sphere.

Other terms used in discussing ocular hazards are explained briefly in the following two paragraphs. The technical definitions are given in Appendix A of this text. Appendix A also provides a translation table of the more common terms into French, German, and Russian. Figure 2-33 gives simple conceptual drawings of some radiometric forms.

2.16.3 Photometric Analogues of Radiometric Terms

The terms "luminance" and "illuminance" are "photometric" terms which are related to the visual response of the eye; whereas "radiance" and "irradiance" are "radiometric" terms which are related to absolute measurements of radiation. Terms in the "photometric" system are valuable to illuminating engineers in describing levels of visible light in a given situation; whereas terms in the radiometric system are a part of the fabric of physical units and are not dependent on the response of the eye. There are no fixed methods for translating light levels measured in one system to corresponding levels in the other system, since such factors would depend upon the spectral distribution of the radiant source, i.e., how much of the source energy is infrared and ultraviolet radiation not visible to the eye, and how the source energy is distributed in the spectral band to which the eye is most sensitive.

Review of Optical Radiation Physics

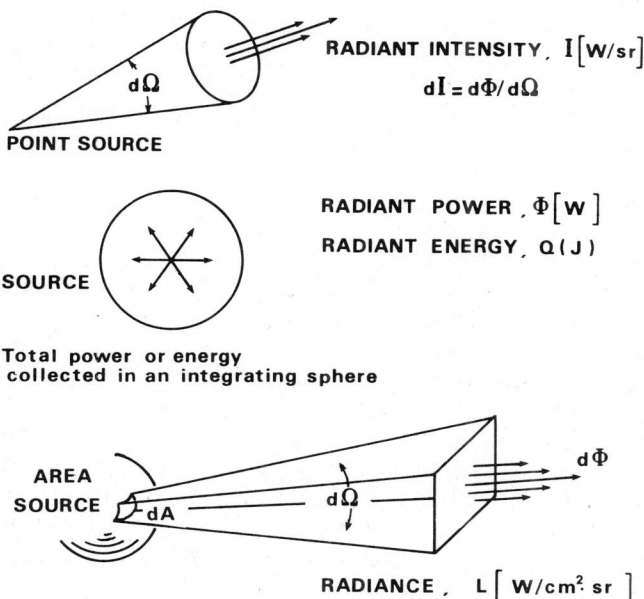

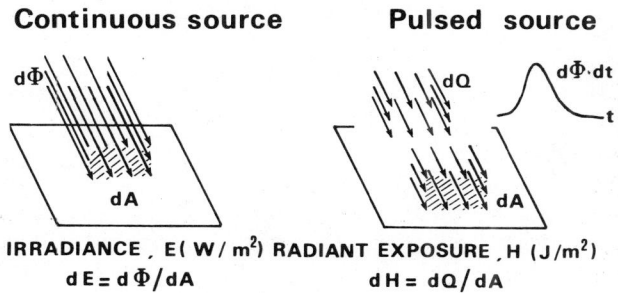

Figure 2-33. Simple conceptual drawings of some radiometric terms.

2.16.3.1 Brightness

The terms "radiance" and "luminance" are used to describe the rate of light or radiant energy leaving the source per solid angle, i.e., the "brightness" of the source. Alternatively, the terms "irradiance" and "illuminance" are used to describe the level arriving at a given point in space, i.e., the level measured by detector which measures the number of photons falling upon a unit of surface. As we shall see later, the concept of radiance shall play a very important role in the evaluation of light sources. We shall see in 15.5.7, Diffuse Reflection, that radiance is conserved.

2.16.3.2 Intensity

The radiometric quantity most often used to define the optical output of a point source or a highly collimated beam is the radiant intensity or which corresponds to the photometric *luminous intensity* (candle power). Since the solid angle (Figure 2-32) of the beam remains constant with distance as is shown in Fig. 2-30, the ratio of the total power to the solid angle remains constant. This ratio is known as the *radiant intensity* and is expressed in watts per steradian (W/sr). One lumen of luminous power per steradian is called a *candela*; thus a 1,000,000 candle-power searchlight has a luminous intensity of 1,000,000 candelas. If the source had a radiant efficacy of 100 lumens per watt then the radiant intensity of that searchlight would be 1,000 W/sr. Measurements of the radiant intensity or the candlepower of a searchlight must be made in the so-called "far field" where the inverse square law is in effect. As long as the source is a point source or sufficiently far away that the inverse square law appears to apply, then the radiant intensity permits a quick calculation of the beam irradiance at any point located at range r from the source. For instance, a source with a beam intensity of 10,000 W/sr has a beam irradiance E at a range r equal to:

$$E = I/r^2 \qquad (2\text{-}31)$$

2.17 REVIEW QUESTIONS

It cannot be overemphasized that time spent now assuring oneself that he or she fully understands these basic radiometric and photometric concepts, terms, and units will be time well repaid.

1. What is the frequency of a light wave of wavelength 600 nm? What is the wavelength of electromagnetic radiation which corresponds to a frequency of 300 GHz (3×10^{11} Hz)?

2. Which one of the following radiations is not part of the electromagnetic

spectrum: (a) radiofrequency; (b) ultraviolet; (c) infrared; (d) ultrasonic; (e) X rays; (f) light.

3. What is the energy of a single ultraviolet photon at 200 nm?

4. Which of the following wavelengths is in the vacuum ultraviolet; the UV-A; UV-B; UV-C; IR-A; IR-B; light? (a) 210 nm; (b) 22 μm; (c) 2210 nm; (d) 1064 nm; (e) 694 nm; (f) 334 nm; (g) 22 nm; (h) 254 nm.

5. What is the total radiance of a 2800°K blackbody? The radiant exitance? The wavelength of maximal spectral radiance?

6. What is Brewster's angle for a plastic having an index of refraction of 1.45? of diamond which has an index of refraction of 2.4195?

7. What percentage of an incident beam of light is reflected for normal incidence from water?

8. What is the reflected irradiance of a 1-joule laser beam from a $MgCo_3$ block (reflectance of 0.9) at 1 m at an angle of 30° from the block's surface?

9. What is the solid angle subtended by a circular source 2 cm in diameter at a distance of 2 m?

10. A ribbon filament of tungsten at 2900°K has a spectral radiance of 0.031 W/(cm^2·sr·nm) at 900 nm. What is the emissivity at that wavelength?

11. What is the speed of light in a glass with an index of refraction of 1.5?

12. What is the approximate absolute temperature of the human body? At what wavelength would be the peak of spectral radiance? What is the radiant exitance of the human body if the emissivity in the infrared is 0.94?

13. A beam of light passing through a 1-m thickness of an attenuating medium loses 90% of its initial power. What is the coefficient of this medium?

14. Atmospheric scientists sometimes refer to attenuation factors in terms of decibel loss (one log unit reduction - 10 dB) per kilometer (dB/km). If a laser beam at 694.3 nm experiences a loss of 2 dB/km, what is the attenuation coefficient?

15. What is the velocity of light in a glass material having a refractive index of 1.5?

2.18 REFERENCES

Allen, L. and Jones, D. G. C., 1967, "Principles of Gas Lasers," Plenum Press, New York.
Arnaud, J. A., 1976, "Beam and Fiber Optics," Academic Press, New York.
Basov, N. G., 1965, Semiconductor lasers, *Science* 149:821–827.
Beran, M., and Parrent, G., Jr., 1964, "Theory of Partial Coherence," Prentice Hall, Englewood Cliffs, New Jersey.
Bitt, S., Weaver, E. G., Rabson, T. A., and Tittel, F. K., 1978, Continuous wave UV radiation tunable from 285 nm to 400 nm by harmonic and sum frequency generation. *Appl. Opt.* 17(5):721–723.
Born, M. and Wolf, E., 1965, "Principles of Optics," 3rd revised edition, Pergamon Press, Oxford.
Carlson, F. P., 1977, "Introduction to Applied Optics for Engineers," Academic Press, New York.
Charschan, S. S., 1972, "Lasers in Industry," Van Nostrand Reinhold Co., New York.
Commission International de l'Eclairage (International Commission on Illumination), 1970, International Lighting Vocabulary, Publication CIE No. 17 (E-1.1) Paris.
Ditchburn, R. W., 1963, "Light," 2nd ed., Interscience Publishers, London.
Dudley, W. W., 1976, "CO_2 Lasers," Academic Press, New York.
Eaglesfield, C. C., 1967, "Laser Light," St. Martins Press, New York.
Eden, G., Burnham, R., Champagne, L. F., Donohue, D., and Djeu, N., 1979, Visible and UV lasers: problems and promises, *IEEE Spectrum* 15(4):50–59 (April 1979).
Ellenbass, W., 1972, "Light Sources," Crane, Russak and Co., New York.
Feynman, R. P., Leighton, R. B., and Sands, M., 1963, 1964, & 1965, "The Feynman Lectures on Physics," in 3 Vols., Addison-Wesley Publishing Co., Reading MA.
Fishlock, D., 1967, "A Guide to the Laser," American Elsevier Publishing Co., New York.
Fowles, G. R., 1968, "Introdu ction to Modern Optics," Holt, New York.
Francon, M., 1963, "Modern Applications of Physical Optics," Interscience Publishers, New York.
Garbuny, M., "Optical Physics," Academic Press, New York.
Gorog, I., Goedertier, P. V., Knox, J. D., Ladany, I., Wittke, J. P., and Firester, A. H., 1976, Information scanning technology: applications of CW A1GaAs injection lasers, *Appl. Opt.* 15(6):1425–1430.
Halliday, D., and Resnick, R., 1974, "Fundamentals of Physics," rev. ed., Wiley, New York.
Herzberger, M., 1958, "Modern Geometrical Optics," Interscience Publishers, New York.
Hudson, R. J., Jr., 1969, "Infrared System Engineering," John Wiley and Sons, New York.
International Standards Organization (ISO), 1978, "Units of Measurement," ISO Handbook 2, ISO, Geneva (Available from the American National Standards Institute, New York).
Jenkins, F. A., and White, H. E., 1957, "Fundamentals of Optics," 3rd ed., McGraw-Hill, New York.
Kingslake, R., 1965-1967, "Applied Optics and Optical Engineering," Volumes I-IV, Academic Press, New York.
Klauder, J. R. and Sudashan, F. C. G., 1968, "Fundamentals of Quantum Optics," W. A. Benjamin, Inc., New York.
Kline, M. V., 1970, "Optics," John Wiley and Sons, New York.
Kline, M. V., and Ray, I. W., 1965, "Electromagnetic Theory and Geometrical Optics," Interscience Publishers, New York.
Koechner, W., 1976, "Solid-State Laser Engineering," Springer-Verlag, New York.
Kogelnik, H. and Li, T., 1966, "Laser Beams and Resonators," *Appl. Optics* 5:1550.
Koller, L. R., 1965, "Ultraviolet Radiation," 2nd ed., John Wiley and Sons, New York.
Kruse, P. W., McGlauchlin, L. D., and McAquistan, R. B., 1962, "Elements of Infrared Technology," John Wiley and Sons, New York.

Lengyel, B. A., 1966, "Introduction to Laser Physics," John Wiley and Sons, New York.
Levi, L., 1968, "Applied Optics," Vol. 1, John Wiley and Sons, New York.
Linfoot, E. H., 1964, "Fourier Methods in Optical Image Evaluation," Focal Press, London.
Longhurst, R. S., 1967, "Geometrical and Physical Optics," 2nd ed., Longmans, Green and Co., London; John Wiley and Sons, New York.
Meyer-Arendt, J. R., 1968, Radiometry and photometry: units and conversion factors, *Appl. Opt.* 7:2081–2084.
Mooradian, A., Jaeger, T., and Stokseth (eds.), 1976, "Tunable Lasers and Applications," Springer-Verlag, New York.
Pohl, R. W., 1967, "Optik and Atomphysik," 12th edition, Springer-Verlag, Berlin.
Polanyi, T., and Tobias, I., 1971, Principles and Properties of the Laser, American Optical Corporation Research Laboratory, Framingham Center, MA.
Pressley, R. J., 1971, "Handbook of Lasers," Chemical Rubber Co., Cleveland.
RCA Corporation, 1974, "RCA Electro-Optics Handbook," EOH 11, RCA, Harrison, New Jersey.
Ross, D., 1969, "Lasers, Light Amplifiers and Oscillators," Academic Press, New York.
Ross, M. (ed.), 1971-77, "Laser Applications," Academic Press, New York, 1971, Vol. 1; 1974, Vol. 2; 1977, Vol. 3.
Siegman, A. E., 1971, "An Introduction to Lasers and Masers," McGraw Hill, New York.
Sinclair, D. C. and Bell, W. E., 1969, "Gas Laser Technology," Holt Rinehart and Winston, New York.
Smith, F. G., and Thomson, J. H., 1971, "Optics," Wiley, London.
Smith, P. W., 1970, Mode-locking of lasers, *Proc. IEEE* 58(9):1342–1357, (Sept. 1970).
Smith, W. J., 1966, "Modern Optical Engineering," McGraw-Hill, New York.
Smith, W. V., and Soronkin, P. P., 1966, "The Laser," McGraw-Hill, New York.
Sommerfeld, A., 1964, "Optics," Lectures on theoretical physics, Vol. IV, Academic Press, New York.
Strong, J., 1958, "Concepts of Classical Optics," W. H. Freeman and Company, San Francisco.
Stroke, G. W., 1969, "An Introduction to Coherent Optics and Holography," Academic Press, New York.
Svelto, O., 1976, "Principles of Lasers," Plenum Press, New York.
Townes, C. H., 1965, Production of coherent radiation by atoms and molecules, *Science* **149**: 831–840.
U.S. Naval Research Laboratory, 1963, "Military Infrared Applications Handbook," Washington.
van de Hulst, H. W., 1957, "Light Scattering by Small Particles," John Wiley and Sons, New York.
Walsh, J. W. T., 1965, "Photometry," 3rd edition, Constable and Company, London, 1958; Dover Publishing Company, New York.
Welford, W. T., 1962, "Geometrical Optics," North-Holland Publishing Company, Amsterdam.
Williams, C. S., and Becklund, 1972, "Optics, A Short Course for Engineers and Scientists," Wiley Interscience, New York.
Wolf, E. (ed.), 1966, "Progress in Optics," North-Holland Publishing Company, Amsterdam.
Wolf, E., and Zissis, G. W., 1979, "Infrared Applications Handbook," Office of Naval Research, Washington, DC.
Wood, Robert W., 1934, "Physical Optics," 3rd edition, MacMillan and Company, New York.

Chapter 3
Review of Anatomy and Physiology of the Eye and Skin

3.1 INTRODUCTION

The material in this chapter is provided as an introduction to those aspects of the anatomy and physiology of both the eye and skin which should be familiar to those working extensively in the field of optical radiation safety. This chapter is neither a comprehensive nor a detailed treatment of these subjects. It is primarily intended for those who have not had specialized training in the life sciences and it can be conveniently bypassed by anyone who is familiar with the subject. Hopefully, it may also serve as a review of the anatomy and physiology of the skin and eye for those who have not studied this subject for some time. The eye in itself and the subject of vision in general are fascinating subjects about which there are vast bodies of literature. However, in this chapter, emphasis will be placed upon those aspects of ocular anatomy and physiology which are important to this study: the optical properties of the ocular media (cornea, aqueous, lens, and vitreous), retinal structure, and image formation.

3.2 THE EYE

3.2.1 The Structure of the Eye

3.2.1.1 General

The adult human eye is roughly the size of a 25-cent U.S. coin (approximately 25 mm in diameter). Figure 3-1 shows a simplified drawing of the human eye which

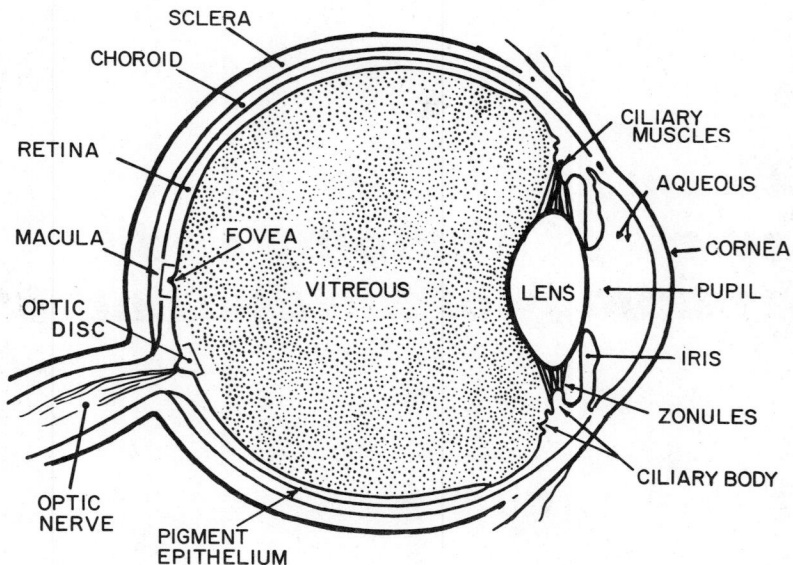

Figure 3-1. The general structure of the eye showing the principal structures referred to in this text. This cross-section is for a horizontal section as seen from above for a standard left eye. The physical dimension and optical parameters based upon the Gullstrand normal eye are given in Appendix B.

names the principal structures of the eye. The optical constants for a standard eye are given in Appendix B. Light passes through the various ocular structures to fall upon the retina where it triggers a photochemical process which evokes the neural impulses that lead to vision. In this journey the light first passes through the structures in the anterior portion of the eye–the cornea, the aqueous humor in the anterior chamber, the pupil (and sometimes the iris), the somewhat pliable crystalline lens, and into the posterior part and the vitreous humor and the numerous layers of the retina. Each eye is nearly a sphere and its movement within the bony socket is controlled by six muscles. Together, the two eyes can be directed at a distant point in space to provide stereoscopic depth perception out to approximately 580 m or a disparity angle of 24 arc seconds. The eye is protected from external blows (and from optical radiation from above) by the brow ridge (supraorbital ridge).

3.2.1.2 The Cornea

The cornea of the eye is living tissue which is exposed directly to the environmental elements. It is protected from drying out only by the tear film. In comparison with the epithelial (epidermal) cells of the skin which have a dead horny layer to protect them, the corneal epithelial cells must survive a very harsh environment. Perhaps for this reason, the corneal epithelial cells have only a very short lifetime--approximately 48 hours. The corneal epithelium has one of the highest metabolic rates in the entire body. The tear layer of 6-10 μm thickness which protects this cell layer and maintains wetness is fairly finely balanced (Fig. 3-2). The outermost surface of the tear layer is a superficial lipid mono-multilayer less than 0.4 μm in thickness, then beneath this are mucin layers with gradually increasing concentrations of mucin. The constant blinking of the lids spreads the mucins which can adsorb onto the epithelium, thereby creating a hydrophilic surface upon which tears will spread without beading. Maintenance of a smooth optical interface obviously depends upon adequate mucin production by the conjunctival goblet cells, sufficient tear secretion, and blinking.

The inhomogeneous cellular corneal structure has caused some physicists to wonder how it can be so transparent. The subject of corneal transparency and the apparent importance of maintaining an orderly mosaic of cells is complex and will not be further discussed here. It is sufficient to indicate that this inhomogeneous system must maintain a very delicate balance between parts to retain transparency. The interested reader is referred to Benedek (1971) for an extended discussion. The corneal epithelial cells are constantly being created in the germinative stromal layer as others are continually sloughed off in the tear layer. Injury to the stroma or deeper layers seems to be required before permanent irreparative change can occur in the cornea; injury limited to the epithelium would be expected to be repaired within two days by normal cell turnover.

3.2.1.3 The Aqueous

The aqueous, as its name implies, is essentially water; hence one cannot speak of "injury" to the aqueous. The aqueous slowly drains out of the eye through a filtration bed at the base of the ciliary body. It is replinished largely by secretion from the ciliary body. The aqueous as well as the cornea serves as a heat-absorbing water filter for the lens, protecting it from IR-B and IR-C thermal radiation. Of course in this role any significant elevation of the temperature of the aqueous will be transferred to the lens by conduction. The pressure within the eye is determined by the balance between inflow and outflow. As the eyeball is a more or less rigid container, increases above the physiological level within the eyeball (so-called *glaucoma*) may inhibit blood flow into the eye, leading to injury and atrophy of the retina. Injury to the eye can also result in pressure changes which will in time produce glaucoma. Thus glaucoma, like cataract, may be a response to chronically renewed trauma of any type. Another result of injury to the eye is the collection of floating debris--cell remains, blood, etc.--in the aqueous. These can compromise the optical pathway

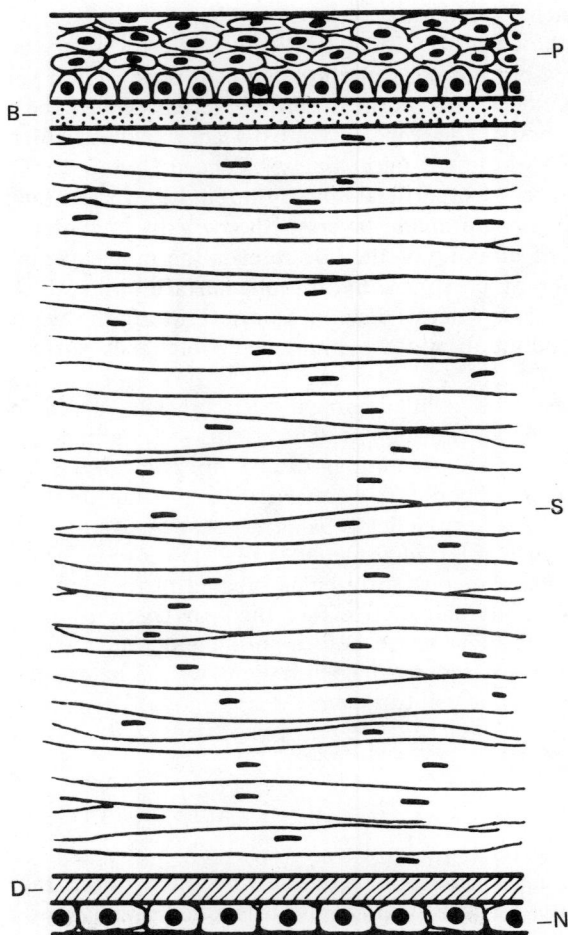

Figure 3-2. An artist's conception of the structure of different layers of the cornea. The epithelium (50-100 μm thick) is the structure facing the environment (P); Bowman's membrane (B) is 8-14 μm thick; stroma (S) is about 500 μm in thickness near the visual axis; Descemet's membrane (D) is 5-10 μm thick and the corneal endothelium (N) is about 5 μm thick. Adapted from Duke-Elder (1937).

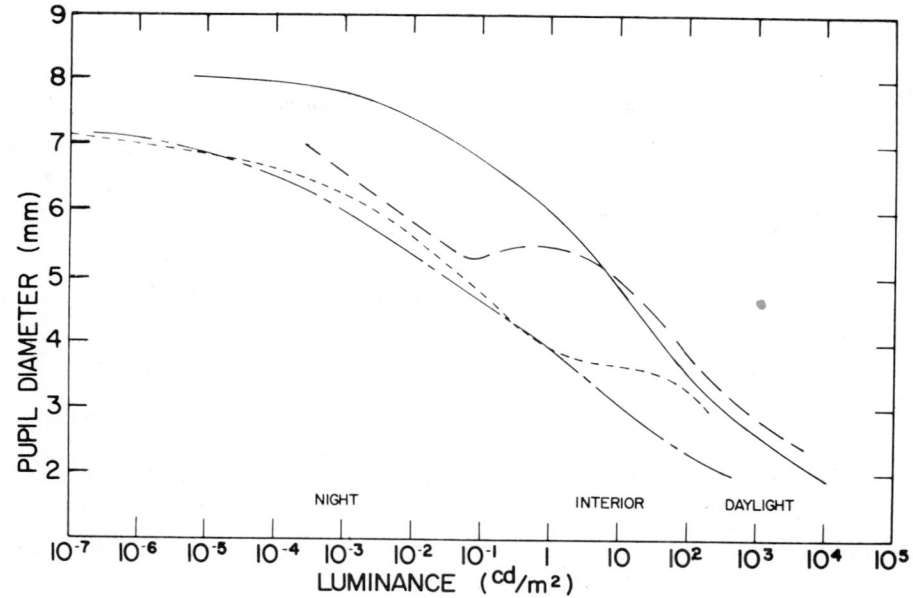

Figure 3-3. Variation of human pupil size with ambient light conditions. The abscissa provides the luminance of the adapting field with pupil diameter measured in 4 studies from Crawford (1936), ---; Reeves (1921), ———; Flamant (1948), – – –; and the average of 8 studies by de Groot and Gebhard (1952), ——–--——–-, (from Sliney, 1971, with permission).

and be responsible for changes in optical function if sufficient amounts accumulate.

3.2.1.4 The Iris

The iris is a normally heavily pigmented layer of muscular tissue which adjusts the pupil of the eye. Opposing radial (dilator) and circular (sphincter) muscles adjust the size of the pupil from approximately 2 to 7 mm as a function of the average brightness of the subject being viewed. *Myosis* (pupil contraction) is most marked for rapid changes in retinal illumination. Gradual changes in ambient lighting has only a weak effect. The myosis is more pronounced if the central areas of the retina (fovea and macula) are illuminated than if peripheral areas are illuminated at the same level. *Mydriasis* (dilation of the pupil) is slower. The pupillary response is wavelength dependent in accord with adaptation of the retina. Figure 3-3 shows the variation of pupil size as determined by several different studies. The organic pigments of the iris are similar to pigments in the skin and retina and do not strongly absorb in the near-infrared spectral band (IR-A). Upon exposure to a very bright light source, a dilated pupil will constrict within about 20 ms (Davson, 1962).

3.2.1.5 The Lens

The crystalline lens (termed "crystalline" by the early anatomists through its resemblance to rock crystal or glass) is supported in place by fine ligaments (zonules) which are connected to the ciliary body. The ciliary muscles control the eye's focusing ability and their excessive use may result in eye fatigue. The outer enclosure of the lens is the non-cellular laminated membrane known as the lens capsule to which the supporting zonules are attached. The inner portion is termed the lens cortex, and the most dense, central region is termed the nucleus.

The lens, like the cornea, is an inhomogeneous material, yet it is clear in the visible range of the spectrum. This clarity is the result of a precise relation of the various minute, optically active constituents. Damage to the lens disturbs this relation and destructive interference of light rather than the normal constructive interference results with increased light scattering. The lens becomes milky or looks like it has in it a miniature waterfall or cataract.

There are several geometric references useful in discussing the lens. An axial line, drawn through the center of the pupil, running back through the lens along the optical pathway, passes through the anterior (facing the cornea) and the posterior (facing the retina) poles. The equator is perpendicular to this axis around the fattest part of the lens.

The lens fibers come from the transparent ribbon-like lens cells which run from the anterior to the posterior pole attaching at the sutures, as shown in Fig. 3-4. Each lens fiber runs completely around from the front of the lens to the back. The bulging posterior surface is accomplished by having the lens fibers fatter in the back than in the front. Thus, injury to any single fiber which in time extends through that entire fiber will be more apparent in the thicker part of the lens. If surface lens fibers are injured the injury will appear to be more concentrated in the posterior portion of the lens immediately adjacent to the capsule (posterior subcapsular cataract).

The capsule, a tough membranous coating surrounding the lens, molds the semiplastic lens into shape, rather flat along the anterior pole and bulging along the posterior pole. Since the tough capsule prevents the lens from growing any larger, as new cells are added the older cells in the center of the lens become squeezed into a smaller volume by loss of water. This loss of water decreases the pliability of a nucleus relative to the more pliable cortex. The lens in youth has a small nucleus. With age the nucleus increases in size. This increase is a reliable gauge of age and the corresponding loss of overall elasticity of the lens by an increase of the nucleus in proportion to the cortex is accompanied by a loss of the ability of the lens to change its shape with changes in tension. The ability of the lens to focus or accommodate depends upon the changes in shape with changes in tension from the ciliary muscle. This continual growth of the nucleus is the cause of loss of accommodation with age, or presbyopia.

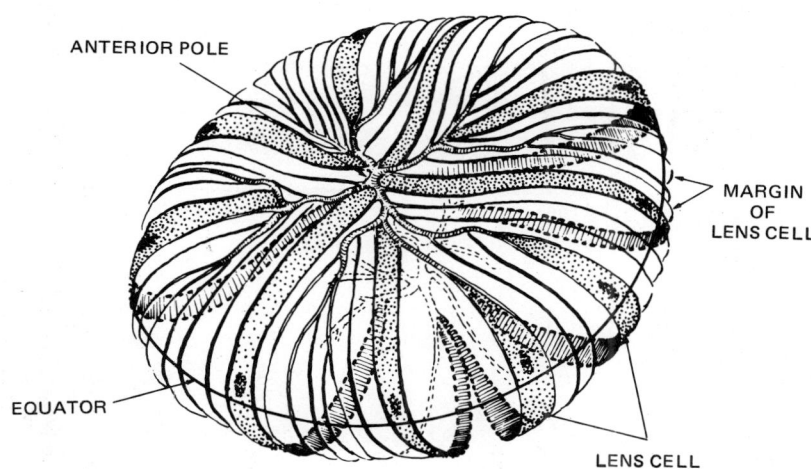

Figure 3-4. The human lens. Although the lens appears largely transparent, a very careful analysis reveals cells which stretch from the anterior to the posterior pole. Cell nuclei are generally located near the equator. Dissection of the lens reveals layers much like an onion, although the lens' layers grow from the inside out as opposed to those in an onion where the newer cells are located in the center. The center of the lens is known as the nucleus and the outer layer is the cortex. The membranous capsule surrounding the lens is attached to the outermost growing layer of lens cells. The capsule is attached to the suspensory ligaments which control accommodation (adapted from Hogan, Alvarado and Wedell, 1971).

3.2.1.6 The Vitreous Body

The vitreous body, a colorless gel formed by collagen fibers with only a few cells, more or less fills the posterior chamber. The vitreous is attached both to the retina and to the ciliary body. The retinal attachments change with age and frequently are lost completely as the vitreous body shrinks with age. The vitreous is largely water, but because of the gel-like nature of the vitreous there is very little circulation. Trauma to the vitreous, especially contact with blood, can cause the vitreous to shrink with resulting traction on the retinal attachments which can lead to a detachment of the retina followed by loss of retinal function.

3.2.1.7 The Retina

The retina, in contrast to other peripheral sense organs, is actually an extension

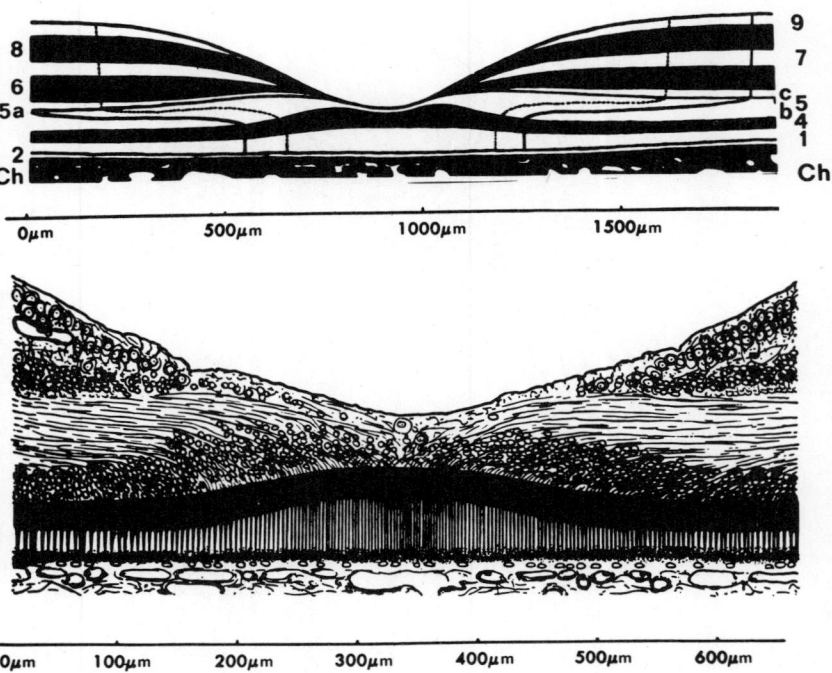

Figure 3-5. The Retina. This drawing of the layered structure of the retina illustrates the constriction of the neural layers near the fovea and their absence in the foveal pit (adapted from Polyak, 1941, *in* Adler, 1970, p. 425).

of the brain and consists of several very complex layers of nerve cells. Figure 3-5 shows a schematic drawing of the retina emphasizing the nerves and their interconnections. There are two types of photoreceptor cells: rods and cones, names for the shape of the distal (away from the synaptic end) extension of the photoreceptor cell. In the retina there are probably 120 million rods averaging 60 μm and 2 μm in diameter and 6 million cones approximately 50 μm long and 3 to 5 μm in diameter. These receptor cells are interconnected by other specialized cells. The organization of the retina will be discussed in greater detail in section 3.2.6. The specific anatomical aspects of the retina of particular importance in a study of retinal injury from light sources are the retinal pigment epithelium (RPE) and adjacent layers. The outer segments of the rods and cones are immediately anterior to the RPE. As shown in

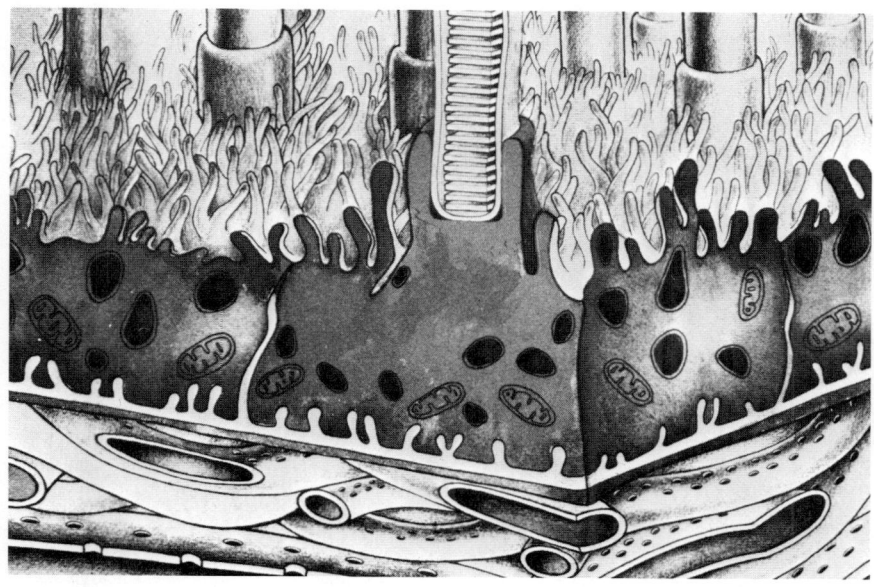

Figure 3-6. The outer segments of the rods. Notice the discs (made up of two lamellar membranes) stacked in the outer segments of the rod. The outermost discs are shed daily and are consumed by the pigment epithelium. The microvilli reach up from the retinal pigment epithelium to assist in this process. (Drawing courtesy J. Marshall and M. Raynor, Institute of Ophthalmology, London.)

Fig. 3-6 there are very small protrusions (*microvilli*) of the RPE which extend upward around the outer segments. As the cones do not extend as near to the RPE as do the rods, the microvilli extend out further to the cone outer segments. It is known that the RPE plays a critical role in the retinal metabolism and photochemistry, hence proper function of the RPE is essential for normal vision. The orderly array of the outer segments is shown in Fig. 3-6A. The cone outer segments are at a higher level than the rod outer segments. In this figure the pigment epithelium has been stripped off to allow good visualization of the outer segments. The outermost discs (made up of lamellar membranes) of the rod outer segments (Fig. 3-7) are continually shed and consumed (phagocytized) by the RPE cells; the rate of shedding is greatest in early morning. The cone lamellar membranes do not form complete discs and do not appear to shed in the same manner as in the rods. Most of the renewal activity in the cones occurs at night.

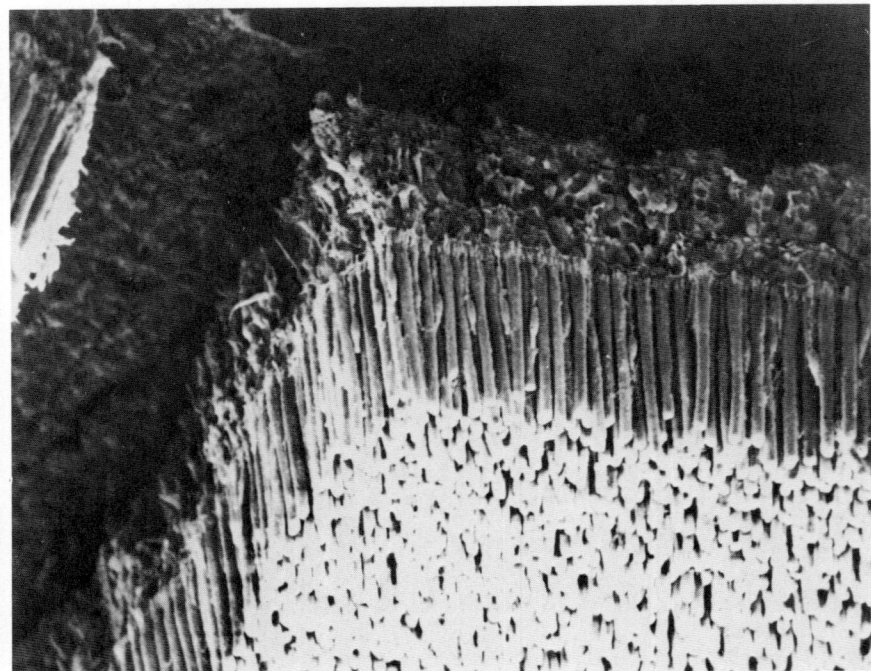

Figure 3-6A. The photoreceptor layer as seen by the scanning electron microscope. This three-dimensional view of the rods and cones in the frog retina was made by peeling away the pigment epithelium. The orientation of the retina is the same as in Figs. 3-5, 3-6 and 3-7--up is toward the front of the eye, or light enters the eye from the top. (Original electron micrograph courtesy Dr. R. Steinberg, University of California, San Francisco.)

Bruch's membrane separates the RPE from the blood supply in the capillary layer of the choriocapillaris and serves as an analogue of the blood-brain barrier.

The neural retina and RPE have different embryonic origins and there is not a strong attachment between them. As a result of any kind of trauma producing a hole in the retina, such as by mechanical shock--often resulting from a strong blow to the head--the neural retina will separate or detach from the RPE. This retinal detachment is quite serious unless quickly repaired, as loss of function and atrophy of the retina inevitably follows. Additional details of the organization and other characteristics of the retina will be given later in this book.

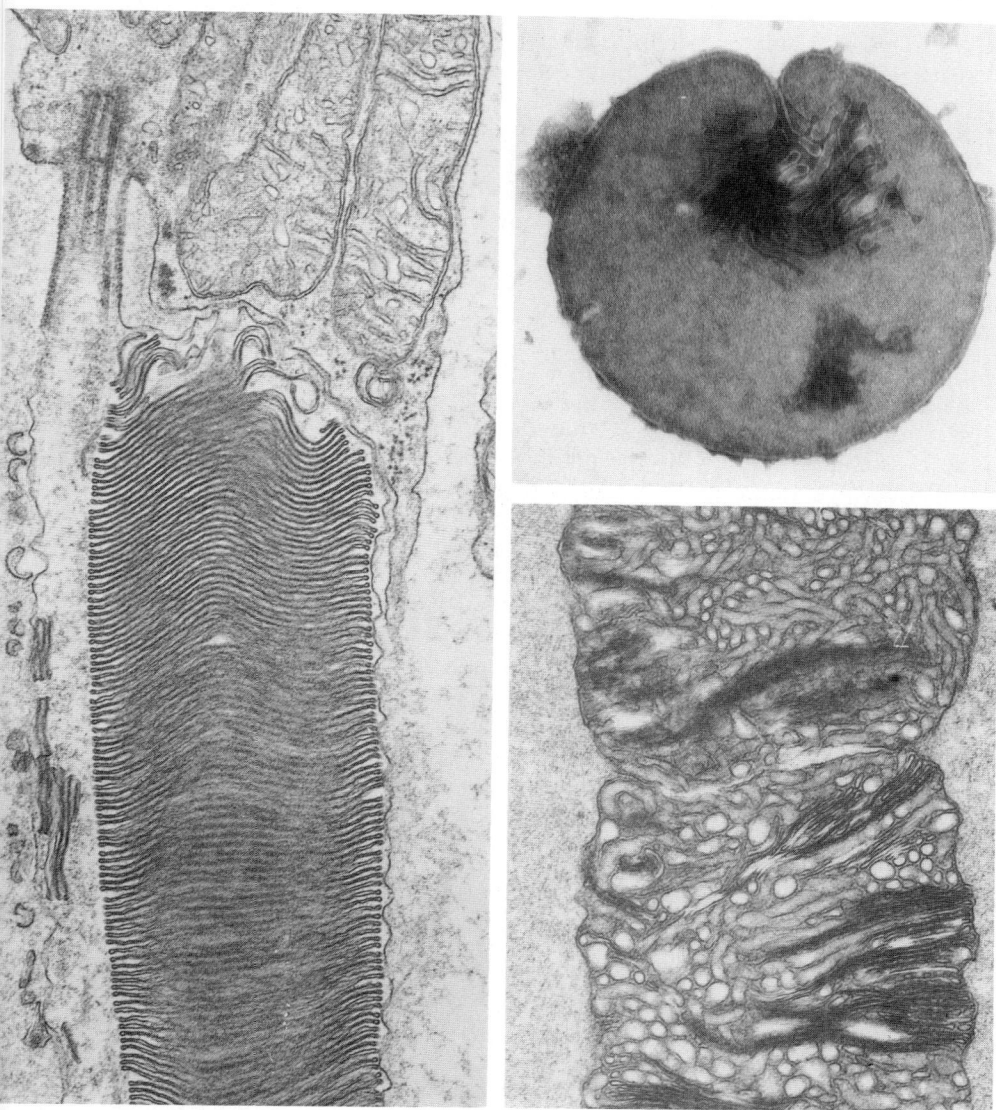

Figure 3-7. Ultrastructure of the rod outer segment in the retina. The left panel shows the junction of the discs with the inner segment. Upper right is a cross-section of a single disc and lower right is an expanded view of the discs following exposure to a high intensity laser which caused complete disorganization of the usual orderly stacked array. (Electron micrographs courtesy Dr. J. Marshall, Institute of Ophthalmology, London.)

3.2.1.8 The Choroid

The choroid is an extremely vascular spongy tissue with many pigment granules scattered throughout it. The thickness is variable; the average is about 250 μm. The blood vessels are very large in the choroid, and even in the choriocapillaris (the portion of the choroid closest to the retina) where the smallest vessels are found, the capillaries are 10 to 30 μm in diameter as compared to the 8 μm or less of the normal capillaries. Only a single blood corpuscle can move at a time through a typical capillary in other parts of the body and then the corpuscles often must suffer considerable distortion in the process. However, in the capillaries of all parts of the choroid several corpuscles can move through at the same time. This indicates some modification to allow a very high flow rate for the blood. Indeed the large blood flow through the choroid in proportion to the small amount of metabolically active tissue, accompanied by the data that only 4% of the blood oxygen is lost while the blood is in the choroid suggests that the oxygen supply of the tissue may be only a secondary function of the circulation in the choroid. Perhaps, as has been suggested by Ernest and Potts (1971) the primary function of the blood in the choroid is to keep the eye warm and at a uniform temperature. This extreme vascularity also indicates that heat from laser exposures introduced in this region under steady-state conditions will do little to elevate the temperature unless high power levels are used. In any case, the temperature regulation in the choroid differs markedly from the generally poorly regulated peripheral portions of the body.

Between the choroid and the pigment epithelium is Bruch's membrane. This is the basement membrane separating the retina from the cellular components of the blood which tend to leak out of the vessels in the choriocapillaris into its interstitial tissue. It is possible that breaks in Bruch's membrane are among the most deleterious effects from exposures to lasers and other optical sources and can result in magnification of an originally slight trauma into serious retinal injury.

3.2.1.9 The Sclera

The sclera is the dense, fibrous shell of the eye and is roughly spherical in shape. In the front of the eye it blends into the cornea, which might be considered as a transparent part of the sclera. The sclera is a little over 1 mm thick where the optic nerve enters and is approximately 0.5 mm at the equator or middle, and is again almost 1 mm thick in front where it blends into the cornea. The sclera is almost uniform in character, although the most superficial or outer portion has some blood vessels and the inner surface is laced with melanin particles. The shape of the eyeball is maintained by the rigidity of the sclera to some degree, but mostly by the internal pressure (about 10 mm Hg).

3.2.2 Refractive Power of the Eye

Most of the refractive power of the eye rests in the air-to-cornea interface, as the cornea has a refractive index of 1.376 as compared with a refractive index of 1.00 for air. The cornea also has a slightly higher index of refraction than the aqueous humor and therefore the cornea's posterior surface subtracts slightly from the refractive power of the front surface. The lens of the eye actually provides only a 30% additional refractive power since the changes in indexes of refraction between the aqueous humor and the lens and between the lens and vitreous humor are not nearly as great as the change from the air to the cornea.

The refractive power of the cornea and lens is often expressed in terms of diopters. A *diopter* (D) is the reciprocal of the effective focal length expressed in meters. The focal length is the distance from a simple lens to the point of focus. A simple lens with a focal length of 10 cm (0.1 m) has a refractive power of 10 diopters (10 D) since the reciprocal of the focal length expressed in meters is 1/0.1 or 10. The total refractive power of the relaxed normal eye is approximately 59 D. The cornea alone provides a refractive power of approximately 45 D. When the eye is under water, the cornea has practically no refractive power as its refractive index is nearly the same as water. The loss of the refractive contribution by the cornea increases the focal length of the eye as only the refractive power of the crystalline lens is left, and the image is focused far behind the retina.

To bring near objects into focus on the retina, the lens changes the radius of curvature of its anterior surface by contracting the ciliary muscle. Also, the refractive index of the lens is not uniform. It varies from approximately 1.41 at the center to 1.39 at the periphery. The approximate effective refractive index of the lens is 1.4.

3.2.3 The Standard Eye

The physical constants of the eye, the actual dimensions, refractive indices, etc. vary considerably over the human population and therefore attempts to standardize a set of parameters for the eye have often started some debate. Nevertheless, for dealing with the population as a whole and for general safety calculations, a set of values that seems to be widely accepted are those of Gullstrand (given in Appendix B). A discussion of the parameters of interest from the Gullstrand schematic eye and a simplified (reduced) model may be found in almost any book on physiological optics (such as Adler, 1970). Listed in Table 3-1 are physical dimensions of different layers of the cornea and retina that are used in assessing optical radiation hazards and particularly in the comparison of the human eye with that of the rhesus monkey.

3.2.4 Image Formation and Accommodation

For most calculations important in optical hazard analysis such as retinal image size it is permissible to use the optical constants of the standard eye and assume that the eye is a camera with a simple 59-diopter thin lens having a focal length equivalent to 17 mm for the relaxed emmetropic eye. (The reciprocal of 59 D is 0.017 m =

17 mm.) Although the refractive power of the lens is around 20 D at rest, with accommodation it may be as great as 32 D. As mentioned earlier (section 3.2.1.5) the human eye is able to *accommodate* for viewing objects at different distances by contraction of the ciliary muscle to release the tension on the suspensory ligaments of the lens and allow the front surface of the lens to become more curved (the change in the rear surface is much less pronounced) during accommodation. The normal human eye is able to focus by this method of accommodation from roughly 10 cm (the near point in youth) to infinity. When the ciliary muscle relaxes, then the suspensory ligments which are also attached to the periphery of the lens place tension on the lens to flatten it and reduce the radius of curvature to give a refractive power of 20 D. This is termed the *relaxed* state of the eye.

When the sphincter ciliary muscle constricts, the iris also constricts somewhat which eliminates the more peripheral rays passing through the lens. This both decreases spherical aberrations, and increases the depth of focus, thus tending to make near vision clearer.

3.2.4.1. Defects in Image Formation

As one grows older the ability of the lens to undergo the change of shape attendant upon accommodation becomes hampered as discussed in Section 3.2.1.5. The loss of this ability of the lens to change shape as one grows old with the corresponding loss in the ability to accommodate is called *presbyopia*.

Many persons of all ages have a deviation from normal in length of the eye, or in the curvature of the cornea. Either of these can result in an inability of the lens to change its shape sufficiently to permit a sharp image to be formed on the retina. These optical defects are illustrated schematically in Fig. 3-8. *Hyperopia* (farsightedness) and *myopia* (nearsightedness) are compared along with *emmetropia* (normal vision). Corrections for these abnormalities are also shown in the form of external lenses. If either the cornea or the lens has a different radius of curvature in one axis than in another, then an astigmatic or non-spheric optical surface is formed. In an extreme case there may be a combination of hyperopia along one axial plane and myopia along another axial plane. This astigmatism must be corrected (neutralized) by a cylindrical lens. The shape of the cornea with advancing age follows a certain trend. In infancy it is nearly spherical, in childhood, astigmatic, in middle age spherical again and then in old age tends again towards astigmatism. The lens also changes slightly.

3.2.4.2 Chromatic Aberration

In addition to the spherical aberrations which are exaggerated by a large pupil, chromatic aberrations also tend to blur the retinal image. Chromatic aberrations result from the change in the refractive index of the constituents of the human eye as a function of wavelength. Rays of red light tend to be focused behind rays of blue light since in the eye the average refractive index for the short wavelength end of the

TABLE 3-1. Average Physical Dimensions of the Eye for Man and the Rhesus Monkey

Structure	Rhesus Monkey	Man
Thickness of:		
Tear Layer	6 μm	6 μm
Cornea	516 μm	600 μm
— epithelial layer	--	50 μm
— Bowman's membrane	--	10 μm
— stromal layer	--	530 μm
— Descemet's membrane	--	7 μm
— Endothelium	--	5 μm
Aqueous humor	2.9 mm	3.1 mm
Lens	3.5 mm	3.6 mm
Vitreous humor	11.57 mm	16.97 mm
Retina	300 μm	250 μm
— nerve fiber layer	19 μm	22 μm
— ganglion cell layer	56 μm	37 μm
— inner nuclear layer	65 μm	44 μm
— pigment epithelium	11 μm	13 μm
— choriocapillaris	10 μm	11.5 μm
— choroid	162 μm	125 μm
Diameter of optic disc	1.6 mm	2500 μm
Diameter of macula	1.5 mm	2500 μm
Diameter of foveola	275 μm	150 μm
Distance from edge of disc to margin of foveola	1578 μm	1723 μm

The source for most of the above data was Coogan et al. (1974) and personal communications from W. T. Ham, Jr., and J. J. Ruffolo at the Medical College of Virginia, and D. Egbert, USAF School of Aerospace Medicine.

TABLE 3-2. Angular Dimensions at the Retina of the Human Eye*

Dimension	Angle (mrad)	Angle (arc-min)	Lateral Dimension (μm)
Image of source subtending one arc-min	0.289	1.0	4.9
Movement of retinal image corresponding to one arc-min	0.289	1.0	4.9
Image of source subtending one mrad	1.0	3.46	17
Image of source subtending 1°	17.5	60.6	297
Image of source subtending 3.4°	595	206	1000
Average distance between center of adjacent cones in the foveola	0.1	0.35	1.75
Average distance between center of adjacent cones in the fovea	0.18	0.6	3.0
Diameter of smallest cones at tip	0.06	0.2	1.0
Diameter of smallest cones at base	0.09	0.3	1.5
Diameter of fovea	34.7	120	590
Diameter of foveola	5.8	20	100
Distance between centers of retinal images of parallel lines which are just resolved	0.26	0.9	4.4
Vernier acuity	0.02	0.08	0.4

*Adapted from data in Polyak (1941) and Ditchburn (1973).

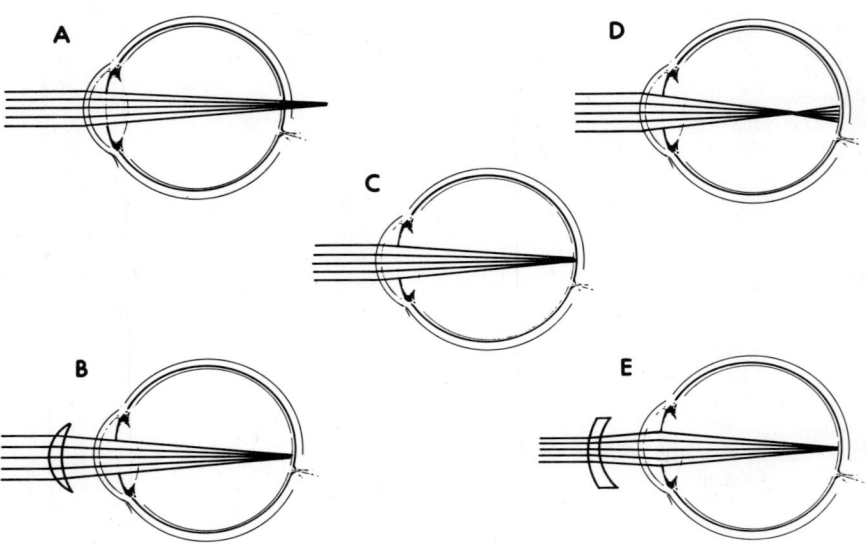

Figure 3-8. Illustration of optical defects of the human eye and the corresponding spectacle lens corrections. The simple ray diagrams illustrate how the rays from a collimated point source at infinity would be imaged at the retina. In hyperopia shown in panel A (farsightedness), the rays are imaged behind the retina. Panel B shows how a positive lens is used to correct this problem. The middle panel, C, illustrates emmetropia, the normal eye. Panel D shows myopia, or nearsightedness, where the rays are imaged in front of the retina. Panel E illustrates how a negative lens corrects this problem.

spectrum is larger than at the long wavelength end. It is interesting to note that the crystalline lens filters out most of the near ultraviolet and some shorter wavelength visible light which, if allowed to pass through to the retina, introduce even more severe chromatic aberration and would probably hamper vision. There is a yellowish pigment which filters out blue light in the area of the retina known as the *macula lutea* (the yellow spot) where the highest resolution vision takes place and where chromatic aberration from blue light would most severely hamper acute vision. This leads to another very interesting aspect of the eye to be considered later—the retina is not at all homogeneous.

3.2.5 Ocular Performance and Minimal Image Size

The discussion of the structure of the eye up to this point has been highly simplified. The eye is certainly one of the most fascinating structures of the human body and even the titles of the literature on its function would fill a large collection of books. There are many conflicting claims as to optical performance and the mechanisms involved in the function of the eye. Even at the risk of being somewhat superficial the description that follows is an attempt to provide those aspects of the human visual system which should be known by health and safety personnel concerned with optical radiation hazards. Many excellent textbooks on the physiology of the eye exist and the reader is directed to the general reference list at the end of this chapter for more detailed, in-depth discussions.

One of the most fundamental parameters for describing the functional ability of the human eye is *visual acuity* and there are several different methods to test this. A commonly encountered measure is the Snellen chart which has letters or other symbols formed in a standard way. In the Snellen chart, the capital letter E and other letters are so constructed that the width of all lines and the separation between lines are equal. Furthermore, the visual angle subtended by the width of each line in a letter is one minute of arc for the reference viewing distance, usually 20 feet (6 meters). Normal vision is expressed as 20/20 (or metrically 6/6) vision, which means that the same letters can be discerned at a distance of 20 feet (6 meters) which the average person can read at that distance. If the vision is less than average, for instance 20/40 (or 6/12), then only those figures can be read at 20 feet which the normal individual can read at 40 feet.

The average person can detect the separation between two point images separated by a visual angle of approximately one minute of arc. This visual angle (one minute of arc) corresponds to about 4.5 μm to 5 μm on the retina as shown in Table 3.2. This is quite an impressive achievement when the structure of the eye is analyzed. Diffraction theory indicates that the human eye, or any other optical system such as a telescope, is theoretically limited in its ability to separate any two adjacent point objects (such as two stars in close proximity). Figure 3-9 shows the point spread functions (the distribution of light created by diffraction effects) of two point images in the image plane of an optical system. Because of diffraction at the circular aperture (the pupil in the case of the human eye) each point image has a certain diameter. The diffraction limit to the point image is termed the *Airy disc*. The Airy disc diameter d_r (min) can be calculated (from Eq. 2-16) for an optical system if the focal length and the wavelength of light are known. The Airy disc diameter corresponds to the diameter of the first minimum around the central bright spot of the diffraction pattern. The formula is:

$$d_r = 2.44 \cdot \lambda \cdot f_e / d_e \qquad (3\text{-}1)$$

where d_e is the diameter of the eye's pupil, λ is the wavelength of light, and f_e is the eye's effective focal length. All of the parameters should be expressed in the same units, for instance in centimeters (cm). As an example the Airy disc diameter

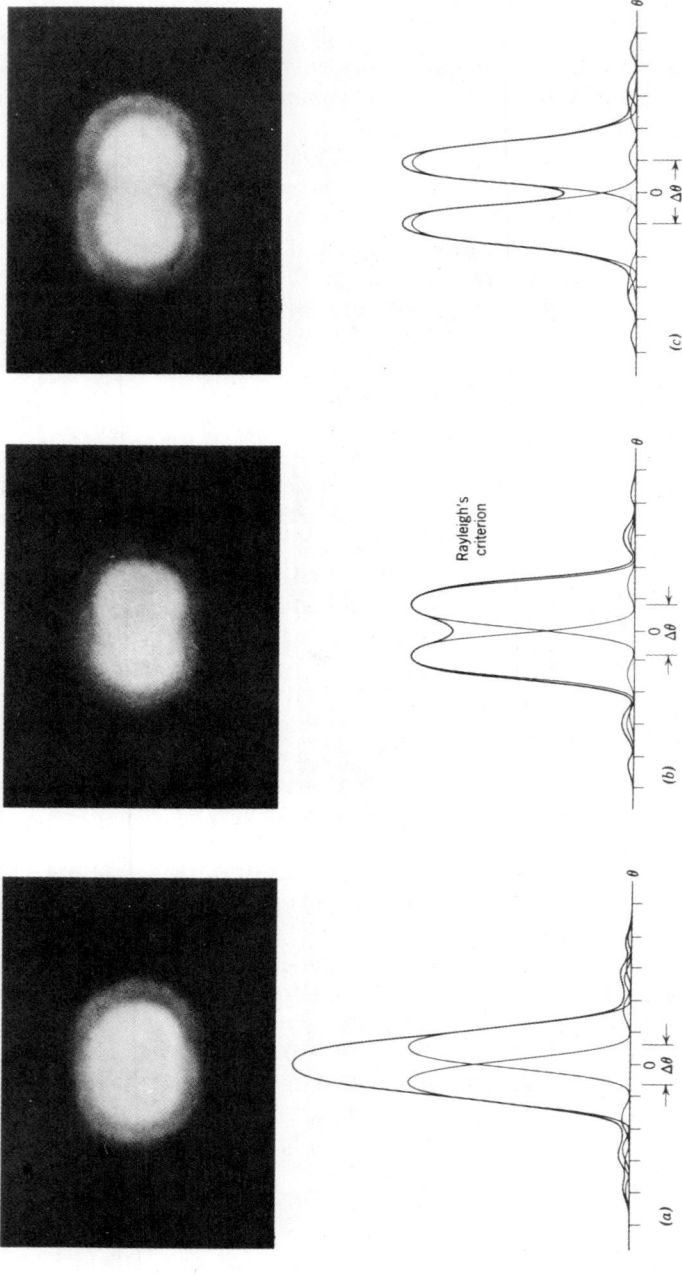

Figure 3-9. The point spread function for two point images in an image plane of an optical system. By Rayleigh's criterion, two point images are considered separate and distinct if they are separated by one diameter of the Fraunhofer diffraction pattern as defined by the first minima of the Fraunhofer diffraction pattern. In reality it has been shown that the eye is able to resolve two points which are in fact closer (from Halliday and Resnick, 1974, with permission).

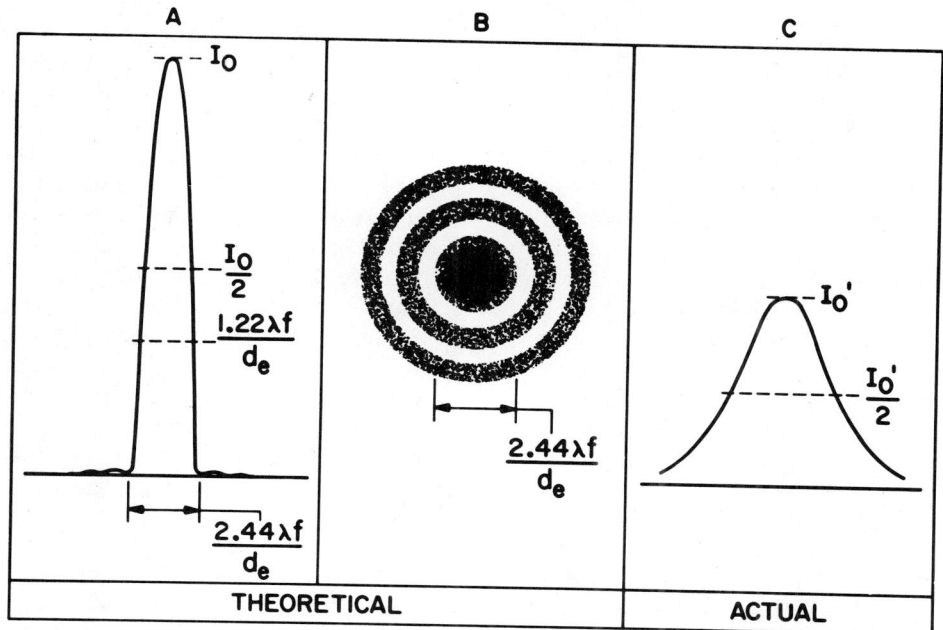

Figure 3-10. The retinal point image. The light from a point source is not imaged as a geometrical point on the retina. Theoretically this point spread distribution should appear as shown in A and B, but actually it appears as shown in C. The ratio of I_O in the actual image to that in the theoretical image is known as the Strehl ratio and is a parameter sometimes used in evaluating the performance of an optical system (from Sliney, 1971, with permission).

for a 3-mm pupil at a wavelength of 500 nm (green light) is calculated by Eq. (3-1) as follows:

$$d_r \text{ (min)} = 2.44 \ (5 \times 10^{-4} \text{ mm}) \ (17 \text{ mm})/(3 \text{ mm}) \quad (3\text{-}1)$$

$$= 6.91 \times 10^{-3} \text{ mm or } 6.9 \ \mu\text{m}$$

In actual practice (as shown in Fig. 3-10) there is always some spherical aberration that tends to prevent the human eye from quite reaching a theoretical Airy disc diameter. However, at small pupil sizes of the order of 2 mm (corresponding to vision in bright daylight) the image on the retina is nearly diffraction limited. The visual system actually exceeds the performance defined by the so-called *Rayleigh criterion,* named after the British physicist. Rayleigh felt that an optical system permitted one to distinguish between two adjacent stars if the image separation was one Airy disc (or blur circle) diameter. That is to say that the two Airy-disc functions would meet at their 50-percent-peak-irradiance points. In reality, the performance of the human eye is such that two points can be detected as different when their blur circles overlap with perhaps only a 10-percent variation in irradiance between the two central points and the minimum between them is 60 arc-seconds. The two-point discrimination is dependent on illumination and with high luminance some subjects achieve 15 arc-seconds difference. Because of the neural processing that takes place in the retina and in the higher visual pathways, two adjacent lines can be distinguished to an even more refined degree of acuity. *Vernier acuity* exceeds two-point discrimination with the ability to detect a dislocation of 4 to 10 arc-seconds. The detection of disparity between the images in the two eyes also exceeds two-point discrimination. A good and extensive review of this subject is given by le Grand (1967). The diameters of individual cones vary, but the smallest are approximately 1 μm at the tip and 1.5 μm at the base.

The whole point of this discussion of visual acuity is to emphasize that the functional interpretation of the retinal image by the brain differs from the retinal image itself. However, in a laser safety calculation the physical properties of the retinal image are important, not the image hypothesized on the basis of the functional ability of the retina/brain system. Figure 3-11 illustrates the minimal diameter reported by several different investigators and gives a comparison of these values to the theoretical diffraction-limited performance of a "standard" eye with a focal length of 17 mm at the ruby laser wavelength of 694.3 nm. As the pupil size becomes larger, the retinal image would theoretically be expected to become smaller due to diffraction theory. However, reports of visual performance and actual measures of light images on the retina for various pupil sizes indicate that the blur circle on the retina actually gets larger.

There is an important consequence of this increase in blur circle with increase in pupil diameter. This is illustrated in Fig. 4-5. When viewing a point source of light, such as a laser or a distant star, the retinal irradiance is greatly "amplified" over that at the cornea. That is, the "optical gain" of the eye (the ratio of the corneal-to-retinal irradiance) is of the order of 100,000 times (as pointed out in Chapter 1, section 1.1). Figure 4-15 shows that the theoretical optical gain would generally be in excess of 1,000,000 for larger pupil sizes. This curve is based on actual measurements of the retinal image profile for line images since the point image is too difficult to measure directly. Fortunately, the point image is related to the line image by a known factor. The profile of the point image can be calculated by measuring a function known as the optical *modulation transfer function* (MTF). Figures 3-11 and 4-15 show that the eye's best performance occurs for a pupil size of approximately 3 to 4 mm and that the optical gain of the eye remains relatively constant over a range of pupil sizes from 3 to 6 mm.

3.2.6 Retinal Function and Organization

3.2.6.1 Lateral Organization of the Retina

A not uncommon question of a child to his parents is: "Why is it that when I read a column of print in the newspaper my eyes scan back and forth, and I can see the entire newspaper sheet at one time?" The answer is that reading is only done

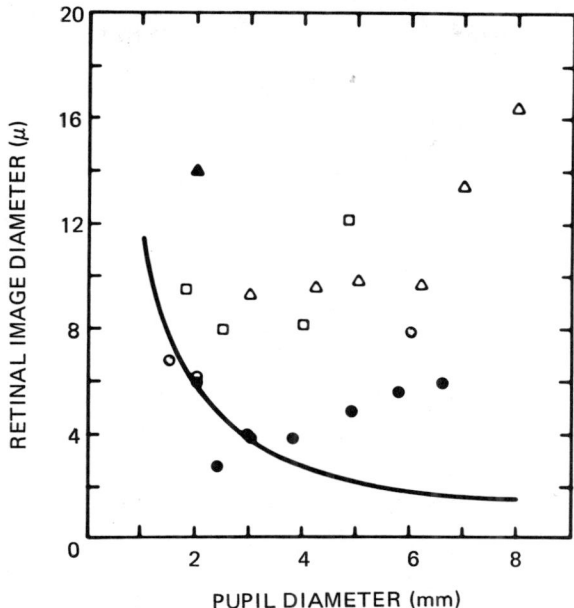

Figure 3-11. Comparison of minimal disc diameters to theoretical performance of optical system with focal length of 1.7 cm at 694 nm. Retinal image size is given at half-peak-intensity points for theoretical diffraction limited eye (line) and for values derived from data of Krauskopf (1962), △ ; Arnulf and Dupuy (1960), □ ; van den Brink (Vos, 1966), ▲ ; Westheimer and Campbell (1962), ○ ; Campbell and Green (1965), ▵ ; and Campbell and Gubisch (1966), ●. All data are for white light, except Cambell and Green (632.8 nm) and theoretical curve (694.3 nm). Redrawn from Sliney (1971).

by the one small central area in the retina known as the *fovea centralis*. This area is responsible for the highest acuity. The fovea is the center of a larger, specialized region known as the *macula lutea* ("yellow spot") or more simply, the *macula*. As shown in Fig. 3-5 the fovea is a depression in the retina in which many of the retinal layers are reduced in thickness and is sometimes termed the foveal pit. The pit is the highest concentration of the cone receptors which are responsible for not only color vision but also vision of greatest acuity. In the fovea these cones are packed very tightly. In the 100-μm diameter central fovea (termed the *foveola* by Polyak) there are perhaps only 7,000 cones. It is estimated that there are probably 100,000 cones in the entire rod-free region, the fovea, and over 4,000,000 in the macula. In the more peripheral parts of the retina beyond the macula, the receptors

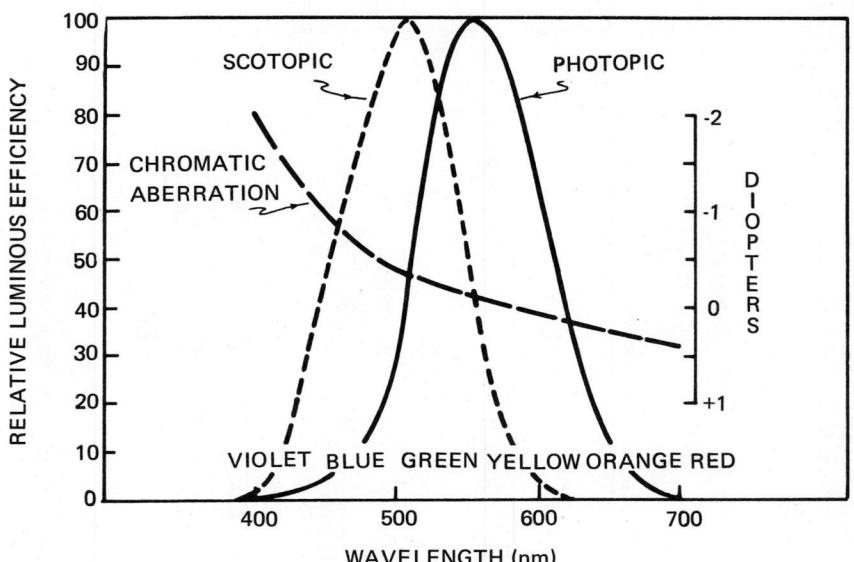

Figure 3-12. The scotopic (night) and photopic (day) responses of the eye. The CIE Function V_λ (photopic) and V'_λ (scotopic) for the CIE standard observer are illustrated as a function of wavelength. Peak rod sensitivy (scotopic) occurs at approximately 500 nm. Also shown is the variation of chromatic aberration as a function of wavelength. Notice the strong chromatic aberration existing in the short wavelength (blue) end of the spectrum. (Adapted from the Military Optical Design Handbook, 1962).

are mostly rods. In the entire retina it is estimated that there are 7,000,000 cones and 125,000,000 rods which eventually feed into the 800,000 to 1,000,000 nerve fibers in the optic nerve.

3.2.6.2 Spectral Sensitivity to Light

Rods play the major role in night vision and are responsible for the eye's ability to respond to very low light levels. A single flash of less than 100 photons (perhaps only 10) can be seen by the human eye. The peak wavelength of the visual response is approximately 500 nm for night vision (scotopic vision). Figure 3-12 shows the variation of scotopic (nighttime—rod vision) and photopic response of the eye (daylight—color vision) with the wavelength of light entering the eye. The fact that the two curves are not the same was first noticed by the physiologist, Purkinje, who found that as the eye adapted to a darker environment the peak sensitivity of the eye was spectrally shifted towards the blue (the so-called "Purkinje shift"). The scotopic response of the eye is due to rod cell activity, whereas the photopic response of the eye is generally agreed to be the sum of three different cone mechanisms—a blue cone, a green cone, and red cone mechanism. Also shown in Fig. 3-12 is the variation in chromatic aberration as a function of wavelength. The strong chromatic aberration in the blue wavelengths was discussed in Section 3.2.4.2.

3.2.6.3 *Visual Sensitivity in the UV and Near Infrared*

Although the visual response is limited largely to wavelengths between 400 and 760 nm, it is necessary to point out that there is some limited sensitivity of the retina in the near ultraviolet (UV-A) and near infrared (IR-A). If it were not for the absorption properties of the crystalline lens, most near-ultraviolet radiation could be readily perceived. When the lens is removed after a cataract operation the resulting *aphakic* eye is able to respond to ultraviolet radiation between approximately 320 and 400 nm. Even with our ultraviolet-absorbing crystalline lens in place, an extremely small fraction (less than one percent) of the incident ultraviolet radiation from 320 to 400 nm is imaged on the retina. For instance, it is possible to see the slit source in an ultraviolet double-monochromator even when stray light has been removed. However, as the monochromator is dialed to wavelengths below 310 nm it is no longer possible to see the exit slit image of the source. The image of the slit is very much blurred because of chromatic aberration and intraocular scattering, but is nevertheless present. In addition, there exists—particularly at wavelengths near 350 nm—a considerable haze over the image which results from fluorescence of the crystalline lens.

In the infrared portion of the spectrum it is possible to see wavelengths at least as far out as 1064 nm, the wavelength of the neodymium: YAG laser (Sliney, et at., 1976). Figure 3-13 shows the response of the photopic mechanism of the human eye out to 1064 nm. As the visual threshold for 1064-nm radiation is approached, the maximum permissible exposure level for this radiation is also approached. There is a ratio of nearly 11 orders of magnitude between the sensitivity of the fovea to the wavelength of 550 nm and to the wavelength of 1064 nm. In the near-ultraviolet the sensitivity threshold increases with age because of yellowing of the lens, whereas the curve shown in Fig. 3-13 for the IR appears to be relatively independent of age.

3.2.6.4 *Spectral Characteristics of the Ocular Media*

The ocular media of the normal eye transmit at least 1% of the radiation over the entire range from 400 nm to 1400 nm. At wavelengths beyond 1400 nm, water absorbs very heavily, and essentially all incident radiation is absorbed very superficially, principally within the cornea. Figure 3-14 illustrates in a simplified fashion the optical transmission of the human eye (as reported by Geeraets and Berry, 1968) and shows the fraction of light actually absorbed in the retina throughout

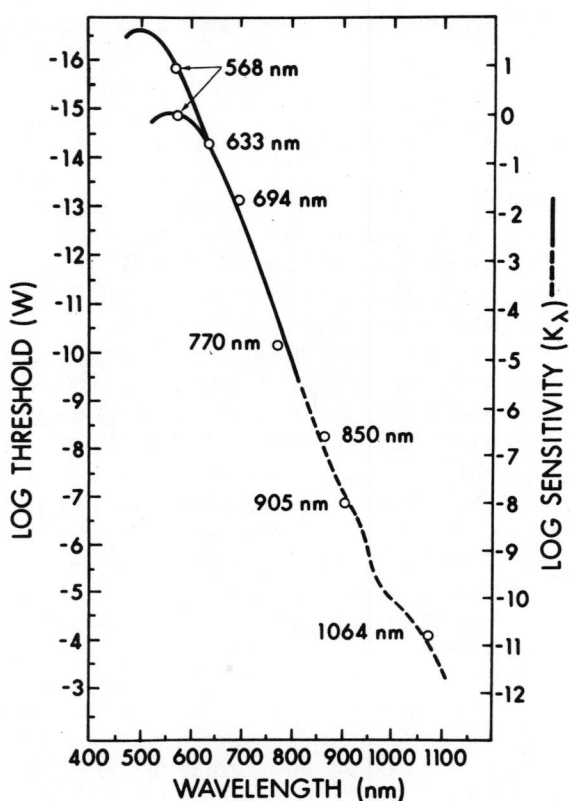

Figure 3-13. Spectral sensitivity curve for point source viewed by the fovea, V_λ, and for rod vision (through uppermost 568-nm point). In contrast with Fig. 3-12, which was plotted on a linear scale, we see that the eye in actuality responds over many log units and its response can be plotted over many wavelengths, as is shown in this plot for wavelengths greater than 500 nm. The solid line, to 770 nm, is the CIE luminous efficacy, V_λ function. The broken line beyond 770 nm is the extrapolated function proposed by Walraven and Leebeek (1963), which was based upon previous infrared visibility studies and absorption properties of water. The circles are data from the study of Sliney *et al.* (1976) as plotted against the left-hand ordinate (redrawn from Sliney *et al.*, (1976).

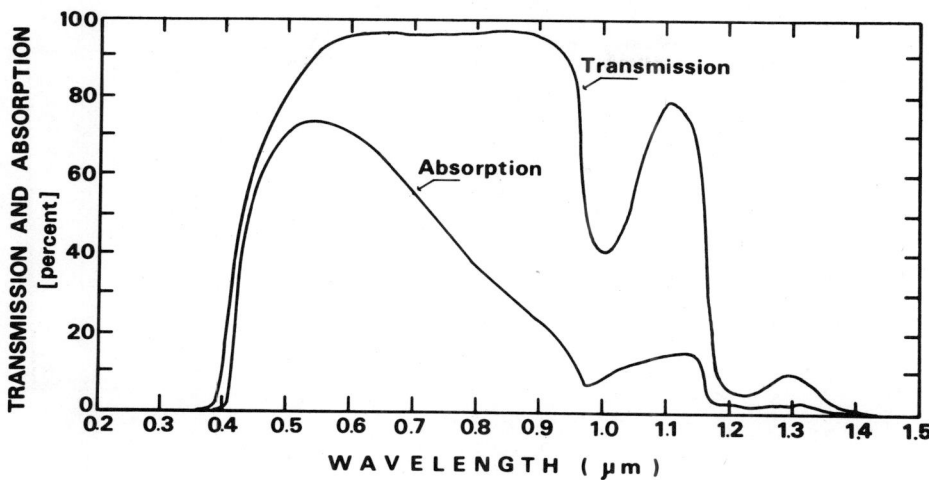

Figure 3-14. Optical spectral transmission of the human eye and absorption of light energy in the retina and choroid as a function of equal corneal spectral irradiance. The upper curve of spectral transmission would be used in calculating a retinal irradiance. The lower curve would be used to calculate retinal absorbed dose rate (from the data of Geeraets and Berry, 1968).

this wavelength region. The spectral region between 400 to 1400 nm is often termed the *retinal hazard region,* but clearly the spectral characteristics of the ocular media play an important role in assessing optical hazards to the retina. The adverse effects of optical radiation upon the different structures of the eye and a more detailed discussion of the spectral characteristics of absorption in the various ocular structures will be discussed in Chapter 4.

3.2.6.5 *Retinal Processing*

Before this discussion of the eye is complete, some additional material must be included on the retina. An optical engineer who might set about to design a system somewhat like the eye would probably build a mosaic of detectors with coaxial cables leading from behind the detectors to some central processing station. Strangely enough to a modern-day optical engineer, the human retina is not constructed quite in this fashion. Instead of the coaxial cables leading from behind the mosaic of detectors, the cables in the human eye—the nerve cells—actually lead out

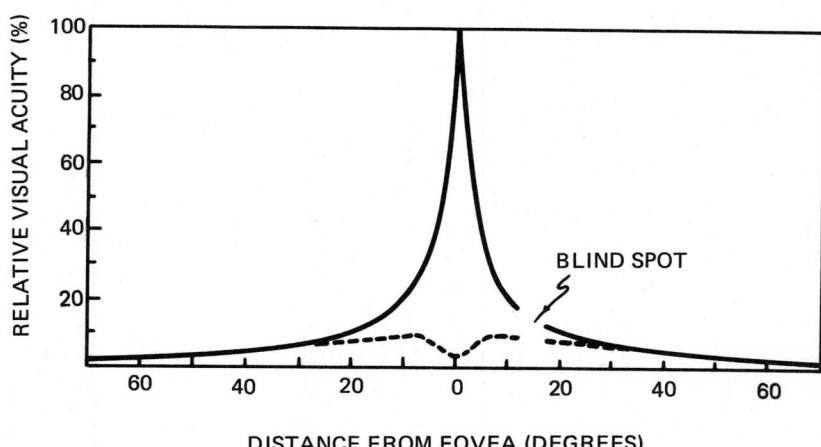

Figure 3-15. Variability of visual acuity as a function of visual angle. Solid line is for photopic (daylight) response; dashed line is for scotopic (nighttime) response. Adapted from data in Walsh (1959) and Randall, Brown and Sloan (1966).

in the opposite direction. That is, to say, before the light enters the receptor layer of rod and cone cells it must pass through layers of blood vessels, nerve fibers, and specialized nerve cells such as ganglion cells and bipolar cells. Only within the macula, and particularly within the fovea where the receptors are most densely packed, are all of these extra layers pulled aside. The central processing system in the human visual system is the *visual cortex* in the brain but there are many intermediate processing centers, some of which are located within the neural retina itself. All receptor cells in the retina are interconnected in a variety of circuits to make use of *horizontal cells* and *bipolar cells* in the retina that send a highly processed signal back to the visual cortex. Still, even in the face of the anatomical and electrophysiological evidence, some scientists believe that the receptors within the fovea have almost a private and direct-access line to the visual cortex. The problem is best illustrated in the eagle or hawk fovea which has a resolving ability equal to (or even much better than) the human fovea, but has many fewer ganglion cells (or optic nerve fibers) than receptors.

Figure 3-15 illustrates the widely variable visual acuity as a function of visual angle. The dotted line which represents scotopic vision decreases practically to zero at the fovea (where there are essentially no rods) but peaks not far away. The photopic curve behaves in quite the opposite manner with the best visual acuity along the optic axis at the fovea.

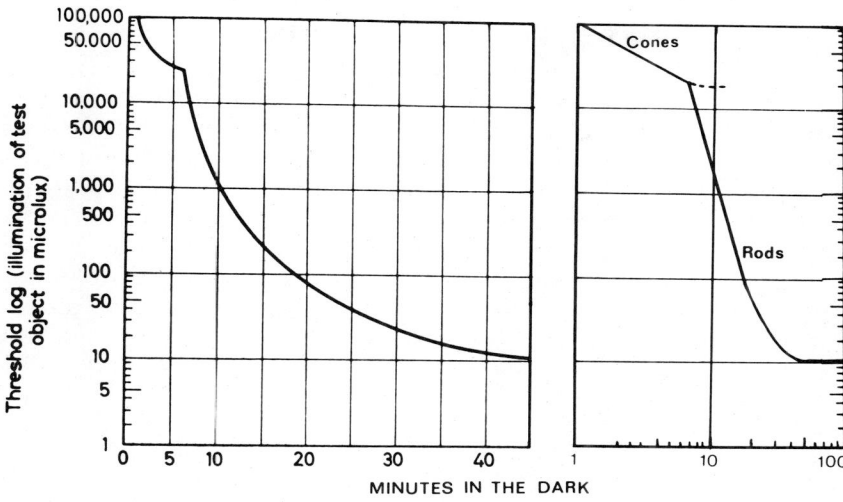

Figure 3-16. The threshold sensitivity of the eye for a point source of light varies as a period of adaptation to the dark. Note that the cones reach a plateau within a matter of 10 minutes, whereas the rods continue to adapt up to periods sometimes exceeding 30 minutes. The dark-adaptation curves are plotted in two panels—one with semi-logarithmic scales (left) and the other with log-log scales. For an extended source the cone plateau is approximately 500 td and the rod plateau is approximately 5×10^{-4} td. These retinal illuminances correspond to source luminances for an 8-mm pupil of 10 cd/m^2 and 10^{-5} cd/m^2 respectively. The unit of troland (td) is often used in these plots since it indicates the retinal illuminance and can be calculated easily from source luminance; i.e., the source luminance in cd/m^2 is multiplied by the pupillary area in mm^2 to obtain trolands.

3.2.6.6 Eye Movements

Some of the remarkable processing that takes place in the retina apparently depends upon eye movements. There are several levels of eye movements ranging from a very fine ocular tremor where the eye's visual axis vibrates over visual angles of only a few seconds-of-arc to widely ranging *saccades* (greater movements) of the eye which have the fovea scanning over areas in object space of several degrees. Such eye movements may be important to note as they may have a role in calculations on the dwell time of a laser beam on a particular spot on the retina during intrabeam viewing. However, the worst case should be kept in mind for it has been shown that if a person wishes to stare at an object, the retinal image can be stabilized onto one very small area of the retina for several seconds.

3.2.6.7 Dark Adaptation

Another remarkable characteristic of the retina is its ability to dark adapt. Figure 3-16 shows how the visual threshold changes as a function of time within the dark. A person placed in a darkened room suddenly will not at first be able to discern any objects in the room even if there is a small amount of light. After a time in the dark, various objects can be perceived. Sometimes this process takes as long as 20 to 30 minutes. Figure 3-16 illustrates the fact that the dark adaptation process goes through two periods—first an adaptation of the cones where the threshold of photopic vision gradually decreases and then reaches a plateau, and then the scotopic visual threshold rapidly decreases. Note that plots in Fig. 3-16 have a logarithmic scale for threshold luminance. The straight lines in the log-log presentation show the exponential character of dark adaptation. The slope of the line is a function of the level of light adaptation.

3.2.6.8 The Visual Field

In addition to the description of visual acuity and spectral sensitivity of the eye, the visual field of each eye is also of interest. The *visual field* is the map of the eye's visual capability in terms of object space. The extent of the visual field is limited by anatomical features such as the nose and the supraorbital ridge above the eyes. The visual field extends roughly 50 degrees upward, 80 degrees downward, 60 degrees nasally and more than 90 degrees temporally.

In certain diseases of the retina there is a constriction of the visual field. There may also be localized losses of vision due to retinal lesions. These losses of visual field are termed scotomas (or scotomata) or blind spots. A *scotoma* often develops after a person stares at the sun during an eclipse without adequate eye protection—an eclipse scotoma. Scotomas resulting from laser-induced lesions of the retina will be described at length in Chapter 26. There are two natural blind spots, one in each eye, which are due to the optic disc, the point in the retina where the optic nerve enters the eye. Light falling on these areas are not perceived. Fortunately, since each optic nerve exits the eye nasally, the two blind spots do not overlap. The brain also tends to "fill in" areas of the visual field blanked out by scotomas. An example of a visual field chart with a scotoma marked is shown in Figure 26-5.

One curious characteristic of retinal sensitivity is an angular dependence of cone retinal sensitivity which is known as the *Stiles-Crawford Effect* (Fig. 3-17). The rods do not exhibit this characteristic that is often attributed to waveguide properties of the cones. A very small beam of light entering the edge of an 8-mm pupil would evoke only one-fifth the visual response of an axial ray of light entering at the center of the pupil.

Safety considerations for the eye and various aspects of vision will be discussed in more detail in various subsequent chapters. Any reader who is interested in an in-depth discussion of any particular point is directed once again to the list of general references at the end of this chapter.

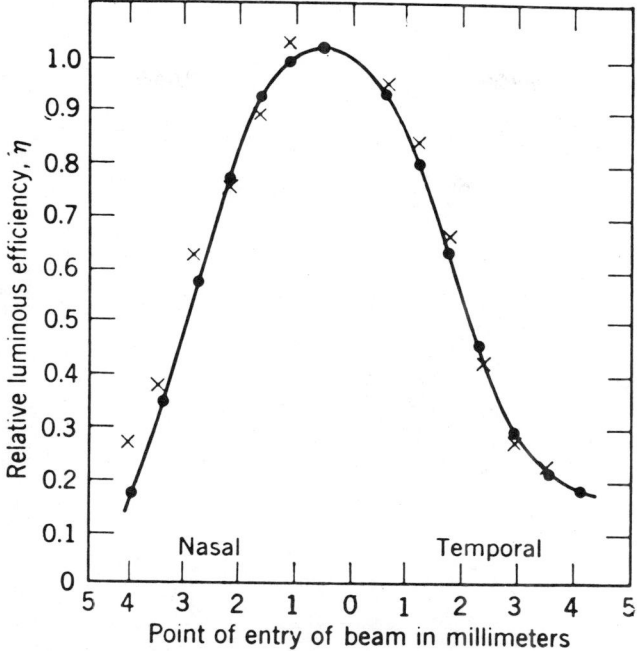

Figure 3-17. The Stiles-Crawford effect. In 1936 Stiles and Crawford discovered that light entering the pupil near the edge of the aperture is greatly reduced in its effectiveness for eliciting a visual response. This effect has been interpreted by many as an indication of the waveguide nature of the cones (adapted from Graham, 1956).

3.3 THE SKIN

3.3.1 Anatomy

Although the skin is normally of less interest than the eye when optical radiation hazards are considered, it is nonetheless more vulnerable in certain conditions where the eye is protected by the blink reflex or by protective equipment. Additionally, the biological effects of ultraviolet radiation upon the skin increases our need to know some basic facts about the skin, which incidentally is the largest organ of the body.

Figure 3-18 shows the anatomical structure of the skin. This organ is not at all homogeneous, but consists of a variety of cells including sweat (eccrine) glands, sebaceous glands, hair follicles and other specialized cells.

The outermost layer, the stratum corneum or horny layer, consists of flattened, dead, epidermal cells. These epidermal cells or keratinocytes, originate in the

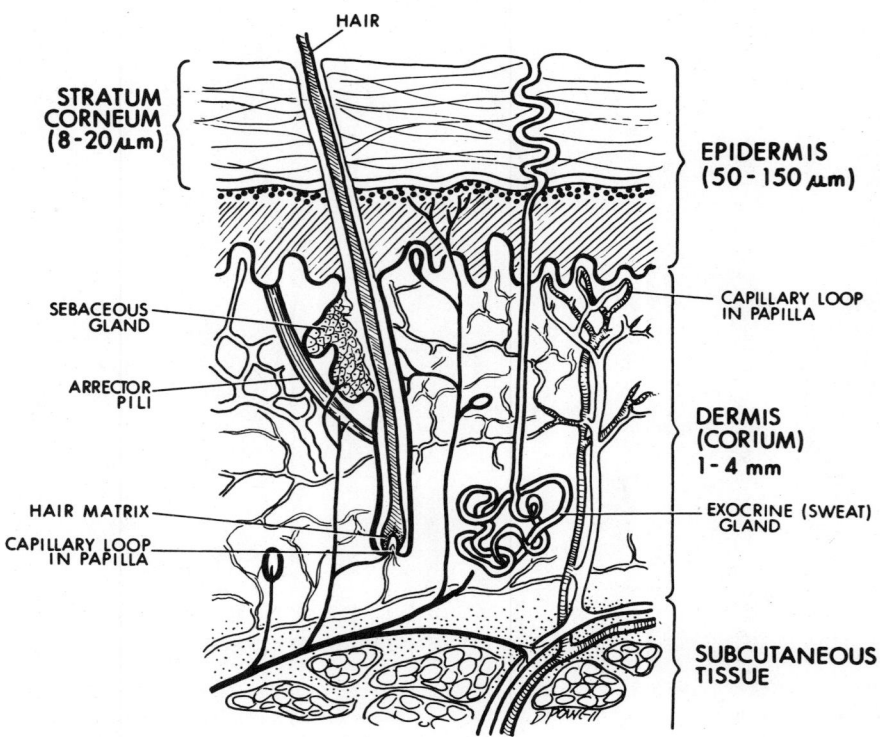

Figure 3-18. Anatomical structure of the skin. The actual thicknesses of different layers vary with individuals and depend upon the region of the body. See Table 3-3 for thickness of various layers of human skin.

germinative layer (a single cell layer of collumnar germinative basal cells) at the bottom of the epidermis, grow, and are gradually pushed outward until they die and are flattened to form a protective layer over the living cells. Individual cells and groups of dead cells are continuously worn off in daily activity to be replaced by the continual regenerative process in the skin. The stratum corneum provides the skin with a protective covering which not only protects the living tissue against water loss and against injury by physical objects, by abrasions, and from direct exposure to air and dust, but it also protects against injury from radiant energy. The stratum corneum is approximately 10-20 μm thick over most parts of the body, except in the soles of the feet and the palms of the hand where it is much thicker (500-600 μm).

The epidermis is the outermost layer of the skin and is relatively uniform in thickness throughout the body (50-150 μm). The fibrous proteins known as keratin are produced in the keratinocytes of the epidermis. It is keratin that serves as a major protective tough substance in the skin; hair and nails are composed almost entirely of keratin. The daughter cells of the keratinocytes differentiate and become "prickle cells" of the malpighian layer of the epidermis—the *stratum malpighii*. As these cells migrate outward, changes continue to occur; granules appear in the cytoplasm of each cell; the cells tend to flatten (i.e., squamous cells), and the cells now form the *stratum granulosum*. Still later, the cells lose their nuclei, die, dehydrate and flatten out to form the tough stratum corneum. It is generally agreed that the entire process of cell migration from the basal layer of the epidermis to final soughing off the surface of the stratum corneum takes 28 days in normal skin. Of this 28-day period, the cell spends about 14 days in the epidermis and 14 days in the stratum corneum.

A tanning process takes place in the epidermis. Melanocytes—specialized cells which produce melanin pigment granules—are located in the basal layer of the epidermis. The melanocytes send out dendritic processes which interdigitate within the keratinocytes. Melanosomes (the pigment granules) are then transferred into the keratinocytes. The pigment is thus distributed throughout the epidermis and stratum corneum by cell migration. The structural detail of melanin is not well known. Chemically, the protein melanin is derived largely from the white amino acid tyrosine. It is important to remember that melanin is not chemically inactive but plays a role as a scavenger of free radicals and may serve as a catalytic surface. The melanin in the skin is not identical to the melanin in the retinal pigment epithelium.

A detailed discussion of the specialized sensory cells and tiny glands in the skin is quite beyond the scope of this text. The millions of tiny glands include: apocrine (sweat) glands which discharge sweat into hair follicles, eccrine (sweat) glands which carry saline water from the dermis and subcutaneous layer directly to the skin surface, and sebaceous glands which secrete sebum—an oily substance which lubricates hairshafts and maintains the slightly acidic, oily film over the stratum corneum. Of primary interest to the reader is the collection of eccrine sweat glands which play a major role in the body's thermoregulatory mechanism, since evaporative cooling is the most efficient means the body has as its disposal for ridding itself of excess body heat as long as the humidity is not 100%. More than two liters of sweat can be discharged in one day. On the average, the skin contains about as many sebaceous glands as eccrine sweat glands, except that there are few sebaceous glands on the palms of the hands and soles of the feet compared to the number of eccrine glands in those regions. It is the relative absence of the sebaceous glands in those regions which accounts for ready penetration of water into these regions of the skin when the body is immersed for some period in pure water, causing that skin to develop a wrinkled appearance.

The dermis, or corium, is much thicker than the epidermis, but consists of much larger cells. The dermis is largely connective tissue which gives the skin its elasticity and supportive strength. Nerve cells, blood vessels and lymphatic glands are found in the outermost dermal layer—the papillary dermis. Unlike the epidermis, the thickness of the dermis is not at all uniform throughout the body; it varies from 1 mm to 4 mm.

The innermost layer of the skin is generally known as the subcutaneous layer. It is composed largely of fatty tissue that serves a shock-absorbing and insulating role. The thickness of this layer varies considerably from one body region to another and from one person to another.

The following general summary may be helpful. One square centimeter of normal skin contains on the average: 3 million cells, one meter of capillaries, 15 sebaceous glands, 10 hair follicles, 100 eccrine glands, 4 meters of nerves and 3000 sensory cells at the ends of nerve fibers (including 25 tactile sensors, 200 pain endings, 12 heat sensors and 2 cold sensors), although many if not all of these sensors may have several sensory functions.

3.3.2 Optical Properties

The stratum corneum is highly absorbing at the actinic ultraviolet wavelengths which cause sunburn and is also highly absorbing at far-infrared wavelengths. At wavelengths in the near-infrared, radiant energy has a considerable depth of penetration as shown in Fig. 5-3. The thickness of the stratum corneum varies throughout the body depending upon whether callous layers are present such as on the tips of the fingers and heel of the foot, or are totally absent such as on the abdomen. There is little difference between the thickness of the stratum corneum in different parts of the body for Caucasian and black which confirms that pigmentary difference is primarily responsible for the difference in susceptibility to ultraviolet effects between the two races.

The tiny particles of organic pigment *(melanin)* help shield the dermis from harmful ultraviolet radiation and provide color to the skin. The melanin granules are produced by melanosomes in the dermis and migrate up into the epidermis. This process is stimulated by ultraviolet radiation. Melanin not only protects the dermis by absorption of ultraviolet radiation but also by scattering optical radiation. Melanin, like most organic dyes, does not absorb very much in the near-infrared spectral region. Also, the melanin granules are small (1 μm in diameter) and scatter rather than absorb in the near infrared. For these reasons, near-infrared radiation penetrates deeply into the tissue. Since the index of refraction of the stratum corneum is 1.5, the Fresnel reflective component is somewhat similar to glass (Fig. 2-6). Optical radiation incident upon the skin at grazing angles of incidence is hardly absorbed at all. For this reason and because of scattering, the relative effectiveness of optical radiation in penetrating into the epidermis (and dermis) varies approximately as the cosine of the angle of incidence. Since light penetrates the outermost layers of the skin, undergoes multiple scattering, and some light is scattered back out of the skin, the skin has an appearance that cannot easily be duplicated by a non-translucent surface. Indeed, most of the reflected light from the skin is not due to a surface reflection at all.

3.3.3 Body Heat Regulation

The skin plays a major role in the thermoregulatory system of the human body. At incident irradiances less than those that cause thermal skin burns, the body can be subjected to *heat stress*. When internal body temperature reaches a certain level, the eccrine glands (pores of the skin) dilate, producing sweat. This permits evaporative cooling as well as conductive cooling. The reflectance of human skin in the far infrared is also very low with a correspondingly very high emissivity for wavelengths in the 8-to-13 μm infrared region. These are the major wavelengths of emission for radiative cooling of the skin at body temperature. Since 8-to-13 μm IR-C radiation is not transmitted by water, the skin surface must be warm to radiate this energy. The capillaries in the dermis dilate to increase blood flow and improve heat loss by radiative and conductive cooling when the thermoregulatory system senses too great an internal body temperature. Skin color is changed to a red flush when these capillaries dilate.

A comparison of the reflectance of human skin (in Fig. 5-4) with the solar spectrum (in Fig. 6-11) shows a striking similarity. The skin reflects largely in the visible part and near-infrared parts of the spectrum where solar radiation is greatest, and absorbs heavily in the ultraviolet and far-infrared where there is very little solar radiation. A basic law of thermal physics requires that any good radiator of infrared energy must have a very high absorptance, hence a very low reflectance. The skin does indeed have a low reflectance in the far-infrared. Indeed, the skin seems well adapted to the natural environment. The skin both reflects direct solar radiation and reradiates internally generated infrared radiation with the greatest possible efficiency. However, the human body is less capable of reflecting the infrared radiation from man-made sources such as a fire, or more specifically from molten steel in a steel mill. This type of heat stress is a greater problem than that outdoors in the sun. It is interesting to note that for wavelengths greater than approximately 1000 nm, melanin plays little or no role in the absorption and reflection properties of the skin. Hence skin pigmentation as the human eye perceives it is limited largely to the visible spectrum. Beyond the visible one could not detect the color differences of race. We are all black, in the far infrared.

The reader who is interested in studying the anatomy and physiology of the skin to greater lengths is directed to the list of references on the skin at the end of this chapter.

3.4 REVIEW QUESTIONS

1. What is the refractive power of the relaxed normal human eye? What is the effective focal length of the relaxed human eye in air?

2. In which part of the visible spectrum does the eye have the greatest chromatic aberration?

3. What is the retinal Airy disc diameter for a point source of 450-nm light entering a 7-mm pupil?

4. Approximately what fraction of incident 488-nm laser radiation that enters the eye is actually absorbed in the retina?

5. Would you expect a neodymium laser operating at 1064 nm to be more hazardous or less hazardous than a laser operating at 530 nm?

6. What is the function of the stratum corneum?

7. What is the penetration depth of 1064-nm radiation in the skin?

8. Compare the peak spectral response of the photopic system of the human retina to the peak of the solar spectrum. Do they coincide? Would they coincide if the solar spectrum were expressed in quantum units rather than in normal terms of irradiance?

9. What is the range of refractive power for a young human lens?

10. Explain why the image of an ultraviolet source at 350 nm is very blurry.

11. Explain what is meant by visual acuity.

12. What is the smallest sized image on the human retina?

13. What is the dermis?

14. On white paper draw two lines—one with black ink, one with blue ink. Can you detect the difference in color? Now draw two small dots. Can you detect the difference in color? Why?

3.5 REFERENCES

3.5.1 General References: EYE

Adler, F. H., 1970, "Physiology of the Eye," fifth ed., St. Louis, Mosby.
Cornsweet, T. N. (ed.), 1970, "Visual Perception," Academic Press, New York.
Davson, H. (ed.), 1962, "The Eye" (in four volumes), Adademic Press, New York.
Ditchburn, R. W., 1973, "Eye Movements and Visual Perception," Clarendon Press, Oxford.
Duke-Elder, S. (ed.), 1939, "Textbook of Ophthalmology" (in seven volumes), C. V. Mosby, St. Louis.
Duke-Elder, S. (ed.), 1960, "Transparency of the Cornea," Charles C. Thomas, Springfield, IL.
Duke-Elder, S., 1961-72, "System of Ophthalmology" (in twelve volumes), Kimpton, London.
Emsley, H. H., 1939, "Visual Optics," 2nd edition, Hatten Press, London.
Graham, C. H., 1965, "Vision and Visual Perception," J. Wiley & Sons, New York.

Graham, C. H., 1951, Visual perception, in "Handbook of Experimental Psychology" (S. S. Stevens, ed.), Wiley and Sons, New York.
Graymore, C. N. (ed.), 1970, "Biochemistry of the Eye," Academic Press, New York.
Harrington, D. O., 1964, "The Visual Fields," 2nd edition, C. V. Mosby, St. Louis.
Hogan, M. J., Alvarado, J. A., and Waddell, J. E., 1971, "Histology of the Human Eye: An Atlas and Textbook," W. B. Saunders, Philadelphia.
Jameson, D., and Hurvich, L. M., 1972, Visual Psychophysics, Vol. VII (4): "Handbook of Sensory Physiology," Springer-Verlag, New York.
Langer, H., 1973, "Biochemistry and Physiology of Visual Pigments," Springer-Verlag, New York.
Le Grand, I., 1967, "Form and Space Vision," Indiana University Press, Bloomington.
Polyak, S., 1941, "The Retina," University of Chicago Press, Chicago.
Polyak, S., 1957, "The Vertebrate Visual System," University of Chicago Press, Chicago.
Snyder, A. W., and Menzel, R., 1975, "Photoreceptor Optics," Springer-Verlag, New York.
von Helmholtz, H., 1962, "Physiological Optics," (1866 original in German), translation by Southhall, Optical Society of America, 1927, republished by Dover, New York.
Warwick, R., 1976, "Wolff's Anatomy of the Eye," H. K. Lewis and Co., Ltd., London.
Wyszecki, G. and Stiles, W. S., 1967, "Color Science," Wiley and Sons, New York.
Zinn, K. M., 1972, "The Pupil," Charles C. Thomas, Springfield, IL.

3.5.2 General References: SKIN

Fitzpatrick, T. B., Arndt, K. A., Clark, W. H., Jr., Eisen, A. Z., Van Scott, E. J., Vaughn, J. H. (eds.), 1971, "Dermatology in General Medicine," McGraw-Hill, New York.
Fitzpatrick, T. B., Pathak, M. A., Harber, L. C., Seiji, M. and Kukita, A. (eds.), 1974, "Sunlight and Man," University of Tokyo Press, Tokyo.
Hardy, J. D., 1968, "The Skin Senses," Charles C. Thomas, Springfield, IL., pp. 444–456.
Magnus, I. A., 1976, "Dermatological Photobiology," Blackwell Scientific Publications, London.
Montagna, W. and Lobitz, W., 1964, "The Epidermis," Academic Press, New York.
Montagna, W. and Parakkal, P. F., 1975, "The Structure and Function of the Skin," 3rd edition, Academic Press, New York.
Parrish, J. A., 1975, "Dermatology and Skin Care," McGraw-Hill, New York.

3.5.3 Specific References

Arnulf, A., and Dupuy, O., 1960, La transmission des contrastes par le systeme optique de l'oeil et les sueils de contrastes retiniens, *Comp Rend Hebdomadaires des Seance de l'Academe des Sciences,* **250**:2757–2759.
Benedek, G. B., 1971, Theory of transparency of the eye, *App. Opt.,* **10**(3):459–473.
Bettelheim, F. A., and Kumbar, M., 1977, An interpretation of small-angle light-scattering patterns of human cornea, *Invest. Ophthal. Vis. Sci.,* **16**(3):233–236.
Campbell, F. W., and Green, D. G., 1965, Optical and retinal factors affecting visual resolution, *J Physiol.,* **181**:576–593.
Campbell, F. W., and Gubisch, R. W., 1968, Optical quality of the human eye, *J. Physiol.,* **186**: 280–299.
Coogan, P. S., Hughes, W. F., and Mollsen, J. A., 1974, Histologic and Spectrophotometric Comparisons of the Human and Rhesus Monkey Retina and Pigmented Ocular Fundus, Final Report, Rush-Presbyterian St. Luke's Medican Center, 1753 W. Congress Parkway, IL, Contract No. F41609-71-C-0006 (January 1974).
Crawford, B. H., 1936, The dependence of pupil size upon external light stimulus under static and variable conditions, *Proc Roy Soc,* **121**(B):376–395.
DeGroot, S. G., and Gebhard, J. W., 1952, Pupil size as determined by adapting luminance, *J. Opt. Soc. Am.,* **42**:492–495.

Ernst, J. R., and Potts, A. M., 1971, Paraphysiology of the distal portion of the optic nerve: IV. Local temperature as a measure of blood flow, *Am. J. Ophth.*, **73**: 435–444.

Fender, D. H., 1964, Control mechanisms of the eye, *Sci. Am.*, **211**(1):24–33.

Flamant, F., 1948, Variation du diametre de la pupille de l'oeil en fonctuion de la brillance, *Rev. Opt.*, **27**:751.

Geeraets, W. J., and Berry, E. R., 1968, Ocular spectral characteristics as related to hazards from lasers and other light sources, *Am. J. Ophth.*, **66**:15–20.

Goodeve, C. G., 1934, Vision in the ultraviolet, *Nature* **134**:416–417.

Halliday, D., and Resnick, 1967, "Physics for Students of Science and Engineering," 2nd edn., John Wiley & Sons, New York.

Hollyfield, J. G., and Rayborn, M. E., 1979, Photoreceptor outer segment development: light and dark regulate the rate of membrane addition and loss, *Invest. Ophthal. Vis. Sci.*, **18**(2): 117–132.

Krauskopf, J., 1962, Light distribution in human retinal images, *J. Opt. Soc. Am.*, **52**:1046–1050.

Randall, H. G., Brown, D. J., and Sloan, L. L., 1966, Peripheral visual acuity, *Arch. Ophth.*, **75**: 500–504.

Reeves, P., 1920, The response of the average pupil to various intensities of light, *J. Opt. Soc. Am.*, **4**:35–43.

Said, F. S., and Weale, R. A., 1959, The variation with age of the spectral transmissivity of the living human crystalline lens, *Gerontologia*, **3**:213–231.

Sliney, D. H., Wangemann, R. T., Franks, J. K., and Wolbarsht, M. L., 1976, Visual sensitivity of the eye to infrared laser radiation, *J. Opt. Soc. Am.*, **66**(4):339–341.

Sliney, D. H., 1971, The development of laser safety criteria—biological consideration, M. L. Wolbarsht (ed.), *in* "Laser Applications in Medicine and Biology," Vol. 1, Plenum Press, New York.

Snyder, A. W., 1974, Light absorption in visual photoreceptors, *J. Opt. Soc. Am.*, **64**(2):216–230.

Stiles, W. S., and Crawford, B. H., 1933, The luminous efficiency of rays entering the pupil at different points, *Proc. Roy. Soc.*, **112**(B):428–450.

Thoss, F., and Bourzina, S., 1976, The influence of adaptation and field area on the exponents of Stevens' Power Functions and the light reaction of human pupil, *Vis. Res.*, **16**:317–320.

Vos, J. J., 1966, Some considera ions on eye hazards with lasers, Report No. IZF 1966-4, Institute for Perception RVO-TNO, National Council for Applied Research in the Netherlands, Soesterberg, the Netherlands (AD800156).

Vos, J. J., Walraven, J., and Meeteren, A., van, 1976, Light profiles of the foveal image of a point source, *Vis. Res.*, **16**:215–219.

Walraven, P. L., and Leebeek, H. J., 1963, Foveal sensitivity of the human eye in the near infrared, *J. Opt. Soc. Am.*, **53**:765–766.

Walsh, J. W. T., 1958, "Photometry," 3rd ed., Dover Publications, Inc. New York.

Westheimer, G., and Campbell, F. W., 1962, Light distribution in the image formed by the living human eye, *J. Opt. Soc. Am.*, **52**:1040–1045.

Wolbarsht, M. L., 1976, The function of intraocular color filters, *Fed. Proc.*, **35**(1):44–49.

Yarbus, A. L., 1967, "Eye Movements and Vision," Plenum Press, New York.

Young, R. W., 1976, Visual cells and the concept of renewal, *Invest. Ophthal.*, **15**(9):700–725.

Chapter 4
Effects of Optical Radiation on the Eye

4.1 INTRODUCTION

The attendant hazards of laser operations vary greatly depending upon the exact type of laser and its application. The optical radiation hazards also vary greatly, from the small lasers used for alignment and leveling to high-powered pulsed ruby and neodymium lasers used for microdrilling and microwelding systems to still more powerful CO_2 laser systems used for welding and cutting.

The literature on the effects of optical radiation upon the skin and eye is enormous (Sliney, Krial, and Ryan, 1978). There are many effects—some are considered beneficial, others are considered marginal or possibly "potentially" hazardous, and the remainder are always considered hazardous. Since this book is largely concerned with safety it will focus on those interactions which are potential hazards to the eye (in this chapter) and to the skin (Chapter 5). Other internal structures of the human body are affected by optical radiation but these effects are chiefly of interest to surgeons and can be found in other texts (e.g., Goldman and Rockwell, 1971). Likewise the damages to tissue far in excess of the threshold effects that are of interest in setting safety standards will not be described in great detail. The detailed discussion of effects that are far below threshold of injury will be omitted for similar reasons.

The effects of optical radiation on the eye vary significantly with wavelength. For this reason the subject will be discussed in three sections. First the effects of ultraviolet radiation which are generally photochemical on the lens and cornea will be considered, but the main concentration will be on the retinal hazard region where the eye is particularly vulnerable to injury because of its imaging characteristics. Finally IR effects upon the anterior structures of the eye will be covered.

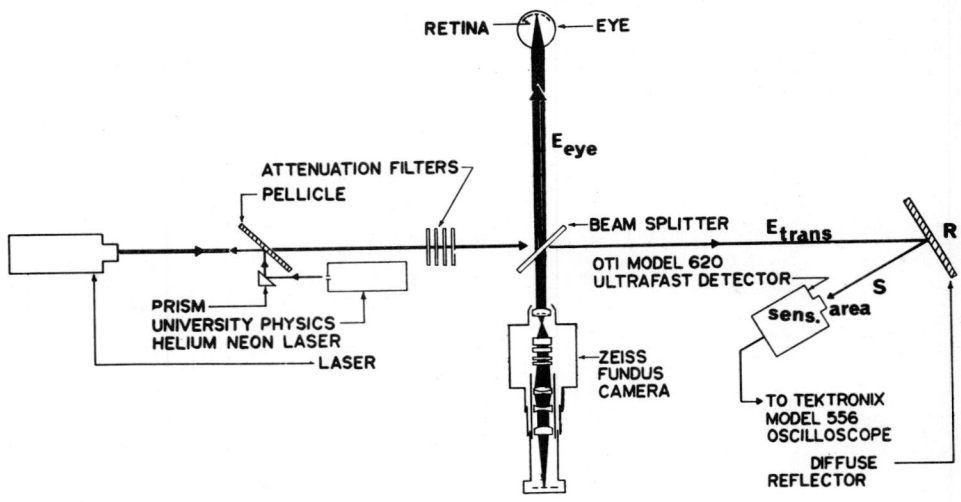

Figure 4-1. The experimental arrangement frequently used to deliver laser radiation to the eye of an anesthetized monkey. The specific arrangement shown is that of Frisch *et al.* (1971). The investigator views the retina during the experiment by means of a Zeiss fundus camera. Photographs are taken before and after the laser exposures. The exposures are placed in a regular grid of small lesions across the retina in order to facilitate identification during a later ophthalmoscopic or histologic examination. Figure courtesy of Dr. Edwin A. Beatrice, Letterman Army Institute of Research, San Francisco.

4.2 DETERMINING THRESHOLDS

The mere matter of what constitutes a threshold for a biological effect would require a full chapter for an in-depth discussion. There are many end points that can be used in establishing a threshold of injury. For instance, damage to the retina of the eye from visible radiation can be the appearance of a tiny white patch on the retina visible upon *ophthalmoscopic examination*. This technique (Fig. 4-1) has been used in most threshold of injury studies. The end point could be any *histologically-defined* injury seen with the light microscope; or it could be consistent *ultrastructural changes* only visible with an electron microscope (transmission or scanning EM). *Histochemical techniques* can also serve to document an end point for injury. Finally, there are the detection of *functional alterations* in sensory (behavioral) responses by task oriented animal subjects, e.g., visual acuity, color vision, dark adaptation. These functional changes can also be detected by electrophysiological recordings of *altered neural function* within the visual system. To add to the problem different investigators would define different threshold levels for any one of these end points.

The most reliable statistical method for describing any biological threshold is probit analysis. Figures 7-3, 7-4 will show this method applied to the data collected from one animal or several animals when an ophthalmoscopically visible lesion in the retina resulting from exposure to an argon laser is used as the end point. One point on this curve, the 0.5 damage probability (ED_{50} dose), is often assigned a special significance. This point is the exposure dose required to produce an ophthalmoscopically visible lesion in 50-percent of the exposures in a group of animals or in a single animal where multiple exposures have taken place. The ED_{50} point has in the past been termed a "threshold" point by some investigators although clearly the use of the term "threshold" in describing a 50-percent probability of injury seems rather inappropriate. In toxicological studies of the effects of chemicals upon biological systems the term threshold has often been used to define the 10-percent probability of a biological response. The whole question of how biological thresholds must be translated into exposure safety levels which includes the rationale of the probit method is the subject of Chapter 7 and shall be dealt with in detail there. This chapter will consider somewhat more qualitatively, and with less refinement of the exact details of threshold, the general biological effects of incoherent and coherent optical radiation upon ocular tissues.

4.3 THE EFFECTS OF DIFFERENT OPTICAL SPECTRAL BANDS

4.3.1 Retinal Injury

The eye is the most sensitive end organ and is generally the most vulnerable to laser exposure, particularly in the case of pulsed laser radiation. This is true for all spectral regions, but most particularly in the visible and near-infrared parts of the spectrum, indeed together they are known as the *retinal hazard region*. Light and near-infrared (IR-A) radiation is sharply focused onto the retina. When an object is viewed directly, the light forms an image in the fovea, the center of the macula. This central area, approximately 0.25 mm in diameter for humans, has the highest density of cone photoreceptors, as described in Chapter 3. The typical result of a retinal injury is a blind spot or *scotoma* within the irradiated area. A scotoma due to a lesion in the peripheral retina may go unnoticed. However, if the scotoma results from a lesion located in the fovea, which accounts for central vision, a severe visual handicap is the result. A central scotoma would occur if an individual were looking directly at the source of the incident laser radiation during the exposure. The size of the scotoma would depend upon whether the injury was near to or far above the threshold irradiance, the angular extent of the source of radiation, and the extent of accommodation.

Laser lesions of the retina resulting from exposures in the visible range cause many alterations in structure which can only be seen microscopically. The histological assessment of the retinal injury may be accomplished in many ways. Fig. 4-2 shows the displacement of the pigment granules in the pigment epithelium. In Fig. 4-3 is a conventional cross-section of a laser lesion in the peripheral retina of a human eye, while Fig. 4-4 gives a scanning electron micrographic view of a similar

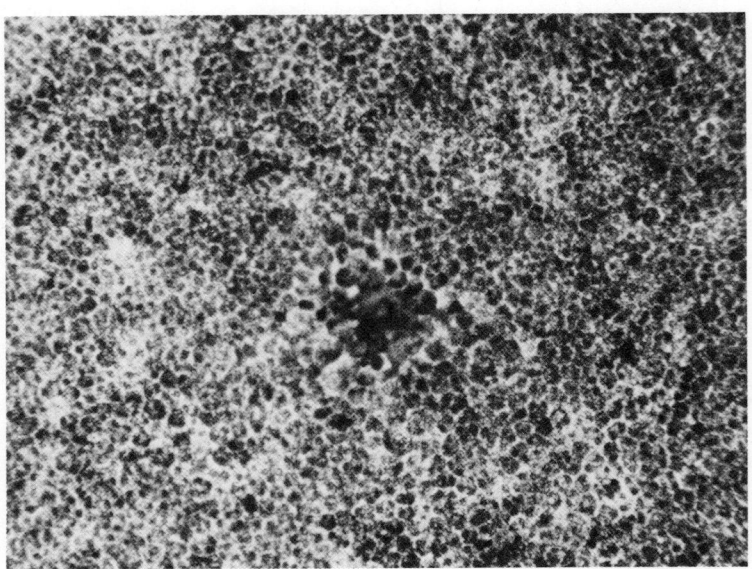

Figure 4-2. Histological changes seen in the retina following laser exposure. Flat-mount preparation of the rhesus pigment epithelium following exposure to ruby laser (694.3 nm), 23 µJ, 30 ns; 3 weeks old, original magnification X100 (from Frisch, Beatrice and Holst, 1971, with permission).

cross-section in a rabbit eye. Recent research into the protein synthesis of the photoreceptors by Young (1976) shows that the cone may not renew its photosensitive structures in the same manner and at the same daily period as do the rods. The cone is a highly specialized photosensitive light reactive cell. Therefore, alteration of these photoreceptors by a laser or other high intensity light source may be permanent, or recovery may be slower than from similar injury to rod outer segments.

There has been recent evidence to suggest that there can be partial repair of some segments of the visual cells following laser retinal injury (Tso, et al., 1972). This probably occurs only within a narrow zone between non-injury and permanent injury.

4.3.2 Injury to the Anterior Portion of the Eye

The anterior structures of the eye are the cornea, conjunctiva, aqueous humor, iris and lens. The cornea, aqueous and lens are part of the optical pathway and as such must retain transparency. One of the more deleterious effects of injury

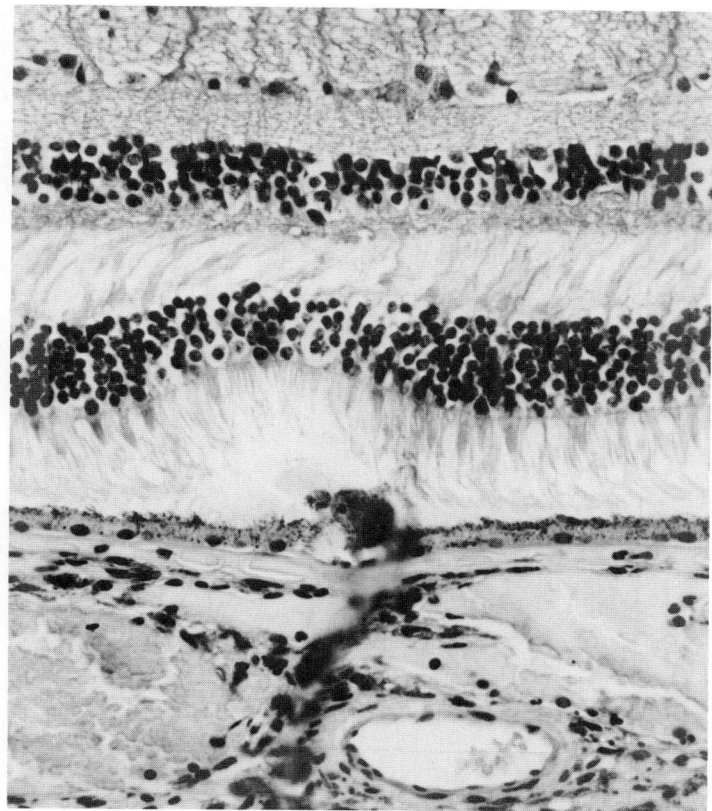

Figure 4-3. A cross-section histological preparation of retina and choroid. Lesion is in human retina resulting from argon laser exposure not in the macula (as indicated by the 1-cell-thick-ganglion-cell layer). There is marked disturbance of the pigment epithelium layer, some derangement of the outer segments and of the outer nuclear layer. The inner layers of the retina appear to be undamaged. This lesion resulted from a 0.2-s exposure at 60-mW argon radiation into the eye with a retinal spot size of 100 μm. It was well above threshold and was visible immediately after exposure (from Landers *et al.*, 1976, with permission).

to them is a loss of transparency.

At very short wavelengths in the ultraviolet and long wavelengths in the infrared, essentially all of the incident optical radiation is absorbed in the cornea. The cornea is exposed directly to the environment save for the thin lipid film—tear film. This is unlike any other living tissue (the skin is protected by dead stratum corneum), and the surface corneal cells must of necessity have a high turnover rate. Indeed, the corneal epithelium, the outermost living layer of the cornea upon which the tear layer flows, is completely renewed in almost a 48-hour period.

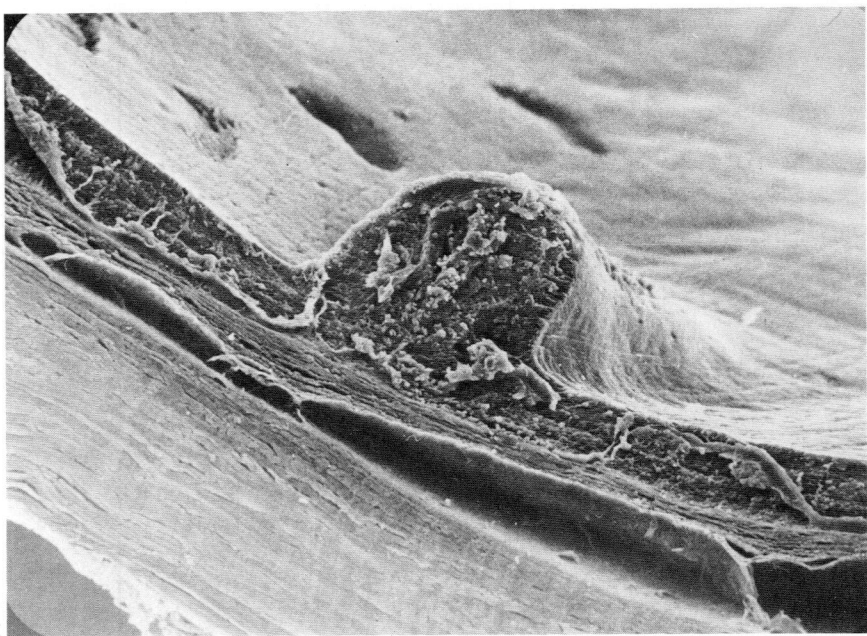

Figure 4-4. Scanning electron micrograph of a laser lesion (dye laser at 585 nm) in a rabbit retina. The retina is sectioned through the full thickness and is humped up and folded so that the photoreceptor layer (PR) comes to lie in a central vertical line. Choroid (Ch) and sclera (S) are both included. The internal limiting membrane (ILM) is only slightly disturbed (from Borwein *et al.*, 1976, with permission).

Hence damage limited to this outer corneal layer can be expected to be temporary. Indeed, injury to this tissue by short ultraviolet radiation, as occurs in ultraviolet *photokeratitis* or *photophthalmia* (known also as *welder's flash*), seldom lasts more than one or two days. Unless deeper tissues of the cornea are also affected, surface epithelium injuries are rarely permanent injuries.

Near-ultraviolet and near-infrared radiation (UV-A, IR-A, and possibly IR-B) are absorbed heavily in the lens of the eye. Damage to this structure is of great concern in that the lens has a very long memory. An exposure from one day may result in effects which will not become evident for many years. This is known to be true in the case of glassblower's or steel puddler's cataract and in cataracts caused by ionizing radiation. New tissue is continually added around the outside of the lens but the interior tissues remain in the lens for the lifetime of the individual. Hence chronic exposures may result in delayed effects. This is of great concern whenever the lens absorbs a substantial fraction of the incident radiation.

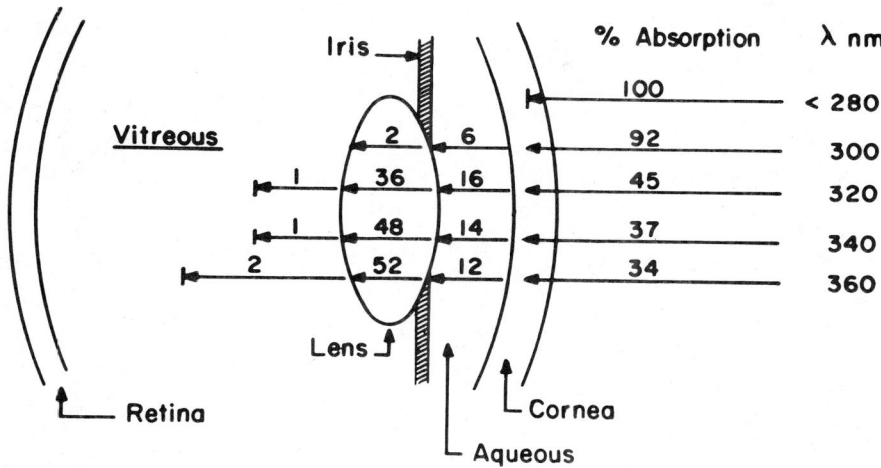

Figure 4-5. Schematic of absorption of ultraviolet radiation in the ocular media. Values represent the percent of ultraviolet radiation incident upon the corneal surface that are absorbed by various layers, redrawn from a figure by Matelsky, 1969. Based on data by Boettner and Wolter, 1962.

Absorption of optical radiation in the aqueous would not be expected to damage the aqueous *per se* as it is not a cellular structure, although a photochemical reaction within the aqueous solution theoretically could affect some metabolites and affect the cornea or lens secondarily. Such a theory has never been proposed in detail or tested but this example points out that in addition to spectral absorption of optical radiation within any ocular structure, the relative *sensitivity* (called "radiosensitivity" when speaking of ionizing radiation effects on tissue) must be considered. With this consideration in mind the reader should study Fig. 4-5 which shows the relative absorption of the different ocular media at several UV wavelengths. These absorption values are particularly useful in considering direct thermal effects upon these structures but are of limited value where photochemical effects are possible.

Now that the effect of radiation on the eye has been introduced all of these effects will be considered in greater detail. The remainder of this section will be organized by spectral bands, using the CIE photobiological designations.

4.4 ULTRAVIOLET RADIATION EFFECTS

4.4.1 Photochemical Injury

The ultraviolet spectral band designations recommemded by the CIE are: UV-A (315-400 nm) which is a relatively less photobiologically active band than the rest of the ultraviolet; UV-B (280-315 nm) which is of most severe concern for skin exposure; and UV-C (100-280 nm) which is particularly effective as germicidal and viricidal radiation. Essentially all of the significant adverse effects of UV have now been shown to result initially from a photochemical reaction rather than by a thermal damage mechanism. This is aptly demonstrated by the fact that a reciprocity relation between irradiance (dose rate) and exposure duration exists, i.e., a constant radiant exposure (dose) is required to elicit the response over a wide variation of exposure durations. An additional characteristic of any photochemical reaction is a rather steep drop-off of the action spectrum in the long wavelength end. Here the energy of a single photon is generally insufficient to produce an effect.

Until the advent of the laser the principal hazard problem recognized in the use of optical sources was the potential for injury of the skin and eye from ultraviolet radiation at wavelengths less than 320 nm. The spectral band less than 320 nm is often called the "actinic ultraviolet" and consists principally of the two bands known as UV-B and UV-C. The high attenuation afforded by many optical materials such as glass in the spectral range 200-320 nm generally encouraged the empirical safety approach in which optical sources are enclosed in glass, plastic or similar materials to absorb this actinic radiation. If injurious effects were noted the source enclosure or eye filter protection was increased in thickness.

The photochemical effects of ultraviolet radiation upon the eye are still not completely understood. The relative spectral effectiveness of radiation in eliciting any particular biological effect is referred to by photobiologists as an *action spectrum*. The steep slopes of many ultraviolet action spectra demonstrate the importance of not routinely extrapolating biological data of injury developed from one wavelength to another wavelength, or of not assuming that any smooth curve does not have fine structures. The development of a wavelength tunable laser source in the ultraviolet region has, by making a spectacular increase in spectral irradiance in any narrow wavelength band over that afforded by present ultraviolet sources, provided a dramatic new tool for ultraviolet photobiology that has yet to be fully exploited.

4.4.2 Effects Upon The Retina

The visual spectral sensitivity of the retina includes the near ultraviolet radiation, UV-A, as well as the visible range from 400 nm to 700 nm. However, the lens of the eye is a strong absorber of wavelengths shorter than 400 nm down to 315 nm while the cornea absorbs heavily at wavelengths below 300 nm (Fig. 4-5). As a result, visual sensitivity is markedly decreased between 420 nm and 380 nm.

Nevertheless the fraction of a percent of UV-A which reaches the retina can have adverse effects as has been demonstrated by Zuclich and Connolly (1976). Zuclich and Taboada (1978) found retinal lesions following exposure to a HeCd mode-locked laser at 325 nm. The lesion threshold was about 0.4 J/cm^2 at the cornea for a beam diameter of 1.6 mm. Because of the heavy scattering of UV-A in the ocular media it is difficult to estimate the retinal exposure. Young rhesus monkeys were used, hence the transmission of the ocular media was still relatively high (perhaps 1%) whereas in adult humans this transmission is much less.

Aphakics (persons with the crystalline lens removed) are a special exception to this rule and one would expect that they would be particularly susceptible to UV-A effects upon the retina.

4.4.3 Effects Upon the Cornea

UV-B and UV-C radiation are absorbed in the cornea and conjunctiva and sufficiently high doses will cause keratoconjunctivitis—that painful effect known to most as *snow blindness* or *welder's flash*. The fine structure of the cornea is shown in Fig. 3.2. The initial effect of UV exposure is damage to or destruction of the epithelial cells. Under normal conditions the corneal epithelial layer is completely replaced in a matter of a day or so. It can even be removed completely and will grow back quickly. Although injury to the epithelium is extremely painful as there are many pain fibers located among the cells in the epithelial layer, it is usually temporary because of the enormous recuperative powers of the epithelial layer. Damage to Bowman's membrane, the stroma, Descemet's membrane and the endothelium are more of a problem. Damage to the stroma is usually followed by invasion of the entire cornea by blood vessels which turns the cornea milky and is difficult to treat except by grafting of a donor cornea. As the cornea is insulated from the usual immunological responses of the body, grafts from unselected donors are not rejected as they are in other parts of the body. After exposure, as in other photobiological responses, there is a characteristic latency period without subjective symptoms which varies inversely with the exposure dose. The period is generally between 6 and 12 hours, being longer for longer wavelengths. At exposures well above threshold this period may be less. The reddening of the conjunctiva (conjunctivitis) within the *palpebral fissure* (area between the eyelids) is accompanied by *lacrimation* (heavy tear flow), *photophobia* (discomfort to light), *blepharospasm* (painful uncontrolled excessive blinking) and a sensation of "sand" in the eye. Corneal pain can be quite severe and the major treatment is the use of a corneal anesthetic. An epithelial haze often accompanies these subjective symptoms. Recovery takes one to two days.

Comparative studies show that animals are less sensitive to ultraviolet than humans. This difference must be kept in mind when any mechanism for UV damage in humans is extrapolated from animal models and used as a basis for setting levels. A study on human volunteers (Pitts and Tredici, 1971) produced discomfort and photophobia, but not all levels of exposure gave both of these symptoms to an equal degree. No experiments were conducted which gave high levels of tearing or acute discomfort sufficient to cause blepharospasm. The first noticeable physical sign in all trials was epithelial haze (Pitts and Gibbons, 1973). This seemed responsible for the slight decrease in visual acuity measured at the same time. Perhaps some test for intraocular light scattering, such as that proposed by Wolbarsht et al. (1977) for glare sensitivity, might demonstrate this corneal haze well enough to be used as a test for overexposure to ultraviolet. It is possible, however, that by the time any such test would show a positive result there may have already been an injury from UV exposure.

The action spectrum and threshold dose of ultraviolet keratoconjunctivitis have been investigated by several groups. General agreement may be found in the results of the different investigators if the differences in experimental techniques, instrumentation, and optical sources, as well as subjects are considered. Of the published studies those particularly relevant to human exposure were those on primate and human eyes by Pitts and his collaborators (Pitts and Tredici, 1971; Pitts, 1974; and Pitts and Cullen, 1977). Using a 40-kW argon transpiration arc and a xenon-arc source with monochromators they obtained data for 10-nm bands between 200 and 300 nm and for 5-nm bands between 300 and 330 nm. They found the peak of the photokeratitis action spectra to be located within the 265-275-nm band and reported a threshold for photokeratitis at that band of approximately 4 mJ/cm^2 for both human and primate eyes and a somewhat similar response in the rabbit cornea (Fig. 4-6). This is somewhat different from earlier studies on rabbits by Cogan and Kinsey (1946) which demonstrated a peak in the action spectrum at 288 nm and from Sherashov (1970) who had similar findings. Cogan and Kinsey used a high pressure mercury arc with its characteristic, irregularly spaced lines, and a monochromator adjusted to pass broader wavelength bands.

The reciprocity of irradiance and exposure duration probably holds for time periods similar to those that hold for ultraviolet erythema (reddening) of the skin. Specifically, it matters little whether the radiant exposure of the cornea occurs in one microsecond or in two hours. The product of the irradiance and the duration of exposure required for the same effect is a constant. These studies did not reveal an action spectrum for conjunctivitis different from keratitis, although some reports in the earlier literature seem to suggest this. The action spectra reported by Pitts and Cullen (1977) and Cogan and Kinsey (1946) are provided in Figure 4-6 for direct comparison thresholds shown for each band. The action spectra in the 200-300-nm bands are probably quite accurate. In the range between 300 and 320 nm they may be somewhat less accurate since the very steep slope of the curves makes it very difficult to provide precise points in this region. Earlier experiments by Pitts (1974) suggested a much shallower slope action spectrum in the 300-320-nm range at 10-nm intervals. This difference demonstrates that thresholds averaged over 10-nm intervals and weighted against an action spectrum which changes rapidly in a sensitive region can lead to serious error, especially if, as in this case, sufficiently narrow wavelength intervals cannot be used because of the lack of spectral intensity in the arc.

Individuals develop keratoconjunctivitis from daylight ultraviolet radiation but only under unusual circumstances, such as following prolonged exposure to ultraviolet reflected from snow. Snow is essentially the only material found in the

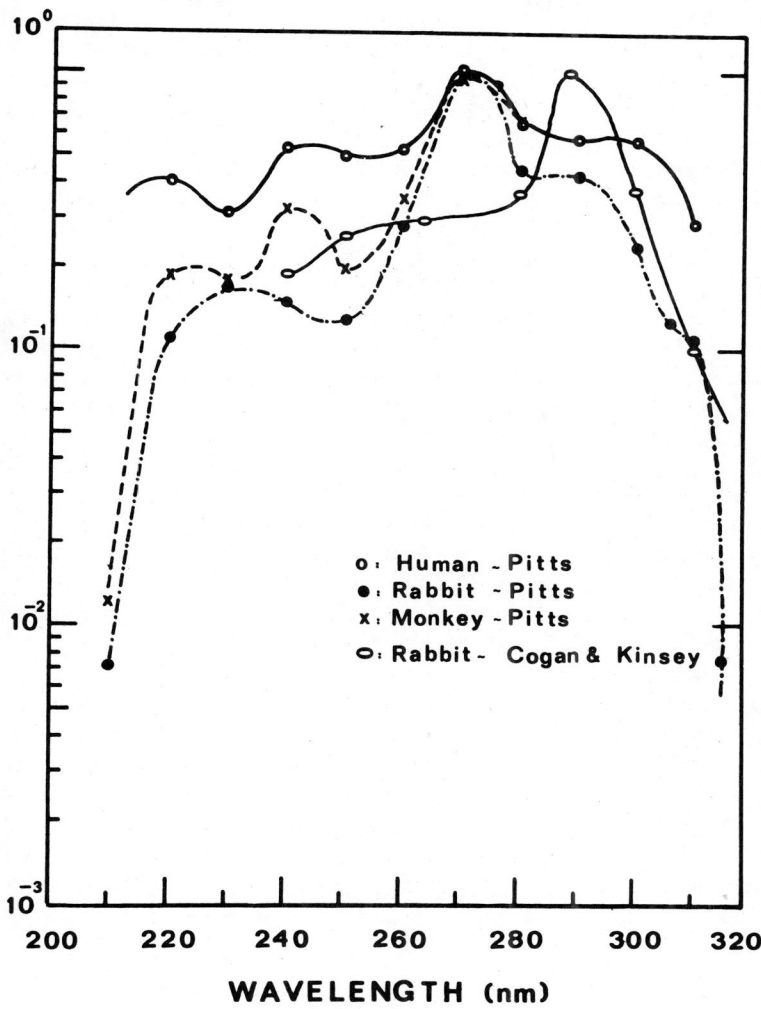

Figure 4-6. Action spectra for photokeratitis by ultraviolet radiation. Data reploted from Pitts (1974) and Cogan and Kinsey (1946). The abscissa shows the relative sensitivity of the cornea to ultraviolet injury for humans and primates (monkeys). The sensitivities are not significantly different from 270 nm to 300 nm.

natural environment with a high reflectance in the actinic ultraviolet spectral region. Water reflects very little and transmits a large percentage. Eskimos who have had to live with this situation have evolved a type of eye protection using whale bone with slits cut into it to provide a highly restricted field of view which eliminates upwelling ultraviolet radiation from nearby snow and still permits viewing of distant objects. Skiers who fail to wear protective goggles often develop ultraviolet photokeratitis. Additionally, accidental exposures to ultraviolet radiation from germicidal lamps, which emit principally at 253.7 nm occasionally occur. These accidents have confirmed the human threshold for keratitis at this wavelength of approximately 10 mJ/cm^2.

The widespread use of optical sources which have high levels of UV-C and UV-B in industry is the cause of many corneal injuries. The growing availability of UV lasers will increase these hazards. The UV-rich industrial sources circumvent the natural defenses of the body by allowing direct exposure of the cornea at normal angles of incidence unshielded by the brow or eyelids. In many cases these UV-rich sources have increased hazards as they are incorporated into optical systems whose elements are selected for either high transmission or high reflection in the UV. Welding is a prime example of a potentially hazardous industrial exposure, but the use of UV in the chemical industry for the manufacture of plastic is potentially much more dangerous due to the presence of possible photosensitizers.

The exact photochemical and biochemical mechanism of photokeratitis is still not well understood; however, in recent years some understanding has developed. The shape of action spectra obtained by Cogan and Kinsey (1946) led them to suggest that albumins and globulins may serve as the active chromophores, whereas the 265-275-nm maximum of Pitts led him to suggest that nucleoproteins were primarily involved because of some similarity of absorption spectra of nucleoproteins such as DNA to the action spectrum. Of particular interest recently has been the work of Hamerski and colleagues in Poland, who have studied the biochemical changes occurring in the corneal proteins (β and γ globulins) during the asymptomatic period following UV exposure. Cysteine topical solutions increased the asymptomatic period and a glycerol solution apparently prevented the normal clinical symptoms of photokeratitis (Hamerski 1969). Tapaszto and Vass (1969) in other biochemical studies also suggested changing the tear film to counteract the symptoms.

4.4.4 Lenticular Effects

The lens has much the same sensititity to ultraviolet as the cornea. However, the cornea is such an efficient filter for UV-C that little if any reaches the lens except at levels where the cornea is also injured. In the UV-A the cornea has substantial transmission while the lens has high absorption (Fig. 4-5).

As mentioned in Chapter 3 (3.2.1.5) the lens cells reach from front to back and meet at the lens sutures. The parts of the cells around the sutures are far away from the metabolizing part of the cells and are especially liable to injury. Also, injury to the thin part of the individual cells on the anterior surface usually involves the thicker parts of the same cells at the posterior pole, which gives a greater visual disturbance. In distinction to the corneal epithelium, the lens cells, especially those in the nucleus, have a very slow rate of renewal.

Some scientists have long speculated that the near-ultraviolet radiation, generally the UV-A from the sun, may play a causal role in senile cataract and other forms of cataract. The arguments in favor of this thesis largely rested on the high incidence of cataracts in people living near the equator where the total solar exposure is rather large. This argument, however, has been largely speculative. Bachem (1956) was one of the first scientists to attempt to achieve an ultraviolet cataractogenesis action spectrum. As he reported a UV-B action spectrum for rabbits and guinea pigs which peaked near 297 nm, many other scientists were very skeptical; after all, practically no 297-nm radiation reaches the lens.

As the lens ages it loses its elasticity. There has been speculation that exposure to both UV-A and IR can hasten this hardening of the lens. The formation of brunescent cataracts has been linked to UV-A and/or UV-B exposure (Kurzel et al., 1977), but no clear evidence has accumulated that brunescent cataract hastens the loss of accommodation.

The low transmission of the lens for UV-A is due to a pigment which accumulates throughout life. This pigment apparently shields the retina from near-ultraviolet radiation, particularly because of a possible damaging effect upon the retina, but perhaps primarily because the retinal photoreceptors have fairly high sensitivity in this range. The eye is an optical system essentially uncorrected for chromatic aberrations and visual acuity would be decreased if the lens transmitted UV-A wavelengths to blur the retinal image which is in focus for the longer wavelength visible range.

The UV-A absorbing pigment in the lens is itself a photodegradation product of other molecules which absorb in the UV-B, although some photodegradation may also occur from absorption in the UV-A. The exact pathways of degradation have not been worked out completely but it is most likely that tryptophan is the molecule involved either by direct absorption of the UV-B or by radiationless transfer of energy from other absorbing molecules. Tryptophan is degraded through N-formylkynurenine into the higher oxidative states of kynurenine which at one stage form a brownish material that often becomes dense enough to turn the lens almost black.

Although biochemical mechanisms for long-term photodegradation of lens constituents, particularly tryptophan, have been more or less experimentally determined (see Kurzel et al., 1977 for review), it is only recently when acute exposures at very high radiant exposures were used to produce cataracts in experimental animals that Bachem's work has been substantiated. A study by Pitts and Cullen (1977) and also by Zuclich (1977) have shown that doses of the order of 10 to 300 J/cm^2 do indeed cause corneal opacities in the UV-A (320 nm to 400 nm), but only the exposures in the UV-B appear to be strongly effective in causing lenticular opacities. The lenticular opacity may last only for a few days, then disappear if the exposure is sufficiently low. If the exposure is well above this level, the opacity, which first appears at the anterior polar region, gradually progresses to the posterior cortex. The action spectrum reported in these recent studies of cataractogenesis is shown in Fig. 4-7. Figure 4-7 also presents the collective data for UV-A

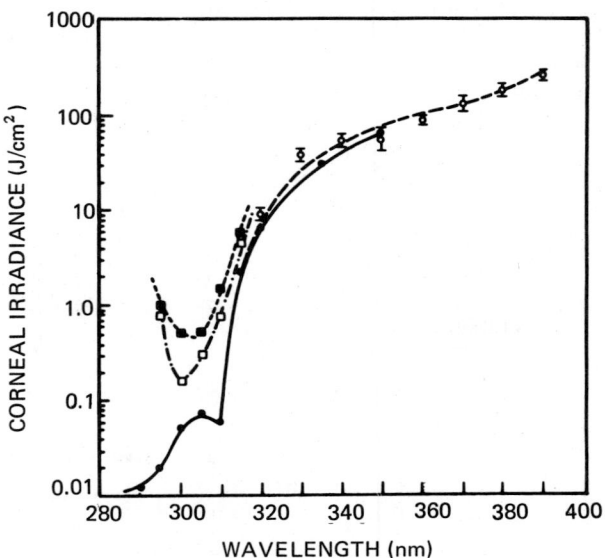

Figure 4-7. Action spectra for injury to the lens and cornea by near-ultraviolet radiation. Lower solid curve is the data of Pitts, Cullen and Hacker (1977), for photokeritis; upper dashed line is the data for permanent lenticular opacities; intermediate dot-dash line with open squares is the threshold for temporary lenticular opacities. The open circles with dashed lines represent threshold for corneal injury by Zuclich and Kurtin (1977).

induced corneal injury while Fig. 4-8 shows that this effect at the 350/357-nm lines of the krypton laser has a reciprocal relationship with power for exposure durations from 0.1 ms to 100 s. This certainly supports the contention that the damage process is photochemical in nature. At what duration additivity fails and recovery overcomes injury is not yet known. A note of caution should be given here. The corneal area exposed in the study by Zuclich of corneal injury in experimental animals (rhesus monkeys) was quite small—only 1.4 mm in diameter, and the exposure durations were often quite long—up to 100 s. If there were substantial movement of the animal during these periods of exposure these values may actually be high, since the exposures may have covered larger areas of the cornea. Nevertheless, since reciprocity holds, this represents probably the best data available at this time for wavelengths greater than 330 nm. The Pitts studies were performed with a much larger exposure area. Ebbers and Sears (1975) created cataracts with 325-nm HeCd laser radiation in the rhesus lens at levels of 260 J/cm^2.

The additivity of the UV-B cataractogenesis is unknown. Although photokeritis would occur before cataractogenesis (Fig. 4-7) following UV-B exposure, one cannot rule out additivity over many days of exposure for the cataractogenetic mechanism. The lens metabolism is very slow and UV-B exposure rates might have to be very low to be below the threshold where the biochemical recovery process overwhelms the photochemical damage process.

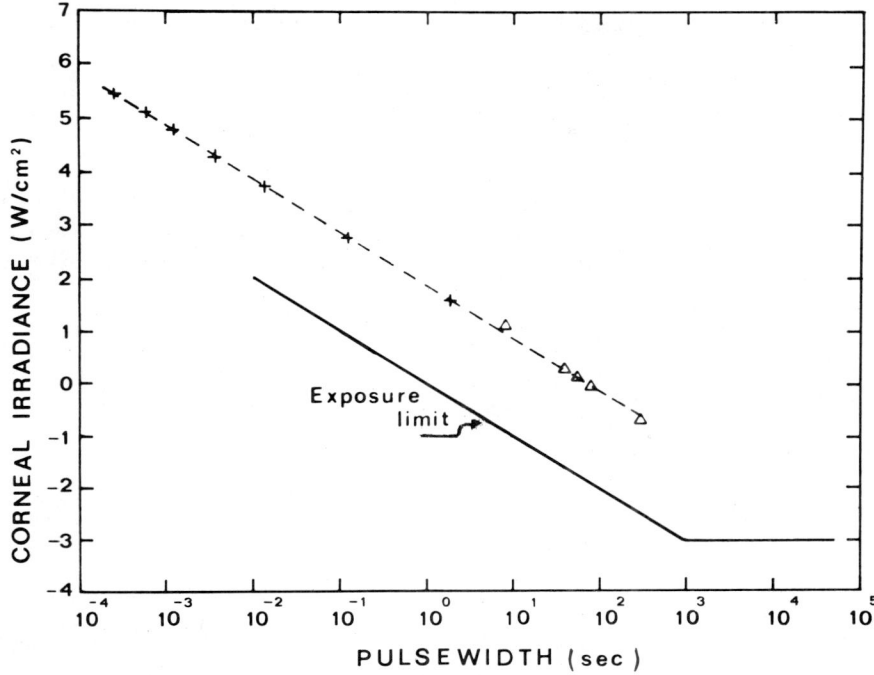

Figure 4-8. Comparison of threshold data for corneal injury as a function of exposure duration between a 350-nm argon laser (Δ) and pulsed UV sources (+) (adapted from Zuclich, 1978).

Pirie (1972) in Great Britain, and Kurzel *et al.* (1973) and Lerman (1972) in the United States have shown how the amino acid tryptophan which is present in the lens of the eye can be photo-oxidized by ultraviolet radiation, particularly effectively at UV-B wavelengths, and have speculated on the role of ultraviolet radiation in the production of senile cataract. The whole subject of ultraviolet induced cataractogenesis has been reviewed by Kurzel *et al.* (1977) and particularly for chronic exposures is a subject of great interest for future investigation. There is still much to be learned on this subject but effects of ultraviolet radiation on the lens of the eye are sufficiently documented to suggest caution in chronic, repeated exposures.

Sunlight itself contains potentially hazardous levels of both UV-A and UV-B. The reflectivity of a few natural environments such as sand and snow are high enough in the UV-A and UV-B regions to pose a formidable problem. However, not all who are exposed to high levels of sunlight seem to be sensitive to it, and the role of photosensitizers either in the diet or as abnormal products of metabolism must always be considered. To date the only UV-A photosensitizer that has been clearly incriminated is 8-methoxy-psoralen. Thus in the industrial environment chronic exposures to UV radiation must be considered hazardous. Certainly some types of cataracts appearing in welders could be caused by this portion of ultraviolet. Also many of the so-called IR cataracts such as those found in glass blowers, steel smelters, or furnacemen may have an UV-B contribution as well.

4.4.5 Effects on the Iris

It is likely that ultraviolet passing through the cornea could irritate the iris. For chronic exposures the possibility of melanoma exists, although the documentation for this possibility is not convincing. However, the high concentration of melanin pigments in the iris should protect against melanoma very much as the high concentrations of melanin apparently protect Negroes against skin cancer. Melanomas of the iris are usually found in blue eyes, which lack melanin pigment in the iris. No quantitative data exists on the sensitivity of the iris to damage from the UV. It is likely that other structures such as the cornea would be more sensitive to UV than the iris.

4.5 THE RETINAL HAZARD REGION (400-1400 nm)

4.5.1 Background

Injury to the retina, generally termed "retinal burns," resulting in a loss of vision following observation of the sun, has been described throughout history. Even Socrates, in Plato's *Phaedo* (Plato, 1892), discussed eclipse blindness (solar retinitis or eclipse scotoma) and suggested that a suitable precaution was to observe the eclipse by viewing the sun's reflected image in water. As was discussed in Chapter 2, water reflects only 2% at normal incidence, so this recommendation could have the effect of looking at the sun through goggles having a 50-fold attenuation factor. Man-made optical radiation sources, comparable to the sun in luminance and capable of causing chorioretinal injury, have been developed chiefly in this century. The incidence of injury from man-made sources is no doubt far less than the incidence of eclipse blindness. Until recently it was felt that chorioretinal injury would not result from exposure to visible light in industrial operations. Indeed, this is still largely true, since the normal aversion response to high brightness light sources (the blink reflex and movement of the head and eyes away from the source) provides adequate protection from most bright visual sources. However, recent increases in the use of high intensity, high radiance optical radiation sources having output parameters significantly different from those encountered in the past may present serious potentials for chorioretinal injury. In industry, besides lasers, one may encounter sources of continuous optical radiation such as compact arc lamps (as in solar simulators), quartz-iodide-tungsten lamps, gas and vapor discharge tubes, electric welding units, and sources of pulsed optical radiation such as flash lamps used in laser research and photolysis, exploding wires, and super-radiant light. While ultraviolet radiation from most of these devices has been considered and may remain the principal concern, the potential for chorioretinal injury should not be overlooked.

Reports of accidental and experimentally produced retinal injury from intense man-made radiant sources, such as electric arcs and the nuclear fireball, form an extensive literature. Experimental attempts to produce retinal injury from light sources originated in the middle of the nineteenth century with the Austrian investigator Czerny, who used a magnifying glass to focus the rays of the sun onto the rabbit retina. Verhoeff, Bell and Walker (1916) performed the classical studies of injury to the eye by optical radiation and provided a fascinating review of injuries to nineteenth-century scientists who first developed a variety of electric light sources. Recent review of the subject may be found in several references which are given at the end of this chapter.

Quantitative studies of retinal injury conducted since the late 1950's used principally rabbits and monkeys and have made use of both arc lamps and lasers as the optical source for exposure. These studies provide most of the information required to evaluate hazards from all sorts of optical sources. Many of these studies reviewed casually might appear to contradict one another; however, general trends and closer agreement become evident when it is realized that different experimental conditions—different retinal image sizes, wavelengths, experimental animals, and source distributions—have been used. In addition, the data from studies of the optical performance of the human eye are required to estimate the absolute retinal irradiance profile for small image sizes.

To summarize all of the results of these many studies is difficult; however, several general points are important to understand when evaluating optical radiation sources. First, however, we should consider the means of estimating the retinal exposure.

4.5.2 Determining the Retinal Exposure

The optical properties of the eye play an important role in determining retinal injury. Such factors as the image quality, pupil size, spectral absorption and scattering by the cornea, aqueous, lens, and vitreous, as well as the spectral reflectance of the fundus and absorption and scattering in the various retinal layers must be known for a definitive description. These will be considered separately.

4.5.2.1 *Pupil Size*

The limiting aperture of the eye determines the amount of radiant energy entering the eye and therefore reaching the retina. The energy transmitted is proportional to the area of the pupil. For the normal dark-adapted eye, pupil sizes range from approximately 7 to 8 mm; for outdoor daylight the normal pupil will constrict to approximately 1.6 mm. The ratio of areas between a 2-mm and 8-mm pupil is 1:16; hence, a 2-mm pupil accepts one-sixteenth the light admitted by an 8-mm pupil. The angle subtended by the source also plays a role; thus a light source of a given luminance causes a different pupil size dependent upon viewing distance (i.e., the image area on the retina) and the luminance of the surrounding field. It is

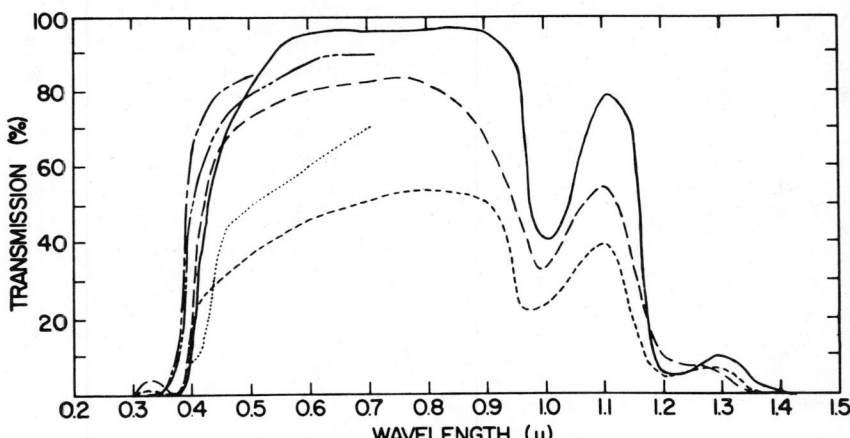

Figure 4-9. Comparison of experimentally measured spectral transmissions of the ocular media. Human eye data are from Ludvigh and McCarthey (1938), ...; Geeraets and Berry (1968), ———; and Boettner and Wolter (1962), - - - - direct, and — — — total. Bovine eye data from Pitts (1959), —— —— ——; and rabbit eye data from Kinsey (1948), - — —. Rabbit eye data of Geeraets and Berry (1968) which are not shown are very close to their human eye data (from Sliney, 1971).

important to remember that pupil size for a given environment varies with age, emotional state, and other factors—notably the use of some medications which create abnormally large pupil sizes. Therefore, in a large population, the pupil size will vary greatly under the same environmental exposure conditions. It is also known that although the total amount of light entering the eye varies as the area of the pupil varies, the light as actually perceived by the retina does not vary so simply. An effect first reported by Stiles and Crawford (1933) is that rays from the periphery of the pupil are less effective in producing the same visual stimulus as light rays entering through the center of the pupil. This is partially an optical effect due to the structure of the receptors and to pupillary vignetting, and partially results from neurological processing.

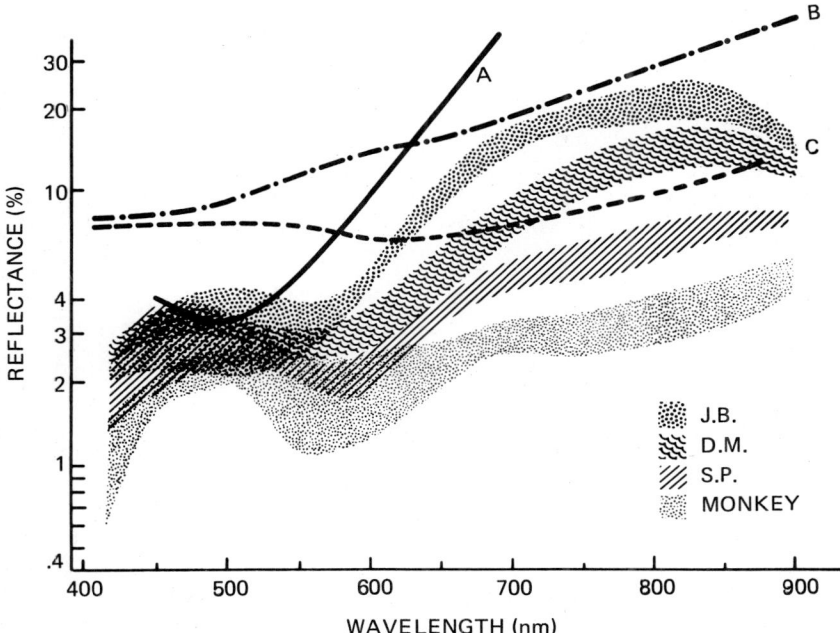

Figure 4-10. Spectral reflectance of the fundus (redrawn from Flowers *et al.*, 1977). Envelopes containing reflectance curves of 4 subjects are shown in shaded areas. JB a 30-year-old female Caucasian (blond); DM, a 22-year-old male Caucasian (brunette); SP, 23-year-old female Negro; monkey adult male (monkey). Curve A represents human fundus data of Vos, Munnik and Boogaard (1965); Curve B, human fundus data of Geeraets and Berry (1968); Curve C, monkey fundus data of Geeraets and Berry.

4.5.2.2 Spectral Transmission of the Ocular Media

The transmission of the ocular media between 300 nm and 1400 nm has been studied by several investigators. Two groups of studies are most often used, those of Geeraets and Berry (1968) and those of Boettner (1967) and Boettner and Wolter (1962). Figure 4-9 presents the results of these two studies along with earlier reports. The highest transmission values, from Geeraets and Berry, were obtained using intact enucleated (removed) human eyes and measuring total spectral transmission. Boettner and Wolter measured the spectral transmission of the cornea, aqueous, lens, and vitreous separately, which could account for the lower total transmission. They also measured the direct transmission, which limited the amount of scattered light accepted by the detector. The highest transmission values may be considered maximum even for large image sizes, while the lower values are probably more reasonable for smaller image sizes where forward scattering tends to limit the peak retinal irradiance. Unfortunately the experimental techniques used

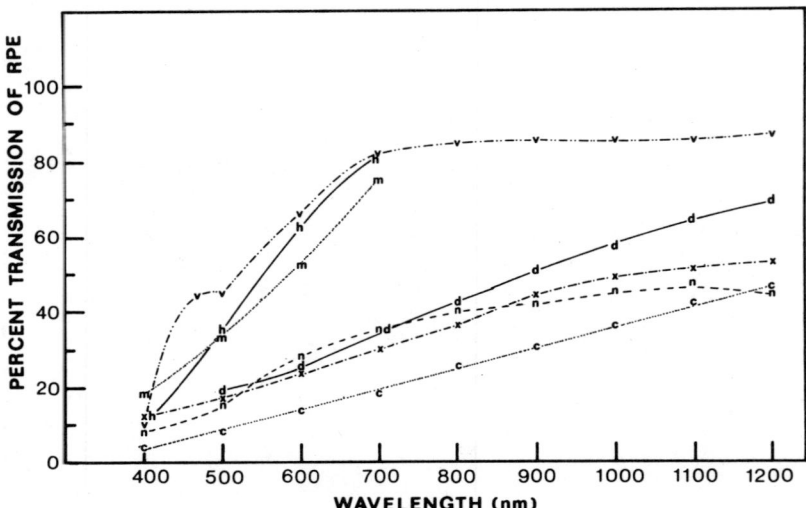

Figure 4-11. Transmission of retinal pigment epithelium. The upper 3 curves are data which include all transmitted scattering which may be used to obtain true spectral absorption values for the RPE. The lower 4 curves obviously do not include, or correct for, diffuse transmission. The trend in all of these spectral transmission values show that relatively little radiant energy is absorbed at the long wavelength end of the retinal hazard spectrum. In this plot (v) is data of Geeraets et al. (1962), for a human eye; (h) is data for a human retina and (m) for a macacus (monkey) retina obtained by Gabel et al. (1976); (c) is data for lightly pigmented human (Caucasian) retina; (n) is data for heavily pigmented (Negro) human retina; and (x) is data for the rhesus monkey obtained by Coogan et al. (1974); and (d) is data of Hayes and Wolbarsht (1968) for dog pigment epithelium. From the best (upper curves) the following absorption coefficients for a 5-μm RPE were calculated: 4240 cm^{-1} @ 400 nm, 2100 cm^{-1} @ 500 nm, 920 cm^{-1} @ 600 nm, 400 cm^{-1} @ 700 nm, and 140 cm^{-1} @ 1060 nm.

did not permit a clear indication of the comparable image sizes for each curve. Whatever the case, it is known that there is a large individual variability and this must be kept in mind by anyone desiring to use these data in a highly quantitative calculation. The other factor which must not be forgotten is the shift of the short-wavelength cutoff at 390-410 nm with age. The lens transmits less UV-A and blue light with increasing age (i.e., the lens yellows with age).

4.5.2.3 Spectral Absorption by the Retina and Choroid

Geeraets and Berry (1968), Gabel and associates (1976), and Flower et al. (1977) measured the fundus reflection and absorption in human retinal pigment epithelium and choroid. Figure 4-10 shows the small spectral reflectance of the human retina and indicates that this factor can almost be neglected. Figure 4-11 shows the spectral transmission data of the retina (essentially the RPE) which has been used by several groups to calculate retinal absorption. Note that very little is absorbed in the IR-A band. The uppermost curves are valid since they include the

Effect of Optical Radiation on the Eye

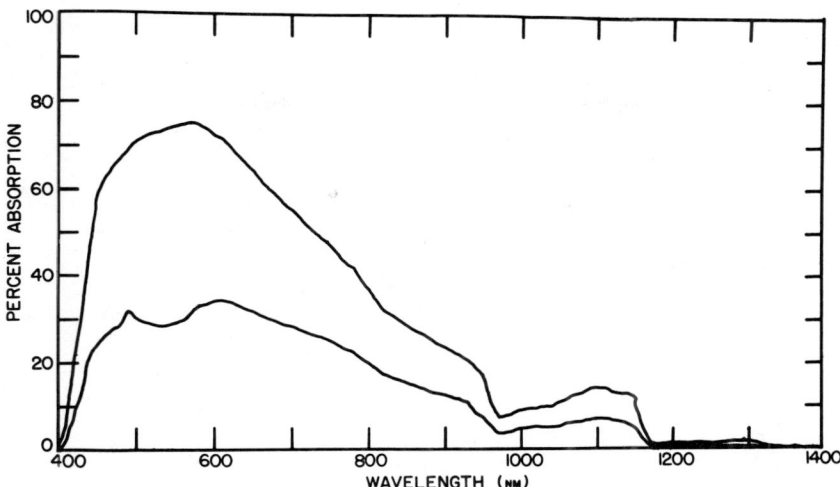

Figure 4-12. Relative spectral effectiveness curve for retinal thermal injury. Shown above is the spectral absorbed dose in retina and choroid relative to constant corneal exposure as a function of wavelength. Retina and choroid spectral absorption values corrected for fundus reflectance (upper curve) obtained by Geeraets and Berry (1968) were multiplied by corresponding direct transmission spectral factors of the ocular media, Boettner and Wolter (1967), to give relative spectral effectiveness (lower curve).

measurement of scattered radiation. When all of these factors are taken into account it is possible to multiply the spectral absorption data of the retina by the spectral transmission data for the ocular media to arrive at an estimate of the *relative absorbed spectral exposure dose in the retina and choroid* for the same spectral radiant exposure at the cornea. This should provide a relative spectral effectiveness curve for retinal thermal injury, at least for exposure times less than approximately 10 seconds. Figure 4-12 provides two such curves using the maximum and minimum transmission values shown in Fig. 4-9. Comparison of actual threshold retinal burn data obtained at different wavelengths generally support the upper curve for large image sizes and the lower curve for smaller image sizes.

4.5.2.4 Optical Image Quality

The retinal image size can be calculated for most extended sources by geometrical optics. As shown in Fig. 4-13, the angle subtended by an extended source defines the image size. If the effective focal length of the relaxed normal eye (f_e is approx. 1.7 cm) is known, the retinal image size d_r can be calculated if the viewing distance r and the dimension of the light source D_L are also known:

$$d_r = D_L \, f_e / r \qquad (4\text{-}1)$$

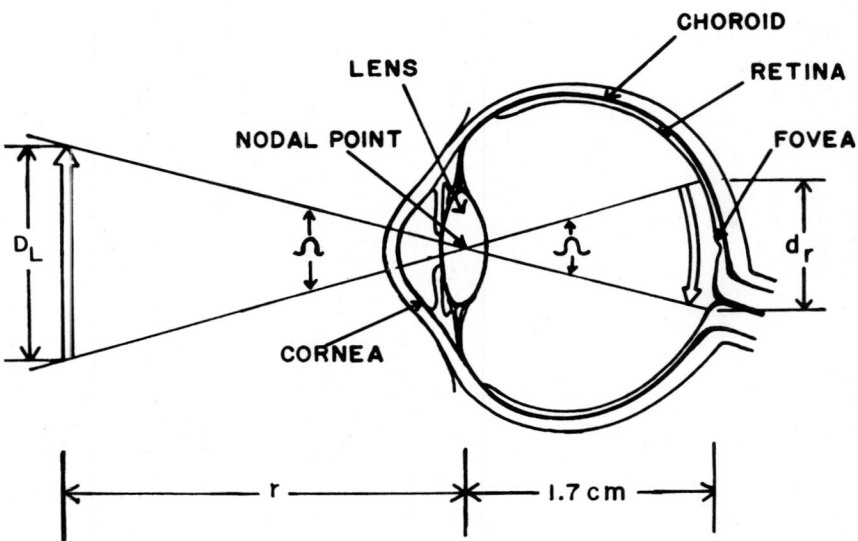

Figure 4-13. The source angle at the eye. An extended source is imaged at the retina; the approximate size of the image is determined using the simple geometric relation that both the object and image subtended an angle (Ω) measured at the eye's nodal point (approximately 1.7 cm in front of the retina) (from Sliney and Freasier, 1973).

This formula was derived from Fig. 4-13 using similar triangles and applying the approximation that the arc and the chord of a circle are approximately the same for small angles. This approximation breaks down for very large image angles. For example, an error in d_r of nearly 5 percent results when the source subtends an angle of 60°. By similar arguments the solid angle Ω_s subtended by either the source or the image as measured at the nodal point of the eye is the same (Fig. 4-13), hence for small angles the source area A_L and the image area A_r are always proportional in the ratio of the square of the viewing distance to the square of the eye's focal length f_e. Again, a small error is introduced for large angles (e.g., an error of A_r of about 5 percent for a circular source area subtending an angle of 20°). The retinal irradiance and source radiance are likewise proportional. Indeed, the radiance L of the source can be defined from the irradiance at cornea E_c for small angles since the solid angle of the source Ω_s is determined by A_L and r:

$$L = E_c / \Omega_s$$
$$= E_c \, (r^2 / A_L) \qquad (4\text{-}2)$$
$$= E_c \, (f_e^2 / A_r)$$

Likewise, the total power Φ_r entering the eye (through the pupil of area A_c) that actually reaches the retina (for a transmission τ) must be the product of the retinal image area A_r and retinal irradiance E_r:

$$\Phi_r = E_r \cdot A_r$$
$$= \tau \cdot E_c \cdot A_c \quad (4\text{-}3)$$
$$= \tau \cdot E_c [(\pi \cdot d_e^2)/4]$$

where the pupil diameter is d_e.

From this we obtained the quantitative relation for small angles of retinal irradiance to source radiance (or retinal illuminance to source luminance):

$$E_r = (\pi \cdot d_e^2 \cdot L \cdot \tau)/4 f_e^2$$
$$= 0.27 \, d_e^2 \cdot L \cdot \tau \quad (\text{for } d_e \text{ in cm}) \quad (4\text{-}4)$$

Equation (4-4) is of great practical value, since it permits the definition of a permissible radiance (luminance) from a permissible retinal irradiance for any source of known radiance or luminance without concern for the viewing angle or viewing distance. Ignorance of this formula has caused many people to waste time trying to calculate with high precision the retinal image size of extended sources by measuring the total power entering the eye with allowances for the effect of pupil size. All of this effort could have been averted had they simply understood that for each point in the source there is a corresponding point at the retinal image plane. Although the effective nodal point, hence f, varies slightly for the accommodated eye (i.e., for viewing distances less than 6 m), the formula is not significantly affected even for very short viewing distances. The above derivation assumes a source of uniform radiance; however, since each source point has a corresponding image point, the retinal irradiance in an incremental area of the image is likewise related to the radiance of a corresponding incremental area of the source. This would be shown by a more rigorous derivation of equation (4-4) in differential form.

As an aside, it may be pointed out that formula (4-4) is also useful in photographic radiometry. A similar equation that would relate film plane illuminance or irradiance E_f to source luminance or source radiance L can be derived by using equation (4-3) and simply replacing the ratio of d_e/f with the f-number (f#) of the camera which gives the formula:

$$E_f \cdot t = H_f$$
$$= (\tau \cdot L \cdot t)/4(f\#)^2 \quad (4\text{-}5)$$

where t is the exposure duration and H_f is the exposure at the film plane, f# is the

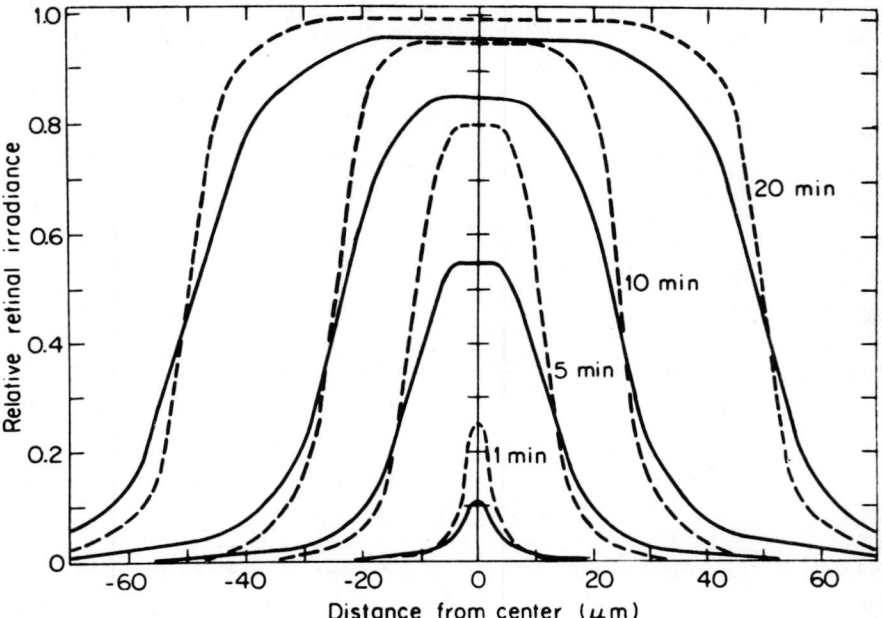

Figure 4-14. Approximate retinal irradiance profile for circular images at the retina for disc sources. The disc source has subtended viewing angles of 1, 5, 10 and 20 minutes of arc corresponding geometrically to retinal image diameters of 5 μm, 25 μm, 50 μm, and 100 μm respectively (obtained by Gubisch, 1967) for the normal human eye. As the source angle decreases appreciably below 20 minutes of arc the peak retinal irradiance falls further below the normal eye's value of 1 calculated by geometrical optics of Equation (4-4). The dashed line profiles are for 7-mm pupil (from Sliney and Freasier, 1973).

ratio of focal length f to the aperture d_e and is termed the *focal ratio* or *f-number* of the lens. Equation (4-5) will be used later in the discussion on photographic radiometry in Chapter 11 on measurement.

4.5.3 Small Images

Formula (4-4) breaks down for very small image sizes (or for very small hot spots in an image) where the source or source element in question subtends an angle of less than 10 min-of-arc. Figure 4-14 shows the approximate retinal irradiance profile for circular sources subtending angles of 1, 5, 10, and 20 min-of-arc. One minute-of-arc corresponds geometrically to approximately 5 μm on the retina. Note that for a given source radiance the image irradiance decreases as the image size decreases to a "point" image. This decrease results from image blur due to diffraction of light at the pupil, aberrations induced by the cornea and lens, and by

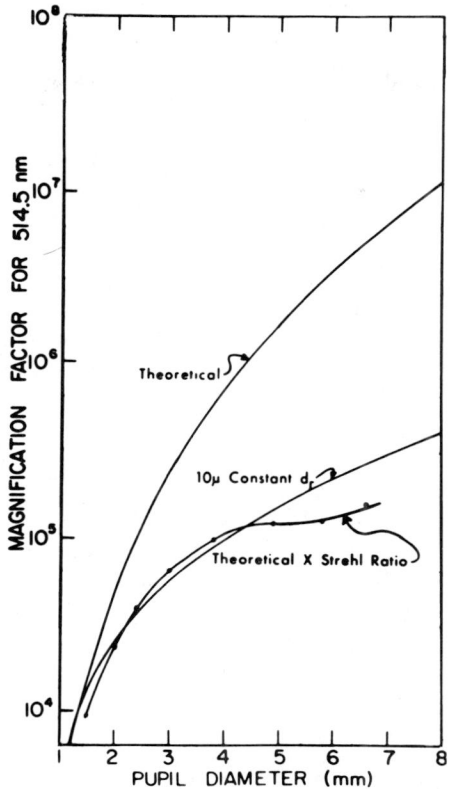

Figure 4-15. Optical gain of the eye for a point source as a function of pupil size. Influence of pupil size is demonstrated upon the optical gain or magnification factor of corneal to retinal irradiance for a point source viewed by the normal human eye. A theoretical curve was obtained using Airy formula for peak retinal irradiance. A second curve shows the optical gain for constant retinal image diameter of 10 μm. The final curve is believed to more accurately represent the actual optical gain and was derived by multiplying the theoretical values by the Strehl ratios reported by Gubisch (1967). The Strehl ratios used may be high due to experimental difficulties in measuring low levels of forward scatter (from Sliney and Freasier, 1973).

scattering from the cornea and the remainder of the ocular media. Since the effects of aberrations increase with increasing pupil size, greater blur (hence reduced peak retinal irradiance) is noted for larger pupil sizes. This effect is also evident in Fig. 4-15 which shows the optical gain (i.e., peak E_r/E_c from knowledge of the Strehl ratio) as a function of pupil size for a point source. This relation is useful in evaluating intrabeam viewing of a laser where the collimated light can produce a "point image" in a relaxed normal (emmetropic) eye. When a laser is directly viewed from within the beam or when an extended source is viewed at a great distance by the normal eye (i.e., the source angle is less than approximately 1 min-of-arc), the retinal image profile is essentially the same regardless of the source angle. This fact requires the determination of the potential hazard for intrabeam viewing of a laser by the corneal irradiance rather than by the source radiance. For these reasons, investigators studying retinal injury using a collimated laser beam to produce a minimal image size should also report not only the total power entering the eye in presenting their retinal injury thresholds, but also the beam size, profile and divergence.

The accuracy of the Strehl ratio data upon which Fig. 4-15 is based is difficult to ascertain. Several arguments can be given, such as the use of theoretical modulation transfer functions (MTFs) of imaginary retinal image profiles which suggest that the Strehl ratios upon which Fig. 4-15 are based are quite reasonable (Sliney and Freasier, 1973). With these optical gain figures, effective retinal image sizes of ~ 22 μm in diameter can be calculated for most larger pupil sizes. However, if the retinal image profiles are defined in terms of the half-peak power points the actual diameter is only 5 to 10 μm in diameter. Thus, care must be exercised in the use of simple figures such as effective diameter when defining the retinal image profile. In actuality the retinal image profile is a sharp central distribution surrounded by some widely scattered radiation such that a fair percentage of the total radiation is in the outer veiling corona.

4.5.4 Retinal Pigment Epithelium Absorption

As pointed out previously in this chapter (section 4.5.2) the visible and near-infrared radiation is transmitted through the ocular media and is absorbed principally in the retina. However it must first pass through the neural layers of the retina before reaching the retinal pigmented epithelium (RPE) and choroid. The visual pigments in the rods and cones absorb only a small fraction of light to initiate the visual response—perhaps only 5 percent of the total energy entering the eye. The retinal pigment epithelium (RPE) absorbs about 50 percent of the light and is optically the most dense absorbent layer. As the absorption takes place in a highly concentrated layer of melanin granules in a layer of approximately 3 to 4 μm, the greatest temperature rise exists in this layer (Figure 4-16). Many mathematical models assume the retinal pigment epithelial thickness to be approximately 10 μm. This is the cell thickness. However, the thickness of the absorbing layer of melanin granules at any selected location is probably only 3 to 4 μm. The melanin granules are normally clustered near the junction with the receptors. The RPE layer is sufficiently uneven that in a cross section of any great thickness the pigmented granules are apparently distributed over a 10 μm width due to folding and depressions in the layer of pigmented cells. The pigment granules are spherical or ellipsoidal with a diameter (or major axis) of approximately 1 μm. The actual size, shape, and physical characteristics of individual melanin granules become quite important for a thermal model adequate to describe the behavior of this layer during very, very short pulse exposures. The granules may be heated to incandescence during Q-switched exposures.

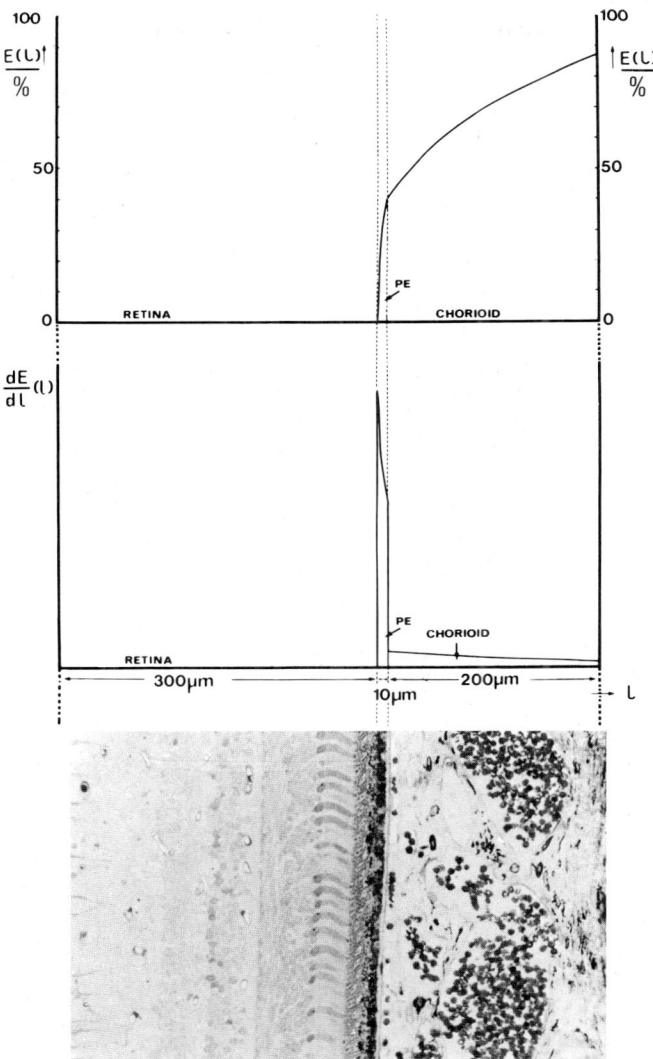

Figure 4-16. Relative absorption and temperature rise in different layers of the retina and choroid. This figure from Gabel, Birngruber and Hillenkamp (1976), dramatically illustrates that although more of the total energy is absorbed in the choroid, as shown in the upper graph, the energy absorbed per unit length dE/dL (L) is far greater in the pigment epithelium. The lower panel shows a light microscopic cross section of the same layers of neural retina pigment epithelium, and choroid.

4.5.5 Chorioretinal Thermal Injury

The mechanism of injury is considered to be largely thermal for accidental exposures from arc lamps, CW lasers, or the sun for durations on the order of 0.1 s to ~ 10 s or from exposures from long-pulsed lasers or flashlamps on the order of 1 ms to 10 ms. Since injury appears to result principally from protein denaturation and enzyme inactivation, the variation of temperature with time of the retinal tissue during and following the insult must be considered. Several efforts to develop mathematical models for the light absorption, heat flow, and the rate-process injury mechanisms within the complex structure of the retina have been moderately successful within the general pulse exposure duration time frame of 1 ms to 10 s. Figure 4-17 shows the calculated temperature elevation for small retinal image sizes and the temperature-time history for different pulse durations for threshold injury based on a retinal thermal model developed by White (1975). Of particular interest is the fact that for pulse durations less than 1 ms there is actually a smaller peak temperature rise in the overall retinal pigment epithelium than for longer pulses. This suggests a different mechanism of injury and may be related to the thermal relaxation times of the pigment granules (Hayes and Wolbarsht, 1968, 1971). The greatest value in retinal thermal models has been to gain a broader understanding of the damage mechanism and provide the direction for future experimental studies. Such analyses of injury mechanism make it possible to draw some general, but tentative, conclusions. Since thermal injury is a rate process, no single critical temperature exists above which injury will take place independent of exposure duration. For narrow ranges of exposure duration, a critical temperature should predict injury thresholds if photochemical effects are not present. Shorter exposures require greater temperature elevations for the same degree of retinal injury—at least for exposure durations greater than 1 ms (as shown in Fig. 4-17). Welch and Priebe (1976) have experimentally measured the variation in critical peak temperature rise as a function of exposure duration.

Since the very large complex organic molecules absorbing the radiant energy would have broad spectral absorption bands, one would not expect the monochromatic nature of laser radiation to create any different effects from radiation from conventional sources, and indeed experimental evidence strongly supports this conclusion. The coherence of laser radiation is also not considered to affect the hazard potential for chorioretinal thermal or photochemical injury. Although a speckle pattern resulting from interference effects of laser light at the retina does exist, the very fine gradations in retinal irradiance resulting from this effect (Considine, 1966) would certainly be lost as soon as the pulse duration is greater than a few microseconds. Both thermal conduction and ocular tremor would smooth out the distribution of light and localized temperature elevations resulting from the 1 μm to 10 μm gradations in the speckle pattern and these nonuniformities would be blurred. Chorioretinal injury from either a laser or a non-laser source should therefore not differ if image size (retinal irradiance distribution), exposure duration, and wavelength are the same. Non-thermal, non-photochemical effects of a uniform speckle pattern could however produce adverse behavioral effects following very long-term exposures (Zwick and Jenkins, 1978).

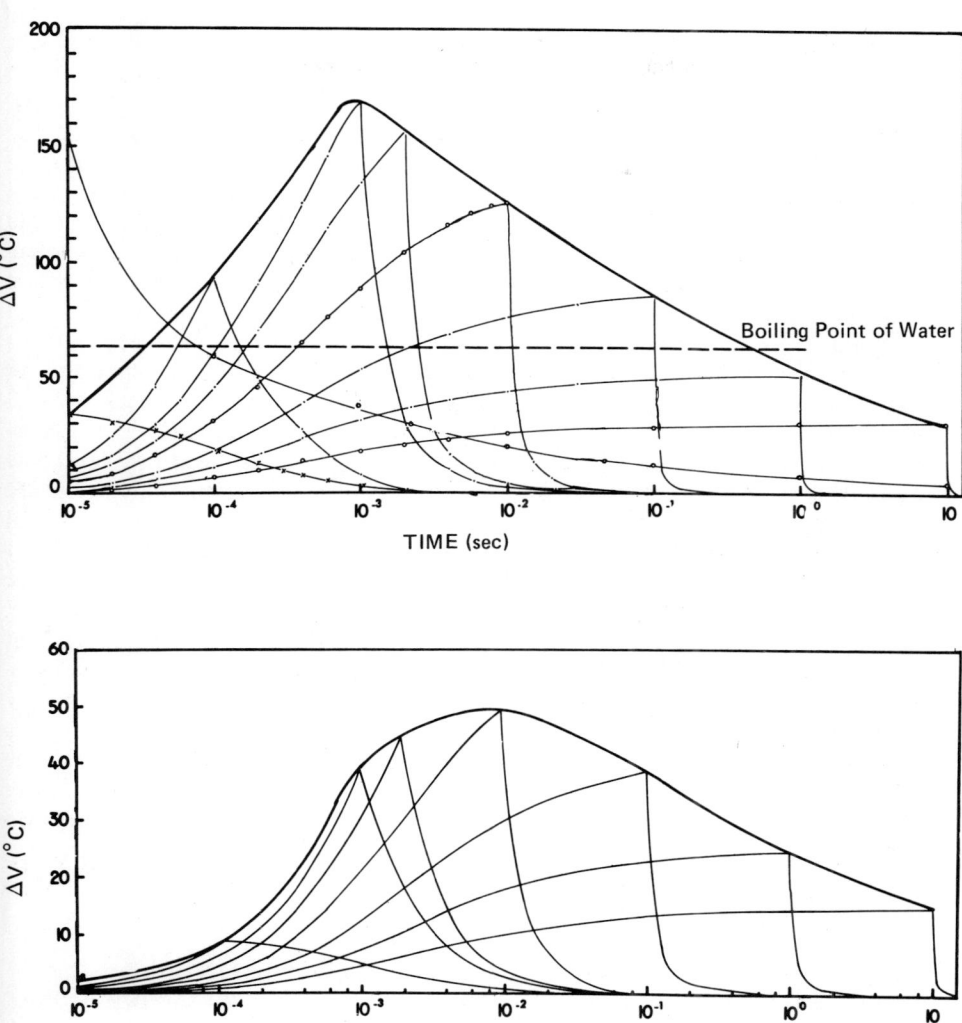

Figure 4-17. Time-temperature histories for injury thresholds as calculated by a thermal model. The upper set of curves are calculated for 0.01-ms to 10-s exposures for minimal image size lesions in the rhesus monkey. The temperature increases are for the center of a 10-μm-thick RPE at the center of a 16-μm image. The lower set of curves are for the same minimal threshold irradiance data in the rhesus monkey with the temperature calculation still at the center of the 10-μm-thick RPE, but moved 20 μm radially from the center of the image. These points indicate the time-temperature history of cells just adjacent to the exposed retinal area; note that the peak of the temperature envelope is displaced to 10 ms, and the boiling point of water is never reached by any of the curves. In each set, the bold upper curve is an envelope of the peak temperatures reached for that time-temeperature history. (Calculated by T. P. White and D. H. Sliney.)

4.5.6 The Effect of Retinal Image Size

The tissue surrounding the absorption site can much more readily conduct away the absorbed heat for image sizes of 10 µm to 50 µm in diameter than it can for large image sizes of the order of 1,000 µm (1 mm). Indeed, retinal injury thresholds for the same time domain of 0.1 s to 10 s show an enormous dependence upon image size as would be expected from calculations of heat flow in the retina. For example 1 to 10 W/cm^2 results in a minimal threshold for a 1,000-µm image, but an irradiance of 1 kW/cm^2 is required to produce that same type of threshold lesion in a 20-µm image. It is this dependence that explains the fact that momentary viewing of the sun (160-µm image) by the unaided eye does not produce a retinal burn; however, viewing the sun through a binocular or telescope, while not increasing the retinal irradiance, does greatly increase the retinal image size, and a retinal burn is likely to result. This dependence is not so marked for much shorter exposure durations and some thermal models would suggest that no such dependence should exist for exposure durations shorter than approximately 1 ms. However, this is not borne out in animal experiments. The retinal burn threshold data for limiting-case, small image diameters of 20 µm to 70 µm are normally presented as total energy or total power entering the eye. This appears reasonable at first since the exact image size in the retinal exposure distributions cannot be confidently determined for point sources. The only flaw is that the beam diameter at the cornea does influence the retinal image size and the injury threshold (Frisch, Beatrice and Holsen, 1971). Figure 4-18 shows the retinal image size dependence of threshold lesions as observed ophthalmoscopically for a wide range of pulse durations and for two or three wavelengths. At one time it was believed that injury thresholds for pulse durations of the order of 1 µs were reasonably constant as a function of image size. However, recent studies to better understand the damage mechanism have revealed that there appears to be no pulse duration whereby the threshold of injury does not vary for image size. Only for very long exposures do (non-thermal) injury thresholds not vary with size.

4.5.7 The Effect of Pulse Duration

The spot-size dependence of threshold for short pulse durations is baffling. The expectation when exposure durations are of the order of 1 µs is that injury will take place before there is significant heat flow. Indeed, the variation of threshold with pulse duration itself (Fig. 4-19) is also rather puzzling, especially the increase in threshold for 20-ns Q-switched pulses over those of 1 µs duration. Obviously, the Q-switch-pulse energy is being dissipated in some mechanism such as an acoustical transient which does not contribute to the normal thermal injury process which determines the minimum threshold.

Experiments conducted at the Letterman Army Institute of Research with image distributions that were non-circular, such as line images on the retina, produced lesions which for long exposure durations were circular in nature, as would be predicted by thermal injury calculations and heat flow calculations, but the

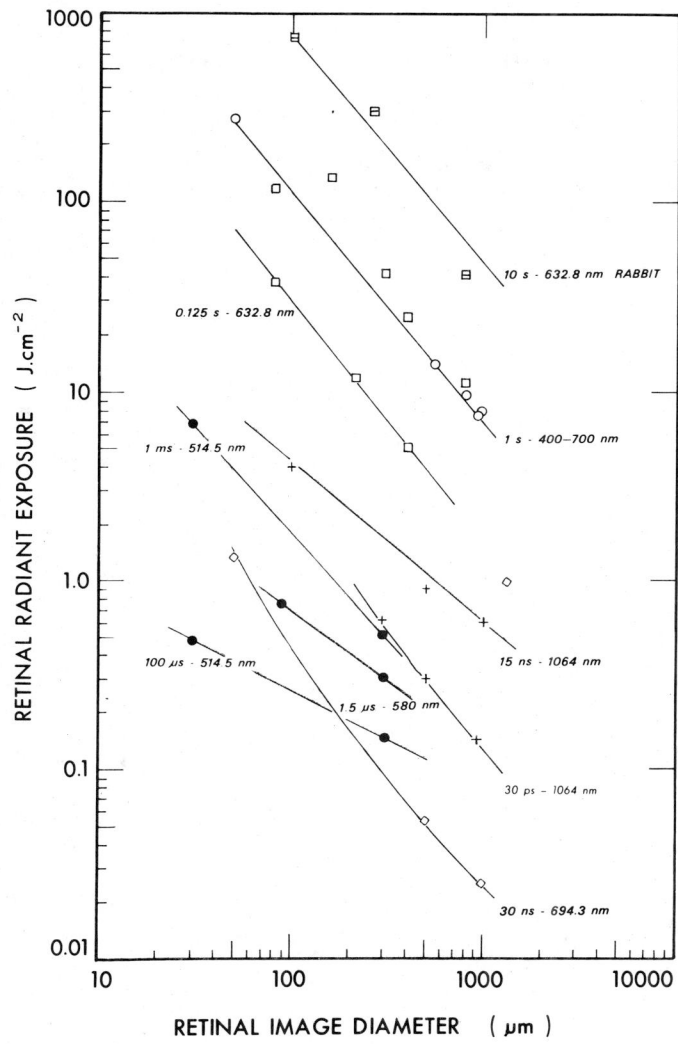

Figure 4-18. The dependence of retinal lesion threshold on image size. Although the thermal model would predict a strong spot-size dependence for exposures from 0.125 s to 10 s (the upper 3 curves) the dependence of Q-switched and millisecond exposures as shown in the lower 6 curves cannot be explained by a simple model of thermal injury. Notice that—largely independent of pulse duration—the spot size dependence very roughly approximates a function that is inversely proportional to the image diameter. Principal sources of data were: Frisch, Beatrice and Holsen, 1971, Ham et al., 1970, Goldman, Ham and Mueller, 1977 and private communications with E. Beatrice and D. Lund of the Letterman Army Institute of Research and with F. Hillenkamp of the University of Frankfurt.

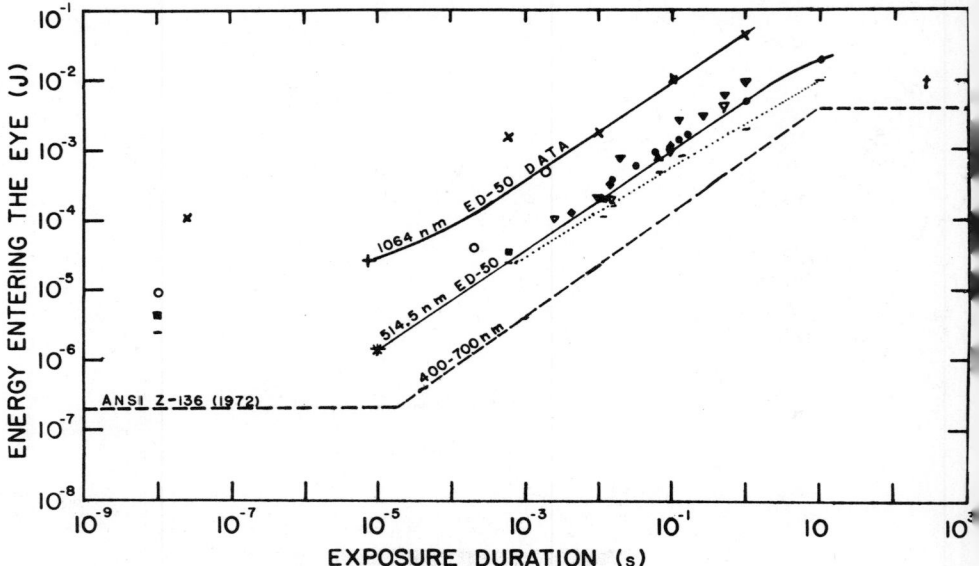

Figure 4-19. The dependence of retinal injury threshold upon pulse duration. The injury thresholds are in the rhesus monkey as a function of laser energy entering the eye and duration of exposure. The dashed line shows exposure limits in the ANSI Z-136 standard. Notice the anomalous increase of threshold for shorter durations below 10 μs (adapted from Wolbarsht and Sliney, 1975).

same image distributions had lesions which were very elongated for very short Q-switched pulses which would be predicted by a thermal model of injury for short pulses (Beatrice and Lund, 1976). On the other hand, the peak temperature elevation as shown in Fig. 4-17 suggests that the short pulse injuries may not be thermal. Perhaps the best explanation might be that the damage occurs at the immediate site of the pigment granules as suggested by Hayes and Wolbarsht (1968) and Vassiliadis (1971). In those models the peak temperature elevation of the entire retinal pigment epithelial cell does not reach more than a few degrees Centigrade elevation for nanosecond and microsecond pulses although the peak temperatures in the melanin granules themselves can be in excess of 1,000°C. Therefore, any long-chain organic molecules, enzyme systems and other microscopic biological subcellular components could be damaged if adjacent to the melanin granules. This, then, would produce a chance for the death of that cell. Photoacoustical effects as discussed by Cleary (1977) and Barnes (1974) certainly make a large contribution also; but whether the acoustic transient adds to or subtracts from the injury mechanism is not yet clear. Experiments by Hayes and Wolbarsht (1968) indicated that the melanin granules themselves are not like inorganic metallic particles which when heated to incandescence may not change structure or appearance. The melanin granules are very complex organic molecules which serve a biological function other than serving as an absorber of light. If, for instance, the melanin granules serve as a catalytic surface for a biochemical reaction then the alteration of this surface by very high heating of the melanin granules could obviously have a substantial effect on cellular metabolism. The low water content of the granules is against this hypothesis. On the other hand, the biological effect from a Q-switched laser exposure to the retina at threshold may be an almost immediate appearance of a lesion. If the only cause of cell death is the initial damage to only a few melanin granules then such a rapid appearance of injury in the cells is unexpected. Perhaps membrane damage from the adjacent hot melanin granules plays a role.

There have been surprisingly few serious laser injuries of the eye reported in the last fifteen years from pulsed lasers. This low accident rate cannot be accounted for by assuming that the ocular exposure limits are overly conservative—they are not. The explanation lies largely in the fact that the accidental exposure of the eye to a collimated beam is normally an extremely remote possibility, if only a few rudimentary, common-sense precautions are followed to keep the eye out of the beam. There are only a few situations where the probability of hazardous exposure is great. The laboratory is one, and each year there are a few retinal injuries reported. However, it is difficult to ascertain the exposure conditions in sufficient detail to allow useful threshold or injury data to be derived. There is always a suspicion that the injury was caused by deliberate viewing, and that the reported "accidental" exposure conditions are fabricated by the victim to support the claim of non-intentional viewing.

However, some data have been gathered by the use of human volunteers. Many people whose otherwise healthy eyes are removed for melanomas have consented to have laser exposures prior to surgery. Figure 4-3 shows a lesion resulting from such an exposure (Landers et al., 1976).

For the short exposure durations resulting from Q-switched lasers, exploding wires, super-radiant light, and mode-locked lasers, the exposure thresholds of injury are lowest. Although it is believed that in a Q-switched exposure durations the injury mechanism is largely thermal, the effect of acoustic transients due to the rapid heating and thermal expansion in the immediate vicinity of the absorption site (each melanin granule) may play a role as mentioned above. For still shorter exposure durations, direct electric field effects, Raman, and Brillouin scattering, and multi-photon absorption could play a role in the damage mechanism. The actual electric field strength of the incident retinal threshold irradiance at threshold (25 μm image) for a 30-ps mode-locked Nd:YAG (1064 nm) laser pulse is 9×10^{10} V/m^2 and for a frequency-doubled pulse (532 nm) from the same laser is 1.3×10^{11} V/m^2. These are both in excess of the electric field strength required to cause breakdown in biological membranes (Goldman et al., 1975, 1977; Hayes and Wolbarsht, 1971).

4.5.8 Location of Retinal Burns

The different regions of the retina (the fovea, the remainder of the macula, and the peripheral retina) play different roles in vision, and the significance of functional loss of all or part of any one of these regions due to retinal injury varies. The greatest visual acuity exists only for central (foveal) vision (Figure 3-16) and the loss of this retinal area dramatically reduces vision. The loss of an area of similar size located in the peripheral retina could be subjectively unnoticed. Depending upon wavelength and damage mechanism, the relative sensitivity to injury varies as has been shown by Lappin and Coogan (1970) and Lawwill et al. (1977). Most studies also indicate that detectable retinal functional loss occurs at about half the level for the ophthalmoscopically visible thermal damage (Geeraets et al., 1970; Ham et al., 1978). There are some exceptions to this general statement for very lengthy exposures (Lawwill et al., 1977; Harwerth and Sperling, 1975).

4.5.9 Very Long Exposure Durations

The human retina is normally subjected to irradiances below 10^{-4} W/cm^2 (see Fig. 4-20) except for occasional momentary exposure to the sun, arc lamps, welding arcs, photoflash lamps, incandescent filaments, and similar high radiance sources. The retinal images resulting from viewing such sources are quite small, for example 150 μm for the sun, and exposure durations are short, normally limited to the duration of the blink reflex (0.15 to 0.2 s). The natural aversion to bright light normally limits further retinal exposures above 10^{-4} W/cm^2. Until recently, a few studies of adverse retinal effects existed for the irradiance range of 10^{-4} W/cm^2 to 1 W/cm^2. Studies in this range have generally centered on flash blindness effects following light exposures lasting up to 1 s. As flash blindness effects are related to "bleaching" of retinal visual pigments (or more properly photopigment absorption) photometric units have most commonly been used. The range of 10^{-4} W/cm^2 to 1 W/cm^2 generally falls within 10^{-2} lm/cm^2 to 300 lm/cm^2 or 3×10^4 to 1×10^9 trolands. A CW laser at a level of approximately 1 μW/cm^2, a periodically pulsed flashlamp, or a high radiance near-infrared source can be viewed without a significant aversion response.

Exposure of large areas of the retina to moderately high luminance light on the order of 1 cd/cm^2 ($\sim 10^{-4}$ W/cm^2 at the retina) for durations of one to several hours has been investigated in experimental animals. Generally the light sources employed in these studies were fluorescent lamps. A thermally-enhanced photochemical mechanism of injury or phototoxic effects appears to be most likely (Kuwabara, 1970; Noell and Albrecht, 1971). It is doubtful that the early studies which were conducted principally with nocturnal animals, can be related to any possible conditions of human exposure. These studies taken collectively suggest that abnormally high environmental levels of retinal illumination for apparently any species (particularly albinos) can cause retinal degeneration. The effects are particularly dramatic when the normal, diurnal cycle of light and dark is eliminated by constant illumination (Williams and Baker, 1979). The levels and durations of

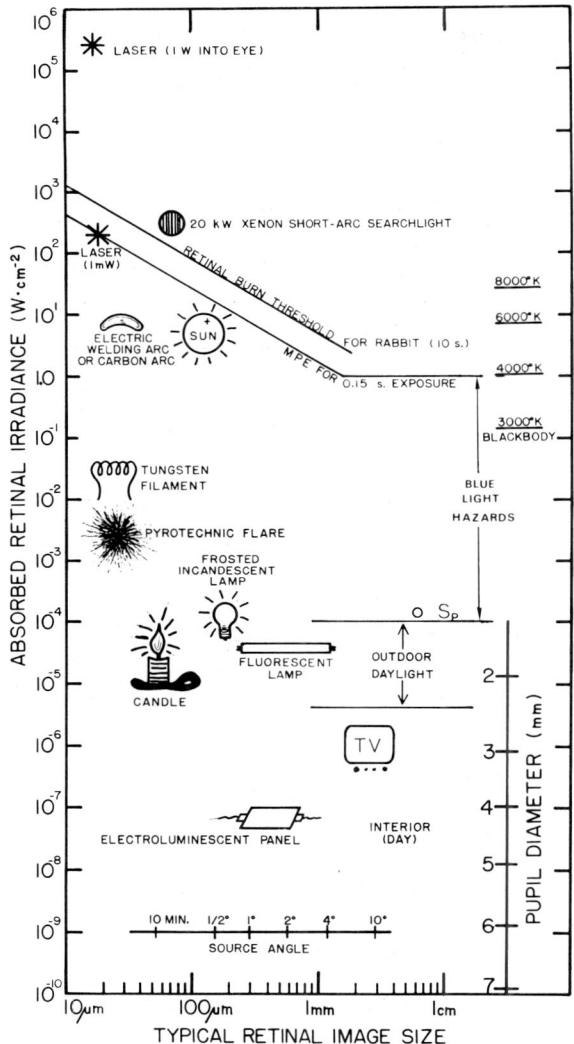

Figure 4-20. Range of retinal irradiances from a variety of conventional optical sources. The eye is exposed to light sources having radiances varying from approximately 10^4 W/cm^2·sr to approximately 10^{-6} W/cm^2·sr and even less for reflected lights. The resulting retinal irradiances vary from approximately 200 W/cm^2 down to 10^{-7} W/cm^2 and lower. Retinal irradiances are shown for typical image sizes for a variety of sources. The minimal pupil size was assumed for intense sources except for the searchlight (7-mm pupil). The retinal burn threshold for a 10-s exposure of the rabbit retina is shown as the upper solid line (Ham *et al.*, 1966). The threshold for permanent shift of blue cone sensitivity in monkeys obtained by Harworth and Sperling (1975) is shown as a short-solid line labelled O-Sp, at 3×10^{-4} W/cm^2. The approximate pupil sizes are shown at lower left based upon exposure of most of the retina to light of the given irradiance.

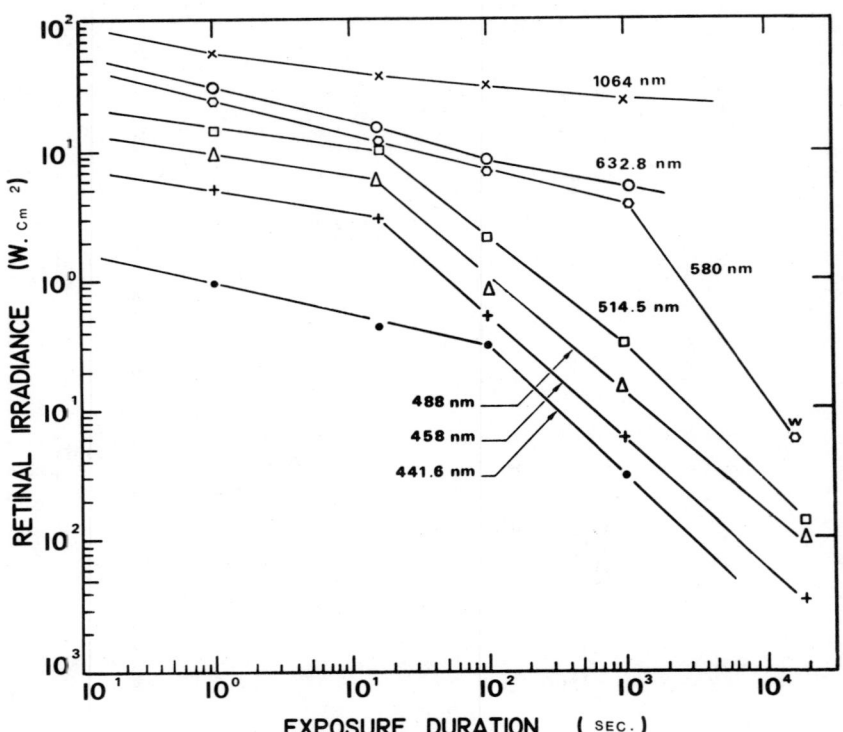

Figure 4-21. Retinal thresholds irradiances for several wavelengths for long-term retinal injury. All data are for retinal injury from long-term exposures of the rhesus monkey retina to extended sources. Data points for exposures less than 1.4×10^4 s are from Ham et al. (1976) and data points for 4-hr exposures (1.44×10^4 s) are from Lawwill et al. (1977). All data points are for laser lines except for one point, marked W, which is for a white-light source just above the 580-nm threshold for 4 hr (from Lawwill). Note the obvious change in the slope of the curves which is presumed to indicate a change from predominantly thermal injury from purely photochemical injury. The line at 632.8 nm probably turns down for longer exposures; however the purely thermal effect of 1064-nm infrared neodymium laser radiation would not be expected to ever turn down.

these retinal exposures exceed those of normal human experience. Only rarely have investigators reported that continual exposure to high luminance levels in the natural environment (or work environment) have elicited significant functional changes in the human retina (Livingston, 1932; Peckham and Harley, 1951; Smith, 1944; Medvedovskaya, 1970).

An exposure of the monkey retina by Tso (1973) to an irradiance of approximately 15 min from a clinical indirect ophthalmoscope resulted in damage to the retinal pigment epithelium. This damage threshold for a 4.5-mm diameter retinal image from the tungsten filament closely agrees with the 12-min exposure threshold of 0.42 W/cm^2 reported by Verhoeff and Bell in 1916 for 3-mm diameter image in the rabbit. It has generally been suggested that the damage mechanism for these comparatively long exposure durations of 10 to 30 min may be a thermally enhanced phototoxic effect. More recently it has been shown that wavelengths, particularly at the short-wavelength end of the spectrum are most effective in causing some type of photochemically induced lesion of the retina (Ham et al., 1976; Ham et al., 1978; Lawwill et al., 1977) as shown in Fig. 4-21. Instead of the adverse effect being highly centralized around the pigment layer and adjacent outer receptor layer, the photochemical effect appears to act upon all of the layers of the retina. The effect does appear first at locations of the pigment granules—particularly in the ellipsosomes where cytochrome-C is located (MacNichol et al., 1978). At 442 nm the threshold for visible retinal lesion is $\sim$ 30 J/cm^2 and is independent of exposure duration for $t > 100$ s. Threshold lesions were not apparent until 48 hours post-exposure. Recovery was noted within 11-30 days, but a hypo-pigmented area remained. The threshold was elevated by a factor of two in the macula, and three times the threshold created permanent retinal injury (Ham et al., 1978, 1979). These findings agree with eclipse-burn experience (Sliney, 1971). For instance, Hatfield (1970) and Penner and McNair (1966) reported significant numbers of patients who recovered within 30 days. It is not completely clear whether the photochemical type of lesion, which results from exposures to the rhesus monkey retina for durations of the order of 15 sec to 4 days, at levels as low as 10^{-4} W/cm^2 is directly related to a functional loss of vision. Moon et al. (1979) showed a close relation at 442-nm; however, there is some evidence based upon ERG techniques to suggest that there may not be such a direct relationship with functional loss for blue light injury to the retina (Lawwill et al., 1977).

Repeated exposures from incoherent light of large areas of the retinas of trained monkeys at retinal irradiances just above those experienced in a bright natural outdoor environment showed a permanent decrease in functional sensitivity to the blue range (Harwerth and Sperling, 1975). Exposure of the monkeys to narrow bands of wavelengths from the green to the red elicited a similar, but not a lasting, response. These types of studies repeated by Zwick et al. (1978) showed more dramatic changes with coherent light having a speckle pattern. Prolonged *erythropsia* (red vision) in aphakics has also been reported following exposure to large-area, high luminance sources with large amounts of ultraviolet such as snow fields (MacDonald and Fordon, 1971). The adverse effect produced by long-term exposure from repeatedly flashed electronic flashlamps probably poses the only type of chronic retinal exposure hazard that could actually exist under any realistic conditions, since all of the other retinal effects occur only at levels greater than those which normally produce discomfort ($\sim$ 1 cd/cm^2) for such large sources.

The blue light injury effect has an interesting implication for incandescent lamps which are very low in blue light output. For instance, the resulting retinal irradiance from viewing a 60-W incandescent tungsten filament lamp with a 2-mm pupil would normally not exceed 0.04 W/cm^2. Even a dilated (8-mm) pupil would only raise the retinal irradiance to 0.6 W/cm^2, which is insufficient to create a thermal injury, but possibly could exceed levels for the long-term photochemical injury mechanism. Fortunately tungsten source spectra contain very little blue light. Vassiliadis *et al.*, 1969, showed that monkeys exposed to 10-Hz repetitively flashing xenon arc lamps for more than 17 min developed ophthalmoscopically visible lesions at an average retinal irradiance of approximately 0.2 W/cm^2, a value well below that expected to be required for acute thermal injury. But it should be remembered that xenon flashlamps are relatively rich in their output of blue light. Mercury lamps are richer yet in blue light output (see Fig. 22-1, p. 696).

There is growing concern among some investigators who have studied the adverse retinal effects of intense light sources that life-long exposure to light plays a role in retinal aging. Certain age degenerative retinal effects may be light initiated. This opinion is prompted by the strong similarity between histological and ultrastructural changes in aged retina and those in retinae experimentally exposed to intense light sources. These changes are all disorganization of the outer receptors; depigmentation of the RPE, and decrease in the total number of receptors. Clearly, considerably more research will be required before this opinion can be validated or be shown to be in error.

Studies were conducted during and following World War II of the effects of prolonged exposures of individuals to bright outdoor environments upon night vision and retinal sensitivity. Lifeguards exposed to the high luminance environment (approximately 1 cd/cm^2) encountered at the seashore have shown both a short-term depression in photopic sensitivity and a marked long-term loss of scotopic (night) vision (Peckham and Harley, 1951). Flying officers in Iraq prior to World War II were exposed to very bright outdoor desert environments for their period of service and appeared to have more ocular symptoms than the normal population (Livingston, 1936). Welders, glass blowers and others working in bright light environments also may have color vision abnormalities which some investigators relate to the exposure to these bright light sources (Gupta and Singh, 1968).

To place these chorioretinal injury data in better perspective, Figure 4-20 shows the retinal irradiance for many CW sources. It is re-emphasized that several orders of magnitude in brightness (radiance or luminance) exist between sources that cause chorioretinal burns and those levels to which individuals are continuously exposed. The retinal irradiances shown are only approximate and assume minimal pupil sizes, accompanied by squinting for all of the very high luminance sources, except the xenon searchlight for which a 7-mm pupil was assumed for the case of nighttime turn-on.

4.5.10 Large Temporary Changes in Visual Sensitivity; Flashblindness

Intensive investigation has been carried on in flashblindness, both in anticipating functional loss that might be expected from a given exposure and in design of protection devices. The response times of present-day devices range from a few milliseconds down to several microseconds. Even within this long delay great difficulty has been encountered in producing a device which can attenuate the light source by more than 1,000. The flashblindness produced within this short time

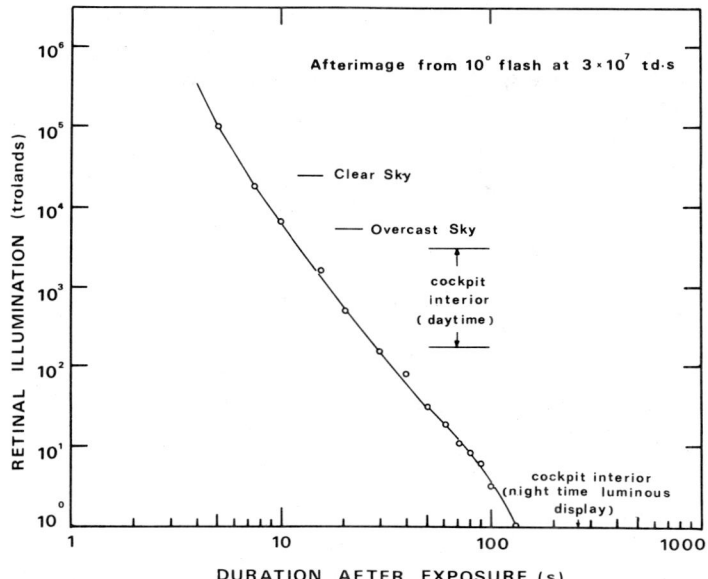

Figure 4-22. Flashblindness. Studies of flashblindness recovery were directed largely at determining the time course of visual loss for military pilots exposed to an atomic flash. Shown above is the duration that the afterimage remains above a level equivalent to the retinal exposure to normal level of approximately 2×10^4 td. The curve shows the data for only one experiment of Norma D. Miller (1966).

domain shows many nonlinearities. The reciprocity between time and energy (Block's law) and between area and intensity (Ricco's law) does not always hold. The site of these deviations from linearity has not been clearly defined. It may be in the photoreceptors, in the intermediate retinal cells, or elsewhere in the nervous system. The spectral distribution of an exposure that produces flashblindness of the lamp is itself important, as chromatic adaptation may change the apparent target contrast and visibility. Most of these aspects are predictable, however (Miller, 1965, 1966; Chisum, 1973).

In dealing with the enormous amount of data on flashblindness and attempting to relate it to retinal mechanisms, it is well to keep in mind the ideas originally expressed by J. L. Brown (1964). He shows that recovery from flashblindness does not involve a single, simple mechanism. It involves those parts of the visual system which usually govern dark adaptation as it is measured conventionally, but it may also reflect neurophysiological effects whose influences are not usually seen in studies of dark adaptation. When the adapting flash energies are sufficiently high it may also reflect recovery from actual retinal injury. Although an empirical equation fits

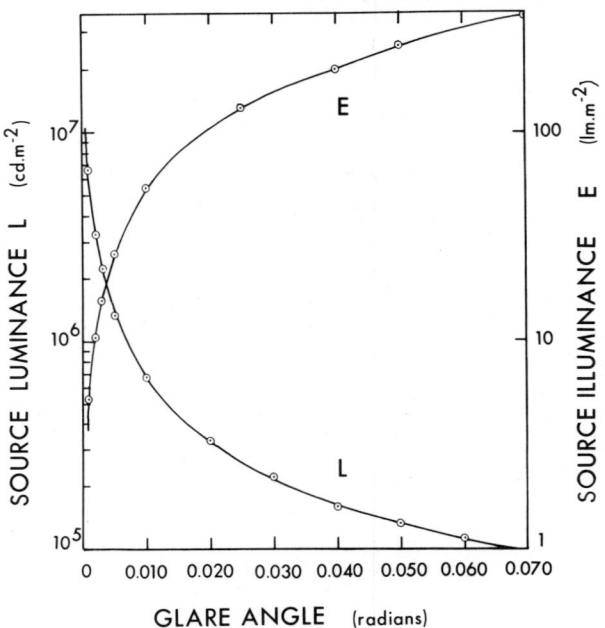

Figure 4-23. Discomfort Glare. The illuminance E at the cornea and luminance L of a souce which causes discomfort when an individual is suddenly exposed to it after being adapted to a luminance of 1000 cd·m^{-2}.

the data for a wide range of conditions, the equation is an empirical one and cannot be expected to cover the extremes.

At the present time, it is exactly these extreme cases that are of concern. Their relationship to most former psychophysical studies of flashblindness is very difficult to assess. It is only work such as that by Chisum (1973) in which extremely short flashes and high energy levels were used that will be related to the physiological changes attendant upon intensity levels near the threshold for injury.

To date, the studies of flashblindness have concentrated on retinal exposures from relatively large extended sources having angular extents ranging from 1° to 15° as viewed by the subject. Figure 4-22 illustrates the recovery time necessary from a bright flash of 3×10^7 troland-seconds (td·s) which corresponds for a 7-mm pupil to a source luminance of 78 cd·s/cm^2 or about 0.5 J/(cm^2·sr) for a xenon flash lamp. As can be seen from the figure, the afterimage which interferes with visual performance would be significant for about 10 s in daylight and 1-2 minutes at night for a military pilot exposed to an atomic flash.

4.5.11 Discomfort Glare

If a very bright light source is suddenly switched on after the eye has been adapted to a luminance much lower than that of the source, the viewer experiences a discomforting sense of shock blinks, and tends to turn his head or squint. This effect is much more dramatic when the ambient luminance is low. Out-of-doors in full daylight, the luminance of a large extended source required to elicit this phenomenon is of the order of 100,000 cd·m^{-2} (10 cd·cm^{-2} or 29,000 foot-lamberts); however, the luminance of this source must be far greater to elicit this response if the source subtends an angle less than ¼° as shown in Figure 4-23. In terms of illuminance, however, the level required is less for smaller source sizes. For a searchlight or laser viewed at great distances, this discomfort should apparently be experienced at levels as low as 10 lm·m^{-2} (corresponding to 10 μW·cm^{-2} from a searchlight or 1.5 μW·cm^{-2} from the 568 nm krypton laser). This effect is only temporary. The formula of Petherbridge and Hopkinson for determining discomfort glare for small sources of luminance L_s is:

$$L_s \leq \frac{1}{\theta} \left(\frac{1076 \, L_o}{0.824} \right) 0.625 \qquad (4\text{-}6)$$

where θ_s is the angular subtense of the source in radians and L_o is the background luminance in cd·m^{-2}. In glare tests at the US Army Environmental Hygiene Agency, the blue and green laser wavelengths appeared somewhat more discomforting than the yellow or red wavelengths.

4.5.12 Veiling Glare

A related interference with normal vision, which is present with a glaring light source in the field of view, is termed "veiling glare." A luminous veiling haze appears to surround the source and tends to obscure objects in the vicinity of the glare source. This phenomenon has been the subject of extensive study and the classical equation of Halladay (1927) which describes the veiling luminance, β (cd·m^{-2}) as a function of the source illuminance (lm·m^{-2} at the viewer) and the angle away from the point source θ (in degrees) is:

$$\beta = 10 \, E/\theta^2 \quad (\text{for } 1° < \theta < 30°) \qquad (4\text{-}7)$$

and it has sometimes been expressed by LeGrand (1937) as:

$$\beta = 10 \, E^{0.9}/\theta^{1.9} \quad (\text{for } 1 < \theta < 25°) \qquad (4\text{-}8)$$

or most recently by Walraven (1973) as:

$$\beta = 29 \, E/(\theta - 0.13)^{2.8} \quad (\text{for } 0.5° < \theta < 8°) \qquad (4\text{-}9)$$

These functions are plotted in Figure 4-24. [See also Section 26.3.3 page 886.]

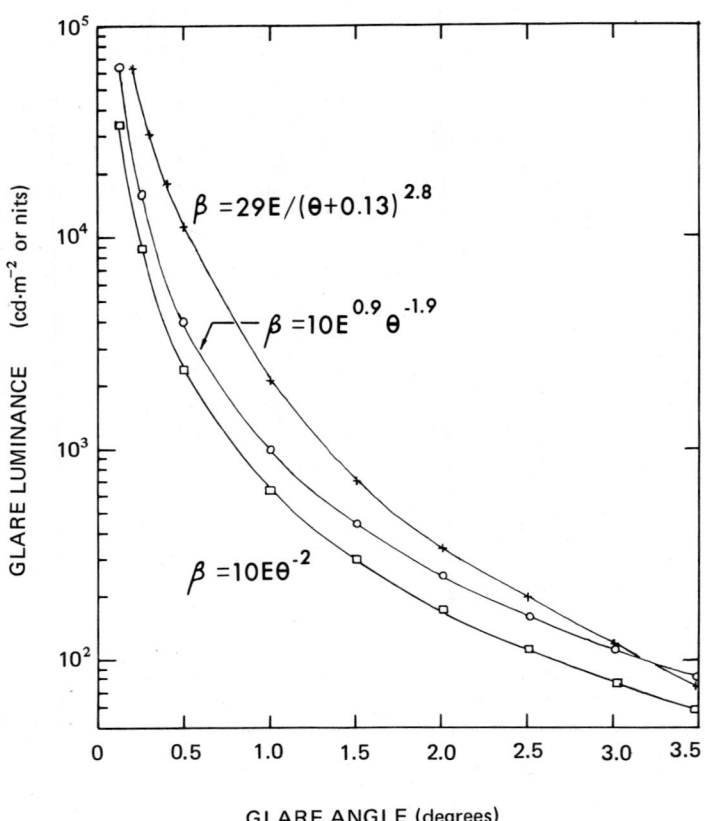

Figure 4-24. Disability or Veiling Glare. The effective luminance of a point glare source is plotted as a function of glare angle θ for three formulas described in the text. Although wavelength is not supposed to affect this type of glare, studies at the US Army Environmental Hygiene Agency showed some dependence when using CW lasers as the glare source. Blue light created more glare than red.

4.5.13 Flashing Lights

Classical studies of vision suggest that a strobe operating at 10 Hz can appear brighter than a CW source of the same peak brightness due to the Bartley effect for flashing light sources. Similarly, the brightness of a single pulse appears brighter than it really is; this phenomenon is termed the Broca-Sulzer effect.

Strobelight sources produce little annoyance during daylight. However, at night if a strobe illuminates an area which would otherwise be dark at a frequency of 5-10 Hz, the objects illuminated by the strobe will appear to float around because of loss of a fixation point during off-periods of the light. This effect is often taken advantage of for various entertainment purposes, and intense strobes operating at these frequencies may be found in many nightclubs. Sources of strobe light systems for entertainment purposes reveal that complaints of headaches are common for total exposure period greater than 1 minute. For example, a dance hall would be advised to operate the strobe only for less than 1 minute at a time (usually less than 30 s). Despite the annoyance of the light, most tasks can normally be carried out if the ambient illumination is increased.

An extensive survey of the medical literature suggests that epileptic seizures in susceptible individuals represent the only well-documented health hazard from exposure to low-frequency intermittent light. The most sensitive frequency range is from 8 to 16 Hz. Various estimates indicate that approximately 1.0 percent of the epileptic population (which is less than 1.0 percent of the general population) will experience these "flicker-induced" seizures; therefore, the probability that a photosensitive epileptic employee is present in a particular work force is quite remote. Such individuals usually are aware of their susceptibility.

A variety of vague physiologic and behavioral symptoms resulting from exposure to low frequency intermittent light have been described. These include headaches, drowsiness, vertigo, visual illusions, anxiety, apprehension, irritability, and impaired ability to concentrate; however, these effects are poorly documented and have occurred only under carefully controlled laboratory conditions (Ulett, 1953).

4.5.14 Injuries to the Iris at Retinal Hazard Power Levels

Little quantitative data exists for damage to the iris by visible radiation (light). The high absorption of the melanin pigment within the visible range suggests an action spectrum for damage similar to that in the retina. The RPE spectral transmission which indicated the spectral absorption is shown in Fig. 4-11 for several wavelengths. The argon laser (448 and 514.5 nm) has a very low threshold as compared with a Nd:YAG laser (1064 nm). The ruby laser (694.3 nm) thresholds lie between the Nd:YAG and the argon laser thresholds, as would be expected (Dannheim and Rassow, 1976; van der Zyppen et al., 1978). The iris has been considered to be very sensitive to infrared radiation due to the heavy pigmentation. This is probably a misconception. The absorption by melanin pigment decreases markedly after 700 nm and at 1060 nm melanim absorbs very little more than other tissues, due both to the specific absorption of melanin and the inefficiency of absorption of the small particles of melanin. When sufficient radiation is absorbed to affect the iris the result is constriction of the pupil and formation of an aqueous flare. In this instance an aqueous flare is the dilation of blood vessels near the aqueous uveal border (the term "aqueous flare" has been used by others to refer to light scatter from proteins floating in the aqueous).These symptoms have all been well characterized by Duke-Elder and McFaul (1972). Higher level exposures may result in severe injury with muscle paralysis, hemorrage and thrombosis, and inflammation of the iris stroma. These symptoms are followed within a few days by necrotic spots in the iris which appear to be bleached and atrophic.

A generalized mechanism for damage of the iris by simple heating has been proposed by Goldmann (1933) but details of the actual physiological changes are lacking. Few quantitative studies are available to support any damage model, and none have attempted to show why the sensitivity to the Nd:YAG laser at 1060 nm is one-tenth that for an argon laser at 488 nm. Although this difference roughly follows the absorption spectrum of melanin, it is not certain that the high absorption of the iris in the blue is due to the pigment or to the presence of some other substance within the tissue.

As the threshold for injury of the iris is very high compared to the other anterior structures, it is not often injured. The major problem associated with the iris is the high optical absorption by the melanin granules in both the vessel layer and the pigment epithelium, as heat generated in the iris may be transferred to the lens and injure it. Also, inflammation of the iris by overheating can cause adhesions to either the cornea or the lens. These adhesions can be very painful and may also give rise to unwanted pathological changes in either the lens or the cornea.

4.6 INFRARED RADIATION AND THE EYE

4.6.1 Infrared Spectral Bands

The CIE committee E-2.1.2 defined three biologically significant infrared bands. These bands—IR-A, extending from 760-780 nm to 1400 nm; IR-B, from 1.4 μm to 3 μm; and IR-C from 3 μm to 1 mm—are useful in considering the biological effects of infrared optical radiation.

The principal adverse biologic effects attributed to infrared radiation are infrared cataracts (also known as glass blowers', glass workers' or furnaceman's cataracts), flash burns of both the skin and the cornea of the eye from various intense sources, and heat stress from less intense thermal radiation. Hazardous levels for the eye and skin are comparable in the infrared beyond 1.4 μm since the injury mechanism is largely thermal and since IR-B and IR-C are absorbed by the ocular media. The effects of infrared radiation on the iris are discussed in section 4.5.14.

4.6.2 Infrared Cataract

As explained in Chapter 3, the ocular media absorb an increasing amount of the radiant energy incident upon the cornea for increasing wavelengths in the near infrared (IR-A). For infrared wavelengths greater than 1.4 μm (IR-B and IR-C) the cornea and aqueous absorb essentially all of the incident radiation, and beyond 1.9 μm the cornea is considered the sole absorber (Figure 4-25). The absorbed energy may be conducted to interior structures of the eyes and elevate the temperature of that tissue as well as the cornea itself. Heating of the iris by absorption of visible and near-infrared radiation is considered to play a role in the development of opacities in the crystalline lens, at least for short exposure times. Hence one would expect the spectral absorption and reflectance of the iris to determine the action spectrum for this effect for such exposure times.

During the first half of this century there was a major debate between two ophthalmologists on the cause of infrared cataract. Vogt (1919) argued that infra-

Effect of Optical Radiation on the Eye

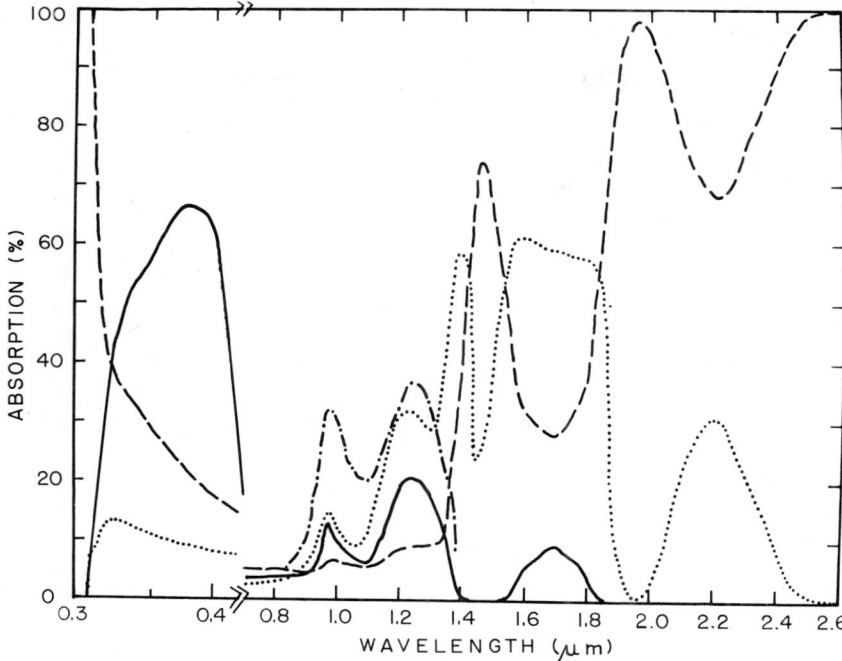

Figure 4-25. The spectral absorption of the Ocular Media for the Human Eye. Each portion of the ocular media, the cornea (- - - -), the aqueous humor (• • • •), the lens (———), and the vitreous humor (- • - •), absorb different portions of the incident optical radiation at different wavelengths. Very little is absorbed in the visible region, hence the break in the curves. Note the strong absorption of the lens in the near-ultraviolet region and the absorption of the vitreous in the 0.86-1.35 μm infrared region.

red cataract was the result of direct absorption of infrared wavelengths in the crystalline lens. On the other hand, Goldmann (1933) later was able to demonstrate that the opacities tended to develop first near the periphery adjacent to the iris and argued that at least for short exposure durations the mechanism was the heat transfer from the elevated temperature of the iris. Most recently Wolbarsht and associates (1977) have demonstrated that Goldmann's findings can be confirmed for short exposure times but direct radiation is a major cause for long-term, low-level exposures.

Direct absorption by the lens produces damage by direct degradation of the lens proteins (Wolbarsht *et al.*, 1976). For example, a CW Nd:YAG laser at 1 W/cm² at the cornea for 60 seconds will elevate the temperature immediately behind the iris sufficiently to form a cataract on the anterior surface of the lens. However, radiation of the lens alone at lower levels for longer exposures produces cataracts in the part of the lens not covered by the iris (Wolbarsht *et al.*, 1976,

1977). Furthermore, the portion of the lens behind the iris does not develop a cataract at these lower irradiances for longer exposures.

The primary step in cataract formation from direct IR-A (Nd, 1060-nm) irradiation appears to be the breakdown of the α- and γ-crystallins to smaller subunits. Secondly, after prolonged exposure the lower molecular weight subunits of β-crystallin disappear by agglutination to form higher molecular weight insoluble albuminoids. These agglutinated and insoluble β-crystallins appear to disturb the ultrastructural organization of collagen fibrils in the lens which leads to loss of transparency by increased light scattering. As yet no data have been collected to connect the experiments on the acute effects of IR-A exposure to the cataracts from chronic exposures (lasting for months to years) as may occur in environmental or industrial situations. The forms of IR cataract that have been documented in humans following industrial exposures consist of patches of light-scattering material diffusely scattered throughout the lens rather than dense patches located at the posterior pole (Szafran, 1965). An action spectrum of cataractogenesis in the infrared is needed along with research to determine whether any focusing of the radiation that may take place within the lens would cause the posterior pole to be affected preferentially over other parts of the lens. For example, if longer wavelengths at which the focal properties of the lens and cornea do work were as effective in cataractogenesis as the shorter wavelengths, then a diffuse type of cataract would be expected at longer wavelengths but not at shorter wavelengths. Furthermore, since IR is seldom present in the working environment in the absense of UV and visible light, the combined effects of all of these spectral bands must be evaluated.

By noticing the dilation of blood vessels near the aqueous which would be responsible for conducting heat away from the anterior part of the eye, Fischer and coworkers (1936) demonstrated that wavelengths near 900 nm appeared to be the most effective in heating the anterior portion of the eye. Other than this study of the "aqueous flare," and that of Langley, Mortimer and McCulloch (1960), there have been no serious attempts to try to determine the action spectrum for IR cataractogenesis.

Jacobson and co-workers (1963) found that significant corneal doses of nearly 10 J/cm^2 are required to produce lenticular changes within the duration of the blink reflex (i.e., up to 100 W/cm^2). The sensory nerve endings in both the cornea and iris are quite sensitive to small temperature elevations, and a temperature elevation of 47° corresponding to approximately 10 W/cm^2 absorbed in the cornea elicits a painful response in humans. Hence it is generally considered that the blink reflex provides protection against infrared radiation up to levels in excess of that causing flash burns of the skin. Indeed, it has been reported that in some accidents involving explosions where skin injury might be attributed to the infrared flash, the skin was injured, while the cornea was not. The explanation has normally been given that this was the result of the protective action of the blink reflex (Duke-Elder, 1972).

Quantitative data for the production of lenticular opacities following exposure to infrared are very limited. It is not known whether the principal factor responsible for the development of a cataract in a worker after many years of exposure to nearby radiant sources such as molten glass or metal may result from very moderate intraocular temperature rise during chronic exposure, from greater temperature elevations experienced during very occasional exposures to the sources at very close range, or from both conditions, and whether trace levels of UV or blue light must be present.

To understand the development of infrared effects in the lens it is useful to compare the infrared corneal dose rate experienced in other environments. In temperate climates the cornea is exposed to near-IR and far-IR radiation of approximately 1 mW/cm². Some workers exposed for 10 to 15 years to infrared irradiances of 80 to 400 mW/cm² encountered in the glass and steel industries have developed lenticular opacities. Such irradiances, even if only from visible radiation, definitely produces a marked sensation of warmth, provided that a significant area of the skin is exposed (greater than a few square centimeters). A corneal infrared irradiance of 0.1 W/cm² is well below the level required to cause acute injury of the anterior ocular structures and is often used as a guideline for occupational exposure to far-infrared radiation (see Chapter 9). However, safe chronic ocular exposure values, particularly to IR-A, probably are of the order of 10 mW/cm² or below. Before this discussion of infrared cataractogenesis is closed, it is appropriate to point out that one industrial physician (Dunn, 1950) argued that his experience with a large number of workers exposed to infrared radiation showed no evidence of infrared cataract. Additionally, although Wallace and Colleagues (1971) found an increase in what they called "Type I cataract" among Welsh steel workers exposed to high IR levels, they pointed out that this type of lens change would not really affect visual function and perhaps would not even be called a cataract by some. Of course, it should be noted that many industrial methods now used, as well as protective clothing and equipment, probably reduce the level of this type of radiation to which the eye is exposed. For instance, the openings to higher temperature furnaces are a great deal smaller than they have been in past years, which would reduce the total irradiance of the eye from infrared radiation. There are sufficient data and cases of a very specific form of cataract in these types of workers which certainly suggest that infrared does indeed cause glass-blower's or furnaceman's cataract. Duke-Elder (1972) gives many illustrations of the characteristic posterior cortical opacity which is known in German as the *Feuerstar* or *fire* cataract because of its appearance. It should, however, be remembered that this appearance can be due to the structure of the lens as discussed in section 4.4.4.

4.6.3 Infrared Radiation and the Cornea

The cornea is quite transparent in the IR-A. In the IR-B there are some fairly narrow water absorption bands at 1430 nm and 1959 nm. Above 2000 nm absorption is very high, making the cornea very susceptible to far-infrared radiation heating. As might be expected the threshold for damage therefore parallels the absorption bands. Radiation in the IR-C band can induce a burn on the cornea similar to that on the skin. It has been suggested that following IR exposure the posterior corneal surface shows more damage than the anterior surface (Verhoeff, Bell and Walker, 1916). This differential has rarely been documented following industrial

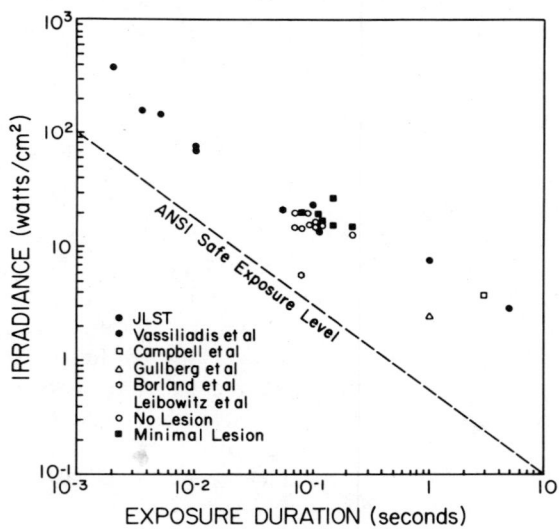

Figure 4-26. Thresholds for corneal injury from CO_2 laser radiation. The collected data of Stuck and colleagues of the US Army (JLST), much of it unpublished, is compared to the published threshold data of Vassiliadis (1971), Campbell *et al.* (1968), Goldberg *et al.* (1966), Borland *et al.* (1971), and Liebowitz and Peacock (1969). The range of data for the same exposure durations is thought to be due largely to the use of different corneal image sizes, and the two lowest points are believed the result of hot spots in a multimode laser irradiance pattern. Collation of data courtesy of Mr. Bruce Stuck, Letterman Army Institute of Researcch.

exposures. Levels of infrared radiation high enough to give corneal damage cause such immediate and severe corneal pain that the eye's aversion response is activated as quickly. For this reason corneal burns are rarely seen from industrial exposures. The sensory nerve endings of the cornea are quite sensitive to all temperature elevations and an elevation of 10°C causes a pain response. There is some data which indicates that the temperature rise can be felt before the pain appears (Sliney, 1972).

Infrared lasers such as the CO_2 laser (10.6 μm), the HF and DF lasers (2.7 to 4.0 μm), or the CO laser (5 μm) having CW output irradiances of the order of 10 W/cm² or greater could produce corneal lesions by delivering at least 0.5 to 10 J/cm² before the blink reflex is operative. Exposure limits for infrared (IR-B and IR-C) lasers are 100 mW/cm² for CW exposure based upon CO_2 laser studies. However, this limit assumes a relatively small area of irradiation. The level would certainly have to be lowered for exposures from very large infrared laser beams or other incoherent sources of far-infrared radiation. Studies with pulsed lasers such as the erbium laser (1.54 μm) shows that the thresholds of injury may be tens or hundreds of J/cm^2 for short pulses where wavelengths penetrate deep within the aqueous. On the other hand, for CO_2 lasers where the absorption half-value layer is only 10 μm and surface heating in the cornea is the main cause of injury, the threshold can be a fraction of 1 J/cm^2. A 1 to 100-ns exposure from an HF (2.7–3.0 μm) laser or from a CO_2 laser (10.6 μm) has been shown by Ham to have an injury threshold of the order of only 0.005 to 0.01 J/cm^2. Figure 4-26 presents the reported corneal damage thresholds for 10.6 μm laser radiation as a function of longer exposure durations. The curve follows that predicted for thermal injury (Vassiliadis, 1971).

4.7 UNCERTAINTIES

The quantity of biologic data and understanding of optical radiation effects upon the eye are particularly weak in the near-UV and in the infrared. This is largely the result of the fact that lasers and optical sources operating in the retinal hazard region have previously been the cause of greatest concern. It is important to note in any discussion of the general concern. It is important to note in any discussion of the general effects of infrared on the eye, that the diagrams in Fig. 1-2 must be considered only very schematic. A detailed study of the relative absorption coefficients of the different ocular structures in the near-infrared and the near-UV strongly supports this. As shown in Fig. 4-25 the different structures vary greatly in the ratio of absorptance at any given wavelength. It will remain for future research to fully understand the damage mechanisms and to determine the exact thresholds of injury for chronic exposure between 0.3 μm and 0.4 μm and for both acute and chronic exposure from 1 μm to 2.7 μm.

4.8 REVIEW QUESTIONS

1. List the sequence of ocular structures that light must pass through prior to reaching the retina.

2. Name the ocular structure which is the principal absorber of the laser radiation from:

    (a) HeCd laser at 441.6 nm; at 325 nm;

    (b) HeNe laser at 632.8 nm; at 1.15 μm; at 3.39 μm;

    (c) Argon laser at 488 nm; at 514.5 nm;

    (d) Neodymium: YAG laser at 1064 nm;

    (e) CO laser at 5 μm;

(f) CO_2 laser at 10.6 μm;

(g) Ruby laser at 694.3 nm.

3. For what reason is there a sharp demarcation at 1.4 μm between IR-A and IR-B?

4. Would you expect any significant difference in biological effects and thresholds of injury for the eye between IR-B radiation and IR-C radiation?

5. List the dividing lines between the seven CIE biologically-significant spectral bands.

6. What is known about the role of the pigment granules within the pigment epithelium? Of what are they composed?

7. Does heat flow within the retina play a significant role in determining the threshold of injury?

8. Can one see IR-A laser wavelengths or UV-A laser wavelengths? If one were using three lasers for laser display purposes—one argon 488-nm laser, an argon 514.5-nm green laser, and a helium-neon 632.8-nm red laser for display purposes and it was determined that the maximum power of the helium-neon laser was 50 mW, how much power would be necessary for the argon laser lines in order to meet equal brightness requirements limited by the helium-neon laser?

9. What wavelength may be considered the most dangerous from an IR cataractogenesis standpoint? What wavelength is probably the most hazardous from a retinal thermal injury standpoint? What wavelength is considered the most hazardous from a long-term chronic exposure standpoint? What wavelength of infrared is considered the most hazardous to the cornea?

10. What wavelength in the ultraviolet is considered most hazardous for the effect of photokeratitis? Why is it difficult to determine an action spectrum for injury of the skin and eye within the spectral region 300 to 315 nm? If the threshold for injury from a pulsed laser at the retina is 0.8 J/cm^2 for a 100-μs retinal exposure, what is the retinal irradiance?

11. What is the retinal irradiance from a 500-nm laser extended source which has a radiance of 1,000 $W/(cm^2 \cdot sr)$ if the pupil diameter is 3 mm? What is the retinal image size when viewing the sun? What is presently believed to be the primary damage mechanism for retinal injury induced by staring at the sun? A light source is located 3 m from the eye and is a disc 3 cm in diameter. What is the retinal image size?

12. In terms of threshold of injury expressed in terms of radiant exposure for a 1-s exposure to the eye, what wavelength, is the most hazardous and what is the threshold at this wavelength?

13. If an individual sustains a threshold, a superficial injury to the cornea, what cells are injured and how long will recovery be expected to take?

14. There can be some partial recovery of visual loss suffered as a result of a laser-induced retinal injury. T or F?

15. Why is the eye the structure of greatest concern from a laser hazard standpoint?

4.9 REFERENCES

Adams, D. O., Beatrice, E. S. and Bedell, R. B., 1972, Retina: ultrastructural alterations produced by extremely low levels of coherent radiation, *Science* 177:58–60.

Bachem, A., 1956, Ophthalmic ultraviolet action spectra, *Am. J. Ophth.* 41:969–975.

Barnes, F. S., 1974, Biological damage resulting from thermal pulses, *in* "Laser Applications in Medicine and Biology," (M. L. Wolbarsht, ed.) Vol. 2, pp. 205–221, Penum Press, New York.

Bartley, S.H., and Ball, R. J., 1968, Effects of Intermittent illumination on visual acutiy, *Amer. J. Optom. and Arch. Amer. Acad. Optom.* 45:458–464.

Beatrice, E. S., and Lund, D. J., 1976, Characteristics of Damage Produced by Non-circular Retinal Laser Irradiation, Letterman Army Inst. of Res. Non-ionizing Rad. Div., Institute Rpt. #31 (October 1976).

Berggvist, T., Hartmann, B., and Kleman, B., 1978, Imaging properties of the eye and interaction of laser radiation with matter, *in* "Current Concepts in Ergophthalmology, (B. Tengroth and D. Epstein, eds.), pp. 55–71, Department of Ophthalmology, Karolinska Institute, Stockholm.

Bernstein, H. N., Curtis, J., Earl, F. L. and Kuwabara, T., 1970, Phototoxic corneal and lens opacities, *Arch. Ophth.* 83:336–348.

Birngruber, R., Gabel, V. P., and Hillenkamp, F., 1978, Threshold criteria and derivation of safe levels for laser radiation, *in* "Current Concepts in Ergophthalmology," (B. Tengroth and D. Epstein, eds.), pp. 73–80, Department of Ophthalmology, Karolinska Institute, Stockholm.

Boettner, E. A., 1967, Spectral Transmission of the Eye, Final Report, AF 41 (609)–2996, USAF School of Aerospace Medicine, AD 663246 (July 1967).

Boettner, E. A., and Wolter, J. R., 1962, Transmission of the ocular media, *Invest. Ophth.* 1: 776–783.

Boettner, E. A., and Dankovic, D., 1974, Ocular absorption of Laser Radiation for Calculating Personnel Hazards, Univ. Michigan, Ann Arbor, MI; School of Aerospace Med., Brooks AFB, TX, Contract F41609-74-C-0008, Project AF-6301 (November 1974).

Borland, R. B., Brennan, D. H., and Nicholson, A. N., 1971, Threshold levels for damage of the cornea following irradiation by a continuous wave carbon dioxide (10.6 micron) laser, *Nature (London)* 234:151–152.

Borwein, B., Sanwal, M., Medeiros, J. A., and McGowan, J. W., 1976, Scanning electron microscopy of normal and lased rabbit retina, *Canad. J. Ophth.* 11:(4)309–322.

Boynton, R. M., Rinalducci, E. J., and Sternhein, C., 1969, Visibility losses produced by transient adaptational changes in the range from 0.4 to 4000 footlamberts, *Illum. Eng.* **64**: 217–227.

Bresnick, G. H., Frisch, G. D., Powell, J. O., Landers, M. B., Holst, G. E., and Dallas, A. G., 1970, Ocular effects of argon laser radiation, Part I: Retinal damage threshold studies, *Invest. Ophth.* **9**(11):901–910.

Brown, J. L., 1973, Experimental investigations of flash blindness, *Human Factors* **6**:503–516.

Cain, C. P., and Welch, A. J., 1974, Measured and predicted laser-induced temperature rises in the rabbit fundus, *Invest. Ophth.* **13**(1):60–70.

Campbell, C. J., Rittler, M. C., Bredemeier, H., and Wallace, R. A., 1968, Ocular effects produced by experimental lasers. I. Carbon dioxide laser, *Am. J. Ophth.* **66**:604–614.

Cavonius, D. R., Elgin, S., and Robbins, D. O., 1974, Thresholds for damage to the human retina by white light, *Exp. Eye Res.* **19**:543–548.

Chisum, G. T., 1973, Flashblindness recovery following exposure to constant energy adaptive flashes, *Aerospace Med.* **44**:407–413.

Chisum, G. T., 1967, "Recent Research in Flashblindness with Human Subjects," in Proceedings of the US Army Natick Laboratories Flashblindness Symposium, US Army Natick Laboratories (November 1967) (AD 697–793).

Chisum, G. T., and Hill, J. H., 1967, Flashblindness: The effects of preflash adaptation and pupil size, *Aerospace Med.* **38**:395–399.

Chisum, G. T., Hill, J. H., and Smith, F. K., 1961, "Flashblindness Recovery Time Following Exposure to High-Intensity, Short-Duration Flashes," Aerospace Medical Research Department, US Naval Air Development Center, Report No. NADC-MA-6142 (November 1961).

Chisum, G. T., and Morway, P. E., 1974, Flashblindness following double flash exposures, *Aerospace Med.* **45**:1013–1016.

Cleary, S. F., 1977, Laser pulses and the generation of accoustic transients in biological material, in "Laser Applications in Medicine and Biology," (M. L. Wolbarsht, ed.) Vol. 3, Plenum Press, New York.

Cloud, T. M., Hakim, R., and Griffin, A. C., 1960, Photosensitization of the eye with methoxsalen, *Arch. Ophth.* **64**:346.

Cloud, T. H., Hakim, R., and Griffin, A. C., 1961, Photosensitization of the eye with methoxsalen. II. Chronic effects, *Arch. Ophth.* **66**:689.

Cobb, S., 1947, Photic driving as a cause of clinical seizures in epileptic patients, *Arch. Neurol. Psychiat.* **58**:70.

Cogan, D. G., 1950, Lesions of the eye from radiant energy, *J. Am. Med. Assoc.* **142**:145–151.

Cogan, D. G., 1961, Photosensitization and cataracts, *Arch. Ophth.* **66**:28–29.

Cogan, D. G., and Kinsey, V. E., 1946, Action spectrum of keratitis produced by ultraviolet radiation, *Arch. Ophth.* **35**:670–677.

Considine, P. S., 1966, Effects of coherence on imaging systems, *J. Opt. Soc. Am.* **56**(8):1001–1009.

Coogan, P. S., Hughes, W. F., and Mollsen, J. A., 1974, Histological and Spectro-Photometric Comparisons of the Human and Rhesus Monkey Retina and Pigmented Ocular Fundus. Final Report, Rush-Presbyterian St. Luke's Medical Center, 1753 W. Congress Parkway, Chicago, IL, Contract #F41609-71-C-0006 (January 1974).

Cushman, W. H., 1971, Effect of flash field size on flashblindness in an aircraft cockpit, *Aerospace Med.* **42**(6):630–634.

Dannheim, F., and Rassow, B., 1978, Laser lesions of the anterior segment of the rabbit eye: studies of cornea, iris, lens and sclera using argon, ruby and YAG laser, *Albrecht von Graefes Arch. Klin Ophth.* **205**(3):175–205 (English abstract, German).

Davidoff, R. A., and Johnson, L. C., 1963, Photic activation and photoconvulsive responses in a non-epileptic subject, *Neurology* **13**:617–631.

Davidson, S. and Watson, C. W., 1956, Hereditary light sensitive epilepsy, *Neurology* **6**(4):235.

Davies, J. R., and Randolph, D. I., 1967, "Proceedings of the US Army Natick Flashblindness Symposium," US Army Natick Laboratories, Natick, MA, November 1967 (AD 697–793).

DeGroot, S. G., and Gebhard, J. W., 1952, Pupil size as determined by adapting luminance, *J. Opt. Soc. Am.* **42**:492–495.

Delmelle, M., 1979, Possible implication of photooxidation reactions in retinal photo-damage, *Photochem. Photobiol.* **29**(4):713–716.

Dewan, E. M., Menkin, M. F. and Rock, J., 1978, Effect of photic stimulation on the human menstrual cycle, *Photochem. Photobiol.* **27**:581–585.

Duke-Elder, S., 1954, Injuries, *in* "Textbook of Ophthalmology," Vol. 6, C. V. Mosby, Co., St. Louis, Missouri.

Duke-Elder, S. and McFaul, P., 1972, Non-mechanical injuries, *in* "Sytem of Ophthalmology," Vol. 14, Part 2, C. V. Mosby, Co., St. Louis, Missouri.

Dunn, K. L., 1950, Cataracts from infrared rays (glass worker's cataracts). *Arch. Ind. Hyg. Occup. Med.* **1**:166–180.

Ebbers, R. W. and Sears, D., 1975, Ocular effects of a 325 nm ultraviolet laser, *Am. J. Opt. & Physiol. Opt.* **52**(3):216–223 (March 1975) (DDC AD A-016-194).

Fischer, F. P., Vermuellen, D. and Eymers, J. G., 1936, Uber die zur Schadigung des Auges notige Minimalquantität von ultravioletten und infrarottem licht. *Arch. Augenheilk* **109**:462-467.

Flower, W., McLeod, D. S., and Pitts, S. M., 1977, Reflection of light by small areas of the ocular fundus, *Invest. Ophthal.* **16**:981–985.

Foulks, G. N., Friend, J. and Thoft, R. A., 1978, Effects of ultraviolet radiation on corneal epithelial metabolism, *Invest. Ophthal. & Vis. Sci.* **17**(7):694–697.

Frisch, G. D., Beatrice, E. S., and Holsen, R. C., 1971, Comparative study of argon and ruby retinal damage thresholds, *Invest. Ophthal.* **10**:911–919.

Fry, G. A., 1965, Distribution of focused and stray light on the retina produced by a point source, *J. Opt. Soc. Am.* **55**:333–335.

Fry, G. A., Pritchard, B. S., and Blackwell, H. R., 1963, Design and calibration of a disability glare lens, *Illum. Eng.* **58**:120–123.

Gabel, V. P., Birngruber, R., and Hillenkamp, F., 1976, Die lichtabsorption am augenhintergrund, GSF-Bericht A 55, Gessellschaft für Strahlen-und Umweltforschung, MbH, München (August 1976).

Geeraets, W. J., 1969, Radiation effects on the eye, *The Sight Saving Rev.* **39**:181–196 (Winter 1969-70).

Geeraets, W. J., and Berry, E. R., 1968, Ocular spectral characteristics as related to hazards from lasers and other light sources, *Am. J. Ophth.* **66**:15–20.

Geeraets, W. J., Williams, R. C., Chan, G., Ham, W. T., Jr., Guerry, D., III, and Schmidt, F. H., 1962, The relative absorption of thermal energy in retina and choroid, *Invest. Ophth.* **1**:340–347.

Geeraets, W. J., Burkhart, J., and Guerry, D., 1963, Enzyme activity in the coagulated retina: a means of studying thermal conduction as a function of exposure time, *Acta. Ophth. (Suppl.)* **76**:79–93.

Gerathewohl, S. J., and Strughold, H., 1953, Motoric responses of the eyes when exposed to light flashes of high intensities and short durations, *J. Aviat. Med.* **24**:200–207.

Gibbons, W. D., and Allen, R. G., 1978, Retinal damage from Suprathreshold Q-switched laser exposure, *Health Phys.* **35**(3):461–469.

Gibbons, W. D. and Allen, R. G., 1977, Retinal damage from long-term exposure to laser radiation, *Invest. Ophthal.* **16**(6):521–529.

Ginsburg, B. L., 1952, Rotation of the eye during involuntary blinking, *Nature* **169**:412.

Goldman, A. I., Ham, W. T., Jr. and Mueller, H. A., 1975, Mechanisms of retinal damage resulting from the exposure of rhesus monkeys to ultrashort laser pulses, *Exp. Eye Res.* **21**:457–469.

Goldman, A. I., Ham, W. T., Jr. and Mueller, H. A., 1977, Ocular damage thresholds and mechanisms for ultrashort pulses of both visible and infrared laser radiation in the rhesus monkey, *Exp. Eye Res.* **24**:45–56.

Goldman, H., 1933, Genesis of heat cataract, *Arch. Ophth.* **9**:314–316.

Goldman, H., König, H., and Mader, F., 1950, The transmission of the lens of the eye for infrared, *Ophthalmologica* **120**:198–205.

Goldman, L., and Rockwell, R. J., Jr., 1971, "Lasers in Medicine," Gordon and Breach, New York.

Green, J. B., 1969, Photosensitive epilepsy, *Arch. Neurol.* **20**:191-198.

Grover, D., and Zigman, S., 1972, Coloration of human lenses by near ultraviolet photo-oxidized tryptophan, *Exp. Eye Res.* **13**:70–76.

Gubisch, R. W., 1967, Optical performance of the human eye, *J. Opt. Soc. Am.* **57**:407–415.

Gupta, M. N., and Singh, H., 1968, Ocular Effects and Visual Performance in Welders, Gov't. of India Ministry of Labour Employment and Rehabilitation. Department of Labour and Employment, Report No. 27.

Ham, W. T., Jr., Ruffolo, J. J., Mueller, H. A., Clarke, A. M., and Moon, M. E., 1978, Histologic Analysis of Photochemical Lesions Produced in Rhesus Retina by Short-Wavelength Light, *Invest. Ophthal., Vis. Sci.* **17**(10):1029–1035.

Ham, W. T., Jr., Williams, R. C., Mueller, H. A., Guerry, D., Clarke, A. M., and Geeraets, W. J., 1966, Effects of laser radiation on the mammalian eye, *Trans. N. Y. Acad. Sci.,* Series 2, **28**:517–526.

Ham, W. T., Jr., Geeraets, W. J., Mueller, H. A., Williams, R. C., Clarke, A. M., and Cleary, S. F., 1970, Retinal burn thresholds for the helium-neon laser in the rhesus monkey, *Arch. Ophth.* **84**(12):797–808.

Ham, W. T., Jr., Clarke, A. M., Geeraets, W. T., Cleary, S. F., Mueller, H. A., and Williams, R. C., 1975, The health problem in laser safety, *Arch. Environ. Health* **20**(2):156–160.

Ham, W. T., Jr., Mueller, H. A. and Sliney, D. H., 1976, Retinal sensitivity to damage from short wavelength light, *Nature* **260**:153–155.

Ham, W. T., Jr., Mueller, H. A., Ruffolo, J. J., Jr., and Clark, A. M., 1979, Sensitivity of the retina to radiation damage as a function of wavelength, *Photochem. Photobiol.* **29**(4):735–743.

Hamerski, W., 1969, Investigations on histochemical changes in experimental corneal lesions induced with UV radiation and on the prevention of photophthalmia, *Pol. Med. J.* **8**:1469–1476.

Hansson, H. A., 1971, A histochemical study of cellular reactions in rat retina transiently damaged by visible light, *Exp. Eye Res.* **12**:270–274.

Harwerth, R. S., and Sperling, H. G., 1975, Effects of intense visible radiation on the increment threshold spectral sensitivity of the Rhesus monkey eye, *Vis. Res.* **15**:1193–1204.

Hatfield, E. M., 1970, Eye injuries and the solar eclipse, *Sight Sav. Rev.* **40**:79–85.

Hayes, J. R., and Wolbarsht, M. L., 1968, Thermal model for retinal damage induced by pulsed lasers, *Aerospace Med.* **39**:474–480.

Hayes, J. R., and Wolbarsht, M. L., 1971, Models in pathology mechanisms of action of laser energy with biological tissues, *in* "Laser Applications in Medicine and Biology," (M. L. Wolbarsht, ed.) Vol. 1, pp. 255–274, Plenum Press, New York.

Hillenkamp, F., Birngruber, R., and Gabel, V. P., 1978, Physical considerations of laser injury to the eye, *in* "Current Concepts in Ergophthalmology," (B. Tengroth and D. Epstein, eds.), pp. 47–54, Department of Ophthalmology, Karolinska Institute, Stockholm.

Holladay, L. L., 1927, Action of a light-source in the field of view in lowering visibility, *J. Opt. Soc. Amer.* **14**:1–15.

Hudnell, A. B., Jr., and Chick, E. W., 1962, Corneal ultraviolet therapy, *Arch. Ophth.* **62**:304.

Jacobson, J. H., Cooper, B., Najac, H. W. and Kohtiao, A., 1963, The Effects of Thermal Energy on Anterior Ocular Tissues. AMRL-TDR-63-53, 6570th Aerospace Medicine Research Laboratory, Wright-Patterson Air Force Base, OH (AD 412730) (June 1963).

Katz, M. L., Stone, W. L., and Dratz, E. A., 1978, Fluorescent pigment accumulation in retinal pigment epithelium of antioxidant-deficient rats, *Invest. Ophthal., Vis. Sci.* **17**(112):1049–1058.

Khitun, V. A. Korzun, P. A., Shostak, V. I., and Obukhova, Ye. A., 1971, Restoration of visual acuity after a bright light flash of short duration, in "Problems of Physiological Optics," (V. G. Samsonova, ed.), NASA Tech. Translation F-650, pp. 169–171.

Klang, G., 1948, Measurement and studies of the fluorescence of human lens in vivo, *Acta. Ophthal., Suppl.* **31**:1–152.

Konig, H., 1970, Die Blendwirkung Monochromatischen Lichtes auf das Menschliche Auge, *Vis. Res.* **10**:875–885.

Kurzel, R. B., Wolbarsht, M. L., and Yamanashi, B. S., 1977, Ultraviolet radiation effects on the human eye, in "Photochemical and Photobiological Reviews," (K. C. Smith, ed.), Vol. 2, pp. 133–167, Plenum Press, New York.

Kurzel, R. B., Wolbarsht, M. L., and Yamanashi, B. S., and Borkman, R. F., 1973, Tryptophan excited states and cataracts in the human lens, *Nature* **241**:132–133.

Kuwabara, T., 1970, Retinal recovery from exposure to light, *Am. J. Ophth.* **70**(2):187–198.

Landers, M. B., III, Wolbarsht, M. L., and Shaw, H. E., 1976, The current status of laser usage in ophthalmology, in "Third Conference on the Laser," (L. Goldman, ed.), *Ann. N. Y. Acad. Sci.* **267**:230–246.

Langley, R. K., Mortimer, C. B., and McCulloch, C., 1960, The experimental production of cataracts by exposure to heat and light, *Arch. Ophth.* **63**:473–488.

Lappin, P. W., and Coogan, P. S., 1970, Relative sensitivity of various areas of the retina to laser radiation, *Arch. Ophthal.* **84**:350–354.

Lawwill, T., Crockett, S., and Currier, G., 1977, Retinal damage secondary to chronic light exposure, *Documenta Ophthalmologica* **44**(2):379–402.

LeGrand, Y., 1937, Recherches sur la diffusion de la lumiere dans l'oeil humain, *Revue d'Optique* **12**:201–214, 241–266.

Leibowitz, H. M., and Peacock, G. R., 1969, Corneal injury produced by carbon dioxide laser radiation, *Arch. Ophth.* **81**:712–721.

Lerman, S., 1976, Progress of lens biochemistry research. Lens fluorescence in aging and cataract formation. *Documenta Ophthalmologica, Proceeding Series,* pp. 41–60, (W. Junk, ed.), B. V. Publishers, Hague.

Lerman, S., Kuck, J., Borkman, R., and Saker, E., 1976, Acceleration of an aging parameter (fluorogen) in the ocular lens, *Ann. Ophth.* **8**:558–561.

Lerman, S., 1972, Lens proteins in aging and cataract formation, in "Contemporary Ophthalmology-Honoring Sir Stewart Duke-Elder," (J. G. Bellows, ed.) Williams and Wilkins, Baltimore, MD.

L'Esperance, F. A., Jr., 1968, An ophthalmic argon laser photocoagulation system: Design, construction and laboratory investigations, *Trans. Am. Ophth. Soc.* **66**:827–904.

Livingston, P. C., 1932, The study of sun glare in Iraq, *Brit. J. Ophth.* **6**:577–625.

Ludvigh, E., and McCarthy, E. F., 1938, Absorption of visible light by the refractive media of the human eye, *Arch. Ophth.* **20**:37.

MacDonald, J. E., and Fordon, L., 1971, Erythropsia and light toxicity thresholds, Annual Meeting of the Association for Research in Vision and Ophthalmology, Sarasota, FL (April 1971).

MacKeen, D., Fine, S., and Fine, B. S., 1973, Production of cataracts in rabbits with the ultraviolet laser, *Ophth. Res.* **5**:317–324.

MacNichol, E. F., Jr., Kunz, Y. W., Levine, J. S., Harosi, F. I., and Collins, B. A., 1978, Ellipsosomes: organelles containing a cytochrome-like pigment in the retinal cones of certain fishes, *Science* **200**:549–552.

Mainster, M. A., 1929, Ophthalmic applications of infrared lasers–thermal considerations, *Invest. Ophthal. Vis. Sci.* **18**(4):414–420.

Marshall, C., Walker, A. E., and Livingston, S., 1953, Photogenic epilepsy: Parameters of activation, *AMA Arch. of Neurol. and Psychiatry* **69**:760–765.

Marshall, J., 1978, Retinal injury from chronic exposure to light and the delayed effects from retinal exposure to intense light sources, in "Current Concepts in Ergophthalmology," (B. Tengroth and D. Epstein, eds.), pp. 81–104, Department of Ophthalmology, Karolinska Institute, Stockholm.

Matelsky, I., 1968, The non-ionizing radiation, in "Industrial Hygiene Highlights," (L. V. Cralley, ed.) pp. 140–178, Industrial Hygiene Foundation of America, Pittsburgh, PA.

Mayyasi, A. M., Johnston, W. L., and Burkes, W. T., 1971, Variability of depth perception under conditions of intermittent illumination, in "The Perception and Application of Flashing Lights," pp. 55–60, University of Toronto Press.

Medvedovskaya, T. P., 1970, Data on the condition of the eye in workers at a glass factory, *Hygiene and Sanitation* **35**:446–447.

Mellerio, J., 1971, Light absorption and scatter in the human lens, *Vis. Res.* **11**(2):129–141.

Meyer-Schwickerath, G., 1960, Chapter 1: The historical and experimental background of radiation damage to the retina, in "Light Coagulation," C. V. Mosby, Co., St. Louis, Missouri.

Miller, N. D., 1965, Visual recovery from brief exposures to high luminance, *J. Opt. Soc. Amer.* **55**:1661–1662.

Miller, N. D., 1966, Positive afterimage following brief high-intensity flashes, *J. Opt. Soc. Amer.* **56**(6):802–806.

Miller, N. D., 1966, Positive afterimage as a background luminance, *J. Opt. Soc. Amer.* **56**(11):1616–1620.

Moon, M. E., Clarke, A. M., Ruffolo, J. J., Jr., Mueller, H. A., and Ham, W. T., Jr., 1978, Visual performance in the Rhesus monkey after exposure to blue light, *Vis. Res.* **18**:1573–1577.

Newsome, D. A., 1971, Afterimage and pupillary activity following strong light exposure, *Vis. Res.* **11**:275–288.

Noell, W. K., 1979, Effects of environmental lighting and dietary vitamin A on the vulnerability of the retina to light damage, *Photochem. Photobiol.* **29**(4):717–723.

Noell, W., and Albrecht, R., 1971, Irreversible effects of visible light on the retina–role of vitamin A, *Science* **172**:76–79.

Ogilvie, J. C. and Ryan, M. L., 1955, Threshold sensitivity to light measured with an extraneous ultraviolet source in the visual field, *J. Opt. Soc. Am.* **45**:206–209.

O'Steen, W. K., 1979, Hormonal and dim light effects in retinal photodamage, *Photochem. Photobiol.* **29**(4):745–753.

Parrish, J. A., Fitzpatrick, T. B., Tanenbaum, L., and Pathak, M. A., 1974, Photochemotherapy of psoriasis with oral methoxsalen and longwave ultraviolet light, *New Engl. J. Med.* **291**:1207–1211.

Pathak, M. A., Dall'Acqua, F., Rodighiero, G., and Parrish, J. A., 1974a, Metabolism of psoralens, *J. Invest. Dermatol.* **62**:347.

Pathak, M. A., Kramer, D. M. and Fitzpatrick, T. B., 1974b, Photobiology and photochemistry of furocoumarins (psoralens), in "Sunlight and Man: Normal and Abnormal Photobiologic Responses," (M. A. Pathak, L. C. Harber, M. Seiji et al., eds.) University of Tokyo Press, Tokyo, pp. 335–368.

Peckham, R. H., and Harley, R. D., 1951, The effect of sunglasses in protecting retinal sensitivity *Amer. J. Ophthal.* **34**:1499–1507.

Penner, R., and McNair, J. N., 1966, Eclipse blindness, *Am. J. Ophth.* **61**:1452–1457.

Pirie, A., 1972, Photooxidation of proteins and comparison of photooxidized proteins with those of the cataractous human lens, *Isr. Med. Sci.* **8**:1567–1573.

Pitts, D. G., 1974, The human ultraviolet action spectrum, *Am. J. Optom. Physiol. Opt.* **51**:946–960.

Pitts, D. G., 1959, Transmission of the visible spectrum through the ocular media of the bovine eye, *Am. J. Optom. Arch. Am. Acad. Optom.* **36**:289–298.

Pitts, D. G., and Cullen, A. P., Hacker, P. E., and Parr, W. H., 1977, Ocular ultraviolet effects from 295 nm to 400 nm in the rabbit eye, Univ. of Houston, College of Optometry, TX, Contract CDC-99-74-12, DHEW, NIOSH (October 1977).

Pitts, D. C., Cullen, A. P., and Hacker, P. D., 1977, Ocular effects of ultraviolet radiation from 295 to 365 nm, *Inv. Ophthal. and Vis. Sci.* **16**(10):932–939.

Pitts, D. G., and Tredici, T. J., 1971, The effects of ultraviolet on the eye, *Am. Ind. Hyg. Assn. J.* **32**(4):235–246.

Pitts, D. G., and Gibbons, W., 1973, Corneal light scattering measurements of UV radiant exposures, *Am. J. Optom.* **50**:187–194.

Plato, 1892, Phaedo, *in* "The Dialogues of Plato," (B. Jowett, translator) 3rd edition, pp. 159–266 (99 D), Oxford University Press, London.

Projector, T. H., 1958, Efficiency of flashing lights, *Illum. Eng.* **53**:600–604.

Rapp, L. M. and Williams, T. P., 1979, Damage to the albino rat retina produced by low intensity light, *Photochem. Photobiol.* **29**(4):731–733.

Reeves, P., 1920, The response of the average pupil to various intensities of light, *J. Opt. Soc. Am.* **4**:35–43.

Said, F. S., and Weale, R. A., 1959, The variation with age of the spectral transmissivity of the living human crystalline lens, *Geontologica* **3**:213–231.

Semmlow, J. and Stark, L., 1973, Pupil movements of light and accommodative stimulation: A comparative study, *Vis. Res.* **13**:1087–1100.

Sherashov, S. G., 1970, Spectral sensitivity of the cornea to ultraviolet radiation, *Biofizika* **15**: 543–544.

Sliney, D. H., 1971, The development of laser safety criteria, *in* "Laser Applications in Medicine and Biology," (M. L. Wolbarsht, ed.) Vol. 1, pp. 163–238, Plenum Press, New York.

Sliney, D. H., 1972, Non-ionizing radiation, *in* "Industrial and Environmental Health: The Worker and the Community," (E. D. Cralley, ed.), pp. 171–241, Academic Press, New York.

Sliney, D. H. and Freasier, B. C., 1973, Evaluation of optical radiation hazards, *Appl. Opt.* **12**: 1–23.

Sliney, D. H., Krial, N. P., and Ryan, L., 1978, Laser Hazards Bibliography, US Army Environmental Hygiene Agency, Aberdeen Proving Ground, MD (August 1978).

Sliney, D. H., Wangemann, R. T., Franks, J. K., and Wolbarsht, M. L., 1976, Visual sensitivity of the eye to infrared laser radiation, *J. Opt. Soc. Am.* **66**(4):339–341.

Smith, H. E., 1944, Actinic macular retinal pigment degeneration, *U.S. Naval Med. Bull.* **42**: 675–680.

Spitznas, M., 1971, Morphogenesis and nature of the pigment granules in the human adult retinal pigment epithelium, *Zeitschrift für Zellforschung und Microskopische Anatomie* **122**:378–388.

Stiles, W. S. and Crawford, B. H., 1933, The luminous efficiency of rays entering the pupil at different points, *Proc. Roy. Soc.* B **112**:428–450.

Stone, W. L., Katz, M. L., Lurie, M., Marmor, M. F., and Dratz, E. A., 1979, Effects of dietary vitamin E and selenium on light damage to the rat retina, *Photochem. Photobiol.* **29**:725–730.

Szafran, L., 1965, A lens opacity with the morphological features of smelting cataract in a welder, *Medycynz. Pracy* **16**(3):246–249.
Tapaszto, I., and Vass, Z., 1969, Alterations in mucopolysaccharide compounds of tears and of the corneal epithelium caused by ultraviolet radiation, *Ophthalmologica (Add.)* **158**:343–347.
Tso, M. O. M., 1973, Photic maculopathy in the Rhesus monkey, a light and electron microscopy study, *Invest. Ophthal.* **12**:17–34.
Tso, M. O. M., Fine, B. S. and Zimmerman, L. E., 1972, Photic maculopathy produced by the indirect ophthalmoscope, *Am. J. Ophth.* **73**:686–699.
Tso, M. O. M. and LaPiana, F. G., 1975, The human fovea after sun gazing, *Trans. Am. Acad. Ophth.* **79**:788–795.
Tso, M. O. M., Wallow, I. H. L., Powell, J. O., and Zimmerman, L. E., 1972, Recovery of the rod and cone cells after photic injury, *Trans. Amer. Acad. Ophthal. and Otol.* **76**:1247–1262.
Twersky, V., 1975, Transparency of pair-correlated, random distributions of small scatterers, with applications to the cornea, *J. Opt. Soc. Am.* **65**(5):524–530.
Ulett, G. A., 1953, Flicker sickness, *AMA Arch. Ophthal.* **50**:685–687.
Urbach, F., (ed.), 1969, "The Biologic Effects of Ultraviolet Radiation," Pergamon Press, New York.
van der Zypen, E., Frankhauser, F., and Bebie, H., 1978, On the effects of different laser energy sources upon the iris of the pigmented and the albino rabbit, *Int. Ophthal.* **1**(1):39–48.
van Norren, D., and Vos, J. J., 1974, Spectral transmission of the human ocular media, *Vis. Res.* **14**:1237–1244.
Vassiliadis, A., Rosan, R. C., Hayes, J. and Zweng, H. C., 1969, Investigation of retinal hazards due to pulsed xenon lamp radiation, SRI Report 7112 Stanford Research Inst., Menlo Park, CA.
Vassiliadis, A., 1971, Ocular damage from laser radiation, in "Laser Applications in Medicine and Biology," (M. L. Wolbarsht, ed.) Vol. 1, pp. 125–162, Plenum Press, New York.
Vassiliadis, A., Chang, H., Peabody, R. R., Peppers, N. A., Honey, R. C., Rose, H. W., Rosan, R. C., Zweng, H. C., Flocks, M., and Dedrick, K., 1968, Investigations of Laser Damage to Ocular Tissues, Stanford Research Institute, Menlo Park, CA (March 1968).
Verhoeff, F., Bell, L., and Walker, C. B., 1916, Pathological effects of radiant energy on the eye, *Proc. Am. Acad. Arts Sci.* **51**:630–811.
Vogt, A., 1919, Experimentelle Erzeugung von Katarakt durch isoliertes kurzwelliges Ultrarot, dem Rot beigemischt ist, *Klin. Mbl. Augenheilk* **63**:230–231.
Vos, J. J., and van Meeteren, A., 1971, Visual Processes Involved in Seeing Flashes, in "The Perception and Application of Flashing Lights," pp. 3-28, University of Toronto Press, Toronto.
Vos, J. J., Munnik, A. A., and Boogard, J., 1965, Absolute spectral reflectance of the fundus oculi, *J. Opt. Soc. Amer.* **55**:573.
Vos, J. J., Walraven, J., and van Meeteren, A., 1976, Light profiles of the foveal image of a point source, *Vis. Res.* **16**:215–219.
Wallace, J., Sweetnam, P. M., Warner, C. G., Graham, P. A., and Cochrane, A. L., 1971, An epidemiological study of lens opacities among steel workers, *Brit. J. Ind. Med.* **28**:265-271.
Walraven, J., 1973, Spatial characteristics of chromatic induction; the segregation of lateral effects from straylight artifacts, *Vis. Res.* **13**:1739–1753.
Westheimer, G. and Campbell, F. W., 1962, Light distribution in the image formed by the living human eye, *J. Opt. Soc. Am.* **52**:1040–1045.
White, T. J., 1975, Unpublished computer program.
White, T. J., Mainster, M. A., Tips, J. H., and Wilson, P. W., 1970, Chorioretinal thermal behavior, *Bull. Math Biophys.* **32**:315–322.
Williams, T. B., and Baker, B. N. (eds.), 1980, "The Effects of Constant Light on the Visual Process," Plenum Press, New York.

Wolbarsht, M. L. and Sliney, D. H., 1974, Needed: More data on eye damage, *Laser Focus* **10**: 10–13.

Wolbarsht, M. L. and Landers, M. B., 1972, "Laser Exposures in the Maculas of Human Volunteers," I. CW He-Ne, CW Argon, Pulsed Ruby Laser Measurements, Technical Report N00014-67-A-0251-0011 (December 1972).

Wolbarsht, M. L., Orr, M. A., Yamanashi, B. S., Zigler, J. S., and Matheson, I. B. C., 1977, The origin of cataracts in the lens from infrared laser radiation, Ann. Report contract DAMD 17-74-C-4143, US Army Research and Development Command, Washington, D.C.

Wolbarsht, M. L., Yamanashi, B. S., and Orr, M. A., 1977, The origin of cataracts in the lens from infrared radiation, Report 7-20-1977: 62772A 3E62772A813.00.013, Duke Univ. Eye Center, Durham, NC, Contract DAMD 17-74-C-4133 US Army Med. Rsh. and Dev. Command, Washington, D.C.

Wolbarsht, M. L., 1978, The effects of optical radiation on the anterior structures of the eye, *in* "Current Concepts in Ergophthalmology," (B. Tengroth and D. Epstein, eds.) pp. 29–46, Department of Ophthalmology, Karolinska Institute, Stockholm.

Yarbus, A. L., 1967, "Eye Movements and Vision," Plenum Press, New York.

Young, R. W., 1976, Visual cells and the concept of renewal, *Invest. Ophthal.* **15**:700–725.

Young, R. W., 1978, The daily rhythm of shedding and degradation of rod and cone outer segment membranes in the chick retina, *Invest. Ophthal., Vis. Sci.* **17**:105–116.

Zigman, S. and Vaughan, T., 1974, Near-ultraviolet light effects on the lenses and retinas of Mice, *Invest. Ophthal.* **13**(6):462–465.

Zigman, S., Yulo, T. and Schultz, J., 1974, Cataract induction in mice exposed to near-UV light, *Ophth. Res.* **6**:259–270.

Zuclich, J. A. and Connolly, J. S., 1976, Ocular damage induced by near-ultraviolet laser radiation, *Invest. Ophth.* **15**:760.

Zuclich, J. A. and Kurtin, W. E., 1977, Oxygen dependence of near-UV induced corneal damage, *Photochem. Photobiol.* **25**:133–135.

Zuclich, J. A. and Taboada, J., 1978, Ocular hazard from UV laser exhibiting self-mode-locking, *Appl. Opt.* **17**:1482–1484.

Zweng, H. C., Little, H. L. and Peabody, R. R., 1969, "Laser Photocoagulation and Retinal Angiography," C. V. Mosby, Co., St. Louis, Missouri.

Zwick, H. and Beatrice, E., 1978, Long-term changes in spectral sensitivity after low-level (514 nm) exposure, *Mod. Probl. Ophth.* **19**:319–325.

Zwick, H., and Jenkins, D., 1978, Effects of coherent light on retinal receptor processes of pseudemys, *Invest. Ophth., Vis. Sci.* **17**(Suppl):172.

Chapter 5
Optical Radiation Hazards to the Skin

5.1 INTRODUCTION

Laser radiation injury to the skin is normally considered secondary to injury of the eye despite the fact that thresholds of injury to the skin and eye are comparable except in the retinal hazard region (400-1400 nm). In the far-infrared and the ultraviolet spectral regions where optical radiation is not focused on the retina, skin injury thresholds are approximately the same as corneal injury thresholds. The probability of exposure of the skin is greater than for the eye because of the skin's greater surface area, and yet we still consider injury to the eye of greater significance. Threshold injuries resulting from short exposure to the skin from far-infrared (IR-C) and UV-C radiation are also very superficial and may only involve changes to the outer dead layer—the "horny layer"—of the skin cells. A temporary injury to the skin may be painful if sufficiently severe; but eventually it will heal, often without any sign of the injury. Injury to larger areas of skin are far more serious as they may lead to serious loss of body fluids, toxemia, and systemic infections.

After eye protection has been provided to personnel who may be exposed to hazardous levels of optical radiation it is often necessary to analyze potential exposure to the skin. Injury to the skin can result either from thermal injury following temperature elevation in skin tissues or from a photochemical effect (e.g., "sunburn") from excessive levels of actinic ultraviolet radiation.

5.2 THERMAL INJURY

5.2.1 Critical Temperatures

Thermal injury of the skin has been the subject of many studies in this century. Hardy and his coworkers (1956) found that severe pain could always be induced in human skin tissue when the tissue temperature was elevated to 45°C. This temperature also corresponds to an injury threshold if the exposure to optical radiation lasts for many seconds.

Skin injury resulting from momentary but very intense heat exposures are generally termed "flash burns." Flash burns of the skin following exposure to optical radiation in industry are practically unknown. Most conventional sources such as open arc processes and industrial furnaces do not possess significant irradiances in occupied areas where skin injury could occur in a duration shorter than a natural protective reaction time to intense heat. The flash burns that do occur are more often the result of conductive heating of the skin by exceedingly hot gases or steam.

Studies of flash burns from simulated nuclear weapons have produced a considerable amount of data (Buettner, 1952). Ham and his colleagues (Evans et al., 1955) used a carbon arc source and exposed 2-cm^2 patches of skin for 0.5 s in their studies of thermal injury. A first-degree burn (very superficial reddening of the skin) resulted from exposure of normal skin to a white light source at an irradiance of 12 W/cm^2. A second degree burn (a blistering) occurred at an irradiance of 24 W/cm^2. The severest type of skin injury, a third degree burn (where the entire outer layer of the skin, the epidermis, was destroyed), occurred at an irradiance of 34 W/cm^2. These irradiances are now quite possible to achieve with high-powered CW lasers and focused xenon arcs. However, it should be noted that these thresholds depend upon the area of irradiated tissue. For a much smaller area (e.g., 1 mm^2) of irradiated tissue, the heat conduction is far greater and would permit higher irradiances prior to injury. For whole-body irradiation a far lower irradiance could be expected to cause injury. Hazardous exposures to larger areas of skin are hardly likely to be encountered in the normal work environment. Even if they are, the heat stress alone from the source would require protective measures at lower power levels.

5.2.2 Dependence Upon Exposure Duration

The threshold of injury obviously depends also upon exposure duration. The previously mentioned thresholds are for just one exposure duration—0.5 s. For exposure durations less than 0.5 s the irradiance required for an injury would significantly increase as the exposure duration decreases. Henriques and associates (1947) studied this *rate process of thermal injury* in skin tissues and noted that for greater exposure durations a lower temperature was required to coagulate proteins and destroy tissue by elevated temperature. Figure 5-1 shows this time dependence of

Optical Radiation Hazards to the Skin

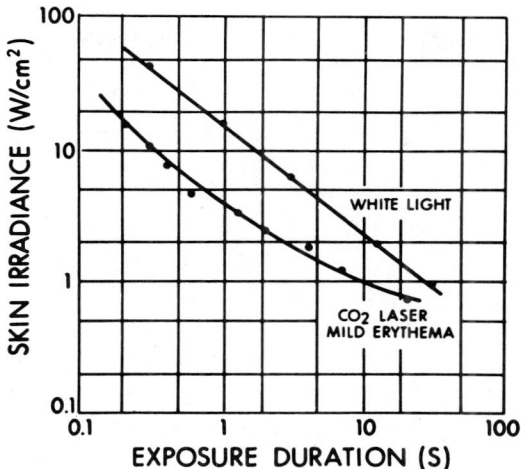

Figure 5-1. Thresholds of injury for pigskin. Lower curve is for mildest erythema for 10.6 μm infrared laser radiation (Parr, 1969). Upper curve is for white-light first-degree burn thresholds based upon the studies of Davies (1959).

threshold for white-light, arc-source burns (upper curve) and for far-infrared laser radiation (lower curve). The explanation for these threshold differences lies in the fact that thermal injury depends upon energy absorbed per unit volume (or mass) to produce a critical temperature elevation. Skin reflectance and penetration greatly influence this absorption.

5.2.3 Penetration Depth

The studies of the effects of pulsed laser radiation upon pig skin performed in the 1960s provided single-wavelength thresholds of injury for very short exposure durations of the order of 1 ms and 20 ns. For such short exposure durations the influence of heat flow from the absorbing site is not a major factor. For this reason these studies aptly showed that the threshold of injury depended upon the reflectance of the skin and the penetration depth of the optical radiation into the skin tissue. The outermost, dead, horny layer, the *stratum corneum,* is approximately 8 to 20 μm in thickness except in calloused areas, and (as described in Chapter 3) is composed of flattened, dead cells which have migrated from the inner layers of the *epidermis.* The dead tissue serves as a filter which is particularly effective in filtering out ultraviolet and far-infrared radiation, thereby protecting the deeper living tissue.

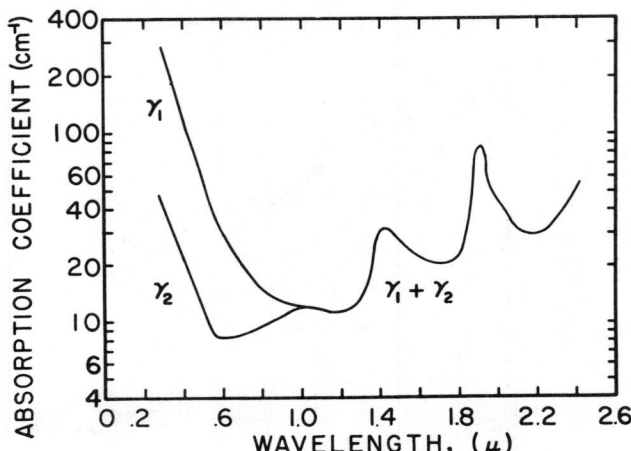

Figure 5-2. The linear absorption coefficients of fair skin, from *in-vitro* measurements. The upper curve γ_1 refers to the superficial layers and the lower curve γ_2 to the deeper tissues. Beyond 1.0 μm the skin follows Beer's law, with $\gamma_1 = \gamma_2$ (from Davis, 1963, with permission).

Figure 5-2 presents the smoothed curves of the linear absorption coefficients of two skin layers versus wavelength. It must be admitted that this Figure is compounded of about equal parts of freehand art and literature research. It is hoped, however, that it represents the best estimates available as to the true values of these coefficients. Figure 5-3 shows schematically the penetration depth of different optical wavelengths. Note that far-infrared (IR-C) radiation as represented by the CO_2 laser wavelength (10.6 μm) penetrates only to very shallow skin tissue before 99% of the incident optical radiation is absorbed. Near-infrared (IR-A) radiation such as 1.06 μm from neodymium laser penetrates well into the dermis before being largely absorbed. In comparison to an irradiance of 1 W/cm^2 of 10.6-μm radiation, the irradiance of 1 W/cm^2 of 1.06-μm radiation would be unable to raise the absorbing tissue layer to as great a temperature since the absorbing volume is much greater for the same incident irradiance. IR-A wavelengths have long been used to deliver "deep heating." Heat lamps used for physical therapy are designed to have their primary spectral emission in the IR-A spectral region. Light at other laser wavelengths in the blue end of the visible spectrum is absorbed more superficially, but nevertheless does reach the dermis.

5.2.4 Reflection

The reflectance of the skin also plays a role in determining how much radiation can be effectively absorbed. Figure 5-4 shows the skin's spectral reflectance throughout most of the optical spectrum. It varies with pigmentation significantly only in the visible and near-infrared spectrum. The shape of the spectral reflectance

Optical Radiation Hazards to the Skin

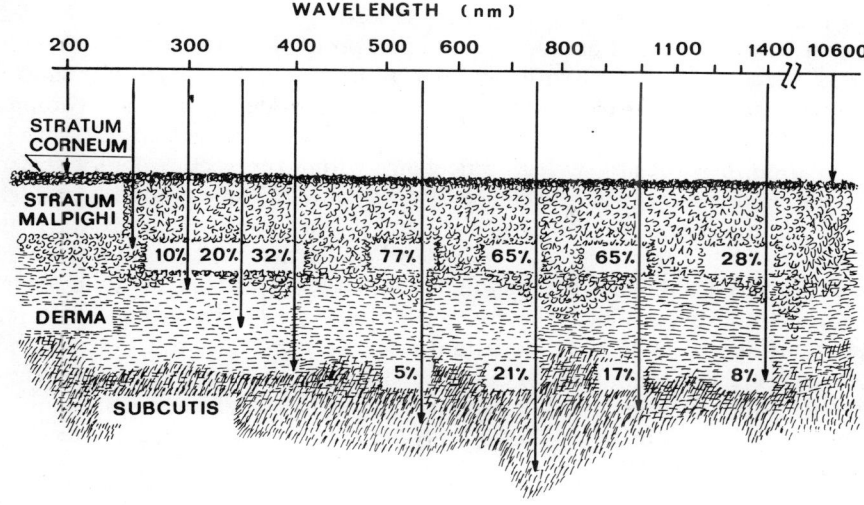

Figure 5-3. Schematic showing penetration depth into the skin for different wavelengths (after Ippen, in Urbach, 1969, p. 683).

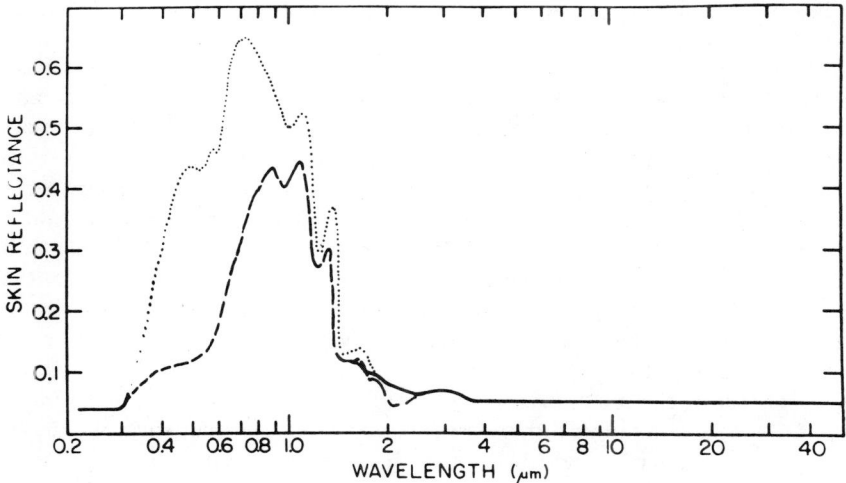

Figure 5-4. Spectral reflectance of human skin. Dotted line and dashed line are data of Jacquez and coworkers (1955) for individuals having a very fair complexion (••••) and for individuals having heavily pigmented (---) skin. Spectral reflectance for skin in the UV and IR regions reported by Hardy and coworkers (1956) and Buettner (1937) is shown by the solid line.

curve illustrates how the skin reflects most solar radiation which is in the visible and near-infrared spectral bands. This comparison of the reflectance of the skin in the visible and near-infrared with the solar spectrum shows a remarkable similarity and how the optical properties of the skin are adapted for the natural environment. Even the lower curve in Fig. 5-3, which represents the reflectance of skin with high pigmentation, has a relatively high reflectance within the peak region of the solar spectrum. Because the skin reflectance is so very low and absorption is very high in the far-infrared region, the skin has a spectral thermal emissivity of nearly 1 which enhances its ability to rid the body of excess heat by thermal radiation. A basic law of thermal physics requires that any material that has a high emissivity in the infrared must also have a very high absorptivity in that same spectral region. This almost total absorption of IR-C radiation is, however, a disadvantage to workers in industries where high ambient levels of far infrared radiant heat exist. Likewise although more than 40% of a neodymium laser beam would be reflected from most skin surfaces only approximately 4% of a 10.6-μm CO_2 laser beam would be reflected from skin.

5.2.5 The Warmth Sensation and Heat Flow

The warmth sensation resulting from absorption of radiant energy normally provides adequate warning for an avoidance reaction to prevent thermal injury of the skin from almost all sources except the nuclear fireball and some high-powered, far-infrared lasers. The spot size dependence of this sensation is nicely illustrated by irradiating human skin with a beam of CO_2-laser radiation at 10.6 μm. An irradiance of 0.1 W/cm^2 produces a definite sensation of warmth if the beam diameter is not much larger than 1 cm in diameter. On the other hand, one-tenth this level (0.01 W/cm^2) can readily be sensed only if the whole body or a large portion of the body is exposed. The dependence upon the size of the irradiated area results from conduction of heat away from the absorbing area thus limiting surface temperature rise, the sensation of heat being a function of temperature rise. As noted previously the skin temperature elevation required to elicit persistent pain (as well as thermal injury after several seconds) is approximately 45°C. Since the reflectance of the skin at a wavelength of 632.8 nm is nearly 10 times greater than that at a wavelength of 10.6 μm, even for a very heavily pigmented individual, the effective irradiances would have to be increased by nearly that same factor to elicit the same thermal response.

The face is the most sensitive exposed portion of the body to infrared radiation. CO_2-laser communications researchers often place their head in the beam to locate a low irradiance beam. Although this practice is not considered hazardous if the beam irradiance is below 100 mW/cm^2 it is clearly not advisable unless the size of the beam is well known.

Optical Radiation Hazards to the Skin

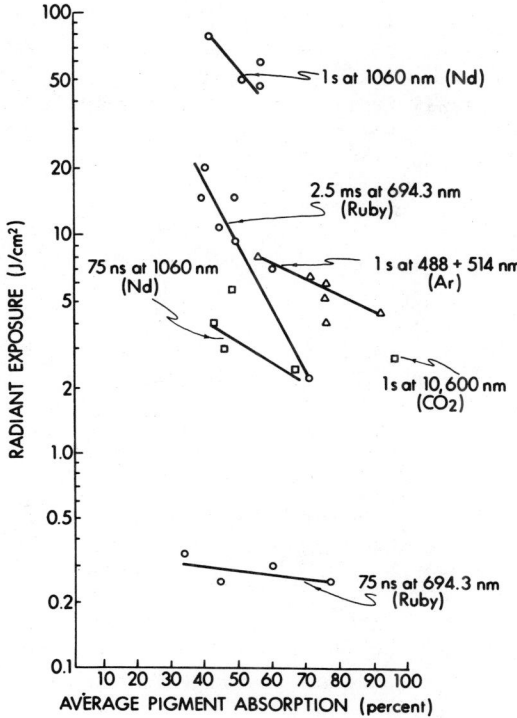

Figure 5-5. Collection of laser injury threshold data for skin (from Rockwell and Goldman, 1974).

5.3 LASER INJURY THRESHOLDS FOR THE SKIN

5.3.1 Thermal Injury

A considerable number of studies of skin injury from laser radiation were conducted by the U.S. Army at Fort Knox and at the University of Cincinnati School of Medicine during the 1960s. Figure 5-5 shows the collection of much of the human threshold data. It is noted that skin injury thresholds for high energy pulsed lasers generally range from approximately 0.2 J/cm^2 to 0.4 J/cm^2 for Q-switched ruby lasers depending upon skin pigmentation. As in the retina, the thresholds of injury for CW (> 0.25 s) exposures are greater than 1 W/cm^2, and are highly dependent upon exposure duration. High-power CW lasers operating in the visible and near-infrared spectrum that are capable of producing significant burns to the skin in less than 1 s have only been developed in recent years. Table 5-1 is a tabulation of some thresholds of injury from lasers upon the skin.

TABLE 5-1. Summary of Reported Laser Skin MRD-50's [†]

Laser Type	Exposure Method and Skin Type	Wavelength (nm)	Exposure Time (s)	MRD_{50} (J/cm^2)
RUBY	Normal Mode Pulse Human (Caucasian) Human (Negro)	694.3	2.5×10^{-3}	11-20 [a] 2.2-6.9 [a]
	Q-Switched Pulse Human (Caucasian) Human (Negro)	694.3	75×10^{-9}	0.25-0.34 [a] 0.25-0.30 [a]
ARGON	Shuttered Pulse Human (Caucasian) Human (Negro)	488-514	1.0	4.0-8.2 [a] 4.5-6.0 [a]
CARBON DIOXIDE	Shuttered Pulse Human (Caucasian) Human (Negro) White Pig	10,600	1.0 0.001 1.0 1.4×10^{-9}	2.8 [a] 2.8 [a] 1.0 [b] 3.0 [c] 0.23 [d]
NEODYMIUM GLASS	Q-Switched Pulse Human (Caucasian) Human (Negro)	1,060	75×10^{-9}	4.2-5.7 [a] 2.6-3.0 [a]
Nd:YAG	Shuttered Pulse (CW) Human (Caucasian) Human (Negro)	1.064	1.0	48-78 [a] 46-60 [a]
HYDROGEN FLUORIDE	White Pig	2,900	10^{-7}	0.3 [d]

REFERENCES

[a] Rockwell and Goldman (1974)

[b] Brownell et al. (1969)

[c] Parr (1969)

[d] Rockwell, R. J., Jr., Private Communication (1977)

[†] MRD-50 — The minimal reactive dose (MRD-50) which results in a visible reaction following 50 percent of the exposures.

Figure 5-5 presents a variety of threshold data reported by Rockwell and Goldman (1974) which illustrate the dependence upon skin pigmentation for some wavelengths and the independence for far-infrared wavelengths, as would be expected. In the far infrared all tissue absorbs heavily, not just melanin pigment granules.

5.3.2 Delayed Effects

The possibility of adverse effects from repeated or chronic laser irradiation to the skin has been suggested, although it is normally discounted (Goldman et al., 1971). Only optical radiation in the ultraviolet region of the spectrum has been shown to be a cause of long-term, delayed effects. These effects are: accelerated skin aging, and skin cancer. At present, laser safety standards for exposure of the skin do attempt to take into account all of these adverse effects.

5.4 AMBIENT ENVIRONMENT AND HEAT STRESS

The temperature of the ambient environment can play a role in adding or subtracting to the temperature rise from continuous exposure of the skin to optical radiation, particularly if whole-body exposure is possible. Although whole-body exposure to laser radiation is uncommon, it is not impossible. Just as whole-body exposure to far-infrared radiation from furnaces can cause heat stress, so also could far-infrared laser radiation. As was explained in Chapter 3, radiant absorption is only one factor in defining heat stress.

A formulation known as the WBGT Index has been developed for dealing with heat stress that includes heat stress from radiant energy. It was developed to protect personnel from several types of injuries while working in hot environments. It is designed to maintain the deep internal body temperature of an acclimatized worker below $38^{\circ}C$. Since internal body temperature is normally impractical to monitor, the WBGT Index is based upon ambient measurements. This index weights radiant energy less than high humidity and high air temperature as the latter is of greater concern. The formula recommended by ACGIH to determine the WBGT Index differs according to the environment:

$$WBGT = 0.7\ WB + 0.3\ BG \quad \text{for indoors, no solar load} \quad (5\text{-}1)$$

$$WBGT = 0.7\ WB + 0.1\ DB + 0.2\ BG \quad \text{for sunlight, outdoors} \quad (5\text{-}2)$$

where WB is the static wet bulb temperature, DB the dry bulb temperature, and BG is the black globe temperature. In addition to the WBGT index, a similar scheme—the wet globe thermometer (WGT) is also in use. Both indices suffer from the same drawback. Neither index accounts for the spectral variation in skin reflectance;

TABLE 5-2. ACGIH Permissible Heat Exposure Threshold Limit Values
(Values are given in °C. WBGT)

Work–Rest Regimen	Work Load		
	Light	Moderate	Heavy
Continuous Work	30.0	26.7	25.0
75% Work – 25% Rest, Each hour	30.6	28.0	25.9
50% Work – 50% Rest, Each hour	31.4	29.4	27.9
25% Work – 75% Rest, Each hour	32.2	31.1	30.0

Higher heat exposures than shown in the Table are permissible if the workers have been undergoing medical surveillance and it has been established that they are more tolerant to work in heat than the average worker. Workers should not be permitted to continue their work when their deep body temperature exceeds 38.0° C. The determination of WBGT requires the use of a black globe thermometer, a natural (static) wet-bulb thermometer, and a dry-bulb thermometer (from ACGIH TLV Book, 1978).

both systems could if the BG absorber surface were grey instead of black in the visible range. A detailed discussion of protection of personnel in hot environments is beyond the scope of this text. Such a discussion can be found in any number of texts on industrial hygiene and occupational health.

To give the reader an idea of the effect of CO_2 laser radiation, or any far-infrared radiation, upon the WBGT Index, an irradiance of 0.1 W/cm^2 from a CO_2 laser incident on the black globe thermometer in a typical indoor laboratory environment of constant air temperature and humidity will raise the WBGT from 21°C (70°F) to 27°C (85°F). This latter temperature exceeds the recommended level for exposure to thermal radiation for some conditions as given in Table 5-2.

5.5 ULTRAVIOLET RADIATION EFFECTS ON THE SKIN

5.5.1 Ultraviolet Erythema

Everyone is familiar with sunburn. The medical term for this well-known reddening of the skin by ultraviolet radiation (or by other means) is *erythema* (red = erythros in Greek). Erythema from ultraviolet radiation is a difficult process to describe in simple terms. Photobiologists and dermatologists normally describe ultraviolet erythema in terms of an action spectrum; that is, a graph which shows

Optical Radiation Hazards to the Skin

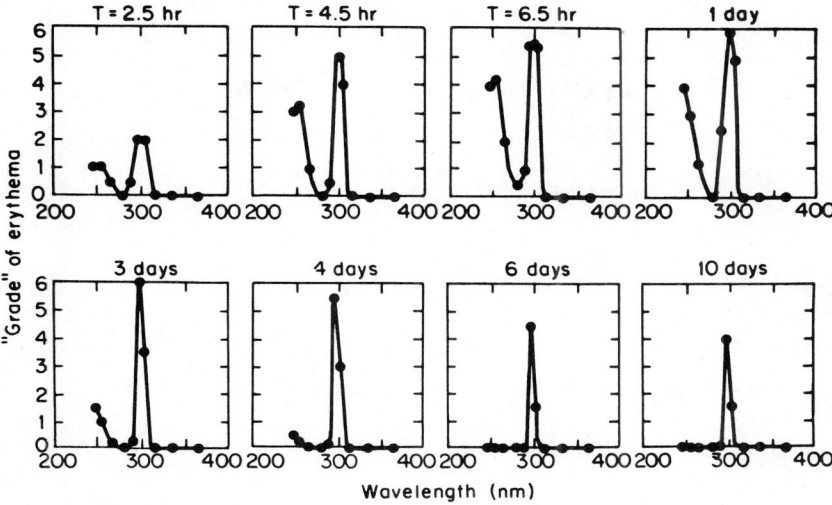

Figure 5-6. Time course of moderate ultraviolet erythema. Ultraviolet erythema action spectra obtained by Hausser (1928) for eight different observation times (from Sliney and Freasier, (1973).

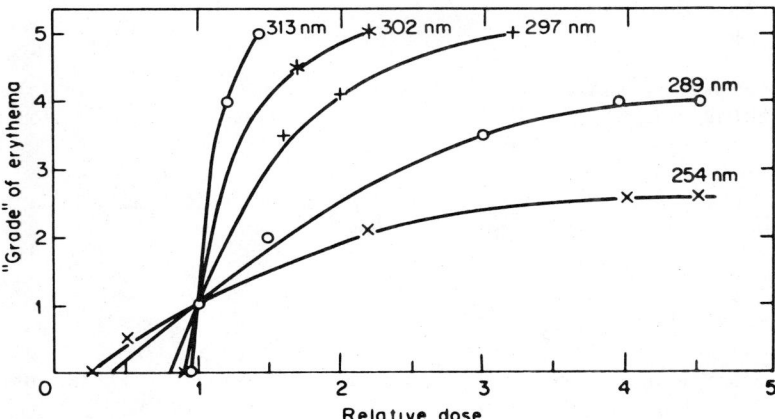

Figure 5-7. The degree or *grade* of erythema (skin reddening) for increasing dose. The monochromatic UV-B radiation penetrates more deeply into the skin than UV-C radiation and is far more effective in producing serious erythema (as well as longer-lasting tan). The grading system of Hausser and Vahle (1921) consisted of a comparison of skin redness with a logarithmic density scale obtained with red dye solutions. An erythema grade of 1 was above minimal erythema (based on Hausser and Vahle, 1921; from Sliney and Freasier, 1973).

TABLE 5-3. Reported Minimal Erythema Dose (MED) Values for Normal, Untanned, Human Skin

Reference	MED (mJ/cm^2)			
	297-300 nm Wavelength		254-260 nm Wavelength	
	at 6-8 hrs	at 24 hrs	at 6-8 hrs	at 24 hrs
Berger, Urbach and Davies, 1968	14	14	6.3	10
Blum and Terus, 1946		29.2		4.2
Coblentz, Stair, and Hogue, 1932		50		17
Cripps, Ramsey and Ruch, 1971	7†-13*	7†-12*	3.7	3.9
Freeman, Owens, Knox, and Hudson, 1966		12		8.5
Luckiesh, Holladay, and Taylor, 1930		4.3		3.4
Magnus, 1964	50		25	
Rottier and van der Leun, 1960		25		
Sayre, Olson, and Everett, 1966	16†-23*		7.2	

† at 297 nm
* at 300 nm

NOTE: The substantial variation in the MED's can be explained by variation in experimental methods, biologic variability and definition of MED. The earlier investigators used low pressure Hg lamps and attempted to use isolated lines, whereas the recent studies generally used monochromators with xenon-arc lamps and significant bandpass (e.g., 10 nm). The uniformity of the beam, cleanliness and location of the untanned skin, and radiometric measurement and calibration techniques can also affect the result.

the relative effectiveness of various wavelengths of ultraviolet radiation in eliciting the response. The action spectrum of ultraviolet erythema was investigated by several teams of physicists in the 1920s and early 1930s. Figures 5-6 and 5-7 illustrate some of the key findings of Hausser and Vahle (1927) which represent the classical work on this subject. These are generally summarized in many textbooks by a single graph representing a "standard" action spectrum for obtaining a minimal erythemal dose (MED). All investigators emphasized the importance of noting the length of time following the exposure for the various degrees of erythema to develop and the value of defining the action spectrum at a well-defined degree of redness and not at a "just perceptible erythema." They all chose to work with exposure doses above those where the highly transitory erythema produced by UV-C radiation played a significant role. Some representative MED's of several investigators are given in Table 5-3.

More recent dermatological investigations (Everett et al., 1965, Freeman et al., 1966) revealed that the action spectrum for this "just perceptible erythema" was quite different from the classical curve, which is not at all surprising. Erythemal thresholds vary significantly with the skin pigmentation and with the thickness of the stratum corneum over at least one order of magnitude. Erythemal thresholds for very dark skin may be more than ten times greater than those for very light Caucasian skin. Erythemal thresholds for skin of intermediate pigmentation will fall in between these extremes. The erythema threshold for skin stripped of its stratum corneum is approximately 3 mJ/cm^2 from 250 to 290 nm which is similar to photokeritits thresholds (Everett et al., 1965).

Clearly, to choose the proper action spectrum from a health hazard standpoint is dependent upon how it would be applied. An action spectrum used to develop hazard criteria for occupational exposure to incoherent and coherent ultraviolet radiation requires a judgement of the exposures that result in acute as well as chronic effects. Erythema production for a given spectral source is dependent only upon the total radiant exposure dose. *Reciprocity* exists in this relationship; the product of irradiance and exposure duration (the radiant exposure) is a constant over the total exposure duration range. This reciprocity for UV skin erythema has been shown to exist over a wide range of exposure durations, from microseconds to more than an hour.

The exact reactive mechanism of ultraviolet erythema is still not really understood. Despite the many studies which have described the wavelength specificity, character, and time course of the response, there have been few studies of the exact chain of events which transpire from the absorption of a UV photon by a chromaphore to the delayed response. To date any description is largely a matter of speculation. Ultraviolet erythema *per se* is a general inflammatory reaction and differs only slightly from other erythemal reactions due to chemical and physical insults. The available responses of any biologic tissue is, after all, quite limited. The actual red appearance of the skin is due largely to vasodilation (enlargement of blood vessels, especially capillaries) in the dermis. Accompanying the vasodilation is an increase in capillary permeability which permits larger serum proteins to enter the dermis, shifting the osmotic pressure at the capillary wall such that edema (swelling) takes place from increased water entering the dermis. Other biological protective and reparative processes involving lymphocytes and leukocytes also are associated with the inflammation. One popular theory has the UV chromophore in the epidermal keratinocytes. Upon UV exposure some intracellular substances are released and gradually diffuse to the dermis where vasodilation is triggered. This would explain the latent period of several hours. Suffice to say that erythema is only the outward appearance of a complex reaction involving many cellular and subcellular responses, and that the chain of events, triggered initially by the absorption of UV photons by some, as yet unclear chromophore, is little understood.

Indeed, the wavelength dependence of the delay in erythema suggests that at least two (one in the UV-C and another in the (UV-B), if not more, chromophores are involved in the erythemal response (van der Luen, 1965; Fitzpatrick *et al.*, 1974; Parrish *et al.*, 1978).

The skin, unlike the cornea of the eye, does develop its own protection against ultraviolet radiation. Indeed, there are two self-protective effects that occur in the skin following exposure to actinic UV radiation (UV-B and UV-C: melanogenesis (tanning) and skin thickening. The exact mechanism of melanogenesis is not well understood; several theories have been put forward. Although a very slight immediate pigment darkening (IPD) or immediate tanning (IT) is sometimes observable, it is only transient, lasting perhaps for 3 to 36 hours. The explanation often given for IPD is that it is photooxidation (darkening) of preformed melanin. Melanogenesis, or delayed tanning (DT) does not become evident for several days following the exposure. Although IPD is most strongly stimulated by UV-A, and DT most strongly by UV-B and somewhat by UV-A, an individual with a greater pigmentation baseline (often called "constitutive" pigmentation) will have a greater ease in achieving IPD and DT than a very fair-skin individual. Melanogenesis occurs in the melanocytes; melanosomes within the melanocytes produce melanin granules which are then transferred to adjacent keratinocytes. The melanin then is carried through the layers of the epidermis for the life of the keratinocyte (Fitzpatrick *et al.*, 1974).

As the skin becomes more pigmented, the melanin granules in the skin tend to absorb and scatter the incident ultraviolet radiation to decrease the dose to the sensitive tissue. In addition to increased pigmentation, the stratum corneum thickens (Kligman, 1969). At one time it was thought that the stratum corneum thickness varied with race, but this is now known to be untrue (Table 3-3). Since the layer of dead horny tissue has a high absorptivity for ultraviolet radiation, far less ultraviolet radiation reaches the living tissue to cause injury after the stratum corneum thickens (Everett *et al.*, 1966).

Although actinic ultraviolet radiation (in the UV-C and UV-B ranges) is normally considered to be the cause of sunburn and other forms of UV erythema, radiation in the near ultraviolet spectrum (UV-A) can also cause erythema (Parrish *et al.*, 1976). The thresholds for UV-A erythema are quite high—typically of the order of 20 to 60 J/cm^2, whereas thresholds for producing mild erythema on the untanned Caucasian skin from 297-nm radiation are typically near 10-20 mJ/cm^2 (Table 5-3). As described above Melanogenesis, or suntanning, begins to occur shortly after exposure to UV-B and UV-C radiation. Part of the UV-A radiation also aids in this process.

The erythemal response is independent of the size of the area irradiated except for very small areas where the scattering and diffusion of the stratum corneum and the epidermis create a larger effective irradiated area within the inner layer of the epidermis and the corneum. It is generally accepted that for irradiated spot sizes exceeding 2-3 mm in diameter, the MED does not vary with spot size. A common notion that wet skin is more susceptible than dry skin does not appear to have any basis in fact. Although one could theorize a focusing effect by water droplets, the internal scattering in the skin should counter this effect. Perhaps the

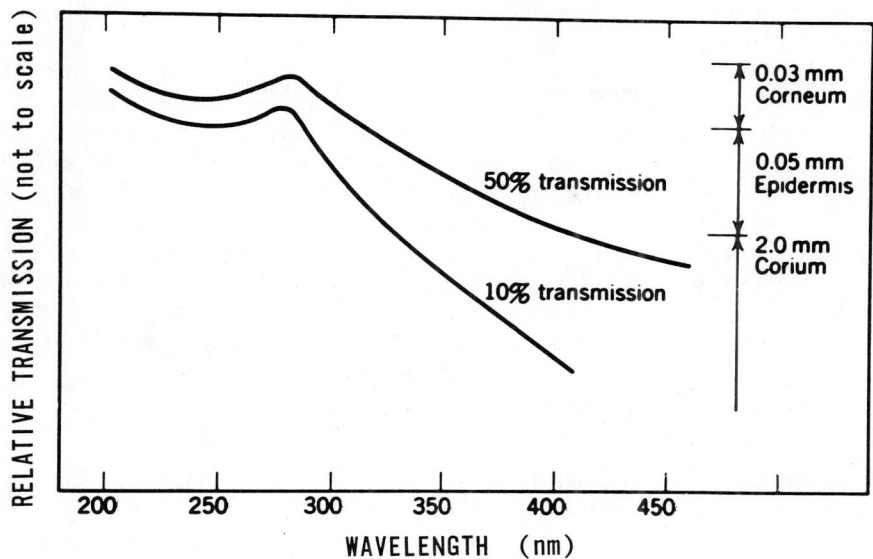

Figure 5-8. Quantitative spectral measurements of the penetration of human skin by ultraviolet radiation (adapted from E. Fischer and S. Solomon, "Ultraviolet Radiation," E. Licht, New Haven, 1959).

creation of a smooth surface of water increases the optical coupling, but this could produce only a marginal variation.

5.5.2 Delayed Effects

Chronic exposures to ultraviolet radiation are known to accelerate skin aging and it is now generally agreed that such exposures increase the risk of certain types of skin cancer. Such skin cancers show up only upon the exposed areas of skin, such as the face, hands, and back of the neck, which are chronically exposed to sunlight. Individuals in outdoor occupations, such as farmers, have the highest incidence of this type of skin cancer (Urbach, 1969).

The exact action spectrum of UV skin carcinogenesis is unknown because of the enormous and lengthy laboratory study that would be required to develop definitive spectral thresholds. Some limited information for UV carcinogenesis in rats points largely toward UV-B, as the UV-B radiation penetrates more deeply into the skin (Fig. 5-8) than radiation in the rest of the actinic ultraviolet spectrum: UV-C radiation (Rusch, Kline, and Baumann, 1941). For this reason UV-B is the most effective in affecting living tissue, as is attested by its capability of producing the more severe grades of erythema. Several epidemiologic studies of skin cancer incidence reveal a very strong correlation with terrestrial solar UV-B radiation levels found at given latitudes and ground elevations. These correlations will be illustrated further in Chapter 6 (Figs. 6-5 to 6-7).

In setting an exposure limit for ultraviolet radiation including that from ultraviolet lasers, it has generally been assumed that the probability of skin carcinogenesis would be remote if chronic radiation levels were kept below those required to cause even the slightest barely perceptible erythema. A quantitative definitive threshold for carcinogenesis by ultraviolet radiation appears to be very difficult to define, if indeed such a threshold does exist. A "qualified threshold" (see section 7.3.1) probably does exist. A practical threshold obviously does exist in that all individuals receive a daily UV exposure dose due to UV-B transmission through clothing. This dose is only two or three orders of magnitude less than the dose to exposed parts of the body. Epidemiologic studies correlating solar and ultraviolet exposure with skin cancer may shed some light on whether quantitative thresholds can be defined for human skin cancer.

5.6 PHOTOSENSITIVITY AND PHOTOALLERGY

Some rare individuals are hypersensitive to irradiation from specific optical spectral bands and may develop skin reactions (described as "photosensitivity") following suberythemal exposure. Quite often UV-A exposure will cause a skin reaction similar to that of UV-B (Cripps et al., 1970). In the industrial environment it is highly unusual for the symptoms of photosensitization to be elicited solely by a limited emission spectrum from industrial optical sources, such as "black light" and certain UV lasers. Sunlight will usually elicit or aggravate any skin response. Certain systemic drugs (for example tetracycline and the psoralens) induce hypersensitivity to ultraviolet radiation in many individuals. Topical agents such as lime oil or lime juice applied to skin will also lower the threshold for erythema from ultraviolet radiation. Some rare individuals also have photoallergic reactions, but these individuals are well aware of their problem from exposure to sunlight and would therefore be expected to be cautious whenever in a laser or ultraviolet radiation environment. Table 5-4, prepared by Fitzpatrick and coworkers, summarizes such reactions and the wavelengths which elicit them. Table 5-5 lists common photosensitizers.

5.7 PHOTOTHERAPY

In recent years dermatologists have made use of specialized UV-A sources in phototherapy with orally administered psoralens. Such phototherapy has been shown to be quite effective in eliminating the symptoms of psoriasis and several other skin diseases. The patient is exposed to a controlled dose of UV sunlight or more often to artificial sources arranged in a special cabinet (Figure 5-9).

As a result of the great interest in UV phototherapy (Chapter 22) and its possible delayed effects, there has been an accelerated effort to understand all of the basic interactions of ultraviolet radiation in skin tissue. Hopefully all of this interest will foster the development of UV protection standards worthy of confidence.

TABLE 5-4. Some Examples of Action Spectra of Normal
and Abnormal Reactions in Man

Condition	Wavelength Range (nm)	Maximum Reaction (nm)
Normal sunburn	290-320	297-307
Artificial light sources	250-320	250
Melanin pigmentation	290-320	290-310
	320-480	
Vitamin D production	290-310	290
Hyperbilirubinemia of prematurity	Blue visible spectrum	440-470
UV carcinogenesis	290-320	290-310
Solar urticaria	290-320	varying
	320-400	
	400-600	
Porphyris photosensitivity	380-600	400-410
Xeroderma pigmentosum	290-340	293-307
Polymorphic photodermatitis	290-320	290-320
	320-400	
Lupus erythematosus (LE) and discoid LE	290-320	
Solar (actinic) degeneration	290-400	?
Photoallergic reactions to halogenated salicylanilides and other related compounds	320-380	330-360
Phototoxic reactions to drugs	320-400	320-400
	290-320	
Psoralens (8-methoxy-and trimethylpsoralen)	320-380	330-360

[from T. B. Fitzpatrick *et al.*, 1974, with permission]

TABLE 5-5a. Contact Photosensitizers: Chemicals that Induce Photosensitivity in Man

Name	Use
Halogenated salicylanilides; 3,3',4',5-tetrachlorosalicylanilide; 3,4',5-trichloro- and 3,3',5-trichlorosalicylanilide; 3,3',5-tribromo- and 3,3',5-tribromosalicylanilide; 3,5-dibromo- and 4',5-dibromosalicylanilide	Deodorant, bacteriostatic agents in soaps
Hexachlorophene	Antimicrobial, antiseptic
Bithionol or bis-(2-hydroxy-3,5-dichlorophenyl) sulfide	Antimicrobial, antiseptic
Fentichlor (2,2'-dihydroxy-5,5'-dichlorodiphenyl sulfide); multifungin (bromchlorsalicylanilid); jadit (4-chloro-2-hydroxybenzoic acid-N-n-butylamide)	Antifungal
5-Flurouracil	Antineoplastic
p-aminobenzoic acid (PABA) and esters of PABA	Sunscreen
4,4'-Bis(3-phenylureido)-2,2'-stilbenedisulfonic acid) or blankophor	Fluorescent brightening agent for cellulose, nylon, or wool fibers
Cadmium sulfide	In tattoos
Furocoumarins: psoralen, 8-methoxypsoralen, 5-methoxypsoralen 4,5',8-trimethylpsoralen	In vitiligo for increased pigment formation and sun tolerance
Essential oils: oil of bergamot, oil of lime, oil of cedar, oil of lavender, oil of citron, oil of sandalwood	Cosmetics and beauty aids
Plants: Umbelliferae, Rutaceae	Used in perfumes or flavorings or as spices
Dyes: fluorescein, rose bengal, eosin, erythrocine, trypaflavin, blue, trypan blue	Cosmetics and dye industry
Coal tar and coal tar derivatives containing anthracene, phenanthrene, naphthalene, thiophene, and many phenolic agents; pitch	In therapy for psoriasis and chronic eczema: in hair shampoos

[from T. B. Fitzpatrick et al., 1974, with permission]

TABLE 5-5b. Systemic Photosensitizers: Chemicals that Induce Photosensitivity

Name	Uses
Sulfonamides Sulfanilamide, sulfathiazole, sulfapyridine, sulfamethazine sulfaguanidine, sulfisoxazole, monochlorphenamide	Chemotherapy, antibacterial agents
Sulfonylurea Carbutamide, tolbutamide (Orinase), chlorpropamide (Diabinese)	Hypoglycemic or antidiabetic drugs
Chlorthiazides 6-Chlor-2H-1,2,4-benzothiadiazine-7-sulfonamide-1,1-dioxide (Hydrodiuril)	Diuretics, antihypertensive
Quinethazone (Hydromox)	Antihypertensive
Phenothiazines Chlorpromazine (Thorazine), promethazine (Phenergan), mepazine, Stelazine, trimeprazine, Compazine, promazine (Sparine)	Tranquilizer, nematode infestation agent, urinary antiseptic, antihistamine
Antibiotics Demethylchlortetracycline (Declomycin), chlortetracycline, oxytetracycline, doxycycline	Broad spectrum antibiotic
Griseofulvin	Antimycotic
Nalidixic acid (NegGram)	Antibacterial
Furocoumarins 4,5′,8-Trimethylpsoralen, 8-methoxypsoralen, psoralen	In vitiligo for sun tolerance and increased pigment formation
Estrogens and progesterones Mestranol and norethynodrel, diethylstilbesterol	Oral contraceptives
Chlordiazepoxide (Librium)	Tranquilizer, psychotropic
Triacetyldiphenolisatin	Laxative
Cyclamates, calcium cyclamate, sodium cyclohexylsulfamate	Artificial sweeteners

[from T. B. Fitzpatrick *et al.*, 1974, with permission]

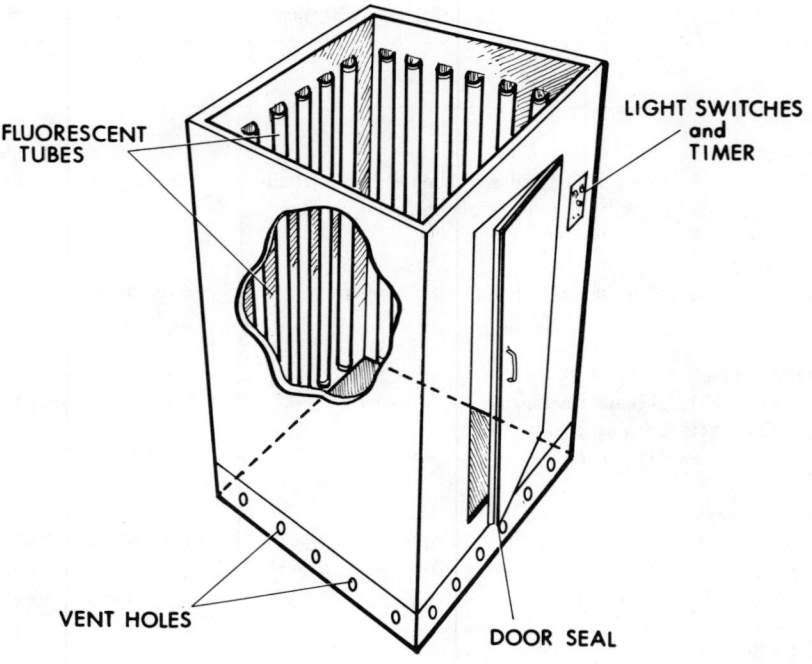

Figure 5-9. Medical UV source for controlled therapy of psoriasis. The safety aspects of this form of therapy are discussed in Chapter 22.

5.8 REVIEW QUESTIONS

1. The thickness of the stratum corneum is approximately: (a) 0.1 mm; (b) 1 mm; (c) 0.03 mm; (d) 0.5 mm.

2. Skin cancer is most often caused by: (a) intense visible light from the sun; (b) infrared radiation; (c) ultraviolet radiation; (d) none of the above.

3. At the 10.6 μm wavelength of the CO_2 laser the skin is: (a) highly reflective; (b) highly absorptive; (c) reflects 50% of the incident radiation; (d) does not absorb any radiation.

4. The threshold of injury from thermal radiation incident upon the skin is dependent upon irradiated area because of: (a) difference in penetration depth; (b) conduction of heat away from small spot sizes; (c) photochemical effects; (d) the rate process of thermal injury.

5. The temperature at which persistent pain occurs in the skin is: (a) 37°C; (b) 45°C; (c) 55°C; (d) 100°C.

6. The maximum recommended internal body temperature to prevent heat stress is: (a) 34°C; (b) 98.6°C; (c) 27°C; (d) 38°C.

7. Does heat flow within the skin play a significant role in determining the threshold of thermal injury of the skin?

5.9 REFERENCES

Bachem, A., 1929, The ultraviolet transparency of the various layers of human skin, *Am. J. Physiol.* **91**:58–64.

Bachem, A., 1955, Time factors of erythema and pigmentation, produced by ultraviolet rays of different wavelengths, *J. Invest. Dermatol.* **25**:215–218.

Berger, D., Urbach, F., and Davies, R. E., 1968, The action spectrum of erythema induced by ultraviolet radiation, preliminary report, "Proceedings, XIII, Congressus Internationalis Dermatologiae – München, 1967," pp. 1112–1117, Springer-Verlag, New York,

Blum, H. F., and Terus, W. S., 1946, Inhibition of erythema of sunburn by large doses of ultraviolet radiation, *and* The erythemal threshold for sunburn, *Am. J. Physiol.* **146**:97–106, 107–117.

Bode, H. G., and Witte, E., 1947, Uber den Zusammenhang zwischen absorierter Strahlenergie und biologischen Effeckt bei Bestrahlung mit Licht verschiedener Wellenlangen, *Strahlentherapie* **76**:627–663.

Brownell, A. S., Parr, W. H., and Hysell, D. K., 1969, Skin and carbon dioxide laser radiation, *Arch. Environ. Health* **18**:437–442.

Brownell, A. S., Hysell, D. K., and Parr, W. H., 1971, Millisecond exposure to simulated CO_2 laser radiation, Report 953, USAMRL Ft. Knox, KY.

Bücker, H., 1965, Zur Erythemwirkung optischer Strahlung, UV-Erythem–Wärmeerythem, *Strahlenther.* **115**:136–142.

Buettner, K., 1952, Effects of extreme heat and cold on human skin. Numerical analysis and pilot experiments on penetrating flash radiation effects, *J. Appl. Physiol.* **5**:207.

Buettner, K., 1937, Thermal radiation and the reflection properties of human skin, *Strahlenther.* **58**:345–360.

Claesson, S., Juhlin, L., and Wettermark, G., 1958, The reciprocity law of UV-irradiation effects, *Acta. Derm. Venereol.* (Stockh.) **38**:123–136.

Clark, C., Vinegar, R., and Hardy, J., 1953, Goniometer spectrometer for the measurement of diffuse reflectance and transmittance of skin in the infrared spectral region, *J. Opt. Soc. Am.* **43**:993–998.

Coblentz, W. W., and Stair, R., 1934, Data on the spectral erythemic reaction of the untanned human skin to ultraviolet radiation, *Bur. Stand. J. Res.* **12**:13–14.

Coblentz, W. W., Stair, R., and Hogue, J. M., 1931, The spectral erythemic reaction of the human skin to ultraviolet radiation, *Proc. Nat. Acad. Sci.* **17**(6):401–405, July 1931.

Cripps, D. J., Ramsay, C. A., and Ruch, D. M., 1971, Xeroderma Pigmentosum, *J. Invest. Derm.* **56**(4):281–286.

Daniels, F., Jr., Post, P. W., and Johnson, B. E., 1972, Theories of the role of pigment in the evolution of human races, *in* "Pigmentation: Its Genesis and Biologic Control," (V. Riley, ed.), pp. 2–22, Appleton Century Crafts, New York.

Davies, J. M., 1959, The Effect of Intense Thermal Radiation on Animal Skin. A Comparison of Calculated and Observed Burns. Report T-24, Army Quartermaster Research and Engineering Command, AD 456794, Natick, MA, (29 April 1959).
Davis, T. P., 1963, The heating of skin by radiant energy, in "Temperature, its measurement, and control in Science and Industry," (C. M. Herzfeld and J. D. Hardy, eds.) Vol. 3, pp. 149–169, Reinhold Publishing Corporation, New York.
Edwards, E., Finkelstein, N., Duntley, S. Q., 1951, Spectrophotometry of living human skin, the ultraviolet range, *J. Invest. Dermatol.* **16**:311.
Epstein, J. H., and Winkelmann, R. K., 1967, Ultraviolet light-induced kinin formation in human skin, *Arch. Dermatol.* **95**:532–536.
Evans, E., Brooks, J., Schmidt, F., Williams, R., and Ham, W. T., Jr., 1955, Flash burn studies on human volunteers, *Surgery* **37**:280.
Everett, M. A., Doran, C. K., Everett, H. D., and Anglin, J. H., Jr., 1963, Modification of sunburn by infrared rays, *J. Am. Med. Assn.* **186**(8):778–779.
Everett, M. A., Olson, R. L., and Sayre, R. M., 1965, Ultraviolet erythema, *Arch. Dermatol.* **92**: 713–719.
Everett, M. A., Waltermire, J. A., Olson, R., and Sayre, R., 1965, Modification of ultraviolet erythema by epidermal stripping, *Nature* **205**:812–813.
Everett, M. A., Yeargers, E., Sayre, R. M., Olson, R. L., 1966, Penetration of epidermis by ultraviolet rays, *Photochem. Photobiol.* **5**:533–542.
Findlay, G. H., 1967, An automatic fractionator for light dosage on the skin, its application to the polychromatic minimal erythema dose, *Brit. J. Derm.* **79**(3):148–152.
Fisher, E. and Solomon, S., 1959, "Ultraviolet Radiation," E. Licht, New Haven, Conn.
Fitzpatrick, T. B., Pathak, M. A., Harber, L. C., Seiji, M. and Kukita, A., 1974, "Sunlight and Man, Normal and Abnormal Photobiologic Responses," University of Tokyo Press, Tokyo.
Freeman, R. G., Owens, D. W., Knox, J. M., and Hudson, H. T., 1966, Relative energy requirements for an erythemal response of skin to monchromatic wavelengths of ultraviolet present in the solar spectrum, *J. Invest. Derm.* **64**:586–592.
Freeman, R. G., Owens, D. W., Knox, J. M., and Hudson, H. T., 1966, Relative energy requirements for an erythemal response of skin to monchromatic wavelengths of ultraviolet resent in the solar spectrum, *J. Invest. Dermat.* **47**(6):586–592.
Goldman, L., Rockwell, R. J., and Richfield, D., 1971, Long-term laser exposure of a senile freckle, *Arch. Environ. Health* **22**:401–403.
Green, A. E. S., Findley, G. B., Klenk, K. F., Wilson, W. M., and Mo, T., 1976, The ultraviolet dose dependence on non-melanoma skin cancer incidence, *Photochem. Photobiol.* **24**:353–362.
Hardy, J. D., 1968, Pain following step increase in skin temperature, in "The Skin Senses," (D. R. Kenshalo, ed.), pp. 444–456, Charles C. Thomas, Springfiled, IL.
Hardy, J. D., Hammell, H. T., Murgatroyd, D., 1957, Spectral transmittance and reflectance of excised human skin, *J. Appl. Physiol.* **9**:257–264.
Hasselbalch, K. A., 1911, Quantitative Untersuchengen uber die Absorption der menschlichen Haut von ultravioletten Strahlen, *Skandinav. Archs. Physiol.* **25**:55.
Hausser, I., 1939, Uber Einzel-und Kombinationswirkungen des kurzwelligen und langwelligen Ultravioletts bei Bestrahlung der menschlichen Haut, *Naturwissenschaften* **33**:563–566.
Hausser, K. W., 1929, Einfluss der Wellenlänge in der Strahlenbiologie, *Strahlenther.* **28**:25–44.
Hausser, K. W., and Vahle, W., 1922, Uber die Abhängigkeit des Lichterythems und der Pigmentbildung von der Schwingungszahl (Wellenlänge) der erregenden Strahlung, *Strahlenther.* **13**: 41–71.
Hausser, K. W., and Gauer, O., 1933, Die absolute Empfindichkeit der Lichterythembildung, *Strahlenther.* **48**:230.

Hausser, K. W., and Vahle, W., 1969, Sonnenbrand und Sonnenbräunung, *Wiss. Veröff. Siemens* **6**:101-120, (Transl. in Urbach, 1969).

Henriques, F. C., Jr., 1947, Studies of thermal injuries, V. The predictability and the significance of thermally induced rate processes leading to irreversible epidermal injury, *Am. J. Path.* **23**:489–502.

Henriques, F. C., Jr. and Moritz, A. R., 1947, Studies of thermal injury, I. The conduction of heat to and through skin and the temperatures attained therein. A theoretical and an experimental investigation, *Am. J. Path.* **23**:531–549.

Jacquez, J. A., Huss, J., McKeenan, W., Dimitroff, J. M., and Kuppenheim, H. F., 1956, Spectral reflectance of human skin in the region 0.7 - 2.6 µm, *J. Appl. Physiol.* **8**:297–299.

Jacquez, J. A., Kuppenheim, H. F., Dimitroff, J. M., McKeenan, W., and Huss, J., 1955, Spectral reflectance of human skin in the region 235–700 mµ, *J. Appl. Physiol.* **8**:212–214.

Jacquez, J. A., and Kuppenheim, H. F., 1956, Spectral reflectance of human skin in the region 235–1000 mµ, *J. Appl. Physiol.* **8**:212.

Johnson, B. E., and Daniels, F., Jr., 1969, Lysosomes and the reactions of skin to ultraviolet radiation, *J. Invest. Dermatol.* **53**:85–94.

Johnson, B. E., Mandel, G., and Daniels, F., Jr., 1972, Melanin and cellular reactions to ultraviolet radiation, *Nature & New Biol.* **235**:147–149.

Kligman, A., 1969, Comments on the stratum corneum, *in* "The Biological Effects of Ultraviolet Radiation," (F. Urbach, ed.), pp. 165–167, Pergamon Press, Oxford.

Logan, G., and Wilhelm, D. L., 1966, The inflammatory reaction in ultraviolet injury, *Br. J. Exp. Pathol.* **47**:286–299.

Loomis, W. F., 1970, Rickets, *Sci. Am.* **223**:77–91.

Lucas, N. S., 1930, The permeability of human epidermis to ultraviolet radiation, *Biochem. J.* **25**:57–70.

Luckiesh, M., Holladay, L. L., and Taylor, A. H., 1930, Reactions of untanned skin to ultraviolet radiation, *J. Opt. Soc. Amer.* **20**(8):423–432.

Luckiesh, M., 1946, "Application of Germicidal, Erythemal and Infrared Energy," Van Nostrand, New York.

Magnus, I. A., 1976, "Dermatological Photobiology," Blackwell Scientific, Oxford.

Magnus, I. A., 1964, Studies with a monchromator in the common idiopathic photodermatoses, *Brit. J. Dermat.* **76**:245–264.

Magnus, I. A., 1969, Biologic action spectra, introduction and general review, *in* "The Biologic Effects of Ultraviolet Radiation," (F. Urbach, ed.) pp. 175–179, Pergamon Press, New York.

Moritz, A. R., and Henriques, F. C., Jr., 1947, Studies of thermal injury, II. The relative importance of time and surface temperature in the causation of cutaneous burns, *Am. J. Path.* **23**:695–710.

Ogura, R. M. and Knox, J. M., 1974, Biochemical changes in ultraviolet light-irradiated epidermis, *in* "Sunlight and Man," (M. A. Pathak, L. C. Harber, M. Seiji, A. Kukita, eds.; T. B. Fitzpatrick, consulting ed.) pp. 147–156, University of Tokyo Press, Tokyo.

Olson, R. L., Sayre, R. M., and Everett, M. A., 1966, Effect of anatomic location and time on ultraviolet erythema, *Arch. Dermatol.* **93**:211–215.

Olson, R. L., Sayre, R. M., and Everett, M. A., 1965, Effect of field size on ultraviolet minimal erythema dose, *J. Invest. Dermat.* **45**(6):516–519.

Owens, D. W., Knox, J. M., Hudson, H. T., and Troll, D., 1975, Influence of humidity on ultraviolet injury, *J. Invest. Dermat.* **64**:250–252.

Parr, W. H., 1969, Skin Lesion Threshold Values for Laser Radiation as Compared with Safety Standards. Report 813, US Army Medical Research Laboratory, Fort Knox, KY (AD688871) (24 February 1969).

Parrish, J. A., Anderson, R. R., Urbach, F., and Pitts, D., 1978, "UV-A, Biological Effects of Ultraviolet Radiation with Emphasis on Human Responses to Longwave Ultraviolet," Plenum Press, New York.

Parrish, J. A., Anderson, R. R., Ying, C. Y. and Pathak, M. A., 1976, Cutaneous effects of pulsed nitrogen gas laser irradiation, *J. Invest. Dermatol.* 67:603–608.

Parrish, J. A., Ying, C. Y., Pathak, M. A., and Fitzpatrick, T. B., 1974, Erythemogenic properties of long-wave ultraviolet light, in "Sunlight and Man," (M. A. Pathak, L. C. Harber, M. Seiji, A. Kukita, eds.; T. B. Fitzpatrick, consulting ed.) pp. 131–141, University of Tokyo Press, Tokyo.

Pathak, M. A., Hori, Y., Szabo, G., and Fitzpatrick, T. B., 1971, The photobiology of melanin pigmentation in human skin, in "Biology of Normal and Abnormal Melanocytes," (T. Kawamura, T. B. Fitzpatrick, M. Seiji, eds.) pp. 149–167, University of Tokyo Press, Tokyo.

Pathak, M. A., and Stratton, K., 1968, Free radicals in human skin before and after exposure to light, *Arch. Biochem. Biophys.* 123:468–476.

Rockwell, R. J., Jr., and Goldman, L., 1974, Research on Human Skin Laser Damage Threshold. Final Report, Contract F41609-72-C-0007, USAF School of Aerospace Medicine, Brooks Air Force Base, TX, prepared by Department of Dermatology and Laser Lab Med. Center, University of Cincinnati (June 1974).

Rottier, P. B., and van der Leun, J. C., 1960, Hyperaemia of the deeper cutaneous vessels after irradiation of human skin with large doses of ultraviolet light and visible light, *Brit. J. Derm.* 72:256.

Rusch, H. P., Kline, B. E., and Baumann, C. A., 1941, Carcinogenesis by ultraviolet rays with reference to wavelength and energy, *AMA Arch. Path.* 31:135–146.

Sans, W. M., Jr., 1974, Inflammatory mediators in ultraviolet erythema, in "Sunlight and Man," (M. A. Pathak, L. C. Harber, M. Seiji, A. Kukita, eds.; T. B. Fitzpatrick, consulting ed.) pp. 143–146, University of Tokyo Press, Tokyo.

Sayre, R. M., Olson, R. L., and Everett, M. A., 1966, Quantitative studies on erythema, *J. Invest. Derm.* 46(3):240–244.

Schmidt, K., 1963, Vergleich intermittierender und kontinuierlicher UV-Bestrahlung bei der Hauterythembildung, *Strahlenther.* 121:383–391.

Schmidt, K., 1964, Zur Hauterythemwirkung von UV-Blitzen, *Strahlenther.* 124:127–136.

Schmidt, R. H., Williams, R. C., Ham, W. R., Brooks, J. W., and Evans, E. I., 1954, Experimental production of flash burns, *Surg.* 36:1163.

Seidl, E., 1963, Uber Erythem– und Pigmentwirksamkeit berschiedener UV-Strahler, *Strahlenther.* 121:450–463.

Snyder, D. S., 1975, Cutaneous effects of topical indomethacin, an inhibitor of prostaglandin synthesis, on UV-damaged skin, *J. Invest Dermatol.* 64:322–325.

Stern, W. K., 1972, Anatomic localization of the response to ultraviolet radiation in human skin, *Dermatologica* 145:361–370.

Thomson, M. L., 1955, The relative efficiency of pigment and horny layer thickness in protecting the skin of Europeans and Africans against solar ultraviolet radiation, *J. Physiol.* 127:236–246.

Treagar, R. T., 1966, "Physical Functions of the Skin," Academic Press, New York.

Urbach, F. (ed.), 1969, "The Biologic Effects of Ultraviolet Radiation," Pergamon Press, New York.

Valtonen, E. J., 1965, Studies of the mechanism of ultraviolet erythema formation, the role of histamine and histadine, *Acta Derm.-Venereol.* 45:199–202.

van der Luen, J. C., 1966, "Ultraviolet erythema: a study on diffusion processes in human skin," Thesis, Utrecht.

van der Leun, J. C., 1965, Observations on ultraviolet erythema, *Photochem. Photobiol.* 4:447–451.
van der Leun, J. C., 1965, Theory of ultraviolet erythema, *Photochem. Photobiol.* 4:453–458.
Willis, I. and Cylus, L., 1977, UV-A erythema in skin: is it a sunburn? *J. Invest. Derm.* 68:128–129.
Willis, I., Kligman, A., and Epstein, J., 1972, Effects of long ultraviolet rays on human skin: photoprotective or photoaugmentative? *J. Invest. Derm.* 59:416–420.
Ying, C. Y., Parrish, J. A., and Pathak, M. A., 1974, Additive erythemogenic effects of middle– (280-320 nm) and (320-400 nm) long-wave ultraviolet light, *J. Invest. Derm.* 63:273–278.

Chapter 6
Optical Hazards from the Ambient Environment

6.1 INTRODUCTION

A proper appreciation of eye and skin hazards from optical radiation requires an understanding of man's exposure in his natural environment. A knowledge of biological thresholds as determined in the laboratory and clinic provides only an incomplete understanding of the relative importance of different adverse effects. It must be remembered that mankind has evolved over many millenia the natural, inborn protective reactions and social habits for protection against a rather harsh natural environment. Hence a prior understanding of this environment and normal exposure conditions is necessary before considering exposure limits and safety standards.

By far the most commonly encountered injury due to optical radiation in man's normal outdoor environment is sunburn (erythema solare), which results from the small fraction of actinic UV-B radiation in the terrestrial solar spectrum. Although man and other forms of life on this planet are largely protected from the short-wave ultraviolet radiation (UV-B and UV-C) by the ozone layer in the upper atmosphere, a harmful amount of UV-B nevertheless reaches the earth. The ocular counterpart of sunburn is the very painful aspect of snow blindness. This combination of photokeratitis and conjunctivitis can result from the reflection of the actinic ultraviolet radiation from snow. Less obvious effects from chronic exposure to solar ultraviolet radiation are cancer and accelerated aging of the skin, and corneal degeneration and lens cataract in the eye.

The etiology of each of those latter effects is still debatable. Nevertheless a growing contingent of the scientific world are beginning to link ultraviolet radiation with one type of spheroidal degeneration of the cornea as well as with brunescent and other types of senile cataracts.

In addition to these effects of ultraviolet radiation upon the eye and skin most people are aware of the effects upon the retina of staring directly at the sun. Throughout history, cases of eclipse blindness have been associated with every solar eclipse. Also, recent reports have suggested that the short wavelengths within the visible spectrum (400 to 500 nm) may be responsible for certain types of retinal degeneration and for accelerating other retinal disease states. A discussion of all of these effects will be helpful prior to considering the hazards of man-made optical sources.

6.2 SUNBURN

The characteristics of ultraviolet erythema (skin reddening) were discussed in detail previously (Chapter 5). It is interesting that the classic work on this subject was performed by a German physicist, K. W. Hausser in the 1920's, as a result of his own experiences with sunburn while walking on a glacier in the Alps. Dr. Hausser, a radiological physicist for the Siemens Corporation in Germany, was afflicted with tuberculosis and had to spend some time at a sanitarium in the Alps. Late one afternoon he walked for several hours on a nearby glacier and experienced no difficulties. Several days later he took a brief walk for less than an hour at noontime and developed a severe sunburn. Puzzled as to why he had been sunburned in a short time on the second day, he hypothesized that the sun's ultraviolet radiation, which was already known to be linked with sunburn, varied in intensity as a function of the time of day. This led him to his classic experiments with W. Vahle (Hausser and Vahle, 1927) which showed the ability not only of different irradiance levels but also of different wavelengths to elicit different degrees of erythema. They also found that even the time course of erythema was a function of wavelength. The normal, untanned Caucasian skin will have a noticeable erythema after an exposure of 30 minutes to the noonday summer sun at mid lattitudes. To acquire the same dose of ultraviolet radiation at 4 p.m. on a summer day would require an exposure of 3 to 4 hours, since the ultraviolet spectral irradiance at 300 nm decreases by a factor of 10 from noontime to 4 p.m. (Fig. 6-1).

Because of the great interest in skin cancer induced by solar ultraviolet radiation, there have been many studies of the variations of actinic ultraviolet radiation as a function of daytime, cloud cover, geographical location, and latitude. One of the more interesting results is that the total ultraviolet dose for a day in the arctic during the summer is at least twice that in the middle latitudes, such as Washington, DC. Figure 6-2 provides a plot of the solar spectral irradiance for different solar zenith angles in the northern hemisphere. For the same zenith angle the sun actually delivers slightly more radiation in the winter time because the distance between the earth and the sun is shorter. However, because of the lower solar elevation angles (greater zenith angles) in winter, the daily ultraviolet dose is far less than in the summer. The increase in atmospheric pathlength for the direct rays with the increase in the sun's zenith angle is accompanied by a dramatic decrease in the ultraviolet radiation reaching the earth. Thus the total solar irradiance may decrease by only 20% as the sun goes from zenith to 50° below zenith (40° elevation

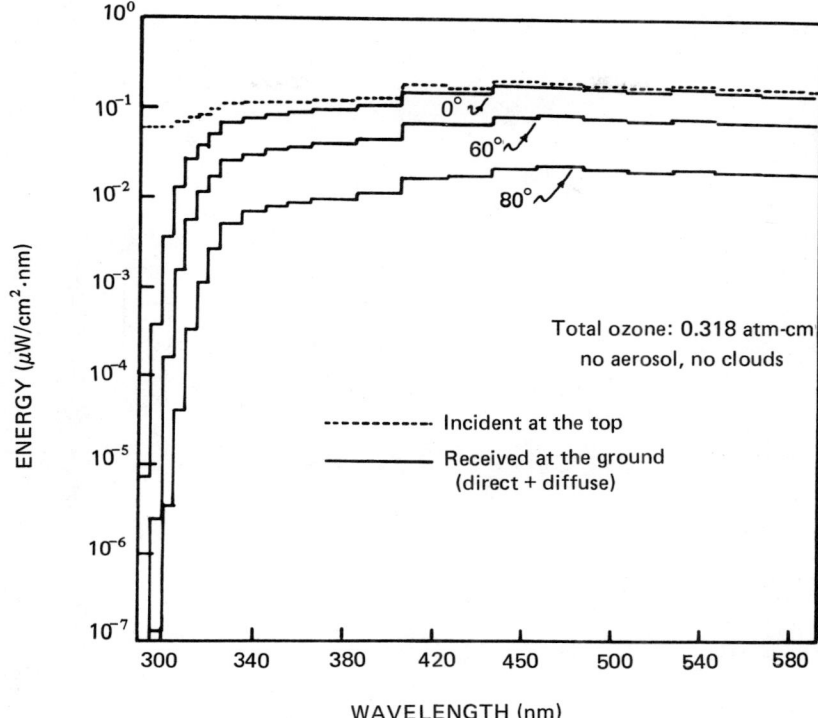

Figure 6-1. Solar spectral irradiance for zenith angles in the northern hemisphere as calculated by Gates (1966). Note the substantial change at 300 nm with change in zenith angle, and the rapid increase in spectral irradiance from 300 to 310 nm. The unit microwatts-per-square-centimeter-per-nanometer is equivalent to milliwatts-per-square-centimeter-per-micrometer.

angle) but the actinic ultraviolet irradiance drops by nearly an order of magnitude. Figure 6-3 illustrates the variation in the average daily total ultraviolet energy reaching the earth on a horizontal surface for each month in the Washington, DC area and in the arctic at Point Barrow, Alaska. There is no ultraviolet and indeed no solar radiation at Point Barrow, Alaska during part of December and January, since the sun never rises there during that period.

6.3 SKIN EFFECTS FROM CHRONIC EXPOSURE

Accelerated skin aging and skin cancer have been linked with ultraviolet radiation for some time, although a large sector of the public still seems unconcerned or even ignorant of this. Each year millions flock to the beaches to seek their share of actinic ultraviolet radiation. To avoid severe sunburn these people would be prudent

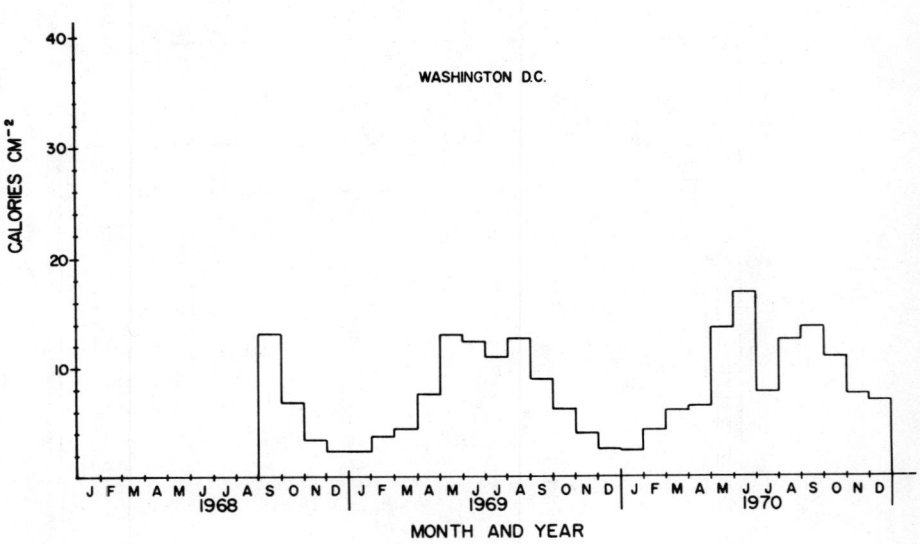
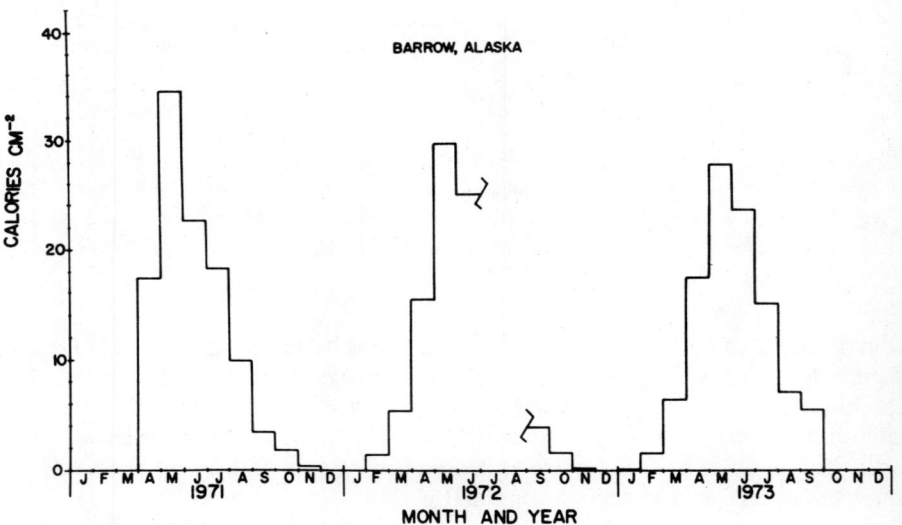

Figure 6-2a. Variation in monthly ultraviolet energy. The two panels show the average daily total ultraviolet energy from the sun and sky (global radiant energy) incident upon a horizontal surface for each month in Washington, DC and in the Point Barrow, Alaska areas. Notice that although the total accumulated ultraviolet radiant exposure in Washington, DC probably exceeds that at Point Barrow, Alaska, there are higher monthly doses in summer months at Point Barrow than in Washington (from Klein and Goldberg, 1974).

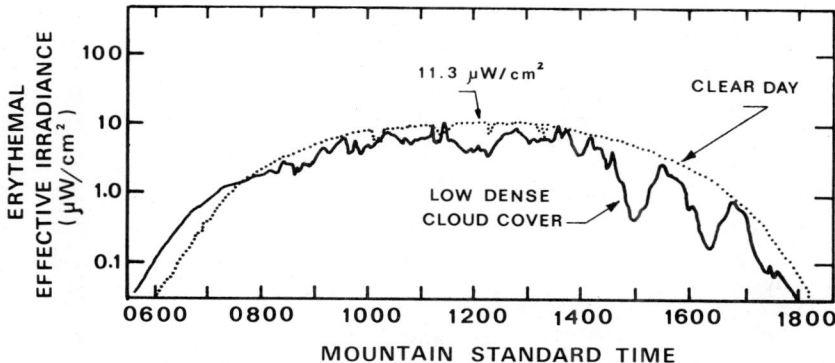

Figure 6-2b. Daily variation in ultraviolet energy. The erythemal effective irradiance is shown in microwatts-per-square-centimeter falling on a horizontal earth surface at Denver, Colorado for one summer day. Notice the strong change as a function of time of day (from Machta *et al.*, 1975).

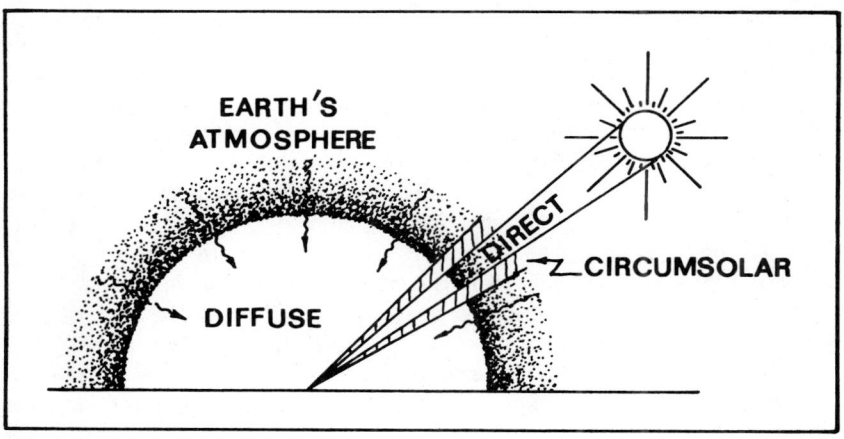

Figure 6-3. The direct and global components in sunlight. This is an artist's highly schematic diagram of the different components in sunlight falling on an observation point on earth. Direct and circumsolar radiation from the sun occupies a small solid angle whereas global diffuse radiation comes from all directions in a "hemisphere." Adapted from Urbach, 1969.

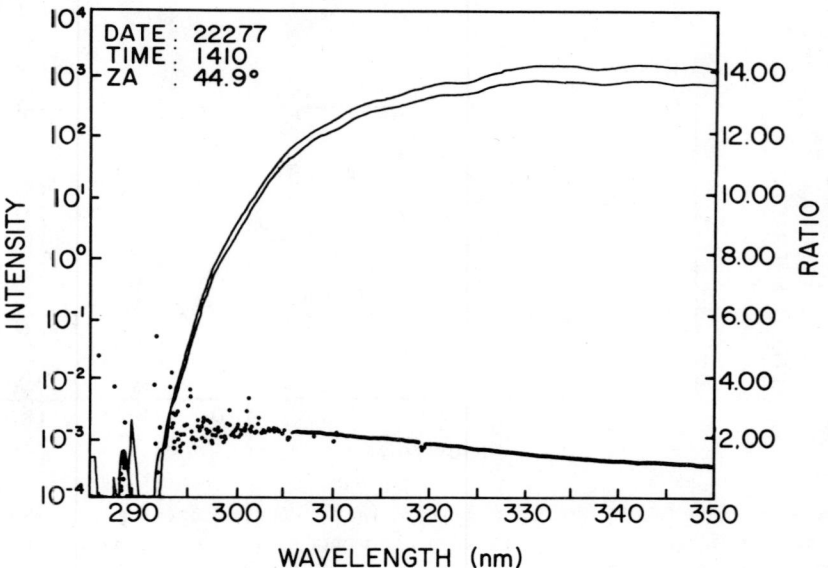

Figure 6-4. Ultraviolet spectral irradiance—global and direct. This is a high resolution plot of the spectral irradiance in Gainesville, FL (measured by Garrison et al., 1978), with a very high resolution double monochromator system. Note the dramatic change in spectral irradiance from 295-305 nm. The intensity units are arbitrary. The lower line is the ratio of diffuse to direct solar radiation.

to sunbathe only before 10 a.m. or after 4 p.m. In the Soviet Union the practice of "sky bathing" has been encouraged because of the fact that the *diffuse component* of ultraviolet radiation is nearly as great as the *direct component* (Figs. 6-3 and 6-4). Thus one can actually shield oneself from the direct sun and thereby remain cooler while still receiving sufficient ultraviolet radiation to produce suntanning. The diffuse ultraviolet irradiance in the UV-B is comparable to the direct irradiance in contrast to visible and IR-A wavelengths. Table 6-1 presents characteristic values for global (direct plus diffuse) UV spectral irradiance.

It is still not known whether levels of ultraviolet radiation exist that are sufficient for suntanning and yet safe from the standpoint of chronic effects. The leathery and wrinkled appearance of exposed areas of the face and the back of the neck and back of the hand are very noticeable on those individuals who work outdoors most of their life, particularly fishermen and farmers. Dermatologists have long noted that most types of skin cancers (especially the squamous epitheliomas) occur only in these exposed areas of people who have spent much of their life outdoors. The susceptibility is also dependent on ethnic factors. People of Celtic origin are most susceptible. Figure 6-5 shows a map of the variation in yearly ultraviolet dose from the sun. Figure 6-6 and 6-7 show the correlation of the incidence of skin cancers with latitude and dose. The high frequency of cloudless days in Arizona gives that state the highest yearly dose level (350 on the map) in the U.S.A. Despite

TABLE 6-1. Approximate Spectral Irradiance for Global Ultraviolet For Cloudless Days at Sea Level, STP, and 3.2 mm Atmospheric Ozone Based upon the Measurements of Bener (1972) *

Wavelength (nm)	Global (Direct + Diffuse) Spectral Irradiance in $\mu W/(cm^2 \cdot nm)$ for Solar Zenith Angle in Degrees					
	0°	30°	60°	70°	80°	85°
297.5	0.218	0.107	0.0116	0.00	0.00	0.00
300	0.720	0.404	0.0766	0.0023	0.00	0.00
302.5	2.08	1.29	0.363	0.0116	0.0018	0.00072
305	4.97	3.43	1.17	0.0661	0.0079	0.00253
307.5	8.22	6.04	2.48	0.220	0.0293	0.00934
310	13.0	9.66	3.99	0.523	0.0706	0.0208
312.5	18.6	14.6	7.46	1.36	0.242	0.0613
315	24.1	18.9	10.2	2.51	0.492	0.131
317.5	29.3	23.7	13.2	3.56	1.01	0.267
320	33.9	27.7	16.6	5.06	1.44	0.449
325	46.5	37.9	22.0	7.71	2.71	1.03
330	53.5	44.1	28.1	11.5	4.62	1.92
340	57.8	47.5	30.9	12.5	5.32	2.32
360	62.4	51.5	33.1	13.5	6.34	3.03
380	72.7	60.0	37.4	14.2	6.65	3.35

* The data in TABLE 6-1 are from an empirical equation developed by Diffey (1977) based upon the measurement of Bener (1972) performed over a period of years at Davos Switzerland for different atmospheric ozone concentrations. The atmospheric ozone concentration fluctuates, but follows a general yearly cycle. For midlattitudes (30° to 50°) this concentration varies from 2.7 to 4.0 mm being highest in the spring and lowest in the fall. A concentration of 3.2 mm is probably a good value for 40° N Lattitude in the summer, i.e., at Washington/Baltimore. Actual measurements of Sliney at Edgewood, MD, are in rough agreement with the above calculations, albeit slightly lower. The values are probably no better than ± 30% near 300 nm. These values are generally higher than those calculated with empirical equations of Green, Sawada and Shettle (1974) and McCullough (1970). One should remember that it is rare to find a cloudless sky in Northern Europe and most of North America, and apparent cloudless skies actually have wisps of clouds that can only be readily detected by a direct spectroradiometric measurement at ~ 300 nm which will fluctuate as these diaphanous wisps pass overhead.

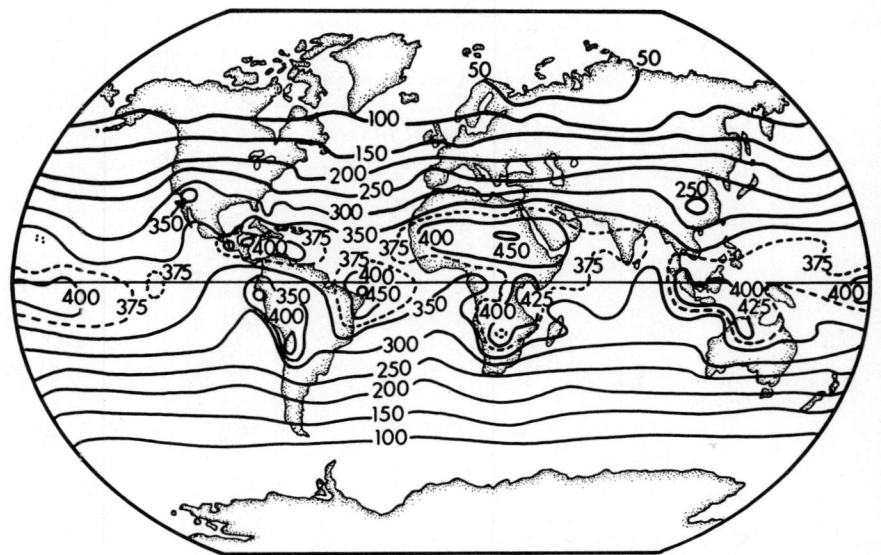

Figure 6-5. Map of variation in yearly UV exposure dose from the sun. This map of the world distribution of "sunburn" ultraviolet radiation is corrected for latitude, cloud cover, and altitude, and was prepared by Professor Rudolph Schulze of Hamburg, Germany. The highest dose in the USA was located in Arizona (350). The values are based on annual values in J/cm^2 of the 10-nm-wide band of ultraviolet radiation centered at 307.5 nm (adapted from Urbach, 1969, p. 647).

this epidemiological evidence and despite laboratory studies (Blum, 1968) both the quantitative threshold and the action spectrum for carcinogenesis by ultraviolet radiation are very difficult to define, if indeed such an effect even exists. Figure 6-8 shows the erythema action spectrum and the DNA absorption spectrum which are sometimes used as the working hypotheses for the carcinogenic action spectra. Such action spectra when compared with the solar spectrum (also shown in Figure 6-8) illustrate the great difficulty of performing carcinogenic studies. There is only a narrow band of wavelengths between 300 and 315 nm where the sun's rays are apparently really effective. For this reason, the spectral irradiance (photon flux) centered at 307.5 nm was used in Figure 6-5.

There is general agreement that a threshold exists above which cellular repair processes cannot any longer overtake the injury processes of ultraviolet radiation, but until both injury and repair processes are understood better, accurate guidance for avoiding solar-radiation-induced skin cancer cannot be provided. It seems proper to question whether not only sunburn and severe erythema should be avoided, but also strong suntanning as well. Obviously no sunlight at all may be as bad, for these deleterious actions should be balanced against the beneficial effects of sunlight exposure, such as the production of Vitamin D in the skin and the indirect effects upon biologic rhythms, gonadal growth and ovulation (Wurtman, 1974).

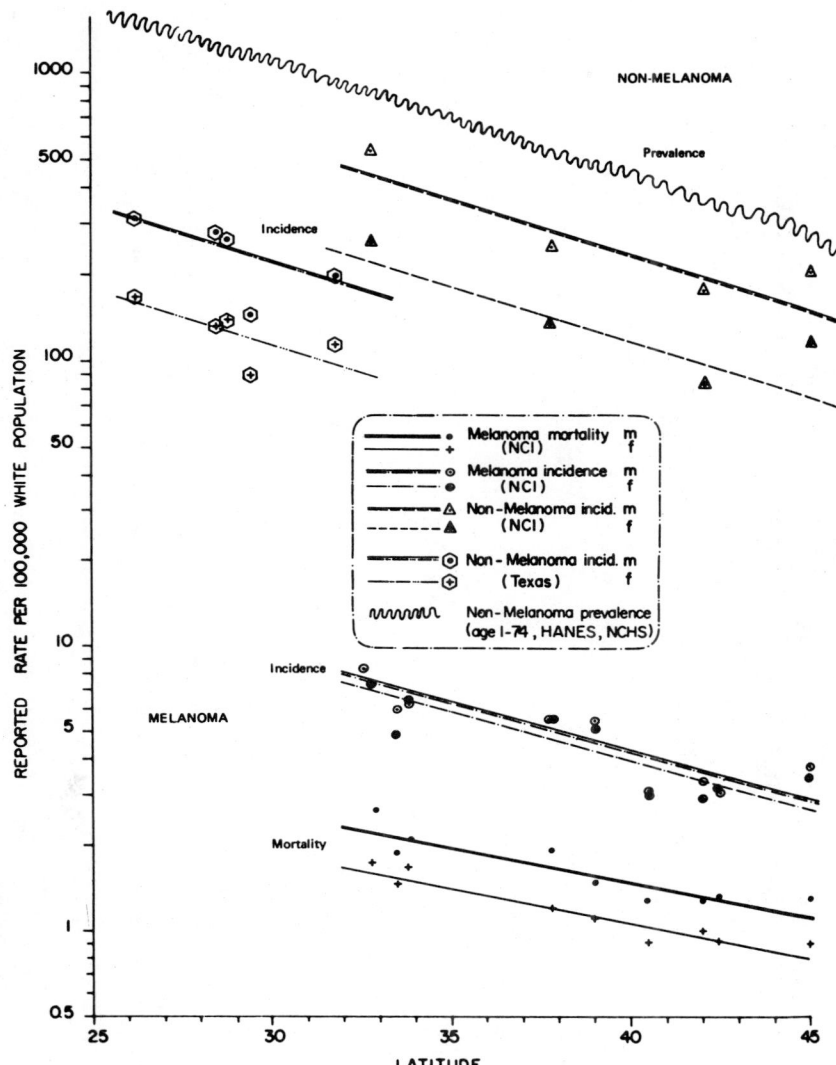

Figure 6-6. Variation of skin cancer incidence with latitude. Both melanoma and non-melanoma incidence and melanoma mortality rates show a clear dependence on latitude (from National Academy of Sciences, 1975).

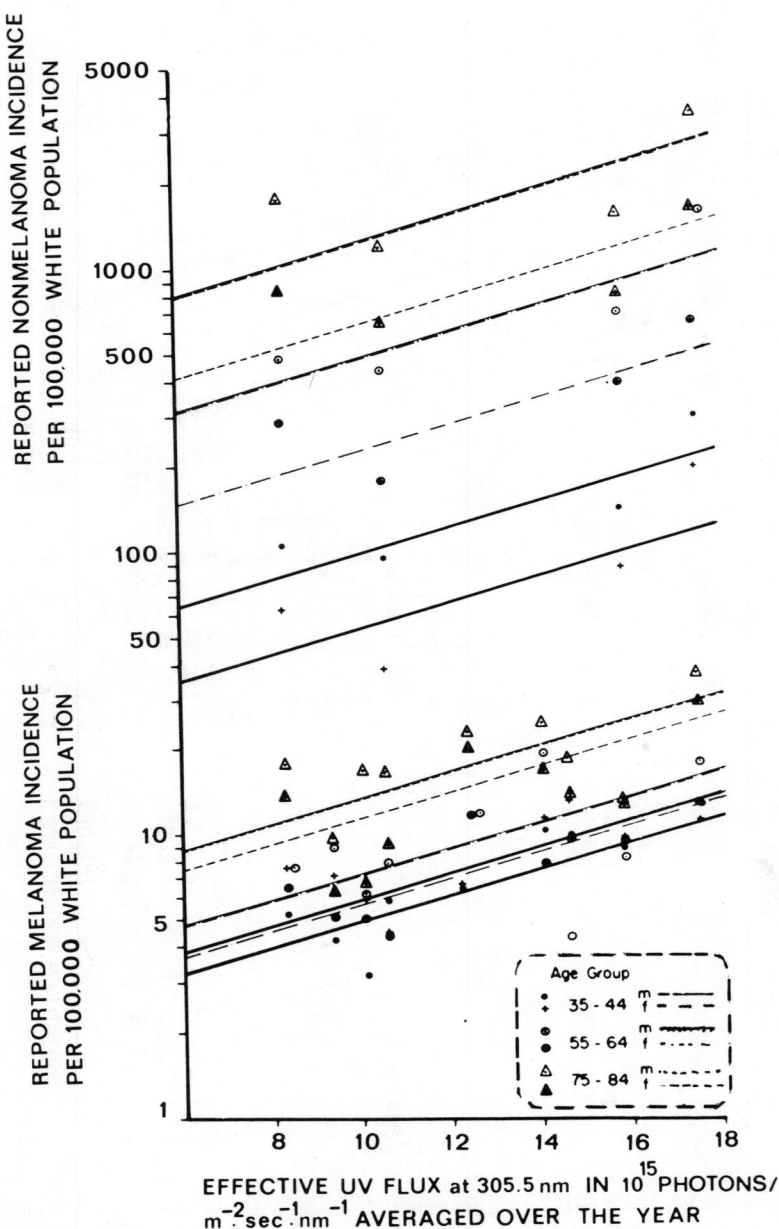

Figure 6-7. Reported skin cancer incidence rates per 100,000 white population among 3 age groups as a function of ultraviolet photon flux. The computations of ultraviolet flux used to prepare this figure were not adjusted for altitude but still show the same trend as Fig. 6-6. A photon rate of 10^{15} photons/s is equivalent to 6.5×10^{-4} W at 305.5 nm (from National Academy of Sciences, 1975).

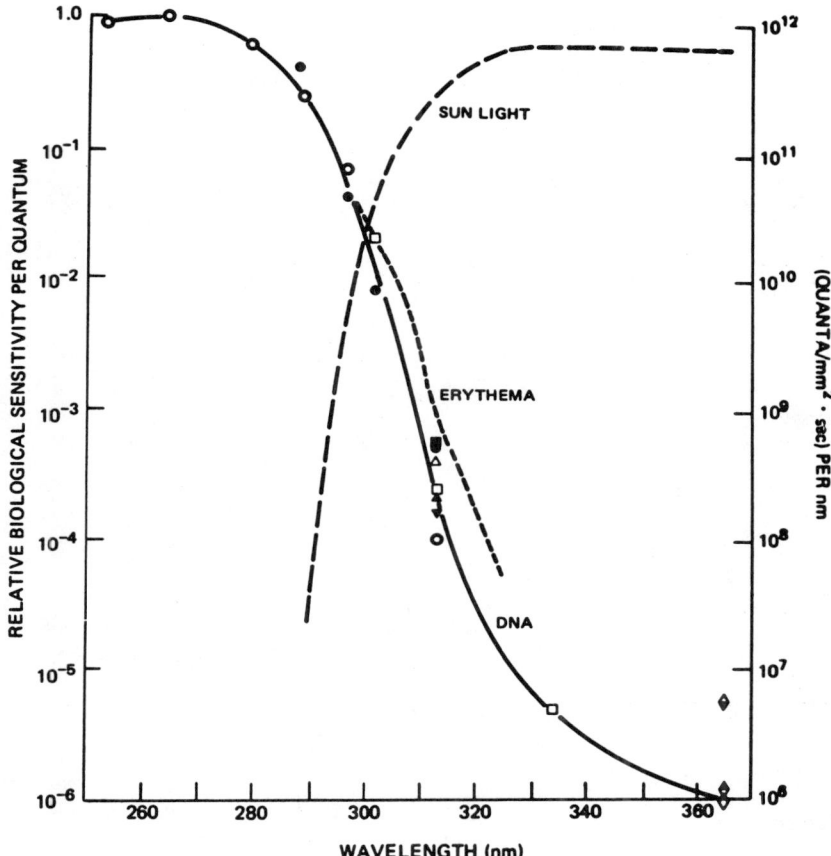

Figure 6-8. Action spectra of erythema and absorption spectra of DNA as compared with ultraviolet solar spectrum. The solid curve represents the action spectra for affecting DNA. The dotted curve is the long wavelength portion of a recent erythemal action spectrum normalized to the DNA spectrum at 297 nm. The sun's spectrum at the earth's surface was calculated by Green for Gainesville, FL, for 2.3 mm of ozone and a zenith angle of 25° (from National Academy of Sciences, 1975).

Many people have the mistaken impression that water strongly reflects ultraviolet radiation. This impression may originate from the deep suntans (and even strong sunburns) of enthusiasts of water sports. But in all likelihood this results from the seemingly rapid passage of time during enjoyment of a sport as contrasted to a sweltering and unpleasant time spent with the usual sunbathing and the high UV reflectivity of the beach sand. Dr. Urbach and his associates at Temple University (1969) in Philadelphia have given an excellent demonstration of the fact that water does not strongly reflect ultraviolet radiation. Figure 6-9 shows photographs of mannequins coated with a photosensitive material which darkened upon exposure to ultraviolet radiation. The eyes and other normally protected parts of the

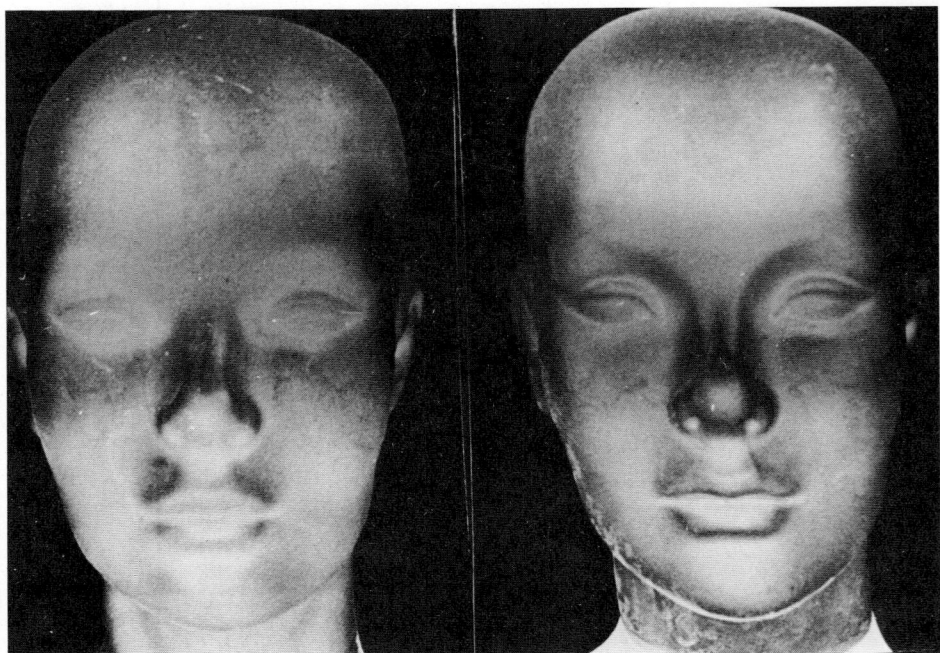

Figure 6-9. Mannequins coated with an ultraviolet-sensitive dye demonstrate the areas of the face exposed to ultraviolet radiation in environmental conditions. The mannequin on the left was exposed to ultraviolet radiation from above without a reflective ground and the mannequin on the right was exposed to ultraviolet radiation from above and ultraviolet reflection from light sand. Areas of the face normally protected from the sun's rays coming from above are exposed by reflections from sand below (from Urbach, 1969).

face of these mannequins were darkened by exposure to ultraviolet radiation only when the background was white sand or aluminum foil. The diffuse reflections from this background exposed these areas to significant ultraviolet doses. Otherwise the eyes were shielded by the brow ridge. In connection with this effect, it should be noted that aside from some sand and snow almost all natural terrain has very poor reflective characteristics in the UV-B (Table 6-2).

TABLE 6-2. Reflectance of Some Natural Surfaces †

Surface	Total Solar Reflectance (Diffuse) (percent)	UV-B Reflectance (Diffuse) (percent)
Fresh snow	89	85
Old snow	50	50
Bright Dry Sand Dune	37	17
Bright Wet Sand	24	9
Sandy Grass Area	17	2.5
Heather, berries	9	2
Water at 60° Zenith * Angle	9	5
Skin	35	1

*NOTE: The reflectance of water depends a great deal upon the angle of the sun and the point of measurement, and whether an integrating sphere reflectance meter was used.

† Based upon the data of Büttner and Sutter, *Strahlentherapie* 54:156 (1935) and Urbach p. 239 (1969).

6.4 CORNEAL EFFECTS

Several epidemiological studies (studies which link disease states and other abnormalities with environmental agents and working conditions) show a high correlation between high levels of natural ultraviolet radiation and the abnormality of the cornea known as *spheroidal degeneration*. For example, this type of corneal degeneration has been cited as the major cause of blindness in the inhabits of the Dahlak Islands in the Red Sea. These islanders are exposed to high levels of reflected ultraviolet from the unusually light-colored sand which covers much of the island (Roger, 1973). In Newfoundland and Nova Scotia the day-long ultraviolet dose is quite high during the summer (Fig. 6-3), and ultraviolet radiation levels are also high from winter snow. These high UV levels are accompanied by an increased incidence of spheroidal degeneration (Fraunfelder and Hanna, 1973). A similar correlation between environmental UV and spheroidal degeneration has also been shown in the southwestern United States.

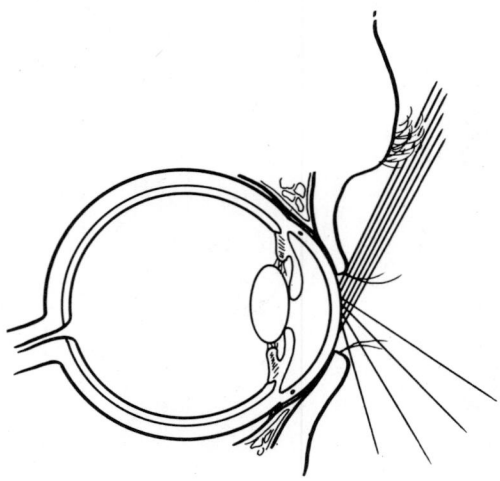

Figure 6-10. Oblique rays of direct sunlight are largely reflected from the cornea and are not absorbed significantly in comparison to ultraviolet rays incident directly along the visual axis. This explains why ultraviolet radiation from overhead lamps and from the sun would not normally cause ultraviolet photokeratitis at levels greatly exceeding those which cause photokeratitis when the irradiation is nearly normal to the visual axis (from Sliney, 1972).

6.5 SNOW BLINDNESS

The most highly reflecting natural-occurring surface for the ultraviolet spectral region is snow. As mentioned in section 6.4, the cornea is naturally shielded from direct solar rays by the brow ridge (Fig. 6-10). For this reason photokeratitis from ultraviolet solar radiation normally occurs only following a walk on snow. This effect is aggravated by looking down toward the ground while walking which causes the reflected ultraviolet radiation to strike the cornea directly and not obliquely (Figure 6-7). In this position, the corneal UV-B irradiance from snow is as high as 10% of the direct solar UV-B irradiance. Oblique angles of incident radiation are not absorbed nearly as effectively as direct incident radiation due to the angular dependence of Fresnel reflection (Fig. 2-6). Eskimos have classically protected their eyes with whalebone goggles with horizontal slits to permit viewing, while at the same time greatly reducing the reflection from the snow.

After snow, the next most reflective material in man's natural environment is sand. Certain types of sand are far more reflective than others. Most people do not experience photokeratitis from the radiation reflected from most varieties of sand, but in some tropical areas such ocular effects may be a problem. Sunburn is also enhanced by these same increased reflections.

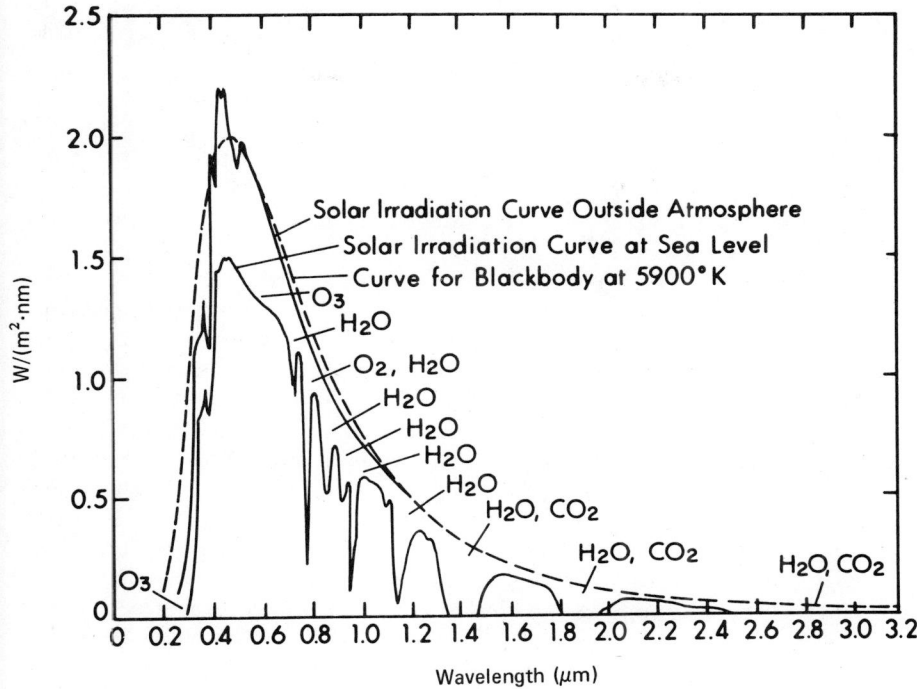

Figure 6-11. Comparison of terrestrial solar spectrum with that outside the atmosphere. The solar spectrum at sea level differs from that outside the atmosphere largely due to absorption by atmospheric molecules in the infrared and absorption and scattering by ozone in the ultraviolet. The total irradiance outside the atmosphere averages 135.3 ± 2.1 mW/cm^2 (based upon the data of Valley, 1965).

6.6 SOLAR RETINITIS

6.6.1 A New Understanding

The literature on solar retinitis or "eclipse burns" is quite extensive. The damage mechanism has been difficult to understand until quite recently. Until the studies of Ham and colleagues (1976) it was generally believed that solar retinitis was a chorioretinal thermal injury. Based on those data it appears reasonable that the short-wave component of the sun's radiance causes a photochemical injury to the retina and choroid which has been called solar retinitis.

6.6.2 Retinal Irradiance

Most clinical reports of solar retinitis do not discuss the quantitative aspects of viewing the sun. The sun, if viewed on the earth, subtends an angle varying from 32 minutes, 36 seconds (9.48 mrad) in January to 31 minutes, 31 seconds (9.17 mrad) in July. These angles correspond to image sizes of 161 μm and 156 μm at the retina respectively. The total solar irradiance at sea level rarely exceeds 0.11 W/cm^2, although the solar constant outside of the earth's atmosphere is 0.137 W/cm^2. Figure 6-11 compares the active solar spectrum outside the atmosphere with that at sea level.

The solar irradiance at sea level, if limited to the spectral region between 400 and 1400 nm, is approximately 70 mW/cm^2. The irradiance of a 160-μm retinal image for a pupil size of 2 mm is approximately 8 W/cm^2, and for a 3-mm pupil is 18 W/cm^2. If the pupil were to dilate during a solar eclipse, an increased irradiance is incident upon the retina. Even though only a portion of the sun is imaged, the radiance of the unobscured portion remains constant. If the sun is viewed through dark glasses without an infrared filter (characteristic of many plastic filters) this also allows the pupil to dilate. This allows most of the sun's infrared radiation to reach the retina, and the total retinal irradiance would not decrease as dramatically as expected. This led some writers (Cogan, 1963) to warn against the use of such filters for eclipse viewing. Fortunately the infrared component of the sun's spectrum does not seem to play a significant role in solar retinitis. At one time it was argued that the pupil dilated with continued staring at the sun (Clarke and Behrendt, 1972). This argument was developed when it was recognized that the temperature rise in the retinal image of the sun for a 2-3 mm pupil would not be expected to cause thermal injury.

6.6.3 Clinical Reports

The reports of eclipse blindness, although generally qualitative, are the largest and most significant group of data on optical retinal injury in humans and thus provide some points for comparison with research data from animals. Some of the more recent reports provide some quantitative information.

A useful report is that of Penner and McNair (1966), which describes clinical findings in 52 eyes of individuals observing an eclipse in Hawaii on February 4, 1962. The eclipse was only partial with a maximum occlusion of one-half of the solar disk. They classified the retinal changes observed ophthalmoscopically into the same three stages used in earlier reports. However, they did not find an increased incidence of solar retinitis in the eyes of deeply pigmented individuals as had often been reported in the past.

Agarwal and Malik, in 1959, presented data on 57 patients who incurred solar retinitis as a result of viewing the sun normally or during an eclipse. Their report described four grades of clinical injury. The more serious injuries were found in individuals who viewed the sun for extended periods of time. In three reported cases of scotomas (blind spots) no ophthalmoscopically visible lesion could be found. In one case the retinal injury resulted from viewing an eclipse by the reflection from a shallow metallic pot of water. Such a reflection could produce a retinal irradiance only one tenth of that from a direct view of the sun. Indeed, viewing the reflection from a pool of water was the recommended procedure among the ancient Greeks for looking at a solar eclipse. Ten years ago this report would have sounded somewhat suspicious, although not impossible, since the retinal irradiance would have been far below thermal injury thresholds. Now we can believe this report since present theory indicates that a very lengthy exposure at this level could indeed result in injury.

In trying to summarize the mass of clinical reports relating to solar retinitis, several important points appear. Retinal injury has occurred from a lengthy observation of the sun without optical aids and with or without filters. Several degrees of retinal injury have occurred ranging from a "tiny white patch" to a "retinal hole." The magnitude of the injury appeared to be dependent upon both duration of exposure and environmental factors, as would be expected from a physical standpoint. Scotomas have been reported to exist without ophthalmoscopically visible lesions, yet lesions have also been observed in sungazers with no apparent associated functional loss of vision. This latter point is significant since the "thresholds" of retinal injury produced in laboratory animals are almost always based upon the appearance of an ophthalmoscopically visible retinal lesion within a specified period (e.g., five minutes, one hour, or 24 and 48 hours). These reports also indicate the possible limitation to valid medical surveillance of individuals exposed to high levels of optical radiation. Another point that should not be neglected is the effect of optical radiation upon the "nutritional" processes in the retina which has frequently appeared in the literature.

Tso (1975, 1976) studied the retinal effects of four malignant-melanoma patients who volunteered to stare at the sun for periods of one half to one hour between noon and 3 p.m. Their loss in visual function did not appear to be substantial. After the eyes were enucleated (removed) because of the retinal cancer, severe retinal injury from photostress was seen histologically.

6.6.4 Damage Mechanisms

Until very recently it was argued that solar retinitis was principally a thermal injury with many experiments interpreted to support this theory. Nevertheless, as more has been learned about the temperature increases required to cause thermal injury in the retina, it seems that thermal retinal injury thresholds for a 158-μm retinal image are ten times higher than the retinal irradiance calculated for direct viewing of the sun. To account for this apparent discrepancy, one group postulated that the patients who developed solar retinitis had unusually large pupils or that their pupils dilated after several seconds of staring at the sun (Clarke and Behrendt, 1972). However, a more likely hypothesis implicates the photochemical effect of short-wavelength, blue light. This latter explanation suggests that solar retinitis would occur only at small zenith angles where the blue components of the sun's radiance is still substantial. The human retina is rarely exposed to the direct image of the sun except at large zenith angles. Measurements of the spectral radiance of skylight and of direct sunlight for a number of solar elevations in Maryland and California are shown in Fig. 6-12. During clear weather the blue component of

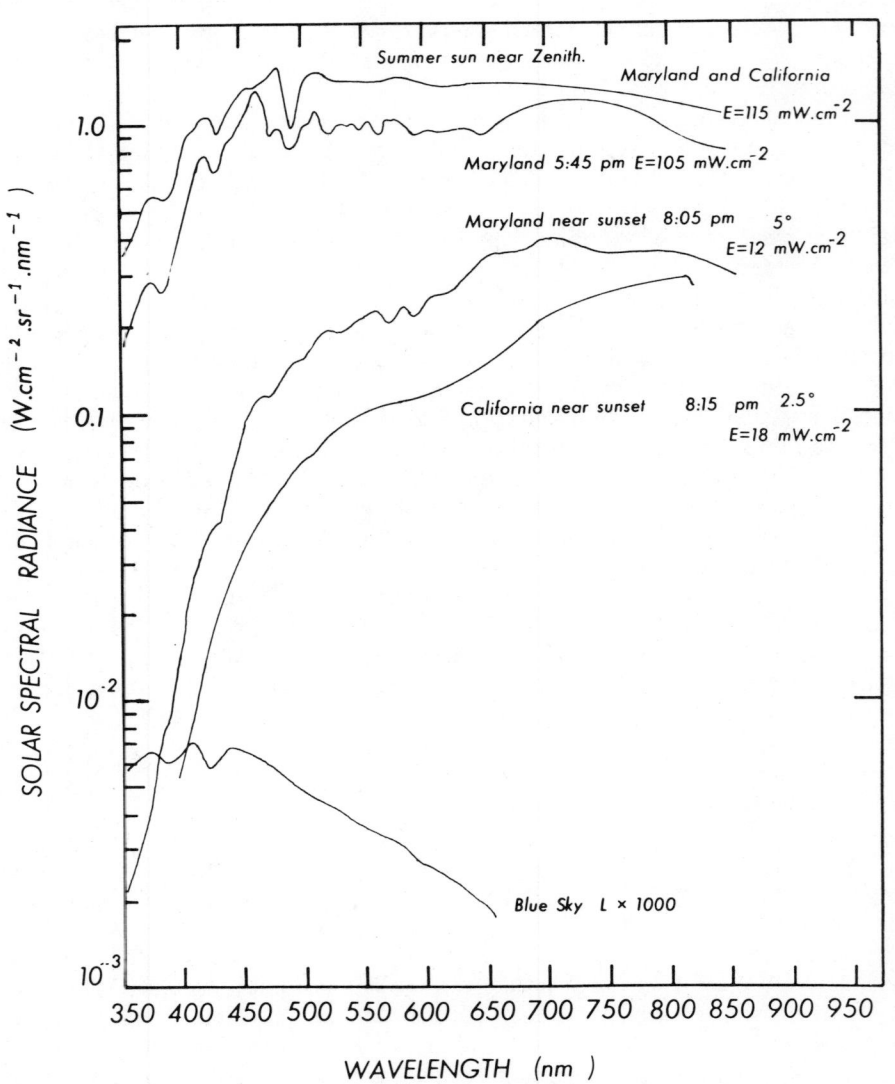

Figure 6-12. Spectral radiance of skylight and direct sunlight for several solar elevations measured in Maryland and California. The radiance which is important in terms of retinal effects is very low for the blue sky as compared to the radiance of the sun itself even at sunset. Note the dramatic change in spectral radiance at 350 nm as a function of solar altitude (from Sliney, 1977).

Optical Hazards from the Ambient Environment—The Sun and Daylight   205

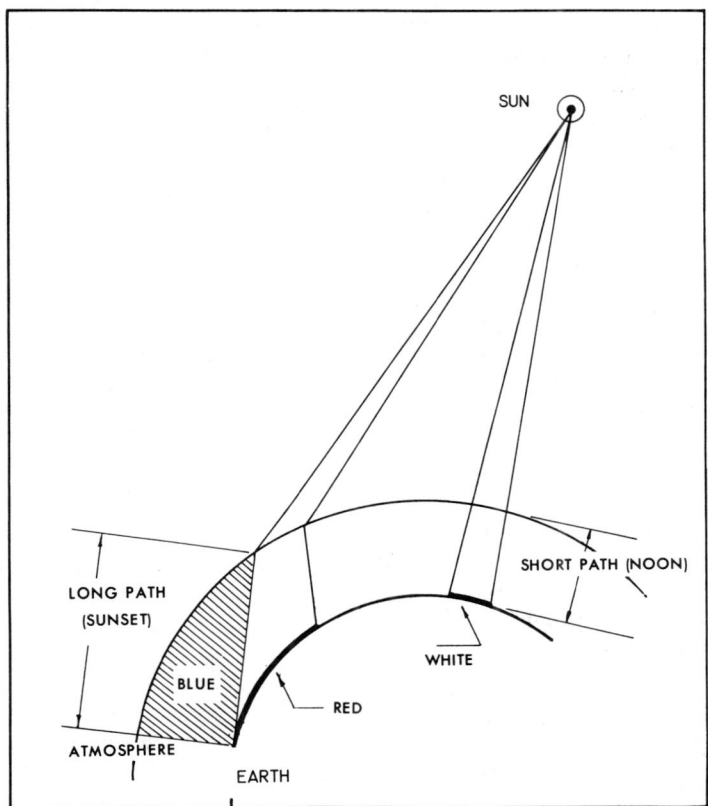

Figure 6-13. The spectral shift of the solar spectrum as the sun sets. The sun appears white when viewed through a short atmospheric path at noontime. The sun's spectral appearance shifts towards the red as the atmosphere pathlength increases (from Sliney, 1977).

direct sunlight varies little for solar elevation angles greater than 20°, which accounts for the sun's position during the middle of the summer day.

The sun is rarely described as white. It is more often termed yellow or even orange, e.g., with a relatively small blue component. As sunset approaches, the relative fraction of blue light in this direct solar spectrum dramatically decreases as the sun nears the horizon (Fig. 6-13). As long as the total solar irradiance exceeds 10 mW/cm^2, it is very difficult to look directly at the sun. It is even unpleasant to have the sun imaged on the peripheral retina. However, once the total irradiance falls below 3 mW/cm^2 (corresponding to an elevation angle of less than 5° at sunset in relatively clear weather), most people find it reasonably comfortable to look at a sunset which lasts for less than 10 minutes. If a 60-nm bandwidth for this blue-light injury mechanism is assumed, the effective blue-light irradiance on the retina can be compared with the experimentally determined 442-nm injury threshold. The retinal irradiance (for a constricted pupil) for a 60-nm spectral band centered at 442 nm is approximately 0.36 W/cm^2 at midday and 0.01 W/cm^2 near sunset. These latter values compared with the 442-nm injury threshold of 30 mW/cm^2 for 10^3 s determined recently by Ham and his colleagues (1976). Therefore, the midday solar retinal irradiance corresponds to a threshold duration of less than 100 s in the region equivalent to a 442-nm laser. From this data it is reasonable that the blue-light damage mechanism alone is responsible for solar retinitis. This would also explain why an individual who drives toward the sun at low elevation angles as he goes to and from work does not receive a retinal injury. When viewing a solar eclipse it would be best to look at a diffusely reflected image as illustrated in Fig. 6-12 or to view it only through very dense neutral filters (with a neutral density of 5.0 to 6.0) as described in section 6.6.6.

6.6.5 Optically Aided Viewing

Although a thermal mechanism does not seem to cause most cases of solar retinitis, it cannot be ruled out as a contributing factor (or even the major one) when the sun is viewed through magnifying optics. Galileo Galilei was the first victim of this type of retinal injury in one eye when he directly viewed the sun through his newly invented refracting telescope. During World War II a number of cases were reported of aircraft lookouts who developed central scotomas after staring into the sun with binoculars. It was characteristic for attacking fighter pilots to dive towards naval ships from the direction of the sun. They followed this pattern to reduce their chances of being detected as the aircraft lookouts were handicapped by solar glare in this direction of view. This was in the days before fire-control radar was on all naval ships. Eccles and Flynn (1944) reported several such cases of retinal injury in Australia. Cordes (1944) reported other cases in the U.S. Navy generally associated with the aircraft spotters using a 20-power long-glass telescope that increases the sun's image size on the retina by 20 times. The telescope reduces the retinal irradiance only slightly—by the factor of the transmittance of the telescope's optics. Because of the reduced heat loss in the center of the 20-fold larger retinal image, the temperature elevation is increased nearly 20 times over the normal image for a 1-s exposure. Figure 6-14 illustrates the temperature-time history of viewing the sun with the unprotected eye and with different optical instruments.

During and following WW II, U.S. Navy doctors reported a type of retinal lesion in large numbers of enlisted personnel (Cordes, 1944; Smith, 1944). The cause of this disorder has been widely debated. Sun gazing is only one cause which has been suggested. Ewald and Ritchey (1970) concluded that this foveomacular retinitis lesion was self-inflicted solar retinitis for the purpose of secondary gain such as release from the service with a pension, or it may have occurred during the non-therapeutic use of narcotic drugs. Epileptic seizures while sunbathing could also be a contributing factor.

6.6.6 Safety in Viewing the Sun

To safely and comfortably view the sun neutral density eye protective filters with an optical density of nearly 6 should be used. This is most easily accomplished using welding filters of Shade No. 14. An alternative (and cheaper) method is to use a pinhole aperture and project the sun's image on a white screen in a dark room (Fig. 6-15). Find a room with a sunbeam entering one window. Block any other windows and cover the one window with a cardboard sheet having a pinhole. The pinhole provides a pinhole camera. A larger pinhole will even make the sun's image visible outdoors.

6.7 REFLECTED SUNLIGHT AND THE EYE

The brightest extended source to which the retina can be exposed except for direct observation of the sun is noontime sunlight reflected from freshly fallen snow (Fig. 6-16). This source has a radiance of approximately 18 mW/(cm$^2 \cdot$sr) with a corresponding retinal irradiance for a 60-nm blue light band centered at 440 nm of 3.6×10^{-4} W/cm^2 for a 2-mm pupil. Assuming that reciprocity holds for photochemical injury during a period of at least 24 hours, then this retinal irradiance from snow would produce injury for an exposure duration of 8×10^4 s, or approximately 23 h.

One aspect of snow blindness, occasionally reported in addition to the characteristic photokeratitis, is a substantial reduction in *night vision*. MacDonald and Fordon (1971) have reported that *erythropsia* occurs in aphakics exposed to such bright sources as sunlight reflected off snow. Erythropsia is red-colored vision possibly due to reduced sensitivity of the blue cones. One cannot help but wonder if the cases of prolonged erythropsia in aphakics approach the level of permanent retinal injury (Mainster, 1978). The removal of the crystalline lens does, after all, substantially change the environment to which the retina is exposed (Kurzel *et al.*, 1977). The reports of experimental retinal injury in animals from blue light suggest the need for further research on the effects of near-ultraviolet radiation which reaches the retina in aphakics. Aphakics often use ultraviolet-absorbing or yellow spectacle lenses to reduce the adverse visual effects of chromatic aberrations at these short wavelengths (Wolbarsht, 1976). However, these yellow lenses have not often been prescribed to protect the retina from the increased exposure to ultraviolet radiation. Actually, as much as 1% of the near ultraviolet reaches the retina in young people while less than 0.1% reaches the retina in adults.

In recent years permanent functional changes in vision have been reported in studies of welders and foundry workers. This suggests that man has adapted to his environment with very little tolerance above the natural levels. During and shortly after World War II there was a great deal of interest in maintaining optimum night vision for nighttime watch standers on ships at sea and at observation posts elsewhere. The military services sponsored research to study the occurrence of reduced vision both at night and in the daytime. These studies demonstrated that individuals exposed to seashore environments such as lifeguards sustained a substantial

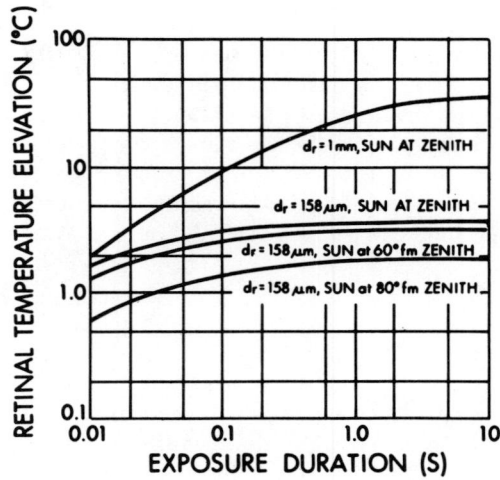

Figure 6-14. Retinal temperature history when viewing the sun directly. The temperature was calculated at the retinal pigment epithelium interface for a 3-mm pupil for two different retinal image sizes d_r (the maximal solar irradiance of approximately 18 W/cm^2 on the retina). The upper curve for a 1-mm retinal image would correspond to viewing the sun through magnifying optics having a magnifying power of 6.3. The retinal temperature increase is greatly increased due to poor heat flow properties for a larger image. A 15-20°C temperature elevation is required for retinal thermal injury (White *et al.*, *Bulletin of Mathematical Biophysics* 33:1–17, 1971).

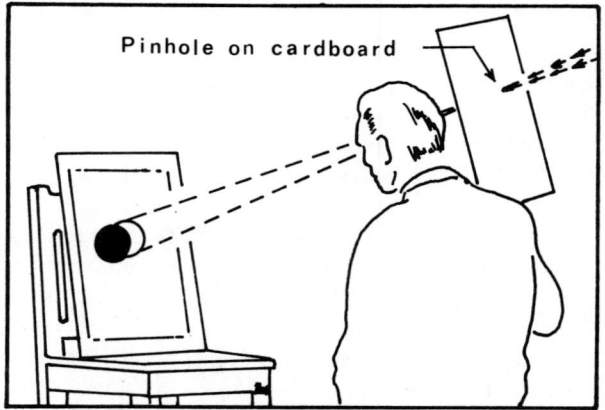

Figure 6-15. Safety in viewing a solar eclipse. This obviously safe approach requires using a pinhole to form an image of the sun. However, with this method the sun's image is sometimes difficult to observe (with too small a pinhole) except in a darkened room by the dark adapted eye (adapted from Flynn, 1952).

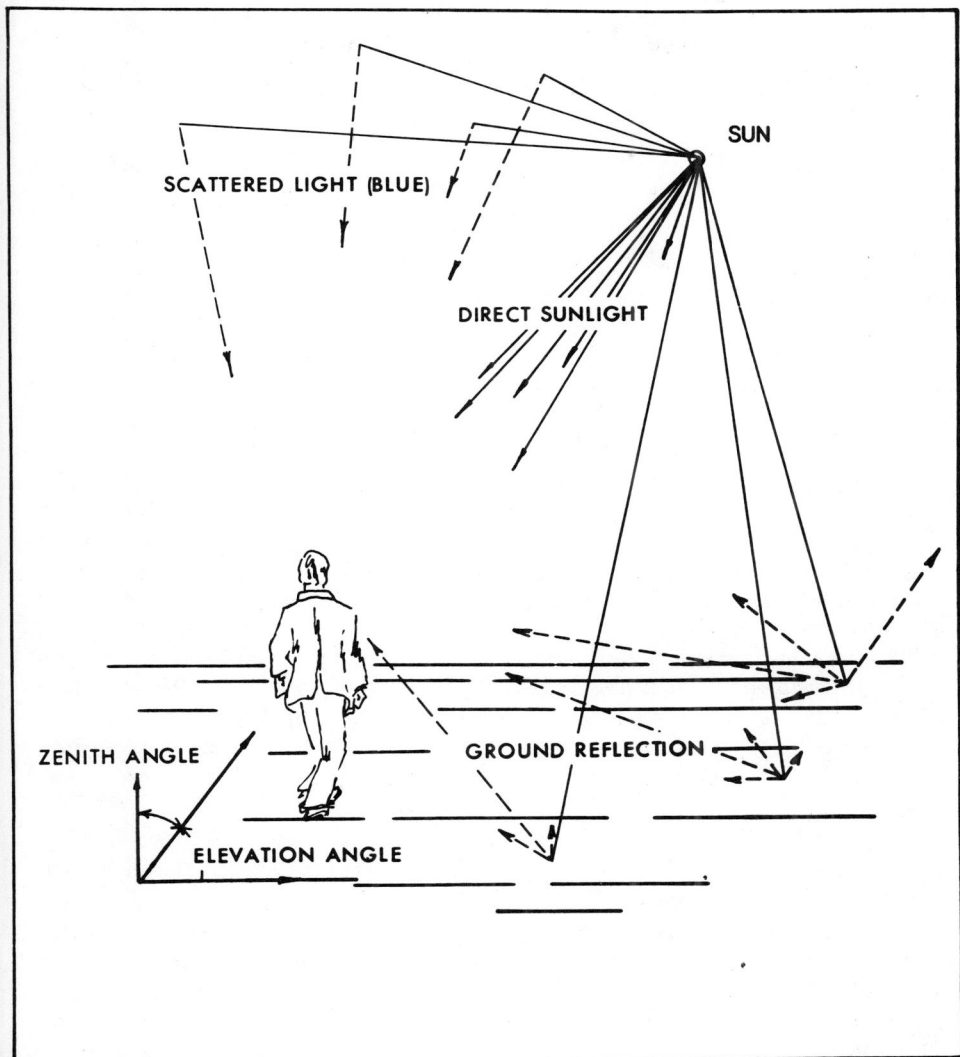

Figure 6-16. Indirect reflected light from the sun as viewed under different conditions. All of the parameters shown here may play a role in retinal effects. The sun's spectrum shifts with zenith angle and the scattered blue light radiance and irradiance change. Additionally, characteristics of ground reflection as from ice, snow or sand will also change with the sun's zenith angle (from Sliney, 1977).

TABLE 6-3. Luminance of Some Natural Sources

Source	Luminance (cd/cm^2 or stilbs)	Luminance (cd/m^2 or nits)
Noonday Sun	1.6×10^5	1.6×10^9
Snowfield at Noon	1	1×10^4
Turf on a Sunny Day	0.1	1×10^3
Clear Day Bright Sky	1	1×10^4
Overcast Sky	0.1	1×10^3
Heavily Overcast Sky	1×10^{-2}	1×10^2
Moon	0.25	2500
Overcast, moonless sky	1×10^{-8}	1×10^{-4}

loss of night vision and color visual sensitivity after day-long exposures to the bright light reflected off the seashore sand. A degree of loss actually lasted for periods of weeks (Peckham and Harley, 1951). More permanent effects were recorded by Marlor and colleagues (1973) in military personnel, by Homer Smith (1944) in U.S. Navy personnel during World War II, and by Livingston (1932) in Royal Air Force flying crews in Iraq in the 1930's. These reports open the question as to the true magnitude of the buffer between levels present in the natural environment and those producing permanent changes in the retina.

Most welders, when asked to select a comfortable shade of welding filter to use with a variety of arcs and gas torches almost always reduced the luminance of the bright source to approximately 1 cd/cm^2. This luminance corresponds to that of bright sand in full sunlight, yet is somewhat less than the brightness of sunlight reflected off snow. Table 6-3 provides characteristic luminance levels of natural environments. As previously noted, to view the sun directly at a comfortable level would require a dark neutral density filter with an optical density of 6 (i.e., an attenuation factor of 10^6).

6.8 SUNLIGHT AND CATARACT

Excessive ultraviolet exposure has also been implicated in cataractogenesis, particularly in the case of brunescent (brown-colored) cataract which is one of the many forms of the senile cataract (Kurzel *et al.*, 1977). An epidemiologic study by

Hiller and colleagues (1977) of cataract in the U.S.A. showed a strong increase in brunescent cataract incidence where annual average sunlight hours were greatest. The dividing line between a senile cataract and the normal yellowing of the lens with age is hard to define. Brunescent cataract may actually be merely an exaggerated form of lens aging. Studies of the ultraviolet photooxidized products of the amino acid tryptophan suggest this as a possible mechanism of brunescent cataract. Throughout the equatorial regions of the world where ultraviolet radiation levels are quite high throughout the year, as in India (Chatterjee, 1973), there is an unusually large incidence of brunescent cataract. Although in the future some other factor such as diet may be found to be the major cause, a contribution from ultraviolet radiation cannot be ruled out. In connection with this, yogurt has been suggested as the dietetic factor. Although yogurt is a staple of some diets in the mideast and India, it is not as large a part of the diet among the lowest income people among whom this cataract has a high incidence. However, on a restricted diet such as is found in the low income groups, each portion of yogurt may be more effective than the same dose coupled with a normal diet. A possible synergism between UV exposure and yogurt in the diet could conceivably explain all.

6.9 SUNLIGHT AND HEAT STRESS

The sun's irradiance on a clear day may vary from 50 to 110 mW/cm^2 at midday. The sun delivers from 3(winter) to 7(summer) kW·hr/(day·m^2) [1kW·hr/(day·m^2) = 86 Ly/day; 1 Ly(Langley) = 1 cal/cm^2]. As noted in Chapter 5 the human body is nicely designed to reflect direct solar radiation as can be seen by comparing the solar spectrum in Fig. 6-11 with the skin's reflectance in Fig. 5-4. In the far infrared the skin's low reflectivity and high emissivity permit the body to both radiate and absorb strongly 10-μm radiation. The ambient radiant exitance of surrounding structures and the ground may vary from 1 to 40 mW/cm^2.

6.10 CONCLUSIONS

Any one of the observations that has been made in this chapter about the dangers of chronic ultraviolet exposure is not too striking in itself; however, taken as a whole they support strongly an argument that mankind has adapted in a narrow fashion for the average natural environment. Any substantial alteration of this environment by man: the use of artificial sources, the removal of the crystalline lens of the eye, a change in the skin or corneal angle of incidence, indeed any change in the spectrum of light which strikes the skin or enters the eye—must be carefully viewed as a potential hazard. This review also illustrates that a true characterization of the hazards of any artificial optical source requires consideration of all of the geometrical and spectral factors discussed in this chapter.

6.11 REVIEW QUESTIONS

1. List the adverse effects of sunlight.

2. The fraction of solar radiation which is below 400 nm (ultraviolet component) is: (a) greater than 30%; (b) between 20 and 30%; (c) between 10 and 20%; (d) between 0 and 10%.

3. Would it be a simple matter to construct a sunburn meter? Give reasons.

4. Is it possible to use an ordinary light meter relating the amount of visible light to the ultraviolet radiation that causes erythema?

5. The solar constant is: (a) 137 mW/cm^2; (b) 100 mW/cm^2; (c) 1.3 W/cm^2 (d) 70 mW/cm^2.

6. What is the spectral irradiance of the sun for a zenith angle of 30° at 500 nm? The peak sensitivity of the daylight response of the eye is at 550 nm. Does this correspond to the peak in solar irradiance in watts-per-square-centimeter? in photons-per-square-centimeter?

7. Spheroidal degeneration of the cornea may be due to what radiation?

8. What is the focal irradiance in a 7-cm diameter magnifying glass (focal length 10 cm) when a young boy decides to use it to focus the sun's rays on some paper at noontime?

9. By what factor does the global UV spectral irradiance at 300 nm vary as the sun goes from zenith to a zenith angle of 60°.

10. The 300-nm solar spectral irradiances for the sun at a zenith angle of 60° would generally be identical in the spring and fall for an instrument located at a fixed latitude. T or F

6.12 REFERENCES

Agarwal, L. P. and Malik, S. R. K., 1959, Solar retinitis, *Brit. J. Ophth.* **53**:366–375.

Bener, P., 1972, "Approximate Values of Intensity of Natural UV Radiation for Different Amounts of Atmospheric Ozone," Final Tech. Rept., Contract DAJA37-68-C-1017, European Research Office, US Army, London.

Berson, E. L., 1973, Experimental and therapeutic aspects of photic damage to the retina, *Invest. Ophth.* **12**(1):35–44.

Chatterjee, A., 1973, Cataract in Punjab, *in* "Symposium on the Human Lens in Relation to Cataract," pp. 265–279, Ciba Foundation Symposium 19, Amsterdam, Associated Scientific Publishers.

Clarke, A. M., and Behrendt, T., 1972, Solar retinitis and pupillary reaction, *Am. J. Ophth.* **73**(5):700–703.

Cogan, D. G., 1963, On viewing the eclipse, *Arch. Ophth.* **69**:690–692.

Cordes, F. D., 1944, A type of foveo-macular retinitis observed in the US Navy, *Am. J. Ophth.* 27:803–815.
Coulson, K. L., 1975, "Solar and Terrestrial Radiation, Methods and Measurements," Academic Press, New York.
Davies, J. M., 1959, The Effect of Intense Normal Radiation on Animal Skin; A Comparison of Calculated and Observed Burns. Report T-24, Army Quartermaster Research and Engineering Command, Nadick, Mass., (29 April 1959) Defense Documentation Center AD456794.
Diffey, B. L., 1979, The calculation of the spectral distribution of natural ultraviolet radiation under clear day conditions, *Phys. Med. Biol.* 22(2):309–316.
Eccles, J. C. and Flynn, A. J., 1944, Experimental photoretinitis, *Med. J. Australia* 1:339–342.
Ewald, R. A. and Ritchey, C. L., 1970, Sun gazing as the cause of foveomacular retinitis, *Am. J. Ophth.* 70(4):491–497.
Fitzpatrick, T. B., (ed.), 1974, "Sunlight and Man," Proceedings of the International Congress on Photosenstitization and Photoprotection, Tokyo, Japan, November 6-8, 1972, University of Tokyo Press, Tokyo.
Flynn, J. A. F., 1959, Retinal burns after sun's eclipse, *Trans. Ophth. Soc. Australia* 20:90–96.
Flynn, J. A. F., 1952, Eclipse blindness: Prevention is better than cure, *Trans. Ophth. Soc. Australia* 12:7–14.
Fraunfelder, F. T. and Hanna, C., 1973, Spheroidal degeneration of cornea and conjunctiva. III. Incidences, classification and etiology, *Am. J. Ophth.* 76(1):41–50.
Garrisson, L. M., Murray, L. E., Doda, D. D., and Green, A. E. S., 1978, Diffuse–direct ultraviolet ratios with compact double monochromator, *Appl. Opt.* 17(5):827–836.
Gates, D. M., 1966, Spectral distribution of solar radiation at the earth's surface, *Science* 151:523–529.
Geeraets, W. J., Nooney, D. W., Svoboda, J. R., and Ching, F. C., 1970, Solar retinopathy following the eclipse of March 7, 1970, *Med. College of Va. Quarterly* 6(1):3–7.
Gerathewohl, S. J. and Strughold, H., 1953, Motoric responses of the eyes when exposed to light flashes of high intensities in short durations. *J. Aviation Med.* 24:200–207.
Goody, R. M., 1964, "Atmospheric Radiation," Clarendon Press, Oxford.
Green, A. E. S., Mo, T., and Miller, J. H. 1974, A study of solar erythema radiation doses, *Photochem. Photobiol.* 20:473–482.
Green, A. E. S., and Hedinger, R. A., 1978, Models relating ultraviolet light and non-melanoma skin cancer incidence, *Photochem. Photobiol.* 28:283–291.
Hadley, M. E., 1972, Functional significance of vertebrate integumental pigmentation, *Am. Zoologist* 12:63–76.
Ham, W. T., Jr., Mueller, H. A., and Sliney, D. H., 1976, Retinal sensitivity to damage from short wavelength light, *Nature* 260:153–155.
Ham, W. T., Jr., Mueller, H. A., Williams, R. C., and Geeraets, W. J., 1973, Ocular hazard from viewing the sun unprotected and through various windows and filters, *Appl. Opt.* 12(9):2122–2129.
Hardy, J. D., Jacobs, I., and Meisner, M. D., 1953, Thresholds of pain and reflex contraction as related to noxious stimulation, *J. Appl. Physiol.* 5(12):724–739.
Harwerth, R. S. and Sperling, H. G., 1975, Effects of intense radiation on the increment threshold spectral sensitivity of the rhesus monkey eye, *Vis. Res.* 15:1193–1204.
Hatfield, E. M., 1970, Eye injuries and the solar eclipse, *Sight Sav. Rev.* 40(1):79–85.
Hausser, K. W., 1928, Influence of wavelength in radiation biology, *Strahlentherapie* 28:25–44.
Hausser, K. W. and Vahle, W., 1969, Sunburn and suntanning. Wissenschaftliche Veröffnungen des Siemens Konzern 6(1):101–120 (1927); translated in "The Biologic Effects of Ultraviolet Radiation," (F. Urbach, ed.), Pergamon Press, New York.
Henderson, S. T., 1970, "Daylight and Its Spectrum," American Elsevier Publishers, New York.

Hiller, R., Giacomotti, L. and Yuen, K., 1977, Sunlight and cataract: an epidemiologic investigation, *Am. J. Epidemiol.* **5**:450–459.

Johnson, F. S., Mo, T., and Green, A. E. S., 1976, Average latitudinal variation in ultraviolet radiation at the earth's surface, *Photochem. Photobiol.* **23**:179–188.

Klein, W. H. and Goldberg, B., 1974, Solar Radiation Measurements: 1968–1973, Smithsonian Radiation Biology Laboratory, Rockville, MD; published by the Smithsonian Institution, Washington, DC.

Knudtzon, 1948, The prognosis of scotoma heliocliptom, *Acta. Ophth.* **26**:470.

Kurzel, R. B., Wolbarsht, M. L., and Yamanashi, B. S., 1977, UV radiation effects on the human eye, in "Photochemical and Photobiological Reviews," (K. C. Smith, ed.) Vol. 2, pp. 133–167, Plenum Publishing Corporation, New York.

Kuwabara, T., 1970, Retinal recovery from exposure to light, *Am. J. Ophth.* **70**:187–193.

Lawwill, T. E., 1973, Effects of prolonged exposure of rabbit retina to low intensity light, *Invest. Ophth.* **12**:45–51.

Livingston, P. C., 1932, The study of sun glare in Iraq, *Brit. J. Ophth.* **6**:577–525.

MacDonald, J. E. and Fordon, L., 1971, Erythropsia and light toxicity thresholds. Presented at the Annual Meeting of the Association for Research in Vision and Ophthalmology, Sarasota, FL.

Machta, L., Cotton, G., Hass, W., and Komhyr, W., 1975, CIAP Measurements of Solar Ultraviolet Radiation, US Department of Transportation Final Report, Interagency Agreement DOT-A5-20082, Washington, DC, August, 1975.

Mainster, M. A., 1978, Solar retinitis photic maculopathy and the pseudophakic eye, *Am. Intraocular Implant Soc. J.* **4**:84–89.

Marlor, R. L., Blais, B. R., Preston, F. R., and Boyden, D. G., Foveomacular retinitis, an important problem in military medicine: epidemiology, *Invest. Ophth.* **12**(1):5–16.

McCullough, E. C., 1970, Qualitative and quantitative features of the clear day terrestrial solar ultraviolet radiation environment, *Phys. Med. Biol.* **15**(4):723–734.

McFaul, P. A., 1969, Visual prognosis after solar retinopathy, *Brit. J. Ophth.* **53**:534–541.

National Academy of Sciences/National Academy of Engineering, 1973, Biological Impacts of Increased Intensities of Solar Ultraviolet Radiation. A Report of the Ad Hoc Panel on the Biological Impacts of Increased Intensities of Solar Ultraviolet Radiation to the Environmental Studies Board of the National Academy of Sciences, National Academy of Engineering, Washington, DC.

Noell, W. K., and Albrecht, R., 1971, Irreversible effects of visible light on the retina—role of Vitamin A, *Science* **172**:76–79.

Peckham, R. H., and Harley, R. D., 1951, The effect of sunglasses in protecting retinal sensitivity, *Am. J. Ophth.* **34**(11):1499–1507.

Penner, R., and McNair, J. N., 1966, Eclipse blindness, *Am. J. Ophth.* **61**:1452.

Pirie, A., 1972, The effect of sunlight on proteins of the lens, in "Contemporary Ophthalmology, Honoring Sir Stuart Duke-Elder," (J. G. Bellows, ed.), pp. 494–501, Williams and Wilkins, Baltimore, MD.

Robinson, N., 1966, "Solar Radiation," American Elsevier, New York.

Roger, F. C., 1973, Clinical findings, course and progress of biatis corneal degeneration in the Dahlak Islands, *Brit. J. Ophth.* **57**:657–661.

Rundel, R. D., and Nachtwey, D. S., 1978, Skin cancer and ultraviolet radiation, *Photochem. Photobiol.* **28**:345–365.

Schmidt, R. H., Williams, R. C., Ham, W. T., Jr., Brooks, J. W., and Evans, I. E., 1954, Experimental production of flash burns, *Surgery* **36**:1163.

Schulze, R., 1962, Zum Strahlungsklima der Erde, *Strahlungther.* **119**:321–348.

Scotto, J., Fears, T. R., and Gori, G. B., 1975, Measurements of Ultraviolet Radiation in the United States and Comparisons with Skin Cancer Data, National Cancer Institute Report No. DHEW (NIH) 76-1029, US Dept. Health Education and Welfare, Washington, DC.

Sliney, D. H., 1972, The merits of an envelope action spectrum for ultraviolet radiation exposure criteria, *Am. Indust. Hyg. Assoc. J.* **33**:644–653.

Sliney, D. H. and Freasier, B. C., 1973, The evaluation of optical radiation hazards, *Appl. Opt.* **12**:1-22.

Smith, H. E., 1944, Actinic macular retinal pigment degeneration, *U.S. Naval Medical Bulletin* **42**:675–680.

Thekakara, M. P., 1976, Solar irradiance: total and spectral and its possible variations, *Appl. Opt.* **15**(4):915–920.

Tso, M. O. M., 1976, Photic injury to the human retina, *in* "Retinitis Pigmentosa: Clinical Implications of Current Research," (M. B. Landers, M. L. Wolbarsht, J. E. Dowling, and A. M. Laties, eds.), pp. 257–259, Plenum Publishing Corporation, New York.

Tso, M. O. M. and La Piana, F. G., 1975, The human fovea after sun gazing, *Trans. Am. Acad. Ophth.* **79**:788–795.

Urbach, F., 1969, Geographic pathology of skin cancer, *in* "Biologic Effects of Ultraviolet Radiation," (F. Urbach, ed.), pp. 635–650, Pergamon Press, New York.

Valley, S. L., 1965, "Handbook of Geophysics and Space Environments," USAF Cambridge Research Laboratories, Hanscom Field, MA; published in New York, McGraw Hill.

White, T. J., Mainster, M. A., Wilson, P. W., and Tips, J. H., 1971, Chorioretinal temperature increases from solar observation, *Bull. Math. Biophys.* **33**(1):1–17.

Wolbarsht, M. L., 1976, The function of intraocular color filters, *Fed. Proc.* **35**(1):44–49.

Wright, R. E., 1936-37, The possible influence of solar radiation on the production of cataract in certain districts of southern India: a preliminary investigation, *Indian J. Med. Res.* **24**:917.

Wurtman, R. J., 1974, The action of light on man and mamals: Normal physiologic and pathologic extracutaneous effects, *in* "Sunlight and Man," (T. Fitzpatrick, ed.) pp. 231–246, University of Tokyo Press, Tokyo, Japan.

Young, J. D. H., and Finley, R. D., 1973, Primary spheroidal degeneration of the cornea in Labrador and Northern Newfoundland, *Am. J. Ophth.* **71**(1):129–134.

Chapter 7
Laser Safety Standards: Evolution and Rationale

7.1 INTRODUCTION

Laser safety standards may take several forms. The standard may be simply a list of guidelines—the do's and don'ts of laser operation or of equipment design with no mention of exposure limits. Some standards may simply be a list of personnel exposure limits or product emission limits. Today most safety standards incorporate all of the above aspects to some extent. This chapter will give the history of laser standard development and explain the scientific and philosophical problems encountered in the development of today's standards. The distinction between occupational exposure standards and equipment performance standards will also be discussed.

Exposure limits may be reflected in three general categories of standards: occupational safety and health standards, environmental quality, or equipment performance standards. Such standards can be either mandatory, regulatory standards published by governments (either state or local), or they may be advisory, recommended standards of professional or technical organizations. Within the United States Government, occupational exposure standards are issued and enforced by the Occupational Safety and Health Administration (OSHA) of the U.S. Department of Labor. Environmental quality standards are issued and enforced by the Environmental Protection Agency (EPA). Federal product performance standards are enforced by the Bureau of Radiological Health (BRH) of the Federal Drug Administration (FDA) in the U.S. Department of Health, Education and Welfare. Federal standards for occupational exposure to nonionizing radiation have existed for microwaves and for the visible CW lasers used in the construction industry since 1971. During 1975 to 1978 OSHA worked on several drafts of an occupational safety standard for personnel employed in laser work which would be far more comprehensive than the 1971 code. However, promulgation of such an OSHA standard has had a low priority. Also in 1975 BRH introduced the first comprehensive classification and performance standard of laser products, which became effective August 2, 1976. This was designed to promote safer products and also safe use of these laser products by requiring certain labeling and performance features. EPA has not proposed any environmental standards for lasers or optical radiation.

7.2 HISTORICAL DEVELOPMENT

7.2.1 Early History of Exposure Limits

In the United States the first safety limits for exposure to laser radiation were formulated during 1962-1963 for use in the military services, since these were the only large organizations using lasers extensively at that time. Several drafts for national "standards" were circulated during the mid-1960's, but not until 1968-1969 were the first group of widely accepted safety exposure limits printed in the United States. By that time the three military services in the U.S. had each published safety codes governing laser usage; in addition, many separate military bases, industrial organizations and research laboratories had found it necessary or convenient to formalize their own safety requirements and practices. Most of these early standards were limited to a few types of lasers operating at several discrete exposure durations because of the limited biological data. A somewhat more sophisticated set of exposure limits was developed by the British Ministry of Aviation in a code of practice for lasers published in 1965. This British standard defined limits for continuous laser exposure which varied with retinal image size and was largely based upon the data of Ham et al. (1963) and Bredemeyer et al. (1963). In the United States, the exposure limits of the American Conference of Government Industrial Hygienists (ACGIH) were first given widespread publicity when they were recommended by the First International Laser Safety Conference held in Cincinnati, Ohio in 1968.

The ACGIH (and U.S. Army) format of 1968 presented three types of exposure limits: Q-switched lasers, normal pulsed lasers, and CW lasers. Exposure limits were given for three different pupil sizes, and additional values were included for viewing extended sources such as diffuse reflections (Sliney and Palmisano, 1968). For purposes of simplification, a set of nine limits for visible and near-infrared radiation was given which could be adjusted slightly for different wavelengths based upon the relative absorption of the laser radiation at the retina. One of the chief complaints leveled at this simplified set of values was its use of step functions. Specifically, the values jumped by a factor of 10 at several points (Figure 7-1). For example, at 1 μs the exposure limit was 10^{-7} J/cm^2 based upon Q-switched exposure data and 10^{-6} J/cm^2 based on normal pulse data. As no lasers then in use had a pulse duration in the neighborhood of 1 μs, this sudden change in the exposure limit at 1 μs presented no problems. When lasers began to appear that had pulse durations of 1 μs, questions naturally arose as to the validity of either criterion. This was not the only problem presented by the simplified set of criteria. The

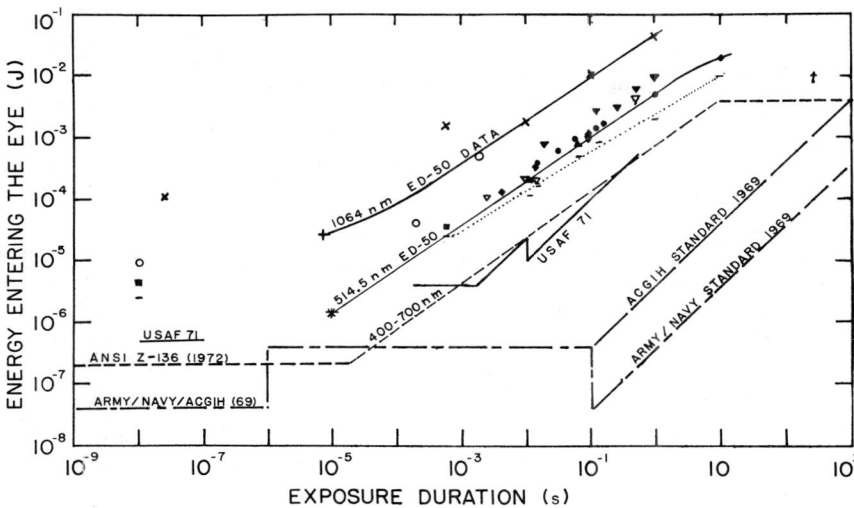

Figure 7-1. Intrabeam exposure limits for visible and infrared laser exposures. Evolution of intrabeam exposure limits for visible and IR-A laser radiation. The ED_{50} (50% probability of damage) values for ophthalmoscopically visible retinal lesions are shown for two wavelengths: 514.5 and 1064 nm. Data points are for minimal image sizes from: Ham et al. (1970) for 632.8 nm (▼); Dunsky and Lappin (1971) for 568 nm (●); Bresnick et al. (1970) for 514.5 nm (▲); Vassiliadis et al. (1971) for 532 nm (■), and for 694.3 nm (○); Vassiliadis et al. for 514.5 nm (◇); Lappin (1970) for 632.8 nm (▽); Naidoff and Sliney (1973) for a welding arc point source (+); Skeen et al. (1972a) for 1064 nm (x); and Skeen et al. (1972b) for 514.5 nm (*). Points marked (−) indicate lowest reported injury values. Note how the later exposure limits fitted the trends of injury data more closely. From Wolbarsht and Sliney, 1974.

CW laser exposure criteria of 1 to 10 $\mu W/cm^2$ did not allow for a momentary exposure but was based on the extrapolation of certain effects from long-term chronic exposure experiments.

The ACGIH limits were in agreement with those of the U.S. Army and Navy but were not adopted by the Air Force. Scientists within the U.S. Air Force felt that biologic data based upon direct minimum-image-size thresholds furnished a more accurate criterion for intrabeam viewing, and they felt that no individual would continuously stare into a CW laser for longer than 1 s. The U.S. Air Force ocular exposure limits in 1969 were therefore much higher (less conservative) than the ACGIH, U.S. Army and U.S. Navy limits (Carpenter et al., 1970). These and other values are compared in Figure 7-1. Aside from the differences in the exposure limits for the eye, these 1969-vintage standards were similar and contained much of the same safety measures, medical surveillance and skin exposure limits.

Since the U.S. Armed Services and other parts of the federal government had sponsored most of the biologic research and were responsible for much of the laser development in the United States during the 1960's their standards were to a large extent followed by industry. The ACGIH standard, although national in scope, was developed and controlled by governmental industrial health personnel. Nongovernmental industrial health and safety personnel did not play a significant role. However, by 1969 it had become clear that a national consensus standard on laser safety was needed.

7.2.2 The ANSI Z-136 Development

In 1969 an effort was initiated by the American National Standards Institute (ANSI) at the request of the U.S. Department of Labor, to develop a consensus standard for the "safe use of lasers and masers." This project was later redefined as "Safe Use of Lasers" and designated as Standards Committee Z-136. A corporate group member of the Institute, the Telephone Group, became the sponsoring activity and Mr. George M. Wilkening of Bell Laboratories was designated chairman; Mr. Sidney S. Charschan of Western Electric was secretary. The committee organization was initiated in 1969 with the formation of subcommittees and hope was expressed that a final standard could be completed in one year if all subcommittees worked diligently. History was to prove that this was an overly optimistic assessment. General consensus was not achieved until the committee approved the last official draft, dated February 29, 1972. In May 1972, the ACGIH proposed a revision of their threshold limit values (TLV's) for laser radiation which incorporated essentially all of the ANSI Z-136 maximum permissible exposures (MPE's). The ANSI standard, however, was not issued in 1972 because many of the ballots on the February 29, 1972 draft contained suggestions for editorial changes to clarify particular points. The final draft was considerably revised and in November, 1972 was submitted to the Board of Standards Review of ANSI. The Review Board finally approved the document on April 26, 1973 and it was issued in October, 1973. The military services and other Federal and State agencies of the United States that made use of laser protection standards adopted most parts of the new ANSI protection standard. Many groups in other countries also accepted this major modification of exposure limits that had been accomplished by ANSI. In 1976 the ANSI standard was slightly revised to take into account more recent biological data and to convert to the four-class system of BRH.

Most of the Committee work was accomplished by correspondence within subcommittees. The Committee Chairman (Wilkening) and Secretary (Charschan) along with the Chairman of the Subcommittee on Special Considerations (Sliney), who was on each of the major subcommittees, aided in coordination of the separate sections of the proposed standard. Meetings of the entire Z-136 Committee were held only about once each year, while executive committee meetings of the subcommittee chairmen were held every two or three months. This approach worked well in drafting this complex document which was remarkably consistant throughout.

The greatest departure in the ANSI standard format from previous standards was the use of smooth curves to express the exposure limits. Step functions were generally avoided. Also, all previous exposure limits were expressed as values of radiant exposure (J/cm^2) or irradiance (W/cm^2) for a specific range of pulse durations. With the advent of lasers having all possible pulse durations it was necessary to provide a sliding scale without discontinuities. Indeed, such an approach permitted a closer approximation of actual biological injury thresholds. However, since the biologic data could not be expressed as a constant radiant exposure or a constant radiant exposure or a constant irradiance, the time dependence of the exposure limits became quite complex. The methods of setting the limits will be discussed in greater detail in Section 7.3 in this chapter.

Many laser manufacturers and users were concerned that if exposure limits were too conservative, lasers would not be used in many important applications. However most of them eventually understood that the exposure limits themselves were not as important as the standards which applied to laser design, installation, and safety procedures. If these latter standards were too restrictive then laser use would falter. The greatest attention was therefore redirected from exposure limits to user procedures and hazard analysis. For this reason, the evolution of hazard classification will now be discussed in an historical context prior to considering exposure limits in finer detail.

7.2.3 Historical Development of Hazard Classification

The initial realization that some form of risk classification was necessary came out of many complaints of research scientists in the early 1960's that they were being needlessly constrained in their use of small helium-neon lasers by safety officers who had read guidelines intended for high-powered ruby and neodymium lasers. During the period of 1966-1968 radically different guidelines were being proposed for each type of laser (Sliney and Palmissano, 1968; ACGIH, 1968). For instance, there were guidelines for high-power ruby lasers, another set of guidelines for argon lasers, another set for low-power helium-neon lasers, and finally a set for low-power semiconductor lasers. This approach was the result of the Sliney and Palmisano (1968; Sliney, 1969) study of hazards connected with nearly 1,000 different laser installations. Previous experience in the field of ionizing radiation made it natural to attempt to adapt some standard methods from health physics. Initially, an installation classification scheme similar to that used with industrial x-ray machines (e.g. enclosed protective, exempt protective, open protective from NBS Handbook 93) was tried. Indeed, there may still be some merit in this approach for grouping arc-source hazards. This approach of using concepts such as "enclosures" and "controlled areas" broke down because of the fact that laser beams presented a very localized hazard, often extending over a great distance. In addition there was widespread use of lasers out-of-doors.

7.2.3.1 High-Power Lasers—Class IV Limits

The early concepts suggested a distinction (Sliney and Palmisano, 1968) between the so-called "high-powered" lasers (which would cause hazardous diffuse reflections) and these low-powered lasers without hazardous diffuse reflections. This was a useful dividing line since it could be shown that a high-power laser gives a severe risk (i.e., a high probability) of retinal injury if an individual viewed a diffuse reflection; whereas low powered lasers (which did not produce hazardous diffuse reflections) would be unable to cause retinal injury unless an individual's eye was within the beam path—a very low probability event. At this time most lasers were still being used in laboratory environments or were completely enclosed, hence there appeared to be little need to provide further breakdowns of hazard categories. The high-power laser category later became Class IV.

By 1971 there were many complaints regarding the lack of subtle distinctions and exclusions for certain types of laser systems in the 1968-vintage guidelines. There were corresponding criticisms of a lack of a sliding scale of exposure limits to correct for different exposure durations and different wavelengths then available. It was during this period that the Committee on the Safe Use of Lasers of the American National Standards Institute developed standard Z-136.1 (1973). Their effort made great improvements on the previous, simplified breakdown of laser categories.

7.2.3.2 Medium-Power Lasers—Class III Limits

The ANSI committee consisted of representatives from research laboratories, governmental agencies, and industrial manufacturers and users of lasers. Hence there were several special-interest groups, each insisting on certain provisions. The manufacturers and users of small helium-neon alignment lasers were one of the most vocal and forceful groups. They pointed to the 100,000 small helium-neon lasers being used for alignment (mostly in the construction industry) with no known reports of injury from such lasers. Therefore they felt that even the control measures required for a lower-power laser category were still too severe for their application. It was therefore suggested that the two general categories, high-power (diffuse reflection hazard) and lower-power (no diffuse reflection hazard) lasers be further broken down into high power, medium power and low power. The small helium-neon lasers would hopefully fall into the low-power category. Since all such alignment lasers marketed at that time were less than 5 mW, it was proposed by this group that a limit of 5 mW be provided as the dividing line between low-power and medium-power lasers.

7.2.3.3 Low-Power Lasers—Class II Limits

The biologically oriented members of the ANSI committee balked at the 5-mW value since existing biological data suggested that a 5-mW exposure of the retina for a brief momentary exposure, even shorter than the blink reflex, might be injurious. Most of the committee agreed that the guiding principle for the dividing line should be the power of a continuous-wave visible laser which would not be injurious for an exposure of less than the eye's aversion response (the blink reflex). Low power lasers would be those that could not cause injury unless the person intentionally stared directly into the dazzling light source. The natural aversion response had been timed in a number of laboratory experiments. The normal blink reflex resulting from unexpected exposure to a short duration bright light source such as an atomic flash or an electronic flash, was shown to vary between 150 ms and 200 ms (Gerathewohl and Strughold, 1953). Therefore, to be slightly conservative, the committee selected an "aversion response" duration of 0.25 s (250 ms). For visible lasers the "Biological Effects of Lasers on the Eye" subcommittee (M. L. Wolbarsht, Chairman) recommended a MPE of 2.5 mW/cm^2 for a 0.25-s exposure.

The next question, then, was whether or not to define the maximal output of the low power category in terms of output irradiance (2.5 mW/cm^2.) or in terms of radiant power. The output characteristic most often specified by laser manufacturers was power, while the beam irradiance was rarely mentioned. Additionally, the irradiance was variable as it depended on the collimating optics used in the laser. One could always assume that the entire beam of the laser could be collected and directed into the eye through the use of survey transits and other optical instruments available at construction sites. Hence it was decided that total power entering the eye would be the most conservative and, at the same time, a realistic definition for the dividing line. It was later (in 1972) decided that the maximum realistic collecting aperture for common optical instruments (e.g. binoculars and telescopes) was 80 mm and this value was used for power and energy measurements in classification.

The question then before the "Laser Measurements and Hazards Evaluation" subcommittee (Dr. R. C. Honey, Chairman) was the selection of the limiting aperture or pupil size to use in translating the irradiance level of 2.5 mW/cm^2 into a power level entering the eye. In bright daylight at a construction site, the typical pupil size is 2 to 3 mm in full sunlight, or 5 to 7 mm in a deep ditch or tunnel. The power entering a 2 mm pupil would only be 79 μW, a level so low that the beam could only be seen in a dark room or mining tunnel. On the other hand, the corresponding level entering a 7-mm (reasonably dark-adapted) pupil would be 1 mW—a useful value, and a value which was easy to remember and specify. This value, however, was still too low for some committee members, inasmuch as the great majorityof lasers actually being used on construction sites had a typical output of 2 mW. With use, after a period of time, the 2-mW laser output normally decreased to approximately 1 mW or slightly less.

Another fact considered was that the beam diameter at the emerging optics of a construction laser was typically large enough that only 1 mW would enter a 7-mm aperture. This would fulfill the general concept of safety except for the case of optically aided viewing where collecting optics would gather the total energy and direct it into the eye.

7.2.3.4 Class I Limits

The dividing line between "totally safe lasers" and low-power, low-risk visible lasers would obviously be the maximum permissible exposure (MPE) but again the concept of collectability was introduced. The standard was written such that if it were possible for all of the energy or power output of the laser to be directed by optics into the limiting aperture, then the total irradiance of the MPE for intra-beam viewing would be translated into an optical power output of the laser. This limiting aperture was the 7-mm pupil of the eye for the retinal hazard region (visible and IR-A) and 1-mm in the UV and most of the IR.

It should be emphasized that there is conceptually a possibility that a laser's output quality would be so poor that no optics, even approaching theoretical perfection, would be able to collect the output of the laser. For this reason it is necessary to consider a radiance limit as well as an irradiance limit. For instance, it is surprising to many that a 1-J neodymium laser, obstensibly a very high-risk, Class IV laser, can be made in the extreme case into a Class I laser and still emit 1 J into the open. This is possible by running the laser beam through a large diffuser such that the source of the laser output is actually a very large extended source from which collimating optics cannot reimage the original source. In this case the output radiance of the diffusion is limited to the maximum permissible exposure for an extended source.

The lowest power class of laser (non-hazardous) was termed "Class I Exempt" by ANSI, and the low risk laser (hazardous only for continuous viewing) was termed Class II. The ANSI subcommittee on Laser Control Measures (R. J. Rockwell, Chairman) had thus established basically four categories: Class I Exempt; Class II Low Power; Class III Medium Power; and Class IV High Power. These divisions were based solely on risk analysis of visible lasers which presented a retinal hazard. Many of these distinctions did not apply to ultraviolet or far-infrared lasers. The classification concept was therefore still in its infancy.

7.2.3.5 *Class III Limits for CW Lasers*

In section 7.2.3.1 the rationale of the division between Class III and Class IV lasers as a distinction between those lasers which would and those which would not cause hazardous diffuse reflections was shown to rest on a recognition of the increased probability of risk of injury resulting from viewing a hazardous diffuse reflection. Most Q-switched ruby and neodymium lasers could produce hazardous diffuse reflections and therefore fell into the Class IV category. Argon lasers in the 1 to 5-W range could in theory produce hazardous diffuse reflections for momentary viewing but only at very close viewing distances. It was believed at that time the retinal threshold for Q-switched lasers did not vary with spot size, and therefore regardless of viewing distance, and regardless of the corresponding retinal image size of the diffuse reflection, the risk would be more or less equal provided that the beams reflection was an extended source. On the other hand, the safety limits and the biological data available in 1971 suggested that the injury threshold for a 0.25-s exposure varies with retinal image size. A 5-W argon laser might present a hazardous diffuse reflection within an arm's-length viewing distance, but not at greater distances. Therefore, the Committee had to find another basis upon which to divide Class III and Class IV CW-visible lasers. Was there any basis for such a division?

It was pointed out that a 1-W argon laser had caused minor skin burns and had also ignited paper and other combustibles, whereas certainly a 0.1 W argon or helium-neon laser would not produce such effects. Studies performed at the U.S. Army Environmental Hygiene Agency with a number of individuals of different skin pigmentations revealed that the normal level for sensing a CW argon, krypton, neodymium, or CO_2 laser was of the order of 100 to 500 mW total power. Specifically, if a person held his hand or sensitive portion of his forearm in such a laser beam he could remove it before the temperature elevation in the skin tissue was high enough to cause injury. A beam irradiance of 500 mW in a small 1 to 3-mm beam would be far in excess of the recommended CW skin protection levels but would still be less than that required to cause a burn within a second. As a beam power of 500 mW was approached, most subjects found that the sensation was most uncomfortable. Some subjects could just barely withdraw their hand in time to avoid a modest erythema. Varying the beam diameter from 1 mm to 10 mm made essentially no difference in these findings. The explanation for this lack of an area effect was that heat conduction was sufficiently fast in skin tissue and the diffusion sufficient that the irradiance was not the key factor. It was therefore concluded that beam power could be the dividing line. Further experiments revealed that levels somewhat above 0.5 W were required to burn paper and ignite other combustibles; therefore, a 0.5-W total power limitation for CW lasers (regardless of wavelength) seemed to be a very logical dividing line between Class III Moderate Risk lasers and Class IV High Risk lasers.

7.2.3.6 Class V

Attaining consensus among the many members of the ANSI Z-136 Committee and its different subcommittees on the classification scheme was not a simple matter for although these dividing lines in this classification were logical to some on a scientific basis, they did not always fall at the natural divisions between either user or manufacturing categories. However most of the adopted dividing lines have withstood the test of time; only few changes were made in 1976 when the ANSI standard Z-136.1 (1973) was revised. One of the changes in the classification scheme of ANSI that took place at that time concerned the Class V "enclosed laser."

In 1971 there were many Committee members, including the authors, who argued for a fifth category, Class V—for lasers which were "enclosed"—lasers that were safe not because of their output being very low, but because of their adequately protective enclosures. The reason for distinguishing between the two categories of Class I and Class V was that user control measures would differ. Control measures for Class I Exempt lasers would be totally nonexistent as such lasers in theory could not be hazardous even if a child or other unknowledgeable individual decided to collect all of the energy through collecting optics and view the source for a maximal reasonable period (the "classification duration"). On the contrary, an enclosed Class V laser could be hazardous if the user unknowingly moved safety panels, disabled the safety interlocks, or otherwise dismantled the system. A safety measure such as a periodic check of interlocks was recommended for Class V laser systems. From 1971 to 1975 the Bureau of Radiological Health developed their specification modeled in many respects after the ANSI Z-136 document. However, the Bureau did not see the need for distinguishing between Class I and Class V lasers in a performance standard and did not adopt a Class V concept (USDHEW, 1973, 1974, 1975).

Inasmuch as the same tests of emission measurement would be required for either Class I or Class V, and because of a desire for standardization the ANSI Z-136 committee voted in 1976 to abolish Class V. It had become obvious that many of the subcategories of "enclosed lasers" led to some confusion. For instance, a laser could be enclosed and the output reduced from Class IV to Class II, yet no simple relaxation of the safety measures were permitted. Likewise Class IV lasers or Class II lasers could be made into enclosed lasers and the risk to an individual opening the cabinet would be greatly different between the two. There was still another factor: the BRH standard had a lucid section on performance characteristics and accessibility which did not appear in the earlier ANSI standard. The ANSI standard had been more conceptual and less definitive. The accessibility concepts and definitions of protection housings of BRH supported the four-class concept.

7.2.3.7 ANSI Changes in 1976

In addition to the dropping of the Class V category (to conform more closely to BRH), the ANSI committee changed some Class I emission limits (thereby differing further from BRH). In the 1976 ANSI standard the subcommittees on Biological Effects of Lasers on the Eye and Biological Effects of Lasers on the Skin proposed revised maximum permissible exposures which were adopted. Since the emission limits for Class I were directly related to the maximum permissible exposure through the conversion factor of the limiting aperture area, it was considered logical to revise the lower limits for Class I emissions as well.

7.3 EXPOSURE LIMITS

To establish a rationale for developing exposure limits from the biological data required a careful analysis of the physical and biological variables influencing the spread of the laboratory biological data, the variables influencing potential for injury in individuals exposed to laser radiation, the increase in severity of injury for suprathreshold exposure doses, and the possibility of reversibility of injury. In addition, the accuracy of available instrumental measurements and the desire for simplicity in expressing the limits influenced the exposure limits. It was difficult to weigh all these factors against each other; however, most specialists did agree in the interpretation of the final limits, even though they used widely different approaches to derive the limits. Separate military, or other high-risk, occupational limits—in contrast to exposure limits for the general population—were not deemed suitable since, unlike ionizing radiation, there was never any debate whether a threshold of injury actually existed. Although there was always a question as to the exact value of a "threshold" of injury for a specific wavelength and exposure duration, there was no doubt that a threshold did exist. Hence, benefit-versus-risk analysis could not be applied to arrive at the specified values in the same way as in the determination of maximum permissible doses for ionizing radiation. However, a benefit-versus-risk analysis could be applied in the hazard analysis of laser applications based on the relative probability of exposure to the levels in excess of the exposure limits. UV-B and UV-C laser radiation could in theory have delayed effects with no real threshold, but was nevertheless treated like longer wavelength laser radiation in 1972.

7.3.1 The Concept of Threshold

In discussing the use of radioactivity and ionizing radiation in industry, science, and medicine, it is common to speak of benefit versus risk as if every exposure had a finite risk and there was not a finite threshold below which no biological injury occurred. Sometimes this discussion is carried over into considerations of other types of hazards, often causing needless concern where the risk is insignificant or even nil. It is therefore important to clarify the basis for such arguments.

Many scientists in radiobiology in the past have used a worst-case approach which is termed "the linear hypothesis." This hypothesis assumes that a biological injury produced following a short-term exposure in a laboratory study will also occur when the total exposure dose is delivered over a protracted period. Total integration of the exposure is thus assumed for all durations. This approach ignores the operation of any reparative processes which could produce a threshold level of detectable damage below which biological injury is balanced by tissue repair. In recent years, sufficient data has accumulated to show that in most cases, the linear hypothesis usually overstates the risk of low-level radiation exposure, although in spite of this newer evidence, the linear hypothesis is still held to by some. In addition, defects in the DNA repair mechanism following UV and X-ray damage of cells has been implicated in mutagenesis and carcinogenesis—suggesting a second probit curve (Smith, 1978; Trosko and Chang, 1978).

In describing the adverse biological effects of optical radiation at wavelengths greater than 320 nm, few scientists would argue that a linear hypothesis applies with total integration of the lifetime exposure. Optical radiation is usually absorbed in a thin layer of tissue and its effects are thermal in nature except for the ultraviolet and visible photochemical processes. For both of these acute effects tissue repair processes result in a definite threshold; that is, an exposure level exists below which no adverse change will occur and no real risk exists. Of course, the threshold can vary with the individual and with environmental conditions. However, if the safety level is set well below these variations, then the exposure conditions are not hazardous and an extensive (if any) benefit-versus-risk argument is not required.

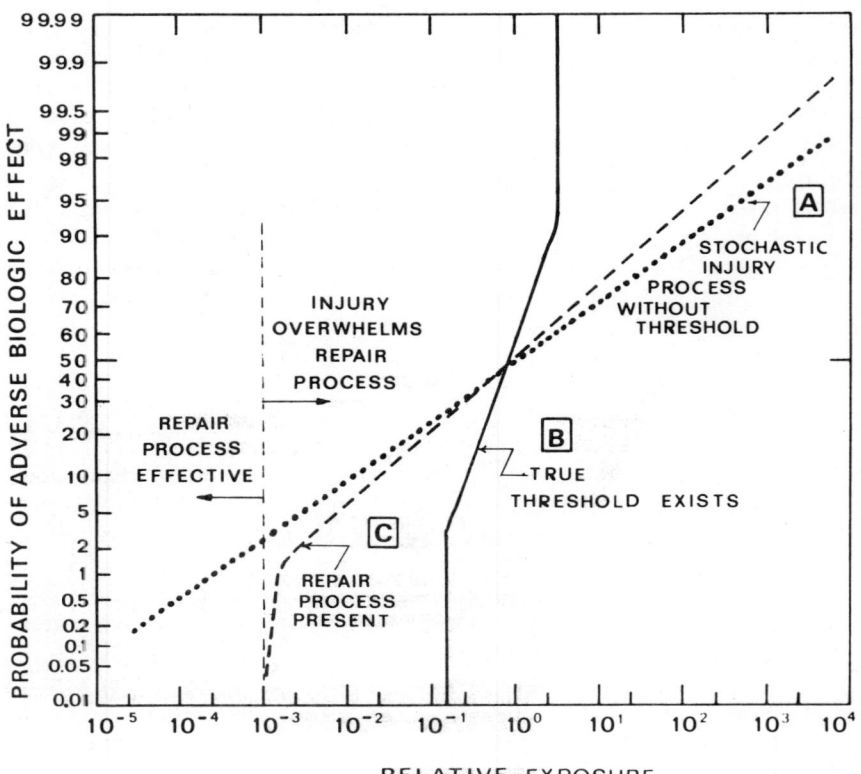

Figure 7-2. Biological thresholds and tissue repair processes. The concept of "threshold" for a biologic effect. Three types of idealized exposure dose response functions are shown. Line A represents an injury process without repair where cumulative exposure would increase the chance of injury and any single exposure would have a finite chance of causing injury. Curve C is similar to A except that a repair process creates a practical threshold; a real threshold does not exist due to errors in repair resulting in injury. Some scientists believe that carcinogenesis results from error-prone repair. Curve C is characteristic of damage produced by a pulse of thermal energy or by a photochemical reaction; a threshold exists and the spread of thresholds is due to biologic variability.

All thermal injury has a threshold. Individual photons in the long-wavelength range do not have sufficient energy to cause more than temporary biological changes at the molecular level. Acute pathological changes can only be demonstrated when a sufficient thermal photon flux exists to overwhelm normal reparative processes, or cause temperature rises so rapid that these processes cannot act. In the case of photochemical injury from shorter wavelengths, individual photons may change or damage an individual molecule. However, it has been shown that critical biomolecules such as DNA have repair mechanisms to correct such damage (Smith, 1978). Therefore, unless there is a very high photon flux density to overwhelm the repair processes the macroscopic damage will not show up. Thus safety limits can be set for any type of radiation in which the reciprocal relation of progressively lower power levels and longer exposure duration seems to show a marked deviation from linearity (Fig. 7-2). At this irradiance level any increases in the exposure duration may not be followed by pathological changes in the exposed tissues. The pessimist would nevertheless be somewhat reluctant to accept this as a true threshold of injury since one could always argue that the repair mechanism could fail. Thus we may yet be forced to admit that there may be some finite, albeit extremely small, risk of injury or delayed effects in a small population.

The first use of the benefit/risk analysis appears to have been by Blaise Pascal in his famous bet (first published in 1620) in which the certainty of a small gain was balanced against a small chance of an infinite gain—that is, certain small pleasures on earth as opposed to even a small chance of eternal bliss. In this benefit/risk analysis Pascal concluded that a small chance of a very large infinite gain outweighed the large chance of a small gain. It must be admitted even today many types of benefit/risk analyses depend upon the same argument with the result that we often choose to make everyone slightly unhappy in order to protect, possibly, one person against his own, often imprudent, behavior.

7.3.2 The Safety Factor and Probit Plots

The margin introduced to account for experimental errors in applying the exposure limits is very difficult to arrive at. This margin is sometimes loosely termed the "safety factor"; in fact, it is not that at all. To illustrate the matter, the interpretation of but one threshold point in a research study will be considered. The threshold of injury is actually the result of considering the probit analysis of many data points.

Probit analysis is a powerful tool in determining safety information but was not originally applied to retinal damage from laser exposure. In the early experiments on retinal damage the experimental design was usually such as to facilitate calculations of the ED_{50} point, that is, the level at which 50 percent of the laser exposures resulted in recognizable injury and 50 percent did not. Then to arrive at the exposure limit or maximum permissible exposure this ED_{50} value was reduced by a fixed "safety" factor. Customarily the practice had been to use a "safety" factor of 2 to 10. However, with probit analysis of the data point a more reasonable approach can be taken. The risk of achieving a particular biological endpoint can be reduced by a known amount or to an acceptable level. This allows those who set safety standards to dispense with arbitrary "safety" factors.

The use and value of probit analysis for calculation of any desired reduction of risk will be clear from the following example. Figure 7-3 shows the data from a 125-ms exposure of an argon laser at different power levels. Two methods (i.e., two endpoints) for assessing the threshold of damage were used—an ophthalmoscopically-visible lesion and a histological examination of a section of the retina in the region of the laser exposure. The judgements of damage or no damage for these criteria are shown in the rows above and below the graph. The curves in the graph

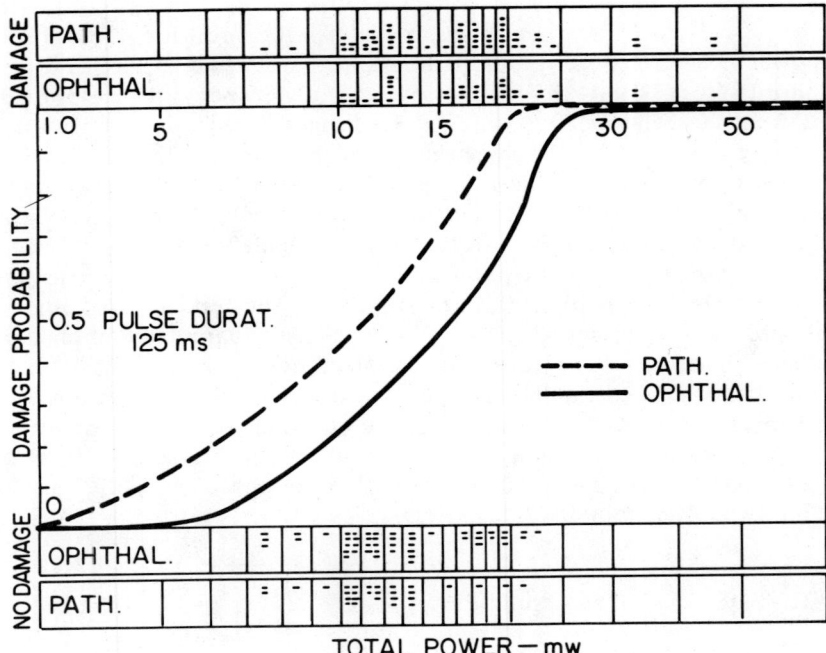

Figure 7-3. Dose response curve for a 0.125-s (125-ms) argon laser exposure. Retinal injury data is shown as a function of radiant power entering the pupil (intraocular power). The upper tally boxes indicate the number of retinal exposures where frank lesions occured at each power level, whereas lower boxes indicate exposures where lesions were not noted. From these tallies the probability of damage curve can be drawn. Note that the ophthalmoscopic-endpoint curve is displaced by approximately 4 mW. A better method of plotting the probability function is shown in Figure 7-5. Adapted from Bresnick et al. (1971).

are best fits for the probability of damage for any particular exposure level as judged by ophthalmoscopic examination or by histological examination. Both curves are somewhat s-shaped, suggesting that the data have a normal probability distribution. Similar data for a different exposure duration (12 ms) are presented in Figure 7-4.

Several questions can now be asked about the data in Figures 7-3 and 7-4. Are the criteria for the ophthalmoscopic and pathologic examination internally consistent, i.e., is the pathological examination in Figure 7-3 merely a more sensitive test of the same process that leads to the ophthalmoscopically-visible lesion (and similarly for Figure 7-4), or is a different factor involved? If both criteria are based on the same process, the displacement of the curves is then a linear one as a function of power, and the two curves should be parallel. It is difficult to judge that by inspection of the curves in Figure 7-3 and Figure 7-4. Furthermore it is pertinent to test if the damage process for the exposure data in Figure 7-3 is the same as for the

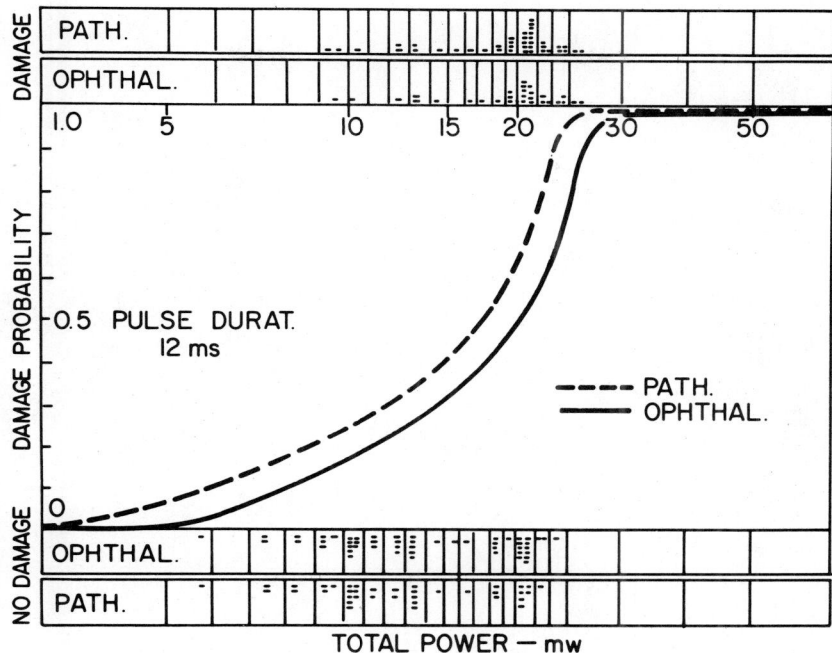

Figure 7-4. Dose response curve for 12-ms argon laser exposure. Note that the shape of the curve is similar to that of Figure 7.3. The corresponding power levels are higher (but energy levels less) than for the 0.125-s curve. A better method of plotting the probability function is shown in Figure 7-5. Adapted from Bresnick *et al.* (1971).

much shorter exposure data in Fig. 7-4. One test would be to examine the dependence on the power level of the exposure, that is, the shape of the curve. However the most important question concerns the "safety factor." How far below the ED_{50} level is risk minimized to a degree that is acceptable, and furthermore is the same safety factor appropriate for both long and short duration exposures? A slightly different presentation of the data gives a simple way to answer all of these questions.

A normally distributed set of data on the percentage probability of damage can be best plotted on normal probability paper. In this type of graph paper the y axis is distorted in such a way as to turn the cumulative s-shaped probability curves shown in Figs. 7-3 and 7-4 into straight lines. Figure 7-5 shows the data from Figs. 7-3 and 7-4 redrawn in such a fashion. It can be easily seen that all four lines are roughly parallel, thus the criteria for both ophthalmoscopy and pathology are the same, and furthermore the mechanism responsible for damage at 12 ms is probably not different from that at 125 ms. Also, the straight lines for probability of damage are easily extrapolated to any desired level. When the data is plotted this way only the slope of the line is needed to perform this extrapolation. Indeed, the experi-

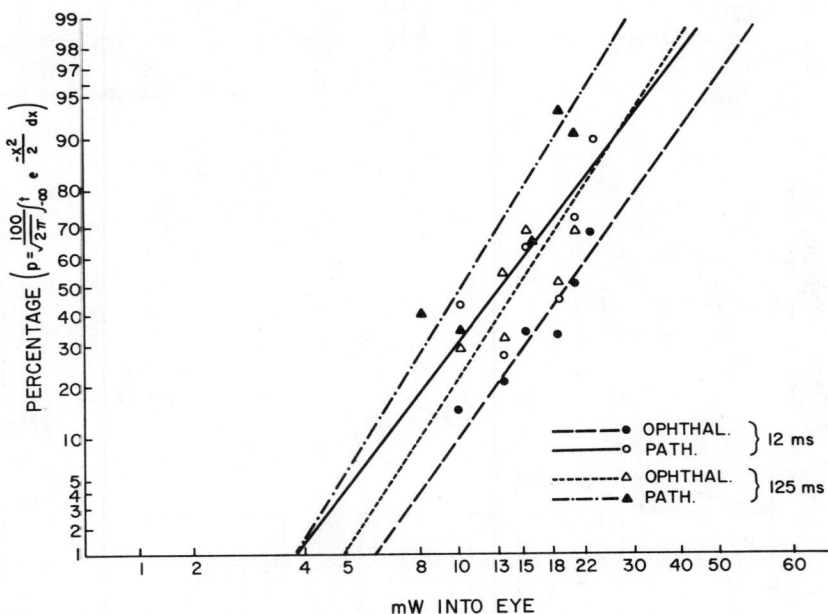

Figure 7-5. Probit plots of damage probability. These data are replotted from Figures 7-3 and 7-4. Note the specialized probit scale. The s-shaped dose-response curves now become straight lines. The parallelism of the different exposure duration criteria indicate that the same mechanism apply to each. The straight lines strongly suggest that the damage probability has a normal distribution.

ments should be designed to give the slope with maximum precision. For this the 20 and 80-percent probability points are more important than the ED_{50} point. Also, careful experimental design will avoid a needless clustering of the points around the 50-percent level and fewer experiments can give more statistically significant information. The fiducial limits of the significance of the slope of the probit plot can be arrived at in similar fashion. For a detailed treatment of the whole subject of probit analysis a standard work on the subject such as Finney (1971) should be consulted, preferably before any experiments are done.

The method of probit analysis has its limits, however. Experimental errors may not always be revealed by the shape of the probit curve; and to the contrary, experimental errors may change the curve and mislead the investigator. One type of error is illustrated in Figure 7-6.

Many laser retinal burn studies have attempted to simulate the "worst-case" exposure from a safety standpoint. That is, the condition of the relaxed normal eye exposed to a collimated beam to achieve the minimal (10-20 μm) retinal image. There are several problems in determining the injury threshold for a 1-s exposure for this minimal image in a monkey from a CW visible laser. First, measurement uncertainties are introduced during the measurement of the laser power and pulse shape entering the eye. If the retinal injury threshold is strongly dependent upon image size, a small error of ± 0.25 diopter in refracting the monkey could result in a far from minimal image of 35-45 µm. A similar error could be introduced if the monkey's accommodation drifted ± 0.25 diopter while under cycloplegia. Furthermore, during a 1-s exposure even shallow breathing and blood circulation of the anesthetized monkey could cause significant movement of the image in comparison to the image size. Also, mydriatic and cycloplegic agents create noticeable corneal haze when applied in overdose. It is only logical to ask whether lesser doses produce a corneal haze not readily evident to the experimenter but still sufficient to scatter much of the laser light entering the animal's eye. Non-uniform retinal pigmentation and other anatomical factors will further spread the data points. If the experimenter made a great effort to place retinal lesions only in sites he or she judged to be of the same uniform pigmentation one would expect a relatively steep exposure dose response probit curve. On the other hand, poor control of these factors would result in a probit curve with a noticeably shallower slope. Minimal retinal lesions placed in the vicinity of the optic disc could require an exposure dose 50 % greater than that required for the same type of lesions of the macula. Still other parameters which may affect the retinal burn threshold such as body temperature have often been overlooked and not controlled during the experiments. Considering these many sources of errors it still seems reasonable that occasionally an experimental data point probably does approach or even achieve the "worst case" exposure conditions. Figure 7-6 shows a hypothetical guess at the position and shape of the actual best case, error-free experimental (bold) curve versus a possible error-ridden experiment curve. It is therefore not at all surprising that the standard deviation for retinal injury thresholds for large retinal images (for example 500 µm) are smaller and hence the slopes of the probability curves are much steeper. The more errors present, the less steep the slope of the curve. Hence, the choice of a sufficiently small probability ordinate point for a safety level is still a conservative standard. In the most recent studies, the investigators have reduced some uncertainties through the use of contact lenses (Fankhauser and Lotmar, 1968) and fluorescein angiography (Borland et al., 1978).

In arriving at a consensus among the members of the ANSI Z-136 subcommittee on "Biological Effects of Lasers on the Eye" for a set of exposure limits, there was no consensus reached on the method of deriving them. Although the members agreed on the final set of limits they each arrived at the limits by somewhat different methods. Some relied upon the dose/response probit curves and a small safety factor; others used a reduction factor of approximately 10 below the experimentally determined ED_{50} point based upon studies of functional impairment and other changes below the visible lesion "threshold." What all of the experimental data revealed was that most reliable data for inter-laboratory comparisons was the ED_{50} point for a visible lesion (Beatrice et al., 1977). For this reason the ED_{50} data points were used extensively in the derivation of limits. However, probit curves of lesion thresholds and electron microscopy are preferred for the derivation of the most natural safety factors or probability of risk.

The value in presenting some of the many difficulties encountered in obtaining retinal injury thresholds from which the exposure limits are derived serves to

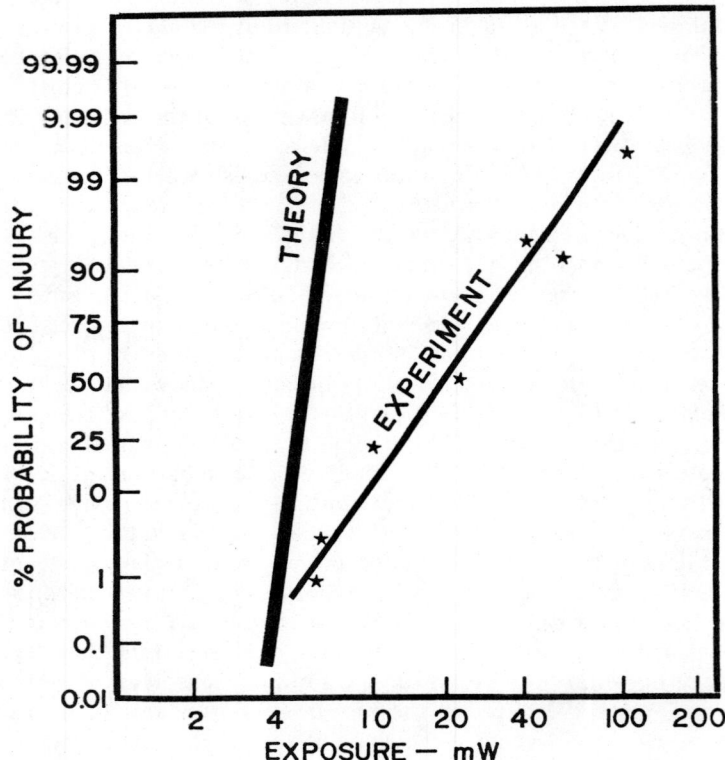

Figure 7-6. Hypothetical and experimental dose response curves. A hypothetical error-free dose response curve (bold line) is compared with an error-ridden curve for an experimental determination of laser retinal burn threshold for the minimal image size. The experimental curve would represent data points where the minimal image size was seldom achieved due to such effects as poor refraction, increased corneal clouding, body movements, etc., that were introduced by the experimental methods.

illustrate that exposure limits should not be considered well defined, sharp lines between safe and hazardous exposure. Considerable judgement and debate were necessary to arrive at a consensus for reasonable exposure levels. To this point we have discussed only thresholds of observed tissue damage. This threshold is only one part of the determination of injury threshold.

7.3.3 Means of Determining Thresholds of Injury

There are several different types of threshold criteria that have been used to study injury in tissue. These are:

(a) direct observation
    (1) without special techniques
    (2) with fluorescein angiography

(b) histology
    (1) light microscopy
    (2) electron microscopy

(c) biochemical studies

(d) electrophysiological tests

(e) functional studies

In setting exposure limits, all of these studies must be taken into account. In studies of skin reaction to optical radiation the first criteria of direct observation of erythema has been used almost exclusively although histological and biochemical techniques have been used in a few studies. The threshold criteria listed above will be discussed briefly as they apply to studies of ocular injury from laser radiation.

7.3.3.1 Direct Observation

In studies of retinal injury, the direct (and occasionally the indirect) ophthalmoscope have been used to observe the appearance of lesions. For thermal injury, the lesion normally appears almost immediately. For photochemical injury mechanisms (as in corneal and skin reactions to UV-B and C) there is a much delayed reaction. A commonly accepted protocol for recording a retinal lesion is five minutes and 24 hours following exposure. Thermal injury will almost always appear within five minutes, whereas the appearance of photochemical injury will be delayed and should normally be seen within 24 hours or 48 hours. A threshold lesion appears as a faint discoloration in the fundus, and will appear as a clearly visible white patch (opacity) at levels above threshold. The exact source of discoloration has often been debated, but is generally assumed to be a rearrangement of pigment granules in the RPE (retinal pigment epithelium) or a slight swelling (edema) at the junction of the RPE and the neural retina. Fluorescein angiography has been used to enhance the sensitivity by a factor of two over regular direct observation (Borland et al., 1978). Because the ophthalmoscopic observation technique is comparatively simple when compared to the alternative methods for determining injury thresholds, it has been used most extensively. There have been a number of studies which have sought to validate the ophthalmoscopic technique by related histological, histochemical and functional studies. Usually these have found the ophthalmoscopically determined threshold never to be more than twice the other thresholds of injury when the exposure duration was between 0.1 ms and 10 s. Several examples of ED_{50} values are given in Table 7.1.

A wavelength effect was also observed. Argon laser thresholds in the macula were elevated by a factor of 2 as compared with other parts of the retina, while no such difference was first found for similarly placed ruby or neodymium laser exposures of large size. Small-size lesion thresholds were typically less in the macula than paramacula, presumably because of better image formation in the macula Lappin and Coogan, 1970).

The biomicroscope, the specular microscope and slit lamp have been used for direct observation of corneal injury. The first appearance of threshold changes normally occurs in the corneal epithelium as a collection of granules. Again the criterian of five minutes and twenty-four hours have been used quite often. Corneal injury from IR-B and IR-C is thermal and the appearance of injury has generally been assumed to be within five minutes, whereas UV-B and UV-C injury (photochemical) to the cornea requires a much more delayed observation. Recently, Mueller and Ham (1975) noted that some corneal lesions from 100-ns IR-B laser exposures did not appear for three or four days; this would suggest accoustic damage to inner layers of the corneal epithelium.

7.3.3.2 Histological Studies

Morphological studies of structural changes in the retina observed under the light microscope or electron microscope always result in a threshold below that which is revealed by direct observation. However, these histological studies were far more tedious and costly and thus were employed more often to study injury mechanisms rather than to establish thresholds. As noted previously, the histologically determined thresholds for 0.1-ms to 10-s exposure retinal exposures are no less than 50% of ophthalmoscopically determined thresholds. For shorter pulsed exposures the histological thresholds are still farther below ophthalmoscopic thresholds (Adams *et al.*, 1972). Hence there are greater "safety factors" for the 10 to 30-ns pulse. Although there is morphologic change following some pulsed exposures, the question must still be asked whether the change is irreversible and whether there would be a functional loss—two questions almost impossible to answer. Also there are always potential misinterpretations of a histological preparation, i.e. artifacts introduced by fixation or staining. Chapter 4 contains an extended discussion of the various types of histopathology with some illustrations of typical lesions.

7.3.3.3 Histochemical studies of Laser Injury

Histochemical studies of laser injury in the retina are rather unusual, although they have been used often in other parts of the eye. An example would be tissue electrophoresis of the lens following laser exposure to document cataractogenesis at an early stage (Wolbarsht, 1978). Geeraets, Burkhart and Guerry (1963) did show an early use of such techniques in studies of thermal injury to the retina.

7.3.3.4 Electrophysiological Studies

Electrophysiological studies aimed at studying changes in retinal function following laser exposure would obviously be of great value if they were sufficiently reliable. Unfortunately the electroretinogram (ERG) and other electrophysiological recordings from large numbers of neurons (mass response) are often open to question. Similar mass responses in other parts of the visual system (the visual evoked response, VER, from the cortex) have a common failing. There is a lack of sufficient sensitivity to show changes in the small portions of the retina affected by a minimal lesion following laser exposure. Most electrophysiological programs have used the ERG and the VER to evaluate that some change has taken place following laser exposure, even if the location of the damage could not be specified. However, Pitts (1967) has made an attempt to localize the damage by single cell recordings in the lateral geniculate body. As a followup to this work studies have been in progress with similar physiological techniques in the retina aimed at distinguishing between flashblindness and permanent retinal damage. This approach may further elucidate the retinal mechanisms involved in laser damage and allow a closer correlation of the appearance of the lesion to the functional loss (Wolbarsht, 1978; Welch and Priebe, 1973).

7.3.3.5 Behavioral Studies

Behavioral studies are designed to detect functional changes or permanent visual loss and have been accomplished using trained primates in most instances. There have also been some human studies. Occasionally patients undergoing retinal coagulation or who are destined to have eyes enucleated, and accident victims of laser retinal injury have volunteered to undergo functional tests. The findings of all of these programs can be interpreted in a number of ways. It is important to distinguish between temporary visual disturbances such as flashblindness and permanent visual loss. Hence such functional tests should be conducted for a period of several days to result in valid data. The results of tests on patient performance within 24 hours of exposure are therefore of limited value. There are instances of functional loss being detected in animals following lengthy exposures to blue light without an ophthalmoscopically visible lesion (Sperling and Harwerth, 1971; Zwick and Beatrice, 1978) (Moon et al., 1978). Trained monkeys have been able to demonstrate high visual acuity despite the presence of a massive thermal lesion over most of the macula (Farrar, Ham et al., 1970). In general, except possibly for extremely long retinal exposures, permanent functional changes correlate quite well (within a factor of two) with the visible lesion threshold. For more detailed discussions of the development of "safety factors," exposure limits and their biological background the reader is directed to the references at the end of this chapter.

TABLE 7-1. Some Representative Injury Threshold Data and ED$_{50}$ Data in Experimental Animals

A. Retinal Injury in the Rhesus Monkey (macaca mulatta) As Determined by Ophthalmoscopic Observation

Wavelength λ (nm)	Site[†]	Exposure Duration t (s)	Image Size (See Note) d_r (μm)	Corneal Intraocular Energy* Q_c (mJ)	Calculated Retinal Rad. Exposure H_r (J/cm^2)	Reference
514.5	EM	0.004	15	0.14	79	Vassiliadis, 1971
514.5	EM	1.0	50	5.5 (3.0)	280	Beatrice & Frisch, 1973
514.5	EM	1.0	540	32(20)	14	
514.5	EM	1.0	940	50(40)	7.3	
514.5	EM & M	1.0	500	16.3	15.3	Ham et al., 1976
514.5	EM & M	16	500	185	165	
514.5	EM & M	100	500	250	220	
514.5	EM & M	1000	500	360	320	
514.5	M	1000	70 ?	120	3100	Gibbons & Allen, 1976
514.5	EM & M	14400	15000	500000	200	Lawwill et al., 1977
532	M	15 × 10^{-9}	40	0.003	0.24	Gibbons, 1973
568.2	M	0.016	40	0.40	32	Dunsky & Lappin, 1971
632.8	EM & M	0.25	50–80	3.3 (1.5)	170	Ham et al., 1970
632.8	M	0.5	40	6.0 (5.5)	400	Lappin & Coogan, 1970
632.8	EM & M	1.0	500	63(58)	30	Ham et al., 1970, 1976
632.8	EM & M	1.0	70	10(9.2)	130	Vassiliadis, 1971
632.8	EM & M	16	500	515	243	Ham et al., 1976
632.8	EM & M	100	500	1780	840	
632.8	EM & M	1000	500	11400	5400	
632.8	M	120	70			Vassiliadis, 1974
694.3	EM	30 × 10^{-9}	40	0.017 (0.008)	1.35	Beatrice & Frisch, 1973

694.3	EM	30×10^{-9}	500	0.104 (0.036)	0.055	Jones & McCartney, 1966
694.3	EM	30×10^{-9}	1000	0.20 (0.13)	0.025	Zweng et al., 1968
694.3	M & EM	0.0015	11000	2900	3.0	Borland et al., 1978
694.3	M	0.0017	70	0.5	11	
694.3	EM	40×10^{-9}	30	0.0029	0.41	
1059	EM	15×10^{-9}	30	0.047	6.6	
1064	M	30×10^{-9}	90	0.15 (0.08)	2.4	Vassiliadis et al., 1969
1064	EM	30×10^{-9}	50	0.22 (0.11)	7.6	
1064	—	6.0×10^{-4}	40	1.8 (1.1)	72	Vassiliadis et al., 1968

* Calculated when not given.

NOTE: Image diameter at 1/e points for all authors except Ham et al. However the calculated retinal exposures for Ham et al., and others are the peak retinal values.

† EM—extramacular exposure
  M—Macular exposure

TABLE 7-1. *Continued*

B. Corneal Injury in the Rhesus Monkey and Rabbit As Determined by Biomicroscope and Slit Lamp

Wavelength λ (μm)	Exposure Duration t (s)	Experimental Subject M—Monkey*	Beam Diameter at Cornea D_c (mm)	Absorption Coefficient in Water α_{H_2O} (cm^{-1})	Threshold or ED$_{50}$ Exposure H_c (J/cm^2)	Reference
10.6	1.4×10^{-9}	R	9.5	937	0.005 (a) 0.20 (c)	Mueller & Ham, 1975
2.61-2.87	45×10^{-9}	M	0.4	3220 (?)	0.62	Egbert & Maher, 1977
1.54	50×10^{-9}	M	0.56	12	21	Lund et al., 1970
2.9	1×10^{-7}	R	6.0	11190	0.004 (a) 0.3 (c)	Mueller & Ham, 1975
3.55-3.98	1×10^{-7}	M	0.48	197 (?)	1.51	Egbert & Maher, 1977
10.6	1×10^{-3}	M	2.5	937	0.8	Brownell & Stuck, 1974
10.6	1×10^{-2}	M	2.5	937	0.73	
2.795	1×10^{-2}	M	0.9	4906	0.86	Egbert & Maher, 1977
10.6	0.1	M	2.5	937	2.34	Brownell & Stuck, 1974
10.6	1.0	M	2.5	937	7.70	
10.6	900	M	10.4	937	220	Fine, 1968
10.6	1800	M	10.4	937	360	
2.7-3.0	4.0×10^{-9}	R		3220 (?)	0.004 (a) 0. (c)	Mueller & Ham, 1975
2.7-3.0	1×10^{-7}	R		3220 (?)	0.009 (a)	

(a) ablation threshold (injury caused by an acoustic transient, or cells were blown off the outer epithelial layer)
(c) coagulation threshold (damage well predicted by a thermal model of Egbert & Maher, 1977)

* The rabbit (R) cornea is considered close to that of humans for this type of study.

7.3.4 Limiting Apertures

One of the difficulties in developing exposure limits for any standard is the specification of the limiting aperture over which the values must be either measured or calculated. For the skin where no focusing effect takes place, the smallest feasible aperture is most desirable. Unfortunately the smaller the aperture the higher the sensitivity required for the measuring instrument and the greater the inaccuracy that will result from calibration problems associated with diffraction and other optical effects.

7.3.4.1 The 1-mm Aperture

A 1-mm aperture is considered the smallest practical aperture size. Under continuous exposure conditions, heat flow and scattering within the layers of the skin tend to eliminate any adverse effects from hot spots smaller than 1 mm. These same arguments hold for corneal exposures at wavelengths greater than 1.4 μm (1400 nm). Furthermore, atmospherically induced hot spots and mode structure variations in beam irradiance patterns in multimode lasers seldom if ever produce peak beam irradiance limited to areas less than 1 mm in diameter.

7.3.4.2 The 11-mm Aperture

Wavelengths greater than 100 μm present a further difficulty. At such far-infrared (submillimeter) wavelengths the aperture size of 1 mm would create significant diffraction effects and calibration would become a problem. However, hot spots must, by arguments from physical optics, be generally larger than at shorter wavelengths. For these reasons, a 1-cm square, or 1.1-cm (1 cm^2) circular aperture was chosen as the limiting aperture for submillimeter wavelengths between 0.1 mm and 1 mm.

7.3.4.3 The 7-mm Aperture

In the retinal hazard region, from approximately 400 nm to 1400 nm, the aperture over which the incident radiation can be averaged is determined by the pupil of the eye if the exposure limits refer to the eye. A pupil size of 7 mm was decided upon, although not without a great deal of debate. As noted earlier, some pre-1969 standards had different exposure levels for different pupil sizes, often expressed in terms of nighttime or daylight environments. However, a detailed study of physiological optics revealed that the intuitive conclusion that a larger pupil increased the retinal hazard was an oversimplification. The work of Gubisch showed that although more energy entered the pupil when it was dilated, much of the additional energy would serve to enlarge the effective image on the retina rather than add much to the retinal irradiance (Sliney, 1971).

This effect was later partially confirmed in some retinal injury studies performed by Frisch, Beatrice and Holsen (1971). The retinal irradiance varies as a function of pupil size as was shown in Fig. 4-15 based on the work of Gubisch (1967). This function is expressed as the optical gain of irradiance from cornea to retina, or the Strehl ratio. As can be seen in Fig. 4-15 the optical gain of the relaxed normal human eye for the intrabeam viewing of a laser varies little with pupil sizes between 3 mm and 7 mm. The theoretical optical gain would be approximately 200,000. According to Gubisch, the peak retinal irradiance is largely unaffected by variation of pupil size (Sliney, 1971).

The independence of peak retinal irradiance from pupil size suggests that the risk of injury from intrabeam viewing of a laser is essentially the same whether the laser is viewed at night with a 7-mm pupil or in daylight with a 3-mm pupil. Based upon this argument a 2-3 mm limiting aperture should be used to define retinal exposure in the 400-1400 nm spectral band. However, this argument is an oversimplification since it tacitly assumes that the retinal injury threshold does not depend upon increasing image size. This is a reasonable assumption. If the exposure duration is less than 0.1 ms there would be insufficient time for the exposed retinal area to cool. On the other hand, it was well known even in 1968 that the retina could withstand an irradiance as great as 1 kW/cm^2 for several seconds if the image diameter was as small as 10 μm—an image area sufficiently small to assure adequate cooling from the surrounding tissue (Clarke et al., 1969).

During the 1960's there was considerable debate about the relation of retinal image size to injury threshold power or threshold energy, particularly for the smaller images. Some argued that small image thresholds were large (Tengroth et al., 1963). Others argued that these results were an artifact in judging the lesion size, that even small images produced what seemed to be a large lesion. Later studies confirmed that there was a real dependence upon image size for most exposure durations and the relation shown in early experiments was not completely an experimental artifact (Fig. 4-18). It became clear during the development of the Z-136 standard that the optimum aperture for retinal injury varied with exposure durations and retinal image size. A detailed analysis is too lengthy to present here, but from it the conclusion was reached that an aperture between 5 and 7 mm was optimum. For several reasons, some of them "political," the 7-mm aperture was adopted. A still larger measuring aperture of 80 mm is used for power and energy measurements as mentioned in section 7.2.3.3. The rationale of this will be explained in more detail in Chapter 9.

7.3.5 Spectral Dependence of Exposure Limits

The injury thresholds for the cornea and retina of the eye and for the skin vary considerably with wavelength. Once again in establishing exposure limits the biological data could only be followed approximately when deriving the spectral dependence of the exposure limits. The exposure limits were adjusted for variation in wavelength by compromise. They did not track the actual biologic data exactly, but in a more simplistic way. Figure 7-7 provides a good example of the

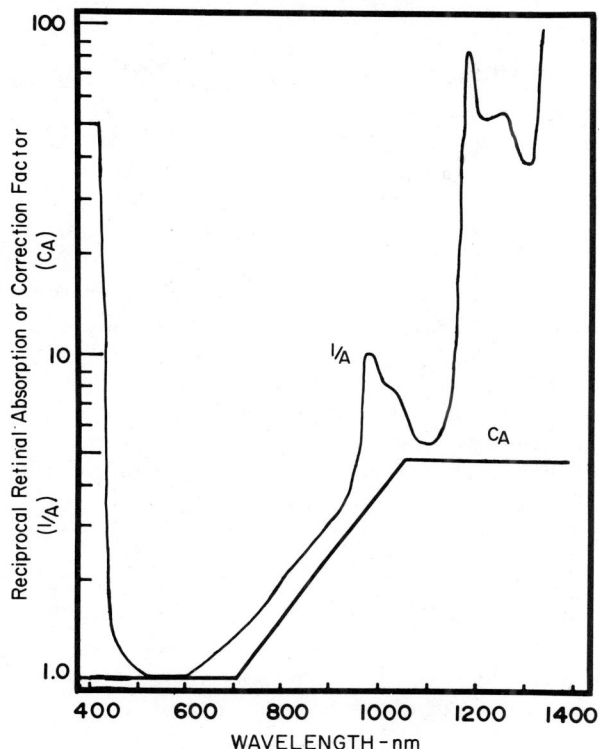

Figure 7-7. The retinal absorption and spectral weighting factor C_A. The upper curve is the reciprocal of the retinal absorption (1/A) spectrum (plotted in Fig. 4-12) relative to corneal irradiance. It may also be thought of as the reciprocal of the action spectrum for retinal thermal injury. A more useful spectral weighting factor, C_A is the lower function composed of straight-line segments to approximate (1/A). From Wolbarsht and Sliney (1974).

way in which a theoretical variation of the exposure limit was slightly modified to provide a spectral correction factor useful in a standard. In this case Fig. 7-7 provides the reciprocal of the product of the relative spectral transmission of the ocular media with the retinal absorption. This indicates the relative effectiveness of different wavelengths for causing retinal *thermal* injury. However, this curve still does not show the relative spectral hazard to the lens of the eye in the near infrared. Also plotted in this graph is the spectral correction factor used for pulsed retinal exposure limits in the Z-136.1 standard. Because of variations of thresholds with image size and variation of image size with wavelength, a further adjustment in this spectral correction factor for the ANSI Z-136.1 standard was made for IR-A wavelengths between 1.06 μm and 1.4 μm, but only for very short exposure durations (less than 0.1 ms).

7.3.6 Repetitively Pulsed Laser Exposure

The values in the initial Z-136 standard for repetitively pulsed lasers were based upon very limited data (Skeen *et al.,* 1972a, 1972b). This was an area where the protection standards were developed from purely empirical extrapolations, as no documented biological background existed. This lack of data pointed the way to later research of considerable magnitude. The cumulative effect of repetitive pulses was considered to be a function of the exposure duration of the individual pulse in a pulse train. For short pulses (duration less than 10 μs) the MPE limit for a single pulse was multiplied by a correction factor to provide a reduced exposure on a per-pulse basis (Fig. 8-5). This value was then compared to the values for the total energy and total "on-time" for the duration of the entire train of exposures to determine which limit would apply. For a train of pulses where the individual pulse duration exceeded 18 μs a criterion based upon total on-time of the train of pulses was applied to each individual pulse. This resulted in a reduced exposure limit for each pulse. However, all of these approaches were based largely on biological experiments which utilized single pulses of "minimal image size" in the rhesus monkey eye. Only a few experiments with repetitive pulses had been performed. For this reason, the ANSI Z-136 document contained a caution to the user on the poor validation of these approaches to repetitive pulse trains. In 1979, these repetitive-pulse guidelines were being altered to reflect the most recent data on this subject (Marshall, 1978; Stuck *et al.,* 1978). The latest threshold data indicated that the total energy threshold for a train of pulses increased as the total exposure ("on-time") raised to the ¾-power [just as single-pulse thresholds do from 10 μs to 10 s (Fig. 7-1)]. This can be seen from a careful examination of the data in Table 7-2.

7.3.7 Special Use Restrictions

The "low-risk" ANSI/BRH Class II is very close to the "no-risk" ANSI/BRH Class I in practice since it applies only to 0.4 μW to 1 mW *visible* lasers which are difficult to stare into because of the aversion response (Section 4.5.10). There is a big increase in risk when the eye cannot protect itself as would apply if a visible laser beam irradiance exceeded 2.5 mW/cm^2 (i.e., a total of 1 mW entering the 7-mm pupil of the eye by unaided or optically aided viewing). The laser classification merely denoted the risk if the laser is viewed under the worst-case condition. In practice if this worst-case condition is seldom experienced, further recommendations can be added for certain *limited applications only*. An example of this is the BRH limit of 5 mW for total power in surveying/alignment lasers, which recognizes that "moderate-risk" (ANSI/BRH Class III) lasers are sometimes needed in this application but that the benefit in this application outweighs this moderate risk of the 1 to 5 mW visible laser group.

7.4 PRESENT STANDARDS

The present standards can conveniently be divided into four major groups

TABLE 7-2. Some Representative ED_{50} Threshold Data for Multiple-Pulse Retinal Exposure in the Rhesus Monkey (macaca mulatta) for a Minimal Image Size

Wavelength	Exposure Duration of Pulse	PRF	Total Number of Pulses	"Threshold" ED_{50} Total Intra-Ocular Energy	Reduction (Ratio to Single-Pulse "Threshold")	Reference
λ (nm)	t (ns)	F (Hz)	n	Q_c (mJ)		
1064	10	N/A	1	0.164	N/A	Ebbers & Dunsky, 1973
1064	10	10	5	0.785	0.96	
1064	10	10	10	1.37	0.84	
1064	10	20	10	1.22	0.74	
1064	10	20	20	2.40	0.73	
1064	180	N/A	1	0.137	N/A	Stuck et al., 1978
1064	180	100	2	0.15	0.55	
1064	180	100	3	0.27	0.65	
1064	180	1000	2	0.16	0.58	
1064	180	1000	3	0.153	0.37	
1064	180	1000	6	0.33	0.40	
1064	180	1000	74	1.014	0.10	
1064	180	1000	1000	10.1	0.074	
1064	180	3000	2	0.121	0.44	
1064	180	3000	3	0.131	0.32	
1064	180	3000	6	0.182	0.22	
1064	270	N/A	1	0.028	N/A	Hemstreet et al., 1973
1064	270	1	5	0.031	0.22	
1064	270	10	5	0.0284	0.20	
1064	270	10	50	0.128	0.091	
1064	270	100	50	0.202	0.14	
1064	270	100	500	1.283	0.092	
1064	270	1000	500	0.918	0.066	
1064	270	1000	5000	5.94	0.042	
1064	730	N/A	1	0.025	N/A	
1064	730	10000	5000	3.65	0.029	
1064	730	10000	50000	19.7	0.016	
1064	700	N/A	1	0.025	N/A	Skeen et al., 1972b
1064	700	10	500	0.77	0.062	
532	15	N/A	1	0.003	N/A	Gibbons, 1973
532	15	5	150	0.076	0.17	
532	15	5	600	0.096	0.053	
514.5	10000	N/A	1	0.0016	N/A	Skeen et al., 1972a
514.5	10000	10	5	0.0033	0.41	
514.5	10000	100	50	0.0105	0.13	
514.5	10000	1000	500	0.0775	0.097	
514.5	10000	10000	5000	0.555	0.070	

Note: Some of the data in this table were adapted from tables in Stuck et al., 1978, and from Marshall, 1978.

which depend upon the organization responsible for them. These groups—state and local, Federal, national (non-US) and international—have many points of similarity, but may differ widely in purpose and effect, to say nothing of clarity or rigor. Many industrial and military organizations have formulated their own standards; however, these have lately been superseded by one or another of the consensus types developed by ANSI or ACGIH. However, many have still retained some type of a code of safe practice with a rather detailed training program.

7.4.1 Local and State Regulations

Table 7-3 gives a reasonably complete listing of state standards, regulations and statutes which apply to laser safety. Attempting to keep such a list current is very difficult and the reader should contact at least two types of state offices to check present status where up-to-date information is essential. Normally state regulations relating to lasers will be enforced by one or both of the following types of agencies:

(a) *Department of Labor*—typically a work safety standard regulating laser users in the work place.

(b) *Department of Health*—typically a general user standard supervised by an industrial health or radiation safety office within a department of health.

The organization of state governments vary and in some cases the Health and Labor agencies may be combined in some way.

Section 360-F of Public Law 90-602 enacted by the Congress of the United States in 1968 (Radiation Control for Health and Safety Act) limits states from regulating the same aspects of radiation safety performance except in the same (or less restrictive) manner as the USBRH regulations.

7.4.2 Present Federal Standards

A hazard-classification scheme was first presented in the American National Standards Institute's Z-136.1 standard on the Safe Use of Lasers. The Bureau of Radiological Health's classification scheme, which took effect August 2, 1976 governs the manufacture of laser devices, as described in Chapter 9. This was a slight modification of the 1973 ANSI scheme. The BRH safety classification has also been used in the drafts of the OSHA (Occupational Safety and Health Administration) standard for laser safety in the workplace. The basic philosophy behind the division into specific classes is based upon human access and potential hazard in the BRH standard. (Classification is also based upon normal use in the ANSI standard.) Maintenance areas have to be interlocked and *routine service* areas have to be labeled. The BRH regulations also aim toward limiting the classification of a laser

TABLE 7-3. States with some form of current laser safety standards or regulations

State	Agency	Title	Date
States with current regulations–including registration			
Alaska	Dept. Envir. Conser.	Title 18, Art 7 & 8	10/71
Georgia	Dept. Health	Ch 270-5-27	9/ 1/71
Illinois	Dept. Pub. Health	Registration Law	8/11/67
Massachusetts	Dept. Pub. Health	Sect 51, Ch 111	10/ 7/70
New York	Dept. Labor	Code Rule 50	8/ 1/72
Pennsylvania	Dept. Envir. Resour.	Ch 203, Title 25, Part 1	11/ 1/71
Texas	Dept. Health	Radiation Control Act Parts 50, 60, 70	7/ 2/74
States with existing regulations–or voluntary regulations with no registration requirement			
Missouri	Dept. Health	Existing Ionizing Regulation applies	
Montana*	Dept. Health & Envir. Sciences	Reg: 92-003	
Virginia	Dept. Health	Voluntary Program	
Washington	Dept. Lab. & Ind.	Ch 296-62-WAC	
States with enabling legislation passed			
Arizona*	———	HB-5	8/11/70
Arkansas*	Public Health	Act 460	
Florida*	Div. Health	Ch 501-122	
Louisiana*	Div. Radiation Control	HB-1165	7/31/68
Mississippi*	Dept. Health	HB-499	4/24/64
Oklahoma*	Health Dept.	HB-1405	4/14/69

* *New Regulations now being drafted or pending passage.*

product to the highest class necessary for its intended function. The classes used by BRH (USDHEW, 1973) are (in a simplistic way):

Class I laser product which can emit optical radiation "at levels at which biological damage has not been established."

Class II (or "low-power" laser devices by ANSI) are those *visible* lasers which do not have enough output power to injure a person accidentally, but which may cause "eye damage from chronic exposure."

Class III laser products emit "at levels at which biological damage to human tissue is possible from acute direct exposure." It has been subdivided into IIIa and IIIb.

Class IIIa covers visible lasers that are not hazardous to the normal person when viewed with the unaided eye but may be hazardous when the energy is collected and directed into the eye, as with binoculars.

Class IIIb consists of lasers which can produce a chance of accidental injury if viewed directly. The primary danger from such a laser is exposure to the direct or specularly reflected beam.

Class IV as conceived by ANSI includes lasers which not only produce a hazardous direct or specularly reflected beam but also can be a fire hazard, a serious hazard to the skin, or produce a hazardous diffuse reflection. BRH states simply that "biological damage is possible from acute direct or diffuse exposure."

In September 1975 the ANSI Z-136 committee voted to increase the permissible exposure limits for the eye for durations greater than 10 s within the spectral region of 550 to 1400 nm. This MPE revision also affected the ANSI Class I limits for such wavelengths. BRH did not move to adopt these less restrictive limits. As an example, the eight-hour limit for viewing the 632.8-nm line of the helium-neon laser was increased by a factor of 17. Skin exposure limits for near-infrared radiation were also increased, and ANSI eliminated Class V to make its classification system more compatible with BRH's.

In 1976 ANSI also adopted limits for short-term exposure to actinic ultraviolet radiation. These were more conservative than the 1976 BRH limits.

7.4.3 Foreign National Standards

Table 7-4 lists some national standards or regulations known to the authors. Because of the present number of countries which could have such standards or regulations it is nearly impossible to maintain a current and accurate list, but hopefully the table will provide the reader wtih a starting point. Once again, the governmental agencies with which to check would be those responsible for radiation safety, for industrial and public health, and for labor safety regulation. Any national standards organizations of the country in question should also be consulted.

7.4.4 International Standards

Table 7-5 lists those international guides or standards that have been formulated to date.

7.5 FUTURE TRENDS

Present eye and skin protection standards in the ANSI Z-136 and ACGIH formats are based upon experimental data available in 1976. However, detailed information was lacking for certain wavelengths and exposure conditions. The extrapolations that were necessary to cover these cases were based on current theories of the mechanism of injury. Unfortunately the publication of these stand-

Table 7-4. Present National Standards Regulations and Guidelines Relating to Laser Hazards

Country	Type of Document*	Document
Canada	A	Radiation Emitting Devices Act, Chap. 34 (1st Suppl., 1970.
	B	Radiation Emitting Devices Regulations, Part VII, "Laser Scanners;" Part VIII, "Demonstration Lasers," Canada Gazette Part II, Vol. 111, No. 22, Nov. 8, 1977. Has some simularities to the BRH performance standards for these types of lasers.
Australia	D	Standards Association of Australia, "Laser Safety," Standard AS-2211, 1978. Comprehensive Standard similar to IEC and draft British Standard.
Denmark	E	Provisional Instructions for Safety Arrangements in Work with Lasers, Feb. 23, 1971.
France	E	National Security (Safety) Institute: Lasers, Cahiers de Notes Documentaires No. 42, pp. 105-109, April 1966; has control measures listed.
	D	Technical Electronics Union: "Portable and Hand-held Laser Pulsed Photocoagulators with a Maximum High Voltage Not Exceeding 5 kV; No. C74-310, March 29, 1973.
Germany (Fed. Republic)	C,D	German Workman's Compensation Insurance (public corporation, Cologne, Union of Professional Association) (Berufsgenossenschaft) "Laser Radiation" VBG-93, April 19, 1973, and "Implementation Regulations and Clarifications of VBG-93, April 1974. Has ACGIH 1968 TLV values and control measures, "high power" lasers are $>$ 10 mW.
	B	State Board of Mines, "Code for Approving CW Laser Systems." Has control measures for He-Ne lasers less than 2 mW.
	D	German Standards Institute, DIN, "Protective Screens and Goggles Against Laser Beams," DIN 58215, September 1974.
	D	German Standards Institute, DIN, VDE Specification 0836 for the Electrical Safety of Laser Equipment and Installations, DIN 57836, 1 February 1977.
United Kingdom	D	British Standards Institution, "Protection of Personnel Against Hazards from Laser Radiation," BS 4083, 1972, but revised draft BS 4803, "Radiation Safety of Laser Products and Equipment," expected to be approved in 1979. General with classification and control measures.

Table 7-4. *Continued*

Country	Type of Document*	Document
United Kingdom	D	British Standards Institution, "Eye Protection Against Laser Radiation," 72/61379 DC.
U.S.S.R.	C	Izd-vo Minzdrava USSR, Moscow, "Temporary Sanitary Regulations When Working With Lasers," 1972. See Kirillov, *et al.*, Kvantovia Elektronika, 3(7), 1976.
United States	E	American Conference of Governmental Industrial Hygienists, Cincinnati, Threshold Limit Values for Chemical Substances and Physical Agents in the Workroom Environment with Intended Changes for 1978 and "A Guide for Control of Laser Hazards," 1976.
	D	American National Standards Institute (ANSI), "Safe Use of Lasers," Standard Z-136.1-1976.
	C	U.S. Department of Labor, OSHA, Washington, D.C.
	B	U.S. Department of Health, Education and Welfare, FDA/BRH, Washington, "Performance Standard for Laser Products," 21CFR1040, 1975, revised 1978.
	A	Public Law 90-602, "Radiation Control for Health and Safety Act of 1968," Washington, DC, 1968. Controls for all radiation from electronic products can be promulgated by FDA/BRH in the form of product performance standards.

*A - Law; Enabling Legislation
  B - Governmental regulation on product performance
    C - Governmental regulation on users (e.g., in the workplace)
      D - Standard (non-regulatory) of the user or manufacturer
        E - Guidelines

ards left the impression among many observers that *all* of the questions involving the hazards of exposure to laser radiation had been answered. This certainly was not the case. Among the major problem areas yet to be dealt with were laser exposures delivered in extremely short periods (sub-nanosecond mode-locked laser pulses) delivered at very low levels of exposure for long periods of time. At present it seems that a different mechanism produces threshold retinal damage for short pulses as opposed to long exposures at much lower levels. However, no data exists to show if interaction between the two mechanisms exists, and whether it is competitive or synergistic. In addition, exposure to infrared and ultraviolet laser radia-

Table 7-5. International Guidelines or Standards Relating to Lasers

Source	Standard or Guide
International Electrotechnical Commission (IEC), Geneva	"Radiation Safety of Laser Products and Equipment" Still in Committee TC-76 as of January 1978. Classification and performance standard similar to BRH regulation, and exposure limits similar to ANSI; applies to both manufacturer and user. Committee Chairman: G. Wilkening, USA
International Radiological Protection Association (IRPA)	"Overviews on Non-Ionizing Radiation," April 1977, published by US Dept. of Health, Education and Welfare, Rockville; a general information booklet explaining the biological effects of all non-ionizing radiations, including radio-frequency radiation. Chairman: H. Jammet, France
International Standards Organization (ISO), Geneva	"Filters and Eye Protectors Against Laser Radiation," ISO standard expected approval by 1979; density limits, optical quality of lenses, standard markings. Chairman of ISO/TC 94/SC 6/WG 3: E. Sutter, Fed. Rep. Germany
World Health Organization (WHO) European Office, Copenhagen	"Optical Radiation, with Particular Reference to Lasers," a chapter in a Manual for Non-Ionizing Radiation, Report ICP/CEP 803, 1977. Authors: Goldman, L., Rockwell, R. J., Michaelson, S. M., Sliney, D. H., Tengroth, B. M., and Wolbarsht, M. based upon a working group meeting held in Dublin in October 1975. Informative, general guidelines on laser bioeffects, hazard evaluation and controls; gives exposure limits that are the same as ANSI Z-136.1, 1976; Available free from WHO European Office.

tion has not been adequately studied. There are still several large gaps in the available data regarding exposure to repetitive pulse trains of laser radiation. There are also some interesting questions remaining with regard to non-circular images, especially when one dimension is small, such as the line images and elliptical images produced by some laser diodes or by a scanning laser.

7.5.1 DELAYED EFFECTS

Much of the available exposure data were collected in an empirical fashion without an adequate attempt to determine in detail the underlying mechanism of injury. The implications of repreated exposures at lower levels than described in present protection standards cannot be evaluated without a far more complete understanding of the applicable mechanisms of injury. Without such studies there can be no assurance that some effects will not occur after a long delay—perhaps years later after the active use of such lasers. The ocular effects are by far the most important, and delayed effects may result from chronic exposure of the lens and anterior portion of the eye to ultraviolet and/or infrared radiation.

7.5.2 Injury Mechanisms

Past studies have revealed that there are probably three principal mechanisms of injury: thermal injury, photochemically induced injury, and thermal-mechanical (acoustic transient) injury. Each type of injury has its own time domain and/or wavelength region in which it is the principal cause of threshold injuries.

Threshold retinal lesions from very short exposures such as from mode-locked and Q-switched lasers may result from some non-linear processes or from self-focusing, two-photon absorption leading to ultraviolet radiation injury, Raman and Brillioun scattering and singlet oxygen production, membrane breakdown, or an acoustic transient from localized heating in the vicinity of absorbing pigment granules. The acoustic energy imparted to tissue does not contribute to localized heating in the RPE and for this reason energy normally available for thermal injury is dissipated. This may explain why retinal exposure thresholds for 30-ns exposures are higher in energy than 1-μs thresholds. Somewhere in the domain of pulse durations between 1 μs and 1 ms the acoustic transient no longer plays a significant role for longer pulses and the process of thermal denaturation begins to dominate the picture. Thus thermal injury is the principal mode of action for medium duration pulses for exposures from a few microseconds to a few seconds.

Exposures to short-wavelength visible laser radiation for durations greater than 10 to 100 s appear to result in injury if exposure levels are well above those encountered in the natural environment. The limiting mechanism in this exposure domain appears to be some variety of photochemical injury to the retina. Several mechanisms have been proposed for damage at this level. Probably several are interrelated, of which the most important appears to be absorption of light by melanin granules or a chromophore distributed throughout the retina. For example, selenium-containing molecules (as in glutathione peroxidase) absorb heavily in the blue and UV-A, and selenium could play an important metabolic role in the retina (Combs and Scott, 1977). Also, oxygen levels altered as a result of some photochemical reactions could create adverse effects (Fridovich, 1977). Likewise, flavoproteins absorb heavily in the blue and would affect some metabolic processes. Although the temperature of the retina is an important factor, it plays a contributory or synergistic role rather than the principal one. When laser exposures occur in several different wavelengths and time domains at the same time it is not possible with present information to predict what the interaction will be, if any. Yet it is certain that there will be some; it would be surprising if each acted independently as if the other were not there.

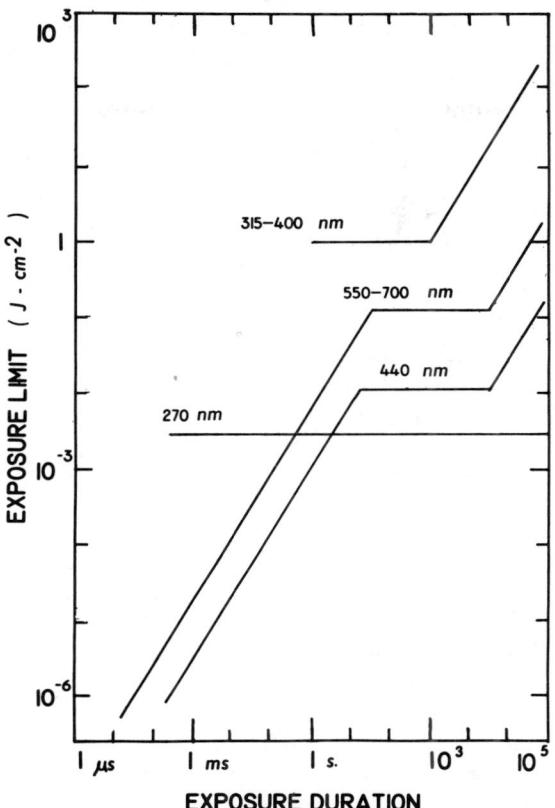

Figure 7-8. Corneal exposure limits as a function of wavelength. A comparison of corneal exposure limits for intrabeam viewing for different spectral regions. The horizontal lines of constant exposure demonstrate where photochemical damage mechanisms predominate.

All photochemical effects known have a strong wavelength dependence. This is especially marked in the long-term exposures for wavelengths less than 550 nm. Figures 4-21 and 8-3 show the wavelength dependent thresholds and the corresponding exposure limits which mimic the threshold curves. Figure 7-8 places the exposure limits for several wavelengths in perspective. The horizontal lines of constant exposure dose illustrate the regions of photochemical injury very well.

Longer-term exposures to infrared radiation result in injury at levels that are well above present exposure limits—as they should be. These effects seem to follow a power dependent thermal injury mechanism as opposed to the exposure dose related photochemical model used for visible radiation in this time domain.

For most exposure durations (i.e., $t > 1ms$), injury to the cornea and lens of the eye from ultraviolet radiation appears to be a photochemical or thermally enchanced photochemical effect.

The need to extend the data base for the ANSI, ACGIH, and BRH exposure criteria that has just been displayed should not alarm any laser user. Based upon the best knowledge available the present exposure limits have adequate safety factors to ensure that no chronic effects will appear if exposure is limited to the recommended values. However, it is only fair to point out that where meager biologic data existed, larger safety factors were used. If these protection standards are to be revised and any remaining unwarranted fears of chronic effects laid to rest, a continuing program on biological effects is still required.

The standards governing the potential exposures encountered by the great majority of laser users who work with visible lasers are based upon a very large accumulation of data. For most commonly encountered visible lasers the potential exposure durations range between 0.1 ms and 1 s. Furthermore, there is no reason to believe there is any danger if the eye is exposed to visible laser radiation which does not appear dazzling. This is the case in laser display systems and holographic viewing systems for the retinal illumination there is no greater than is encountered in the natural environment, i.e. daylight exposures or normal illumination from indoor light sources.

Litte data are available for long-term (chronic) exposures to laser radiation (or even for exposure to non-laser sources such as bright, small-source lamps and high luminance extended sources). Thus, the permissible exposure levels were based on a theory that the total retinal dose from visible illumination levels normally encountered in the natural environment were safe (Chapter 6, section 6.7).

The protection standard levels in the far-infrared region are based upon an understanding of the possible thermal effects on the cornea and a knowledge of exposures which have not resulted in adverse effects upon the eye. Because of the lack of accurate data for the infrared laser exposures of the human eye, worst-case exposure conditions were assumed. Specifically it was assumed that absorption took place in a very thin layer at the anterior surface of the cornea. This condition is best represented by CO_2 laser exposures (or for that matter, exposure of the eye to any wavelength beyond approximately 3 μm). At wavelengths less than 3 μm the radiation penetrates into the cornea more deeply and significant absorption may take place in the aqueous and lens (Fig. 4-24). For some of these wavelengths (1.5 to 1.6 μm) short-term exposures to much greater irradiances are permitted. However, the implications for infrared cataracts are greatest for chronic exposures. The increased interest in certain near-infrared lasers such as carbonmonoxide, hydrogen-fluoride and deuterium-fluoride lasers, holmium, erbium, calcium-fluoride, and even neodymium lasers will require extensive research programs to define in more detail the permissible exposure conditions in the middle and near-infrared regions. At present a thermal model of injury predicts levels required to cause thermal coagulation of the corneal epithelium (Egbert and Maher, 1977) but cannot predict corneal surface ablation thresholds for submicrosecond pulses (Mueller and Ham, 1975).

Only scattered data points are available for damage thresholds to the cornea and lens of the eye from ultraviolet radiation. Extrapolations from studies using non-laser ultraviolet sources were made to arrive at reasonable values. All present data points argue for photochemical damage mechanisms for exposures greater than 1 ms. The previous lack of availability of ultraviolet lasers has not permitted extensive studies of laser injury thresholds and possible special mechanisms of injury. Hopefully the availability in the future of a tunable ultraviolet laser with a continuous-wave or nearly continuous output should permit such studies. In the meantime, persons using the present ultraviolet standards should consider them only the best available guidelines and limit exposure as much as possible.

One may legitimately ask how it is possible to study delayed chronic effects upon the retina and other portions of the eye. Is it necessary that such studies be conducted for 20-30 years before the effect can be known? Fortunately several powerful research tools are becoming more available which permit a study of the ultrastructural changes in tissues soon after exposure. This type of an examination can permit a more fundamental understanding of the mechanism of injury and permit an accurate prediction of chronic effects. The most valuable of such tools are electron microscopes, both scanning and fixed types, and various spectroscopic probes. As a better understanding of retinal physiology and the fundamental photochemical mechanisms of vision develops, the prediction of the existence or absence of chronic effects will be more reliable.

The interpretation of all such studies requires a sophisticated level of experience. It is important to remember in planning research studies that the availability of acute threshold data does not answer all questions. It is hoped that this brief review will permit the reader to assess the need for further biological studies of laser effects, especially where present information is lacking. Also we wish to encourage laser manufacturers and others with lasers of unusual characteristics to make such equipment readily available to institutions presently conducting laser bioeffects research. In addition, and most importantly, this research will assist in a balanced approach to any future revisions of the present exposure limits.

7.6 REFERENCES

Adams, D. O., Beatrice, E. S., and Bedell, R. B., 1972, Retina: ultrastructural alterations produced by extremely low levels of coherent radiation, *Science,* 177:58–60.

ACIGH, 1968, American Conference of Governmental Industrial Hygienists, *A Guide for Control of Laser Hazards,* Cincinnati (1968, revised 1973, 1976).

Anderson, F. A., 1974, Biological Bases for and Other Aspects of a Performance Standard for Laser Products, DHEW No. (FDA) 75–8004, Bureau of Radiological Health, Rockville, Maryland (July 1974).

ANSI, 1976, American National Standards Institute, *Safe Use of Lasers,* Standard Z-136.1, New York.

Beatrice, E. S., and Frisch, G. D., 1973, Retinal laser damage thresholds as a function of image diameter, *Arch. Environ. Health,* 27:322–326.

Beatrice, E. S., Randolph, D. I., Zwick, H., Stuck, B. E., and Lund, D. J., 1977, Laser hazards: Biomedical threshold level investigations, *Mil. Med.,* 14(11):889–892.

Boettner, E. A., and Dankovic, D., 1974, Ocular absorption of laser radiation for calculating personnel hazards: Determination of the absorption coefficients in the rhesus monkey, Final contract report F41609-74-C-0008, University of Michigan, Ann Arbor, MI (Nov. 1974). (Available from NTIS: AD-A009 176)

Borland, R. G., Brennan, D. H., Marshall, J., and Viveash, J. P., 1978, The role of fluorescein angiography in the detection of laser-induced damage to the retina: A threshold study for Q-switched, neodymium and ruby lasers, *Exp. Eye Res.*, 27:471–493.

Bredemeyer, H. G., Wiegmann, O. A., Bredemeyer, A., and Blackwell, H. R., 1963, Radiation thresholds for chorioretinal burns, Institute for Research in Vision and Department of Ophthalmology, Ohio State University, Columbus, OH, Air Force Tech. Doc. Rept. No. AMRL-TDR-63-71, July 1963, (Available from NTIS: AD 416 652).

Bresnick, G. H., Frisch, G. D., Powell, J. O., Landers, M. B., Holst, G. C. and Dallas, A. G., 1971, Ocular effects of argon laser radiation, I. Retinal damage threshold studies. *Invest. Ophthal.* 9:901–910.

Brownell, S., and Stuck, B. E., 1974, Ocular and skin hazards from CO_2 laser radiation, *Army Science Conference Proceedings*, Vol. 1, pp. 123–138, US Military Academy, West Point, NY, NTIS No. AD785609, June 1974.

Carpenter, J. A., Lehmiller, D. J., and Tredici, T. J., 1970, US Air Force permissible exposure levels for laser irradiation, *Arch. Environ. Health*, 20:171–176.

Cavonius, D. R., Elgin, S., and Robbins, D. O., 1974, Thresholds for damage to the human retina by white light, *Exp. Eye Res.*, 19:543–548.

Clarke, A. M., Geeraets, W. J., and Ham, W. T., Jr., 1969, An equilibrium thermal model for retinal injury, *Appl. Opt.*, 8:1051–1054.

Combs, G. F., Jr. and Scott, M. L., 1977, Nutritional interrelationships of Vitamin E and Selenium, *BioScience*, 27(7):467–473.

Cope, F. W., Sever, R. J., and Polis, B. D., 1963, Reversible free radical generation in the melanin granules of the eye by visible light, *Arch. Biochem. Biophys.*, 100:171–177.

Dunsky, I. L., and Lappin, P. W., 1971, Evaluation of retinal thresholds for CW laser radiation, *Vision Res.*, 11:733–738.

Ebbers, R. W., and Dunsky, I. L., 1973, Retinal damage thresholds for multiple pulse lasers, *Aerospace Med.*, 44:317–318.

Egbert, D. E., and Maher, E. F., 1977, Corneal damage thresholds for infrared laser exposure: empirical data, model predictions, and safety standards, Report SAM TR-77-29, US Air Force School of Aerospace Medicine, San Antonio, TX, December 1977. (Available from NTIS)

Fankhauser, F., and Lotmar, W., 1968, Methods of Photocoagulation through the Goldman contact glass, *Mod. Probl. Ophthal.*, 7:256–272.

Fankhauser, F., 1977, Physical and biological effects of laser radiation, *Klin. Monatsbl. Augenheilkd.*, 170(2):219.

Farrer, D. N., Graham, E. S., Ham, W. T., Jr., Geeraets, W. J., Williams, R. C., Mueller, H. A., Cleary, S. F., and Clarke, A. M., 1970, The effect of threshold macular lesions and subthreshold macular exposures on visual acuity in the rhesus monkey, *Am. Ind. Hyg. Assn. J.*, 31(2):198–205.

Fine, B. S., 1968, Corneal injury threshold to carbon dioxide laser irradiation, *Am. J. Ophthal.*, 66(1):1–15.

Finney, D. J., 1971, Probit Analysis, 3rd edn., Cambridge University Press, Cambridge.

Fridovich, I., 1977, Oxygen is toxic!, *BioScience*, 27(7):462–466.

Frisch, G. D., Beatrice, E. S., and Holsen, R. C., 1971, Comparative study of argon and ruby retinal damage thresholds, *Invest Ophthal.*, 10:911–919.

Geeraets, W. J., 1968, Retinal injury from laser and light exposure, in Laser Eye Effects, (H. G. Sperling, Ed.), Armed Forces-NRC Committee on Vision, National Research Council, Washington, DC, pp. 20–56.

Geeraets, W. J., Burkhart, J., and Guerry, D., 1963, Enzyme activity in the coagulated retina, a means of studying thermal conduction as a function of exposure time, *Acta Ophthal (Suppl)*, 76:79–93.

Gerathewohl, S. J., and Strughold, H., 1953, Motoric responses of the eyes when exposed to light flashes of high intensities and short durations. *J. Aviat. Med.*, **24**:200–207.

Gibbons, W. D., 1973, Retinal Burn Thresholds for Exposure to a Frequency-Doubled Neodymium Laser, USAF Report SAM-TR-73-45, US Air Force School of Aerospace Medicine, Brooks Air Force Base, TX.

Gibbons, W. D. and Allen, R. G., 1977, Retinal damage from long-term exposure to laser radiation, *Invest. Ophthal., Vis. Sci.*, **16**(6):521–529.

Gibbons, W. D., and Egbert, D. E., 1974, Ocular Damage Thresholds for Repetitive Pulsed Argon Laser Exposure, Report SAM-TR-74-1, US Air Force School of Aerospace Medicine, Brooks Air Force Base, San Antonio (February 1974).

Gibson, G. L. M., 1970, Retinal Damage from Repeated Subthreshold Exposures Using a Ruby Laser Photocoagulator, Report SAM-TR-70-59, US Air Force School of Aerospace Medicine, Brooks Air Force Base, San Antonio, TX (October 1970) (Available from NTIS: AD 715 210).

Goldman, A. I., Ham, W. T., Jr., and Mueller, H. A., 1977, Ocular damage thresholds and mechanisms for ultrashort pulses of both visible and infrared laser radiation in the rhesus monkey, *Exp. Eye Res.*, **24**:45–46.

Gullberg, K., Hartman, B., Kock, E. and Tengroth, B., 1967, Carbon dioxide laser hazards to the eye, *Nature*, **215**:857–858.

Gubisch, R. W., 1967, Optical performance of the human eye, *J. Opt. Soc. Am.*, **57**:407–415.

Ham, W. T., Jr., Clarke, A. M., Geeraets, W. J., Cleary, S. F., Mueller, H. A., and Williams, R. C., 1970, The eye problem in laser safety, *Arch. Environ. Health*, **20**:156–160.

Ham, W. T., Jr., Williams, R. C., Geeraets, W. J., Ruffin, R. S., and Mueller, H. A., 1963, Optical masers (lasers), *Acta Ophthal (Suppl.)*, **76**:60–78.

Ham, W. T., Jr., Geeraets, W. J., Mueller, H. A., Williams, R. C., Clarke, A. M., and Cleary, S. F., 1970, Retinal burn thresholds for the helium-neon laser in the rhesus monkey, *Arch. Ophthal.*, **84**:797–809.

Ham, W. T., Jr., Mueller, H. A., and Sliney, D. H., 1976, Retinal sensitivity to damage from short wavelength light, *Nature*, **260**(5547):153–155.

Ham, W. T., Jr., Ruffolo, J. J., Jr., Mueller, H. A., Clarke, A. M., and Moon, M. E., 1978, Histologic analysis of photochemical lesions produced in rhesus retina by short-wavelength light, *Invest. Ophthal., Vis. Sci.*, **17**(10):1029–1035.

Hatch, T. F., 1971, Thresholds: do they exist?, *Arch. Environ. Health*, **22**:687–689.

Hatch, T. F., 1973, Criteria for hazardous exposure limits, *Arch. Environ. Health*, **27**:231–235.

Hemstreet, H. W., Bruce, W. R., Altobelli, K. K., Stevens, C. C., and Connolly, J. S., 1974, Ocular Hazards of Picosecond and Repetitive Pulse Argon Laser Exposures, First Annual Report, February 1973-February 1974, USAF Contract for School of Aerospace Medicine, Brooks AFB, TX, Technology Inc., San Antonio, TX.

Holmberg, B., and Winell, M., 1977, Occupational health standards, an international comparison, *Scand. J. Work Environ. Health*, **3**:1–15.

Jones, A. E., and McCartney, A. J., 1966, Ruby laser effects on the monkey eye, *Invest. Ophthal*, **5**:474–483.

Lappin, P. W., and Coogan, P. S., 1970, Relative sensitivity of various areas of the retina to laser radiation, *Arch. Ophthal.*, **84**:350–354.

Laser Institute of America, 1976, *Laser Safety Guide*, LIA, 4100 Executive Park Dr., Cincinnati, OH 45241.

Lawwill, T., Crocket, S., and Currier, G., 1977, Retinal damage secondary to chronic light exposure, *Doc. Ophthal.*, **44**(2):379–402.

Lee, J. A. H., 1972, Sunlight and the etiology of malignant melanoma, In *Melanoma and Skin Cancer*, V.C.N. Blight, Government Printer, New South Wales.

Lund, D. J., Landers, M. B., Bresnick, G. H., Powell, J. O., Chester, J. E., and Carver, C., 1970, Ocular hazards of the Q-switched erbium laser, *Invest. Ophthal.*, 9(6):463–470.

Marshall, W. J., 1978, A proposal for a new method to determine MPE values for repetitive pulse trains, US Army Environmental Hygiene Agency, Aberdeen Proving Ground, MD, June 1978.

Moon, M. E., Clarke, A. M., Ruffolo, J. J., Jr., Mueller, H. A., and Ham, W. T., Jr., 1978, Visual performance in the rhesus monkey after exposure to blue light, *Vis. Res.*, 18:1573–1577.

Mueller, H. A., and Ham, W. T., Jr., 1975, The ocular effects of single pulses of 10.6 μm and 2.5-3.0 μm Q-switched laser radiation, A Report to the Los Alamos Scientific Laboratory L-Division, Virginia Commonwealth University.

Naidoff, M. A. and Sliney, D. H., 1974, Retinal injury from welding arc, *Amer. J. Ophthalmol.*, 77(5):663–668.

Noell, W. K. and Albrecht, R., 1971, Irreversible effects of visible light on the retina, Role of Vitamin A, *Science*, 172:72–75.

Peabody, R. R., Rose, H., Zweng, H. C., Peppers, N. A., and Vassiliadis, A., 1969, Threshold damage from CO_2 lasers, *Arch. Ophthal.*, 82:105–107.

Pitts, D. G., 1967, LGN single cell responses as a function of intense light flashes, *in Proceedings of the US Army Natick Laboratory Flashblindness Symposium* (J. M. Davies and D. G. Randolph, eds.), pp. 92–119, November 8-9, 1967.

Robbins, D. O., Zwick, H., and Holst, G. C., 1974, Functional assessment of laser exposures in an awake, task-oriented Rhesus monkey, *Mod. Probl. Ophthal.*, 13:284–290.

Skeen, C. H., Bruce, W. R., Tips, J. H., Jr., Smith, M. G., and Garza, C. G., 1972a, Ocular Effects of Repetitive Laser Pulses, Technology, Inc., San Antonio, Texas Air Force Contract F41609-71-C-0018 (June 30, 1972) (AD 746795).

Skeen, C. H., Bruce, W. R., Tips, J. H., Smith, M. G., and Garza, C. G., 1972b, Ocular Effects of Near Infrared Laser Radiation for Safety Criteria, US Air Force Contract No. F41609-71-C-0016, Technology, Inc., San Antonio, Texas (June 1972) (AD 746793).

Sliney, D. H., 1969, Evaluating hazards and controlling them, *Laser Focus*, 5(15):39–42.

Sliney, D. H., 1971, The development of laser safety criteria, *in Lasers in Medicine and Biology*, (M. L. Wolbarsht, Ed.), Vol I, pp. 163–238, Penum Press, New York.

Siney, D. H., and Palmisano, W. A., 1968, The evaluation of laser hazards, *Am. Industr. Hyg. Assn. J.*, 29:325–431.

Smith, K. C., 1978a, Symposium on DNA repair and its role in mutagenesis and carcinogenesis, *Photochem. Photobiol.*, 28:119.

Smith, K. C., 1978b, Multiple pathways of DNA repair in bacteria and their roles in mutagenesis, *Photochem. Photobiol.*, 28:121–129.

Sperling, H. G., and Harwerth, R. S., 1971, Red-green cone interactions in the increment-threshold spectral sensitivity of primates, *Science*, 172:180–184.

Stokinger, H. E., 1970, Criteria and procedures for assessing the toxic responses to industrial chemicals, *in Permissible Levels of Toxic Substances in the Working Environment*, pp. 36–52, International Labor Office, Geneva.

Stuck, B. E., Lund, D. J., and Beatrice, E. S., 1978, Repetitive Pulse Laser Data and Permissible Exposure Limits Institute Report No. 58, Letterman Army Institute of Research, Division of Non-Ionizing Radiation, Presidio of San Francisco, San Francisco (April 1978).

Trosko, J. E., and Chang, C., 1978, Relationship between mutagenesis and carcinogenesis, *Photochem. Photobiol.*, 28:157–168.

U.S. Department of the Army, 1975, Control of Hazards to Health from Laser Radiation, TB MED 279, 3rd Edn., Washington, DC (May 1975).

U.S. Department of the Air Force, 1973, Laser Health Hazards Control, Air Force Manual AFM 161–168 (1973, under revision).

U.S. Department of Commerce, National Bureau of Standards, 1963, Safety for Non-Medical X-Ray and Sealed Gamma-Ray Sources, NBS Handbook 93, ANSI Standard Z-9.1-1963, NBS Washington, DC.

U. S. Department of Health, Education and Welfare, Food and Drug Administration, BRH, 1973, Laser Products, Proposed Performance Standard, in: Federal Register, 38(236):34084–34834091, Dec. 10, 1973.

U.S. Deparment of Health, Education and Welfare, Food and Drug Administration, BRH, 1974, Laser Products, Proposed performance Standard, in: Federal Register, 39(172):32094–32109, Sep. 4, 1974.

U.S. Department of Health, Education and Welfare, Food and Drug Administration, BRH, 1975, Performance Standard for Laser Products, Title 21, Code of Federal Regulations, Part 1040, first published in: Federal Register, 40(148):32252–32266 (July 31, 1975); as amended in: Federal Register, 43(229):55387–55393 (November 28, 1978).

U.S. Department of Labor, Occupational Safety and Health Administration, 1976, Title 29, Code of Federal Regulations, Part 1910.

Vasiliadis, A., 1971, Ocular damage from laser radiation, in: "Laser Applications in Medicine and Biology," M. L. Wolbarsht, ed., Vol. I, pp. 125–162, Plenum Press, New York.

Vassiliadis, A., Rosan, R. C., and Zweng, R. C., 1969, Research on ocular laser thresholds, SRI Report No. 7191, Stanford Research Institute, Menlo Park, California (NTIS No. AD 700422).

Vassiliadis, A., Zweng, H. C., and Dedrick, K. G., 1971, Ocular Laser Threshold Investigations, SRI Report No. 8209, Stanford Research Institute, Menlo Park, California (January 1971). (Available from NTIS)

Walkenbach, J. E., 1972, Determination of retinal lesion threshold energies of pulse repetition Nd^{3+}: YAG laser in the Rhesus monkey, M. S. Thesis, Virginia Commonwealth University, Richmond, VA (June 1972).

Wallow, I. H. L., Lund, O. E., and Gabel, V. P., 1974, A comparison of retinal argon laser lesions in man in cynomolgus monkey, Albrecht V. Graefes Arch Klin. Exp. Ophthalm., 189:159–164.

Wallow, I. H. L., Gabel, V. P., Birnguber, R., and Hillenkamp, F., 1975, Clinical and histological studies following argon laser effects on the retina, histopathological evaluation of laser injuries for the assessment of a functional injury threshold for laser, Ber Dtsch. Ophthalmol., 73:360–362, 1975 and Ber Dtsch. Ophth. Ges., 73:374–386, 1975.

Ward, B. and Bruce, W. R., 1971, Chorioretinal burn: body temperature dependence, Ann. Ophthal., 3:898.

Welch, A. J., and Priebe, A., 1973, Changes in the rabbit electroretinogram C-wave following ruby laser insult, Aerospace Med., 44(11):1246–1250.

Wolbarsht, M. L., 1978, Electrophysiological Determination of Retinal Sensitivity to Color After Intense Monochromatic Light Adaptation, Report SAM-TR-78-9, U.S. Air Force School of Aerospace Medicine, Brooks Air Force Base, San Antonio, TX (September 1978).

Wolbarsht, M. L. and Sliney, D. H., 1974, The formulation of protection standards for lasers, in: "Laser Applications in Medicine and Biology," M. L. Wolbarsht, ed., Vol. II, pp. 309–359 Plenum Press, New York.

7.7 REVIEW QUESTIONS

1. Distinguish between occupational health standards and product safety standards. Give two examples of agencies of the U.S. government which have now or could in the future issue standards which apply to laser applications.

2. The British Ministry of Aviation standard for lasers issued in 1965 was the most sophisticated laser safety standard of its time because retinal exposure limits varied with _____ size.

3. Early proposals (e.g., Sliney and Palmisano, 1968) for laser exposure limits varied with pupil size (i.e., separate daytime and nighttime limits). Why was the dependence upon pupil size not retained in the later standards?

4. The ANSI Committee Z-136 was an activity of the U.S. government. T or F ?

5. What are three hazards likely to be produced by a Class 4 laser but not by a Class 3 laser.

6. In which CIE spectral band(s) would it be logical to consider the possibility that a threshold for injury may not exist? Explain.

7. What is a probit curve? What is meant by ED_{50} ?

8. List five different investigative methods to study retinal injury.

9. How can a laboratory investigator who studies the effects of acute laser exposures to tissue predict possible delayed effects of laser exposure?

10. List five states in the U.S.A. which have laser safety regulations. What two types of state agencies might promulgate laser safety standards?

Chapter 8
Current Laser Exposure Limits

8.1 INTRODUCTION

In the previous chapter we examined the evolution of laser safety standards with emphasis on the permissible exposure limits and in this chapter we shall discuss in detail the most recent set of limits, those promulgated by the ANSI Z-136.1 Standard, Safe Use of Lasers 1976. This set of limits is also identical to the threshold limit values (TLV's) of the American Conference of Governmental Industrial Hygienists (ACGIH). These limits are essentially identical to those given in the proposed International Electrotechnical Commission (IEC) Standard being written by Technical Committee #76 of the IEC and are also the values recommended as "best available" in the World Health Organization (WHO) Manual on Non-Ionizing Radiation (1977). If one attempts by some method or other to translate these limits into the BRH classification limits one will find some differences. However, since the BRH standard, as the only Federal standard available, applied to laser emission performance standards and not to occupational exposures it would actually be incorrect to apply the BRH standards in occupational health and safety practice.

It is also likely that if the U.S. Department of Labor, Occupational Safety and Health Administration (OSHA) were to recommend exposure limits they would probably recommend the ANSI Z-136 limits as they are the most up to date. The military services in their laser safety publications generally subscribe fairly closely to the ANSI Z-136.1 1976 limits and although some state standards still exist with exposure limits that date back to the 1968 vintage and 1973 vintage standards these instances are not very common. Therefore, unlike the subject of laser classification where there are a number of subtle differences between the different standards, there appears to be almost universal concensus to be found in recent standards for occupational exposure limits. A discussion of these exposure limits may be

TABLE 8-1. Exposure Limits for Direct Ocular Exposures
(Intrabeam Viewing) from a Laser Beam

Spectral Region	Wave Length	Exposure Time, (t) Seconds	Exposure Limits	
UVC	200 nm to 280 nm	10^{-9} to 3×10^4	3 mJ/cm²	
UVB	280 nm to 302 nm	"	3 "	
	303 nm	"	4 "	
	304 nm	"	6 "	
	305 nm	"	10 "	
	306 nm	"	16 "	⎫
	307 nm	"	25 "	⎪ not to
	308 nm	"	40 "	⎬ exceed
	309 nm	"	63 "	⎪ $0.56\, t^{1/4}$
	310 nm	"	100 "	⎪ J/cm²
	311 nm	"	160 "	⎪
	312 nm	"	250 "	⎪
	313 nm	"	400 "	⎪
	314 nm	"	630 "	⎪
	315 nm	"	1.0 J/cm²	⎭
	315 nm to 400 nm	10^{-4} to 10	$0.56\, t^{1/4}$ J/cm²	
UVA	315 nm to 400 nm	10 to 10^3	1.0 J/cm²	
	315 nm to 400 nm	10^3 to 3×10^4	1.0 mW/cm²	
Light	400 nm to 700 nm	10^{-9} to 1.8×10^{-5}	5×10^{-7} J/cm²	
	400 nm to 700 nm	1.8×10^{-5} to 10	$1.8\,(t/\sqrt[4]{t})$ mJ/cm²	
	400 nm to 549 nm	10 to 10^4	10 mJ/cm²	
	550 nm to 700 nm	10 to T_1	$1.8\,(t/\sqrt[4]{t})$ mJ/cm²	
	550 nm to 700 nm	T_1 to 10^4	$10\, C_B$ mJ/cm²	
	400 nm to 700 nm	10^4 to 3×10^4	C_B µW/cm²	
IR-A	700 nm to 1049 nm	10^{-9} to 1.8×10^{-5}	$5\, C_A \times 10^{-7}$ J/cm²	
	700 nm to 1049 nm	1.8×10^{-5} to 10^3	$1.8\, C_A\,(t/\sqrt[4]{t})$ mJ/cm²	
	1050 nm to 1400 nm	10^{-9} to 10^{-4}	5×10^{-6} J/cm²	
	1050 nm to 1400 nm	10^{-4} to 10^3	$9(t/\sqrt[4]{t})$ mJ/cm²	
	700 nm to 1400 nm	10^3 to 3×10^4	$320\, C_A$ µW/cm²	
IR-B & C	1.4 µm to 10^3 µm	10^{-9} to 10^{-7}	10^{-2} J/cm²	
	1.4 µm to 10^3 µm	10^{-7} to 10	$0.56\,\sqrt[4]{t}$) J/cm²	
	1.4 µm to 10^3 µm	10 to 3×10^4	0.1 W/cm²	

C_A — See Fig. 8-8, Laser EL listing.

$C_B = 1$ for $\lambda = 400$ to 550 nm; $C_B = 10^{[0.015\,(\lambda - 550)]}$ for $\lambda = 550$ to 700 nm.

$T_1 = 10$ s for $\lambda = 400$ to 550 nm; $T_1 = 10 \times 10^{[0.02\,(\lambda - 550)]}$ for $\lambda = 550$ to 700 nm.

For $\lambda = 1.5$ to 1.6 µm increase EL by 100.

TABLE 8-2. Exposure Limits for Viewing a Diffuse Reflection of a Laser Beam or an Extended Source Laser

Spectral Region	Wave Length	Exposure Time, (t) Seconds	Exposure Limits
UV	200 nm to 400 nm	10^{-3} to 3×10^4	Same as Table 8-3
Light	400 nm to 700 nm	10^{-9} to 10	$10 \sqrt[3]{t}$ J/(cm²·sr)
	400 nm to 549 nm	10 to 10^4	21 J/(cm²·sr)
	550 nm to 700 nm	10 to T_1	$3.83 (t/\sqrt[4]{t})$ J/(cm²·sr)
	550 nm to 700 nm	T_1 to 10^4	$21/C_B$ J/(cm²·sr)
	400 nm to 700 nm	10^4 to 3×10^4	$2.1/C_B \times 10^{-3}$ W/(cm²·sr)
IR-A	700 nm to 1400 nm	10^{-9} to 10	$10\, C_A \sqrt[3]{t}$ J/(cm²·sr)
	700 nm to 1400 nm	10 to 10^3	$3.83\, C_A (t/\sqrt[4]{t})$ J/(cm²·sr)
	700 nm to 1400 nm	10^3 to 3×10^4	$0.64\, C_A$ W/(cm²·sr)
IR-B & C	1.4 μm to 1 mm	10^{-9} to 3×10^4	Same as Table 8-3

C_A, C_B and T_1 are the same as in footnote to Table 8-1.

TABLE 8-3. Exposure Limits for Skin Exposure from a Laser Beam

Spectral Region	Wave Length	Exposure Time, (t) Seconds	Exposure Limits
UV	200 nm to 400 nm	10^{-3} to 3×10^4	Same as Table 8-1
Light &	400 nm to 1400 nm	10^{-9} to 10^{-7}	$2\, C_A \times 10^{-2}$ J/cm²
IR-A	400 nm to 1400 nm	10^{-7} to 10	$1.1\, C_A \sqrt[4]{t}$ J/cm²
IR-B & C	1.4 μm to 1 mm	10^{-9} to 3×10^4	Same as Table 8-1

$C_A = 1.0$ for λ = 400–700 nm; see Fig. 8-8 for greater wavelength values.

NOTE: To aid in the determination of EL's for exposure durations requiring calculations of fractional powers, Fig. 4 may be used.

rather dry but an attempt will be made to review the present limits by way of example in as interesting a fashion as possible. The limits will be tabulated first followed by an explanation of the situations where special interpretation is required. Finally, a few examples will be given with the necessary calculations.

8.2 PRESENT EXPOSURE LIMITS

8.2.1 Commonality of Limits

Tables 8-1 through 8-3 provide all of the occupational health and safety limits for laser radiation in the optical spectrum from 0.2 μm (200 nm) to 1mm (1000

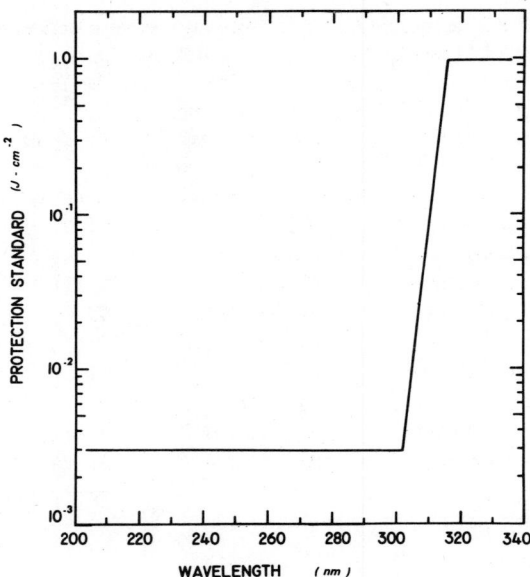

Figure 8-1. Exposure limits for continuous exposure to ultraviolet laser radiation for both the skin and the eye for wavelengths less than 340 nm.

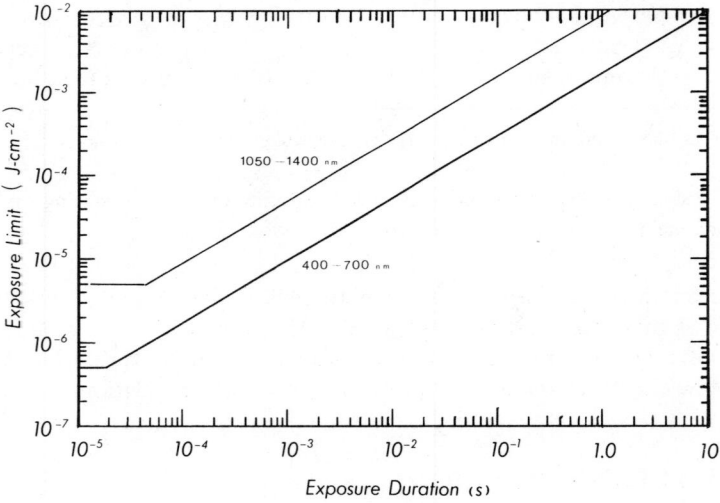

Figure 8-2. Exposure limits for intrabeam (direct) viewing of a laser pulse for visible wavelengths (lower line) and for IR-A wavelengths between 1050 nm and 1400 nm (upper line). Values for pulse durations less than 10^{-5} s and greater than 1 ns are constant.

Current Laser Exposure Limits

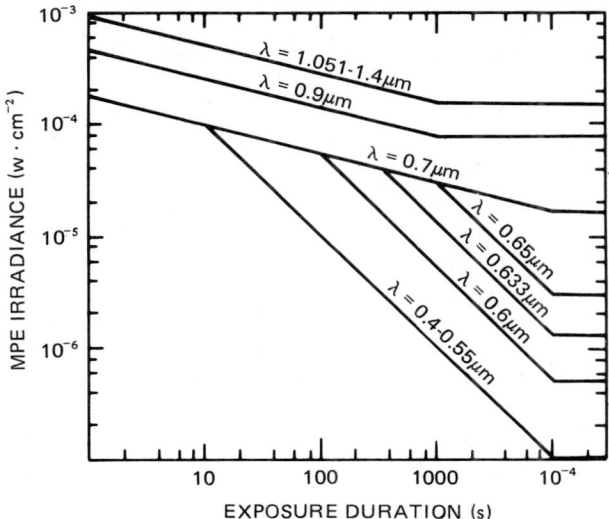

Figure 8-3. Exposure limits for intrabeam (direct) viewing of a continuous (CW) laser source for several wavelengths and wavelength regions between 400 nm and 1400 nm. Values for exposures greater than 10^4 s are constant.

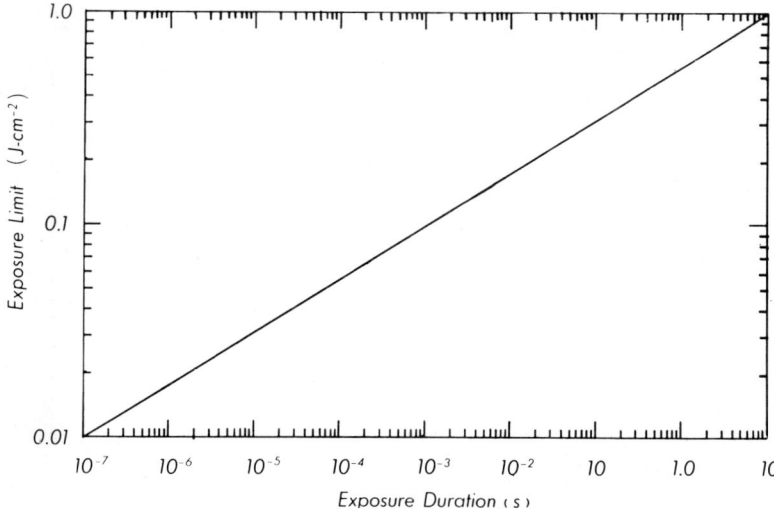

Figure 8-4. Exposure limits for pulsed laser exposure of the skin and eyes to radiation at wavelengths greater than 1400 nm and for wavelengths between 315 and 400 nm. These values are adjusted upward for skin exposure between 400 and 1400 nm.

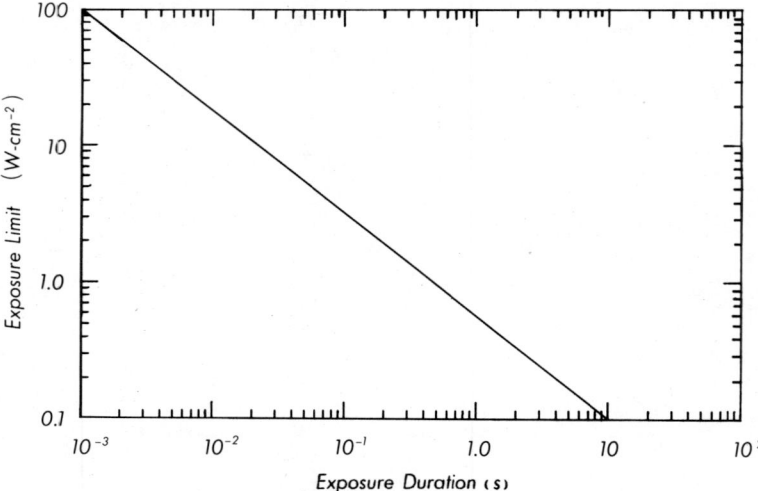

Figure 8-5. Exposure limits for continuous (CW) exposure of the skin and eyes to laser radiation at wavelengths between 1400 nm and 1 mm. Values for skin exposure in the 400-to-1400-nm region are greater by a factor of $2 \cdot C_A$.

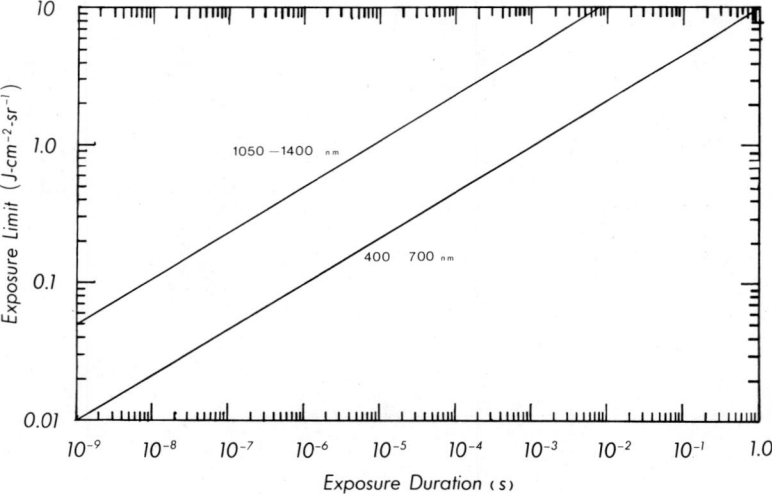

Figure 8-6. Exposure limits for viewing extended sources or diffuse reflections of pulsed laser radiation for wavelengths between 400 nm and 700 nm (lower line) and for wavelengths between 1050 nm and 1400 nm in the IR-A (upper line). For wavelengths between 700 nm and 1050 nm the value of the lower line is increased by the factor C_A.

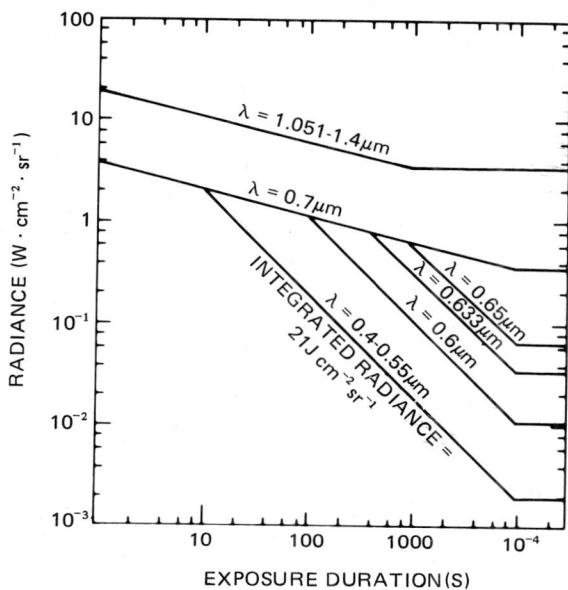

Figure 8-7. Exposure limits for viewing extended sources or diffuse reflections of continuous (CW) laser radiation for certain wavelengths in the retinal hazard region (400 nm to 1400 nm). EL values for durations greater than 10^4 seconds are constant.

μm)—a 5000-fold spectral range. Figures 8-1 through 8-7 provide graphical plots of many representative limits. These limits have been given different terms depending upon the standard. They are called the *maximum permissible exposures* (MPE's) by ANSI, the *threshold limit values* (TLV's) by the American Conference of Government Industrial Hygienists (ACGIH), the *protection standards* by the U.S. Army, the *exposure limits* (EL's) in a World Health Organization Manual on Non-Ionizing Radiation, and finally, as *maximum permissible exposures* (MPE's) by the IEC Technical Committee #76 on Laser Equipment. The actual tables and figures have been adapted from the ACGIH booklet "Threshold Limit Values for Chemical Substances and Physical Agents in the Workroom Environment with Intended Changes for 1978," as modified in the UV in 1979.

It is useful and indeed necessary to quote the TLV preamble of ACGIH: *"The threshold limit values are for exposure to laser radiation under conditions to which nearly all workers may be exposed without adverse effects. The values should be used as guides in the control of exposures and should not be regarded as fine lines between safe and dangerous levels. They are based on the best available information from experimental studies."*

TABLE 8-4. Selected Values of the Limiting Angle to Extended Source
Which may be Used for Applying Extended Source ELs

Exposure Duration(s)	Angle α (mrad)
10^{-9}	8.0 †
10^{-8}	5.4 †
10^{-7}	3.7 †
10^{-6}	2.5 †
10^{-5}	1.7 †
10^{-4}	2.2
10^{-3}	3.6
10^{-2}	5.7
10^{-1}	9.2
1.0	15
10	24
10^2	24
10^3	24
10^4	24

† For exposure durations less than 0.1 ms α min is less for λ = 1050 to 1400 nm.

8.2.2 Limiting Apertures

The EL's expressed as radiant exposure or irradiance in this section may be averaged over an aperture of 1 mm except for EL's for the eye in the spectral range of 400-1400 nm, which should be averaged over a 7-mm limiting aperture (pupil); and except for all EL's for wavelengths between 0.1 - 1 mm where the limiting aperture is 11 mm. No modification of the EL's is permitted by arguing for pupil sizes less than 7 mm.

The EL's for "extended sources" apply to sources which subtend an angle greater than α_{min} (Table 8-4) which varies with exposure duration t. This angle is *not* the beam divergence of the source. These limits expressed as either radiance or integrated radiance may be averaged over an angle as great as α_{min} or sampled over a source area as small as 1 mm in diameter.

8.2.3 Correction Factors A and B (C_A and C_B) For Eye Exposure

All EL's in Tables 8-1 and 8-2 are to be used as given for wavelengths 400 nm to 700 nm. EL's at wavelengths between 700 nm and 1400 nm are increased by a correction factor (which is C_A in the tables) as shown in Fig. 8-8. For certain exposure durations greater than T_1 (shown in Fig. 8-9) at wavelengths between 700 to 800 nm, correction factor C_B is also applied.

Current Laser Exposure Limits

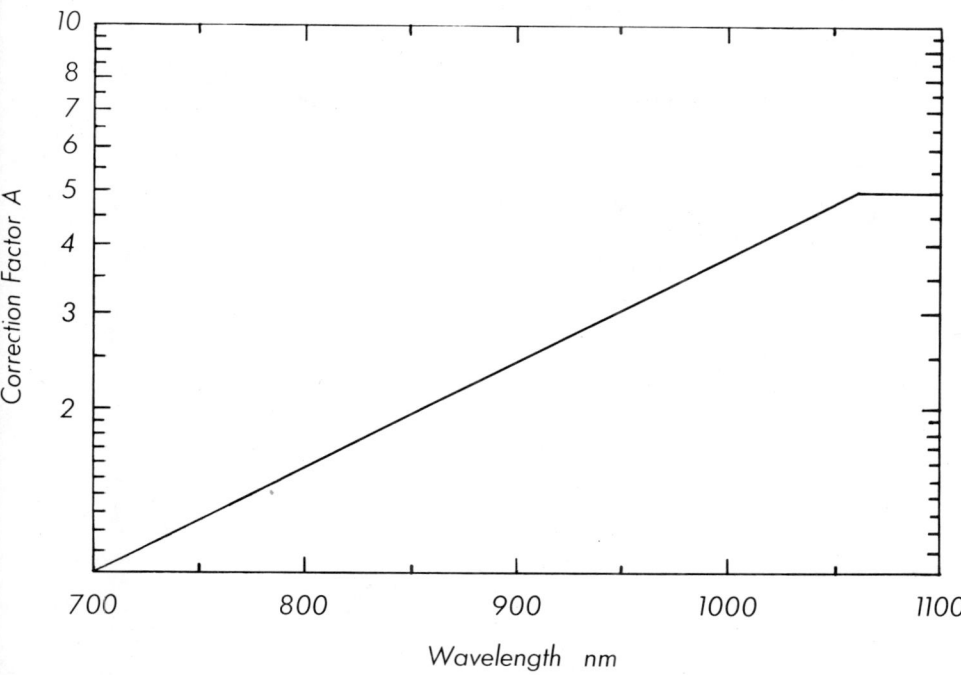

Figure 8-8. Correction Factor A, C_A. The formula for C_A is: $C_A = 1$ for wavelengths (λ) of 400 nm to 700 nm; $C_A = 10^{[0.002 (\lambda - 700 \text{ nm})]}$ for 700 nm $< \lambda <$ 1050 nm; and $C_A = 5$ for 1050 $< \lambda <$ 1400 nm.

8.2.4 Repetitively Pulsed Lasers

Since there are few experimental data for multiple pulses, caution must be used in the evaluation of such exposures. The exposure limits for irradiance or radiant exposure in multiple pulse trains have the following limitations:

(1) The exposure from any single pulse in the train is limited to the exposure limit for a single comparable pulse.

(2) The average irradiance for a group of pulses is limited to the EL as given in Tables 8-1, 8-2 or 8-3 of a single pulse of the same duration as the entire pulse group.

(3) When the instantaneous Pulse Repetition Frequency (PRF) of any pulses within a train exceeds 1, the EL applicable to each pulse is reduced by a factor (C_p) as shown in Fig. 8-11 for pulse durations less than 10^{-5} s. For pulses of greater

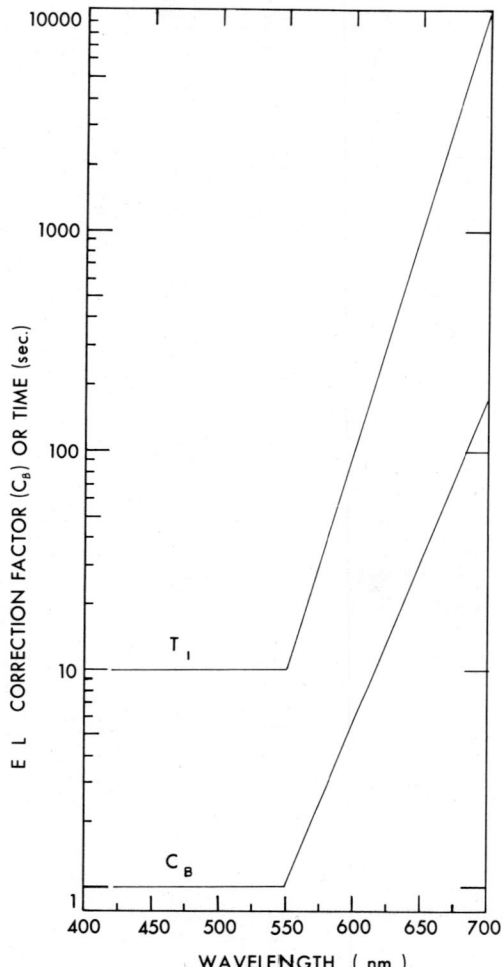

Figure 8-9. Correction Factor B, C_B, and time T_1. These two factors are used for calculating the EL for the eye for wavelengths between 550 nm and 700 nm for CW exposure durations greater than 10 s.

duration, the following formula should be applied:

$$\text{Limit (single pulse in train)} = \frac{\text{Limit (pulse nt)}}{n} \quad (8\text{-}1)$$

where n is the number of pulses in train, t is the duration of a single pulse in the

TABLE 8-5. Additivity of Effects on Eye (o) and Skin (s) from Different Spectral Regions

Spectral Region	UV-C and UV-B 200 to 315 nm	UV-A 315 to 400 nm	Visible and IR-A 400 to 1400 nm	IR-B and IR-C 1400 to 10^6 nm
UV-C and UV-B 200 to 314 nm	o s			
UV-A 315 to 400 nm		o s	s	o s
Visible and IR-A 400 to 1400 nm		s	o s	s
IR-B and IR-C 1400 to 10^6 nm		o s	s	o s

train and Limit (nt) is the exposure limit of one pulse having a duration equal to nt seconds. The "pulse" duration nt is known as the TOTP [total on time pulse] T in the ANSI standard. For a short group of n pulses, the reduced EL shall not be less than the single-pulse EL divided by n.

Using Tables 8-1 through 8-3 one can readily determine the exposure over a long duration. These values can then be checked against Figures 8-2 through 8-4 for corroboration. However, when a laser emits optical radiation at several widely different wavelengths, or when pulses are superimposed upon a CW background, computation of the exposure limit may become quite complex. Exposures from several wavelengths in the same exposure time domain are considered additive as a precautionary basis with due allowance for all spectral effectiveness correction factors. Table 8-5 provides a general guide for the additivity of exposures under different time and wavelength domains. The limits are divided into three tables: exposure limits for direct intrabeam viewing by the eye, for viewing extended sources by the eye, and for exposure limits to the skin. Exposure limits are specified for pulse durations of 1 ns to 0.25 s and for continuous exposures determined by the individual beam exposure condition for a period from 0.25 s to 3×10^4 s (30,000 s is approximately 8 hr).

8.3 POINT SOURCE OR EXTENDED SOURCE?

8.3.1 Dual Limits in the Retinal Hazard Region

One of the first difficulties encountered in applying the exposure limits is to determine whether the extended source criteria Table 8-4 apply. In essentially all viewing conditions where the individual is directly viewing the laser (intrabeam viewing), Table 8-1 is applicable. Indeed it is very unusual that a laser would be considered an extended source.

To calculate the "safe" brightness of an extended source such as a holographic display or a screen illuminated by a static or by a scanning laser beam, would require the use of Table 8-2. The values given in Table 8-2 apply to viewing a diffuse reflection from a laser beam. It is also conceivable that a laser device could be intentionally designed as a diffuse source. If a laser system designer wishes to develop a laser which radiates a great deal of monochromatic optical power and still remain in the Class I category, the only solution is to modify the laser beam. The laser source may be converted to a diffuse source with the commensurate loss in collimation. There are indeed applications for such equipment (e.g., beacons); therefore it is possible to apply the extended source criteria of Table 8-2 to the direct output of the laser system if the source is a diffuser. As another example, a low-quality semiconductor diode laser may actually be an extended source for certain pulsed modes since the source may not actually be an apparent point source but a rectangular or line source. Some semiconductor laser devices are actually an array of diodes and the array is "extended." In this case, the average radiance of the diode array *might* be applied against the extended source criteria. But in almost all instances a single diode source is still a "point source" within definitions of the standard.

8.3.2 Alpha Min (α_{min})

As an aid to determine when extended-source EL's are applicable the concept of α_{min} was invented. The value of α_{min} is a linear angle expressed in mrad and is the minimum viewing angle at which extended source EL's apply. For viewing distances beyond the location where the source angle subtends an angle less than α_{min} the source is considered from a safety standpoint to be a "point source" and the intrabeam viewing criteria of Table 8-1 apply. For close-in viewing of extended sources where a truly extensive image falls on the retina, then the extended source criteria apply. Because of the fact that the extended source EL's and the point source EL's do not vary in exactly the same manner as a function of pulse duration (or exposure duration) t this limiting angle α_{min} varies also with exposure duration (Table 8-4). Indeed α_{min} is nothing more than:

$$\alpha_{min} = [4/\pi] \ [EL \ (point \ source)/EL \ (extended \ source)]^{1/2} \qquad (8\text{-}2)$$

A division of the point source EL by the extended source EL leaves a solid angle which represents the minimum solid angular subtense of a source under consideration as an extended source. Inasmuch as few people work with solid angles, and since most sources are reasonably circularly symmetric, it was decided that the linear angle which corresponds to the apex angle of a right circular cone's limiting solid angle should be derived and presented in the standard. It was in this way that Eq. (8-2) for α_{min} was derived. There is indeed a further argument for the use of a limiting linear angle rather than solid angle: the true retinal hazard for a line source is more dependent upon image length than image area.

8.4 SPECTRAL CORRECTION FACTORS (C_A and C_B)

By looking at the mathematical expressions for the EL's in Tables 8-1, 8-2 and 8-3, it can be noted that for wavelengths in the retinal hazard spectral region (400-1400 nm) the expression often takes the form of one or two correction factors (C_A and C_B) multiplied by a function of the exposure duration t. The function of t indicates how the risk of injury varies with time and the two spectral factors take care of spectral variations in this risk.

Figures 8-1 through 8-7 provide graphical plots of many of the exposure limits. The most refined set of exposure limits where the most correction factors apply are concentrated about the EL's for continuous-wave visible and near-infrared lasers. This results from the fact that for extended exposures there can be either a purely thermal injury mechanism as is the case for a 1064-nm laser irradiation of the retina or there can be a nearly purely photochemical damage mechanism as there is for exposure of the retina by 441.6-nm laser radiation. There can also be a combination of both effects as is the case for irradiation of the retina for extended periods by 632.8-nm laser radiation. This is shown most clearly in Figures 8-3 and 8-5, and Figure 4-21.

There are two sets of correction factors which apply at the red end of the visible and in the near infrared region. Correction factor C_A mimics the change in absorption of optical radiation in the retina and choroid as is shown in Fig. 7-7. This value applies most correctly to thermal injury mechanisms. The second correction factor C_B (Figure 8-9) refers to the time dependent effect as a function of wavelength for the photochemical mechanism of injury. The photochemical effect becomes less dominant for longer wavelengths. These functions mimic the variation in threshold noted in Fig. 4-21 and which are expressed in the exposure limits defined in Fig. 8-3 and Fig. 8-5.

8.5 RESTRICTIONS ON EL's

It is important to keep in mind that the exposure limits were developed for conditions of occupational exposure and the underlying assumption is that nearly all workers may be exposed to the limits without adverse effects, but one must remember that some photosensitive individuals might nevertheless experience adverse effects for wavelengths less than 500 nm.

To quote again from the booklet of ACGIH threshold limit values, the limits are to be used "as guides in the control of exposures and should not be regarded as fine lines between safe and dangerous levels. They are based on the best available information from experimental studies."

8.6 REPETITIVELY PULSED LASERS

As noted in the previous chapter one of the most difficult matters encountered in setting EL's relates to those dealing with repetitively pulsed lasers. Since there are so many parameters, such as overall duty cycle, total length of exposure, PRF, and pulse duration most of the experimental results do not lend themselves to a clear empirical expression. The exposure limits in the 1976 ANSI standard and 1978 ACGIH TLV Book—if given in terms of either irradiance or radiant exposure for multiple pulse trains—were limited by the three restrictions given in paragraph 8.2.4.

In 1977 Lund, Stuck, and Beatrice noted that the minimal-image retinal injury thresholds expressed as total energy delivered in a group of pulses when plotted against the time of the pulse group followed a $t^{3/4}$ relation just as single-pulse thresholds. From this observation it was possible to reformulate the rules of additivity for multiple pulse exposures. Their new C_P would be defined as 10,000/PRF for short pulses. There were several attempts by others to derive similar formulae, but as this book went to press the final resolution of this problem had still not been achieved.

8.7 USING THE TABLES AND FIGURES

To determine the exposure limit for any given exposure condition it is best to calculate the value first using the table, if indeed any calculations are necessary. This value should then be compared with the estimated value found in one of the figures (8-1 through 8-7). This second step of checking the graphical value with the calculated value is an aid to avoid simple calculational errors. When one is dealing with a calculation that may determine the preservation of sight in an individual, it is obviously very important not to make an error. A mere slip of the decimal place or failure to add or subtract exponents correctly could result in a miscalculation of an order of magnitude or more that could result in eye injury if the calculated value were too high. To simplify the process, a four-step method to determine exposure limits is provided.

8.7.1 Step 1.

First determine which table provides the exposure limit being sought. Note that Tables 8-1 and 8-2 both refer to exposure limits for the eye and that Table 8-3 refers to exposure limits for the skin. In some instances it may be desirable to find both an ocular exposure limit and skin exposure limit. Remember that exposure limits for wavelengths outside of the retinal hazard region (400 to 1400 nm) are identical for the skin and eye. The first difficulty encountered in this step is to determine whether Table 8-1 or Table 8-2 applies to the ocular exposure limit. It should be noted that Table 8-1 and Table 8-2 differ only in the retinal hazard region; that Table 8-1 refers to direct intrabeam viewing conditions and that Table 8-2 refers to extended source viewing conditions. Actually these two tables may be thought of as a dual limit; that is, whichever limit is most lenient is the one to choose. In most safety studies the worst-case condition would be of interest; namely, an individual's eye could be located within the beam path of the laser and directed toward the laser source. In this case Table 8-1 almost always is the applicable criteria. On the other hand, if an individual is not located within the beam path and looking toward the laser, but is looking at a diffuse reflection, or if for some reason the laser source is diffused and does not appear as a point source then in many instances Table 8-2 would apply. In all instances for any viewing condition Table 8-1 will provide the most conservative exposure limit, hence one will never be in error on the side of danger if one limits one's analysis to Table 8-1.

It is almost a rule that the exposure limits for the eye are always less than or equal to the exposure limits for the skin. Because there is not always the same ratio between the extended source criteria and the point source criteria a single limiting angle cannot be specified such as would be the case in the definition for point source viewing on a geometrical basis.

Quite logically it could be stated, as the early version standards of 1968 vintage standards did, that any source subtending an angle greater than 1 mrad (17-μm image on the retina) might be considered an extended source. From a standpoint of physiological optics this could be readily defended. However, because of heat flow in the retina and because of eye movement, the same site of the point image is not the only point of energy deposition in the retina; hence the point source from a standpoint of retinal injury is actually translated into a larger site on the retina. This should help to explain why a source size greater than 1 mrad can be just as hazardous as a smaller source.

An angle which defines the crossover point between the point source criteria (Table 8-1) and the extended source criteria (Table 8-2) is the function α_{min} plotted in Fig. 8-10. It should be noted that it varies between 1.6 mrad and 23 mrad depending upon exposure duration t and that the lowest value occurs at 18 μs. Therefore in viewing an extended source such as a diffuse reflection, a laser array, or diffused laser source, part of step 1 includes a determination of the pulse duration of the laser which by reference to Fig. 8-10 gives α_{min}. If this α_{min} is less than the actual angular subtense of the source at the nearest viewing distance then Table 8-2 should be used to determine the applicable exposure limits. If not, as will be the case in most instances, the calculations and analysis for ocular EL's should be limited to Table 8-1. The formula for determining viewing angle α is:

$$\alpha = D_L/r_1 \tag{8-3}$$

where D_L is the diameter of the light source and would be the longest linear dimension. If the light source or reflection is not circularly symmetric and r_1 is the viewing distance, to find maximum viewing distance at which the extended source criteria would apply the formula would be formula 8-3 inverted, namely:

$$r_1(min) = D_L/\alpha_{min} \tag{8-4}$$

It would be emphasized that the source size D_L is *never* the diameter of the laser output beam unless a diffuser is the output aperture. In any collimated laser beam it is always possible to look down the beam toward the laser and see a point image. This is certainly true if the far-field divergence or the intrinsic divergence of the

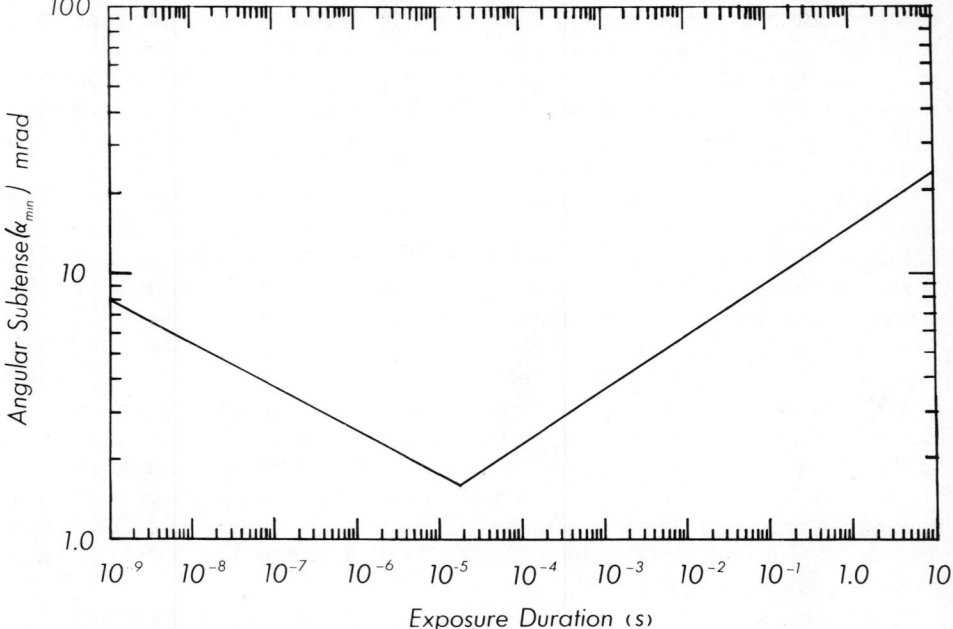

Figure 8-10. Angular subtense α_{min}. For wavelengths between 400 nm and 1400 nm this angle is used as the dividing line between extended source EL's and point source EL's. For wavelengths between 700 nm and 1400 nm α_{min} is greater than the line for $t < 10^{-4}$ s.

laser is less than 1 mrad. It cannot be overemphasized that the extended source criteria do not apply for ordinary intrabeam viewing of collimated laser beams. The only possible exception would be the viewing of a semiconductor diode laser which has been collimated by optics. And even in this case only where $\alpha_{min} \leq \phi$ is the source size sufficiently large for Table 8-2 to apply.

8.7.2 Step 2.

Determine the wavelength of the laser or wavelength band and then proceed to the table of interest and note that the left-hand columns refer to the spectral band and to the actual wavelength.

8.7.3 Step 3.

Determine the pulse duration or exposure duration of the laser and from that

Current Laser Exposure Limits

select the appropriate line in the table. The next column will be a formula for the exposure limit, or if the formula is a constant for that spectral region and exposure domain it will be simply listed as a set value.

8.7.4 Step 4.

Check the limiting aperture and make sure that the beam size is much larger than the limiting aperture. Otherwise one must take the total beam power and divide by the area of the limiting aperture in order to make an adequate comparison with the exposure limit.

8.8 EXAMPLES

8.8.1 Calculate or Determine the Exposure Limits for the Skin and the Eye for a 20-ns Pulsed Ruby Laser (Wavelength of 694.3 nm)

Since no mention is provided of repetitive pulses we shall simply determine the exposure limit for a single pulse exposure from this laser. For "point-source" viewing the exposure limit for looking directly into the source is given in Table 8-1. In the spectral region termed "light" the first row refers to exposure durations of 10^{-9} to 1.8×10^{-5} s (which includes 20 ns). In this case no calculation is necessary. The exposure limit is constant and has a value of 5×10^{-7} J/cm² (5×10^{-3} J/m²).

From Table 8-2 the exposure limit is determined for viewing an extended source (diffuse reflection) created by this laser. It will be a limit expressed as integrated radiance. It is once again the first line under the spectral region termed "light" and it is noted that for exposure durations ranging from 1 ns to 10 s the value is $10 \sqrt[3]{t}$ J/(cm²·sr). With a desk-top or pocket calculator the cube root of 2×10^{-8} is found to be 0.0027. Hence the exposure limit is 0.027 J/(cm²·sr) or 27 J/(m²·sr). To determine the exposure limit for the skin for the 20-ns ruby laser Table 8-3 is used. Once again the first line under spectral region "light" provides limits for the pulse duration domain of 10^{-9} to 10^{-7} s and the value is $2 C_A \times 10^{-2}$ J/cm². The footnote indicates the factor C_A is equal to 1 throughout the visible, and the desired value is 2×10^{-2} J/cm² or 200 J/m². This completes the determination of exposure limits for this laser, unless it is assumed that an individual were to be repeatedly exposed to a very great number of pulses in any one day. In this case the limit to be found for retinal viewing assumes an additive effect up to a certain total radiant exposure for very large values of t up to 10^4 s as measured at the cornea namely a value of 10 mJ/cm². Since the value of 5×10^{-7} J/cm² divided into 10 mJ/cm² would give a total number of pulses of 20,000 it is essentially inconceivable that anyone would be staring into a ruby laser for this many pulses. In fact, anyone familiar with ruby laser technology would know that it would not be easy to build a ruby laser that could provide 20,000 pulses within 10^4 seconds.

8.8.2 Determine the Exposure Limits for a TEA Laser Which has a Pulse Duration of 1 μs (10^{-6} s) and a Wavelength of 10.6 μm

As noted earlier in this chapter all of the exposure limits for *pulsed* far-infrared and for *short-pulsed* ultraviolet lasers are identical. Hence Table 8-1 has all applicable values that would apply to viewing a point source, a diffuse source, or an exposure to the skin. The desired value for the TEA laser is calculated as:

$$\begin{aligned} EL &= 0.56 \sqrt[4]{t} \ J/cm^2 \\ &= (0.56)(10^{-6})^{1/4} \\ &= (0.56)(3.16 \times 10^{-2}) \\ &= 1.77 \times 10^{-2} \\ &= 0.018 \ J/cm^2, \text{ or when expressed as irradiance,} \\ &= (0.018 \ J/cm^2)/(10^{-6} \ s) \\ &= 18 \ kW/cm^2 \end{aligned} \qquad (8\text{-}5)$$

Tables 8-1 to 8-3 show that the same EL applies to direct intrabeam viewing, to extended source viewing, and to skin exposure.

8.8.3 Determine the EL's for an Erbium Q-Switched Laser Operating at 1.54 μm with a 20-ns Pulse

Table 8-1 has a special wavelength region of EL's between 1.5 and 1.6 μm. The EL given in both Tables 8-1 and 8-2 is increased by a factor of 100 for time periods shorter than 1 μs. Hence the exposure criteria for a 20-ns far-infrared laser pulse is calculated and then at the end increased by this special correction factor of 100. From Table 8-1 the direct intrabeam exposure limit for a 20-ns pulse is 10^{-2} J/cm^2. This value applies for all exposure durations between 1 ns and 100 ns. Hence our intrabeam EL is 1 J/cm^2 (or $10^4 \ J/m^2$).

In Tables 8-2 and 8-3 the exposure criteria for diffuse reflection viewing is identical to the values for intrabeam viewing, as would be expected for a far-infrared laser. However, the criteria for skin exposure at this wavelength is not increased by a factor of 100. Hence it may be concluded that the criteria for a single-pulsed exposure to the skin is 10 mJ/cm^2 and 100-fold greater for the eye, i.e., 1 J/cm^2.

8.8.4 Determine the EL for a Gallium-Arsenide Laser Operating at a PRF of 100 Hz at a Wavelength Varying Between 905 and 910 nm with 100-ns Pulses

When encountering a laser which operates over a band of wavelengths, always choose the wavelength correction factor that is smallest. In Fig. 8-8 the correction factor for the wavelength 905 nm is the smallest, most restrictive value and is equal to approximately 2.5. This may be checked by using the formula given at the bottom of Table 8-1 which is that correction factor A is calculated in the following manner:

$$C_A = 10^{[(\lambda - 700 \text{ nm})/500]}$$
$$C_A = 10^{[905-700/500]} \quad (8\text{-}6)$$
$$= 10^{[205/500]}$$
$$= 2.57$$

The next correction factor that must be known is the repetitive-pulse correction factor C_P. And C_P is found directly by looking at Fig. 8-11 and for 100 Hz: the correction factor is 0.1. As a note, the value of C_P from a PRF of 1 to 100 Hz is $1/\sqrt{F}$. Looking at the value for a single pulse in Table 8-1 we notice that the exposure limit for such a short pulse is $5(C_A \cdot C_P) \times 10^{-7}$ J/cm²; hence:

$$\begin{aligned} \text{EL (single pulse)} &= C_A \cdot C_P \cdot 5 \times 10^{-7} \text{ J/cm}^2 \\ &= (2.57)(0.1)(5 \times 10^{-7}) \\ &= 1.3 \times 10^{-7} \text{ J/cm}^2 \text{ per pulse} \\ &= 1.3 \times 10^{-3} \text{ J/m}^2 \text{ per pulse} \end{aligned}$$

For this PRF the easiest measurement could be the average irradiance of the beam. The average irradiance corresponding to this exposure limit is:

$$\begin{aligned} \text{EL (average irradiance)} &= (1.3 \times 10^{-7} \text{ J/cm}^2 \text{ per pulse})(100 \text{ Hz}) \\ &= 1.3 \times 10^{-5} \text{ J/cm}^2 \text{ per second} \quad (8\text{-}7) \\ &= 1.3 \times 10^{-5} \text{ W/cm}^2 \\ &= 0.13 \text{ W/m}^2 \end{aligned}$$

For any repetitively pulsed laser not only the single pulse limitation must be considered but also the average irradiance limitation. The exposure limit for long term exposure to this gallium-arsenide laser for intrabeam viewing is from Table 8-1 listed as $320 \, C_A \times 10^{-6}$ W/cm² for periods greater than 1000 s; hence the average power limitation on the exposure limit equals:

$$\text{EL (avg)} = 320(2.57) \times 10^{-6} \text{ W/cm}^2 = 0.82 \text{ mW/cm}^2 = 8.2 \text{ W/m}^2$$

Since this long-term limit is higher than the average irradiance limit calculated from the single pulse criteria the single-pulse derived limit must be applied under all conditions.

It is characteristic for repetitively pulsed lasers with relatively low PRF's to have exposure limits determined by the single pulse limitation. However if the PRF is extremely great (e.g., several kHz), then the long-term chronic exposure limit would apply. In this particular case, for the gallium-arsenide laser, the cross-over point would occur for a PRF of 10 kHz (in fact the 10 kHz point would be a cross-over for any repetitively pulsed laser with constant PRF and equal pulse intervals based on the 1976 ANSI standard.

In Table 8-2 the exposure limit for an extended source for this type of pulse

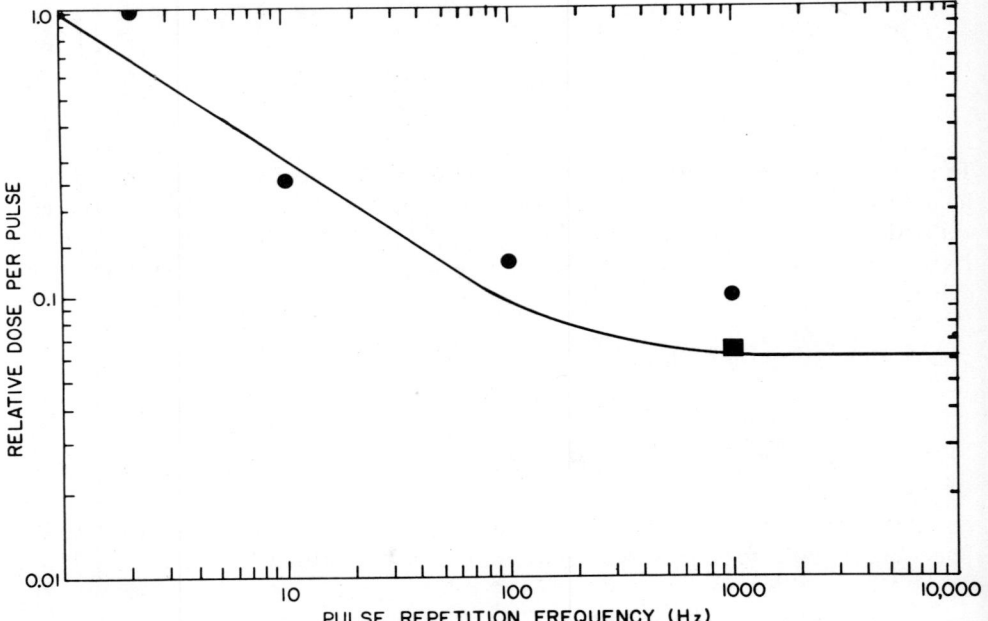

Figure 8-11. Correction Factor. C_P (ordinate) is used for calculating the reduced single-pulse EL of a pulse in a train of pulses if the pulse duration is less than 10^{-5} s. C_P (solid line) is 0.06 for a PRF (F) greater than 1 kHz. Experimental biologic data for argon (●) and neodymium (■) repetitive pulse trains of 0.5 s total exposures by Skeen *et al.* (1972) are shown for comparison.

train is given as:

$$\begin{align} \text{EL (single pulse criteria)} &= 10\, C_A \times \sqrt[3]{t} \ \text{J/(cm}^2 \cdot \text{sr)} \\ &= 10\,(2.57)\,(10^{-8}\,\text{s})^{1/3} \\ &= 2.57\,(4.65 \times 10^{-3}) \\ &= 0.12 \ \text{J/(cm}^2 \cdot \text{sr)} \end{align}$$ (8-8)

The repetitive pulse correction factor is again 0.1, hence the final answer is 0.012 J/(cm² · sr) per pulse or 1.2 W/(cm² · sr) average radiance for the train. Since the single-pulse criteria was the limiting case for intrabeam viewing it will also be the case for extended source criteria. The applicable α_{min} is always determined by limiting criteria: in this case, the single pulse (100 ns).

Finally, the skin exposure limits are given as:

$$\begin{aligned}
\text{EL (skin)} = 1.1\, C_A \times \sqrt[4]{t}\ \text{J/cm}^2 &= 1.1\,(2.57)\,(10^{-7}\text{s})^{1/4}\ \text{J/cm}^2\\
&= 1.1\,(2.57)\,(1.78 \times 10^{-2})\ \text{J/cm}^2 \quad (8\text{-}9)\\
&= 5.0 \times 10^{-2}\ \text{J/cm}^2
\end{aligned}$$

The value of C_P is not applied to repetitively pulsed trains of exposure limits for the skin. However, the average power limitation is applied and the irradiance for long-term exposures greater than 10 s is $0.2\, C_A\ \text{W/cm}^2 = 0.51\ \text{W/cm}^2$. The exposure limit for a single pulse multiplied by a PRF of 100 provides us with an exposure limit of 5 W/cm² based on single-pulse criteria and only 0.51 W/cm² based on the average irradiance criteria. Hence, in this case the average irradiance is the limiting exposure condition for the determination of skin exposure.

8.8.5 Determine the Exposure Limit for a Helium-Neon Laser (632.8 nm) which is Chopped to Produce 1-ms Pulses at a Frequency of 50 Hz

Following the procedure developed in the past examples for repetitively pulsed laser exposure limit determinations, the first step shall be to determine the individual pulse limitation for long exposures. For any pulse durations exceeding 18 μs the exposure limit is based on the total-on-time pulse concept (TOTP concept). In this instance the criteria that would apply to a pulse train must be calculated. Since this is a visible laser the logical viewing duration to apply is the standard aversion duration recommended by ANSI which is 0.25 s. Hence the total-on-time nt [see Equation (8.1)] is equal to:

$$nt = t \cdot F \cdot T \quad (8\text{-}10)$$

where t is the pulse duration, F is the PRF and T is the total duration (0.25 s). Then:

$$\begin{aligned}
nt &= (10^{-3}\text{s})\,(50\ \text{Hz})\,(0.25\ \text{s})\\
&= 1.25 \times 10^{-2}\ \text{s}
\end{aligned}$$

We must now determine the exposure limit for a single pulse lasting 12.5 ms (the TOTP for the train). From Table 8-1 the intrabeam exposure limit is:

$$\begin{aligned}
\text{EL} &= 1.8 \times t^{3/4}\ \text{mJ/cm}^2\\
&= 1.8\,(1.25 \times 10^{-2})^{3/4}\ \text{mJ/cm}^2\\
&= 1.8\,(3.7 \times 10^{-2})\ \text{mJ/cm}^2 \quad (8\text{-}11)\\
&= 6.73 \times 10^{-2}\ \text{J/cm}^2
\end{aligned}$$

To find the value for a single pulse this figure is divided by the number of pulses in the train. Since there are 12.5 pulses, this gives 5.4 mJ/cm². The reduction factor for this as compared with the limit for a single pulse 1 ms exposure is found by calculating the single pulse EL from Table 8-1:

$$\text{EL (single pulse)} = 1.8\,(10^{-3})^{3/4}\ \text{mJ/cm}^2$$
$$= 1.0 \times 10^{-2}\ \text{mJ/cm}^2$$

This gives a modest reduction in the single-pulse criteria because this pulse is in a train. This rather modest reduction factor is characteristic of the additive effect of long pulses greater than 18 μs. The same procedure is followed for the extended source criteria but not applied to the skin exposure limits. Again, the skin exposure limits would be based upon the value of 0.2 W/cm^2 average irradiance.

8.9 FUTURE DEVELOPMENTS

If changes occur in the 1976 vintage EL's they are most likely to occur in one of the following cases: repetitively pulsed lasers–formulas; UV limits for $t > 10^4$ s; and in IR-B EL's. The reader is cautioned to check before applying the EL's in this chapter to be sure that revisions in recognized standards have not taken place since the publication of this manual.

8.10 REVIEW QUESTIONS

1. The laser exposure limits of the American Conference of Governmental Industrial Hygienists and the American National Standards Institute are identical. True or false?

2. At present all exposure limits for all groups in the United States and throughout the world are equal in every detail. True or false?

3. What does the correction factor C_A relate to and does it apply to exposure limits for the skin?

4. Calculate the exposure limit for a carbon-monoxide laser operating at 5.0 μm with a pulse duration of 100 ns.

5. In what spectral regions are the exposure limits for the skin and for intrabeam viewing by the eye and diffuse source viewing by the eye identical?

6. Calculate the exposure limit for a helium-cadmium CW laser operating at 441.6 nm if the exposure duration could be 0.25 s or all day long.

7. Calculate the exposure limit for intrabeam viewing of a helium-neon laser where the viewing duration is estimated to be 1000 s.

8. Calculate the exposure limit for diffuse reflection viewing of a 5-W argon laser which is used as a beacon and the output is diffused evenly over a 4-cm target and the wavelength is 488 nm.

9. Calculate the exposure limit for intrabeam viewing of a 1-kHz gallium-aluminum-arsenide laser operating at 850 nm.

10. Derive Equation 8-2.

8.11 REFERENCES

American National Standard Institute, 1976, Standard Z-136.1-1976, American National Standard for the Safe Use of Lasers, New York, American National Standards Institute, Inc., (March 8, 1976).

American Conference of Governmental Industrial Hygienists, 1978, Threshold Limit Values for Chemical Substances and Physical Agents in the Workroom Environment with Intended Changes for 1978, Cincinnati, ACGIH, 1978.

Goldman, L., Rockwell, R. J., Michaelson, S. M., Sliney, D. H., Tengroth, B. M., and Wolbarsht, M. L., 1977, Optical Radiation, with Particular Reference to Lasers, Document ICP/CEP 803, Regional Office for Europe, World Health Organization, Copenhagen.

International Electrotechnical Commission, 1978, Technical Committee #76, Laser Equipment, Radiation Safety of Laser Products and Equipment Classification, Requirements and User's Guide, Fifth Draft, IEC Geneva.

Skeen, C. H., Bruce, W. R., Tips, J. H., Jr., Smith, M. G., and Garza, C. G., 1972, Ocular Effects of Repetitive Laser Pulses, Technology Inc., San Antonio, TX, Air Force Contract F41609-71-C-0018, June 30, 1972, Available from NTIS, Springfield, VA as AD 746 795).

Stuck, B. E., Lund, D. J., and Beatrice, E. S., 1978, Repetitive Pulse Laser Data and Permissible Exposure Limits, Letterman Army Institute of Research, Division of Non-Ionizing Radiation, Presidio of San Francisco, San Francisco, April 1978.

Chapter 9
Laser Hazard Classification

9.1 INTRODUCTION

The present system of classifying lasers according to their hazard category or risk category evolved between 1965 and 1972. It arose from a need to distinguish between lasers of differing risk, so that hazard control which would be required for very dangerous lasers would not needlessly be applied to small, relatively less hazardous, lasers. At present the laser hazard classification schemes used in standards promulgated by the American National Standards Institute (ANSI), by the Bureau of Radiological Health (BRH) of the United States Food and Drug Administration, by the International Electrotechnical Commission (IEC), by the British Standards Institution (BSI), and by the American Conference of Governmental Industrial Hygienists (ACGIH) are all very similar. Indeed only very minor differences exist. Most regulations of Federal agencies, state, and local governmental that pertain to laser safety generally follow either the ANSI Z-136 or BRH classification scheme. Since all lasers manufactured for use within the U.S. must have a label designating their classification if they were manufactured since August 2, 1976, the BRH classification scheme will generally be followed by most users in the future. It will be discussed in detail in this chapter.

Descpite some differences between the ANSI and BRH standards, it is important to remember that the two are complementary; each is weak without the other. Without the user control measures required by the ANSI standard, the safety control features required by the BRH standard may be inadequate or unused (e.g., the beam shutters or remote control connectors may not be employed by the user). Likewise, the ANSI standard may more readily and effectively be applied when the performance standards are met and the manufacturer labels the correct hazard classification.

It is well to keep in mind that all standards change with time. Both the BRH and the ANSI standards have been revised since first promulgated. These revisions in the past (as well as those to be expected in the future) are based upon new biological injury data, or on an improved understanding of the risks of applications of laser products. This Chapter includes only those revisions made to the BRH regulation in December 1978 and those contemplated by ANSI in 1979. To understand better the differences between the BRH and ANSI standards, the historical development and the underlying rationale which was presented in Chapter 7 should be reviewed.

9.2 DIFFERENCES BETWEEN ANSI AND BRH LASER CLASSIFICATION SCHEMES

There are basically two areas of difference between the 1976 BRH emission limits and the 1976 ANSI classification limits. One set of differences relate to the modified Class 1 limits based upon a revision of the MPE's and AEL's by ANSI in 1976. The other group of differences existed from the start. The BRH felt the need for including classification limits for short-pulsed ultraviolet radiation where ANSI had not imposed limits in 1973. Therefore there is no similarity between the classification divisions for pulsed ultraviolet lasers (lasers having an output pulse duration less than 0.25 s).

The BRH did not adopt a repetitive pulse correction factor. Therefore, where the repetitive pulse correction factor would be applied for a laser's classification, there will be a difference between the ANSI and BRH classification. The ANSI classification will be more restrictive.

Finally, for pulsed visible and near-infrared lasers (400 nm to 1400 nm) the dividing line between Class 3 and Class 4 lasers is based not upon an output energy or power, but upon an output radiant exposure capable of causing a hazardous diffuse reflection. This dividing line differs by a factor of π (3.14) between the two standards. For a uniform beam irradiance this dividing line differs by a factor of π (3.14) between the two standards; but in actuality it is difficult to give a precise difference factor between the two dividing lines. The BRH standard uses a 7-mm aperture and the ANSI standard uses a 1-mm aperture and the two standards could be equivalent for small beams. Both have the same maximal 10 J/cm^2 endpoint. In deriving these limits the ANSI committee set the upper limit of Class 3 pulsed lasers at the radiant exposure required to cause a hazardous diffuse reflection (exceed the MPE) from a 100-percent reflectance, white, diffuse Lambertain surface. By Lambert's Law this radiant exposure would be the extended-source MPE (specified in units of radiance) divided by a factor of π. The important fact to remember is that for the case of the upper limit for Class 3 pulsed lasers, the BRH limits are a factor of π more restrictive than the ANSI limits (for a large beam of uniform irradiance).

The revised 1976 ANSI MPE's were limited to the spectral region between 550 nm and 1400 nm for CW lasers and for exposure durations greater than 10 s. Therefore the BRH and ANSI classification limits for a Class 1 laser differ in this spectral region. These differences are summarized in a table at the end of this chapter (Table 9-3). The reader should not place too much significance upon the fact that the most recent ANSI revision (1979) and the IEC proposed laser standard designated classes as 1,2,3 and 4 rather than the Roman Numerals used by BRH.

9.3 THE BRH PERFORMANCE STANDARD FOR LASER PRODUCTS

9.3.1 General Concepts

The BRH Performance Standard for Laser Products was published on July 31, 1975 in the Federal Register. It became effective for all laser products manufactured for use in the United States after August 1, 1976. The standard was revised effective December 8, 1978 and January 29, 1979 (43FR55387). The regulation (Title 21, Chapter 1, subchapter J, part 1040) appears rather complex at first. The overall philosophy is not difficult to understand and has been explained in the first part of this chapter. A detailed discussion of the philosophy of the BRH standard appeared in two issues of the *Federal Register* (38FR34084, 1973 and 39FR32094, 1974). The detailed requirements for tests, maintenance of records by manufacturers, and certification can become quite complicated and will not be discussed in any detail here. Manufacturers can obtain information from the standard published in the latest *Code of Federal Regulations* (21CFR1040); and in addition, a complete package of booklets and pulbications used for guidance of manufacturers is available to new manufacturers of laser products by writing to the Bureau of Radiological Health, Division of Compliance, U.S. Department of Health, Education and Welfare, Rockville, MD 20850 [Telephone (301) 443-4874].

9.3.2 The Importance of the BRH Regulation

Many people ask about the value of such a Federal regulation. Many manufacturers and users feel that the requirements needlessly add to the cost of a laser product. In defense of the regulation it should be understood that the original intent of classifying lasers was to move the requirement for detailed measurements from the user to the manufacturer. After all, the manufacturer of a laser product knows best the output limitations of his particular laser product and could more correctly ascertain whether measurements made of a laser's output on any particular date would indeed be maximal. Also, the manufacturer of a laser product is far more likely to have some of the costly but necessary radiometric instruments than would the average user. The user, then, would have to follow only a simple set of control-measure guidelines (e.g., those in ANSI Z-136), provided that the laser was adequately classified.

In addition to this measurement concept the Bureau of Radiological Health was charged by the Congress of the United States with the responsibility of ensuring that electronic products manufactured for consumer use in the United States are reasonably safe from faulty design which would constitute a hazard to public health. Lasers, quite obviously, if misused could present such a hazard. Therefore it was incumbent upon the Bureau of Radiological Health to enforce certain performance characteristics which would limit hazardous exposure. The degree of "restrictions" placed upon the designer depends upon how low a class he tries to achieve. The details of some of the performance standards have sometimes been a subject of controversy between manufacturers and the government but as time posses the particular value of certain requirements become more obvious. At the time of publication of this book a second set of changes were being considered by BRH.

The BRH standard requires manufacturers to label each laser product with its class and certain other output characteristics. Additionally, depending upon the class of laser, certain "performance" (generally engineering) features must be present. In the original (1973) ANSI classification standard the only engineering requirements suggested were adequate interlocks for the former Class V laser and a remote control connector on a Class IV laser to disable the laser in the event that the remote control switch (generally mounted on an entrance door) would be opened by an intruder who could be exposed to hazardous direct beams or diffuse reflections. Additional engineering and performance requirements are contained in the BRH Laser Product Performance Standard. Most of the BRH requirements were later adopted by ANSI. The BRH requirements will be listed later in this chapter.

9.3.3 Accessible Emission Limits

The term "accessible emission limit" was introduced by BRH as it was not in the ANSI Z-136 standard. The accessible emission limit (AEL) for a given classification would be the maximum *accessible* emission level permitted within a particular class computable as a function of emission duration, and time—and wavelength—dependent factors k_1 and k_2 as given in AEL tables. In other words a laser might emit a Class IV output power but the radiation would have to be truly accessible to an individual in excess of Class III emission limits before the laser product would be considered to be in Class IV. The means of measuring the class limits and the determination of accessibility will be given later in the chapter.

Accessible emission limits for laser radiation in each class are specified in Tables 9-1a, 9-1b, and 9-1c in terms of the factors k_1 and k_2 which vary with wavelength and emission duration. The k factors are given in Table 9-2a with selected numerical values in Table 9-2b. Figure 9-1 shows some of these limits in perspective.

Unlike the ANSI Z-136 standard and the proposed IEC standard, the BRH emission limits apply not only to laser radiation but to any incoherent electromagnetic radiation produced in the laser product which is "collateral" with the laser beam. Actually the BRH expanded the obvious meaning of "collateral" and defines collateral radiation as "any electronic product radiation except laser radiation, emitted by a laser product as a result of the operation of the laser(s) or any component of the laser product that is physically necessary for the operation of the laser(s)." Effective in January 1979, collateral radiation for wavelengths greater

TABLE 9-1a. Class I Accessible Emission Limits for Laser Radiation

Wavelength (nanometers)	Emission duration (seconds)	Class I – Accessible emission limits
> 250 but ≤ 400	≤ 3.0 × 10^4	2.4 × $10^{-5} k_1 k_2$ J*
	> 3.0 × 10^4	8.0 × $10^{-10} k_1 k_2 t$ J
> 400 but ≤ 1400	> 1.0 × 10^{-9} to 2.0 × 10^{-5}	2.0 × $10^{-7} k_1 k_2$ J
	> 2.0 × 10^{-5} to 1.0 × 10^1	7.0 × $10^{-4} k_1 k_2 t^{3/4}$ J
	> 1.0 × 10^1 to 1.0 × 10^4	3.9 × $10^{-3} k_1 k_2$ J
	> 1.0 × 10^4	3.9 × $10^{-7} k_1 k_2 t$ J
	OR**	
	> 1.0 × 10^{-9} to 1.0 × 10^1	$10 k_1 k_2 t^{1/3}$ J cm^{-2} sr^{-1}
	> 1.0 × 10^1 to 1.0 × 10^4	$20 k_1 k_2$ J cm^{-2} sr^{-1}
	> 1.0 × 10^4	2.0 × $10^{-3} k_1 k_2 t$ J cm^{-2} sr^{-1}
> 1400 but ≤ 13000	> 1.0 × 10^{-9} to 1.0 × 10^{-7}	7.9 × $10^{-5} k_1 k_2$ J
	> 1.0 × 10^{-7} to 1.0 × 10^1	4.4 × $10^{-3} k_1 k_2 t^{1/4}$ J
	> 1.0 × 10^1	7.9 × $10^{-4} k_1 k_2 t$ J

* Class I accessible emission limits for the wavelength range of greater than 250 nm but less than or equal to 400 nm shall not exceed the Class I accessible emission limits for the wavelength range of greater than 1400 nm but less than or equal to 13000 nm with a k_1 and k_2 of 1.0 for comparable sampling intervals.

**Instructions for the Class I dual limits are set forth in paragraph (d)(4) of this section.

TABLE 9-1b. Class II Accessible Emission Limits for Laser Radiation

Wavelength (nanometers)	Emission duration (seconds)	Class II – Accessible emission limits
> 400 but ≤ 710	> 2.5 × 10^{-1}	1.0 × $10^{-3} k_1 k_2 t$ J

TABLE 9-1c. Class III Accessible Emission Limits for Laser Radiation

Wavelength (nanometers)	Emission duration (seconds)	Class III – Accessible emission limits
> 250 but ≤ 400	$\leq 2.5 \times 10^{-1}$ -------	$3.8 \times 10^{-4} k_1 k_2$ J
	$> 2.5 \times 10^{-1}$ -------	$1.5 \times 10^{-3} k_1 k_2 t$ J
> 400 but ≤ 1400	$> 1.0 \times 10^{-9}$ to 2.5×10^{-1} --	$10 k_1 k_2 t^{1/3}$ J cm^{-2} to a maximum value of 10 J cm^{-2}
	$> 2.5 \times 10^{-1}$ -------	$5.0 \times 10^{-1} t$ J
> 1400 but ≤ 13000	$> 1.0 \times 10^{-9}$ to 1.0×10^{1} ---	10 J cm^{-2}
	$> 1.0 \times 10^{1}$ --------	$5.0 \times 10^{-1} t$ J

TABLE 9-2a. Values of Wavelength Dependent Correction Factors k_1 and k_2

Wavelength (nanometers)	k_1	k_2
250 to 302.4	1.0	1.0
> 302.4 to 315	$10^{\left[\frac{\lambda - 302.4}{5}\right]}$	1.0
> 315 to 400	330.0	1.0
> 400 to 700	1.0	1.0
> 700 to 800	$10^{\left[\frac{\lambda - 700}{515}\right]}$	if: $t \leq \frac{10100}{\lambda - 699}$ then: $k_2 = 1.0$ if: $\frac{10100}{\lambda - 699} < t \leq 10^4$ then: $k_2 = \frac{t(\lambda - 699)}{10100}$ if: $t > 10^4$ then: $k_2 = \frac{\lambda - 699}{1.01}$
> 800 to 1060	$10^{\left[\frac{\lambda - 700}{515}\right]}$	if: $t \leq 100$ then: $k_2 = 1.0$ if: $100 < t \leq 10^4$ then: $k_2 = \frac{t}{100}$ if: $t > 10^4$ then: $k_2 = 100$
> 1060 to 1400	5.0	
> 1400 to 1535	1.0	1.0
> 1535 to 1545	$t \leq 10^{-7}$, $k_1 = 100.0$; $t > 10^{-7}$, $k_1 = 1.0$	1.0
> 1545 to 13000	1.0	1.0

Note: The variables in the expressions are the magnitudes of the sampling interval (t), in units of seconds, and the wavelength (λ), in units of nanometers.

TABLE 9-2b

Selected Numerical Solutions for k_1 and k_2

Wavelength (nanometers)	k_1	k_2				
		$t \leq 100$	$t = 300$	$t = 1000$	$t = 3000$	$t \geq 10{,}000$
250	1.0					
300	1.0					
302	1.0					
303	1.32					
304	2.09					
305	3.31					
306	5.25					
307	8.32					
308	13.2					
309	20.9			1.0		
310	33.1					
311	52.5					
312	83.2					
313	132.0					
314	209.0					
315	330.0					
400	330.0					
401	1.0					
500	1.0					
600	1.0					
700	1.0					
710	1.05	1	1	1.1	3.3	11.0
720	1.09	1	1	2.1	6.3	21.0
730	1.14	1	1	3.1	9.3	31.0
740	1.20	1	1.2	4.1	12.0	41.0
750	1.25	1	1.5	5.0	15.0	50.0
760	1.31	1	1.8	6.0	18.0	60.0
770	1.37	1	2.1	7.0	21.0	70.0
780	1.43	1	2.4	8.0	24.0	80.0
790	1.50	1	2.7	9.0	27.0	90.0
800	1.56	1	3.0	10.0	30.0	100.0
850	1.95	1	3.0	10.0	30.0	100.0
900	2.44	1	3.0	10.0	30.0	100.0
950	3.05	1	3.0	10.0	30.0	100.0
1000	3.82	1	3.0	10.0	30.0	100.0
1050	4.78	1	3.0	10.0	30.0	100.0
1060	5.00	1	3.0	10.0	30.0	100.0
1100	5.00	1	3.0	10.0	30.0	100.0
1400	5.00	1	3.0	10.0	30.0	100.0
1500	1.0					
1540	100.0*			1.0		
1600	1.0					
13000	1.0					

*The factor $k_1 = 100.0$ when $t \leq 10^{-7}$, and $k_1 = 1.0$ when $t > 10^{-7}$

Note: The variable (t) is the magnitude of the sampling interval in units of seconds.

than 400 nm had to be sampled only to a maximum duration of 1,000 s (unless from a viewpoint); but for shorter wavelengths, the collateral radiation is sampled for greater than 10^4 s. Collateral radiation does not apply to light emitted by a light bulb or a separate pilot warning light source on the laser product but does apply to radiation emitted as "physically necessary to the operation of the laser," e.g., coming from the laser beam emission port from power supply tubes or from a pump lamp discharge tube. Although collateral radiation was judged a useful concept for ultraviolet radiation and bright pump-lamp light, the ANSI and IEC drafting committees generally felt that including all collateral radiation in the same AEL's probably creates more problems of measurement than it assures safety inasmuch as it is seldom a significant hazard in a commercial laser product. Therefore, collateral radiation is considered entirely separately in the ANSI and draft IEC standards. Many of the laser limits and measurement techniques have a built-in assumption that the radiation is one or a few wavelengths and may be focused to a point—assumptions that seldom apply to collateral radiation.

The dimensions of the radiometric quantities used to specify acceptable emission limits are radiant energy expressed in joules (J); radiant power in watts (W); irradiance expressed in watts-per-square-centimeter (W/cm^2); radiance expressed in watts-per-square-centimeter-and-steradian W/(cm$^2 \cdot$ sr); radiant exposure expressed in joules-per-square-centimeter (J/cm^2); and integrated radiance expressed in joules-per-square-centimeter-and-steradian J/(cm$^2 \cdot$ sr). The factors k_1 and k_2 are dimensionless. The variable t is the duration of emission in seconds. Obviously an accessible emission limit containing joules, when divided by the "sampling interval" or emission duration t, is equivalent to the accessible emission limit if specified in units of watts as average power.

Figure 9-1 is a graph of the accessible limits for CW lasers assuming a potential exposure duration of a full day or periods greater than 10^4 s (2.8 hr = 2 hr, 47 min). Beyond this duration of 2.8 hr there are no further changes in the Class I limits for either the BRH standard or the ANSI standard. In effect the authors of the MPEs assumed that it was highly unlikely that the same area of the retina would be illuminated for that great a duration. The concept of repair processes in equilibrium with the injury producing exposure enter the picture also. A discussion of this problem is given in Chapter 7.

The BRH standard for infrared lasers does not exist beyond 13 μm (an infrared range initially proposed in an ANSI 1971 draft). The ultimate, long-wavelength limit for the ANSI 1973 and 1976 standards was 1 mm. Additionally, the lower wavelength limit of the BRH regulation is 250 nm rather than the 200 nm spectral limit in the ANSI standard. The BRH chose the dividing line of 250 nm because at the time of publication of their standard the National Bureau of Standards did not specify a standard of irradiance at wavelengths less than 250 nm. Collateral radiation limits in the BRH regulation also extend into the x-ray region, "0.5 mR per hour averaged over a cross-section parallel to the external surface of the product having an area of 10 square centimeters with no dimension less than 5 centimeters."

A laser with a single-wavelength (monochromatic) output must have its applicable emission duration defined. Although this emission duration (or classification

Laser Hazard Classification

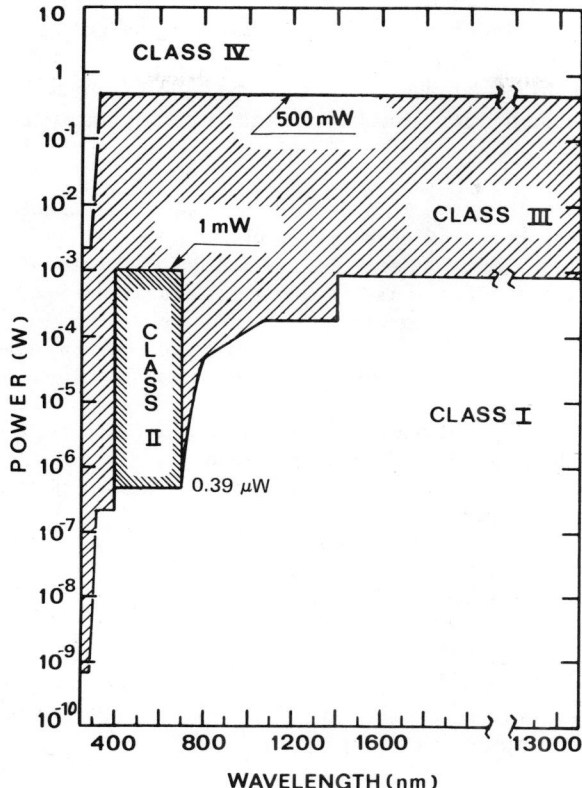

Figure 9-1. Emission Limits in Perspective. The 1978 BRH limits for CW laser emission by class. The ANSI Z-136.1, 1976 limits are the same except for slight differences for upper limits of Class I CW lasers at wavelengths between 550 nm and 1400 nm, and ANSI limits exist between 200 and 250 nm and 13 μm and 1 mm.

duration) may be defined by the Laser Safety Officer in the ANSI standard (and may be a viewing duration in the ANSI standard), the manufacturer must use durations specified in the tables of emission limits in the BRH standard and assure that the emission has been determined "for all sampling intervals within the durations specified (10^{-9} s to $> 10^4$ or $> 3 \times 10^4$ s). In the 1978 revision the BRH did allow a maximum sampling duration of 1000 s for Class IIa laser products. The BRH classification procedures are pegged to measurements, whereas the voluntary ANSI procedures permit some judgement of the use and other factors by the Laser Safety Officer. Since a laser could be an extended source and still emit below the Class I limits during its operational emission duration, it is necessary to have a dual set of limits for Class I lasers emitting in the retinal hazard region (400-1400 nm). Therefore Table 9-1a provides two sets of limits in the retinal hazard region where extended source limits exist. When lasers emit multiple wavelengths then the accessible emission limit is modified. The following paragraphs extracted from the BRH standard, define the classification procedure and the tests for classification.

From 21CFR1040.10(d):

(3) *Beam with multiple wavelengths in different ranges.* Laser or collateral radiation having wavelengths within two or more of the wavelength ranges specified in Tables I–A, I–B, and I–C of this paragraph exceeds the accessible emission limits of a class if it exceeds the applicable limits within any one of those wavelength ranges. This determination is made for each wavelength range in accordance with paragraph (d) (1) or (2) of this section.

(4) *Class I dual limits.* Laser or collateral radiation in the wavelength range of greater than 400 nm but less than or equal to 1,400 nm exceeds the accessible emission limits of Class I if it exceeds both:

(i) The Class I accessible emission limits for radiant energy within any range of emission duration specified in Table I–A of this paragraph and,

(ii) The Class I accessible emission limits for integrated radiance within any range of emission duration specified in Table I–A of this paragraph.

9.3.4 Laser Products Versus Laser Systems

A laser product is defined by BRH as "any manufactured product or assemblage of components which constitutes, incorporates, or is intended to incorporate, a laser or laser system. A laser or laser system which is intended for use as a component of an electronic product shall itself be considered a laser product." Therefore, a laser diode or laser discharge tube alone is a laser and is also termed a "laser product" but not a system. This is an important distinction, since not all BRH performance requirements apply to all laser products: some BRH performance requirements apply only to a laser system and not to a laser alone.

A "laser system" is defined by BRH as "a laser in combination with an appropriate laser energy source with or without additional incorporated components." The "energy source" is meant to be the laser's power supply, but not the "electrical supply mains or batteries."

9.3.5 Tests for Compliance

The BRH standard lists a number of tests for compliance. The tests for compliance are basically radiometric measurements and require the manufacturer to perform the measurements or calculate the applicable parameters under the worst-case conditions without damaging the laser. Additionally the standard requires that the manufacturer take into account all possible measurement uncertainties including statistical variations and account for these in setting a rejection level. If the measured output plus this additional uncertainty factor does not exceed the limits for a certain class, then it would not be rejected in the test for that class. This BRH approach permits the use of an instrument and measurement procedure with a large uncertainty if the laser output is well below the pertinant class limit. Very little uncertainty would be permitted if the laser output were close to a class limit. For example, if a manufacturer only must certify a line of 0.5 mW HeNe lasers as Class II (upper limit of 1.0 mW), he could use a measurement technique with a rather large uncertainty—or 40%— and if he had a laser that "measured" 0.7 mW (i.e., 0.7 mW ± 0.28 mW) he could still certify the product as Class II provided that it met other Class II requirements. On the other hand the manufacturer of a nominal 1.0 mW laser would probably classify the product as Class III. This approach varies from the philosophy of the ANSI document which recognized the same practical difficulties of making the classification measurements but as a consequence allowed a ± 20% error. Hence, it is necessary to specify which classification standard is used when a laser is classified.

In the following paragraphs are the principal BRH measurement requirements. Some of the measurement procedures were changed in the 1978 amendment so that collateral radiation and some fanned beams would not have to be collected if not really of concern from a hazard standpoint. Hence the need for a specification of a solid angle of acceptance and a collecting lens. These concepts will be addressed in Chapter 11.

(e) *Tests for determination of compliance*.

(1) *Tests for certification*. Tests on which certification pursuant to § 1010.2 of this chapter is based shall account for all errors and statistical uncertainties in the measurement process. Because compliance with the standard is required for the useful life of a product, such tests shall also account for increases in emission and degradation in radiation safety with age.

(2) *Test conditions*. Except as provided in § 1010.13 of this chapter, tests for compliance with each of the applicable requirements of this section and § 1040.11 shall be made during operation, maintenance or service as appropriate:

(i) Under those conditions and procedures which maximize the accessible emission levels, including start-up, stabilized emission, and shut-down of the laser product; and,

(ii) With all controls and adjustments listed in the operation, maintenance, and service instructions adjusted in combination to result in the maximum accessible emission level of radiation; and,

(iii) At points in space to which human access is possible in the product configuration which is necessary to determine compliance with each requirement, e.g., if operation may require removal of portions of the protective housing and defeat of safety interlocks, measurements shall be made at points accessible in that product configuration; and,

(iv) With the measuring instrument detector so positioned and so oriented with respect to the laser product as to result in the maximum detection of radiation by the instrument; and,

(v) For a laser product other than a laser system, with the laser coupled to that type of laser energy source which is specified as compatible by the laser product manufacturer and which produces the maximum emission level of accessible radiation from that product.

(3) *Measurement parameters*. Accessible emission levels of laser and collateral radiation shall be based upon the following measurements as appropriate, or their equivalent:

(i) The radiant power (W) or radiant energy (J) detectable through a circular aperture stop having a diameter of 80 millimeters (except for scanned laser radiation) and within a circular solid angle of acceptance of 1×10^{-3} steradian with collimating optics of 5 diopters or less.

(ii) The irradiance (W cm^{-2}) or radiant exposure (J cm^{-2}) equivalent to the radiant power (W) or radiant energy (J) detectable through a circular aperture stop having a diameter of 7 millimeters and, for irradiance, within a circular solid angle of acceptance of 1×10 cm^{-3} steradian with collimating optics of 5 diopters or less, divided by the area of the aperture stop (cm^{-2}).

(iii) The radiance (W cm^{-2} sr^{-1}) or integrated radiance (J cm^{-2} sr^{-1}) equivalent to the radiant power (W) or radiant energy (J) detectable through a circular aperture stop having a diameter of 7 millimeters and within a circular solid angle of acceptance of 1×10^{-5} steradian with collimating optics of 5 diopters or less, divided by that solid angle (sr) and by the area of the aperture stop (cm^2).

(4) *Measurement parameters for scanned laser radiation.* Accessible emission levels of scanned laser radiation shall be based upon the measurement of radiation detectable through a stationary circular aperture stop having a 7-millimeter diameter and within the circular solid angle of acceptance with collimating optics applicable under paragraph (e)(3) of this section, or the equivalent. The direction of the solid angle of acceptance shall change as needed to maximize detectable radiation, with an angular speed of up to 5 radians/second.

9.3.6 Performance Standards

The BRH standards list nine different performance requirements which refer to labelling or engineering design of the laser product (i.e., safety features). A particular design solution is not specified, but characteristics or limitations on product performance which the designer must meet are presented. These performance requirements are compared with those of ANSI in Table 9-4. These performance requirements are reproduced below and are reasonably explicit, although misinterpretation of some of them could result in either non-compliance or needlessly expensive designs to solve these requirements (Laser Focus, 1979). It is wise to make use of the free consultation that is available from the Division of Compliance of BRH once a design is initially planned.

(f) *Performance requirements*

(1) *Protective housing.* Each laser product, regardless of its class, shall have a protective housing which, when in place, prevents human access during operation to:

(i) Laser radiation in excess of the accessible emission limits of Class I wherever and whenever human access to laser radiation exceeding the limits of Class I is not necessary for the performance of the function(s) of the product; and,

(ii) Laser radiation in excess of the accessible emission limits of Class II wherever and whenever human access to laser radiation exceeding the limits of Class II is not necessary for the performance of the function(s) of the product; and,

(iii) Laser radiation in excess of the accessible emission limits of Class III wherever and whenever human access to laser radiation exceeding the limits of Class III is not necessary for the performance of the function(s) of the product; and,

(iv) Collateral radiation in excess of the accessible emission limits specified in Table III in paragraph (d) of this section wherever and whenever human access to collateral radiation in excess of those limits is not necessary for the performance of the function(s) of the product.

Laser Hazard Classification

(2) *Safety interlocks.*

(i) Each laser *product,* regardless of its class, shall be provided with a safety interlock for each portion of the protective housing which is designed to be removed or displaced during operation or maintenance, if removal or displacement of such portion of the protective housing could permit human access to laser or collateral radiation in excess of the accessible emission limits applicable under paragraph (f) (1) of this section. Each required safety interlock, unless defeated, shall:

(a) Prevent such human access to laser and collateral radiation upon removal or displacement of such portion of the protective housing; and,

(b) Preclude removal or displacement of such portion of the protective housing upon failure to prevent human access to laser and collateral radiation as required in paragraph (f)(2)(i)(a) of this section.

(ii) Laser products which incorporate safety interlocks designed to allow safety interlock defeat shall incorporate a means of visual or aural indication of interlock defeat. During interlock defeat, such indication shall be visible or audible whenever the laser product is energized, with and without the associated portion of the protective housing removed or displaced.

(iii) Replacement of a removed or displaced portion of the protective housing shall not be possible while required safety interlocks are defeated.

(3) *Remote control connector.* Each laser system classified as a Class III or IV laser product shall incorporate a readily available remote control connector having an electrical potential difference of no greater than 130 root-mean-square volts between the terminals of the remote control connector. When the terminal of the connector are not electrically joined, human access to all laser and collateral radiation from the laser product in excess of the accessible emission limits of Class I and Table III of paragraph (d) of this section shall be prevented.

(4) *Key control.* Each laser system classified as a Class III or IV laser product shall incorporate a key-actuated master control. The key shall be removable and the laser shall not be operable when the key is removed.

(5) *Laser radiation emission indicator.*

(i) Each laser system classified as a Class II laser product, except Class II laser products that do not exceed the accessible emission limits of Class I for any emission duration less than or equal to 1×10^{-3} seconds, shall incorporate an emission indicator that provides a visible or audible signal during emission of accessible laser radiation in excess of the accessible emission limits of Class I.

(ii) Each laser system classified as a Class III or IV laser product shall incorporate an emission indicator which provides a visible or audible signal during emission of accessible laser radiation in excess of the accessible emission limits of Class I, and sufficiently prior to emission of such radiation to allow appropriate action to avoid exposure to the laser radiation.

(iii) If the laser and laser energy source are housed separately and can be operated at a separation distance of greater than 2 meters, both laser and laser energy source shall incorporate an emission indicator as required in accordance with paragraphs (f) (5) (i) or (ii) of this section.

(iv) Any visible signal required by paragraphs (f) (5) (i) or (ii) of this section shall be clearly visible through protective eyewear designed specifically for the wavelength(s) of the emitted laser radiation.

(v) Emission indicators required by paragraph (f) (5) (i) or (ii) of this section shall be located so that viewing does not require human exposure to laser or collateral radiation in excess of the accessible emission limits of Class I and Table III [Table 9-3].

(6) *Beam attenuator.* Each laser system classified as a Class II, III, or IV laser product, except Class II laser products that do not exceed the accessible emission limits of Class I for any emission duration less than or equal to 1×10^3 seconds, shall be provided with one or

TABLE 9-3. Accessible Emission Limits for Collateral Radiation from Laser Products

Accessible emission limits for collateral radiation having wavelengths greater than 250 nm but less than or equal to 13,000 nm are identical to the accessible emission limits of Class I laser radiation, as determined from Tables I–A and II–A [Tables 9-1a and 9-2a] in this paragraph, for the appropriate ranges of wavelength and emission duration.

Accessible emission limit for collateral radiation within the x-ray range of wavelengths is 0.5 milliroentgen in an hour, averaged over a cross-section parallel to the external surface of the product, having an area of 10 square centimeters with no dimension greater than 5 centimeters.

---

more permanently attached means, other than laser energy source switch(es) electrical supply main connectors, or the key-actuated master control, capable of preventing access by any part of the human body to all laser and collateral radiation in excess of the accessible emission limits of Class I and Table III [Table 9-3].

(7) *Location of controls.* Each Class II, III, or IV laser product shall have operational and adjustment controls located so that human exposure to laser or collateral radiation in excess of the accessible emission limits of Class I and Table III [Table 9-3] of paragraph (d) of this section is unnecessary for operation or adjustment of such controls.

(8) *Viewing optics.* All viewing optics, viewports, and display screens incorporated into a laser product, regardless of its class, shall at all times limit the levels of laser and collateral radiation accessible to the human eye by means of such viewing optics, viewports, or display screens to less than the accessible emission limits of Class I and Table III [Table 9-3] of paragraph (d) of this section. For any shutter or variable attenuator incorporated into such viewing optics, viewports, or display screens, a means shall be provided:

(i) To prevent access by the human eye to laser and collateral radiation in excess of the accessible emission limits of Class I and Table III [Table 9-3] of paragraph (d) of this section whenever the shutter is opened or the attenuator varied.

(ii) To preclude, upon failure of such means as required in paragraph (f) (8) (i) of this section, opening the shutter or varying the attenuator when access by the human eye is possible to laser or collateral radiation in excess of the accessible emission limits of Class I and Table III [Table 9-3] of paragraph (d) of this section.

(9) *Scanning safeguard.* Laser products which emit accessible scanned laser radiation shall not, as a result of scan failure or other failure causing a change in either scan velocity or amplitude, permit human access to laser radiation in excess of the accessible emission limit(s) which are applicable to the scanned laser radiation.

Several of these requirements should be clarified to point out that fulfillment of them need not be very costly.

The *protective housing* obviously should prevent a user from being exposed to hazardous levels (above Class I limits). In many instances housings around lasers need not be opaque simply because the internal workings of the laser do not emit levels in excess of Class I. For instance the gas discharge glow of a HeNe laser seldom exceeds the collateral radiation limit (i.e., the 1,000-s, non-viewport) Class I limit for an extended source of 20 mW/($cm^2 \cdot sr$) in the visible part of the spectrum and may not exceed the limits in the infrared as well.

Laser Hazard Classification

Table 9-4. Laser Product Safety Requirements in the ANSI and BRH Standards

Performance Requirement or Recommendation	ANSI Class 1	BRH Class I	ANSI Class 2a	BRH Class IIa	ANSI Class 2	BRH Class II	ANSI Class 3a	BRH Class IIIa	ANSI Class 3b	BRH Class IIIb	ANSI Class 4	BRH Class IV
Classification label or warning label	no	yes	yes	yes	yes	yes	yes	yes	yes	yes	yes	yes
Protective housing to limit accessible radiation to lowest achievable class required for application.	†	yes	†	yes	†	yes	yes	yes	yes	yes	yes	yes
Safety interlocks for protective housing to assure retention of hazard classification if cover(s) are removed.	†	yes	†	yes	†	yes	†	yes	yes	yes	yes	yes
Scanning safeguard for scanning lasers to maintain class limit in event of scan failure.	*	yes	*	yes	*	yes	*	yes	*	yes	*	no
Remote-control connector to permit use of door or ancillary safety interlocks.	no	no	no	no	no	no	no	yes	no	yes	A	yes
Key-actuated master control so that laser is inoperable when key is removed.	no	no	no	no	no	no	no	yes	A	yes	yes	yes
Laser-radiation emission indicator with no delay.	no	no	no	no	no	yes	no	yes	A	yes	A	yes
Laser-radiation emission indicator with a delay to warn.	no	no	no	no	no	no	no	yes	A	yes	A	yes
Permanently attached attenuator to reduce to Class 1.	no	no	no	no	no	yes	A	yes	A	yes	A	yes
Controls located to reduce the chance of operator exposure.	no	no	no	yes	no	yes	no	yes	no	yes	no	yes
Protective viewing optics so that exposure is less than Class 1.	†	yes	†	yes	†	yes	yes	yes	yes	yes	yes	yes
Safety information must be furnished with the laser system.	no	yes	yes	yes	yes	yes	yes	yes	yes	yes	yes	yes

† — Applicable if higher class is enclosed.
A — Advisory (i.e., a "should" is used by ANSI for advisory recommendations; a "shall" is used to indicate a requirement of the standard).
* — Applicable only to entertainment applications, i.e., laser light shows.

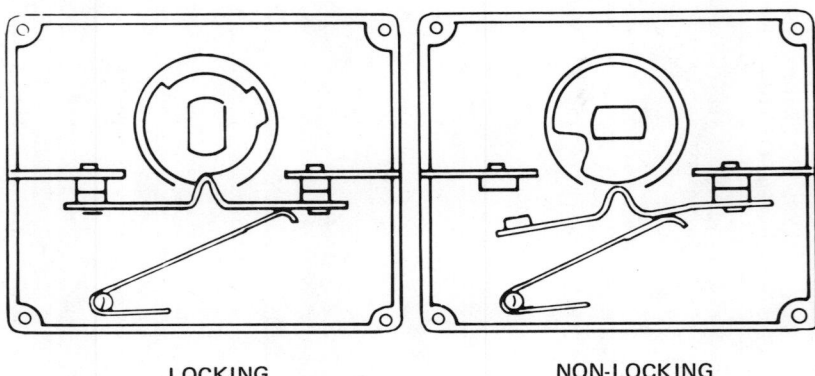

Figure 9-2. Safety Interlocks. For Class I Laser Products, BRH requires interlocks on the protective housing which are failsafe if they are not labeled. The total-disconnect, TV panel plug is acceptable, or the type of switch shown on the right which could not be rotated to open a panel latch (or hinge) if the switch contacts weld together and cannot be broken (after the GW Unimax Switch).

The requirement for *safety interlocks on protective housings* again is not always necessary if Class I limits are not accessible when the protective housing or panel is removed. But, non-defeatable interlocks are required for non-labeled access. Some manufacturers have needlessly interpreted the requirement for an interlocks-defeat warning system as a flashing light or buzzer. In fact, the required visible warning need only be a red warning patch or label which becomes visible when the interlock-defeat mechanism is depressed. It is not necessary to have any electrically activated or mechanically movable part. In many cases, regardless of the class of laser emission, manufacturers routinely put interlocks on access panels to prevent a user from being exposed to high voltages. The BRH has issued a lengthy interpretation on the adequacy of different types of interlocks which will not be discussed in detail here. In essence, BRH requires a *fail-safe* interlock (Fig. 9-2); in general such interlocks are not electrically activated since relays can weld shut in a short circuit; it generally must be mechanically activated. A televison power disconnect plug meets the BRH requirements. Panels intended purely for service need not be interlocked.

As pointed out previously, the *remote control connector* is designed to permit the user to interconnect a door interlock switch to the power supply or beam shutter of his laser. Although ANSI originally required this only for Class IV lasers, BRH extended this requirement to Class III lasers as well. In simple laser devices it has most often been accomplished by the installation on the laser's protective housing of a female jack within the main power supply's AC line circuit. The circuit normally is opened and the laser will remain remotely inoperable unless the line connecting to the circuit (e.g., at the two jack points) is closed by the insertion of the male portion of the connector jack or by a remote interlock switch such as a door switch or other enclosure interlock switch placed in the circuit by the user. On the other hand, where the laser power cannot be suddenly shut off without damage to the laser or without shutting off the cooling system this interlock must be inserted within the high voltage circuit through the use of a relay so that the cooling pump circuit is not opened. The remote control connector could also be designed to activate a beam shutter as long as there is adequate emission delay following the activation by the remote control. A cable from a battery or a power supply may not be considered a remote-control connector.

The *key control* requirement does not literally require an expensive multi-tumbler key switch but can be a very simple key switch. The intent here is to make the operation of the laser difficult at least to the unauthorized user (if the user chooses to remove the key).

The *emission indicator* requirement is most often achieved by the manufacturer with a simple pilot light. In the case of the emission indicator for Class III or Class IV products, a relay is often inserted into the power line which allows a few seconds of delay if such a delay is not already inherent in the laser circuit. Note here that the signal need not be electrically activated. Merely throwing a switch with a visible indicator attached would be one potential solution, provided that the indicator became visible prior to potential lasing and an appropriate delay. The appropriate delay may be as brief as 3-5 seconds for a simple HeNe laser to longer "reasonable" periods for a large Class IV pulsed laser. The intent here is to provide sufficient time for a person to take evasive action if required following his or her alert by the indicator.

The requirement for a *beam attenuator* is sometimes interpreted to mean a filter which just reduces the emission of the beam to a level which is just below Class I limits. Of course the use of the term "attenuator" rather than the term "beam shutter" was used here to permit a manufacturer to make use of a filter instead of an opaque shutter in order to permit a possible alignment mode or to permit the user to check to see if the laser is operating prior to emitting full power. Since a Class I level is often quite low, the beam attenuator is normally made as an opaque beam stop. Some scientists use a different type beam attenuator that can be added by a user for practical use in visible CW laser laboratories that would in itself not provide compliance with the BRH standard. This second attenuator is a filter to reduce the CW visible laser output to a level below 1 mW so that the beam can be seen for alignment but will not be a significant hazard (i.e., be effectively a Class II alignment laser). Although a small metal shield which drops or slides into place over the aperture is the most commonly encountered beam attenuator in present day laser systems, a cap on the end of a chain would also be a permanently attached beam attenuator (Fig. 9-3). Some users, who might be characterized as "not very safety oriented," have found that although they originally objected to the idea of a required "beam attenuator" for safety purposes (not seeing the safety value in it) they later saw its value of as external "attenuator" for keeping the output optics clean when the laser was not in use. For higher power CW lasers, the

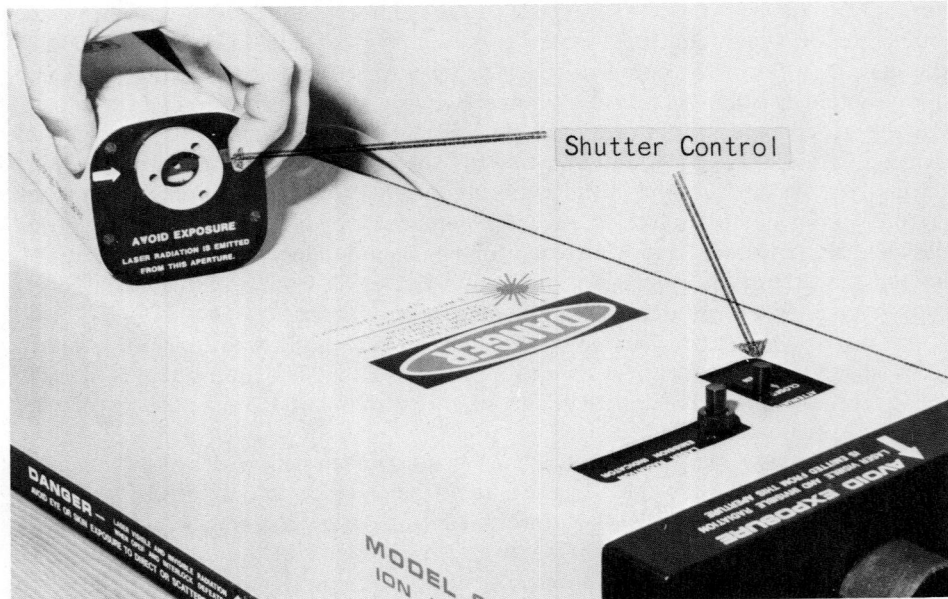

Figure 9-3. Beam Attenuators for CW Lasers. The types of beam attenuators (generally shutters) employed by different manufacturers vary considerably. Shown in the photograph is an external shutter for a 1-2 mW HeNe (small) laser, which is a sliding metal plate with an aperture in it, and an intracavity shutter controlled by a lever on the larger class IV argon ion laser. Note the "Avoid Exposure" warnings at the aperture of each laser and the DANGER label on the larger laser. On the side of the larger laser can be seen another warning label indicating the presence of a defeatable interlock on the protective housing. All of the features mentioned are required by the BRH regulation.

bulky "quick-fix" external beam attenuators of 1976 have been replaced by intracavity attenuators. Unfortunately, some scientific users now complain that the intracavity switches degrade beam performance.

The requirement for protection in *viewing optics* would apply most often to lasers used in materials processing where the eye is routinely viewing the target area and would be exposed to a hazardous reflection were it not for attenuators within the viewing optics. This requirement is also relavent to holographic interferometric viewing systems. BRH has also interpreted this requirement to mean that sighting optics on lasers used for alignment (or surveying) purposes could need a safety filter to preclude hazardous reflections, but the interpretation issued on August 5, 1976, states that the attenuation can apply only to diffuse reflections; and 5-mW HeNe lasers will not present a diffuse reflection hazard for spot diameters > 1 cm. The user instructions should warn against viewing specular reflections. The regulation actually states that the filter is for "accessible levels of transmitted laser and collateral radiation." Figure 19-1 shows an example of such safety controls built

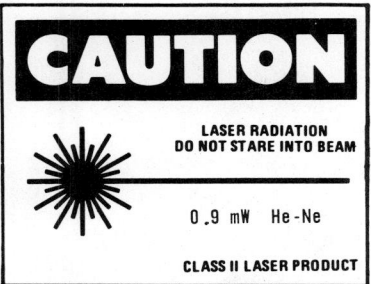 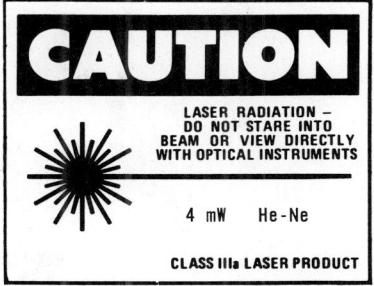

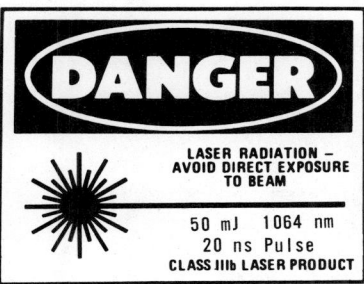 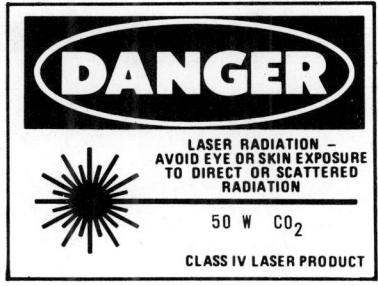

Figure 9-4. Representative BRH Labels. The above caution labels are characteristic of those found on Class II laser products or Class IIIa visible laser products. The danger labels are characteristic of those found on Class IIIb and Class IV products. The wording is in accordance with the BRH performance standard which requires an indication of either the laser medium or wavelength(s), and the maximum output of laser radiation, the pulse duration if appropriate, and a directional sunburst logotype. All must be positioned as shown.

into viewing optics of the material processing laser.

The *scanning safeguard* is obviously necessary when cessation of scanning results in the laser product falling into a higher class. This safeguard is most commonly employed through the introduction of a centrifugal-force-actuated switch which prevent laser emission either electrically or mechanically, i.e., by opening the power circuit or interposing a cutoff beam attenuator. Normally a beamblock or a cover would terminate the output when the angular velocity of a rotating mirror or prism drops below some predetermined value.

It is the *labeling requirement* of BRH that fulfills the principal hazard-evaluation need of the user of the ANSI standard; namely, the manufacturer must indicate the classification of the laser product. We shall not in this chapter go into any great detail on all of the many possible labels. These vary with class, wavelength, and other output characteristics. These labeling requirements can be summarized as

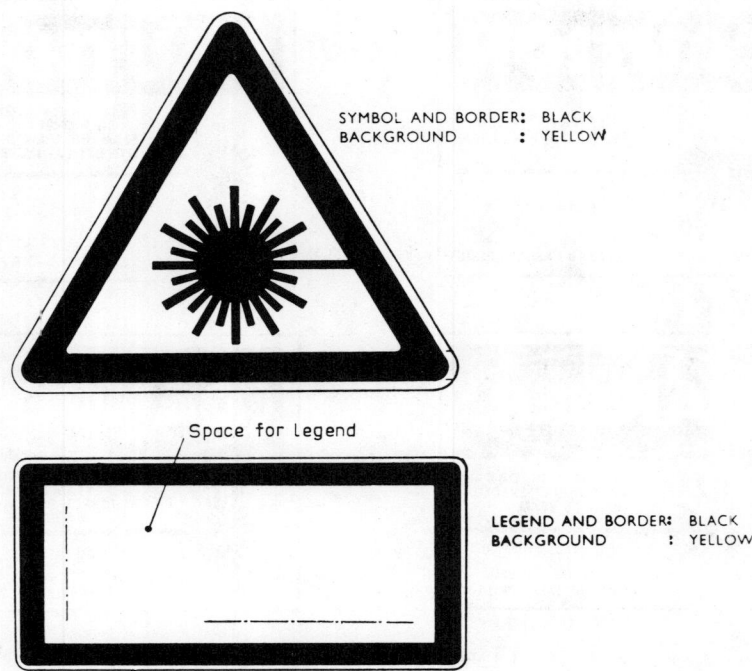

Figure 9-5. IEC Warning Label. The IEC type of label generally uses the BRH wording for laser products. Again the type of information and wording is carefully prescribed in the draft IEC standard.

follows. A danger or caution label such as those shown in Fig. 9-4 which must include a listing of the class; and the laser type or output characteristics are to be provided. In addition to the classification warning label, the manufacturer must also place a warning label near the output aperture of the beam so that the user is clearly informed as to the source of potentially hazardous laser radiation.

The IEC technical committee TC76 adopted basically the same wording and sunburst for their labels. However they followed an internationally accepted format for the label which was triangular. Figure 9-5 shows the IEC label. The words "DANGER" or "CAUTION" and other wording is placed in the rectangular box below the triangle.

9.3.7 User Information

The manufacturer must also provide certain *user information* such as instructions for adequate assembly, operation, and maintenance including any precautions necessary in such operations. Manuals must also include instructions for safe operating procedures.

9.3.8 Servicing and Maintenance

BRH makes an important distinction between servicing and maintenance. *Servicing* refers to the performance of those procedures or adjustments described in the manufacturer's service instruction which would normally be performed by a serviceman representing the manufacturer or another electronics servicing specialist. It does not refer to corrective operations performed by the user. The latter are termed *maintenance*. For instance, if a laser were used in an office copying machine, the addition of toners and other chemicals, the replacement of paper, the adjustment of certain controls for contrast, and the routine cleaning of certain parts as performed by the user is referred to as maintenance. On the other hand, if internal covers must be removed and electrical service performed by a representative of the manufacturer or one who is specially trained for this work, then this activity is termed "service." BRH defines "maintenance" as the "performance of those adjustments or procedures specified in user information provided by the manufacturer with the laser product which are to be performed by the user for the purpose of assuring the intended performance of the product." Figure 9-6 schematically summarizes these distinctions on performance.

9.3.9 Applicability of the BRH Standard

Many questions arise as to whom the BRH standard actually applies. It obviously applies to a manufacturer engaged in the sale of commercial laser products—on a wholesale basis or otherwise. The question naturally arises as to whether it applies to the experimentalist building a laser for his own use in his or her home, or to the research scientists building a "breadboard" laser in his or her laboratory, or to an engineer in a large corporation who builds a laser used in his or her same plant for manufacturing purposes when the laser itself is not sold in interstate commerce. In general the standard does not apply to any of these cases. However, labor safety or occupational health and safety standards may apply to some of the latter cases.

Anyone engaged in the business of modifying laser products is construed as a manufacturer by BRH if his act of modification affects any aspect of the product's performance or intended function for which the BRH regulation applies. After modification, the product must be recertified and reidentified in accordance with the BRH standard. A few examples will help to clarify this matter further. The basement hobbyist may buy laser components such as gallium-arsenide laser diodes or laser modules and build final laser products if he is building only for his own personal use. However, if he sells any of them, then he is a manufacturer and he may sell only certified laser products. If a corporation or a governmental agency

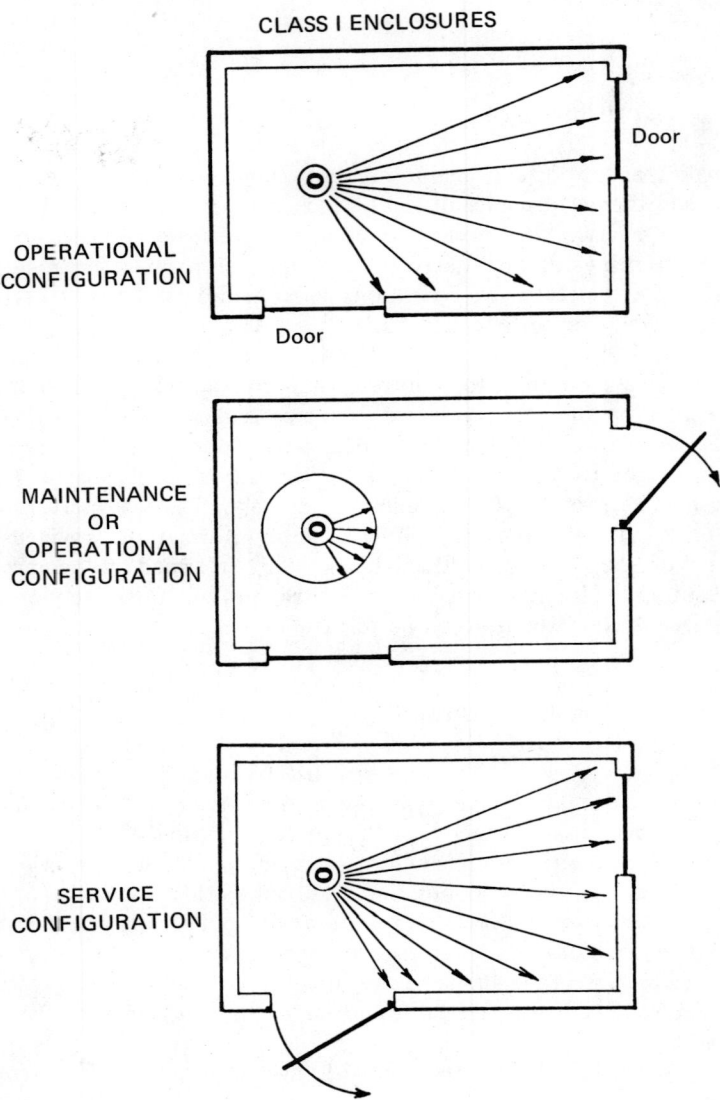

Figure 9-6. Maintenance, Operation, and Servicing Configurations for a laser protective housing. For operation (by the user) laser radiation does not get out of the protective housing enclosure and doors are interlocked to assure this. For maintenance (or operation) laser radiation cannot be accessible to the user if user panels or doors are opened. For service (by trained service personnel—not the user), radiation may be accessible, as through the service panel door.

builds a laser from components, even commercially available ones such as a certified laser without its power supply (and therefore without fulfilling a BRH label requirement, then such activity is not construed as manufacturing laser products if these devices are used solely within the governmental agency or corporate division performing such manufacture. Additionally, a manufacturer or distributor of lasers (o.e.m.) that are uncertified is prohibited from selling such items other than to bonafide manufacturers of certified laser products.

However there is a limitation explained in an interpretation rule by the BRH (issued on November 23, 1976): If one division of a large corporation builds "on a one-time basis" a laser product—one or two or several— and uses them at the same location, this is not considered manufacturing of products which may go into interstate commerce. On the other hand if the manufactured laser goes to another site— especially if that site is another state—then BRH construes that transfer as being in commerce. Then standard reports must be made to BRH and the laser product must be in compliance. If a Federal or state agency, such as a highway survey maintenance shop builds (or modifies) an alignment laser which is used by the same organization in the field, no compliance is required. But if that same shop builds such devices and sends them all over the state (or country) to other divisions, they are considered manufacturers. Other U.S. Government agencies can apply for an exemption from the BRH requirements. To the average reader all of these distinctions may seem rather unnecessary (if not silly), but there is a legal basis for the dividing lines. When in doubt, the potential manufacturer should contact the BRH Division of Compliance either by letter to the previously mentioned address or by telephone (area code 301/443-4874).

The U.S. Department of Defense (DoD) obtained an exemption for a variety of *military laser systems* in August 1976. Lasers intended for use in a tactical environment or tactical simulation or for field training or combat simulation exercises were exempted since camouflage and other military requirements would make complete compliance impractical. Lasers classified on the basis of national security were also exempted. However, lasers used by DoD activities indoors such as for scientific instruments, material processing and alignment or outdoors for any other non-military purposes were not exempted. Military lasers are still required to incorporate as many of the BRH performance characteristics that are practicable.

9.3.10 Reporting and Record Keeping Requirements

It is probably fair to say much of the criticism of the BRH performance standard, where it existed in the laser industry press, centered on the detailed reporting and record keeping requirements. We shall not discuss here the format and reporting requirements for certification record keeping. The manufacturer can obtain this information readily from the Division of Compliance, Bureau of Radiological Health. Presumably, record keeping was originally based upon an attempt by BRH to lessen the need for on-site inspections of laser manufacturers and is written into the Congressional act. The records permit the manufacturer himself to police his own operation, performing routine quality assurance measurements, recording this information and periodically reporting this to the Bureau of Radiological Health. This procedure has also been characteristic of the Food and Drug Administration's regulation of pharmaceutical manufacturers. After the initial adjustment to the record keeping and reporting procedures, complaints appear to have evaporated. BRH has simplified guides to aid the manufacturer in this area (USDHEW, 1976). BRH regional divisions also perform periodic compliance inspections at manufacturer's plant.

9.3.11 Specific Purpose Laser Products

Title 21, CFR 1040.11 deals with specific purpose laser products. This section of the regulation could very well be expanded in the future. At the time of publication of this book there were only three groups of products which had specific requirements: medical laser products; surveying, leveling and alignment laser products; and demonstration laser products. This section of the standard which provides additional requirements is as follows:

§ 1040.11 Specific Purpose Laser Products

(a) *Medical laser products.* Each medical laser product shall comply with all of the applicable requirements of § 1040.10 for laser products of its class. In addition, the manufacturer shall:
   (1) Incorporate in each Class III or IV medical laser product a means for the measurement of the level of that laser radiation intended for irradiation of the human body with an error in measurement of no more than ± 20 percent when calibrated in accordance with paragraph (a) (2) of this section. Indication of the measurement shall be in International System Units.
   (2) Supply with each Class III or IV medical laser product instructions specifying a procedure and schedule for calibration of the measurement system required by paragraph (a) (1) of this section.
   (3) Affix to each medical laser product, in close proximity to each aperture through which is emitted accessible laser radiation in excess of the accessible emission limits of Class I, a label bearing the wording: "Laser aperture."

(b) *Surveying, leveling, and alignment laser products.* Each surveying, leveling, or alignment laser product shall comply with all of the applicable requirements of § 1040.10 for a Class I, Class II, or Class III laser product and, in addition:
   (1) Shall not permit human access to laser radiation in the wavelength range of greater than 400 nanometers but less than or equal to 710 nanometers with a radiant power that exceeds 5.0×10^{-3} W for any emission duration greater than 3.8×10^{-4} second; and,
   (2) Shall not permit human access to laser radiation in excess of the accessible emission limits of Class I for any other combination of emission duration and wavelength range.

(c) *Demonstration laser products.* Each demonstration laser product shall comply with all of the applicable requirements of § 1040.10 for a Class I or Class II laser product and shall not permit human access to laser radiation in excess of the accessible emission limits of Class I and, if applicable, Class II.

The requirements for a beam output monitor for *medical laser products* derives in part from BRH's considerable experience in regulating the use of medical

X-ray equipment. They had found that physicians were often exposing their patients to levels in excess of what they desired or to multiple exposures because of lack of quantitative measurements of the output. In most therapeutic medical laser applications the physician using the equipment needs a general indication of the power output. BRH explained that the physician required the knowledge of output power to permit "day-to-day" reproducibility in patient irradiations. But in most, if not all, cases the actual adjustment of the output during therapy depends upon the reaction of the tissue. This applied to both retinal photocoagulation and surgical cutting and cauterizing procedures. BRH does not require an output power/energy meter for the medical aiming beam. To avoid alarming the patient unduly the required warning label at the exit aperture of a laser has been modified for medical lasers to be simply "laser aperture."

The requirement for an *alignment laser* is intended for CW visible alignment lasers only. One variance has been granted for a pulsed laser system which did not conveniently fall into the conventional categories. Another variance permitted a fan beam to have a power up to 8 mW. In essence, the requirement was to limit construction alignment laser power to 5 mW. This was an upper limit previously endorsed by the manufacturers of such equipment to serve as a dividing line (in the OSHA Construction Safety Standard) above which laser eye protection would be necessary for the user when the OSHA Construction Safety Standards were written.

The requirement for demonstration laser products presents one major problem. Many lasers used in art displays and laser light shows are Class IV lasers. If such displays are "demonstration" then lasers cannot be specifically manufactured for such shows. An artist can purchase a general purpose "research" laser, for example a 10-W argon laser, and modify it with beam scanners and the like for his own purpose. But apparently the artist may not routinely produce laser light shows or sell equipment for them to other artists without being in violation of this paragraph. A BRH Interim Enforcement Policy statement was issued on laser light shows on February 21, 1978. It provided lengthy light show guidelines (see Chapter 20).

9.3.12 The Definition of Accessibility

The definition of accessibility is one of the most difficult areas of the BRH standard. The basic philosophical intent is readily understandable, i.e., if the laser's emission is hazardous but not accessible then why worry about it. On the other hand, a reasonable definition for human access is very difficult to formulate, as anyone can attest who has made such an attempt. Some accessibility concepts in electrical safety standards most often relate to the ability to insert a wire into a crack or hole in a protective housing. It was a similar idea of an unfolded paper clip (10 cm long) that reportedly influenced the writing of one of the requirements in the 1975 standard that was later dropped in the 1978 revised standard. When the BRH standard was first published in July 1975, human access was defined as "access at a particular point to laser radiation or collateral radiation by any part of the human body, by a straight line having an unobstructed length of 100 cm, or by any line having an unobstructed length of 10 cm when the laser or collateral radiation is incident at that point." Since light must travel in a straight line (or in a light guide), the requirement that light could be passed through any area where an unobstructed length of flexible wire of even infinitesimal dimensions could pass seemed reasonable but became untenable in practice. As a recognition of this difficulty the 10-cm (flexible light guide) requirement was dropped in 1978. However, the concept of an infinitesimally thin aperture in the enclosure remains a problem. It could be argued that diffraction effects, particularly for longer-wavelength radiation, would cause rapid divergence of any leakage radiation emitted from a crack or a small hole, but this effect is highly wavelength dependent and is a poor argument. Some manufacturers once complained of difficulties in meeting this requirement since the tolerances for some types of panel closures would have to be extremely stringent. This illustrates a typical problem encountered by the authors in their own experience in writing a military standard or regulation where the concept is sensible, the intent easily understandable, but the practical specification can sometimes be very complicated. Often the attempt to write a requirement which considers every possible exception becomes an incredibly difficult or impossible task.

The ANSI standard allows the user to decide what access is reasonable. The 1977 International Electrotechnical Commission draft standard defined it in the following way:

> *Human access.* **Laser radiation capable of meeting a part of the human body to which it is hazardous, either as emitted from an aperture, by redirection from within a housing to the outside by the use of a reflector or optical guide or by the insertion of part of the body through an enclosure port into the interior of the laser system, or by a failure mode of the laser.**

This may sound better to some but it may be more difficult or impossible to enforce. One application of the BRH definition of accessibility will be considered, for example, the "point-of-sale" application at a supermarket checkout counter with a laser scanner. Normally the laser beam comes through a small horizontal (or tilted and recessed) window in the counter. The beam normally is directed upward by a mirror which can be seen through the output window on the counter. If the output of the laser is along the beam path inside the enclosure before the scanning mirror there almost certainly exists a point where the entire laser power would pass through a 7-mm aperture. At this point the power would typically be Class II or Class III. However, because of the 7-mm aperture measurement criterion for scanned laser radiation, the measurement at the accessible window is very likely to be below the Class I limits. Indeed most manufacturers design it to be Class I. Although the apparent source of laser radiation can be seen deep within the machine it is not accessible because no part of the human body can reach the scanner through the glass window, nor can an "unobstructed" line reach the point. The window is an obstruction for any test probe or for any appendage of the body but is not an obstruction for the light beam itself; thus the BRH definition adequately treats this situation. Of course collecting optics could be used to image the source upon the retina, but in this case they would have to be mounted above the counter a few feet. This is a rather unrealistic possibility and can be ignored. Because of some of the costly timing systems built into these systems to shut off the laser after the accumulation of the daily emission limit, BRH modified the standard in 1978 to include a class IIa with a 1,000-s sampling limit, instead of a "greater than 10^4 s" sampling limit, and no further controls.

A second example is a 500-W CO_2 laser used in the garment industry. Here a computer-directed laser beam is used to cut clothing—several layers at one time—along a predetermined pattern. The beam is directed downward at the cloth from a beam control carriage which moves over the platform holding the cloth. In other models the cloth moves and the beam is stationary. The table may be so large that the nearest point where an individual can stand is 1 m from the closest access point of the beam. Certainly a man's arm is not sufficiently long to reach the beam unless he bends over the table. The manufacturer of such a system obviously can assume that the enforcement agency will not include the case where a person jumps up onto the table and gets down where the cloth is. Would this condition be considered normal use, servicing, or maintenance? Regrettably, the lawyers would probably spend quite some time debating this application which, in fact, is probably a reasonably safe design. Certainly the warning instructions on the equipment or in the instruction manuals should caution the user not to get up on the cutting table or place his hand, eye, or a reflecting metal object in the beam path. The clever equipment designer would probably preclude all of these problems by having a light-weight, clear, plastic cylinder fall down and touch the cloth around the laser beam path.

The next example is a laser scanner used in an aircraft altimeter or obstacle-avoidance device. If the laser can only be activated when the aircraft is in flight, and if the beam is directed toward the ground or toward the front of the aircraft, then by common sense the beam port is not accessible in flight. However the device will probably be classified as a Class III or Class IV, according to the power level with an aperture warning label required on the device. In this case the controls required for a Class III or IV laser would probably cost no more than the controls required for a Class I laser had the manufacturer desired to classify it as such.

Another example is a construction laser device which sends out a plane of light continuously formed by a reflecting cone as shown in Fig. 18-3. This laser device is Class II although the total accessible output in the beam place exceeds 2 mW. This classification is possible because an 80-mm aperture placed immediately adjacent to the exit port can never collect more than 40% of the beam and the safety of a Class II device is achieved. The 80-mm collecting optics is considered the largest optics to be found in any telescope likely to be used by the general population to collect the laser radiation into the human eye or to focus it on the skin.

9.4 PRACTICAL EXAMPLES

At first glance the BRH classification tables appear to be rather complicated. Actually, the number of instances where one must resort to careful calculations are rather few when considering the large number of available lasers. Table 9-5 provides a list of commonly encountered commercial lasers and indicates how they would be classified. For the cases where a question might arise, several examples are given to illustrate the proper use of the tables to find out the exact dividing line between one class and another.

9.4.1 Example 1

Classify a Q-switched ruby laser intended for research which has an output peak power specified by the manufacturer as 30 mW, a pulse duration of 25 ns and a laser rod diameter of one-half inch.

The emission limits for pulsed lasers are given in terms of joules. Table 9-1a shows that the criterion applicable for intrabeam viewing is $2 \times 10^{-7} k_1 k_2$ J, while Table 9-2a gives both k_1 and k_2 as 1.0 for the wavelength interval between 400 and 700 nm (the ruby laser is 694.3 nm). The Class I limit is 2×10^{-7} J; the Class II limit is not applicable because the emission duration is less than 0.25 s, and the Class III accessible emission limit for this range as given in Table 9-1c is $10 k_1 k_2 t^{1/3}$ J/cm^2 to a maximum of 10 J/cm^2 for a pulsed laser; hence the Class III accessible limit is $10 t^{1/3}$ J/cm^2. A pocket calculator or slide rule can easily evaluate $t^{1/3}$ for a t of 25 ns or the cube root of 2.5×10^{-8} s as 2.9×10^{-3}. Hence the upper limit of Class III [AEL (III)] for this type of laser is limited both by the pulse duration and the wavelength and is:

$$\begin{aligned} \text{AEL (III)} &= 10 \, k_1 k_2 \, t^{1/3} \\ &= (10)(1)(2.9 \times 10^{-3}) \\ &= 2.9 \times 10^{-2} \text{ J/cm}^2 \end{aligned} \quad (9\text{-}1)$$

As this value is under the 10 J/cm^2 overall level given in Table 9-1c, the calculated value is within the Class III limit. We may recall that the ANSI limits for pulsed lasers in this region are a factor of π greater.

The task still remains to determine whether the output radiant exposure exceeds the Class III limit. Inasmuch as Table 9-5 has already indicated that the laser will certainly not be Class I the question is whether it is a Class III or Class IV. The output radiant exposure must be calculated to determine if it is above the limit. To do this an emergent beam diameter, a, is assumed which should be between 0.6 and 1.3 cm. The radiant exposure is no less than:

$$\begin{aligned} H &= \Phi \cdot t/a \\ &= Q/A \\ &= 4Q/\pi a^2 \\ &= (3 \times 10^7 \text{ W})(2.5 \times 10^{-8} \text{ s})(4)/(3.14)(1.3 \text{ cm}^2) \\ &= 0.3 \text{ J/cm}^2 \end{aligned} \quad (9\text{-}2)$$

It can be concluded therefore that the laser is Class IV since the lower limit on H exceeds the Class III limit for BRH and ANSI.

Laser Hazard Classification

9.4.2 Example 2

Classify a dye laser having a peak output wavelength at 590 nm which has an output energy of 10 mJ/pulse, an emergent beam diameter of 5 mm, and a pulse duration of 1 μs (10^{-6} s).

From Table 9-5 a pulsed dye laser again may be classed either as Class III or IV. Hence only the output need be calculated under the Class III limit in Table 9-1c. This once again is 10 $k_1 k_2 \ t^{1/3}$ J/cm². For this wavelength range k_1 and k_2 are both 1. The cube root of 10^{-6} s simply is 10^{-2}. Hence the output is 0.1 J/cm² which also does not exceed the 10 J/cm² Class III emission limit. The output radiant exposure of the dye laser must also be calculated as follows:

$$\begin{align}
H_o &= Q/A \\
&= 4Q/\pi a^2 \\
&= 1.27 \ Q/a^2 \tag{9-3} \\
&= 1.27 \ (0.01 \ J)/(0.5 \ cm)^2 \\
&= 0.051 \ J/cm^2
\end{align}$$

Since this value of H_o is below 0.1 J/cm² the laser is Class III provided that its repetition frequency (PRF) is not sufficiently high for the laser's average power output to exceed 0.5 W. Since the PRF was not specified, it is necessary to calculate the PRF required to provide 0.5 W average power:

$$PRF = \Phi_a/Q_p = 0.5 \ W/0.01 \ J = 50 \ Hz \tag{9-4}$$

Such a high repetition rate is somewhat unlikely for a flashlamp-pumped dye laser, although it would not be out of the question for the repetitively pulsed argon laser pump source.

9.4.3 Example 3

Classify a tunable laser which emits between 450 nm and 2 μm at an output of 0.07 J/pulse and a 5-mm diameter beam. The pulse duration is 700 ns and the PRF is 10 Hz or less.

A tunable laser has the most conservative criterion for accessible emission limits in the spectral region between 400 and 700 nm. The calculations for radiant exposure, then, will be essentially the same as the dye laser in Example 2. However, a determination must be made whether the tunable laser which has its peak power output higher than the dye laser will be placed into Class IV. We first calculate the Class III accessible emission limit for a 700 ns pulse. Again k_1 and k_2 are 1.0 for the worst case; although if the laser were adjusted so that it would only emit at some wavelength greater than 700 nm, it is noted from Table 9-2a that the k_1 factor could be larger. Since the pulse duration was 700 ns, k_2 would always be 1.

The radiant exposure output H_o is therefore:

$$H_o = 1.27 \, (0.03 \text{ J})/(0.5)^2$$
$$= 0.15 \text{ J/cm}^2 \qquad (9\text{-}5)$$

The Class III accessible emission limit for a 700 ns visible laser is:

$$\text{AEL (III)} = 10 \, k_1 k_2 \, t^{1/3} = 10(7 \times 10^{-7})^{1/3} \qquad (9\text{-}6)$$
$$= 8.9 \times 10^{-3} \text{ J/cm}^2$$

Since the accessible emission limit in this case is less than H_o this device falls into category IV. It is not even necessary to consider that the multiple-pulse output could be greater than 0.5 W, also placing it in Class IV.

9.4.4 Example 4

A gallium-arsenide laser operating at 905 nm with a specified output peak power of 10 W, a pulse duration of 100 ns, and an emergent beam diameter of less than 1 mm has a PRF of 1 kHz. What is the classification?

The radiant exposure output is calculated in the BRH standard differently from that in the ANSI standard for comparison with the Class III accessible emission limits. The BRH standard specified an instrument which can measure the radiant exposure averaged over a 7-mm aperture and the ANSI document requires that it be measured over a 1-mm diameter aperture. It should be kept in mind that this distinction only applied for measuring radiant exposure. For determining classification ANSI does use a 7-mm aperture in measuring some MPE's in the retinal hazard region. The previous calculations of H_o given in Examples, 1, 2, and 3 with small beam diameters would apply more accurately to the ANSI standard. When working with the BRH standard in this regard the beam diameter a could have been changed to 7 mm if specified at a lower value. The distinction that must be made is that the beam diameter of a laser is normally specified at $1/e$ points (or $1/e^2$ points) and power does exist outside of an aperture equal to the beam diameter. Hence the 5-mm beam diameter probably gave a reasonably good estimation of H_o for problems 2 and 3, albeit somewhat conservative. Thus in calculating the radiant exposure for the gallium-arsenide device, Table 9-5 shows immediately that gallium-arsenide lasers really fall into Class I or III and would not fall into Class IV except for the use of the 1-mm aperture in the case of the ANSI standard, in which case it would be for a raw beam without any collimating optics.

The Class I accessible emission limit for a 905-nm single-pulse is:

$$\text{AEL (I)} = 2 \times 10^{-7} \, k_1 k_2 \text{ J}$$
$$= 2 \times 10^{-7} \, (2.5)(1) \qquad (9\text{-}7)$$
$$= 5 \times 10^{-7} \text{ J}$$

Laser Hazard Classification

The output energy per pulse then is:

$$\begin{aligned} Q_p &= \Phi_p \cdot t \\ &= (10 \text{ W})(10^{-7}\text{ s}) \\ &= 10^{-5} \text{ J} \\ &= 10\ \mu\text{J/pulse} \end{aligned} \quad (9\text{-}7)$$

The average power:

$$\begin{aligned} \Phi_a &= Q_p \cdot F \\ &= (10^{-5})(1000) \\ &= 10^{-2} \text{ W} \\ &= 10 \text{ mW} \end{aligned} \quad (9\text{-}9)$$

Since the output energy per pulse exceeds the single pulse limit it is not necessary to check to see if the average power limitation is exceeded for Class I. Hence the laser is Class III.

9.4.5 Example 5

Classify a helium-cadmium laser which is specified to have an output power of 10 mW at 441.6 nm and an output power of 1.8 mW at 325 nm. The emergent beam diameter is 1.8 mm and the output is continuous wave (CW).

Even if the laser output in the visible were less than 1 mW the laser could not be classified as Class II because of the ultraviolet output. From Table 9-5 it is obvious that the laser is a Class III laser, but to gain experience with the BRH tables we shall go through the calculations. Note that k_1 has a value of 330 at the 325-nm wavelength and a value of 1 at 441.6 nm, and k_2 has a value of 1 in both cases from Table 9-2a. Since the output power is greater than 1 mW the laser is certainly Class III, conceivably Class IV. For a CW laser the limit is:

$$\begin{aligned} \text{Limit (III)} &= 1.5 \times 10^{-3}\ k_1 k_2\ t \text{ J (at 325 nm)} \\ &= 0.495\ (t)\ \text{J} \end{aligned} \quad (9\text{-}10)$$

This is effectively the same as the visible requirement for a CW laser, 0.5 t J. Dividing these formulas by t gives the Class III limit of 0.5 W which is identical to the ANSI limit and which is not exceeded by this laser. Hence the laser is Class III at both wavelength modes of operation.

In fact a general conclusion can be drawn which applies to all CW lasers which are tunable from the visible into either the infrared or the ultraviolet. If the tunable laser is not limited to the visible, then it cannot fall into the Class II category. The laser output would have to be a few microwatts or less to be in Class I; it would have to be less than 1 mW and be limited to the visible to be Class II; and it would have to be less than 0.5 W to be Class III. All CW lasers above 0.5 W would be Class IV.

CW lasers really present no problem whatsoever in classification. The only problems that arise are in the determination of the Class I limits. Since these limits are time-dependent, BRH specified that the "classification duration" (which they term the "maximum sampling interval") must be the greatest duration of potential exposure. If built-in interlocks limit an exposure duration or operating times to less than 10,000 seconds in any one day, the output could conceivably be higher than the Class I limit calculated for a maximal sampling duration exceeding 10^4 s.

9.4.6 Example 6

An aircraft signaler beacon has a 1 J neodymium laser with diffusing optics intended to reduce the total output to 0.3 J directed Lambertially into a solid angle of 2π sr. The diffuser surface area is 17 cm² (if the output is to be below Class I limits), and provided that the interlocks on the diffuser cover meet Class I design requirements, a determination can be made to see if indeed this laser design is indeed Class I. It could very well be a Class IV laser were it not for the diffuser. The Class I emission limits can be calculated from Table 9-1a. Note the dual limits for this range. The second category—for extended sources—for a 25-ns exposure duration from Table 9-2a we find the value for k_1 is 5 and the value for k_2 for such a short exposure is 1.0. The limiting radiance therefore is:

$$\begin{aligned} L \text{ (Class I AEL)} &= (10)(5)(1)(2.5 \times 10^{-8}\text{ s})^{1/3} \text{ J/(cm}^2 \cdot \text{sr)} \\ &= (10)(5)(1)(2.9 \times 10^{-3}) \\ &= 0.15 \text{ J/(cm}^2 \cdot \text{sr)} \end{aligned} \quad (9\text{-}11)$$

This value will probably not be exceeded by the radiance of the source. A guess of the average radiance of the diffuser dome will probably be as much as a factor of 2 below the maximum. In this approach it is assumed that all of the surface area of 17 cm² is equally bright:

$$\begin{aligned} L \text{ (estimated)} &= 0.3 \text{ J}/(17 \text{ cm}^2)(2 \times 3.14 \text{ sr}) \\ &= 2.8 \times 10^{-3} \text{ J(cm}^2 \cdot \text{sr)} \end{aligned} \quad (9\text{-}12)$$

Thus it is obvious that there is a very good chance that the device is a Class I system, at least on a single pulse bases. Measurements must be made to confirm these types of "design-estimate" calculations. The estimated radiance is 52 times less than the Class I limit. The ANSI criterion for the Class I limit is identical.

If the aircraft beacon flashes once every second the integrated total radiance must be calculated to determine if it will exceed the permissible criteria for either ANSI or BRH. The long-term exposure limit from the BRH standard is calculated in the following manner:

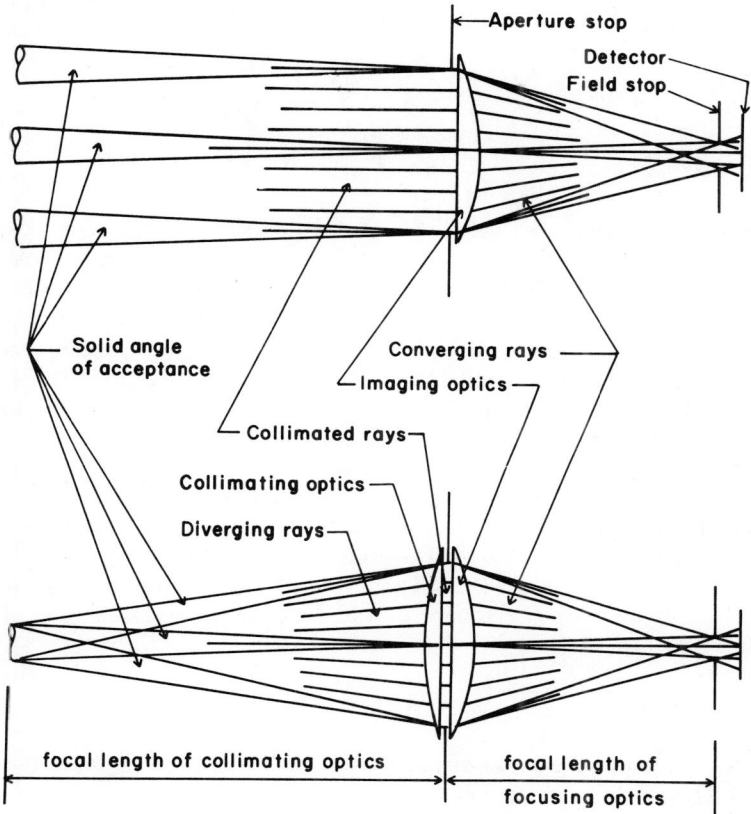

SCHEMATIC DIAGRAM SHOWING CONCEPTS AND TERMINOLOGY OF OPTICAL RADIATION MEASUREMENT

Figure 9-7. Laser Classification Measurement. The above diagram defines the terms used by BRH for accessible emission measurement in section 1040.10 (e) (3). The focal length of the collimating optics may be no shorter than 20 cm (i.e., 5 diopters or less) and the solid angle of acceptance is 10^{-3} sr (2° circular cone) except when measuring radiance or integrated radiance, in which case this solid angle is only 10^{-5} sr (0.22° circular cone). The solid angle of acceptance in the ANSI standard is α_{min}. The BRH standard requires that the solid angle of acceptance track the source at angular velocities up to 5 rad/s.

$$\text{AEL (I) } L_{avg} = 2 \times 10^{-3} \, k_1 k_2 \, t \, J/(cm^2 \cdot sr) \quad (9\text{-}13)$$
$$= 2 \times 10^{-3} \, (5)(100)(t) \, J/(cm^2 \cdot sr) \, (\text{for } t > 10^4 \, s)$$

In terms of average radiance, the limit L for Class I would be:

$$\begin{aligned}\text{AEL (I)} &= 2 \times 10^{-3} \, k_1 k_2 \, t \, J/(cm^2 \cdot sr) \\ &= 2 \times 10^{-3} \, (5)(100)(t) \, J/(cm^2 \cdot sr) \quad (9\text{-}14)\\ &= 1 \, (t) \, J/(cm^2 \cdot sr) \\ &= 1 \, W/(cm^2 \cdot sr) \end{aligned}$$

This value obviously is well below the average radiance of the repetitively pulsed neodymium laser beacon. At 1 pulse per second the beacon would have an estimated average radiance of only $2.8 = 10^{-3}$ W/(cm² · sr). Properly, to determine if the source meets the BRH Class I limit one should measure in accordance with the technique listed for extended sources. The energy per pulse entering a detector would be measured with a 7-mm diameter circular aperture stop and an effective solid angle Ω of acceptance of 10^{-5} sr. This could be accomplished by looking for the brightest spot on the diffuser dome, perhaps by using an infrared image converter or by a camera technique with sensitized Z emulsion. Alternatively, one could place an opaque cover over the diffuser dome with a small aperture covering the bright spot. The 7-mm aperture detector is moved back to a point where the aperture on the diffuser cover had a solid angle of 10^{-5} sr to be set to perform compliance measurements. This distance would be where the area of the aperture in the cover divided by the square of the distance between the source and the detector is equal to 10^{-5}:

$$\Omega = A/r^2 = 10^{-5} \, sr \quad (9\text{-}15)$$

Figure 9-7 illustrates the measurement setup that would be required by the 1978 BRH and ANSI Z-136 standards.

9.4.7 Example 7

Classify a CW water-vapor laser having an average power output of 70 mW at 118.4 μm, and a beam diameter of 8 mm. The BRH standard provides no limits here. However, the ANSI standard makes use of an 11-mm limiting aperture (i.e., A = 0.95 cm²) in this spectral region.

$$\begin{aligned}\text{Class I (ANSI) Limit} &= (0.1 \, W/cm^2)(A \, cm^2) \\ &= (0.1 \, W/cm^2)(0.95 \, cm^2) \quad (9\text{-}16)\\ &= 0.95 \, W\end{aligned}$$

Obviously this far infrared laser is Class I.

9.4.8 Example 8

Multiple Wavelength Laser. A frequency-doubled neodymium laser cloud-height altimeter is designed to emit a beam of two wavelengths: 532 nm and 1064 nm. It is desired to meet the BRH Class III limits. The laser emits one pulse-per-second with a total energy of 0.15 J, specifically: 0.1 J at 1064 nm and 0.05 J at 532 nm in a 10 ns pulse. What output requirements must be met by the laser designer?

To determine if the laser can meet the average-power limitations for Class IIIb lasers of all wavelengths for t > 0.25 s we must convert the pulsed output energy to average power Φ_{avg}:

Output: $\Phi_{avg} = Q \cdot F = (0.15 \text{ J/pulse})(1 \text{ Hz}) = 0.15 \text{ W}$ (9-17)

BRH Limit (IIIb): $\Phi_{avg}(\max) = 5 \times 10^{-1} \text{ t} \cdot \text{J} = 0.5 \text{ W}$

Hence the system will meet the Class III limit for t greater than 0.25 s (repetitive pulsing in this instance).

To determine if the laser can meet the Class IIIb single-pulse output radiant exposure H requirements, we must make use of Table 9-1c and paragraph 1040.10 (d) (3). The additivity concept is similar to those used for chemical contaminant TLV's, i.e., linear additivity. The sum of the ratios of radiant exposures to the AEL's, i.e.:

$$\frac{H_{1064}}{AEL_{1064}} + \frac{H_{532}}{AEL_{532}} < 1 \quad (9\text{-}18)$$

Obviously the designer has several options open. He or she could have a larger beam diameter for the green, 532-nm beam if trying to minimize glass lens sizes. For simplicity, however, a reasonable first approach is to assume common collimator optics with emergent beam diameters equal. With this assumption, the ratio of the two radiant exposures is 2 to 1, i.e.,

$$H_{1064} = 2 H_{532}$$

We now have two equations with two unknowns. Calculating the AEL's from Table 9-1c results in $AEL_{532} = 0.0215 \text{ J/cm}^2$ and $AEL_{1064} = 0.108 \text{ J/cm}^2$. Combining the two results, one has:

$$\frac{2 H_{532}}{0.108} + \frac{H_{532}}{0.0215 \text{ J/cm}^2} < 1$$

which leads to: $H_{532} < 0.0154 \text{ J/cm}^2$

and: $H_{1064} < 0.0308 \text{ J/cm}^2$

TABLE 9-5. Classification for Non-Enclosed, Non-Scanning Lasers†

Type of Laser Device	Wavelength	Temporal Output Mode
Argon Ion (Ar^{3+})	488 nm and 514.5 nm	CW
Carbon-Dioxide (CO_2)	10.6 μm	CW
Carbon-Monoxide (CO)	5 μm	CW
Dye Laser, Argon-Pumped	400 nm to 780 nm	CW
Dye Laser, Xenon-Flashlamp Pumped	450 nm to 780 nm	1 μs
Erbium (Er^{3+})	1540 nm or 1640 nm	20 ns
Gallium-Aluminum-Arsenide (GaAlAs) **	850 nm	100 ns @ 10 Hz to 100 kHz
Gallium-Arsenide (GaAs) **	905 nm	100 ns @ 10 Hz to 100 kHz
Hydrogen-Cyanide (HCN)	115 μm	CW
Helium-Cadmium (HeCd)	325 nm	CW
Helium-Cadmium (HeCd)	441.6 nm	CW
Helium-Neon (HeNe)	632.8 nm	CW
Holmium (Ho^{3+})	850 nm [or 2.06 μm]	100 ns
Krypton Ion (Kr^{+})	568 nm and 647 nm	CW
Neodymium Long Pulse (Nd^{3+})	1060 nm to 1064 nm	1 ms
Neodymium, Q-Switched (Nd^{3+})	1060 nm to 1064 nm	20 ns
Neodymium:YAG (Nd:YAG)	1064 nm	CW
Ruby, Long Pulse (Al_2O_3:Cr^{3+})	694.3 nm	1 ms
Ruby, Q-Switched (Al_2O_3:Cr^{3+})	694.3 nm	20 ns
TEA Laser, CO_2 [or CO]	10.6 μm [or 5 μm]	100 ns
Water Vapor (H_2O) [or HCN]	118 μm [or 337 μm]	CW

† The assumption is made that the laser's output is typical — within the expected laser power outpu
** Assumes a point source which is generally true for a single diode.

k_1	k_2	BRH Standard: 21 CFR 1040 Classification	ANSI Standard Z 136.1 and ACGIH Guide
1.0	1.0	III if $\Phi \leq 0.5$ W IV if $\Phi > 0.5$ W	Same as BRH
1.0	1.0	III if $\Phi \leq 0.5$ W	Same as BRH
1.0	1.0	IV if $\Phi > 0.5$ W	Same as BRH
1.0	1.0	III if $\Phi \leq 0.5$ W	Same as BRH
1.0	1.0	IV if $\Phi > 0.5$ W	
1.0	1.0	III if $H_0 \leq 0.1$ J/cm^2 IV if $H_0 > 0.1$ J/cm^2	III if $H_0 \leq 0.31$ J/cm^2 IV if $H_0 > 0.31$ J/cm^2
100	1.0	III if $H_0 \leq 10$ J/cm^2 IV if $H_0 > 10$ J/cm^2	Same as BRH
1.96	100*	I if $\Phi_a \leq 0.076$ mW and $Q_p \leq 0.4$ μJ III if $\Phi_a > 0.076$ mW or $Q_p > 0.4$ μJ	I if $\Phi_a \leq 0.63$ mW and $Q_p \leq 0.4$ C_p μJ III if $\Phi_a > 0.63$ mW or $Q_p > 0.4$ C_p μJ
2.5	100*	I if $\Phi_a \leq 0.0975$ mW and $Q_p \leq 0.5$ μJ III if $\Phi_a > 0.0975$ mW or $Q_p > 0.5$ μJ	I if $\Phi_a \leq 0.8$ mW and $Q_p \leq 0.5$ C_p μJ III if $\Phi_a > 0.8$ mW or $Q_p > 0.5$ C_p μJ
N/A	N/A	Not defined by BRH	III if $\Phi \leq 0.5$ W IV if $\Phi > 0.5$ W
330	1.0	III if $\Phi \leq 0.5$ W and $\Phi > 0.26$ μW	III if $\Phi \leq 0.5$ W and $\Phi > 8.0$ μW
1.0	1.0	II if $\Phi \leq 1.0$ mW III if $\Phi > 1.0$ mW	Same as BRH
1.0	1.0	II if $\Phi \leq 1.0$ mW III if $\Phi > 1.0$ mW	Same as BRH
1.0	1.0	III if $H_0 \leq 0.91$ J/cm^2 [10 J/cm^2] IV if $H_0 > 0.91$ J/cm^2 [10 J/cm^2]	III if $H_0 \leq 93$ mJ/cm^2 [10 J/cm^2] IV if $H_0 > 93$ mJ/cm^2 [10 J/cm^2]
1.0	1.0	III if $\Phi \leq 0.5$ W IV if $\Phi > 0.5$ W	Same as BRH
1.0	1.0 / I	III if $H_0 \leq 5.0$ J/cm^2 IV if $H_0 > 5.0$ J/cm^2	III if $H_0 \leq 10$ J/cm^2 IV if $H_0 > 10$ J/cm^2
1.0	1.0	III if $H_0 \leq 0.136$ J/cm^2 IV if $H_0 > 0.136$ J/cm^2	III if $H_0 \leq 0.43$ J/cm^2 IV if $H_0 > 0.43$ J/cm^2
1.0	100*	III if $\Phi \leq 0.5$ W IV if $\Phi > 0.5$ W	Same as BRH
1.0	1.0	III if $H_0 \leq 1.0$ J/cm^2 IV if $H_0 > 1.0$ J/cm^2	III if $H_0 \leq 3.1$ J/cm^2 IV if $H_0 > 3.1$ J/cm^2
1.0	1.0	III if $H_0 \leq 0.027$ J/cm^2 IV if $H_0 > 0.027$ J/cm^2	III if $H_0 \leq 0.084$ J/cm^2 IV if $H_0 > 0.084$ J/cm^2
1.0	1.0	III if $H_0 \leq 10$ J/cm^2 IV if $H_0 > 10$ J/cm^2	Same as BRH
N/A	N/A	N/A	I if $\Phi \leq 80$ mW; III if $\Phi \leq 0.5$ W

for present commercial lasers and would normally not fall into Class I.

* $k_2 = 100$ only for sampling intervals greater than 10,000 s (i.e., 2.8 hours)

The minimal emergent beam diameter can now be calculated by:

$$H_{max} = \frac{Q}{\text{Min Beam Area}} \quad (9\text{-}19)$$

$$= \frac{4Q}{\pi a^2} \quad (9\text{-}20)$$

where a is the beam diameter. Then:

$$H_{max} = \frac{1.27 \, (0.05 \, J)}{a^2} < 0.0154 \, J/cm^2$$

$$a < 4.12 \, cm$$

Therefore the designer knows to design for an emergent beam diameter of well over 4.12 cm in order to meet the Class III limits. In fact an emergent aperture size of at least 6 cm would be required for a Gaussian beam.

9.5 CONCLUSIONS

Judging from Table 9-5 there appear to be very few laser systems that would actually be affected by the distinctions between the BRH and ANSI classification schemes. There are a few lasers that might be classified Class IV by BRH that would be classified Class III by ANSI, such as some Q-switched, ruby or neodymium lasers. There may be a few laser checkout counters and other scanning laser products with very low output powers which would be Class II or Class IIa by BRH and Class I by ANSI, but for the most part the standard off-the-shelf lasers used in laboratories or in general purpose applications would probably be classified the same. Therefore except for a few sophisticated products, the distinctions can be considered academic. Hopefully within the next few years the two classification schemes will be made identical.

Although most of the tables appear quite complicated initially, the use of Table 9-5 makes the whole project of determining a laser's classification quite simple. For an individual who wishes to perform many classifications, a careful study first of Table 9-5 and then a comparison of the values in Table 9-5 with Tables 9-1 and 9-2 will be quite helpful. For practice, further problems for classification are given at the end of this chapter.

The individual user who does not care for calculations and measurements of this sort can rest comfortably knowing that the manufacturer will classify any new laser products. Early models are classified in a computerized list of lasers manufactured prior to August 1976 available from the Government Printing Office (Sliney et al., 1976). This list, compiled at the U.S. Army Environmental Hygiene Agency, lists over 2,500 different laser products and provides the classification according to the ANSI standard, which in almost all cases were the same as the BRH classification, and in any case would be applicable to the user environment if

Laser Hazard Classification

the user were following the ANSI Z-136 standard or the ACGIH guide for laser hazard control. Selected examples from this list are given in Appendix E.

9.6 REVIEW QUESTIONS

1. The present classification standards with four classes date back to: (a) 1965; (b) 1968; (c) 1973; (d) 1976.

2. The dividing line between Class III and Class IV CW infrared lasers is what? for CW visible lasers? for CW UV lasers?

3. What is the lowest limit in terms of average power for any CW laser in any region of the spectrum? Give the wavelength or wavelength range that this lowest limit occurs.

4. What are the limiting apertures used by BRH?

5. What are the limiting apertures used by ANSI for classification?

6. Classify a 1.008 mW helium-neon laser.

7. A manufacturer produces a helium-neon laser with an output power of 0.99 mW. How should he classify this laser?

8. Classify a 1-Joule ruby laser rangefinder (694.3 nm, 2 ns pulse).

9. Classify a 1-watt argon laser photocoagulator used in eye surgery.

10. What is the basic distinction between a Class IIIa and Class IIIb laser product.

11. Prove that a He-Ne laser (632.8 nm) with a beam diameter greater than 1 cm and an output power of less than 5 mW does not produce a diffuse reflection radiance greater than the BRH emission limit for extended sources for the maximum sampling interval (i.e., $t > 10^4$ s).

9.7 REFERENCES

American National Standards Institute, Standard Z-136.1, 1976, "Safe Use of Lasers" (in revision, 1979) published by the American National Standards Institute, New York ($9.00).

ACGIH, 1976, "A Guide for the Control of Laser Hazards," American Conference of Governmental Industrial Hygienists, Cincinnati, Ohio ($3.50).

Electronic Industries Association, 1976, "Interpretations of HEW BRH Guide for Submission of Laser Equipment Reports, Laser Engineering Bulletin No. 3, EIA, Washington, DC, ($2.50).

Laser Focus, 1979, Principal violations cited by BRH are interlocks and warning labels, *Laser Focus* 15(4):36–41 (April 1979).

Maxey, M. N., 1978, Radiation protection philosophy: Bioethical problems and priorities, *Am. Ind. Hyg. Assn. J.* **39**(9):689–694.

Mortensen, R. L., 1976, Perspective on laser safety, *Electro-Optical Sys. Design* **8**(8):66–70 (Aug. 1976).

Sliney, D. H., Marshall, W. J., Del Valle, P. F., Franks, J. K., Lyon, T. L., and Krial, N. P., 1976, Laser Classification Guide, NIOSH Publication #HEW (NIOSH) 76-183, available from the Superintendent of Documents, Washington, DC 20402 ($2.50).

Sliney, D. H., and Palmisano, W. A., 1968, The evaluation of laser hazards, *Am. Ind. Hyg. Assn. J.* **29**:325–431.

Sliney, D. H., 1968, The amazing laser, Trans. of the 56th Nat. Safety Congress, Chicago, *Nat. Safety Council* **8**:38–44.

US Congress, 1968, Radiation Control of Health and Safety Act of 1968, Public Law 90–602 (October 18, 1968).

US Department of Health Education and Welfare, 1979, Code of Federal Regulations, Title 21, Chapter 1, subchapter J, part 1040, Performance Standards for Light-Emitting Products.

US Department of Health, Education, and Welfare, 1976a, "Guide for Submission of Information on Lasers and Products Containing Lasers," BRH Publication OMB No. 57 R0068 (July 1976).

US Department of Health, Education and Welfare, 1976b, "National Conference on Measurements of Laser Emissions for Regulatory Purposes," HEW Publication (FDA) 76-8037, BRH, Rockville, MD (April 1976).

US Department of Health, Education and Welfare, 1975, Food and Drug Administration, Laser products, Performance Standards, *Fed. Reg.* **40**(148):32252–32266 (July 31, 1975).

US Department of Health, Education and Welfare, 1978a, "Laser Compliance Measurements Handbook," HEW Publication (FDA) 78-8038, BRH, Rockville, MD (available from NTIS as PB 281 190/AS).

US Department of Health, Education and Welfare, 1978b, Food and Drug Administration, Laser products (amendment to 21CFR1040), *Fed. Reg.* **43**(229):55387–55393 (Nov. 28, 1978)

US Department of Health, Education and Welfare, 1977, Food and Drug Administration, Coherent Radiation, Approval for a variance for laser linemaker, Model 81-11L, *Fed. Reg.* **42**(242):63470–63471 (Dec. 16, 1977).

US Department of Health, Education and Welfare, 1976c, Food and Drug Administration, "Quality Control Practices for Compliance with the Federal Laser Performance Standard," HEW Publication (FDA) 76-8036, BRH, Rockville, MD.

US Department of Health, Education and Welfare, 1976d, Food and Drug Administration, "Tabulated Values of Accessible Emission Limits for Laser Products," HEW Publication (FDA) 76-8029, BRH, Rockville, MD.

Wildavsky, A., 1979, No risk is the highest risk of all, *Amer. Sci.* **67**(1):32–37.

Chapter 10
Protection Standards for Non-Laser Sources

10.1 INTRODUCTION

Although the laser's development has spurred greater interest in potential optical hazards from other conventional nonlaser sources these conventional hazards have not gone unnoticed in the past 75 years. For example, the most commonly recognized potential hazard from arcs and high-intensity lamps was related to erythema and photokeratitis originating from the ultraviolet radiation emitted by lamps and arc processes. Retinal injury from such sources was generally not considered possible, although it was not unheard of. Considering that a good deal was known about optical radiation hazards prior to the development of the laser it seems reasonable to ask the question whether exposure limits and safety standards existed prior to laser safety standards and if not, why not. There was an attempt to standardize an erythemal action curve for dermatologists but this was not really related to safety standards. Additionally, standards were developed for eye protective filters for welders but these were developed empirically and were not based on exposure limits. The only well known safety standard pertained to germicidal ultraviolet lamps used for hospital disinfection and this was established in 1948 by the American Medical Association Council on Physical Medicine.

If this, then, is the history of optical radiation safety standards, then one must logically ask the question why there have been no general standards in the past? Furthermore, why consider them for the future? The answer to these questions lies in several areas. First of all, empirically-developed protective procedures generally prevented injuries. There was also a lack of detailed biologic data. Finally, there was the lack of a real push to establish such standards prior to the great spur of interest in occupational health and safety standards in the 1960's. We shall briefly consider these various aspects since it is important to have such an overview as a proper background for considering protection standards for conventional optical sources.

Since erythema and photokeratitis are acute responses one could always rely on practical experience within a given source. If personnel developed erythema or photokeratitis, then protective procedures would normally be employed without recourse to measurements. Additionally trying to develop an ultraviolet hazard meter was nearly impossible or at the very least was very expensive.

Since continuous visible sources elicit a normal aversion or pain response that can protect the eye and skin from injury, visual comfort has often been used as an approximate hazard index, and eye protection baffles and other controls have been provided on this basis. The determination of shade number for welding goggles is but one example. The architects of the present standards for welding goggle specifications simply relied on a comfort index for viewing the arc, and they specified filtration exceeding the visible filtration values in the infrared and ultraviolet as best as could be accomplished with readily available glass materials. Since ultraviolet and infrared radiation were considered of no value in viewing welding arcs these radiations were filtered out, quite fortunately. Unfortunately, sources rich in ultraviolet radiation provide no aversion response without an accompanying bright visible component in the spectrum and viewing comfort could not always be applied to some arc sources and in particular to germicidal lamps (low pressure mercury gas discharge lamps). Ultraviolet radiation hazards were generally recognized early in the development of a new lamp and any unwanted ultraviolet radiation would be shielded by the choice of an appropriately thick glass envelope based not on measurement of the ultraviolet radiation but merely the absence of acute effects in those people exposed to the prototype lamp systems.

Fortunately, few arc sources are sufficiently large and sufficiently bright to be a retinal injury hazard under normal viewing conditions. Only when an arc or tungsten filament is greatly magnified as in an optical projection system can hazardous irradiances be imaged on sufficiently large areas of the retina to result in a thermal burn. The natural aversion response to bright visible sources would prevent the viewer from receiving a photochemical injury to the retina. Furthermore individuals would normally not step into a projected beam at close range or view an arc with binoculars or with a telescope. Almost all conceivable accidental situations require a hazardous exposure to be delivered within a period of the blink reflect. If an arc were initiated while an individual were located at extremely close viewing range he could conceivably receive a retinal burn. Additionally, if a person viewed a searchlight or a movie projector source at extremely close distances injury could conceivably result. But fortunately all of these conditions are so unusual that the number of accidents have been very, very few and there has been, therefore, no hue and cry for safety standards for such sources. Manufacturers generally took a responsible attitude towards selling optical sources to the public which could be dangerous. Thus we may conclude that the absence of safety standards for light sources has been due to adequate empirically developed protective filters and common sense safety procedures.

The past decade has shown an explosion in optical technology stimulated by the laser. Much higher intensity, higher brightness compact arc lamps and spectral sources have been recently developed, and product engineers have often asked for quantitative guidance with regard to eye safety and skin safety from optical radiation. Although several safety limits for optical radiation have been proposed in the literature within recent years, it is only for the ultraviolet spectral region that there have been any widely accepted standards. Even these standards have provoked controversy. At present there is considerable movement in the direction toward both human exposure limits and product performance standards for nonlaser sources. We shall first consider in this chapter the differences between requirements for laser safety standards and conventional optical source standards, and then proceed to the consideration of ultraviolet exposure limits since most activity in the past has been concentrated on UV hazards.

10.2 CRITERIA FOR BROAD-BAND SOURCES

Exposure criteria for broad-band sources such as arcs and open arc processes, arc lamps, incandescent lamps, and gas discharge lamps may differ considerably from the limits used for the evaluation and control of laser hazards. This difference results from two primary considerations.

The first is that the source normally has a broad spectral band and therefore any coherence effects or narrow wavelength absorption effects that may have gone as yet unnoticed in the understanding of biological effects of lasers are not likely to have any substantial effect upon the hazards from a broad-band source. All of the spectral bands for conventional sources must be evaluated and separate optical bands must be evaluated separately. For instance, the criteria for ultraviolet hazards are completely different from those that apply to visible light hazards.

The second main difference between laser standards and nonlaser hazard criteria results from the fact that most laser exposures that are considered hazardous result from viewing a point source, whereas viewing conditions generally considered hazardous for broad-band sources would in almost all cases result in an extended source viewing condition.

It is also fair to point out that the absolute limit on radiance can be more readily ascertained for a conventional source than for a laser source. Hence the exposure to an individual from a lamp source is seldom likely to greatly exceed the condition of nominal operation. For example, if the current or voltage applied to an arc lamp is drastically increased, the arc is most likely to fail, or else the source will enlarge more than the radiance will increase and the hazard will not increase directly in proportion to the power output of the source as would often be the case for a laser.

10.3 ULTRAVIOLET RADIATION CRITERIA

10.3.1 General

As previously noted the hazards associated with ultraviolet radiation exposure of the eye and skin are often considered separately for each of two spectral regions.

These regions are (a) the *actinic* (or UV-B and UV-C region), where photokeratitis, conjunctivitis and skin erythema are acute health hazards associated with this form of radiation exposure and (b) the near-ultraviolet UV-A region, where the effects are not as well known but cataractogenesis has been suggested as the result of chronic exposure to these wavelengths. Erythema and photokeratitis may also occur in severe acute exposures but only at levels well in excess of those required to elicit the same effect from UV-B or UV-C radiation.

10.3.2 The AMA Standard

Prior to 1971 the only well-known quantitative guidance for exposure of the eye or skin was limited to 254-nm ultraviolet radiation from germicidal lamps covered by the American Medical Association's standard of 1948. The Council on Physical Medicine of the American Medical Association proposed a limit of 0.1 $\mu W/cm^2$ for a 24-hour exposure (8.6 mJ/cm^2) and 0.5 $\mu W/cm^2$ for a 7-hour (13 mJ/cm^2), or shorter, exposure to such lamps. This standard was based on an exposure of 32 mJ/cm^2 delivered from this type of lamp in a 15-minute exposure to lightly pigmented skin (Sliney, 1972). In evaluating other sources, several approaches were followed for the development of UV hazard criteria for the source at hand. The high attenuation afforded by many optical materials in the 200-nm to 314-nm spectral range generally encouraged an empirical approach to ultraviolet hazard problems. The optical source of concern would be enclosed with glass, plastic, or other materials which were known to have high absorptance values at wavelengths below 320-nm rather than analyzing the problem quantitatively. If injurious effects developed in the eye or skin of individual users, the type of source enclosure was changed or the enclosing glass or plastic envelope was increased in thickness.

10.3.3 The Development of the Envelope UV Hazard Criteria

Standards for exposure to the eye and skin recommended by Sliney (1972) and adopted by the U.S. Army, the American Conference of Governmental Industrial Hygienists (ACGIH) and later by the National Institute of Occupational Safety and Health (NIOSH) of the U.S. Department of Health, Education and Welfare (NIOSH, 1972) have generally become accepted to some extent in the U.S.A., particularly where ocular exposure is of concern. Although it is recognized that this criteria appears at first to be rather arbitrary and to assume a single ultraviolet action spectrum (a single chromophore rather than several) the criteria is nevertheless considered by most as the best available and most practical to apply despite some of its theoretical shortcomings. The limit is based upon a single envelope action spectrum which can be applied to both photokeratitis and erythema. In the development of this criteria it was generally assumed that a sliding scale of values varying with wavelength would be required if it were to be applied to a wide variety of conventional light sources and the sun. In applying an action spectrum to the development of hazard criteria for industrial exposure, a judgement had to be made of what exposure limits would obviate unwanted acute and chronic effects; also, simplicity of measurement and application were considered important. If a single instrument which had a spectral response weighted against the envelope action spectrum could be developed then one could make a direct measurement of the ultraviolet hazard. In the 1950's and 1960's some lamp manufacturers did measure the spectral irradiance of broad band ultraviolet sources and weight them against an erythemal action spectrum to get an idea of their risk. This approach was also sometimes performed by research dermatologists, but the spectro-radiometric equipment required for this approach was quite expensive and cumbersome.

It was noted by Sliney that if the threshold data for acute effects obtained from studies of both minimal keratoconjunctivitis and minimal erythema are combined on one graph (Fig. 10-1) then one may draw an envelope curve around this collection of threshold data. The shape of the curve suggests a radiometer detector response with a solar-blind detector with an appropriate absorbing filter. This response could be achieved more readily than an instrument which would try to follow a more accurate action spectrum with its several dips and peaks. This response curve and the associated limit values would appear to be only valid for protecting against acute effects. There is only a limited amount of information to suggest that the limits may also apply to chronic exposure. Epidemiological studies of skin cancer (Chapter 6) suggest that ultraviolet radiation in sunlight is a major causative factor. However, the skin is irradiated by low levels of ultraviolet radiation even through the clothing; but under these conditions erythema is seldom noticed. One therefore could make the tenuous guess that protecting the skin from erythema would either prevent or greatly reduce the chances of the development of skin cancer from that exposure. Studies of skin carcinogenesis in welders show no increased incidence over those working out-of-doors. The validity of such an approach to protect against these delayed effects on the skin will require a great deal of further research to determine the validity of this assumption.

The envelope safety curve does have its limitations when applied to single exposures of the skin. Repeated exposures of the eye to potentially hazardous levels of ultraviolet radiation is not believed to result in increasing the protective capabilities of the cornea, whereas sunburn does result in skin tanning and thickening with increased protection for the deeper skin tissues. Thus the envelope exposure guide is readily applicable to the eye and must be considered as a limiting value for that organ. This curve can only be a starting point for determining permissible acute skin exposures since there are wide variations in thresholds among individuals and races, and even more the threshold for a given individual varies with previous exposure history. The envelope guideline has a built-in safety factor for all but the most sensitive individuals. The magnitude of the safety factor depends on the spectrum of the source, since at least two apparently independent limbs of the curve exist. For example, both the 300-nm and the 254-nm bands may not cause erythema production in an additive fashion. The effects of the two bands certainly do not have the same time course. Sources such as the sun which have a rapidly increasing spectral irradiance in the 300-nm to 315-nm band are difficult to accurately evaluate by using this or any other exposure guidelines. Figure 10-2 provides

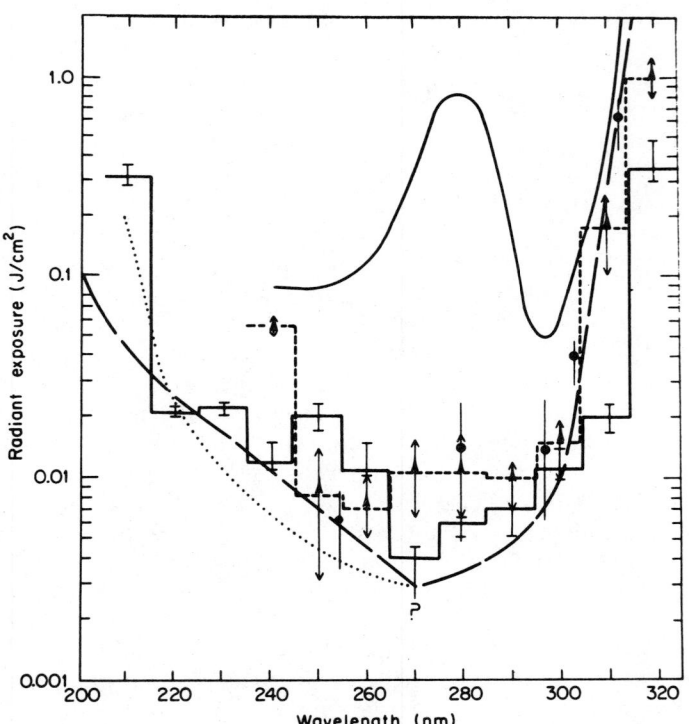

Figure 10-1. Ultraviolet envelope curve. A comparison of minimum thresholds for ultraviolet skin erythema and keratoconjunctivitis with "hazard envelopes" as a function of wavelength. The action spectrum for moderate skin erythema obtained by Coblentz and Stair (1934) is shown as a fine line near the top of the figure. The threshold data for minimal erythema obtained by Freeman et al. (1966) and by Everett et al. (1965) merge into one dotted-line histogram in this semi-logarithmic presentation; one standard deviation is shown by ↕ for each 10-nm band. The range of erythema thresholds obtained by Berger et al. (1968) at several mercury lines are shown as ● representing one standard deviation. Action spectrum for photokeritits thresholds obtained by Pitts and Tredici (1971) is presented as a solid line histogram with approximate range of threshold data shown by I-bars. Bold, dashed curve is an alternative envelope curve for hazard analysis. Note the considerable safety factor between the hazard envelope and the "classical erythema action spectrum (fine line). Action spectra are inverted from the usual presentation (from Sliney and Freasier 1973, with permission).

a comparison of the spectral distributions of several ultraviolet sources. The solar spectral irradiance for the sun at zenith in the tropics increases drastically within a very short wavelength band, making accurate spectral irradiance measurements extremely difficult. On the other hand, open-arc processes such as GMAW (MIG)

Protection Standards for Non-Laser Optical Sources 331

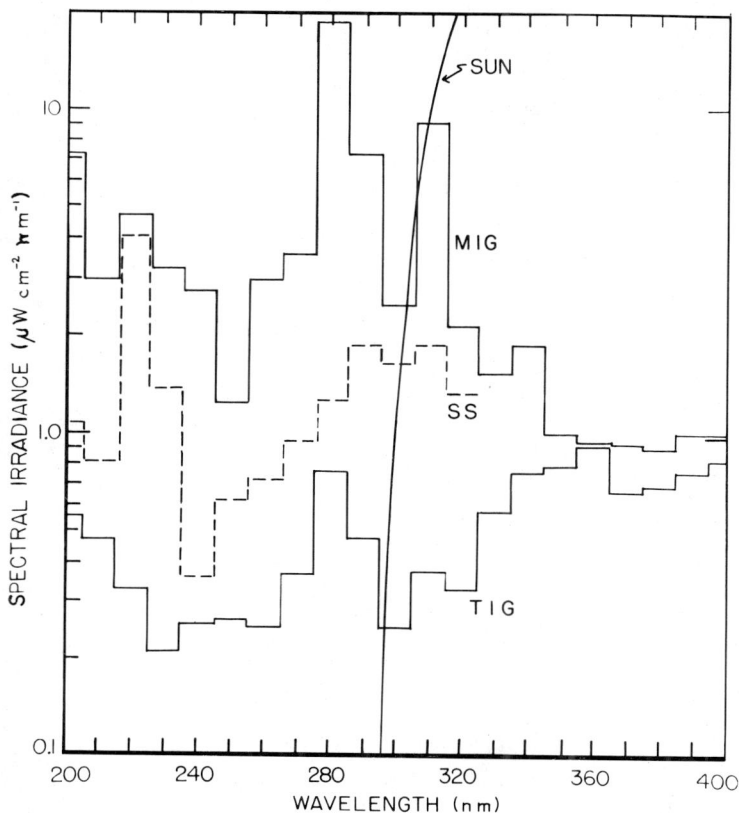

Figure 10-2. Comparison of ultraviolet source spectra. Solar spectral irradiance for the sun at zenith in the tropics is shown to increase drastically within a very short wavelength band, making accurate spectral irradiance measurements extremely difficult. As a comparison, open-arc processes such as welding arcs provide less variation. Welding-arc spectral irradiances are shown for: 80-A DC, TIG (GTAW) welding; 100 A DC, MIG (GMAW) welding; and 70 A AC, stainless steel (SS) welding. All welding measurements were made 200 cm from the arc. Obviously, the exact 300-nm to 315-nm values of the S_λ curve when weighted against the welding spectra would vary the "effective irradiance" very little compared to the same weighting against the solar spectrum if those 300-nm to 315-nm S_λ curve values were slightly inaccurate. Instruments which purport to have a spectral response following S_λ seldom are sufficiently accurate to measure solar radiation (Sliney, 1972).

and GTAW (TIG) welding arcs have less variation. This guideline should be applied with extreme caution to ultraviolet lasers since all the biological data which form its basis were obtained from relatively broad-band sources. Theoretically narrow absorption peaks of an appropriate chromophore, although unlikely, could drastically change the action spectrum of laser sources. However these narrow peaks are not expected for large organic molecules. Nevertheless the laser UV guidelines was made slightly more conservative in the 300-nm to 315-nm band where an error would be most ciritical. Relatively steep long-wavelength cutoffs of an action spectrum are not unreasonable. The accurate measurement of spectral irradiance versus wavelength of a source is discussed in Chapter 14. Suffice to say here, is is very difficult to obtain an accurate measurement of the ultraviolet radiation for most sources and this further complicates the applicability of the standard.

10.3.4 Applying the Ultraviolet Standard

Spectral irradiance from the source of interest can be measured at the point of greatest concern and/or at the nearest point of access. This spectral irradiance E_λ is then weighted by the envelope action curve S_λ (Fig. 10-1, Table 10-1) for wavelengths less than 320 nm. Obviously if one had a calibrated instrument which responded as S_λ then no weighting formulation would be necessary. When the spectral irradiance distribution is used, then it must be weighted by the following formula for determining the effective irradiance of the source normalized at 270 nm:

$$E_{eff} = \sum_{200}^{320} E_\lambda \cdot S_\lambda \cdot \Delta\lambda \qquad (10\text{-}1)$$

The permissible limit for any one day is an accumulated totaled exposure of 3 mJ/cm² (30 J/m²). The standard presumes a total additivity from 1 μs to 24 hr. In point of fact there is a loss of reciprocity for periods greater than 3 or 4 hours.

Most lamps with envelopes constructed of common lime glass or flint glass do not transmit significant levels of potentially hazardous actinic ultraviolet radiation. Nevertheless some concern was expressed at the time of promulgation of the ACGIH ultraviolet TLV as to whether some fluorescent lamps emited effective irradiances of actinic radiation exceeding the 8-hr exposure limit which is 0.1 μW/cm². This was certainly possible for some lamps if one performs the measurement at the surface of the tube. Common fluorescent lamps are low-pressure mercury discharge lamps with phosphor coatings, hence the optical radiation emitted is the visible fluorescence plus characteristic spectral lines of mercury at 254 nm, 280 nm, 297 nm, 303 nm, 313 nm, etc. Therefore the only UV-B or UV-C emissions found for this lamp consist of the first five lines, the last two in the UV-B (the 313-nm line in particular) being the only significant lines that generally pass in this spectral region. The formula required for determining the permissible exposure duration (t_{max}) (in seconds), from a broad-band ultraviolet source, for which the spectral irradiance is known is as follows:

$$t_{max} = 0.003 \text{ J/cm}^2 \Big/ \sum E_\lambda \cdot S_\lambda \cdot \Delta\lambda$$
$$= 0.003 \text{ J/cm}^2 \Big/ E_{eff} \qquad (10\text{-}2)$$

where E_λ is the spectral irradiance in W/(cm²·nm), S_λ is the relative spectral effectiveness (unitless); and $\Delta\lambda$ is the bandwidth in nm. It was hoped that this form of

TABLE 10-1. The ACGIH Threshold Limit Value for Exposure to Actinic Ultraviolet Radiation

Wavelength* (nm)	TLV ($mJ \cdot cm^{-2}$)	Relative Spectral Effectiveness S_λ
200	100	0.03
210	40	0.075
220	25	0.12
230	16	0.19
240	10	0.30
250	7.0	0.43
254	6.0	0.5
260	4.6	0.65
270	3.0	1.0
280	3.4	0.88
290	4.7	0.64
300	10	0.30
305	50	0.06
310	200	0.015
315	1000	0.003

* These wavelength listings are for example, and values for S_λ for each nm are given in Appendix B.

the TLV would encourage the development of an inexpensive instrument to measure all UV sources in relationship to this envelope curve. This would obviate the detailed spectral irradiance measurements in which extended calculations such as those above are now required to evaluate an ultraviolet source. To date this has not been satisfactorily achieved, although some progress is visible.

10.3.5 UV-A Exposure Limits

The envelope action spectra for the actinic radiation limits were first developed in the late 60's by Sliney at USAEHA. At that time there was an almost total lack of information on the adverse effects of UV-A radiation on the eye or skin upon which to base exposure limits for that spectral region. It was known that increasing levels of UV-A were required to elicit an erythema when compared to UV-B radiation. It was known that ultraviolet radiation from a helium-cadmium laser could produce a cataract in a rabbit lens within minutes of exposure but this effect was presumed to be thermal because of the high irradiances in that short exposure duration. Therefore, only the experience with UV-A exposure at that time would be used. Few conventional sources within this spectral region emitted sufficient radiation to create any adverse biologic effects in normal non-photosensitive individuals. The effects on the skin were considered to be principally thermal and the guidelines limiting far-infrared radiation to 10 to 100 mW/cm^2 originally appeared to be acceptable except, of course, for photosensitive individuals. Few sources including the sun, were known to be capable of producing irradiances exceeding 1 to 5 mW/cm^2 in the UV-A band under normal conditions. However guidelines for ocular exposure were considered quite a different matter. The potential role of near-ultraviolet radiation in cataractogenesis had been well documented but the relationship between exposure levels and exposure duration leading to an appreciable cataract had not been sufficiently investigated.

Hence, it was considered reasonable to propose a guideline for ocular exposure below which most conceivable thermal or photochemical injury mechanisms were likely to be demonstrated. To prevent thermal injury it was assumed that for exposure durations less than 1000 s the eye should be protected against exposures above 1 J/cm^2. Because of occupational histories of individuals working with ultraviolet "black light" sources at levels of 1 mW/cm^2 or above it was presumed that a level of 1 mW/cm^2, the approximate outdoor exposure to the eye from UV-A, would be a reasonable upper limit for exposures lasting 1000 s or more. The skin exposure limit presumably could be increased by a factor of 5 for the longer exposure durations. To avoid thermal effects from very short exposure durations the total ultraviolet corneal irradiance was then limited to 1 W/cm^2.

We now know that photochemical effects occur in both the eye and skin and that total daily doses of 20 to 100 J/cm^2 are required to cause acute corneal opacities (Figure 4-7) and skin erythema from UV-A. Acute lenticular opacities at wavelengths greater than 320 nm appear to require much larger doses than could be tested in the laboratory. If an exposure dose of 20 J/cm^2 is spread out over an 8-hour work day the irradiance would be only 0.7 mW/cm^2. Except for reciprocity failure the 1 mW/cm^2 limit could also conceivably be too lenient at the shortest UV-A wavelengths for skin exposure. Possibly 1 mW/cm^2 is too much for chronic ocular exposure, and in the future some adjustments in the UV-A limit may be recommended.

Establishing a product safety limit for ultraviolet-A radiation is a problem inasmuch as use factors are extremely difficult to assess in many applications. In the United States the Bureau of Radiological Health is working on this problem (USDHEW, FDA, 1977). The course of future biologic research of UV-A effects will surely determine how the standards of exposure will be written in future years. One could well imagine a continuation of the envelope action spectrum of Figure 10-1 to wavelengths beyond 315 nm to 380 or even 400 nm since the photochemical injury mechanism appears to be the major factor in injury as was noted in Figure 4-7 and 4-8. At present, to evaluate a broad-band optical source the spectral irradiance E_λ, from 320 to 400 nm, is summed with equal spectral weighting to obtain the total accessible irradiance in the UV-A at the point of measurement. This is compared to the limit of 1 mW/cm^2 for periods greater than 1,000 s or an integrated irradiance of 1 J/cm^2 to determine a permissible exposure duration for periods less than 1000 s.

10.4 VISIBLE RADIATION CRITERIA

The exact boundaries for light ("visible radiation") are often argued. At present the CIE (International Commission on Illumination) sets 380-400 nm to 760-780 nm as "visible." Of particular interest to this study, however, is the effect of all radiation from 400 nm to 1400 nm that reach the retina. For this reason this spectral region is known as the "retinal hazard region." Wavelengths outside this region are not normally considered a retinal hazard except for small children and aphakics (those with the crystalline lens removed by surgery for cataract). So little UV-A radiation reaches the retina that retinal exposure in that spectral region is also generally considered insignificant. In this section we shall consider exposure limits which are designed to protect the retina of the human eye.

Until recently retinal injury from high intensity light sources was thought to be restricted to a thermal injury mechanism in retinal tissues. However in recent years it has become increasingly evident that a photic, i.e., photochemical or phototoxic, effect is responsible for threshold light-induced retinal injury for lengthy exposure durations if short-wavelength light is involved, as was shown in Fig. 4-21. Therefore we must have at least two spectral weighting functions for analyzing a broad-band optical source in the visible and the infrared. In one case we must have a weighting function which is based upon the action spectrum for thermal injury and secondly we must have a weighting function which is based upon the action spectrum for the so-called "blue light" injury mechanism. Such a concept has been in use for evaluating broad-band optical sources in the United States for several years (Sliney and Freasier, 1973). In 1975 the American Conference of Governmental Industrial Hygienists proposed a first step in developing a threshold limit value (TLV) for visible sources. The proposal was a limiting luminance of 1 cd/cm^2 for chronic exposure to a large-field white light source. This is a maximal level for comfort (Sliney and Freasier, 1973). It is below levels which cause either substantial or temporary night blindness or color vision changes. This limit, however, was too simplistic and a new and more complex set of TLV's were proposed in 1976 and 1977. The new limits were somewhat similar to laser exposure limits except that an adjustment for retinal image size was included in the proposal. This followed standards used at the Army Environmental Hygiene Agency (AEHA) for the evaluation of searchlights and similar sources (Sliney et al., 1977). Unfortunately these TLV's proposed in 1976 require many elaborate calculations; in fact the AEHA has formulated a computer program to perform these calculations (Sliney et al., 1978).

It is useful to the reader to remember that the luminance of 1 cd/cm^2, although approximate, is probably a lower limit for hazardous light sources unless the spectral distribution of the visible source is heavily biased toward the blue. A detailed hazard evaluation (with spectral measurements and source size calculations) will almost certainly be below the TLV if the luminance is less than 1 cd/cm^2. This statement applies best to unfiltered high-pressure mercury, argon and xenon arc lamps, carbon arcs, white fluorescent lamps, and incandescent lamps. Although that list appears to apply to almost all lamps, it is possible to have low-pressure gas discharges with a few monochromatic lines. For instance a deuterium arc, which emits mostly in the ultraviolet, or a filtered incandescent lamp, for example a heat lamp which emits enough radiation in the blue end or outside of the visible spectrum for which a luminance criterion would be misleading. The simple luminance guidelines are therefore presented because of the many rugged luminance meters available, whereas field-type spectroradiometers required for a complete hazard analysis are rare.

10.5 APPLYING THE TENTATIVE GUIDELINES OF USAEHA AND ACGIH

Using a blue light hazard function B_λ and a retinal thermal injury function R_λ one may weight the source spectrum to indicate comparative levels of risk to the two types of retinal injury mechanisms. Recalling from Chapter 4 that the retinal irradiance is directly proportional to the radiance L of the source and the square of the pupil size d_e one can calculate the retinal spectral irradiance distribution from the spectral radiance distribution and knowledge of the spectral transmission of the ocular media τ_λ. In the absence of a radiance standard one could use this approach to directly calculate retinal levels and compare them directly to thresholds of injury, as was done at one time (Sliney and Freasier, 1973). However the present approach is to establish exposure limits for the spectrally weighted radiances. These safety weighting functions are given in Table 10-2. Spectral factors weighted against the spectral radiance are then applied in the manner given in 10.5.2 and 10.5.3.

10.5.1 The Retinal Hazard Functions

The R_λ function is basically the reciprocal of the C_A function used in the laser safety standards. It represents the relative fraction of corneal irradiance that is actually absorbed in the retina and choroid (Figure 7-7) and therefore the radiant power that contributes to the temperature elevation in the retina. One temporary modification has been made to a simple function of $1/C_A$; an increased weighting was provided for wavelengths between 400 and 500 nm (as will later be seen in Figure 10-4). This was considered necessary because of the unexpectedly low injury thresholds for 1.0 and 16-s exposures at 440 nm by Ham, Mueller and Sliney (1976) that could not be predicted by a thermal model of injury. Further studies will be required to determine whether the R_λ function must indeed have such large values in this spectral region. Perhaps the hazard limits for the blue light hazard will require further adjustments to apply to exposure durations less than 10 s.

The B_λ function is based upon the data of Ham, Mueller and Sliney (1976) for a 1000-s exposure duration where the thresholds due to the photochemical damage mechanism was most clearly distinguishable from thermal injury thresholds. B_λ is an action spectrum calculated at the cornea and assumes the normal attenuation of UV-A and violet light by the lens. The values of B_λ which were assigned to wavelengths greater than 550 nm are purely arbitrary and were believed to be a best guess at the contribution of the longer wavelengths of visible and IR-A to thermal enhancement of the photochemical injury mechanism.

In addition to the uncertainties associated with the functions R_λ and B_λ, there

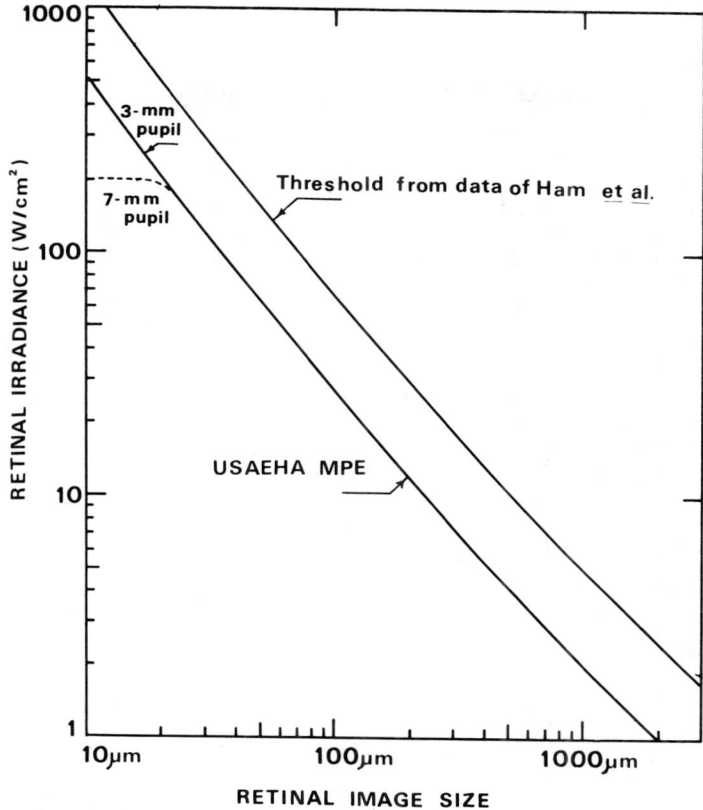

Figure 10-3. Retinal hazard limits of Sliney and Freasier (1973). Prior to the approach of providing a retinal hazard limit in terms of radiance and source size, it was conventional to perform all of the calculations at the retina. The retinal limits shown above were based upon the large image-size retinal injury thresholds of Ham *et al.*, 1966. The present radiance limits are a simplification of the more precise, but more complex methods of Sliney and Freasier to calculate the actual absorbed retinal exposure and corresponding temperature rise in the retinal pigmented epithelium.

are also some uncertainties connected with the time factors in the guidelines. The retinal image size dependence of the thermal exposure limits is basically that used by the USAEHA since 1968 (Figure 10-3). However, some upper limit on the applicable source size (i.e., on the largest applicable retinal image size) will have to be developed. From calculations with a thermal model, the strong dependence upon retinal image size for exposure durations of 0.1 s to 10 s should not exist for image sizes greater than approximately 2 mm, which corresponds to a source angular subtense α of 0.12 rad (6.7°). Hence an upper limit of α must be established, quite possibly at 0.1 rad; but setting this limiting angle must await further

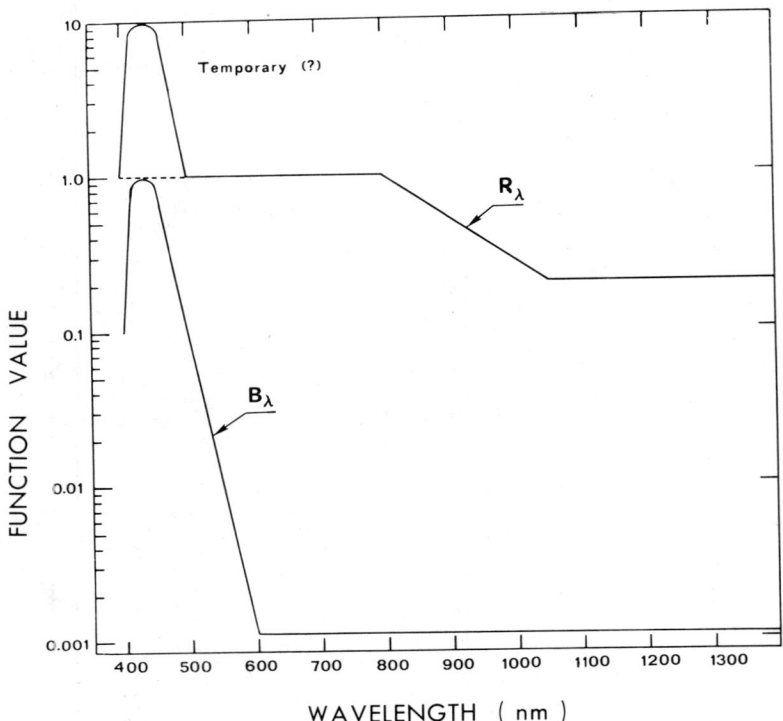

Figure 10-4. The retinal hazard spectral weighting functions. Two spectral weighting functions are R_λ (relative retinal absorption for thermal injury calculations) and B_λ (relative retinal sensitivity to photic injury). These are used in determining the hazard of an optical source in the retinal hazard region (400 nm - 1400 nm). The values of R_λ between 400 and 500 nm were considered a "quick fix" and temporary after the discovery in 1976 that "thermal" thresholds of injury for a 1-second exposure were much lower at 441.6 nm than would be attributable to a purely thermal mechanism.

retinal injury studies. Without a limit on α the TLV would be incredibly over-conservative for very large source angles.

The time dependence of the blue-light hazard criteria assumes perfect reciprocity to a duration of 10^4 s which could be modified in the future to apply to longer exposure durations; however such long exposures to the same retinal area are hard to conceive of other than when protracted over a period of four days. The time dependence of the thermal hazard limit is also open to some modification based upon further research. The exposure dose dependence of retinal thermal injury follows a $t^{0.5}$ function only in a very approximate manner. The laser limits vary as

TABLE 10-2. Spectral Weighting Functions for Assessing Retinal Hazards from Broad-Band Optical Sources*

Wavelength (nm)	Blue-light Hazard Function B_λ	Thermal Hazard Function R_λ
400	0.10	1.0
405	0.20	2.0
410	0.40	4.0
415	0.80	8.0
420	0.90	9.0
425	0.95	9.5
430	0.98	9.8
435	1.0	10
440	1.0	10
445	0.97	9.7
450	0.94	9.4
455	0.90	9.0
460	0.80	8.0
465	0.70	7.0
470	0.62	6.2
475	0.55	5.5
480	.045	4.5
485	0.40	4.0
490	0.22	2.2
495	0.16	1.6
500-600	$10^{[(450-\lambda)/50]}$	1.0
600-700	0.001	1.0
700-1049	0.001	$10^{[(700-\lambda)/500]}$
1050-1400	0.001	0.2

* 1979 Committee on Physical Agents ACGIH and US Army interim guidelines.

$t^{0.75}$ and as $t^{0.33}$ for small images and large images respectively.

With so many possible future changes in these tentative guidelines, the reader is cautioned to check the most current ACGIH guidelines or TLV's. The guidelines provided in the next sections are based upon the best judgement available at the time of the publication of this book.

10.5.2 Retinal Thermal Hazard Evaluation

To protect against retinal thermal injury from short duration exposures, the spectral radiance of the lamp weighted against the function R_λ (Table 10-2 and Figure 10-4) should not exceed:

$$\sum_{400}^{1400} L_\lambda R_\lambda \Delta\lambda \leqslant L\,(\text{Haz}) = \sqrt{t}\ /\ \alpha t \quad W/(cm^2 \cdot sr) \tag{10-3}$$

where L_λ is given in $W/(cm^2 \cdot sr)$, t is the viewing duration (or pulse duration if the lamp is pulse limited) which is limited to 1 ms to 10 s, and α is the angular subtense of the source in radians, and which should be limited to approximately 0.1 radian. If the lamp is oblong, α refers to the longest dimension (1) that can be viewed. For instance, at a viewing distance (r) of 500 cm from a tubular lamp 50 cm long, the viewing angle α is 1/r or 0.1 rad.

10.5.3 Retinal Blue Light Hazard Evaluation

To protect against retinal injury from blue light exposure, the integrated spectral radiance of the lamp weighted with the blue light hazard function B_λ of Table 10-2 (Fig. 10-4) should not exceed $100\ J/(cm^2 \cdot sr)$ for durations less than 10^4 s or exceed $10\ mW/(cm^2 \cdot sr)$ for $t > 10^4$ s:

$$\sum_{400}^{1400} L_\lambda \cdot t \cdot B_\lambda \cdot \Delta\lambda \leqslant 100\ J/(cm^2 \cdot sr) \quad \text{for } t \leqslant 10^4\ s \tag{10-4}$$

or:
$$\sum_{400}^{1400} L_\lambda \cdot B_\lambda \cdot \Delta\lambda \leqslant 0.01\ W/(cm^2 \cdot sr) \quad \text{for } t > 10^4\ s \tag{10-5}$$

and for a point source ($\alpha < 11$ mrad):

$$\sum_{400}^{1400} E_\lambda \cdot t \cdot B_\lambda \cdot \Delta\lambda \leqslant H\,(\text{Haz}) = 10\ mJ/cm^2 \quad \text{for } t \leqslant 10^4\ s \tag{10-6}$$

or:
$$\sum_{400}^{1400} E_\lambda \cdot B_\lambda \cdot \Delta\lambda \leqslant E\,(\text{Haz}) = 1\ \mu W/cm^2 \quad \text{for } t \geqslant 10^4\ s \tag{10-7}$$

It must be emphasized that these levels assume a constricted pupil as would occur with fixed viewing of any type of extended source with a radiance approaching the TLV. For a spectrally weighted source radiance (L) which exceeds 10 mW/$(cm^2 \cdot sr)$ in the blue-light spectral region the permissible exposure duration t_{max} in s is simply:

$$t_{max} = 100\ J/(cm^2 \cdot sr) \bigg/ \sum_{400}^{1400} L_\lambda \cdot B_\lambda \cdot \Delta\lambda \quad \text{for } t \leqslant 10^4\ s \tag{10-8}$$

The extended-source limits are greater than the 1976 maximum permissible exposure (MPE) limits for a 440-nm laser radiation source given by either ANSI or ACGIH, which assume a 7-mm pupil rather than the 3-mm used for the broad-band source analysis.

NOTE: The formulas (10-4) through (10-9) are empirical and are not, strictly speaking, dimensionally correct. To make these formulas dimensionally correct, a dimensional correction factor must be inserted into each formula. It is therefore important to use only the units specified in this chapter.

10.5.4 IR-A Hazard Analysis

The proposed ACGIH TLV also limited the IR-A and IR-B infrared radiation beyond 770 nm to 10 mW/cm² to avoid possible damage (which may be delayed in appearance) to the lens (cataractogenesis). For an infrared heat lamp or other source which lacks a strong visual stimulus the radiance for wavelengths between 700 and 1400 nm for extended-duration viewing conditions should be limited to:

$$\sum_{700}^{1400} L_\lambda \cdot \Delta\lambda \leqslant L\,(\text{Haz}) = [0.6/\alpha]\text{W}/(\text{cm}^2 \cdot \text{sr}) \qquad (10\text{-}9)$$

This limit is also based upon a 7-mm pupil diameter.

10.6 ANSI EFFORTS

The ANSI, in addition to its laser safety standards effort by the Z-136 Committee, has also had a subcommittee (C-78.4) work on high-intensity mercury fluorescent (HID) lamp safety. Spurred on by the BRH, this subcommittee of lamp industry representatives proposed a standard in 1976 requiring rapid burnout of HID lamps when the outer lamp envelope (glass) was broken. The rapid burnout was necessary to prevent personnel injury by actinic ultraviolet radiation emitted by the inner discharge lamp. But this was not a standard for personnel exposure; it was to be a performance standard.

The ANSI Z-311 Committee on general lamp photobiology safety was organized in 1977 to provide much broader lamp safety criteria. A standard from this committee probably will include criteria for personnel exposure. This committee was under the chairmanship of Mr. I. Matelsky of the General Electric Company and was sponsored by the Illumination Engineering Society.

10.7 BRH STANDARDS

At the time of publication of this text the BRH had only one performance standard for non-laser optical sources, but work was well under way on a sunlamp standard and also to develop other standards. Bostrom and Coakley (1976) at BRH recommended a formal technique for indexing the relative risk from ultraviolet of the mercury lamp (HID lamp) safety standard, ANSI C-78.4 and then formally published an HID lamp self-extinguishing requirement if the outer bulb was to be broken (USDHEW, 1978).

10.8 INFRARED STANDARDS

There are no non-laser, infrared (IR) protection standards *per se* that are well known. However, the laser limits can be applied for broad-band sources if in addition the whole-body irradiation is evaluated. Even irradiances as low as 10 mW/cm² can place an uncomfortable thermal load on the human body especially when the irradiation is not confined to one side of the body and this radiant heat load occurs along with high ambient air temperatures. By contrast, the IR laser limit for periods exceeding 10 seconds is 100 mW/cm², which assumes that the total irradiated area of the skin or the eye will be small. It generally is small in the case of laser exposure, but not so likely when the body is exposed to the optical radiation from non-laser sources, and heat stress must be evaluated.

The procedure now generally followed for evaluating heat stress makes use of the WBGT Index, *i.e.*, the wet-bulb-globe-temperature index. There are two formulae which permit the determination of a condition of heat stress in which the contribution of a dry-bulb temperature (DB) is combined with a wet-bulb temperature (WB), which varies with humidity and wind speed, and the black-globe temperature (BG) which includes the radiant (predominantly infrared) contribution. Unfortunately, the developers of the WBGT index used a copper globe painted black instead of a copper globe painted an off-white color or grey. The grey globe would have simulated the reflectance of skin more closely since any such paint becomes highly absorbing in the far-infrared spectral region. As a result, we must now have two formulae for evaluating the heat stress factors—one for sunlight and outdoor workers, and another for infrared sources or for indoor workers. The nature of the skin's reflectance is such that visible and IR-A are reflected, whereas IR-B and IR-C are absorbed (See Figure 5-4). The spectral reflectance of much clothing is somewhat similar to that of skin in the infrared. Obviously, any IR hazard evaluation would use the latter formula. The ACGIH formula for indoor heat stress is:

$$WBGT = 0.7 \, WB + 0.3 \, GT \qquad (10\text{-}10)$$

A heat-stress condition exists when this WBGT value exceeds 25° to 30°C depending upon work load (Chapter 5).

A major problem in any infrared safety standard that would consider wavelengths beyond either 1.4 μm or 3.0 μm is ambient IR-C. The black-body radiant exitance at 273 K (0°C) is 32 mW/cm² and at 300 K (81°F) is 46 mW/cm². A whole-body irradiance of 20 to 50 mW/cm² from radiant warmers on a cold (0°C) winter day is comfortable; but the same irradiance on a hot summer day could bring on heat stress. Therefore any IR safety standard should best distinguish between all the IR bands, and IR-C limits would have to vary with ambient conditions at the very least.

10.9 CONCLUSION

Although there are few present standards for non-laser sources, the existing

Protection Standards for Non-Laser Optical Sources

laser standards can be used to provide an initial estimate of the hazard. It is, however, important to remember that these laser protection standards incorporate several simplifications which depend on the single-wavelength and point-source characteristics of lasers, and may provide the analyst with an overly conservative estimate of the real hazard.

10.10 REVIEW QUESTIONS

1. The AMA UV limit of 1948 was limited to which type source? What was the limit?

2. The envelope UV hazard limit has which of the following disadvantages:
   (a) The limit can only be used for the skin;
   (b) The limit can only be used for the eye;
   (c) The limit is overly conservative for tanned skin;
   (d) The limit is difficult to fit with a safety meter;
   (e) The limit is overly conservative for all types of exposure.

3. What is the permissible exposure duration for a lamp whose effective irradiance in the UV-B and C is $10\ \mu W \cdot cm^2$?

4. What is the permissible exposure duration of a source where the UV-A irradiance at the point of interest is $25\ mW/cm^2$?

5. What are the advantages and disadvantages of using a laser protection standard for evaluating a lamp?

6. Why is the UV-B *laser* safety limit more conservative than the UV-envelope safety limit applicable to broad-band sources?

7. Are UV limits really necessary if glass protective enclosures are used?

8. What is the WBGT for an indoor foundry environment with the following temperatures: WB = 72°F; DB = 79°F; BG = 100°F?

9. When should the $10\ mW/cm^2$ limit be an IR guide?

10. A filtered mercury vapor lamp has a radiance contribution of $0.08\ W/(cm^2 \cdot sr)$ at 405 nm and $0.2\ W/(cm^2 \cdot sr)$ at 436 nm. Other lines are not measurable. Is this 10-cm diameter lamp source hazardous to view at a distance of 100 cm, and if so, is there a maximum safe exposure duration?

10-11 REFERENCES

American Conference of Governmental Industrial Hygienists, 1979, Threshold Limit Values for

Chemical Substances and Physical Agents in the Workroom Environment with Intended Changes for 1979, ACGIH, Cincinnati, OH.

American National Standards Institute, 1977, Draft Standard C78.4, New York, ANSI.

AMA Council on Physical Medicine, 1948, Acceptance of ultraviolet lamps for disinfecting purposes, *J. Amer. Med. Assn.* **137**:1600-1603.

Ashby, L., 1977, The risk equations, the subjective side of assessing risks, *New Scientist* **74**:398–400.

Berger, D., Urbach, F., and Davies, R. E., 1968, The action spectrum of erythema induced by ultraviolet radiation. Preliminary Report, in "XIII, Congressus Internationalis Dermatologiae–München 1967" (W. Jadassohn and C. G. Schirren, eds.), pp. 1112–1117, Springer-Verlag, New York.

Bostrom, R. G., and Coakley, J. M., 1976, Guide number for light sources that emit ultraviolet radiation, *Appl. Opt.* **15**(3):574–575.

Clark, J. H., 1935, The effect of ultraviolet radiation on lens protein in the presence of salts and the relation of radiation to industrial cataract, *Amer. J. Physiol.* **113**:539–547.

Coblentz, W. W., and Stair, R., 1934, Data on the spectral erythemic reaction of the untanned human skin to ultraviolet radition, *Bur. Stand. J. Res.* **12**:13-14.

DIN, 1979, Strahlungsphysik im optischen Bereich und Lichttechnik: Grössen, Formeln und Kurzzeichen für photobiologisch Wirksame Strahlung, Vornorm DIN 5031, Teil 10, Deutsches Institut für Normung, Berlin.

Dunster, J., 1977, The risk equations, virtue in compromise, *New Scientist* **74**:454–456.

Everett, M. A., Olsen, R. L., and Sayer, R. M., 1965, Ultraviolet erythema, *Arch. Derm.* **92**:713–719.

Freeman, R. G., Owens, D. W., Knox, J. M., and Hudson, H. T., 1966, Relative energy requirements for an erythemal response of skin to monochromatic wavelengths of ultraviolet present in the solar spectrum, *J. Invest. Derm.* **47**:586–592.

Gehring, P., 1977, The risk equations, the threshold controversy, *New Scientist* **74**:426–428.

Hazzard, D. G., 1977, Symposium on Biological Effects and Measurements of Light Sources, HEW Publication (FDA) 77-8002, Bureau of Radiological Health, Rockville.

Kletz, T. A., 1977, The risk equation, what risks should we run? *New Scientist* **74**:320.

Illuminating Engineering Society (New York), 1966, "I.E.S. Lighting Handbook," 4th ed., Waverly Press, Baltimore.

Matelsky, I., 1968, The non-ionizing radiations, in "Industrial Hygiene Highlights" (L. V. Cralley, ed.) pp. 140-178, Industrial Hygiene Foundation of America, Pittsburgh.

NIOSH, 1972, A Recommended Standard for Occupational Exposure to Ultraviolet Radiation, U.S. Department of Health, Education, and Welfare, Washington, D.C., (U.S. Government Printing Office No. 017-033-00012).

Parrish, J. A., Anderson, R. R., Urbach, F., and Pitts, D., 1978, "UV-A, Biological Effects of Ultraviolet Radiation with Emphasis on Human Responses to Longwave Ultraviolet," New York, Plenum Press.

Piltingsrud, H. V., Odland, L. T., and Fong, C. W., 1978, An evaluation of ultraviolet radiation personel hazards from selected 400 watt high intensity discharge lamps, *Amer. Ind. Hyg. Assn. J.* **39**(5):406–4B.

Pitts, D. G., and Tredici, T. J., 1971, The effects of ultraviolet on the eye, *Amer. Ind. Hyg. Assn. J.* **32**(4):235–246.

Ramsey, J. D., 1978, Abbreviated guidelines for heat stress exposure, *Amer. Ind. Hyg. Assn. J.* **39**(6):491–495.

Schmidt, K., 1964, On the skin erythema effect of UV flashes, *Strahlentherapie* **124**:127–136.

Sliney, D. H., and Freasier, B. C., 1973, The evaluation of optical radiation hazards, *Appl. Opt.* **12**(1):1–24.

Sliney, D. H., 1972, The merits of an envelope action spectrum for ultraviolet radiation exposure criteria, *Am. Ind. Hyg. Assn. J.* **33**:644–653.

Sliney, D. H., Marshall, W. J., Carothers, M. L., and Kaste, R. C., 1977, Hazard Analysis of Broad-Band Optical Sources, U.S. Army Environmental Hygiene Agency, Aberdeen Proving Ground, MD, December 1977, (available from NTIS as ADA 054-802/4GI).

Sliney, D. H., Bason, F. C., and Freasier, B. C., 1971, The measurement of ultraviolet, visible and infrared radiation, *Am. Ind. Hyg. Assn. J.* **32**:415–431.

U.S. Department of Health, Education and Welfare, 1972, Criteria for a Recommended Standard, Occupational Exposure to Ultraviolet Radiation, Report (HSM 73-11009), National Institute of Occupational Safety and Health, Rockville, MD.

U.S. Department of Health, Education and Welfare, Food and Drug Administration, 1977, Sun Lamp Products, Performance Standard (proposed rule), *Fed. Reg.* **45**(251):65189–65193 (December 30, 1977).

Vassiliadis, A., Zweng, H. C., and Dedrick, K. G., 1971, Ocular Laser Threshold Investigations, Contract F41609-70-C-0002, Stanford Research Institute, Menlo Park, California (Jan. 1971).

Chapter 11
Laser Output Measurements: Radiometry and Calorimetry

11.1 INTRODUCTION

There are many types of measurements which can be made to characterize a laser's output. The types of measurements considered in this chapter fall under the broad term of "radiometric;" that is, measurements of a radiometric quantity such as *radiant power* or *radiant energy, irradiance* or *radiant exposure*. The two quantities radiant power and radiant energy are by far the most important and probably more fundamental for laser measurement. The reader should note that the term "radiometric" when applied to a method of measuring power or energy has often been used in a limited sense—referring to the use of instruments calibrated against a radiometric scale derived from a standard *blackbody*. The contrasting method of measurement under this narrow meaning would be calorimetric measurement where the temperature elevation in an absorber is in itself the final calibration reference. In this chapter the term *radiometry* is meant to apply to all techniques of measuring *optical* radiometric quantities such as radiant power or energy.

11.2 RATIONALE FOR MEASUREMENT

In any discussion of the measurement of laser radiation for purposes of evaluating health hazards it is important first to clarify the conditions and requirements for the measurements. Industrial and environmental health specialists and health physicists usually rely heavily upon measurement in their appraisal of such environmental hazards as toxic chemicals or injurious sound levels. They generally must detect or measure a chemical or physical agent which their own human senses often cannot detect. It is not surprising, then, that one of the first questions asked by such specialists when encountering a potential lazer hazard is: "What instrument do I use to measure laser radiation and how do I use it?" All who have been in this position and asked this question have learned that the answer is quite complex.

Unlike most noxious agents whose hazard potential decrease greatly with distance, a high-powered laser beam is almost always hazardous for a considerable distance. Also its hazard generally exceeds exposure limits by orders of magnitude, typically by a factor of 1,000 or even 1,000,000 times. The presence of the beam can generally be detected by the human eye or through the use of an image converter. Therefore, the question that should have been posed is: "Why should I measure this laser beam?" Clearly no one should place his eye—or in some instances, even his skin—into a laser beam. In many cases there is in fact no requirement for individuals to be located within the laser beam. In some instances reflections of the laser beam may be hazardous and here measurements or calculations may be in order. But again definitive calculations or measurements may appear to be impossible. For example, the slightest change in position or flatness of a reflecting surface, the insertion of a different surface into the beam, the change of mode in the laser beam, or any of a myriad of other environmental changes can greatly affect the calculations or measurements. It soon becomes evident that in most cases even routine monitoring of either an area or an individual by instrumentation is a hopeless task. A more logical approach to hazard assessment is to develop a means of analyzing the potential hazards of a laser based upon the laser's output parameters. For this reason the scheme of laser hazard classification discussed in Chapter 9 was developed.

The laser beam's hazard can be compared closely to an exposed high voltage conductor—a highly localized hazard. Unless an individual touches the conductor (or places his eye in a laser beam) no injury results. The laser beam does not present an area hazard as general as would be presented by a contaminated atmosphere unless a hazardous diffuse reflection or multiple specular reflections are present (see Fig. 17-4). However, any hazard analysis and thus by implication any measurements of laser radiation must reflect the need for determining all potential future exposure conditions.

As a general rule, the present standards in the U.S.A. require only measurement of the laser-output characteristics for the determination of laser classification. Routine monitoring is seldom considered necessary and all measurements are normally performed only one time by or for the manufacturer of the laser equipment. It is true that for certain lasers which are near the borderline between two classes in the hazard classification, periodic measurements may be considered by some to be worthwhile. Additionally, field measurements may be considered by some to be worthwhile. Additionally, field measurements of outdoor laser propagation paths have often been found useful, particularly in military applications. Diagnostics of the beam profile and measurements of beam divergence will be discussed in Chapter 12. The present chapter will be devoted to the measurement of *radiant power* and *radiant energy*, and, to a lesser extent, *irradiance* and *radiant exposures*.

11.3 LASER PARAMETERS TO MEASURE

To illustrate the need for determining certain geometric parameters of the beam and radiometric output considerations it is necessary first to consider which laser output characteristics must be known to predict the beam irradiance E or radiant exposure H at the distance r from the particular laser to be examined from a safety standpoint. The generalized formula for determining E and H will be developed in Chapter 12. Suffice it to say here that if the emergent beam diameter (or beam waist) and beam divergence are known along with the power output of a CW laser or with the energy output of a pulsed laser, then E and H may be calculated for any distance r from the laser (Table 11-1).

A calorimeter or other type of energy or power meter is useful to measure the output radiant energy or radiant power. The measurement of the geometrical characteristics of the beam, specifically the output dimensions of the beam and divergence, can be more involved. One beam parameter measurement procedure which has enjoyed widespread acceptance for safety evaluations has been the use of calibrated apertures or ribbons with a power or energy meter (section 12.6). Table 11-1 lists the essential parameters whose measurements characterize a given type of laser. A power meter with aperture may also be calibrated to measure irradiance directly.

11.4 MEASURING OUTPUT BEAM RADIANT EXPOSURE OR IRRADIANCE

Regrettably, the beam profile is not always single-mode which would facilitate correspondingly simple measurements of diameter and divergence. This is particularly a problem with the ruby solid-state lasers. Figure 11-1 shows several profiles of an emergent beam from a ruby laser. Notice that the pattern of the emerging beam can vary significantly and is quite dependent upon slight adjustments of the cavity mirrors. The pattern is also dependent upon the quality of the ruby crystal. Even without intentional adjustments of the end mirrors, the operation of the laser for several pulses may heat up the cavity sufficiently to create variations as great as those shown in Fig. 11-1. Clearly the measurement of a beam "diameter" (or other dimensions) or divergence for such a laser can be quite a problem. Normally the manufacturer of such a pulsed laser simply lists the laser crystal diameter and does not attempt to measure the beam diameter. Some have attempted to tune the cavity to an optimum condition and measure the output diameter and divergence cone angle into which 88% of the beam power is emitted. This would define the $1/e^2$-peak-irradiance points in a Gaussian beam profile if the laser were Gaussian. Measurements of divergence and diameter will be discussed in greater detail in Chapter 12.

From a safety standpoint the emergent beam irradiance may be defined as the laser power per unit area averaged over either a 7-mm aperture (within 400 nm to 1400 nm) or a 1-mm aperture (based on several measurements). Unfortunately, there is no simplified method to calculate irradiance from a knowledge of the beam power and an "effective beam diameter," since a laser profile (e.g. ruby) may

TABLE 11-1. Minimum Laser Output Parameters

Term and Symbol	A Beam divergence (ϕ) & beam waist (w) (or emergent diameter) (a)	B Peak power (Φ_p)	C Average power (Φ_a)	D Pulse duration (t)	E Energy output per pulse (Q_p)	F PRF (F)	G Integrated Output Energy (Q_t)	H Output Irradiance (E_o)	I Output Radiance Exposure (H_o)
Repetitively pulsed lasers	Yes	Yes, or C	Yes, or B+D+F	Yes	Yes	Yes	Possibly	or Φ and a or w	or Q and a or w
"Single-pulse" laser	Yes	Yes, or E	No	Yes	or B&D	No	Possibly	No	or Q and a or w
CW laser	Yes	N/A if true CW	Yes	No	No	No	Possibly	Yes or a and Φ	No
Relations	range eqn.	$= Q_p/t$	$= \Phi_p \cdot$(duty cycle)	$= Q_p/\Phi_p = \Phi_p \cdot t$	$= \Phi_a/Q_p$	$= nQ_p$	$1.27\,\Phi/\pi a^2$	$1.27\,Q/\pi a^2$
			$= \Phi_a/$(duty cycle)	$= Q_p \cdot F$			$= \Phi_a \cdot T$		

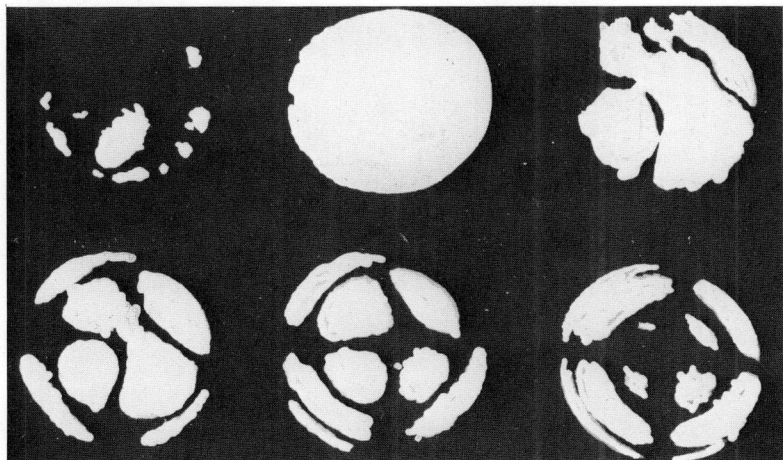

Figure 11-1. Beam Profiles. Photographs of irradiance profiles of the exit beam of a ruby laser having a flat mirror cavity. A relatively uniform beam profile (middle top) is very difficult to achieve (Sliney, 1976).

change rapidly, but an experienced laser physicist or optical engineer may be able to calculate the upper limit of the emergent beam irradiance. This is the value often given by manufacturers in stating the laser characteristics for classification purposes.

From the standpoint of hazard analysis it is necessary to know the maximal output radiant exposure of any pulsed laser to determine if a diffuse reflection hazard exists and to compare the output radiant exposure with the lower limits for a Class IV High Risk laser. One of the most effective techniques devised for this purpose is the use of thermally or photochemically reacting surface emulsions (section 12.6.6). Even ordinary photographic means may be sufficient. If the beam irradiance is insufficient to cause a surface change in special "beam profile paper," or if the output is CW then a radiometric instrument can be used which has a sufficiently small aperture (i.e., 1 mm or less) to intercept only the "hot spot" in a highly collimated beam.

Irradiance and radiant exposure measurements may also be required where it is desirable to indirectly determine the divergence by measuring the variation in peak irradiance or the variation in effective beam diameter over a considerable distance. The atmosphere introduces perturbations of the beam profile which make field measurements difficult. Those are explained in detail in Chapter 13. Where atmospheric perturbations are significant, evaluation of the risk of exposure at great distances from the laser source should be accomplished by irradiance measurements. An instrument is used with a 7-mm or a 1-mm aperture as required by the appropriate exposure limits. A large number of measurements may be necessary to give statistical validity to the determination of a hazardous viewing distance.

Up to this point, the discussion has been concerned with only the relevant

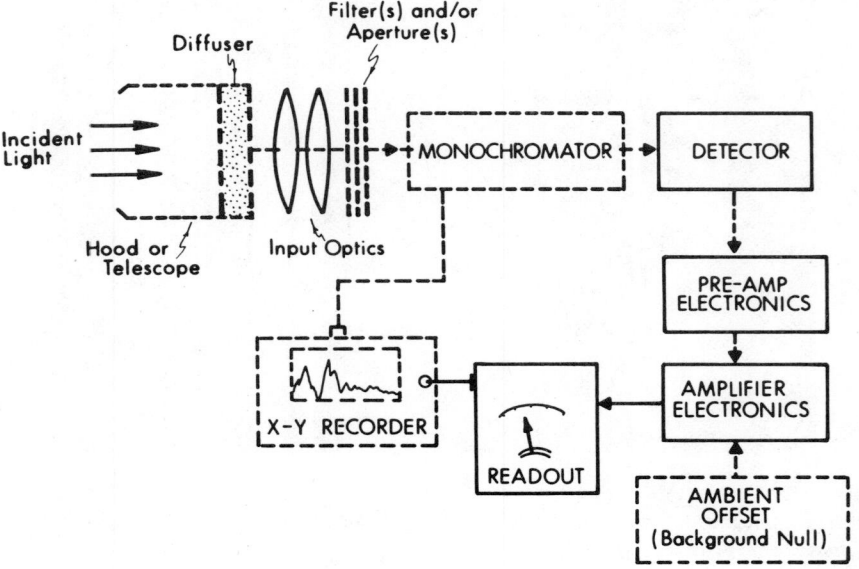

Figure 11-2. General schematic of a radiometer system. Solid lines indicate the essential elements. Other features (dashed lines) are added to operate in certain environments or to provide spectroradiometric information (i.e., the monochromator).

measurements and techniques that are required. It now remains to consider the instrumentation that is available to perform the radiometric measurements.

11.5 TYPES OF RADIOMETRIC INSTRUMENTS

The radiometric instruments of interest in this discussion generally consist of detectors which produce a voltage, a current, a resistance change, or a charge, all of which are measured by a sensitive electronic meter. The exact type of readout meter for the radiometric instrument is normally not of great concern and seldom determines the selection of the instrument. Some experts prefer taut-band galvonometer readouts because they indicate the nature of fluctuations in the radiometric quantity. Others prefer digital meters. However, the reader should be cautioned that digital meters are often difficult to read in daylight illumination and have their greatest value indoors where the ambient illumination does not compete strongly with the luminance of the digital readout. The digital meter is also of principal value when the laser source is stable, as would hopefully be the case for calibration checks and intercomparisons of instruments.

A signal *damping circuit* in the readout electronics is desirable to permit signal averaging of a rapidly changing source output (e.g., a welding arc). The damping

Laser Output Measurements: Radiometry and Calorimetry 353

circuit should have a variable time-constant adjustment to permit selection of an appropriate level.

An *ambient offset* adjustment is a highly desirable feature of any readout meter. If the source being measured is located in a strong ambient (high-light level) environment, the light to be measured may represent only a small fraction of the detector's signal. If fluctuations in the ambient environment are relatively small in comparison with the signal of interest then the ambient-offset, or background compensation adjustment is very useful. However, the effectiveness of such a circuit for measurements out-of-doors in daylight is often inadequate, particularly when clouds are in the sky.

Figure 11-2 gives a general block diagram of a radiometer. Many of the optional features shown in the dashed boxes are available in commercial instruments. Figure 11-3 shows examples of some relatively inexpensive optical power meters which make use of solid-state photodiodes. Figure 11-4 shows two commercially available copper-disc calorimeters.

11.6 DETECTORS

The detector is the primary determining factor in selecting an instrument. Each type of detector, be it a quantum detector (photovoltaic, photoconductive, or photoemissive) or a thermal device has certain characteristics which may be either an advantage or a disadvantage for measuring a certain level of optical radiation in a wavelength range of interest. No single detector is best for measuring all wavelengths and radiant powers of laser radiation. A very sensitive detector can be readily damaged or its response distorted by a high power laser beam, whereas a detector designed to measure very high power laser radiation normally is insensitive to low power irradiation. A detector sensitive to visible light may not respond to infrared radiation—a trait which can be a disadvantage if one must measure an infrared laser, but is an advantage if one must measure a visible laser and does not wish the detector to respond to extraneous thermal radiation sources. Table 11-2 (from Sliney, Bason, and Freasier, 1971) provides the approximate ranges or irradiance, radiant exposure, and radiance of interest to the safety professional in evaluating lasers and non-coherent sources in several spectral bands.

11.6.1 Thermal Detectors

Thermopiles, bolometers, and disc calorimeters are characterized by a relatively flat response as a function of wavelengths. The spectral response of such detectors is dictated by the "black" absorber, such as gold black, carbon black, Parson's black, or Nextal®, which normally are used to coat a metal surface. The temperature rise in the metal is then converted into an electrical voltage or current by one

---

® Trade name of 3M Company for a carbon-particle (microsphere) black paint.

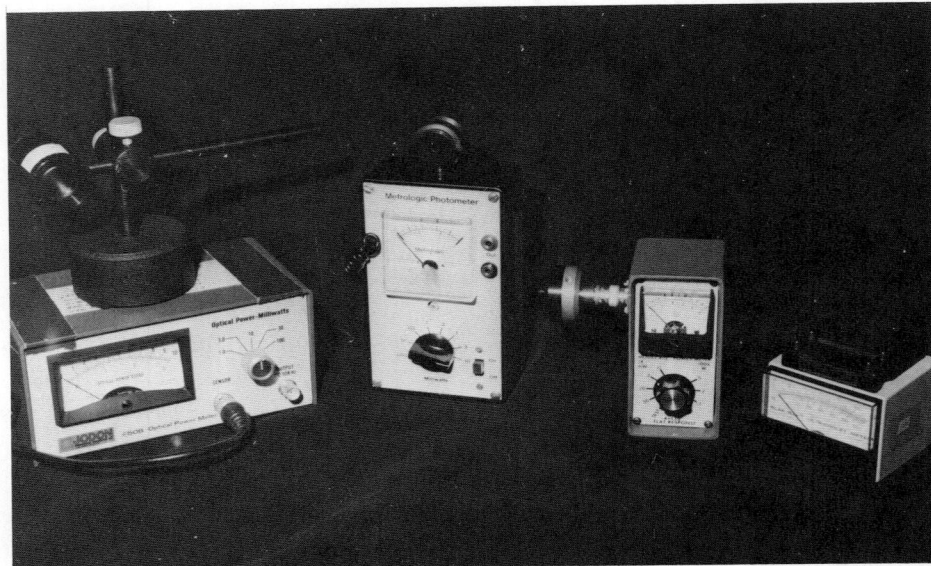

Figure 11-3. Inexpensive ($300) Laser Power Meters. These are used for low-power visible laser measurements (typical range 0.1 to 100 mW). Such instruments typically use a silicon (solar cell) which operates in the photovoltaic mode.

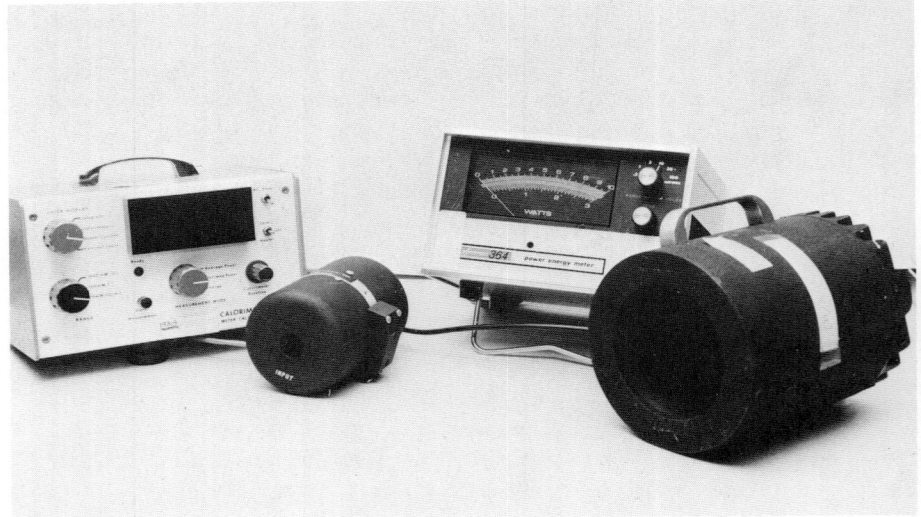

Figure 11-4. Disc Calorimeters. The two commercially available copper disc laser calorimeters shown are manufactured by Calorimetrics and Scientech, both of Boulder, CO.

TABLE 11-2. Approximate Radiometric Ranges of Interest for Hazard Analysis

Wavelength Regions[a]	Irradiance (W/cm^2)	Radiant Exposure (J/cm^2)	Radiance $[W/(cm^2 \cdot sr)]$	Integrated Radiance $[J/(cm^2 \cdot sr)]$
Ultraviolet (0.2–0.4 μm)	10^{-7} to 10^{-2}	10^{-4} to 10^{-1}	NA[b]	NA
Visible (0.4–0.7 μm)	10^{-7} to 10^{-2}	10^{-8} to 10^{-4}	10^{-1} to 10^3	10^{-3} to 10
Metavisible or near infrared (0.7–1.4 μm)	10^{-7} to 10^{-1}	10^{-8} to 10^{-3}	10^{-1} to 10^3	10^{-3} to 100
Far infrared (1.4–20 μm)	0.01 to 1.0	0.001 to 10	NA	NA

[a] Zones of divisions are arbitrary.
[b] Not applicable.

of several effects. Because of the thermal mass of the metal, the time required to heat or cool the detector element limits the response time of the instrument. In recent years the response time of thermopiles has been shortened by using thin-film techniques. Instead of a copper disc or other large metal surface, which is useful for measuring radiant powers on the order of 10 mW to 100 W, a thin film of metal is vacuum deposited on a non-conducting substrate to form a thermopile. Lower powers may be measured (typically 0.01 mW to 100 mW) and the response time can be reduced to fractions of a second as compared with several seconds or even minutes for more conventional thermopiles or disc calorimeters. However, response times of disc calorimeters or even thin-film thermopiles are still too long to measure the peak power of a short-pulse laser.

In recent years a class of detectors which exploit the pyroelectric effect have been introduced. Rather than responding to a final temperature elevation in a metal, pyroelectric detectors actually measure the rate of thermal change in a crystalline material. Pyroelectric materials are crystals which have permanent dipoles (naturally polarized microscopic domains) whose degree of polarization varies with temperature. Any change in polarization results in the generation of a surface charge on the crystal. The surface charge is then measured electronically. Response times of the order of nanoseconds and sensitivities of 10 μJ or less are currently achieved in commercially available pyroelectric detectors. Pyroelectric detectors can be used for measuring CW power by utilizing a beam chopped to give a pulsed input to the pyroelectric crystal so that the crystal temperature is always undergoing change (Figure 11-6). A word of caution should be given regarding CW pyroelectric power meters. They should not be used to measure average power or irradiance of a repetitively pulsed laser unless the chopping frequency is far less than the laser's PRF. The laser pulses may or may not pass through the chopper and the

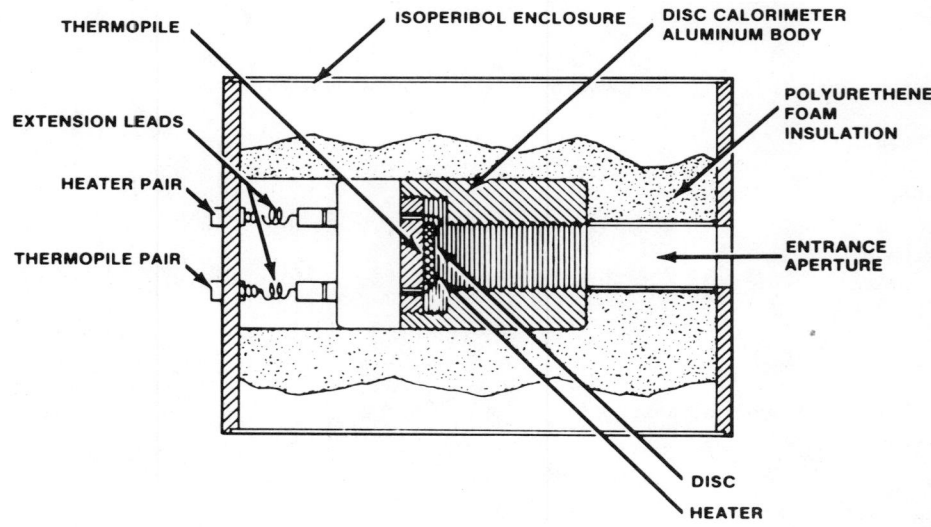

Figure 11-5. Cut-away Diagram of Disc Calorimeter. A scientech isoperibol enclosure is shown with a 36-0001 Disc Calorimeter pressed into position within insulating foam. The laser beam follows an air path through the entrance aperture until it strikes the disc surface where it is absorbed. The heat thus generated on the disc flows through the thermopile where it produces approximately 0.1 volt/watt output signal. The heater attached to the disc permits accurate calibration by electrically generated substitution heat. (Drawing courtesy of Scientech, Inc., Boulder, Colorado).

detector is only calibrated for a true CW source. The light-trapping detector design such as that shown in Figure 11-7 will influence the field of view of the instrument. Another problem introduced in special measurement environments is accoustic response. All pyroelectric crystals respond to accoustic transients, hence measurements near a TEA laser or explosion can result in erroneous response due to the accoustic transient.

Thermal detectors find their greatest application in the measurement of lasers which operate in the infrared region where other detectors do not respond or where other types of detectors require cryogenic cooling. For a single instrument to measure laser power between 10 mW and 100 W at all optical wavelengths disc calorimeters are considered ideal. Through the use of appropriate entrance apertures these instruments can be calibrated to measure irradiance. In many instances the radiant energy output of a pulsed laser can be measured using a disc calorimeter if the beam radiant exposure is below the damage threshold of the absorbing black. Typically this damage threshold is of the order of 1 J/cm^2 or less (e.g., ~ 0.02 J/cm^2 at 20 ns and 0.1 J/cm^2 at 1 ms). For a higher energy pulsed laser a glass

Laser Output Measurements: Radiometry and Calorimetry

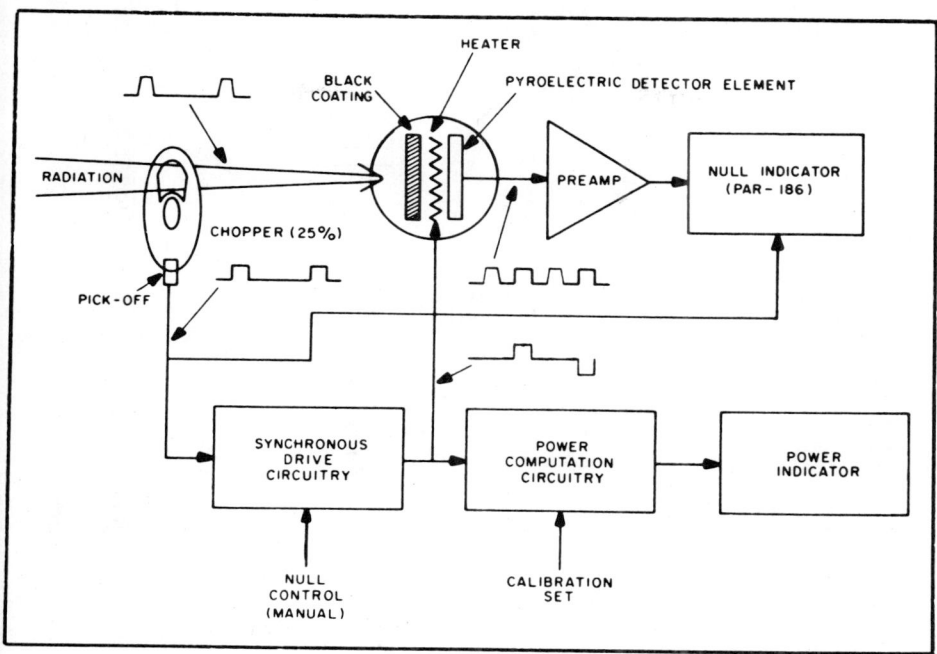

Figure 11-6. Pyroelectric Radiometer. Schematic breakdown of a commercially available pyroelectric radiometer (from Doyle, McIntosh and Geist, 1976, with permission).

absorber in front of the disc, a ballistic thermopile, or a cone calorimeter has often been useful.

The disc calorimeter (Figures 11-4 and 11-5) and the ballistic thermopile (Figure 11-8) are both more suitable for the laboratory than for the field measurements due to the time element required by measurements. Several seconds or even minutes are required for the detector to cool between measurements of pulsed lasers, or for stabilization in CW measurements. Additionally, the changing ambient temperature resulting from air currents in the measuring environment is always troublesome at laser power levels below approximately 10 mW. In the field, one often must move a detector around to find a hot-spot in the beam and a fast response is essential.

All calorimetric detectors have a spectral response dependent upon the absorbing coating (e.g., gold black) and the window material (if any). A typical pyroelectric radiometer response as a function of wavelength (Fig. 11-9) varies only slightly due to minor variations of spectral absorptance of gold black. Gold black has a very high spectral absorptance down to 160 nm in the ultraviolet. Windows are selected based upon environmental constraints and the possible requirement to

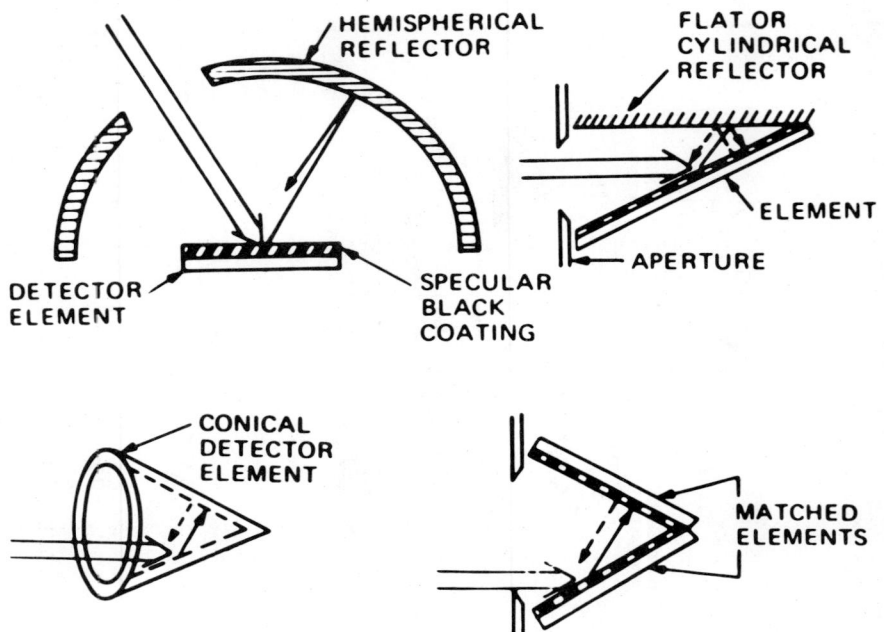

Figure 11-7. Light-Trap Design of Pyroelectric Detectors (after Doyle and McIntosh, 1976). In all cases a black specular coating is used. The lower right design was considered the best approach and was used in a commercial instrument.

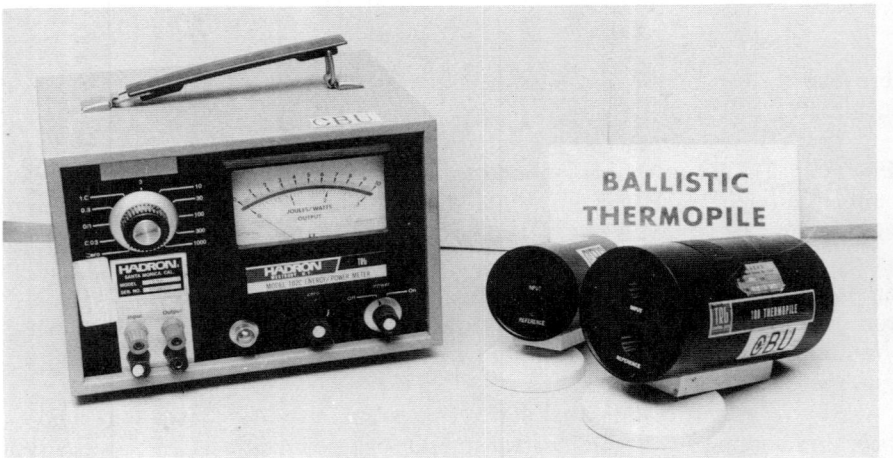

Figure 11-8. Ballistic Cone Thermopile. A photograph of a commercial instrument. The electrical output of the lower reference cone compensates for variation in ambient thermal conditions. Cones are designed with the Mendenhall-wedge angle to trap incident optical radiation.

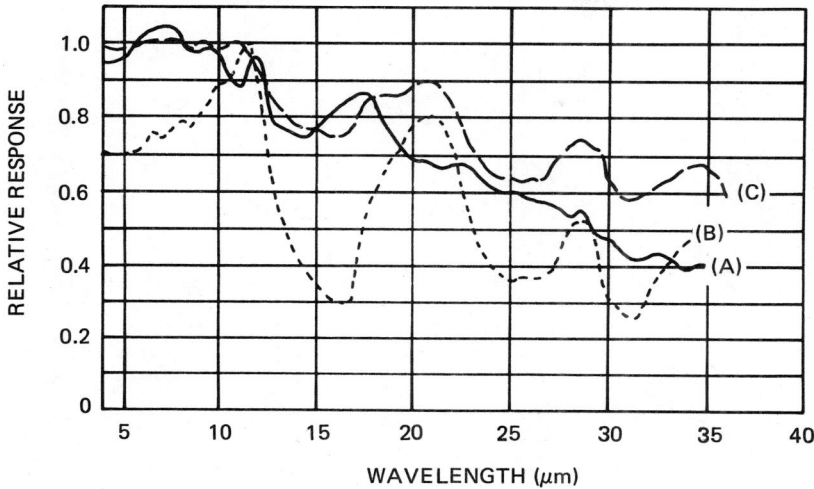

Figure 11-9. Optical Black Coatings. Gold black and 3M Black velvet paint are almost totally absorbing from 300 nm to 4,000 μm. In the IR-C band these coatings vary in spectral reflectance. Curve A is a metallic (nichrome) thin film; Curve B is the organic paint and Curve C is a combination as determined by detector response related to a calibrated detector (from Doyle and McIntosh, 1976, with permission).

reject certain parts of the optical spectrum. Quartz windows are necessary for UV measurements. For specific applications windows are often used to reduce errors introduced by small air currents or to protect the optical coating. Figure 11-10 shows typical window materials for longer wavelength applications. There is probably no optimum window material or optical black which is universally flat from 200 nm to 20,000 nm. The detector user must always consider spectral response.

11.6.2 Quantum Detectors

Quantum detectors which operate normally at room temperature furnish by far the most sensitive way to measure optical radiation in the 200-to-1100 nm spectral region. The spectral sensitivity of photoemissive detectors depends upon the photocathode material used in vacuum photodiodes or photomultiplier tubes (as shown in Figs. 11-11 and 11-12), or in the characteristics of (doped) silicon. All detectors which operate on the photoelectric effect have a characteristic cutoff wavelength λ_c which is related to the intrinsic work function energy of the photoemissive surface. Photons with wavelengths greater than λ_c do not have sufficient

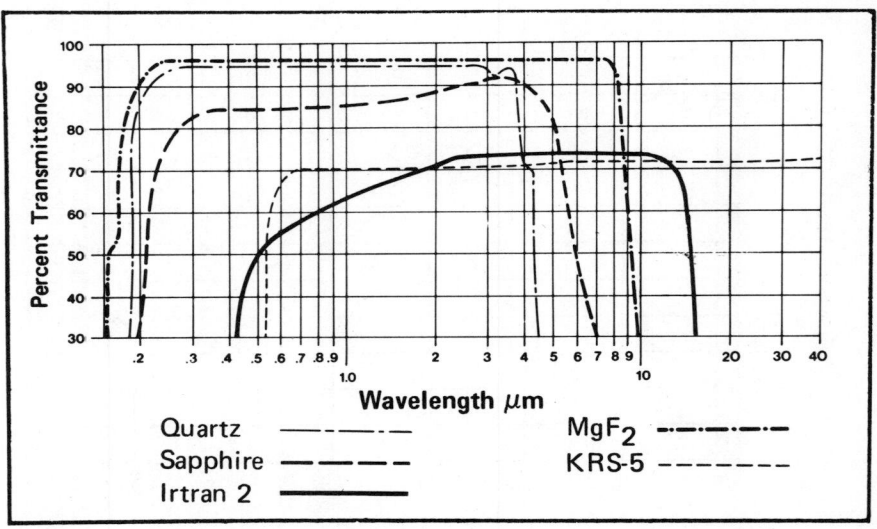

Figure 11-10. Typical Window Materials. A variety of window materials are used for detectors in the infrared. Glass and quartz do not transmit at wavelengths greater than 4 μm.

energy to overcome the critical energy to release an electron. Silicon is employed in solid-state photodiodes which may operate as either photoconductors or photovoltaic detectors. The type of detector chosen normally depends on the wavelengths to be measured but the wavelengths to be excluded are often as important. Response times of less than a nanosecond are possible with some quantum detectors such as biplanar vacuum photodiodes. In recent years GaAs and Germanium detectors have also become popular in specialized applications. Germanium photodiodes have a peak response near 1.5 μm and some useful sensitivity to 1.9 μm. A biplanar vacuum photodiode detector, such as the one shown in Fig. 11-13, has been the most useful to the authors. It has an appropriate selection of input optics, input diffusers, and apertures, which makes it possible to measure radiance, integrated radiance, radiant exposure, radiant power or radiant energy, and irradiance. The chief disadvantage of this type of instrument is the expense (of the order of $5,000 or more) when all of the desirable characteristics have sufficient sensitivity and dynamic range. Because of the strong spectral dependence of the photodiode these instruments are normally not direct reading and the meter reading must be multiplied by one of several calibration factors. Users of this type of equipment eagerly await the arrival of instruments with built-in microprocessors (at additional expense, of course) which would supply an already corrected meter reading.

Simple silicon-detector instruments are quite useful when the natural spectral response of silicon is changed by an appropriate input filter to yield a flat spectral response from 450 to 950 nm. Several instrument manufacturers now market such

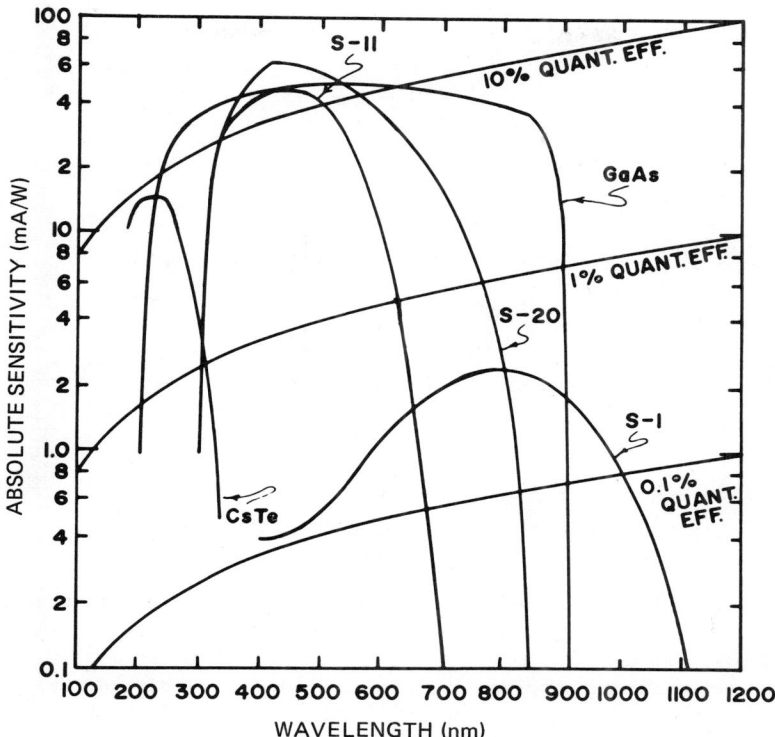

Figure 11-11. Visible/IR-A Detectors. The spectral response curves of several photoemissive materials used in p.m. tubes and vacuum photodiodes in the UV-vis region is shown (courtesy ITT, Fort Wayne).

instruments for $1,000 or less. Figure 11-14 shows such a modified spectral response.

11.6.3 Specifying Detectors

There are several very useful parameters which are used to specify any detector. The most important are the *specific detectivity* D^* (pronounced "dee-star"), the *noise equivalent power* (NEP), and *responsivity* ($\mathcal{R}$). These characteristics will be briefly discussed below.

Responsivity ($\mathcal{R}$) is normally defined by most authorities as the output signal divided by the radiant power input. Sometimes this is referred to as the "gain" of

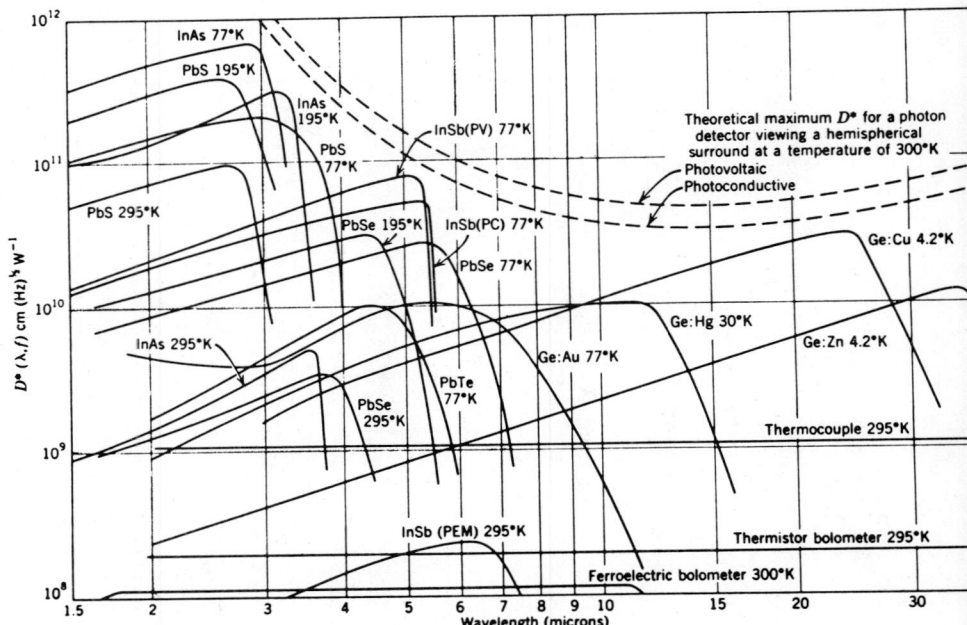

Figure 11-12. Infrared Detectors. The normalized detectivity D* of a variety of detectors used in infrared systems is shown for operation at the indicated temperature. The chopping frequency was 1800 Hz for all detectors except: InSb(PEM) which was 1000 Hz; ferroelectric bolometer, 100 Hz; and the thermister bolometer, 10 Hz. Each detector was assumed to view an hemispherical surround at a temperature of 300°K (from Hudson, Infrared System Engineering, 1969, with permission).

the detector or the efficiency of the detector:

$$\begin{aligned}\Re &= V_s/\Phi(\lambda)\,\Delta\lambda\ (V/W)\\ &= V_s/H(\lambda)\cdot A_d\,\Delta\lambda\ (V/W)\end{aligned} \quad (11\text{-}1)$$

Noise Equivalent Power (NEP). Every detector has some internally produced noise. The NEP is normally defined as:

$$\begin{aligned}\text{NEP} &= \Phi(\lambda)\cdot V_n/V_s\ (W)\\ &= H(\lambda)\cdot A_d\cdot V_n/V_s\end{aligned} \quad (11\text{-}2)$$

where $\Phi(\lambda)$ is the incident radiant power at a given wavelength λ, V_n is the rms value of internal noise and V_s is the signal noise (rms). All of these terms including $\Phi(\lambda)$ are rms values and are wavelength dependent. The NEP can be specified for a single wavelength, as a function of wavelength, or averaged over a band of wavelengths. A variation of NEP is the *noise equivalent irradiance* (NEI) which is:

Laser Output Measurements: Radiometry and Calorimetry

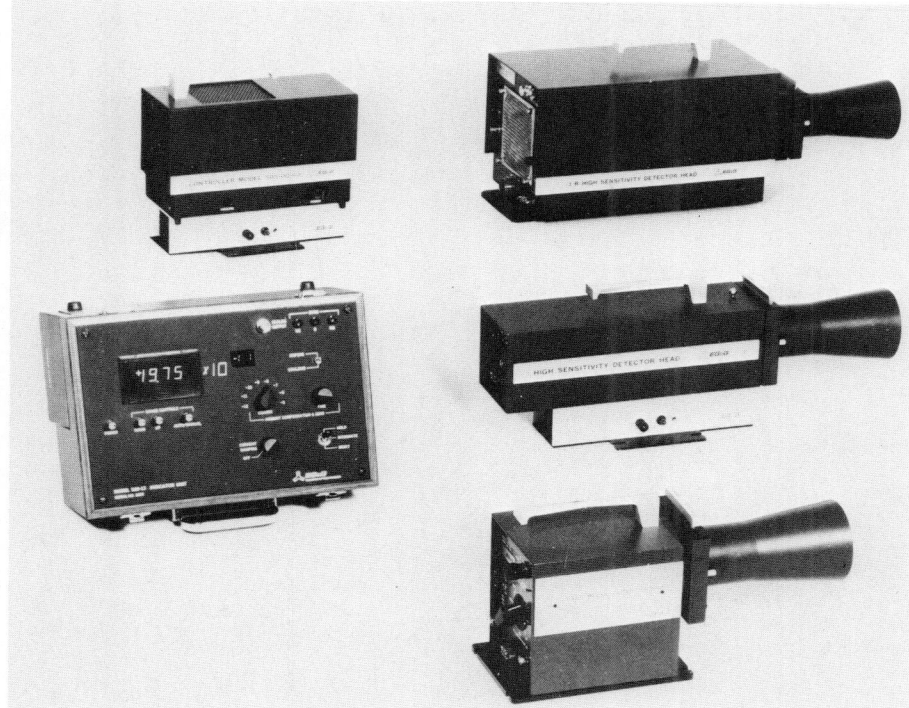

Figure 11-13. An EG & G Radiometer System. A sophisticated general-purpose commercially available radiometer system. Different detector heads contain different vacuum photodiodes or photomultiplier tubes. (Photo courtesy EG & G, Inc., Salem, MA).

$$\text{NEI} = \text{NEP}/A_d \quad (\text{W/cm}^2) \qquad (11\text{-}3)$$

where the detector area A_d is expressed in cm².

Detectivity (D). The simple detectivity (D) is defined as the reciprocal of the NEP. However, a far more useful quantity is the *specific* or *normalized detectivity* D* (D-star), which is most of ten specified by detector manufacturers. The normalized detectivity is:

$$D^* = \sqrt{A_d \cdot \Delta f}/\text{NEP} \quad (\text{cm} \cdot \text{Hz}^{1/2}/\text{W}) \qquad (11\text{-}4)$$

where Δf is the equivalent electrical bandwidth in Hz.

All of these parameters are of primary interest in determining whether a detector will respond with a useful signal at very low levels of irradiance. Of key

TABLE 11-4. Comparison of Detectors and Their Characteristics[a]

Detector Type	Sensitive Material	Configuration	Doping	Operating Temperature (°K)	Peak Response (μm)	Useful Spectral Range	Cutoff Wavelength (μm 50% of peak)	Peak Responsivity (amp/mW)	Response Time (μ sec)	D (λ peak, f, 1 Hz bw) × 10^8 (frequency, Hz)
Photoconductive	PbS	X	I	300	2.1	NIR, IR	2.5	0.001	250	1000 (90)
	InSb	X	P	77	5.0	NIR, IR	5.4	0.001	<2	600 (900)
	Ge: Zn,Sb	X	N	50	12.0	IR, FIR	15.0			30
Photovoltaic	InAs	X	PN	295	3.4	NIR, IR	3.7		<2	25 (750)
	InSb	X	PN	77	5.3	NIR, IR	5.6	0.0003	<1	430 (900)
	Si[b]	X	PIN	300	0.85	V, NIR	1.1	0.0004	0.01	10^4 (1K)
Photomultiplier										
RCA 1P21 (S-4)	CsSb	X	I	300	0.4	V	0.53	4×10^{-5}	<0.01	
RCA 7102 (S-1)	Ag-O-Cs cat. Cu-Be dyn.	F	---	300	0.8	NIR	0.96	3×10^{-6}	<0.01	
Thermocouple detector	chromel-alumel Pt-Rh or Fe-Constantan	S	---	295	Flat	IR-UV NIR, V FIR	40	---	3.6×10^4	14 (5)

Internal photoeffect ——— External photoeffect

Laser Output Measurements: Radiometry and Calorimetry

Golay cell	Air	G	—	295	Flat	IR-UV NIR, V FIR	40	—	2×10^4	16.7 (10)
Superconducting bolometer	NbN	S	—	15	Flat	IR-UV NIR, V FIR	40	—	500	48 (360)
Pyroelectric		S	—	295	Flat	UV-FIR	40	10^9 $1\ \mu A/w$ $10^{-9}/mW$	$1\ \mu s$	2×10^7 (900)

Thermal effect (Golay cell, Superconducting bolometer, Pyroelectric)

- X crystalline
- S solid
- G gaseous
- F thin film

- I intrinsic (undoped)
- P dopant supplies acceptor levels to crystal
- N dopant supplies donor levels to crystal
- PN active area in junction of p- and n-type regions
- PIN p- and n-type crystal region separated by intrinsic crystal region

- UV ultraviolet
- V visible
- NIR near infrared
- FIR far infrared
- IR infrared

[a] This table has been compiled from manufacturers specifications and from Hudson, 1969.

[b] Cells may be operated in either photovoltaic or photoconductive mode by choice of biasing.

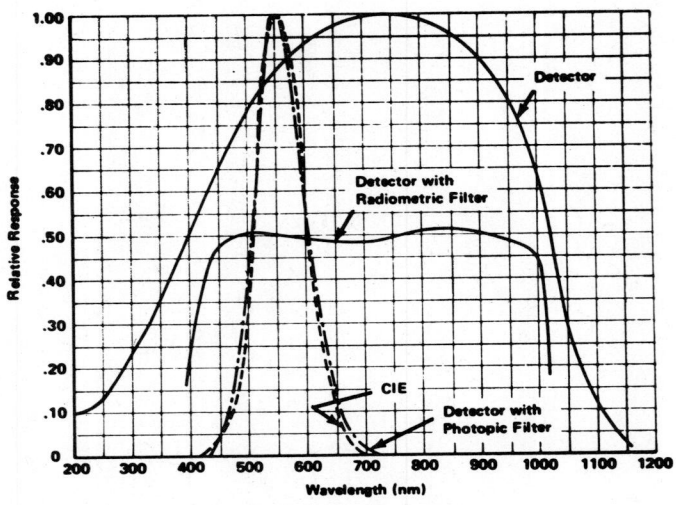

Figure 11-14. Silicon Detectors. The natural spectral response of silicon is adjusted by filters to achieve a photopic response for photometric measurements or a spectrally "flat" response for radiometric measurements between 450 nm and 950 nm. (Courtesy Optronics, Inc., Silver Spring, MD).

importance in radiometry is the detector's linearity. Specifically, will the detector's responsivity remain constant over several orders of magnitude? This factor should be explicit in the specifications of a given instrument. In addition, the relatively minor effects of temperature and an optical "hysteresis" are also pertinent. Temperature can affect the responsivity of some detectors and detector electronics (Landry and Peterson, 1977) and temporary changes in spectral responsivity has been noticed in some silicon detectors. For this reason temperature compensation circuits are now found to some degree in most good instruments. Nevertheless, for the highest accuracy in performing critical radiometric measurements all of the limitations of the various detectors in use must be considered.

Table 11-4 provides a listing of several commonly used detectors and their characteristics. Note that the ambient temperature has a great effect upon the NEP.

11.6.4 Detectors to Resolve Short Pulses

A variety of techniques have been developed to resolve the temporal behavior of short laser pulses. An ultrafast oscilloscope with a solid-state silicon detector or

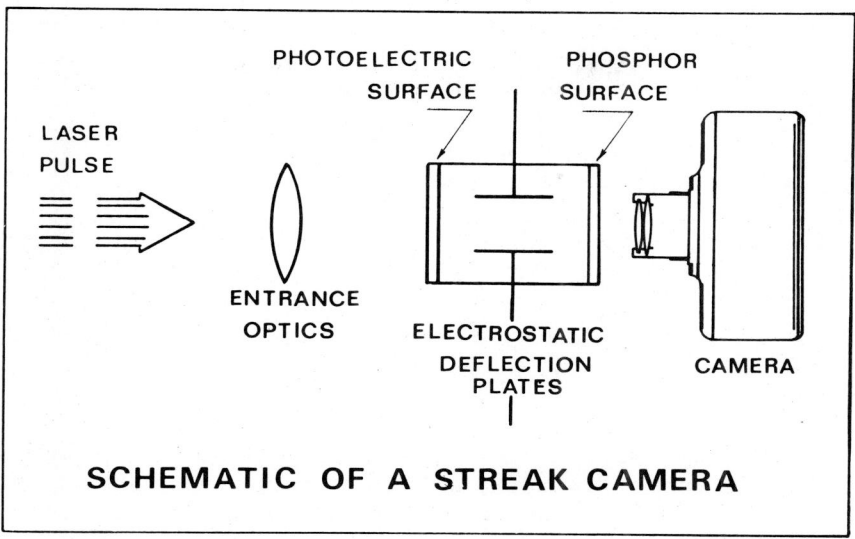

Figure 11-15. Streak Camera. A streak camera is used to display the temporal characteristics of extremely short laser pulses. A light pulse incident upon the photocathode creates a pulse of photoelectrons which are deflected by a varying deflection voltage to provide the display of the pulse shape (see Hadland, 1976).

biplanar vacuum photodiode are most often used to display the pulse shape of a Q-switched (10 ns to 100 ns) pulse. Proper biasing, impedance matching and preamplifier electronics are essential to preclude the distortion of the pulse shape. Although high peak power (kW) ruby or neodymium laser pulses can usually be presented in such a fashion, one is often unable to display the one-watt peak power of GaAs laser pulses because of insufficient sensitivity of the detector/preamplifier system. One must be very careful to avoid a number of pitfalls in using these techniques and those who have not worked with such equipment previously should review some of the references in section 11.13 on this subject (in particular, Bradley and New, 1974).

Still more sophisticated techniques are required to detect and display the temporal characteristics of mode-locked (e.g., 1 ps to 100 ps) laser pulses. One method makes use of two-photon fluorescence, but there are difficulties in interpreting the data from this type of technique and the technique is limited to the laboratory environment. A method which probably enjoys more widespread use makes use of a streak camera (see Figure 11-15). The temporal characteristics of a mode-locked pulse incident upon a photocathode determine the temporal characteristics (pulse shape) of a stream of electrons. The electrons are deflected as a function of time by deflection plates, and the spatial intensity of the phosphor display of the pulse indicates the pulse shape of the original laser pulse. Fortunately for the safety professional, the safety standards do not require much information regarding the exact pulse shape, and research physicists who work with ultrafast shutters, pulse chirping, dynamic spectroscopy, and such lasers generally have a good idea of the laser pulse characteristics.

11.7 SAFETY METERS

At present no radiometric measurement instruments are available which have been designed specifically for hazard analysis of a great variety of lasers. Indeed, it is unlikely that such instruments will be made in the future because of the great variation in exposure criteria for different wavelengths and different exposure durations. The same holds true for non-laser optical source survey instruments. Of course such laser survey instruments could be made for each of the specific categories of lasers but a complete set of these instruments would be quite expensive. For example, such a set of radiometric equipment for hazard analysis assembled from present commercially available items would cost in excess of $20,000. Safety meters designed solely to measure actinic ultraviolet radiation have been constructed, but could not reliably filter out stray light (see Chapter 14).

When the present cost of equipment is considered, the necessity for hazard evaluation measurements must be re-evaluated and alternative techniques sought. Fortunately most high intensity light sources and lasers have fairly consistent maximal output parameters. Because of this consistency and the uncertainties of present exposure limits there is seldom a need for periodic monitoring of a source. Quite often it can be determined by inspection that a source has a radiant output either far exceeding or well below the present exposure limits. Sensitive illuminance meters may be used to measure permissible exposure levels for CW lasers operating in the visible spectrum. For example 1 $\mu W/cm^2$ at the helium-neon wavelengths of 632.8 nm is 0.17 footcandles (1.8 lux), and 1 mW/cm^2 is 170 footcandles (1800 lux). Table 11-3 gives the radiometric-photometric conversion factors for several laser wavelengths. However, when an illuminance meter is used for measurements of a laser that must be calibrated at that specific wavelength, the laser beam must completely fill the detector aperture in order to allow a conversion to irradiance.

11.8 CALIBRATION: THE STANDARD SOURCE OR THE STANDARD DETECTOR

Calibration of all radiometric systems is required periodically. The methods for calibration and calibration check tests vary widely. In the past 15 years the electro-optics revolution which was spawned by the laser has also meant significant advances in radiometric standards. In 1965 the NBS certified standard sources—standard lamps and blackbodies. Today these are being replaced gradually or being supplemented by standard detectors where laser calibration is concerned. These include silicon detectors, electrically calibrated disc calorimeters, and electrically calibrated pyrolectric detectors. Calorimeters which have been calibrated for CW laser use can also be calibrated for pulsed laser use as well (see Thacher, 1976).

TABLE 11-3. Spectral Luminous Efficacy of Laser Wavelengths

λ (nm)	V_λ	k lm/W	$E(\mu W/cm^2)$ equivalent to 100 lm/m²
441.6	2.3×10^{-2}	16	639
457.9	5.4×10^{-2}	37	272
461.9	6.4×10^{-2}	44	230
465.8	7.8×10^{-2}	53	189
472.7	1.07×10^{-1}	73	137
476.2	1.2×10^{-1}	82	123
488.0	1.9×10^{-1}	129	77.4
514.5	6.0×10^{-1}	408	24.5
530	8.5×10^{-1}	580	17.3
568.2	9.6×10^{-1}	653	15.3
632.8	2.5×10^{-1}	170	58.8
647.1	1.4×10^{-1}	95	105
694.3	6.0×10^{-3}	4.1	2450
905*	$\sim 1 \times 10^{-8}$	7×10^{-6}	--
1064*†	$\sim 1 \times 10^{-11}$	7×10^{-9}	--

* Based on measurements of Sliney et al., 1976.
† For Q-switched exposures, threshold of visibility is $\sim 2 \times 10^{-7}$ J/cm².

11.8.1 Spectroradiometric Standards

Spectroradiometric standard lamps are used principally to calibrate spectroradiometers that are used to measure broad-band, non-laser sources and shall be discussed in detail in Chapter 14. However, standards of spectral radiance and spectral irradiance are also available which have been also calibrated in terms of total radiance or irradiance (and luminance or illuminance). Typical standard lamps are the 120-W tungsten-ribbon-filament radiance standard and the 1000-W tungsten-quartz-iodide, irradiance standard. These lamps are generally specified to have an uncertainty of 2% to 10% for the total irradiance or radiance calibration.

One approach would use such a lamp to directly calibrate a standard disc calorimeter or pyroelectric radiometer used for laser power, irradiance, or radiance measurements. The uncertainty of this method is related to the lack of a truly flat spectral response of the instrument, or the lack of a sufficiently broad-band window in the instrument. A further use of a broad-band lamp source makes use of a calibrated, spectrally flat detector, such as a thermopile with a gold black surface, and a monochromator to calibrate other detectors which do not have a spectrally flat response. The two detectors are intercompared against the lamp with an interposed monochromator.

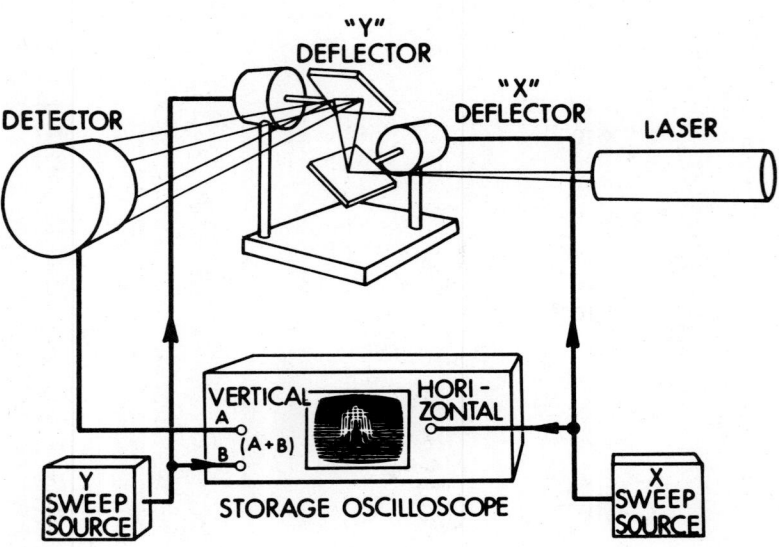

Figure 11-16. Detector Spatial Response. Method of studying the spatial response characteristics of a detector through the use of a pencil laser beam to scan across the detector face in two coordinates (after Boyne, 1976).

11.8.2 Electrical Substitution Method

Some disc calorimeters and pyroelectric radiometers have a built-in electrical heater which can raise the temperature of the copper disc or pyroelectric crystal through an application of a known electrical power which results in the same temperature rise in the disc as from a radiant power input. This approach is termed direct electrical calibration or electrical substitution. Such instruments are rapidly becoming the most favored type of radiometric instrument—particularly in the laboratory. Two such instruments were shown in Figure 11-4.

11.8.3 Broad-Band Calibration

There are a variety of calibration approaches which consider total system performance over a band of wavelengths. For instance illuminance meters are most often calibrated against a broad-band source. Such an approach which does not provide wavelength-by-wavelength calibration factors must rest on an assurance that the relative spectral response of the instrument is actually known and that the response does not vary significantly from the CIE spectral luminosity curve over a useful temperature range. Of course simple illuminance meters generally vary

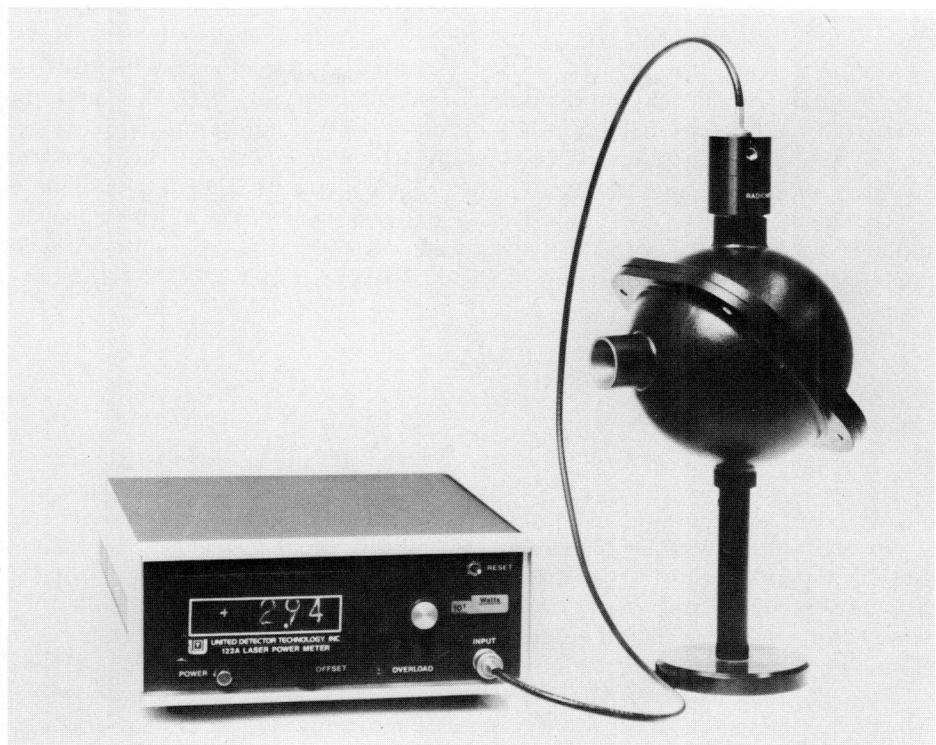

Figure 11-17. Integrating Sphere. An integrating sphere serves two purposes: to provide an aperture with a cosine response, to greatly reduce the irradiance falling on the detector, and to allow the detector to average total intensity through the aperture irrespective of hot spots. Photo shows a commercially available laser power meter using an integrating sphere (courtesy United Detector Technology, Inc.).

significantly at wavelengths greater than 680 nm. Hence such instruments provide widely differing indications of illuminance from LED's which emit in the far-red end of the visible spectrum. In addition to photometric instruments, radiometric instruments are often calibrated for total irradiance. As noted in 11.8.1, the total irradiance of standard lamps is often provided. The use of such a standard lamp where only the total irradiance is specified does, however, require a detector which is "spectrally flat" over the lamp's spectrum.

11.8.4 Acceptance Angle and Surface Uniformity

As previously noted, the world of radiometry is sprinkled with pitfalls. Two of the easiest pitfalls to fall into are to overlook the nonuniformity of detector response with either the angle of orientation or the position on the receiver surface. Figure 11-16 shows how a spatial response scan of one detector may be made to show the lack of uniformity in the response along the surface. The lack of uniform response can lead to errors if a light beam is measured which does not fill the detector. The field-of-view of a detector is normally determined by an entrance aperture, a diffuser and/or integrating sphere (Figure 11-17), or a lens. A diffuser or an integrating sphere can be used to obtain a uniform Lambertian (cosine) angular response, although much sensitivity is lost when these elements are employed. Such input optics are further illustrated in Figure 14-12 as applied to a spectroradiometer.

11.8.5 Calibration Techniques

The calibration of radiant exposure meters is not difficult unless the instrument is nonlinear with changes in exposure duration. In the linear range an irradiance standard and a calibrated shutter may be adequate. However, measurements of ultrashort-pulsed sources as from a Q-switched or mode-locked laser are accompanied by a great deal of uncertainty. Several instruments have been developed for measurement of radiant energy output of pulsed lasers. Such a radiant energy meter can be used to calibrate a radiant exposure instrument designed to measure $\mu J/cm^2$ or even smaller quantities by measuring the output energy of a pulsed laser with two separate methods. The laser output energy Q is measured directly with a ballistic thermopile or disc calorimeter, and indirectly with a radiant exposure meter recording the irradiance reflected from a standard diffuse surface, such as Eastman White, magnesium-oxide, magnesium-carbonate, or barium-sulfate, where the surface reflectance ρ is known at the wavelength(s) of interest. Sulfur is used in the IR-B region (Tkachuk and Kuzina, 1978). The calibration is then determined:

$$H = Q \cdot \rho \cdot \cos \theta \ / \ \pi r^2 \qquad (11\text{-}5)$$

This holds for values of r greater than ten times the laser beam diameter where θ is the angle shown in Figure 11-19.

11.9 BACKGROUND FILTERING

The 400-to-1400 nm spectral region is the retinal hazard region and therefore the levels of optical radiation to be measured can be quite small. Hence the problems of filtering out ambient light and near-infrared radiation can be severe. The use of filters with the usual types of detectors presents great difficulties in the field. Since the transmission of narrow-band filters varies strongly with the angle of incidence of the laser radiation, spectral filtering presents special problems for accurate measurement. The absorption of broader-band color filters is also dependent upon incident angle. In addition to the use of spectral filtering to reduce the

Laser Output Measurements: Radiometry and Calorimetry   373

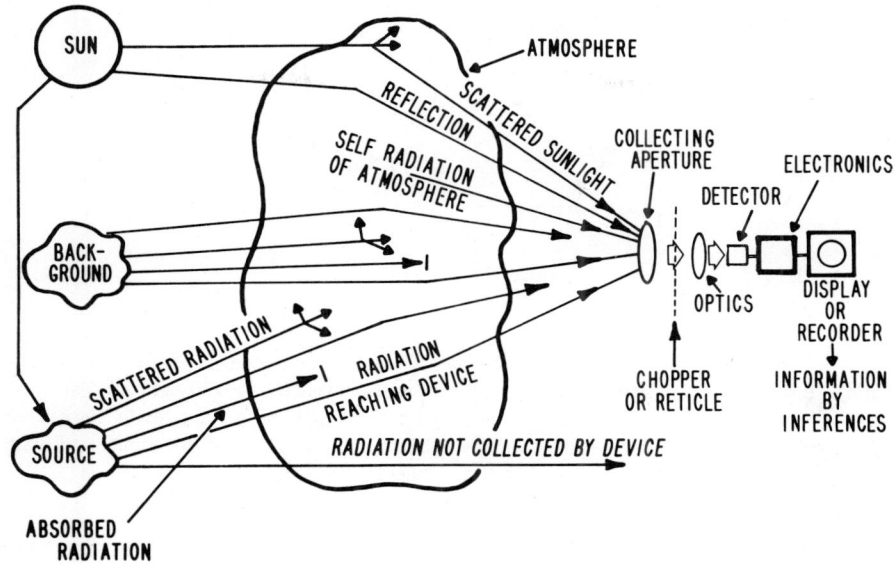

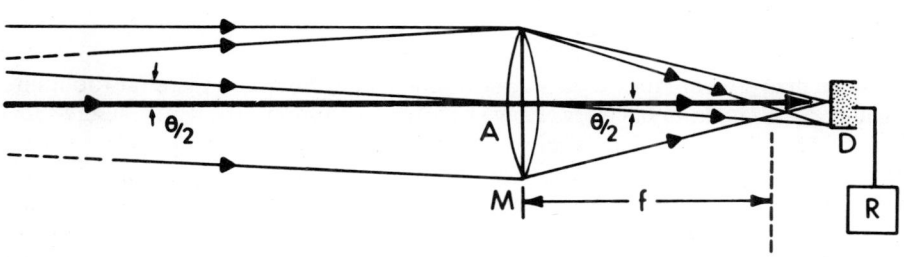

Figure 11-18. Detector Environment. Influence of environmental factors (top) and field of view (bottom) in providing the final radiometric value (after Zissis, 1976).

contribution of ambient light, geometric filtering such as a detector hood or telescopic input optics has been incorporated in some instruments. In the final analysis no technique is as effective as performing the measurements in the dark—which may mean at night.

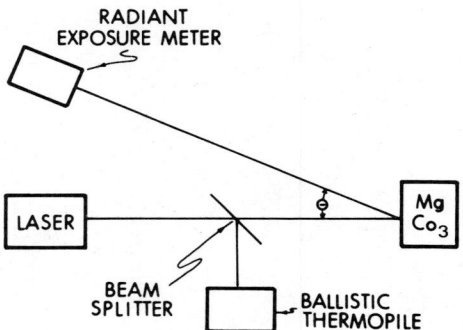

Figure 11-19. Calibration of an Irradiance Meter. The power (or energy) incident upon a standard diffusely reflecting surface produces a known irradiance (or radiant exposure) at distance r. The location of the ballistic thermopile using a 45° beam splitter is poor in this case since polarization changes could create a different beam splitter ratio and introduce a substantial error. Sulfur rather than MgO or $MgCO_3$ is used for IR-B lasers.

11.10 MEASUREMENT TECHNIQUE PITFALLS

11.10.1 Sources of Difficulty

The many techniques used in photometry and radiometry are far too numerous and complex to detail here. However, some common pitfalls do deserve mention. Often a different value from each of two different laboratories is encountered for the output of the same laser. The discrepancy normally arises from a problem of "geometry" or incorrect allowance for pump or ambient light. A measurement of radiant power or energy at two points, each a few meters away from the laser, will often yield sufficient reduction of any error due to pump light or scattered radiation from the cavity as well as laser emission in higher order modes. As noted above, the use of narrow-band transmission filters to reduce ambient light requires enormous care. Measurements performed in a dark room or outdoors at night are far more accurate than using such filters. Also it should be remembered that the baffles required in the measurements of infrared lasers often heat up and emit significant infrared radiation. The use of a chart recorder output from the calorimeter may show breaks in the detector response curves where baffles contribute an erroneous signal (Fig. 11-20). Both readout electronics and detector performance vary with temperature; hence, the use of such equipment outside of the nominal 20°C laboratory condition may produce 20% errors or more (Landry and Peterson, 1977). Detector electronics, e.g., biplanar photodiodes systems will saturate for short pulses. For example an integrating radiometer will have a maximum current handling capability for a given bias and a 20-ns laser pulse may saturate this at a relatively low total photoelectric charge production. Linearity of such systems

Laser Output Measurements: Radiometry and Calorimetry

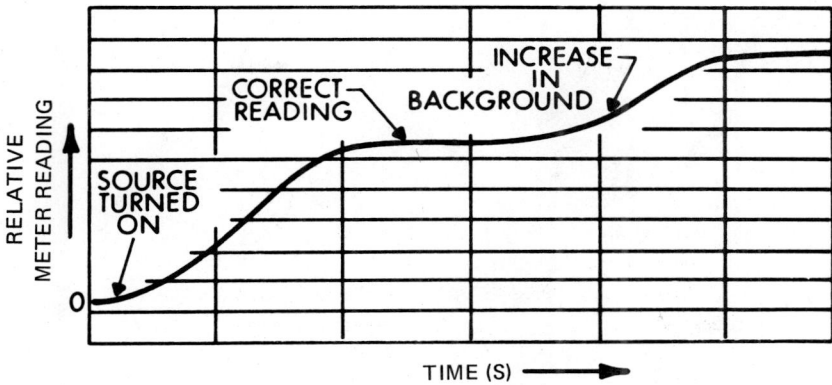

Figure 11-20. Chart Recorder Technique. A chart recorder is used to detect errors introduced by heat baffles in front of a thermal detector. A heater is sometimes employed to provide a third step at a reference level. Correct value is plateau reached prior to significant contribution from the baffles.

must therefore be tested prior to routine use. Radiofrequency interference (RFI) also may introduce errors in readout electronics. Always block the laser beam entrance aperture and turn the laser on and off to check to see that any readout value is not due to interference. Polarization of laser beams sometimes introduces errors, particularly if beam splitters are used in a direct intercomparison between two instruments; for this reason wedges should be used to split a beam into two parts since the differences in reflection resulting from polarization are minimal for small angles (see Fig. 2-6). Ultraviolet laser beams in particular can cause filters to fluoresce and the fluorescence may be detected. The proceedings of a conference sponsored by the National Bureau of Standards (NBS) and by the BRH (James, 1976) contain many hints on how to reduce the uncertainty in laser power/energy measurements.

The use of instruments with different acceptance angles (FOV's) and different aperture sizes (Fig. 11-21) often results in conflicting values for different measurements of the same laser beam. The entrance apertures of the four detectors shown are 2 mm, 1 cm, 1 mm and 5 cm, and one detector has a collimating lens in front.

11.10.2 A Checklist for Good Measurements

One method to avoid some of these pitfalls commonly encountered in both the measurement of lasers and non-laser sources is to make use of a checklist prior to performing a series of measurements. The following checklist was developed originally from a list of items orginally prepared by Mr. Robert Watson of EG&G,

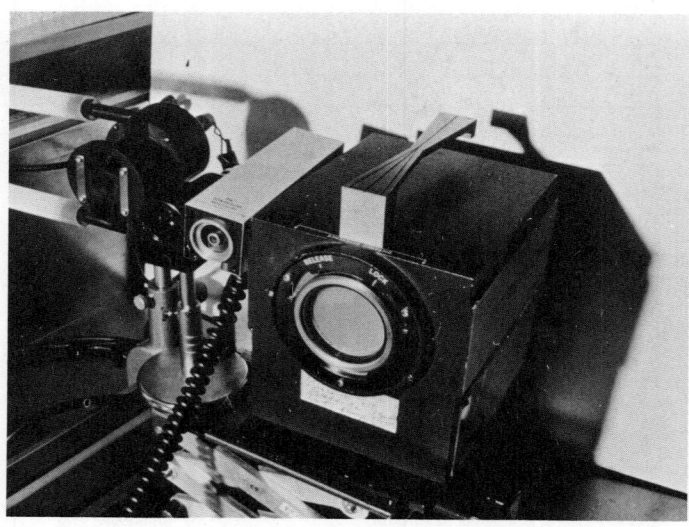

Figure 11-21. Detector Aperture. Photograph of four commercial optical radiation detectors which illustrates the wide variety of entrance aperture sizes.

Inc., Salem, Massachussetts:

1. Make a sketch of the measuring setup to consider geometrical sources of error.

2. Consider the geometry of the source (the source's area, angles into which it radiates, and source uniformity).

3. Consider the geometry of the receiver or radiometer (the size and angular response of the detector or input optics, uniformity of detector response).

4. Consider the effects of polarization at the source, at any beamsplitters, and at the receiver; the ratio of transmitted-to-reflected optical radiation varies with the angle of incidence of the radiation.

5. Consider sources of "stray" radiation within the field-of-view of the instrument; e.g., fluorescence from filters, infrared radiation from baffles and filters, room light, and pump light.

6. Consider the sources of "stray radiation" in the instrument; e.g., stray light scattered from gratings in monochromators, leaks in radiometer housing.

7. Consider the temporal characteristics of the source (pulse-width if pulsed, PRF, source stability if CW, rise-time of pulse, mode locking).

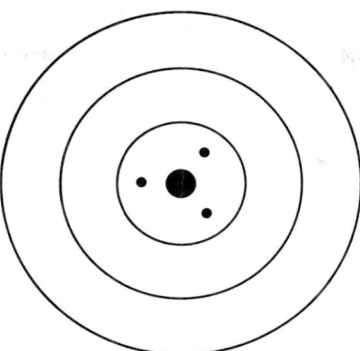

Figure 11-22. Precision vs. Accuracy. The shot group demonstrates the distinction between accuracy and precision. The average value is accurate. The precision is poor.

8. Consider the temporal response of the detector and instrument electronics; e.g., rise-time of the detector, electronics, detector cable impedance matching, etc.). Detectors can saturate at high peak powers, etc.

9. Consider the degree of coherence of the source to preclude errors due to interference phenomena; determine whether coherent radiation will be affected differently at a grating or interference filter?

10. Consider the spectral distribution of the source: Are narrow peaks of high spectral power present in a broad-band source? Is there more than one wavelength in a laser's output? Is there ultraviolet or infrared present when one is measuring visible light?

11. Consider the spectral response of the radiometer and detector element (e.g., type of detector, spectral adjustment filters, uniformity of spectral response with change in viewing angle (a common problem with interference filters), or change with temperature.

12. Consider the repeatability of positioning the source and the detector, and the drift in source output and in instrument response both during the measurement (short-term) and over a long period of time (long-term). These factors determine the repeatability of any measurement.

13. Make use of self-checks or intercomparisons to validate the measurement.

14. Consider sources of "noise." Radio frequency interference (RFI) (e.g., from

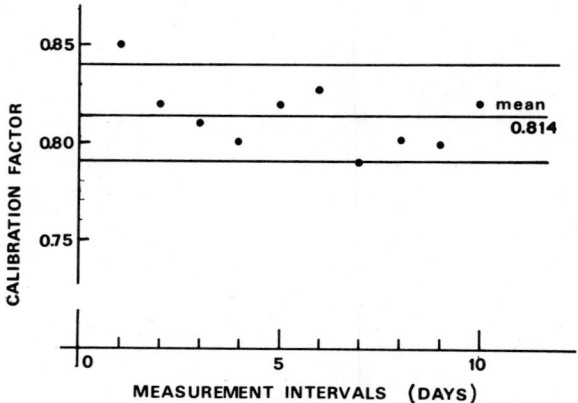

Figure 11-23. Control Chart of Laser Calorimeter Calibration. Only by maintaining such a record is it possible to predict the reliability of a measuring device.

arcs or RF stabilized optical sources) and accoustic transients (for pyroelectric detectors) can wreak havoc on measurements in certain environments.

15. Redesign the measurement arrangement and procedure in light of the analysis (include a statistical study where feasible and relevant).

11.11 THE MEANING OF ACCURACY AND PRECISION

To determine the uncertainty of specific measurements involves both *precision* and *accuracy*. It is very important to fully understand the scientific distinction between these two concepts as these two terms are often used with widely different meaning in everday conversation regarding the uncertainty of measurements. The analysis of a shot group in a bull's-eye target will illustrate these statistical concepts. The shot group as shown in Fig. 11-22 consists of three holes in the target, each situated equidistant from the bull's eye. The accuracy, as defined by the mean of the location of the holes, is excellent; but the precision, which refers to the repeatability of shot after shot, is very poor. Accuracy is dependent upon systematic error; that is, how close the mean value is to the true value to be measured. Precision is related to random or non-systematic errors.

One of the best ways to monitor the reliability of a particular instrument is to maintain a calibration log such as the chart shown in Fig. 11-23. If the calibration factor varies widely over a period of several months, then the instrument's reliability is very poor. If on the other hand the fluctuations are within the range of the imprecision of the calibration method over a long period of time this develops confidence in the meter's reliability.

The subject of statistical analysis of measurement can become very involved and for an in-depth discussion the reader is referred to the procedings of a BRH Conference (James, 1976) and specifically Smith (1976) referenced at the end of this chapter. It is very important that one never uses statistics blindly. Unfortunately superficially sound statistical statements all too commonly give a sense of confidence in a series of measurements. Simply because a series of measurements have good precision, and the instrument was accurately calibrated does not mean that all measurements will be correct. An environmentally introduced error may, for instance, be constant from reading to reading. The greatest pitfall is not finding all of the sources of uncertainty which can produce systematic error. Experience and intercomparison efforts are apparently the only solutions to this problem. Question each measurement as if someone had just stated that the value was incorrect. Be particularly wary of laser output measurements that differ by more than a factor of two from the manufacturer's specifications.

11.12 CONCLUSIONS

Reliable radiometric techniques and instrumentation are presently available to analyze hazards to exposure of the skin and eye to high intensity laser sources. However, the cost of such equipment remains relatively high when compared to survey equipment now available to evaluate many other environmental hazards. Radiometric formulas and manufacturer's specifications of lasers can often be an adequate substitute for measurement. However, more detailed information usually requires some measurements. In this text the characteristics of presently available radiometric equipment have been summarized, but the techniques of radiometric measurements can be quite involved. Not only is a knowledge of the effect of the particular source (geometry, filters, and detector characteristics) required, but good instruments must be available to perform accurate measurements. There are five references which have an asterisk in section 11.14 at the end of this chapter. These present general information for further reading on this subject in addition to the usual bibliography list on specific topics developed in the text.

11.13 REVIEW QUESTIONS

1. What characteristics are desirable in a radiant power meter but are undesirable in a radiant energy meter? Is it possible for the same detector to measure both radiant power and radiant energy?

2. List some common black coatings used with thermal detectors.

3. What radiometric parameters should be required for the hazard analysis of a Q-switched, repetitively pulsed neodymium-YAG laser? What instrumentation might be used to measure these parameters?

4. Define detectivity and responsivity.

5. What room-temperature photocathode would be best suited to detect and measure a laser wavelength of 1060 nm? of 442 nm?

6. Why must light from a CW source be chopped prior to detection by a pyroelectric detector?

7. Why are electrical heaters placed in some disc calorimeters?

8. What must be placed in front of a detector to convert a radiant power meter into an irradiance meter?

9. What window material would have the best characteristics for an infrared radiometer in the 2-30 μm infrared region?

10. Distinguish between accuracy and precision.

11. List five common sources of error in laser beam power or energy measurement.

11.14 REFERENCES

Andreou, D., and Little, V. I., 1973, On the monitoring of laser radiation at 1.06 μm, *J. Phys. E.* **6**:1080-1081.

Baker, H. J., and King, T. A., 1976, An appraisal [of] streak camera operation at the 1.315 μm iodine laser wavelength, *Optics. Commun.* **18**:286–288.

Bartoli, F., Esterowitz, L., Allen, R., and Kruer, M., 1976, A generalized thermal model for laser damage in infrared detectors, *J. Appl. Phys.* **47**(7):2875–2881.

*Bauer, G., 1965, "Measurements of Optical Radiation," Focal Press, New York.

Beck, G., 1976, Operation of a 1P28 photomultiplier with subnanosecond response time, *Rev. Sci. Instrum.* **47**:537–541.

Beck, G., 1976, Photodiode and holder with 60 psec response time, *Rev. Sci. Instrum.* **47**:849–853.

Birnbaum, G., and Birnbaum, M., 1967, Measurement of laser energy and power, *Proc. IEEE* **55**(6):1026–1031.

Blackmon, W., 1973, Laser power and energy measurements, *in* "Electro-Optical Systems Design Conference-1973," available from Industrial and Scientific Conference Management, Inc., Chicago, IL 60606.

Blevin, W. R., and Geist, J., 1974, Influence on black coatings on pyroelectric detectors, *Appl. Opt.* **13**(5):1171–1178.

Block, W. H., and Gaddy, O. L., 1973, Thin film room-temperature IR bolometers with nanosecond response time, *IEEE J. Quantum Elect.* **QE-9**:104–105.

Boivin, L. P., 1978, Reduction of diffraction errors in radiometry by means of toothed apertures, *Appl. Opt.* **17**:3323–3328.

Boivin, L. P., and Smith, T. C., 1978, Electrically calibrated radiometer using a thin film thermopile, *Appl. Opt.* **17**:3067–3075.

Boyne, H. S., 1976, NBS Standards and Measurement Services, *in* "National Conference on Measurements of Laser Emissions for Regulatory Purposes," (James, R. H., ed.) HEW Publication (FDA) 76-8037, U.S. Department of Health, Education, and Welfare, Food and

Drug Administration, Bureau of Radiological Health, Rockville, MD, April 1976.

Bradley, D. J., and New, G. H. C., 1974, Ultrashort pulse measurements, *Proc. IEEE,* **62**:313–345.

Bridges, T. J., Chang, T. Y., and Cheo, P. K., 1968, Pulse response of electro-optic modulators and photoconductive detectors at 10.6 μ, *Appl. Phys. Letters* **12**:297–300.

Bristow, M. P. F., 1979, Fluorescence of short wavelength cutoff filters, *Appl. Opt.* **18**(7):952–955.

Cumin, B., Miehe, J. A., Sipp, B., and Thebault, J., 1976, Picosecond trigger system useful in mode-locked laser pulse measurements, *Rev. Sci. Instrum.* **47**:1435–1440.

Doyle, W. M., and McIntosh, B. C., 1976, Detectors for wavelength independent radiometry, "Procedings 1976 Technical Conference of the Electro-Optical Systems Design Conference," pp 270–276, Kiver Publications, Chicago.

Doyle, W. M., McIntosh, B. C., and Geist, J., 1976, Implementation of a system of optical calibration based on pyroelectric radiometry, *Opt. Eng.* **15**(6):541–548.

*Drummond, A. J. (ed.), 1970, "Precision Radiometry," Vol. 14 of *Advances in Geophysics,* Academic Press, New York.

Duguay, M. A., and Mattick, A. T., 1971, Ultrahigh speed photography of picosecond light pulses and echoes, *Appl. Opt.* **10**:2162–2170.

Edwards, J. G., 1975, A standard calorimeter for pulsed lasers, *J. Phys. E.* **8**:663–665.

Engstrom, R. W. (ed.), 1974, "RCA Electro-Optics Handbook," RCA Corp., Harrison, N. J.

Emmons, R. B., Hawkins, S. R., and Cuff, K. F., 1975, Infrared detectors: an overview, *Opt. Eng.* **14**(1):21–30.

Falconer, I. S., Niland, R. A., and Turk, M. I., 1975, A note on the design of laser beam monitors, *J. Phys. E.* **8**:216–218.

Fligsten, K. G., and Wolbarsht, M. L., 1966, A diffusely transmitting integrating sphere for measuring laser output with a phototransistor, *Proc. IEEE* **54**:1109.

Franzen, D. L., and Schmitt, L. B., 1976, Absolute reference calorimeter for measuring high power laser pulses, *Appl. Opt.* **15**:3115–3122.

Geist, J., 1979, Quantum efficiency of the p-n junction in silicon as an absolute radiometric standard, *Appl. Opt.* **18**(6):760–762.

Geist, J., 1972, Fundamental principles of absolute radiometry and the philosophy of this NBS program (1968-1971), NBS Tech. Note 594–1, Washington, National Bureau of Standards (June 1972).

Geist, J., Dewey, H. J., and Lind, M. A., 1976, Low-level periodic pulsed energy measurements with an electrically calibrated pyroelectric detector, *Appl. Phys. Letters* **28**:171–173.

Geist, J., Schmidt, L. B., and Case, W. E., 1973, Comparison of the laser power and total irradiance scales maintained by the National Bureau of Standards, *Appl. Opt.* **12**(11):2773–2775.

Gibson, A. F., Kimmitt, M. F., Maggs, P. N. D., and Norris, B., 1975, A wide bandwidth detection and display system for use with TEA CO_2 lasers, *J. Appl. Phys.* **46**:1413–1414.

Green, S. I., 1976, 50 picosecond detector laser pulse monitor, *Rev. Sci. Instrum.* **47**:1083–1085.

Greiner, N. R., Arnold, G. P., and Wenzel, R. G., 1973, Rapid recording of infrared spectra from pulsed chemical lasers, *J. Appl. Phys.* **44**:3203–3204.

Gunn, S. R., 1973, Calorimetric measurements of laser energy and power, *J. Phys. E.* **6**:105–115.

Gunn, S. R., 1974, Volume-absorbing calorimeters for high-power laser pulses, *Rev. Sci. Instrum.* **45**:936–943.

Hadland, R., 1976, Recent advances in high speed photography, *in* "Survey of British Electro-Optics," Taylor and Francis, Ltd., London.

Heard, H. G., 1968, "Laser parameter measurement handbook," J. Wiley & Sons, Inc., New York.
Heffner, D. K., 1971, Calibration of lasers—necessity and techniques, in "Laser Applications in Medicine and Biology," (M. L. Wolbarsht, ed.) pp 19—34, Plenum Press, New York.
Hudson, R. D., Jr., 1969, "Infrared System Engineering," Wiley-Interscience, New York.
Hudson, R. D., and Hudson, J. W., 1978, "Infrared Detectors," Academic Press, New York.
Jacob, J. H., Rugh, E. R., Daugherty, J. D., and Northam, N. B., 1973, An absolute method of measuring energy outputs from lasers, Rev. Sci. Instrum. 44:471—479.
*James, R. H. (ed.), 1976, Nation Conference on Measurements of Laser Emissions for Regulatory Purposes, HEW Publication (FDA) 76-8037, U.S. Department of Health, Education, and Welfare, Food and Drug Administration, Bureau of Radiological Health, Rockville, MD (April 1976).
James, R. H., Ellingson, O. L., Peterson, R. W., 1974, Calibration systems for laser power or energy measuring apparatus, Am. Ind. Hyg. J. 35(6):327—332.
Johnson, J. C., and Massey, G. A., 1978, Bolometric laser power meter for sensitive measurements in the ir-vacuum UV spectral range, Appl. Opt. 17:2268—2269.
Joseph, A. S., 1973, Heterojunction PbSnTe detectors solve IR system problems, EOSD 5:24—29 (October 1973).
Kamibayashi, T., Yonemochi, S., and Miyakawa, T., 1973, Superlinear dependence of photon drag voltage on incident power density, Appl. Phys. Letters 22:119—120.
Kimmitt, M. F., Tyte, D. C., and Wright, M. J., 1972, Photon drag radiation monitors for use with pulsed CO_2 lasers, J. Phys. E. 5:239—240.
Kressel, H., and Butler, J. K., 1977, "Semiconductor Lasers and Heterojunction LEDs," Academic Press, New York.
Kruer, M. R., Esterowitz, L., Bartoli, F. J., and Allen, R. E., 1975, Optical radiation damage of SBN materials and pyroelectric detectors at 10.6 μm, J. Appl. Phys. 46:1072—1079.
Labo, J. A., Marston, D. R., and Laudieri, P. C., 1974, Laser Energy Evaluator (LEE): Laboratory and Field Use, USAF School of Aerospace Med., Report SAM-TR-74-50 (December 1974) (DDC AD A-005-294).
Landry, R. J., and Peterson, R. W., 1977, Temperature dependent response of optical radiation measurement instrumentation, Appl. Opt. 16(11):2968—2971.
Lawton, R. A., and Andrews, J. R., 1976, Electrical strobing of a photoconductor cuts sampling oscilloscope's risetime, Laser Focus 12:62—65 (Nov. 1976).
Lind, M. A., and Zalewski, E. F., 1976, Silicon photodetector instabilities in the UV, Appl. Opt. 15(6):1377—1378.
Manes, K. R., Smith, D. L., Haas, R. A., and Glaros, S. S., 1975, Prepulse extinction-ratio measurements on a CO_2 laser system, IEEE J. Quantum Elect. QE-11:635—636.
McCall, G. H., 1972, High speed inexpensive photodiode assembly, Rev. Sci. Instr. 43(6):865.
Melchior, H., Fisher, M. B., and Arams, F. R., 1970, Photodetectors for optical communications systems, Proc. IEEE 58:1466—1486.
Nakatsuka, M., and Kubo, U., 1976, Optical damage threshold of large aperture high power CO_2 laser calorimeter, Japan, J. Appl. Phys. 15:1585—1586.
Nichols, D. B., Wrolstad, K. H., and McClure, J. D., 1974, Time-resolved spectroscopy of a pulsed H_2-F_2 laser with well-defined initial conditions, J. Appl. Phys. 45:5360—5366.
*Nicodemus, F. E. (ed.), 1976-1978, "Self-study Manual on Optical Radiation Measurements," NBS Technical Notes 910 series, National Bureau of Standards, Optical Physics Division, Washington, U.S. Government Printing Office.
Offerberger, A. A., Smy, P. R., and Burnett, N. H., 1975, High power CO_2 laser energy detector Rev. Sci. Instr. 46:317.
Ostertag, E., 1977, Full synchronization of an optical multichannel analyzer for picosecond spectroscopy, Rev. Sci. Instr. 48:18—23.

Penzkofer, A., von der Linde, D., and Laubereau, A., 1972, The intensity of short light pulses determined with saturable absorbers, *Optics Commun.* **4**:377–379.

Penzkofer, A., and Falkenstein, W., 1976, Direct determination of the intensity of picosecond light pulses by two-photon absorption, *Optics Commun.* **17**:1–5.

Peterson, R. W., Coakley, J. M., Mohan, K., and James, R., 1976, The measurement of optical radiations, selected practical considerations, in "NBS SP456, Seminar Proceedings," pp 215–221.

Pierce, R. L., 1975, Fast detectors can measure highpower pulses after attenuation with an integrating sphere, *Laser Focus* **11**(11):62–63 (Nov. 1975).

Pond, C. R., Hall, R. B., and Nichols, D. B., 1977, HF laser spectral analysis using near-field holography, *Appl. Opt.* **16**:67–69.

Rice, R. O., and Macomber, J. D., 1975, Attenuation of giant laser pulses by absorbing filters, *Appl. Opt.* **14**:2203–2206.

Rockwell, R. J., Jr., 1970, Developments in laser instrumentation and calibration, *Arch. Environ. Health* **20**:149–155.

Roundy, C. B., Byer, R. L., Phillion, D. W., and Kuizenga, D. J., 1974, A 170 psec pyroelectric detector, *Optics Commun.* **10**:375–377.

Schaefer, A. R., 1977, Ultraviolet enhanced responsivity of silicon photodiodes: an investigation, *Appl. Opt.* **16**(6):1539–1549.

Schierer, P., 1975, Measuring dye laser pulses with real-time spectrometer, *Laser Focus* **11**:60–62.

Sliney, D. H., 1976, Instrumentation and measurement of laser radiation, in "Laser Hazards and Safety in the Military Environment," LS79, AGARD, Paris.

Sliney, D. H., Bason, F. C., and Freasier, B. C., 1971, Instrumentation and measurement of ultraviolet, visible, and infrared radiation, *Am. Ind. Hyg. Assn. J.* **32**:415–431.

Smathers, S. E., and Maksymonko, G., 1972, Calorimetric measurement of optical power from pulsed lasers, *IEEE Transactions on Instrumentation and Measurement* **IM-21**(4):430–433.

Smith, R. L., and Phelan, R. J., 1973, Limitations of the use of vacuum photodiodes in instruments for the measurement of laser power and energy, *Appl. Opt.* **12**(4):795–798.

Smith, R. L., 1976, Laser power and energy, in "Symposium on Biological Effects and Measurement of Light Sources, " (D. G. Hazzard, ed.), pp 81–86, HEW Publication (FDA) 77-8002, BRH, Rockville, Maryland (October 1976).

Spears, D. L., 1977, Planar HgCdTe quadrantal heterodyne arrays with GHz response at 10.6 μm, *Infrared Phys.* **17**:5–9.

Stimson, A., 1974, "Photometry and Radiometry for Engineers," John Wiley & Sons, New York.

Thacher, P. D., 1976, Calorimeters for pulsed lasers: Calibration, *Appl. Opt.* **15**:1815–1822.

Thomas, S. W., Carman, R. L., Spracklen, H. R., Tripp, G. R., and Coleman, L. W., 1974, Ten-picosecond streak camera for the laser fusion program at LLL, in "Electro-Optical Systems Design Conference—1973," pp 301–309 (available from Industrial and Scientific Conference Management, Inc., Chicago, IL 60606).

Title, A. M., Pope, T. P., and Andelin, J. P., Jr., 1974, Drift in interference filters, *Appl. Opt.* **13**(11):2675–2683.

Tkachuk, R., and Kuzina, F. D., 1978, Sulfur as a proposed near infrared reflectance standard, *Appl. Opt.* **17**:2817–2820.

Treacy, E. B., 1971, Measurement and interpretation of dynamic spectrograms for picosecond light pulses, *J. Appl. Phys.* **42**:3848–3858.

Walker, A. C., and Alcock, A. J., 1976, Picosecond resolution, real-time, linear detection system for 10 μm radiation, *Rev. Sci. Instrum.* **47**:915–920.

*Walsh, J. W. T., 1965, "Photometry," Dover Press, New York.

Watt, B. E., 1973, Calorimeter for picosecond laser pulses, *Appl. Opt.* **12**(10):2373–2377.

West, E. D., and Schmidt, L. B., 1975, Spectral absorptance measurements for laser calorimetry, *J. Opt. Soc. Am.* **65**(5):573–578.
Young, M., and Lawton, R. A., 1978, Saturation of silicon photodiodes at high modulation frequency, *Appl. Opt.* **17**(4):1103–1106.
Zimmerer, R. W., 1976, Theory and practice of thermoelectric laser power and energy measurements, Scientech, Inc., Boulder, CO (May 1976).

Chapter 12
Laser Beam Diagnostics

12.1 INTRODUCTION

It is often necessary to characterize the beam emitted from a laser to define potential exposure conditions. The beam's characteristics may be required near the output of the laser, at some considerable distance from the laser after it has been collimated or focused, or simply at some distance after the beam has left the laser cavity as a "ray beam." The measurement techniques and calculations presented in this chapter assume a non-turbulent medium of propagation; the special problems of characterizing a beam after propagation through the atmosphere is treated in Chapter 13.

The optical radiation emitted by most lasers is confined to a rather narrow beam which slowly diverges or fans out as the beam propagates. Figure 12-1 illustrates the manner in which a circular beam diverges. The divergence angle in this figure is exaggerated to more clearly demonstrate the various beam parameters at a distance (or range r) from the output aperture. The laser beam diameter has increased to a diameter D_L due to its divergence angle, ϕ. Since the divergence of most lasers is so small, it is usually expressed in milliradians. One milliradian is equivalent to 0.001 radian or to 3.44 arc-min.

For a Gaussian beam which is emitted by a laser with a single transverse mode (termed TEM_{00}), there are several well known formulas which can be used to describe the behavior of this beam in the so-called "near field" close to the laser and in the so-called "far field" at some considerable distance from the laser. In actual practice these precise formulas are often not used, and approximations are more common. The simplified approximations used to describe the beam behavior will be discussed first, then several methods for measuring beam diameter, and finally at the end of this chapter, the definitive formulas for Gaussian beams will be provided to give a more complete picture of laser beam propagation. Methods of measuring beam profile will also be discussed.

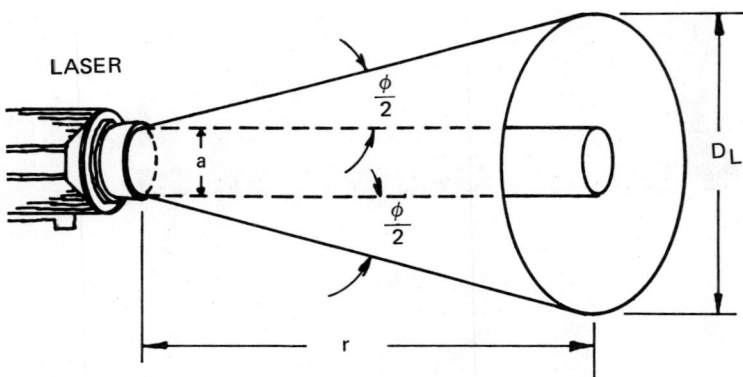

Figure 12-1. Beam divergence. The initial beam diameter and the added diameter $r\phi$ add together at range r to provide the beam diameter D_L.

12.2 THE SIMPLIFIED LASER BEAM

From elementary geometrical considerations a simplified formula can be derived for determining beam diameter at any point downrange from the laser. If it is assumed that the laser beam emitted from the laser cavity has an initial diameter a, and an emergent beam divergence ϕ, the truncated right-angle circular conical beam can be drawn as shown in Figure 12-1. Using the approximation that for very small angles that the sine and tangent of an angle are approximately equal to the angle when expressed in radians,

$$\sin \beta \cong \tan \beta \cong \beta \qquad (12\text{-}1)$$

then from Figure 12-1 the beam diameter D_L at some distance r, is composed of the vertical legs of an upper and a lower right triangle, both defined as:

$$r \cdot \sin(\phi/2)$$

plus the initial beam diameter a. Hence, by using the small angle approximation, D_L is simply:

$$D_L = (r \cdot \phi/2) + (r \cdot \phi/2) + (a)$$
$$= a + r\phi \tag{12-2}$$

As an example, by using Eq. (12-2), a beam with an intial diameter a = 3 mm and a divergence angle of 1 mrad (10^{-3} rad) will have a diameter D_L at a distance of r = 10 m (10^3 cm) of:

$$D_L = 0.3 \text{ cm} + (10^3 \text{ cm})(10^{-3} \text{ rad})$$
$$= 1.3 \text{ cm}$$

It should be noted that to maintain proper units the same dimensions of centimeters are used for both r and a. Of course, meters could have been used as long as the units are consistent. It is also important to note that when an angle is expressed in milliradians it must be changed to radians to apply the small angle approximation. Formula (12-2) may be applied even if the beam were not circular, e.g., elliptical, square-shaped, rectangular, or of any irregular shape. In these cases formula (12-2) could be used to define any cross-sectional dimension of the beam provided that both the emergent dimension a and divergence ϕ were known in the same plane.

12.3 BEAM IRRADIANCE VERSUS RANGE

12.3.1 Circular Beam

Now that the beam diameter is defined as a function of distance from the laser, it is a simple matter to derive a formula which estimates the beam irradiance or radiant exposure at any distance r. The beam irradiance E (in W/cm²) would be the total power Φ in the beam (in watts) divided by the area A_L of the beam (usually expressed in cm²). A *circular* beam area may be defined as:

$$A_L = (\pi/4)(D_L^2)$$
$$= (\pi/4)(a + r\phi)^2 \tag{12-3}$$

Then:

$$E = \Phi/A_L$$
$$= 4\Phi/\pi (a + r\phi)^2 \tag{12-4}$$
$$= 1.27\, \Phi/(a + r\phi)^2$$

Similarly, the radiant exposure H in J/cm² is simply the energy Q in the beam divided by the area of the beam, from which:

$$H = 1.27\, Q/(a + r\phi)^2 \tag{12-5}$$

Unfortunately, this is not the end. Over a large distance r there may be some attenuation of the beam. This attenuation must be expressed by an exponential function. The attenuation of optical radiation could be described by a term $[e^{-\mu r}]$ where μ is termed the *attenuation coefficient* of the medium. It is the sum of scattering coefficients and absorption coefficients of the media through which the laser beam propagates. In the red end of the visible spectrum the attenuation coefficient μ is approximately 1.5×10^{-6} cm^{-1} for conditions of good visibility. This value would apply not only for red light such as the ruby wavelength 694.3 nm, but also to near-infrared wavelengths, e.g., the neodymium-YAG wavelength of 1064 nm. In the blue-green part of the spectrum at the argon wavelengths of 488 nm and 514.5 nm a more characteristic value of the attenuation coefficient would be 2.5×10^{-6} cm^{-1}. The atmospheric effects will be ignored for the remainder of this chapter as this subject will be discussed in detail in Chapter 13.

Equations (12-4) and (12-5) can be modified to include the attenuation term:

$$E_o = 1.27\, \Phi e^{-\mu r}/(a + r\phi)^2 \qquad (12\text{-}6)$$

and

$$H_o = 1.27\, Q e^{-\mu r}/(a + r\phi)^2 \qquad (12\text{-}7)$$

and they can also be further adjusted for other beam profiles. The emergent beam diameter term, a, may be dropped in the far field where $a \ll r\phi$.

12.3.2 Non-circular Beams

For an elliptical beam with major and minor axes a_1 and a_2 and divergences across these major and minor axes of ϕ_1 and ϕ_2 respectively, the equations (12-6) and (12-7) must be modified as follows:

$$E_{ellipse} = 1.27\, \Phi e^{-\mu r}/(a_1 + \phi_1 r)(a_2 + \phi_2 r) \qquad (12\text{-}8)$$

and

$$H_{ellipse} = 1.27\, Q e^{-\mu r}/(a_1 + \phi_1 r)(a_2 + \phi_2 r) \qquad (12\text{-}9)$$

Using tapered prismatic optical elements known as optical integrators, it is possible to produce a nearly perfectly rectangular or square beam. In these cases the formulas for rectangular beam profiles with emergent beam dimensions A and B and divergence angles ϕ_1 and ϕ_2 would be as follows:

$$E = \Phi e^{-\mu r}/(A + r\phi_1)(B + r\phi_2) \qquad (12\text{-}10)$$

and

$$H = Q e^{-\mu r}/(A + r\phi_1)(B + r\phi_2) \qquad (12\text{-}11)$$

12.3.3 Irregular Beam Profiles

These formulas can all be appropriately modified if the beam profile were for a higher order mode or if it were totally irregular as is often the case for a ruby laser. Figures 2-25 and 11-1 show cross-sectional beam profiles for gas lasers and for solid state lasers respectively. In the case of an irregular beam shape the geometric beam parameters "a-effective" (a_{eff}) and "ϕ-effective" (ϕ_{eff}), which would correspond to a perfect circular beam, can be determined by measurements of irradiance or radiant exposure using a small aperture. The aperture obviously must be small compared to the beam cross section. One would first measure the radiant exposure of a pulsed laser beam or the irradiance of a continuous laser beam in at least two or three locations along the propagation path. Then one would insert these values of E and H in the appropriate equation (either 12-6 or 12-7). It then becomes possible to solve for both a_{eff} and ϕ_{eff}.

If either the initial beam irradiance or radiant exposure is measured, then the beam irradiance in the central hot spot can be predicted at much greater distances. It is important to note, however, that the beam irradiance or radiant exposure should be measured at considerable distances from the laser, since many mode profiles overlap one another in the "near field" of the laser. Unless measurements were made in what would truly be called the "far field" this does not reliably produce irradiance or radiant exposure at still greater distances r from the laser.

12.4 HAZARD DISTANCE

It is often desirable to determine the range r to a desired radiant exposure or irradiance. This is particularly true in the case where the radiant exposure H or irradiance E is the permissible exposure limit (H_{EL} or E_{EL}) for that wavelength of laser radiation. This range, although termed by some as the "safe distance," is probably best termed the *nominal hazardous distance* or *nominal ocular hazard distance* (NOHD). By eliminating the exponential term in equations (12-6) and (12-7) we may solve for r = NOHD.

$$\text{NOHD} = (1/\phi)([\sqrt{1.27\Phi/E_{EL}}] - a) \qquad (12\text{-}12)$$

or

$$\text{NOHD} = (1/\phi)([\sqrt{1.27\,Q/H_{EL}}] - a) \qquad (12\text{-}13)$$

Of course a may be disregarded in the far field where $a \ll r\phi$. These formulas are of value if there is little atmospheric attenuation over this distance. Otherwise it is difficult to solve for the NOHD.

The easiest method is to solve for the NOHD through the use of a nomogram, such as the one shown in Figure 12-2. This nomogram, developed by Marshall and Sliney at the U.S. Army Environmental Hygiene Agency, provides a means for solving for any of the unknown terms in the range equation, providing that the

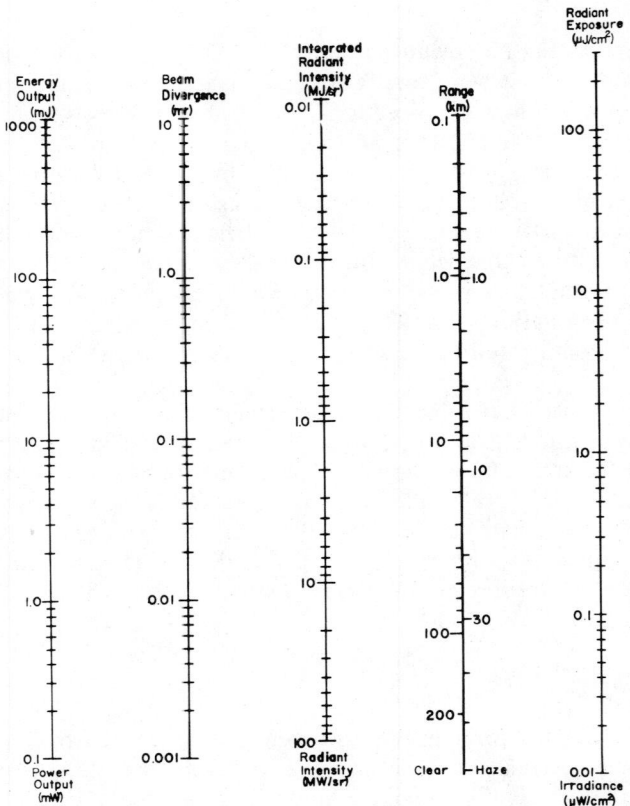

Figure 12-2. Laser range equation nomogram. Either the beam irradiance E (alternatively, radiant exposure H), or hazardous range r (haz) can be calculated with the nomogram if the other values of equation 12-4, 12-5, 12-12 or 12-13 are known. A thin pencil line is drawn through the values of Q (or Φ) and ϕ in the first two columns and extending to the center scale. A second fine pencil line is then drawn between the middle-scale intersect and the known value in either the range (r) scale or the E, H scale. The intersect of this second line with the remaining scale provides the unknown quantity.

As an example, consider a 0.1-J Nd:YAG laser with ϕ = 0.5 mrad (a is ignored); we wish to calculate the range in normal haze ($\mu = 10^{-6}$ cm) to the exposure limit of 5×10^{-6} J/cm². The First line intercepts the middle scale at 0.5 MJ/sr. The second line is drawn from this last intercept through 5 μJ/cm² in the right-most scale. The intercept in the range scale (hazy) is at 2.8 km.

remaining four terms are known. The nomogram is used in the following way. A thin pencil line is drawn from the left-most column (output energy or power) to intersect the second column at the specified divergence and by extending it to the third column to provide the value of radiant intensity. A second thin pencil line is then drawn from the radiant intensity through either the known range of interest (fourth

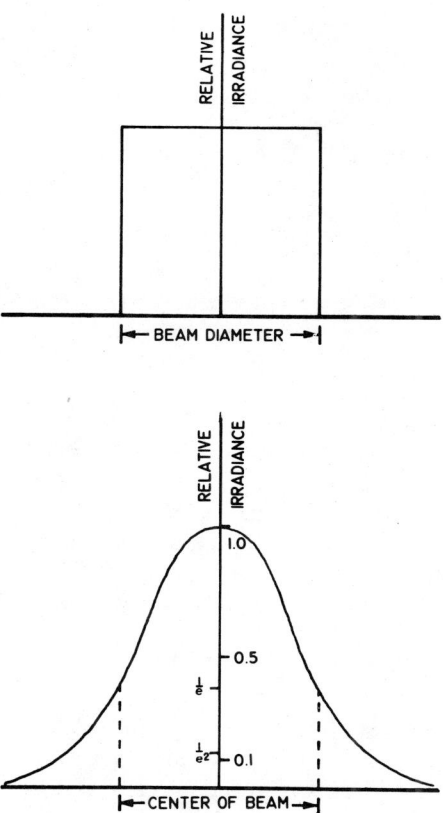

Figure 12-3. Beam Profile. A theoretical Gaussian beam profile is compared with a rectangular profile. There is no problem in defining the beam diameter for the rectangular profile. The Gaussian beam diameter is defined at $1/e$ (for safety) or $1/e^2$ (in industry).

column) or through the known irradiance or radiant exposure of interest (fifth column) to determine the unknown quantity. Likewise, if the output energy were not known or the beam divergence were not known, lines could be drawn through the other known quantities in the same manner, working backwards through the nomogram. There are limits to the accuracy of this approach as will become clear when the effects of atmospheric turbulence are discussed in the next chapter. The fourth column has two scales, one for exceptionally clear weather ($\mu = 10^{-7}$ cm^{-1}) and one for the normal continental ($\mu = 10^{-6}$ cm^{-1}) haze with 25-km visibility to approximate the influence of atmospheric attenuation.

12.5 THE GAUSSIAN BEAM PROFILE

So far the precise cross section of the beam has been arbitrarily ignored other than to describe it as either circularly symmetric, elliptically symmetric, or rectangular. A sharply defined beam is not found in actual practice unless an optical integrator has been used to shape the beam. The most common beam profile is a Gaussian beam profile. Essentially all gas lasers are designed to provide a single-mode (zero-order transverse electromagnetic mode: TEM_{00}) beam profile. Figure 12-3 shows a theoretical Gaussian beam profile and a rectangular cross sectional beam profile to demonstrate the difficulties of defining the diameter of the beam profile. In the lower panel there would be no argument as to the beam diameter since the edges of the profile are very sharply defined. On the other hand, the Gaussian beam profile in the upper panel permits an infinite number of possible ways of defining the beam profile. For instance, the beam diameter can be simply defined as many have done in the past, as that diameter at one half of the peak irradiance point. It is more common today, indeed almost universal, for manufacturers of gas lasers to define the beam diameter at the $1/e^2$-points of peak irradiance. [The term e refers to the base of natural logarithms = 2.72.] On the other hand for laser safety purposes, in order for the terms H and E in equations (12-4) through (12-13) to represent the peak irradiance or peak radiant exposure at the central axis of the beam it is necessary to define the diameter not at the $1/e^2$ points (D_L'), but at the $1/e$ points (D_L). The two diameters differ by a factor of 1.414, i.e., by the square root of 2:

$$D_L = 0.707 \, D_L' \qquad (12\text{-}14)$$

The same arguments apply to the definition of beam divergence. For consistency, one must also define the divergence at either $1/e$ or $1/e^2$ points based upon the diameters downrange. The divergence, as can be shown from manipulating the terms in formula (12-2) is simply:

$$\phi = \Delta D / \Delta r = (D_L - a)/r \qquad (12\text{-}15)$$

Therefore if the two beam diameters—the emergent beam diameter a, and the beam diameter D_L at range r—are defined at $1/e$ points, then the divergence is defined at $1/e$ points. For optically-pumped solid-state lasers, which have profiles not so well characterized, the beam divergence is defined differently. Most manufacturers now consider this divergence as that apex angle defined by a right-angle circular cone into which 90% of the laser beam power is propagated. The value 90% of the total energy is actually an approximation of the value 86.5% of the total beam power which exists within the $1/e^2$ points of a perfect Gaussian beam.

12.6 MEASURING THE BEAM DIAMETER

The fundamental geometrical laser parameter to be measured is beam diameter. From measurements of beam diameters at different points it is possible to calculate

Laser Beam Diagnostics

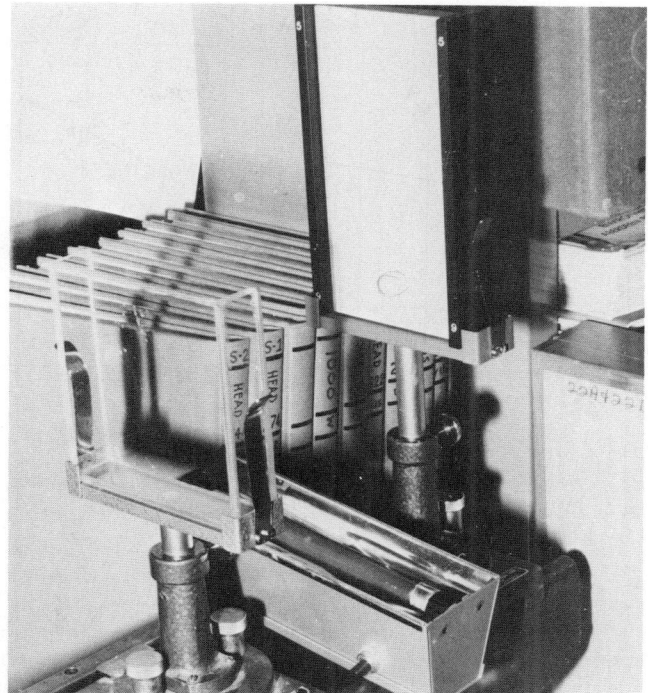

Figure 12-4. Fluorescent screen. A fluorescent screen is used to view an IR or UV beam profile. Note the small fluorescent UV lamp to excite the screen (at the bottom of the picture) and also the water filter to eliminate collateral thermal radiation.

beam divergence and other fundamental parameters such as the "confocal parameter."

12.6.1 By Eye

Of course the most obvious method available to measure a laser's beam diameter is to shine the beam on a large diffuse target board and use a ruler to measure the diameter. If the beam is invisible, a fluorescent panel or phosphorescent screen may be used to visualize it as shown in Figure 12-4. The folly of this scheme becomes readily apparent when the ambient light is adjusted. Since the "edge" of a Gaussian beam as seen by the eye is dependent upon contrast with the surrounding luminance of the target, the beam appears larger when the ambient illumination is reduced. A similar change in appearance occurs when the contrast is adjusted on a TV monitor when a vidicon is used to visualize a laser beam. For this reason, considerable effort is required to calibrate and "linearize" a TV's response to provide an accurate laser beam profile (e.g., see Smith et al., 1978).

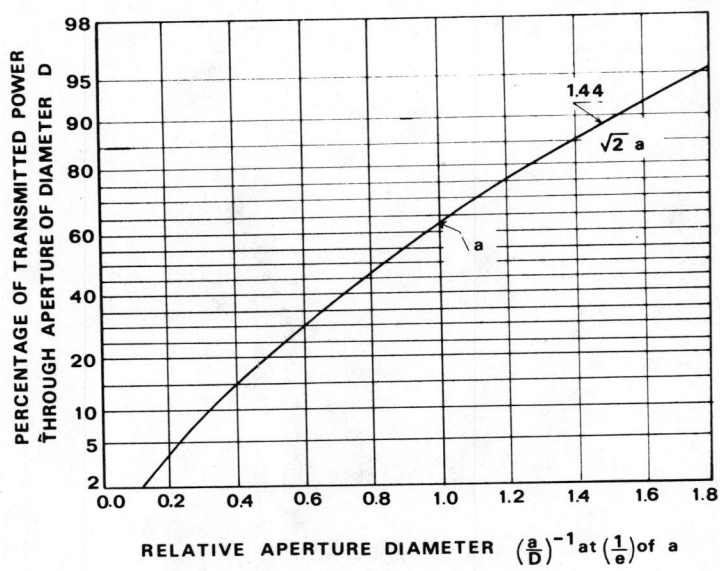

Figure 12-5. Power through an Aperture. Graph of percentage of beam power transmitted through an aperture (Φ) relative to the beam diameter (a) defined at 1/e points. For example, to determine the beam diameter of a beam when 7 mW of a 14-mW beam passes through a 7-mm aperture, note that 50% of a Gaussian beam passes through an aperture of D = 10.80.

12.6.2 The Aperture Method

Figure 12-5 shows a graph of the percentage of beam power transmitted through an aperture relative to the beam diameter as defined at 1/e points. As an example, a 1-W argon laser with 0.5 W entering a 1-mm circular aperture, can be shown by use of this graph to have 50% of the power of a Gaussian beam passing through an aperture having a diameter of 0.79 × a. Therefore, a solution of the simple relation that 0.79 a = 1 mm, gives a = 1.27 mm. Furthermore, a comparison of that value to the manufacturer's specified diameter defined at $1/e^2$ points, requires multiplication of the diameter a by $\sqrt{2}$, which gives a beam diameter at $1/e^2$ points of 1.79 mm. This type of measurement is simply performed by centering the detector aperture within the beam to achieve the highest reading. This method actually does not lead to a serious error for many non-gaussian beams. Equation (12-2), which will be presented in Section 12.7, provides the basis of Figure 12-5.

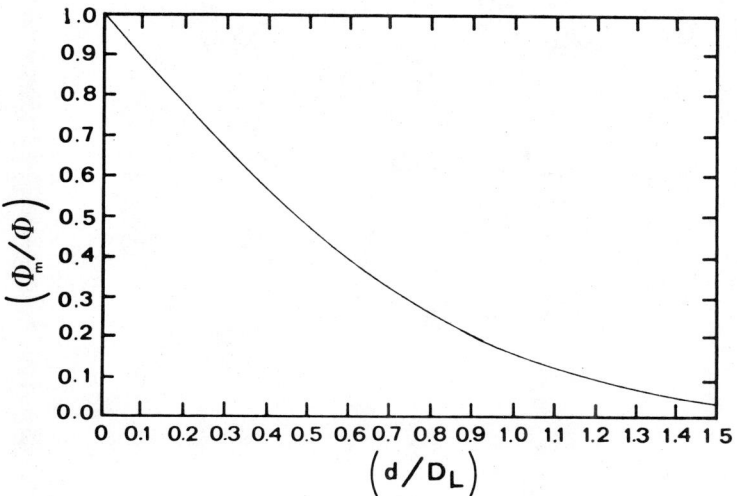

Figure 12-6. The Ribbon Method. Graph of Φ_m/Φ as a function of d/D_L.

12.6.3 The Ribbon Method

Yoshida and Asakura (1976) have described a quick method to measure beam diameter of a Gaussian beam. The beam is directed into a power meter and the power Φ is recorded. A thin ribbon of known width d (or wire of known diameter d) is passed through the beam until a minimum power Φ_{min} is recorded. The ratio of Φ_{min}/Φ can be derived mathematically from the properties of a Gaussian function and is the complementary error function:

$$\Phi_{min}/\Phi = \text{erfc}\,[\,d\,\sqrt{2}/D_L'\,] \qquad (12\text{-}16)$$

where the beam diameter to $1/e^2$-points is D_L'. Obviously formula (12-16) can be rewritten in terms of the beam diameter D_L defined at $1/e$ points since it is ($1\sqrt{2}$) times the diameter D_L:

$$\Phi_{min}/\Phi = \text{erfc}\,[\,d/D_L\,] \qquad (12\text{-}17)$$

Figure 12-6 provides a graph of equation (12-17) for practical use. Table 7B of the *CRC Handbook of Tables of Functions for Applied Optics* lists tabulated values (Levi, 1974). However the ribbon must be sufficiently larger than the wavelength to avoid severe errors from diffraction yet somewhat smaller than the beam diameter for best results.

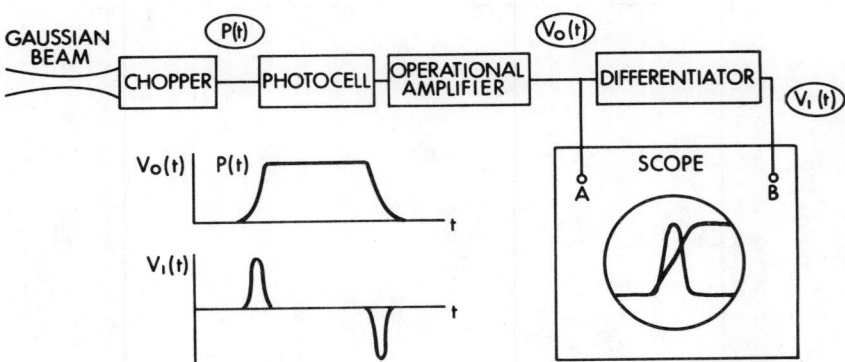

Figure 12-7. Chopper edge technique. Using a chopper, detector and oscilloscope system, one can measure beam diameter.

12.6.4 The Knife Edge Method

Arnaud and colleagues (1971) have described a method similar in some respects to the ribbon technique in that an edge must be moved through the beam. The knife-edge (or razor blade edge) can be rapidly scanned through the beam if it is the edge of a beam chopped blade. The edge must make a steady scan through the beam so that the differential change in transmitted power may be detected in a differential amplifier and displayed on an oscilloscope (Fig. 12-7). The relevant formula applied in this technique is:

$$D_L = (2/\sqrt{\pi})\, v_b \cdot R \cdot C\, [V_{max}/V'_{max}] \qquad (12\text{-}18)$$

where v_b is the blade velocity, R and C are the resistance and capacitance of the differentiating circuit, V_{max} is the maximum voltage from the photodetector and V'_{max} is the maximum voltage from the differentiating circuit. The great advantage to this method is its speed in measuring D_L (at $1/e$ points) which permits rapid motion up and down a beam to find a beam focal point. The disadvantages are that an oscilloscope is required and calibration can be difficult if a known beam diameter is not available.

Firester, Heller and Sheng (1977) have even used a knife-edge scanning apparatus to measure point spread profiles of sub-micron spots in the focal planes of microscope objectives. They made use of an oscilloscope readout and an interferometer to measure the knife-edge displacements.

Laser Beam Diagnostics

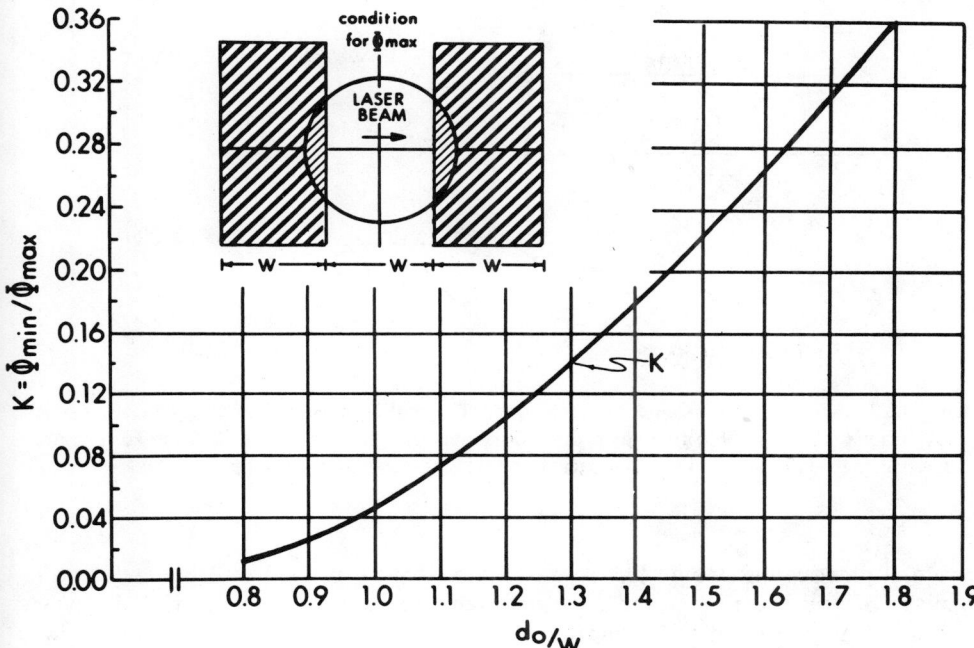

Figure 12-8. Ronchi Ruling Method. The ratio K of minimum vs. maximum power transferred is plotted against the spot-size/ruling-width ratio for the Ronchi ruling method of scanning beam diameter measurement.

12.6.5 The Ronchi Ruling Method

L. D. Dickson (1978) of the IBM Corporation has devised a cute method of measuring the beam diameter of a scanning Gaussian CW beam through the use of a Ronchi ruling (a slit-transmission grating). This is a variation of the Ribbon Method 12.6.3). The beam is directed at the ruling and the sinusoidally varying power is noted. There is no requirement for a precision stage to move a knife edge or ribbon. The basic requirement is a Ronchi ruling with slit ruling width between 60% and 100% of the beam diameter at $1/e^2$ points. For this reason the approximate beam diameter should be known. Figure 12-8 shows the slit-truncated beam (inset) and the ratio K as a function of D_L'/w_s, where D_L' is the beam diameter at $1/e^2$ points and w_s is the width of the slit and also the width of the opaque strips between the slits. The value K is the ratio of the maximum transmitted power Φ_{max} and the minimum transmitted power Φ_{min}:

$$K = \Phi_{min}/\Phi_{max} \qquad (12\text{-}19)$$

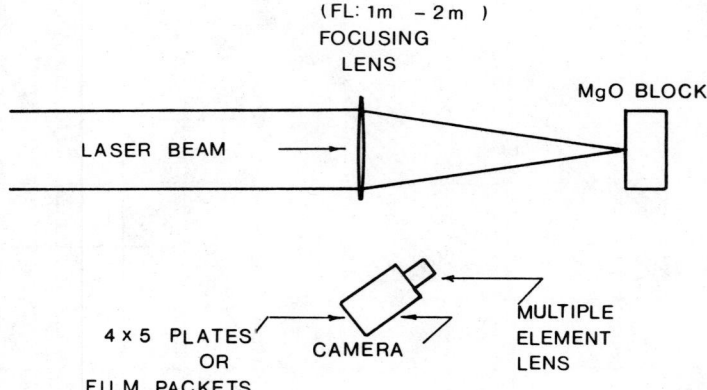

Figure 12-9. Multi-Aperture Camera Arrangement. The multi-aperture camera should be as near the beam path as feasible to reduce distortion, and the target must be diffuse. To measure divergence in this way, the beam divergence should be greater than 0.5 mrad.

In actual practice one would have a number of Ronchi rulings available, a detector to place behind the ruling, and an oscilloscope to monitor the transmitted power function. The power ratio K is plotted as a function of D_L'/w_s as well as for D_L/w_s in Fig. 12-8. As an example, it is desired to determine the diameter of scanning beam in a laser point-of-sale system. The ruling available has N = 2 lines per mm, and the oscilloscope trace shows a power ratio K of 0.2. From Fig. 12-8 the beam-diameter/ruling-width ratio is 1.44 for D_L' and 1.02 for D_L for a K value of 0.2. Hence, by calculating the width w_s as:

$$w_s = 1/2N \quad (12\text{-}20)$$
$$= 1/(2)(2 \text{ mm}^{-1})$$
$$= 0.250 \text{ mm}$$
$$= 250 \text{ }\mu\text{m}$$

Since,

$$K = D_L/w_s$$
$$= 1.02 \text{ and K'}$$
$$= D_L'/w_s$$
$$= 1.44$$

then:

$$D_L = K \cdot w_s$$
$$= (1.02)(250 \text{ }\mu\text{m})$$
$$= 255 \text{ }\mu\text{m}$$

Laser Beam Diagnostics

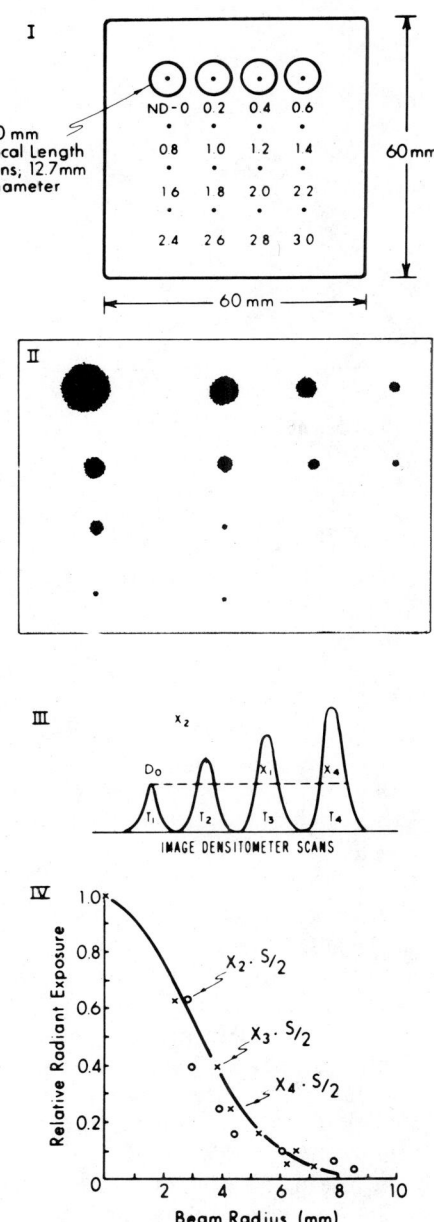

Figure 12-10. Multiaperture camera data reduction method. I. Use sixteen-element lens board to photograph beam spot. II. Develop exposed film. III. Densitometer scan through successive images. IV. Plot relative image dimensions x_1, x_2, x_3, etc. multiplied by scale factors of distance in the object plane to distance in the film plane.

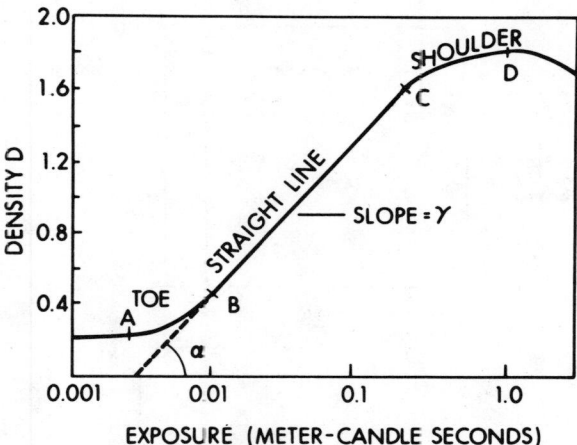

Figure 12-11. An Hurter-Driffield (H-D) or ("characteristic") curve of log luminous or radiant exposure H required to achieve a film density of D_f. Exposures in the linear portion of the curve between B and C are used for radiometry (from Carlson, 1977, with permission).

and

$$D_L' = K' \cdot w_s$$
$$= (1.44)(250 \, \mu m)$$
$$= 360 \, \mu m.$$

12.6.6 The Photographic Methods

All of the previous methods assume a reasonably Gaussian, circularly-symmetric beam. When the beam is irregular as for a higher order mode, the beam must be scanned with a pinhole-aperture detector (if the beam is CW and stable) or the beam pattern photographed. Indeed, photographic or thermally responsive emulsions are practically the only available techniques to measure the profile of a pulsed laser beam. There are a variety of photographic techniques that are useful. All require care in execution since emulsion characteristics vary with exposure characteristics and temperature. The greatest amount of information about the beam profile can be obtained from a series of photographs taken for different film exposures. This can be accomplished through the use of a series of photographs taken one after the other, or best by a multiple-aperture camera developed by Winer (1966) as shown in Fig. 12-9 and 12-10.

There are many characteristics of film that should be known if one wishes to perform photographic radiometry, e.g., "gamma" which is the slope of the H-D (Hurter-Driffield) curve of density-versus-log-exposure (Fig. 12-11) and the reciprocity of the film (Fig. 12-12). One must assure controlled developing techniques. For

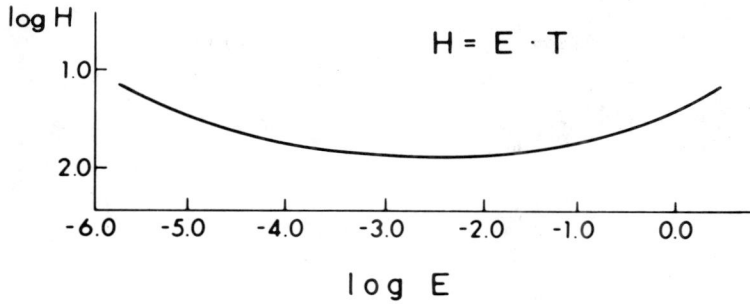

Figure 12-12. Reciprocity Failure of Film. The curved line is a line of constant density. Note that a greater exposure is required for microsecond and 100-s exposures.

this reason the multiple aperture technique is excellent to avoid much of the error introduced when using a series of emulsions.

Gamma curves given by film manufacturers should be regarded as only representative of the type of emulsion and sensitizing from which the characteristic curves were derived. If absolute photometric work is attempted, the following criteria must be met:

1. The response of each emulsion batch of a photographic material must be calibrated at the appropriate wavelengths under processing conditions which are *identical* to the actual measurement condition.

2. In addition, there is the problem of making optical density measurements of the developed emulsion. Care must be taken with microdensitometers that read *specular* or *semispecular* density. These microdensitometers have a collection angle of less than 180° and in general read somewhat higher than *diffuse* microdensitometers. This is due to the scattering by the emulsion. The smaller the grain, the more closely the *specular* density approaches the *diffuse* density.

The maximum density of most common emulsions varies between 2 and 3, and the dynamic range of exposure between the base density and maximum density is only one to three orders of magnitude. Because of this limited dynamic range, a special-purpose film with three emulsions of differing sensitivities was once manufacturered by EG&G for measurement of transient, high luminance events. This special-purpose film is developed in separate stages as is color film.

For measuring pulsed sources it must be remembered that a film's reciprocity failure will require a greater radiant flux density H at the film plane for a q-switched pulse than for a longer pulse to achieve the same film density (Figure 12-12).

Quantitative photographic radiometry can provide reasonable values of radiance or luminance within a precision factor of two. Using stable temperature solutions and uniform development techniques source radiance can be estimated using Eq. (4-5) and calibrated film-density/exposure values. Table 12-1 provides the

TABLE 12-1. Spectroradiometric Data for Photographic Emulsions

	RADIANT EXPOSURE ($\mu J/cm^2$) TO ACHIEVE D = 1.0 AT LASER WAVELENGTH								Contrast
	HeCd 325	HeCd 441.6	Ar 488	Ar 514.5	Nd:YAG 532	HeNe 632.8	Kr 647.1	RUBY 694.3 nm	γ
AGFA-GEVAERT PRODUCT									
10E56 Plate or Film	—	6.0	3.0	2.0	—	—	—	—	7
8375 Plates	—	15	150	25	25	7.5	7.5	5.0	3
10E75 Plates or Films	—	6.0	30	12	6.0	2.0	2.0	2.0	4
KODAK PRODUCT									
High Resolution Plate; Type 1A Film SO-343 (E7B); 649GH (E4AH)	40	100	150	100	80	—	—	—	8
High Resolution Plate; Type 2A	100	300	250	200	200	—	—	—	5
Spectroscopic, Type 649-F Plate or Film		50	80	80	100	90	80	500+	4–5
Holographic Plate, Type 120-02 or Film SO173		50	—	—	—	40	40	40	4–5
Minicard II Film, SO-424 and SO-141	2.0	8.0	5.0	5.0	10	—	—	—	4
Special Plate, Type 125-02	2.0	8.0	5.0	5.0	10	—	—	—	4
High-Speed Holographic Film, SO-253		2.0	4.0	2.5	2.0	0.5	0.35	100+	7
High-Speed Holographic Plate, Type 131-02		2.0	4.0	2.5	2.0	0.5	0.35	100+	7
Direct Positive Laser Recording Film, SO-285		3.5		4.5	7.5	3.0	5.0	—	2

Film									
Recordak Direct Duplicating Print Film, 5468, 8468	0.5	10	10	5.0	4.0	—	—	—	1.9
High Definition Aerial Film, 3414	0.04	0.06	0.3	0.2	0.2	0.2	—	0.5	0.08–3
Technical Pan Film SO-115	—	0.04	0.08	0.07	0.7	0.04	0.03	—	1–3
Linagraph Shellburst Film 2474 and 2476	0.015	0.009	0.03	0.03	0.02	0.015	0.015	0.2	0.5–2
2479 PAR Film	0.01	0.005	0.02	0.03	0.02	0.008	0.008	0.05	0.6–2
2475 Recording Film	0.007	0.003	0.006	0.007	0.006	0.005	0.005	0.005	0.4–2
2485 High Speed Recording Film	0.003	0.0007	0.004	0.005	0.004	0.003	0.003	0.004	0.9–2
*Plus-X Film	—	0.049	0.09	0.098	0.101	0.110	—	—	—
*Panatomic-X Film	—	0.042	0.048	0.068	0.091	0.12	0.28	—	—
*Tri-X Film	0.05	0.047	0.044	0.04	0.036	0.031	—	—	—
*High-Speed Infrared †	0.002	0.003	0.01	0.045	0.033	0.016	0.013	0.01	—

Data for this table is from the catalog of the Newport Research Corporation, Fountain Valley, CA, except for films marked with * which were from Kodak datasheets. Density of 1.0 was obtained at 0.6 above gross fog, except for Tri-X and Plus-X which were at 1.0 above gross fog.
† Exposure at 905 nm was 0.04.

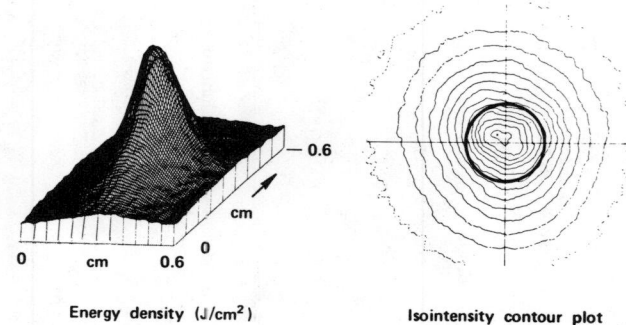

Energy density (J/cm²)   Isointensity contour plot

Figure 12-13. Plastic Block Beam Profile. Using a plastic block, one can produce a three-dimensional profile of radiant exposure from the high-power laser beam imprint into the plastic.

radiant exposure values in $\mu J/cm^2$ at the film for several laser wavelengths and for a variety of holographic and general purpose photographic emulsions. This table is useful in selecting films and for estimating proper exposures. Figure A.2 is a conversion chart for density and exposure values and film sensitivity. In the USA sensitivity relates to an exposure reference line of 1 erg/cm² (i.e., 10^{-7} J/cm²). Thus a film with a sensitivity of 1 requires an exposure 1 erg/cm² and a film with a sensitivity of 100 requires an exposure of 1/100 erg/cm². Also shown in the right column are the actual density values for a gamma of 0.75.

12.6.7 Using Damage Profiles

Black paper and plastic materials are sometimes used to determine approximate beam profiles. Table 12-2 presented thresholds for damage in "black" surfaces. Some surface thresholds change with the upper limits of Class III b pulsed lasers, and they serve the useful purpose of providing the safety specialist with an inexpensive means to check for hazardous diffuse reflections and skin hazards. Figure 12-13 shows the three-dimensional profile imprinted in polymethylmethacrylate plastic (e.g., Plexiglas) by a very high power CW laser beam. This technique is commonly used with high power IR beam profile studies.

12.7 CALCULATING THE TRANSMITTED POWER THROUGH AN APERTURE STOP

The graph in Fig. 12-5 was derived from a general formula which is useful for defining the fraction of radiant power passing through an aperture of known diameter D. The emergent beam diameter a' has already been defined by the manufacturer (at $1/e^2$ points). The ratio of the transmitted power ϕ to the power Φ_0

TABLE 12-2. Radiant Exposures Required to Produce a Visible Change on Various Sensitive Media

Sensitive Surface	Q-Switched Ruby Laser (694.3 nm)		Q-Switched Neodymium Laser (1.06 μm)	
	Threshold (J/cm^2)	Saturation (J/cm^2)	Threshold (J/cm^2)	Saturation (J/cm^2)
Fully developed Polaroid print, black (coated or uncoated)	0.056	0.095	0.07	0.2
Kodachrome II transparency, black (unexposed)[a,b]	0.17	0.21	---	---
Fully developed, fully exposed photographic film (Kodak Panatomic X)[b]	0.08	0.2	0.08	0.18
Dupont Lino-Write 7 direct writing photorecording paper [c]	0.01	0.05	0.02	0.09
Kodak Linagraph direct print paper [c]	0.01	0.05	0.02	0.09
Black paper used to protect sheet film [a]	0.22	0.22	---	---
Black masking tape	0.07	0.08	0.1	0.12
Carbon paper (Tru Rite type I) Grade A, black medium finish[d]	0.024	0.036	0.04	0.06
Black printer's ink on white paper	0.16	0.25	---	---

[a] Both the color transparency and the black paper used to protect photographic film employ dyes which have greatly reduced absorption characteristics in the near-infrared spectrum. The experimental arrangement used at USAEHA did not permit accurate measurement of radiant exposures above 0.7 j/cm^2; hence, threshold data at 1.06 μ could not be obtained.

[b] Both the unexposed color transparency and the fully exposed black and white film had differing thresholds depending on the side exposed. The thresholds listed are for the most sensitive film sides: the emulsion side for the Panatomic X and the nonemulsion side for the Kodachrome II.

[c] The visible response noted was a darkening of the paper. The responses of these papers varied depending on previous exposure to ambient light.

[d] The visible response noted was a change in surface finish from a dull black to a glossy black.

Note: The visible change is normally a lightening of the surface unless noted. Preliminary measurements of the sensitivity of black Polaroid print film to non-Q-switched exposure indicated an increase in threshold of approximately one order of magnitude. Saturation levels are provided only for the minimal type of surface change. In most cases more striking changes occur at still higher radiant exposures.

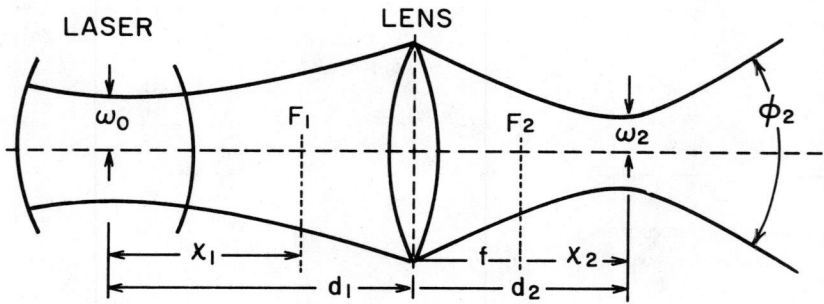

Figure 12-14. Gaussian Beam Wavefront. Notice how the radius of curvature shape changes in the near field. The wavefronts are plane waves at the locations of w_0 and w_2.

entering the aperture Φ/Φ_o is given as follows:

$$\Phi/\Phi_o = 1 - \exp[-2\ (D/a')^2] \qquad (12\text{-}21)$$
$$= 1 - \exp[-(D^2/a^2)]$$

As an example consider a laser beam where a' has been defined by the manufacturer as 1.6 cm and where the radiant power Φ_o is 1 W. From equation (12-21) the amount of power entering the 7-mm pupil is equal to:

$$\Phi/\Phi_1 = 1 - \exp[-2\ \#(0.7^2/1.6^2)] \qquad (12\text{-}22)$$
$$= 1/3$$
$$= 33\%$$

hence $\Phi = 0.33$ W.

12.8 GAUSSIAN BEAM WAVEFRONTS

So far this discussion both the definition of beam divergence and the range equation have been simplified. Those formulas are reasonably accurate for all but "near-field" situations. "Near field" means the region where the wavefront of the emergent laser beam is changing. As the beam reaches the "far field," the wavefront is a circular wavefront whose origin is a point at the laser. However in the near field, as the beam emerges from the laser cavity, the wavefront has quite a different shape, as shown in Fig. 12-14. Some individuals working in laser technology define a distance r_f in the beginning of the far field where the beam has clearly reached the far field:

$$r_f \cong D_a^2/\lambda \qquad (12\text{-}23)$$

where D_a is the laser's exit aperture (laser tube's bore diameter) and λ the wavelength.

As an example, a He-Ne laser which emits at a wavelength of 632.8 nm (i.e., 6.328×10^{-5} cm) and having a 1-mm exit aperture ($D_a = 0.1$ cm) gives us a far-field distance of:

$$r_f \cong (0.1 \text{ cm})^2 / (6.328 \times 10^{-5} \text{ cm})$$
$$\cong 160 \text{ cm}$$

A ruby laser with a wavelength of 6.943×10^{-5} cm and with an exit aperture $D_a = 1$ cm provides a minimal distance to the far field $r_f \cong 140$ m.

However, the value of formula (12-23) is sometimes debated. Other "experts" define r_f by other formulae. What really is of value is a general geometrical formula that permits us to describe a fundamental term known as the "beam waist" dimension w_0 and the Gaussian beam size with distance. First defined by Kogelnick (1966), w_0 is the beam mode dimension or beam *waist*, which is the *radius* of the beam to the $1/e^2$-peak-irradiance point.

12.8.1 Beam Divergence and Diameter

The term w_0 also determines the beam divergence for *higher-order modes*. Bridges (1975) has shown that the limiting full-angle beam divergence $\phi_{\lim}'$ is:

$$\phi_{\lim}' = \sqrt{2 (D_c/d_c)} \, (\sqrt{d_c/R_c}) \qquad (12\text{-}24)$$

which corresponds to the 1/e-point divergence of $\phi_{\lim}$ of:

$$\phi_{\lim} = D_a/d_c \, (\sqrt{d_c/R_c}) \qquad (12\text{-}25)$$

where D_a is the diameter of the confocal cavity (mirror aperture), d_c is the space between the mirrors, and R_c is the radii of the mirrors. Figure 12-15 shows some common resonator configurations that the wavelength λ does not appear in the expression.

If a single-mode laser beam is now considered, then the beam waist w_0 and the beam radius $w(z)$ at any point along the z propagation axis (along which range r is measured) give the following general formulae. The beam diameter as a function of the range along the z axis.

$$D_L = 2w(z) \qquad (12\text{-}26)$$
$$= 2w_0 \sqrt{1 + (\lambda z/\pi w_0^2)^2}$$

The range r could be used instead of z in the far field, but z was retained to maintain

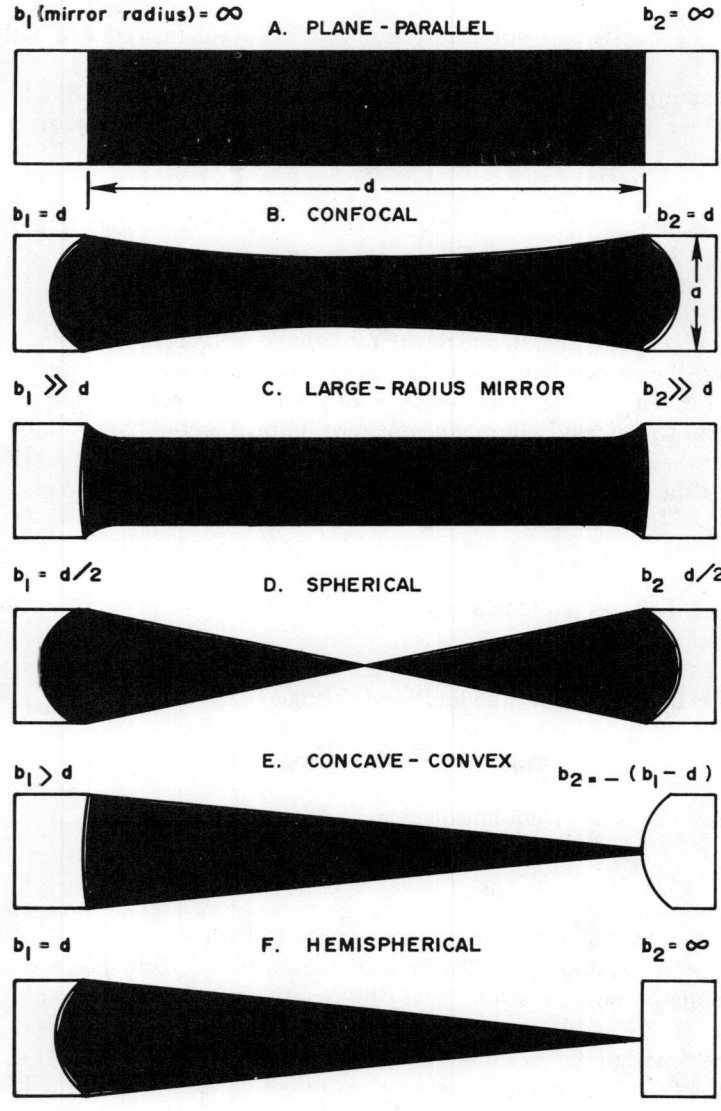

Figure 12-15. Common resonator configurations. Solid state lasers have used plane-parallel resonators. Many modern small HeNe lasers use a hemispherical cavity. Most representative calculations are performed for a confocal cavity. The radii R_c are represented by b_1 and b_2.

Laser Beam Diagnostics

the same symbols as used by Kogelnick and Li (1966). Furthermore, z is measured from the beam waist and r is typically measured from the output mirror.

The full angle beam divergence in the far field is:

$$\phi' = 2\lambda/\pi w_0$$

or

$$\phi = \sqrt{2}\lambda/\pi w_0$$

(12-27)

and the beam waist radius of a confocal resonator is:

$$w_0^2 = d_c \lambda / 2\pi$$

or

$$w_0 = \sqrt{d_c \lambda / 2\pi}$$

(12-28)

These formulae provide the essential characteristics of a Gaussian beam.

12.8.2 Gaussian Beam Front Radius of Curvature

The most fascinating aspect of Gaussian beam propagation is that the wavefront changes in the "near field" (Fig. 12-14). The radius of curvature $R_c(z)$ of the beam's "equiphase" wavefront varies with distance and is given by:

$$R_c(z) = z[1 + (d_c/2z)^2] \text{ for a confocal resonator}$$

or

$$= z[1 + (\pi w_0^2/\lambda z)^2] \text{ in general}$$

(12-29)

12.8.3 Focused Gaussian Beam

Quite often it is desirable to know the beam waist of a focused beam. This new focal spot size w is dependent upon the original w_0 and does not change in magnitude with movement of the lens away from the beam waist. Unfortunately the original beam waist w_0 and its position behind the laser output aperture are not always known and must be determined experimentally by measuring $w(z)$ at several locations or by estimating from the laser's specifications. It is only approximately equal to f and is correctly found only by solving the following formulae for w_1, x_1, x_2 through the use of the "confocal parameters" b_1 and b_2:

$$b_1 = 2\pi \cdot w_0^2/\lambda \quad \text{and} \quad b_2 = 2\pi w_1^2/\lambda \qquad (12\text{-}30)$$

The following equations are employed:

$$(d_1 - f)/(b_2 - f) = b_1/b_2 \qquad (12\text{-}31)$$
$$(d_1 - f) \cdot (d_2 - f) = f^2 - b_1 \cdot b_2/4 \qquad (12\text{-}32)$$
$$x_2/x_1 = b_2/b_1 = 4(f/b_1)^2/[4(x_1 \cdot b_1)^2 + 1] \qquad (12\text{-}33)$$

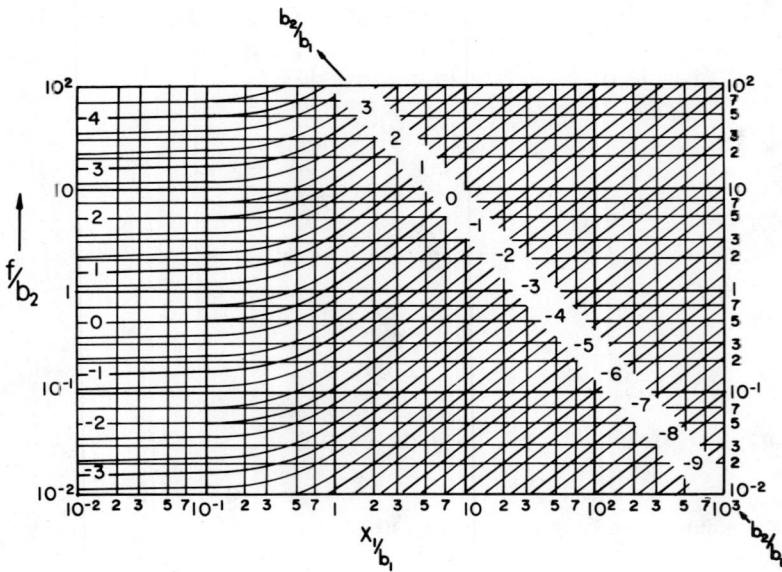

Figure 12-16. Focal Beam Waist. This graph permits one to solve for different values of x_2 and w_2 focal beam waists of equations.

where x_1, x_2, d_1, and d_2 are defined in Figure 12-14. In the case where another lens is placed in a focal beam waist w_1, the next waist w_2 is defined by:

$$w_2 = (w_1 f\lambda/\pi \cdot w_1^2) / \sqrt{1 + (f\lambda/\pi \cdot w_1)^2} \tag{12-34}$$

The new focal distance is:

$$d_3 = f/[1 + (f \cdot \lambda/\pi \cdot w_1^2)^2] \tag{12-35}$$

This formula assumes that the beam is not truncated by an aperture or by the outer edge of the lens.

Figure 12-16 provides a graph from Svetlik (1975) for solving these different values of focal beam waists w and their location along the z (or) r axis after the beam has been transformed (focused) by the lens. The Svetlik graph permits the rapid determination of b_2/b_1 and x_1/b_1. As an example, consider a diverging Gaussian beam with $b_1 = 0.52$ m that is transformed by a lens with $f = 1.0$ m. The lens-to-input-waist distance d_1 is 1.2 m. What is the location of the output waist and what is the confocal parameter b_2?

From these values one calculates $f/b_1 = 1.92$, and since $x_1 = (d_1 - f) = 0.2$ m, the ratio $x_1/b_1 = 0.38$. Using the Svetlik graph, $b_2/b_1 = 8$, hence the other confocal parameter $b_2 = 8 \times 0.52 = 4.16$ m, and from equation (12-33) one calculates $x_2 = 8 \times 0.2$ m $= 1.6$ m and $d_2 = 1.6$ m $+ 1.0$ m $= 2.6$ m.

A focused Gaussian beam, after being transformed by a lens and focused, leaves the focal spot with a final beam divergence of:

$$\phi_2 = 2\pi/\lambda \cdot w_1 \qquad (12\text{-}36)$$

where $2 w_1$ is the focal spot diameter.

12.9 LASER BEAM COLLIMATORS

A simplified formula that comes out of much of the previous discussion is that if one used a collimator immediately in front of the laser the new divergence ϕ_2 and new diameter a_2 have a certain ratio related to the ratio of the initial diameter a_1 and the initial beam divergence ϕ_1, namely:

$$a_1/a_2 \cong \phi_2/\phi_1 \qquad (12\text{-}37)$$

As an example, a laser has an initial beam diameter of 5 mm and a divergence of 3 mrad. It is transformed by a collimator (afocal lens pair) to an emerging diameter of 1.5 cm as would occur with a three-power Gallilean telescope. The divergence would be reduced also by a factor of 3 — to 1 mrad. This approximate formula generally works rather nicely in practice.

12.10 PLANE WAVEFRONTS

As shown above, a Gaussian beam neither propagates over a great distance nor is it focused in the same manner as a plane wave truncated by an aperture. In the latter case the physical optics formulae of Rayleigh serve quite nicely. In some cases, where a laser is of a higher order mode or where the beam is severely truncated by an aperture of diameter D, the approximations calculated from the formula for the Airy disc can be used for defining the far-field divergence ϕ_{ff} and the focal spot size after the beam has been focused by a thin lens of focal length f. The formulae are:

$$\phi_{ff} = 2.44 \, \lambda/D \qquad (12\text{-}38)$$

and for a focused beam the focal spot d_f is defined as:

$$d_f = 2.44 \, \lambda f/D \qquad (12\text{-}39)$$

The values of ϕ_{ff} and d_f are defined at the first minima of the Fraunhofer diffraction pattern which is known as the Airy disc diameter. Figure 2-12 shows a pattern of a plane wave diffracted by a circular aperture of diameter D. The Gaussian beam formulae discussed in the previous section provide the actual beam diameter at $1/e^2$

points for a Gaussian focused beam and these two formulae define this for the plane wave or heavily truncated Gaussian profile.

Before ending the subject of focused beams several important generalities should be noted. First of all, the diffraction-limited beam spot diameter d_f, which in simple terms is the smallest spot size obtainable by means of a given optical system, is larger for longer focal length lenses. Thus to focus a spot at quite a considerable distance it is not sufficient merely to have a long-focal-length lens. This will not provide a very small focal spot diameter unless the lens is enlarged and the initial beam is expanded to fill that lens. Finally, it should be noted that the shorter the wavelength of the optical radiation the smaller will be the diffraction-limited spot according to theory.

12.11 REVIEW QUESTIONS

1. A laser beam has an emergent beam diameter of 1 cm and has a diameter at 1 km of 101 cm. What is the beam divergence?

2. A laser beam has an initial beam diameter of 1 mm and an emergent beam divergence of 0.5 mrad. What is the beam diameter at 50 m?

3. The atmospheric attenuation coefficient is 5.8×10^{-7} cm^{-1}. What is this attenuation coefficient in units of km^{-1}? How would it be expressed in terms of dB/km?

4. Find the irradiance in a He-Ne laser beam at a distance of 300 m where the emergent beam diameter is 2 mm and the beam divergence is 0.3 mrad.

5. What is the Airy disc diameter for a plane-wave incident at a 7-mm aperture and focused with a thin lens having a focal length of 4 cm at the primary He-Ne wavelength in the visible spectrum?

6. A highly irregular laser beam with an emergent beam energy of 1.0 J has an emergent beam peak radiant exposure of 3.4 J/cm^2 and a radiant exposure measured at 1.0 km of 5.6×10^{-5} J/cm^2. What is the effective emergent beam diameter and effective beam divergence?

7. A laser has a Gaussian-beam, single-mode output at 632.8 nm. The beam waist given by the manufacturer of the cavity is 2 mm. Using a thin lens with a focal length of 25 cm located 20 cm from the beam waist, what transformed beam waist will exist at the focal spot and at what distance from the lens will this focal spot be located?

8. What is the beam irradiance in the focal spot of a thin lens with a focal length of 25 cm when the 2-cm diameter lens aperture intercepts the center of a large laser beam of diameter #D_L = 70 mm where the beam irradiance at the lens is 7 mW/cm^2?

9. A diffuse black rod 1 mm in diameter is passed through an argon laser beam. The beam is terminated in a power monitor which reads 1 watt before passage and has a 200 mW minimum as the rod passes through the beam. What is the beam diameter?

10. The manufacturer specifies the beam divergence and emergent beam diameter at $1/e^2$ points of 0.79 mrad and 3 mm. What are these parameters when defined at $1/e$-points?

12.12 REFERENCES

Altman, J. H., Grum, F., and Nelson, C. N., 1973, Photographic speeds based on radiant energy units, *Photog. Sci. Eng.* **17**(6):513–517.

Arnaud, J. A., Hubbard, W. M., Mandeville, G. D., de la Claviere, B., Franke, E. A., and Franke, J. M., 1971, Technique for fast measurement of Gaussian laser beam parameters, *Appl. Opt.* **10**:2775–2776.

Arnaud, J. A., 1976, "Beam and Fibre Optics," Academic Press, New York.

Avizonis, P. V., Doss, T. T., and Heimlich, R., 1967, Measurement of beam divergence of Q-switched ruby laser rods, *Rev. Sci. Instrum.* **38**:331–334.

Bird, G. R., Jones, R. C., and Ames, A. E., 1969, The efficiency of radiation detection by photographic film: State-of-the-art and methods for improvement, *Appl. Opt.* **8**(12):2389–2405.

Birky, M. M., 1969, Simultaneous recording of near-field and far-field patterns of lasers, *Appl. Opt.* **8**:2249–2253.

Bloom, A. L., 1968, "Gas Lasers," John Wiley and Sons, New York.

Boyd, G. D., and Gordon, J. P., 1961, Confocal multimode resonator for millimeter through optical wavelength masers, *Bell System Tech. J.* **40**:489–508.

Bridges, W. G., 1975, Divergence of high order Gaussian modes, *Appl. Opt.* **14**(10):2346–2347.

Burnham, D. C., 1970, Laser beam photography by a multiple beam technique, *Appl. Opt.* **9**:1482.

Carlson, F. P., 1977, "Introduction to Applied Optics for Engineers," Academic Press, New York.

Dickson, L. D., 1979, Ronchi ruling method for measuring a Gaussian beam diameter, *Opt. Eng.* **18**(1):70–75.

Dickson, L. D., 1970, Characteristics of a propagating Gaussian beam, *Appl. Opt.* **9**(8):1854–1861.

Fallon, J. P. and Kellen, P. F., 1973, Film sensitometry with laser sources, *Opt. Eng.* **12**(2):75–79.

Firester, A. H., Heller, M. E., and Sheng, P., 1977, Knife-edge scanning measurements of subwavelength focused light beams, *Appl. Opt.* **16**(7):1971–1974.

Gardiner, H. A. B., Merrill, J. J., Pendleton, W. R., and Baker, D. J., 1969, Systematic errors in emission cross-sections arising in the analysis of laboratory beam measurements, *Appl. Opt.* **8**(4):799–806.

Grimblatov, V. M., Bekshaev, A. Ya., and Kalugin, V. V., 1978, Modulation method of measuring the spatial characteristics of laser radiation, *Sov. J. Quant Electr.* **8**(5):644–648.

Heard, H. G., 1968, "Laser Parameter Measurements Handbook," J. Wiley and Sons, New York.

Hirleman, E. D., and Stevenson, W. H., 1978, Intensity distribution properties of a Gaussian laser beam focus, *Appl. Opt.* **17**(21):3496–3499.

Hoag, A. A., and Miller, W. C., 1969, Application of photographic materials in astronomy, *Appl. Opt.* **8**(12):2417–2429.

Johnson, E. G., 1979, Laser beam profile measurements using spatial sampling, Fourier Optics and Holography, NBS Tech. Note 1009, NBS Boulder, CO.

Kogelnick, H., 1966, Modes in optical resonators, *in* "Lasers," (A. K. Levine, ed.) Decker, New York.

Kogelnick, H. and Li, T., 1966, Laser beams and resonators, *Appl. Opt.* **5**:1550–1567; and *Proc. IEEE* **54**(10):1312–1329.

Laures, P., 1967, Geometrical approach to Gaussian beam propagation, *Appl. Opt.* **6**:747–748.

Levi, L. (ed.), 1974, "CRC Handbook of Tables of Functions for Applied Optics," CRC Press, Inc., Cleveland, OH.

Loewen, E. G., Neviere, M., and Maystre, D., 1976, Optimal design for beam sampling mirror gratings, *Appl. Opt.* **15**:2937–2939.

Moser, H. O., 1974, Instrument for measuring angular intensity distributions of light sources within a few milliseconds, *Appl. Opt.* **13**(1):173–176.

Schell, P. G., and G. Tyrar, 1971, Irradiance from an aperture with a truncated Gaussian field distribution, *J. Opt. Soc. Am.* **61**(1):31–35.

Seka, W., and Zimmermann, J., 1974, Photodiode arrays: A convenient tool for laser diagnostics, *Rev. Sci. Instrum.* **45**:1175–1176.

Sinclair, D. C. and Bell, W. E., 1969, "Gas Laser Technology," Holt Rinehart and Winston, New York.

Smith, W. L., DeGroot, A. J., and Weber, M. J., 1978, Silicon vidicon system for measuring laser intensity profiles, *Appl. Opt.* **17**(24):3938–3944.

Suzaki, Y., and Tichibana, A., 1975, Measurement of the μm-sized radius of Gaussian laser beams using the scanning knife-edge, *Appl. Opt.* **14**:2809–2810.

Suzaki, Y., and Tachibana, A., 1977, Measurement of the laser beam divergence, *Appl. Opt.* **16**(6):1481–1482.

Svelto, O., 1976, "Principles of Lasers," Plenum Press, New York.

Svetlik, J., 1975, Graphical aid to the transformation of a laser beam by a thin lens, *Appl. Opt.* **14**(10):2347–2348.

Thomas, W., Jr., 1973, "SPSE Handbook of Photographic Science and Engineering," J. Wiley and Sons, New York.

Wick, R. V., Saxman, A. C., and Blankinship, E. A., 1973, Real time intensity profiling and beam divergence measurement of a laser beam, *in* "Electro-Optical Systems Design Conference-1973," pp 294–300; (available from Industrial and Scientific Conference Management, Inc., Chicago, Illinois 60606).

Williams, C. S., 1973, Gaussian beam formulas from diffraction theory, *Appl. Opt.* **12**(4):872–876.

Winer, I. M., 1966, A self-calibrating technique for measuring laser beam intensity distributions, *Appl. Opt.* **5**(9):1437–1439.

Wolf, E., 1978, Coherence and radiometry, *J. Opt. Soc. Amer.* **68**(1):6–17.

Woodlief, T., Jr., 1973, "SPSE Handbook of Photographic Science and Engineering," John Wiley and Sons, New York.

Yoshida, A. and Asakura, T., 1976, A simple technique for quickly measuring the spot size of Gaussian laser beams, *Opt. and Laser Tech.* **1**:273–274.

Chapter 13
Atmospheric Propagation of Laser Beams

13.1 GENERAL

To this point lasers and other light beams have been characterized by measurement and by calculation, but the effects of a non-homogeneous or turbulent medium have been ignored. Atmospheric attenuation has been only briefly mentioned. In this chapter these atmospheric effects will be examined in some detail. From a laser-safety standpoint, atmospheric effects are generally only of importance at distances of 300 meters or greater. This chapter may therefore be skipped over by those not concerned with outdoor laser use.

13.2 ATMOSPHERIC ATTENUATION

The effect of atmospheric attenuation may become a major factor in evaluating the irradiance or radiant exposure at distances greater than a few kilometers. This attenuation is the sum of three effects: (1) *Mie (or large particle) scattering,* where the scattering particle's size is much greater than λ (wavelength of the light), and is normally the greatest contributor; (2) *Rayleigh (or molecular) scattering,* where particle size is equal to or less than the wavelength, and is essentially constant for a given wavelength; and (3) *absorption by gas molecules* which is relatively insignificant in comparison to scattering in the visible spectrum and may therefore be disregarded in that region of the optical spectrum. Rayleigh scattering is strongly wavelength dependent; shorter wavelengths are predominantly scattered (Chapter 2).

13.2.1 Scattering

Attenuation due to scattering is much more pronounced at shorter wavelengths, thus red light from a ruby laser is scattered far less than wavelengths in the blue end of the visible spectrum and IR-A wavelengths such as 1064 nm would be scattered still less. A clean atmosphere may therefore be expected to be quite transparent to the ruby or neodymium wavelengths. The atmospheric attenuation effect upon the irradiance E of a non-diverging beam as derived in Chapter 2, section 2.10, is expressed as:

$$E = E_0 \, e^{-\mu r} \qquad (13\text{-}1)$$

where the term E_0 is the emergent beam irradiance at zero range, r is the range expressed in m, cm, or km, and μ is the attenuation coefficient expressed in cm^{-1}, m^{-1}, or km^{-1}. By definition, μ is the sum of the scattering coefficient σ and the absorption coefficient:

$$\mu = \sigma + \alpha \qquad (13\text{-}2)$$

The scattering coefficient is the sum of the Mie and Rayleigh scattering coefficients, σ_M and σ_R; therefore Eqn. 13-2 becomes:

$$\mu = \sigma_M + \sigma_R + \alpha \qquad (13\text{-}3)$$

As an illustration, the Rayleigh scattering effect may attenuate a ruby or neodymium laser beam by as little as 1% (1064 nm) or 4.5% (at 694.3 nm) at 10 km and 10 to 40% at 100 km. Attenuation coefficients are also sometimes expressed in terms of dB per kilometer. A value of 10 dB per kilometer corresponds to an attenuation coefficient of 2.3 km^{-1} or 2.3×10^{-5} cm^{-1}.

The "meterological range" or "visibility range," r_v, based upon the entire visible spectrum may not be readily utilized in arriving at the attenuation coefficient at a given laser wavelength since the ratio of σ_M and σ_R is not constant with changing wavelength. The visibility range is defined as the horizontal distance where the contrast transmission of the atmosphere is 2% (Middleton, 1958). Contrast transmission here refers to the visibility of certain contrast targets at a distance. For broad-band sources such as searchlights, the average value of μ (which we can represent as μ_v) is usually given as:

$$\mu_v = 3.912/r_v \qquad (13\text{-}4)$$

In contrast to μ_v which is an average attenuation coefficient, the spectral attenuation coefficient, μ, varies with wavelength and values range from 10^{-4} per cm in thick fog to 10^{-7} cm^{-1} in air of incredibly good visibility. The Rayleigh scattering coefficient at 694.3 nm is 4.8×10^{-8} cm^{-1}, and is 1.8×10^{-7} cm^{-1} at 500 nm. The general relation for dry air at STP (standard temperature and pressure) if the wavelength λ is in cm and σ_R is in cm^{-1} is:

$$\sigma_R \cong (1.1 \times 10^{-24})/(\lambda^4) \qquad (13\text{-}5a)$$

or, more generally for pure dry air (Middleton, 1958):

$$\sigma_R = 8\pi^3(n_p^2 - 1)^2 \cdot (6 + 3\rho_p)/3\lambda^4 \, N(6 - 7\rho_p) \qquad (13\text{-}5b)$$

or in the most general case:

$$\sigma_R = (4\pi^2 N^2 V^2/\lambda^4)(n_p^2 - n_0^2)/(n_p^2 + 2n_0^2)^2 \qquad (13\text{-}5c)$$

where ρ_p is the factor of depolarization for air ($\rho \cong 0.042$), where N is the number of particles per unit volume (cm³), V is the scattering particle's volume (cm³), n_0 the refractive index of the medium in which particles are suspended, and n_p is the refractive index of the particles. In the far-infrared, water droplets and other aerosols rather than air molecules serve to produce much of the Rayleigh scattering. The effect of aerosols (Mie scattering) in even the cleanest atmospheres raises μ at 694.3 nm to at least 5×10^{-7} cm⁻¹ and more typically to 10^{-6} cm⁻¹.

Rayleigh scattering varies inversely as the fourth power of the wavelength. It is the dominant Rayleigh scattering of short wavelength sunlight that creates the blue sky. Indeed, if one could view the world only through perception of ultraviolet radiation, the world would be eternally hazy due to this type of atmospheric scattering. Rayleigh scattered light has a preferential polarization, which can be readily demonstrated by viewing the blue, daylit sky through polarizing filters at different angles with respect to the sun. Rayleigh scattering is not strongly directional; that is, the angular dependence of scattered radiation is not very dramatic. The angular dependence for an unpolarized beam follows a $(1 + \cos^2 \theta_s)$ function, where θ_s is the angle of the scattered ray relative to the beam axis. Therefore scattering at 0° and 180° (on-axis forward and backward) is only twice as intense as side scatter at 90° from the axis; this side scatter is most polarized. Tricker (1970) provides a nice discussion of atmospheric scattering for the reader interested in further details. The formulae for Rayleigh scattering presented in most texts vary due to different approximations of σ_R. A useful formula from Tricker (1970) for the Rayleigh scattered irradiance E_{rs} from a small collimated beam at a distance r_s to the side, relative to the beam irradiance E_0 is:

$$E_{rs} = (\sigma_R^2 V^2)(1 + \cos^2 \theta_s)(E_0)/r_s^2 \lambda^4 \qquad (13\text{-}6)$$

In contrast to Rayleigh scattering, Mie scattering shows a less marked wavelength dependence and no strong polarizing effect. The scattering profile is dependent upon particle size. Mie scattering has a very strong forward component that is immediately apparent when the beam of a low-power He-Ne laser is viewed at night. The beam path can readily be seen when standing downrange near the beam and looking back toward the laser (section 13.9). Because the magnitude of the backscatter is far, far less, than forward scatter, it is normally not possible to see the beam path while looking downrange and standing near the laser. Mie scattering characteristics can be calculated, but are complex functions of particle index of refraction, of size and shape, of wavelength, and of scattering angle.

Figure 13-1 provides the sea-level atmospheric scattering coefficient at most visible and near-infrared wavelengths as a function of meterological visibility. For instance, at a meterological visibility of 23.5 km the attenuation coefficient at the

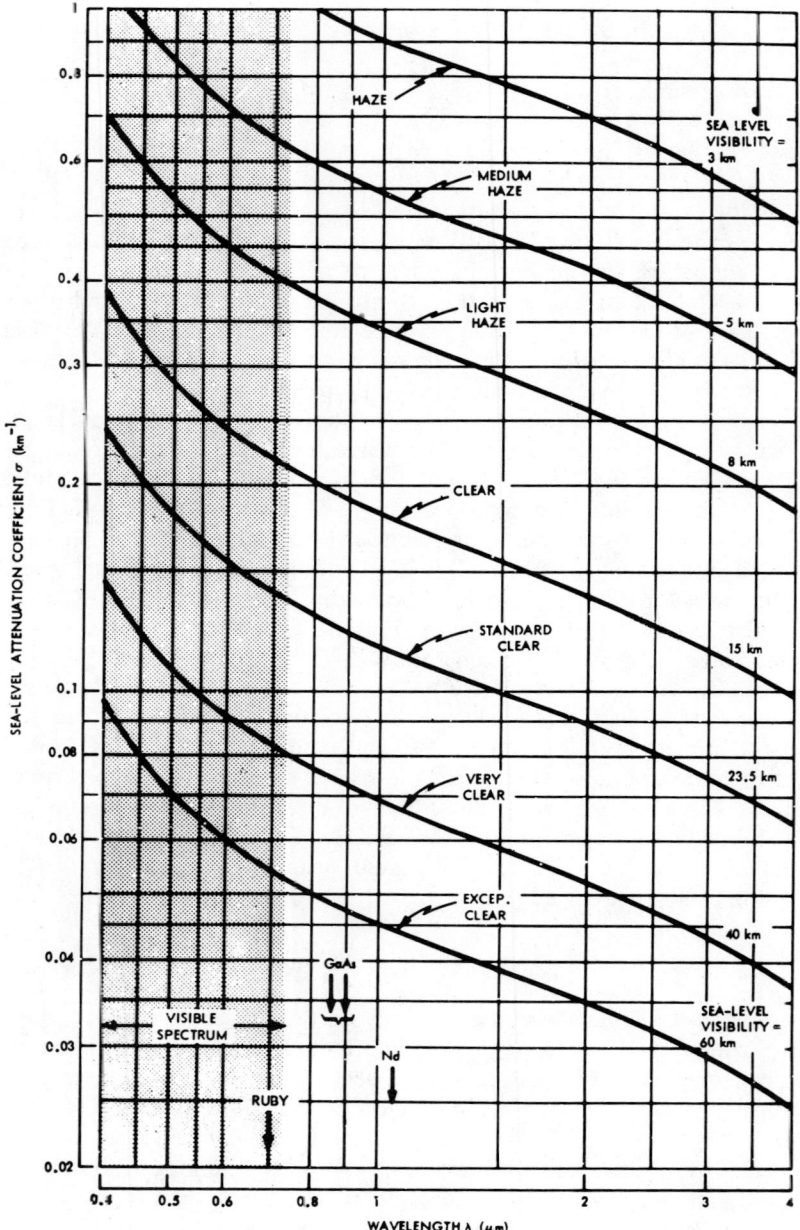

Figure 13-1. Typical values for the total atmospheric spectral scattering coefficient as a function of sea-level meterological visibility. The molecular absorption of water vapour and CO_2 which may be appreciable at some infrared wavelengths is neglected (from Engstrom, 1974, with permission).

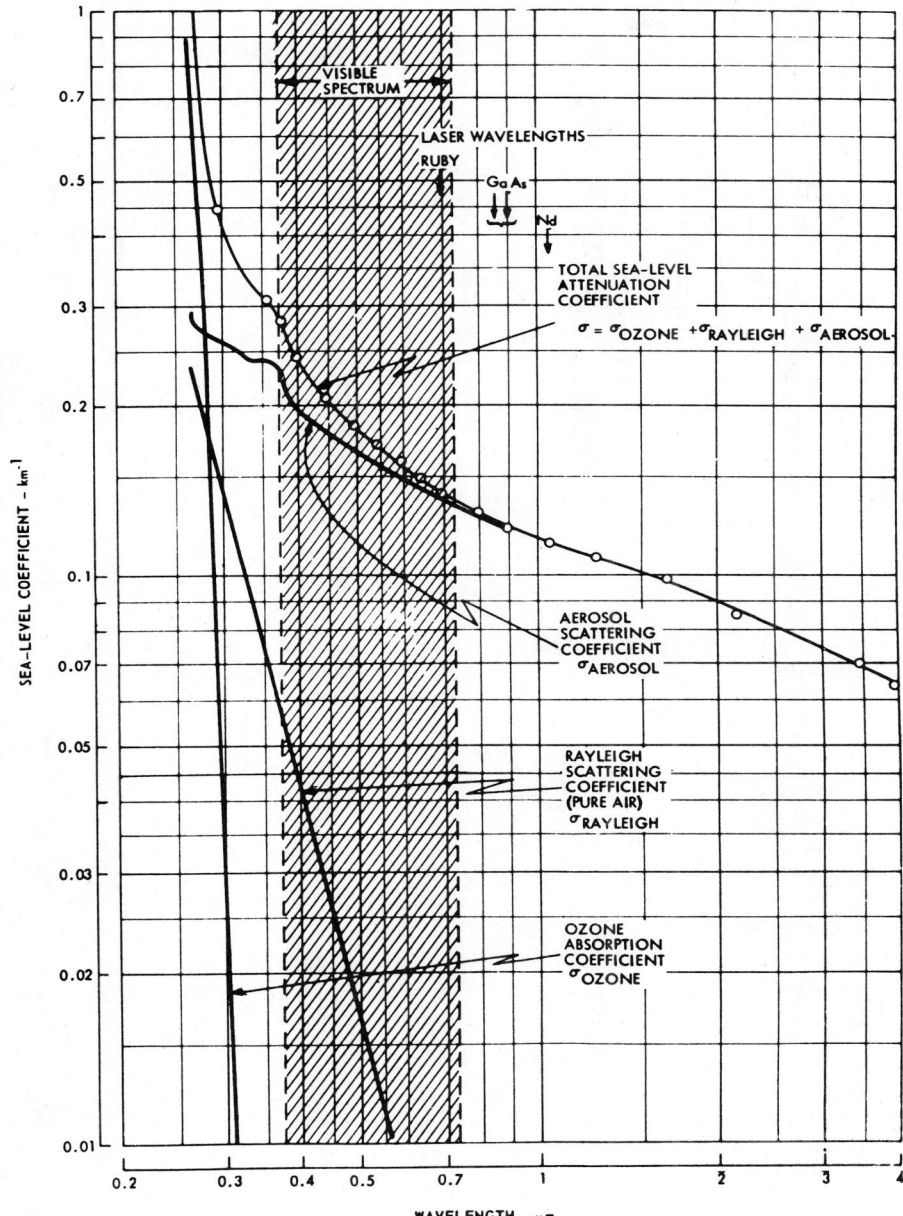

Figure 13-2. The calculated atmospheric attenuation coefficient (neglecting H_2O and CO_2 absorption) is the sum of Rayleigh and Mie scattering coefficients. Ozone absorption dominates in the short ultraviolet region. Circles are calculated points where absorption of H_2O and CO_2 are not significant (from Engstrom, 1974, with permission).

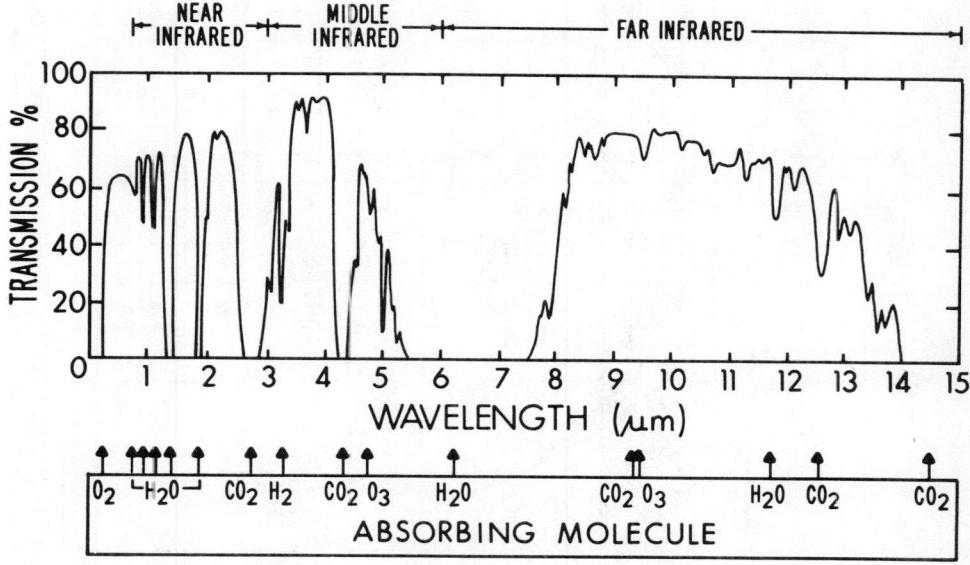

Figure 13-3. Spectral transmission characteristics of the atmosphere in the visible and infrared (low resolution) for a 1830-m path for 17 mm of precipitable water. Note the visible window, the middle IR (3-5 μm) window and the far-IR (8-13 μm) window (adapted from Hudson, 1969).

ruby wavelength 694.3 nm is 1.4×10^{-6} cm^{-1}. The values in Fig. 13-1 are only approximate since the actual scattering coefficient will vary dependent upon the type of aerosol in the atmosphere that determines the meterological visible range. Atmospheric absorption which is negligible in the visible has been neglected. For elevations above sea level the total scattering coefficients are reduced as determined by the approximate formulae listed below for calculating σ as a function of height h (in km) above sea level relative to σ at sea level (σ_o):

$$\sigma_h \cong \sigma_o e^{-0.8 h} \qquad (13\text{-}7)$$

for a horizontal path, and

$$\sigma_{hs} \cong \sigma_o e^{-0.32 h} \qquad (13\text{-}8)$$

for a slant path. Figure 13-2 illustrates the relative contributions of different types of scatter for only one meterological visible range: for $r_v = 23.5$ km which corresponds to the so-called "US model clear standard atmosphere," (Valley, 1965).

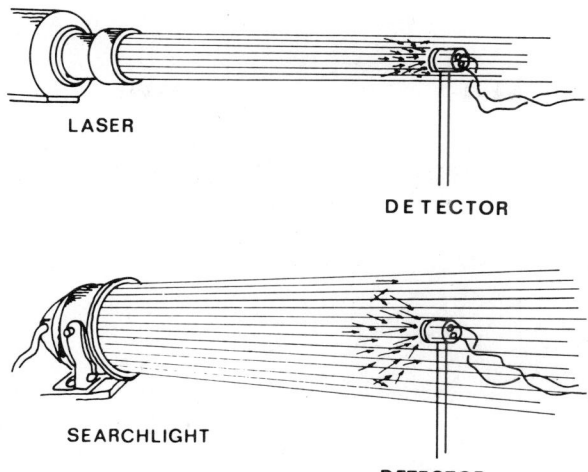

Figure 13-4. Measurements of atmospheric transmission using a laser or a monochromatic searchlight will produce different values because of the larger scattering field in front of the detector when illuminated by the searchlight.

13.2.2 Absorption

At laser wavelengths in the infrared there are many narrow absorption bands due to molecular absorption from gases such as oxygen, carbon-dioxide and nitrogen. At 10.6 μm (carbon-dioxide laser wavelength) the attenuation coefficient in the air is of the order of 10^{-6} cm^{-1}. Atmospheric absorption bands are shown in Fig. 13-3. Figure 13-3 is not sufficiently detailed to permit the resolution of any very narrow transmission bands that may exist at particular laser wavelengths. High resolution transmission data are available from mathematical models and have been tabulated by the Air Force Cambridge Research Laboratories and other organizations (e.g., Valley, 1965; McClatchey and Selby, 1974). Atmospheric absorption in one narrow IR-C region is shown later in connection with section 13.7 (Fig. 13-13).

13.2.3 Measuring Atmospheric Attenuation

The atmospheric attenuation coefficient measured for a broad-beam source may be somewhat less than when measured with a well-collimated laser beam. The explanation of this phenomenon lies in the fact that small-angle forward Mie scattering is quite predominant. For a broad-beam, a detector located at the beam axis measuring the transmitted irradiance would receive scattered light from many angles as shown in Fig. 13-4. On the other hand, if the detector were centered in a well-

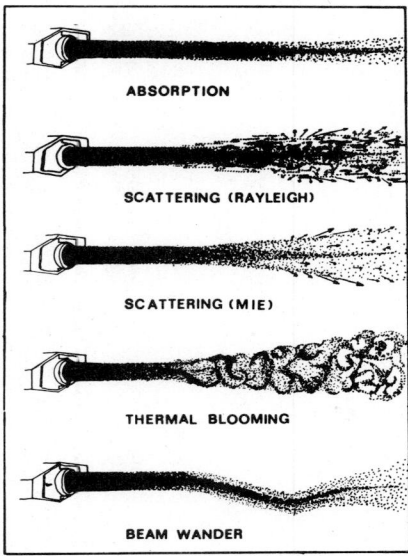

Figure 13-5. Schematic summary of atmospheric effects upon a laser beam. The effects have been exaggerated by the artist for better visualization.

collimated laser beam with a diameter only twice or thrice the detector diameter, with collecting optics, the detector would view very little scattered light. Therefore at a wavelength where Mie scattering is predominant one cannot equate the atmospheric transmittance derived using a searchlight with a narrow-band filtered detector with the transmittance measurement for a collimated laser beam of the same wavelength. There will be less apparent transmittance for the laser beam. To the contrary, Rayleigh scattering does not have a large forward component as it varies as a function of azimuth angle θ_s as a function of $(1 + \cos^2 \theta_s)$. Figure 13-2 (lower left corner) shows the strong wavelength dependence $(1/\lambda^4)$ which is characteristic of Rayleigh scattering and its strong contribution to the attenuation coefficient only in the ultraviolet spectral region. Figure 13-5 summarizes the common attenuating effects upon a laser beam and introduces us to the effects of beam wander and scintillation which result from atmospheric turbulence.

13.3 ATMOSPHERIC TURBULENCE

13.3.1 Irradiance Fluctuations

The safety implications of atmospheric scintillation of laser beams have long

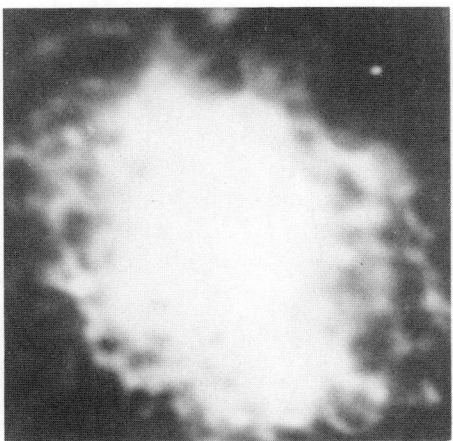 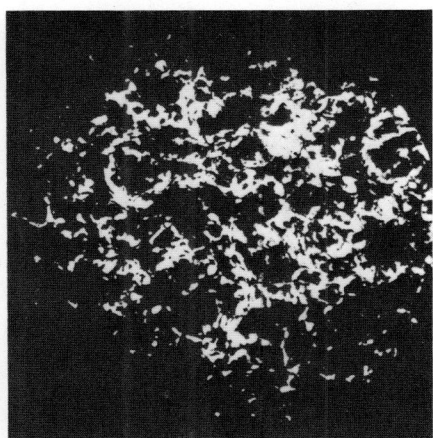

Figure 13-6. Photograph of beam irradiance profiles of ruby laser at 0.5 km (left photo) and at 1.5 km (right photo) taken during a period of moderately strong turbulence. Note the increased breakup of the beam at the greatest distance. Saturation of scintillation will preclude an increased spread of localized irradiances at greater distances.

been recognized. When military laser rangefinders were tested in the field, the "hot spots" (Fig. 13-6) created by atmospheric turbulence near the ground were looked upon as an uncertain variable in determining a laser's hazardous range (Sliney, 1966). In the past ten years several studies have been performed using a variety of lasers, primarily He-Ne, in an effort to quantify this adverse effect (Deitz, 1969, 1970; Dabbert, 1971, 1973). These studies resulted in statistical probabilities of finding an irradiance in a "hot spot" at a certain factor above the mean irradiance. Deitz made the first significant contribution in this area by developing a "nomograph" (Fig. 13-7) for such a purpose (Deitz, 1969). The contribution of turbulence was accounted for by a function of C_N, the *atmospheric refractive index structure constant*, which was dependent largely upon the gradient of air temperature just above the ground. The parameter C_N varies continuously, even on an hourly basis (Fig. 13-8), and with wavelength (Fig. 13-9). There are difficulties in measuring C_N although some simplified optical methods such as that of Weseley and Derzko (1975), and tried by one author (Sliney) have worked reasonably well in the field.

The value of C_N near the ground varies most typically from 5×10^{-8} to 1×10^{-6} $m^{-1/3}$. Turbulence effects (as characterized by C_N) are greatest when the air temperature gradient with height above ground is greatest. It is difficult to generalize, but turbulence appears to be greatest when the sun is out, the sky is cloudless, and the ground is hot (i.e., characteristic of a hot, desert atmosphere). Likewise, on a cold and cloudy day the value of C_N will be low. The temporal frequency will be

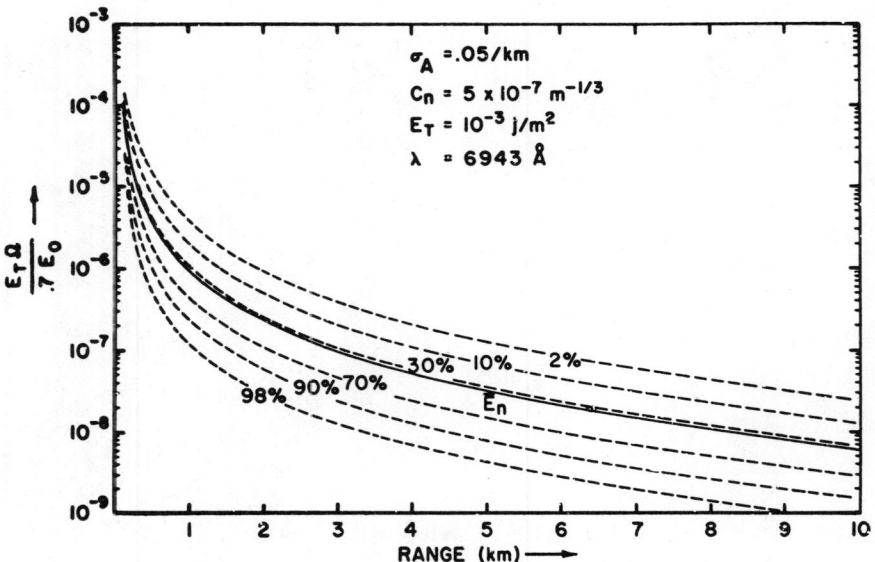

Figure 13-7. Percent probability of beam irradiance exceeding a specified value as affected by atmospheric turbulence (from Deitz, 1969, with permission) for $C_N = 5 \times 10^{-7}$ m$^{-1/3}$ and $\mu = 5 \times 10^{-7}$ cm^{-1}. The ordinate may be thought of as relative radiant exposure. The solid line E_n represents the radiant exposure in a non-turbulent atmosphere. The symbols used by Deitz in this figure are not the same as those used in this text.

lowest and the size of hot spots will be greatest on a still day, and the size of hot spots smallest on a windy day, since the air is mixed by the wind, and turbulons (small pockets of cold air which cause hot spots) are "blown" across the beam rapidly. The smallest pockets of air having uniform temperature are of the order of 0.5 cm ("the inner scale"). The temporal fluctuations of scintillation vary with the wind but have a frequency spectrum up to several hundred Hz. The size of each scintillation spot is often expressed in simple theory as a "transverse correlation distance" or scale length (approximately $\sqrt{\lambda r}$); i.e., it varies as the square root of the range of the propagation beam path (r).

The several theories and the published results of field studies form an extensive literature which is often confusing. Whatever the case, several field observations by the authors down range are worthwhile to remember. The size of hot spots do increase with range although they probably increase very little during strong turbulence beyond the range where "saturation" occurs. At a distance of 800-1200 m the standard deviation of the irradiance distribution no longer increases; this is termed "saturation." A pulsed (~ 1 ms) laser beam profile is frozen when viewed, but the profile of a CW laser beam is constantly changing, and one can see effects of the

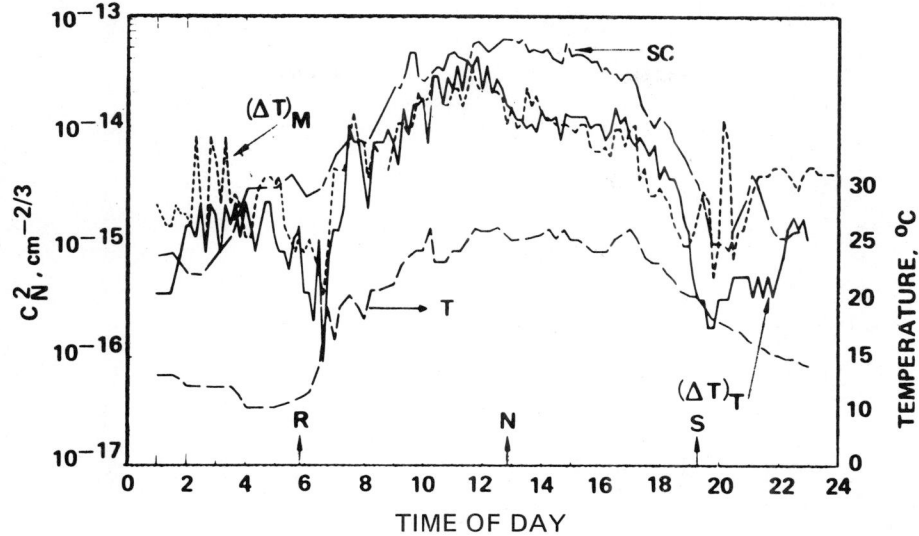

Figure 13-8. Variation of the atmospheric refractive index structure coefficient C_N^2 (left ordinate) in a 24-hr period as measured by three different instruments and the correlation with air temperature T (right coordinate). Note the effects of sunrise (R), solar noon (N), and sunset (S). The three instruments used were an optical scintillometer (SC), and two microthermometers at midrange $(\Delta T)_m$ and at the target $(\Delta T)_T$ (from Pearson, 1975, with permission).

"turbulons" moving across the beam when a cross-wind is present. While the effect of scintillation actually decreases the probability of being exposed to the beam irradiance calculated for the non-turbulent condition, scintillation does indeed present us with a dilemma: that in theory there exists a finite, although very small, risk of being exposed to an instantaneous irradiance that is far in excess of the non-turbulent value. Although some have attempted to calculate statistical risk involved in intrabeam viewing downrange, there has been some debate among laser safety analysts as to the value of using such statistical approaches in establishing "safe" viewing distances, and whether such approaches reveal the full story.

In numerous tests of field lasers by the U.S. Army Environmental Hygiene Agency from 1965 to 1975, the beam irradiance in localized hot spots measured during turbulent conditions appeared to be less on an absolute scale than that predicted by the Deitz nomograph. The most apparent explanation has been that the studies of Deitz and Dabbert did not take into account beam spreading which is always present during periods of strong turbulence. This beam spreading reduces the average beam irradiance so that excursions of localized beam irradiance above the average are not as serious as they appear to be at first glance (Yura, 1971; Ochs and Lawrence, 1971; Whitman and Beran, 1970; Sliney, 1970). Whitman and Beran

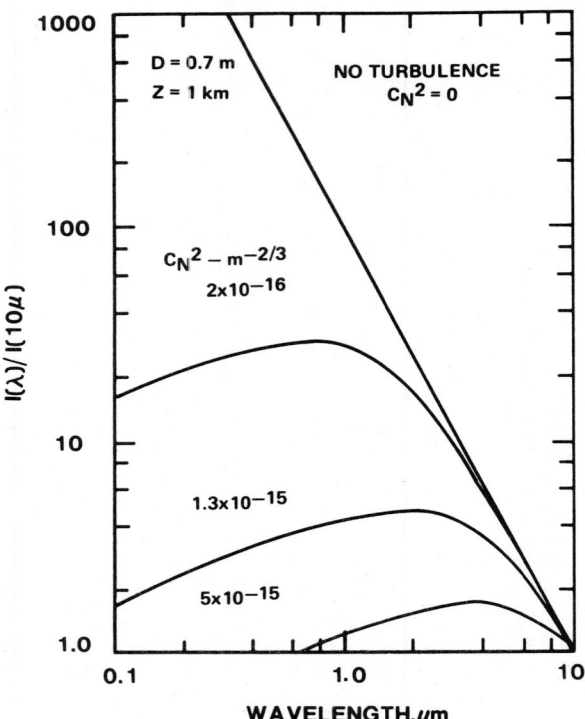

Figure 13-9. Wavelength dependence of turbulence-induced beam spreading and wander effects on the long-term average peak irradiance is shown as normalized by the average irradiance at 10 μm, for different levels of turbulence with an assumed exit aperture diameter of 70 cm and a 1 km beam path (from Gebhardt, 1976, with permission).

predicted that the beam spreading would increase as the $r^{3/2}$ increasing range r and Yura derived a similar dependence (as $r^{8/5}$). As an example, if the turbulence induced beam spread for a 1 mrad beam at 1 km results in a beam diameter of 110 cm (instead of 100 cm) then this 10-cm addition becomes $(3)^{3/2}(10 \text{ cm}) = 90$ cm at 3 km and $D_L = 390$ cm. For strong turbulence ($C_N = 5 \times 10^{-7} \text{ m}^{-1/3}$) the beam spreading at 1 km would be approximately 35 cm by one theoretical prediction (Gebhardt, 1976). Figure 13-10 illustrates the downward displacement of the mean of axial irradiance measurements resulting from ground turbulence. Note that the normal range of irradiance values (bars) seldom exceeds the values calculated for a non-turbulent atmosphere. The estimated attenuation coefficient was 10^{-6} cm^{-1} (10^{-1} km^{-1}).

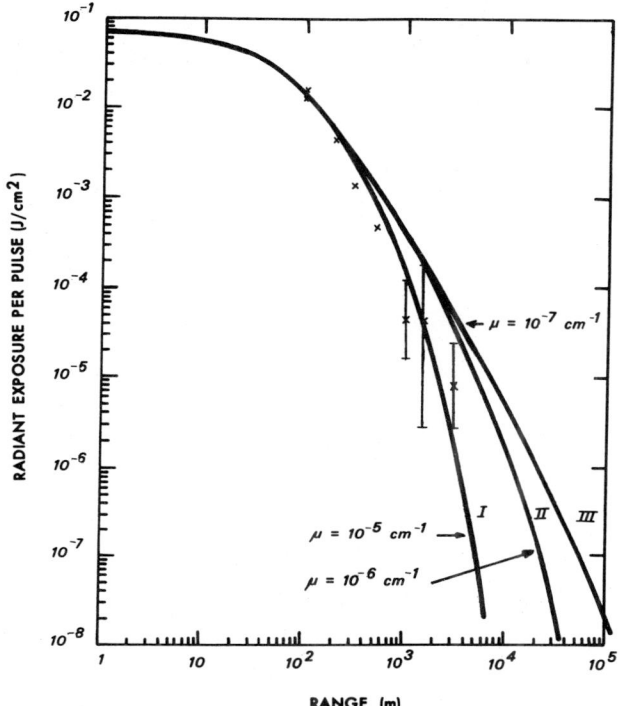

Figure 13-10. Plot of typical range of axial beam radiant exposure measurements under field conditions for a near-earth propagation path for a Q-switched laser rangefinder. Note the spread of readings taken for 100 readings at 1.0, 1.5 and 3.0 km.

13.3.2 Projected Laser Radiance

Most atmospheric propagation studies have been performed by communications engineers and atmospheric physicists who measured the irradiance profile of the laser beam, i.e., the beam "cross section" and did not consider the projected radiance of the laser. The latter parameter is, however, of significance from an eye-safety standpoint. The radiance or "brightness" of an extended light source or IR-A source determines the irradiance falling on the retina (section 3.2.5). The parallel rays from a point source, however, are always imaged on the retina as a minimal image. A source such as a laser is effectively a point source when the intrinsic divergence of the light rays entering the pupil is less than 0.3 mrad. When localized volumes of denser air (turbulons) in the atmosphere tend to focus the collimated rays in a laser beam, the focused rays occasionally can have a divergence greater than 0.3 mrad, and the resulting retinal image is enlarged. The safety question that must

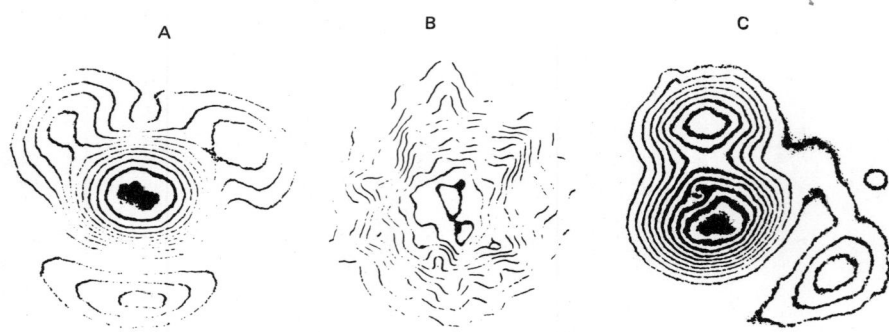

Figure 13-11. Three intrabeam photographic point-spread radiance profiles: (a) weak turbulence; (b) moderate turbulence; and (c) strong turbulence.

be answered when the eye is located within a hot spot of a visible or IR-A laser beam is whether the retinal irradiance will be significantly increased.

For an extended source the law of conservation of radiance can be applied. A telescope (or turbulon) cannot increase the source radiance, and therefore cannot increase the retinal irradiance of a searchlight or other light source that is already resolved by the eye. If, however, the source forms a point image and cannot be resolved into an extended image by either the unaided eye or a telescope because the beam has a very small divergence, then the telescope (or turbulon) can increase the apparent brightness of the laser, and hence its hazard.

13.3.3 Radiance Profiles

The U.S. Army Environmental Hygiene Agency conducted an evaluation of photographic images of a laser viewed over several atmospheric path lengths (Sliney, 1976). This effect on the point image irradiance profile is shown in the microdensitometer scans of Fig. 13-11. Using a beam splitter and an irradiance monitor in front of the camera, beam irradiance could be correlated with each image. The microdensitometer scans also permitted a careful analysis of the irradiance profile on the film. Regrettably it was concluded that only in some instances was this enlarged image on the retina sufficient to offset the effect of increased power entering the eye, and this effect could not eliminate the concern that atmospheric "hot spots" would increase the hazardous range. This image increase could only further decrease the low probability of encountering a hazardous level beyond the nominal ocular hazard distance.

13.3.4 The Influence of Collecting Aperture Size

The scientists and engineers who studied the effects of scintillation upon open-path optical communication links found that the receiver aperture size was very important. Specifically, for a small aperture a few millimeters in diameter, one set of irradiance-distribution statistics applied, but if the entrance aperture were 10 to 20 cm, which might occur if one were to look at a source through a telescope, another set of statistics would apply. This was the case for photograph 13-11b, which was taken through a 10-cm telescope to simulate the retinal profile. For this optically aided viewing situation, many different turbulons contribute to the irradiance profile at the telescope objective and the fluctuations in average beam irradiance become much less when the sampling aperture is increased to such a large area. Therefore the increase in the hazardous range due to turbulence if calculated for very-large-aperture optically aided viewing is minimal when compared to the theoretically increased hazardous range for the unaided eye due to turbulence. A change in pupil size from 3 mm to 7 mm would make little difference in irradiance statistics. A 7-mm entrance aperture (pupil) was used for the other photographs shown in Figure 13-11. For a 50-mm to 80-mm aperture, there is a reduction in the standard deviation of fluctuations but not enough to ignore the scintillation effect during periods of strong turbulence, unless of course the aperture encompasses all or nearly all of the beam.

13.3.5 The Influence of Beam Path Height Above Ground

As a beam path is raised above the ground 10 m or so, it is removed from most of the ground-level turbulence. Therefore the value of C_N decreases rapidly with increasing height. Several years ago when the U.S. Coast and Geodetic Survey was engaged in an extensive project to improve the accuracy of maps through the high-precision satellite-geodesy/laser-geodesy program, laser geodimeters were placed atop towers so that the beam was at least 7 to 10 m above ground level. This effort was necessary to avoid the errors introduced by turbulence. Slant-paths from aircraft-to-ground or mountaintop-to-ground (and vice-versa) also demonstrate a greatly reduced scintillation (Dabbert, 1973). If a laser beam is directed out of a building window where the temperature inside is quite different from the outside, turbulence at the open window will contribute to beam wander. That is, turbulons near the laser may encompass the entire beam and will deflect the entire beam (Fig. 13-5). Turbulons downrange intercept only a portion of the beam and will deflect only a portion of the beam. This results in "hot spots" and beam spreading at locations further downrange.

13.3.6 Conceptual Arguments

The data from many field tests indicate that it is possible to develop a conceptual approach to better understand atmospheric scintillation. For example, consider a very tight, diffraction-limited beam of 1-cm diameter as it leaves the laser. The divergence is of the order of 0.2 mrad. At 1 km the beam diameter should be 21 cm. Along the 1-km beam path the beam will encounter several "turbulons" which can focus or deflect the beam. If a turbulon is strong enough to focus a beam, then it may well be strong enough to deflect all or part of the beam outside of the original 0.2 mrad beam envelope. If this event happens at several locations downrange (with a temporal frequency spectrum extending up to 1 kHz) then the net effect should be beam spreading commensurate with the severity of hot spots.

It can be argued that, simply from the standpoint of diffraction theory, a minimal increase in divergence of the initial beam will be encountered at distances more than a few hundred meters. The law of conservation of brightness was originally considered, not from a standpoint of its effect upon the minimal image size on the retina, but rather from the standpoint of a laser beam being propagated through, say, a multiple collection of lenses. The irradiance should not theoretically be increased beyond a certain limit as defined by the law of conservation of brightness and diffraction limits on focal spot sizes. Unfortunately, a few simple calculations are needed to show that some strong hot spots are indeed possible—at least in the short range of a few hundred meters. Beyond this range these conservation arguments could begin to apply. In fact, this may account for the know effect of saturation of scintillation. The statistical range of beam irradiance values can be described by a standard deviation of a log-normal distribution. This standard deviation increases with range out to a distance of 700-1000 m. Beyond this distance, no further increase in σ_m is observed and it does in fact decrease. The maximum log irradiance standard deviation that has generally been measured is 1.3 (a factor of 20 times).

13.4 PROBABILITIES OF RETINAL INJURY

The slight change in retinal image size and the increased beam spread make it appear that turbulence does not add to the out-of-doors lasers hazard as significantly as was believed in the past. However, there is another factor that has not yet been mentioned. Up to this point in the discussion, it has been tacitly assumed that laser-induced retinal injury is dependent only upon retinal irradiance. This is not the case for many CW or short-pulsed laser exposures, where the injury threshold irradiance decreases for increasing image size (see Figure 4-18). This greatly complicates the determination of the increased retinal hazard due to scintillation. The exposure from a CW laser, of course, becomes averaged over a number of scintillations, and the effect of turbulence does not increase the retinal injury hazard, in contrast to the increase in hazard distance for a pulsed laser.

When all of the probabilities are finally added, one can realize the small chance of an accidental hazardous exposure outdoors. Consider first that an individual is looking into a pulsed laser; second, that his eye is relaxed (focused at infinity) and that his fovea is directed at the laser; third, that his eye is within a significant hot spot; fourth, that the weather provides a high visual range; and furthermore, that his retina is more sensitive (more absorbing) than average. The chance of all of these conditions occurring at the same time beyond the nominal ocular hazard distance is vanishingly small. However, the added risk of someone being located within the beam and viewing the laser with a telescope or pair of binoculars is probably greater. For this reason military laser safety regulations (e.g., those of the U.S. Army) require that the beam be terminated by a backstop such as a hill, within a controlled area (U.S. Army, 1975) unless it is pointed skyward. Fortunately, people in aircraft, being unable to stabilize a binocular do not use them, and atmospheric turbulence is far less for a ground-to-air path. In the latter case one can calculate the hazardous range that has meaning. In Chapter 16 the practical safety problems and control measures for outdoor laser applications will be discussed in much more detail.

13.5 ATMOSPHERIC TURBULENCE AND IR-C LASER BEAMS

The effect of scintillation is dependent upon the degree of variation of the atmospheric index of refraction n_a with variations in temperature. As previously discussed (Fig. 13-9), these variations in n_a are significant at visible and near-infrared wavelengths. The variation of n_a with temperature at far-infrared wavelengths is far less dramatic. But at wavelengths outside of the retinal hazard region, the projected radiance of the laser source obviously plays no role, since corneal injury is related directly to beam irradiance. At the CO_2 laser wavelength (10.6 μm) the scintillation hot spots are rarely detectable.

13.6 THE PROPAGATION OF VERY HIGH POWER LASER BEAMS

To this point it has been tacitly assumed that the laser beam has not affected the atmospheric path through which it passes. But at very high irradiances the atmospheric absorption of laser energy obviously will heat the atmosphere causing further effects upon the beam if the duration of laser operations is sufficiently long. The effect discussed most often is that of "thermal blooming," an effect, as the name implies, which spreads the high energy beam. Figure 13-12 illustrates the effect of thermal blooming and the strong influence of cross wind. If a cross wind exists, then the heated atmospheric molecules will be swept out of the beam along the direction of the wind, but not perpendicular to the wind velocity vector, hence the beam will be reshaped.

13.7 CONCLUSIONS

We have seen that there is virtually no simple or standardized approach available to handle the calculation of atmospheric effects upon a laser beam. Attenuation

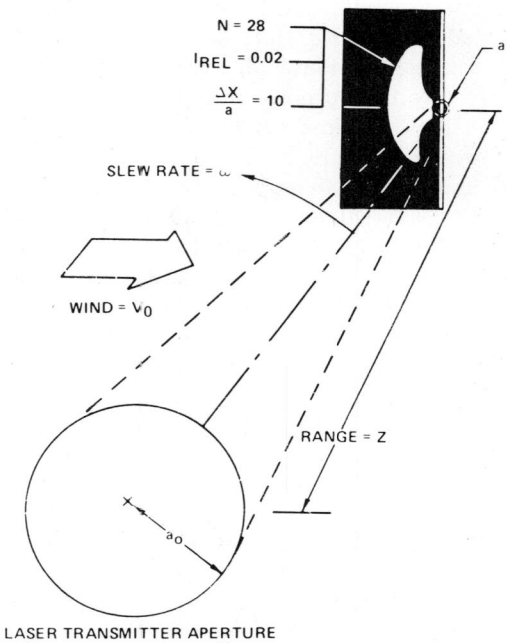
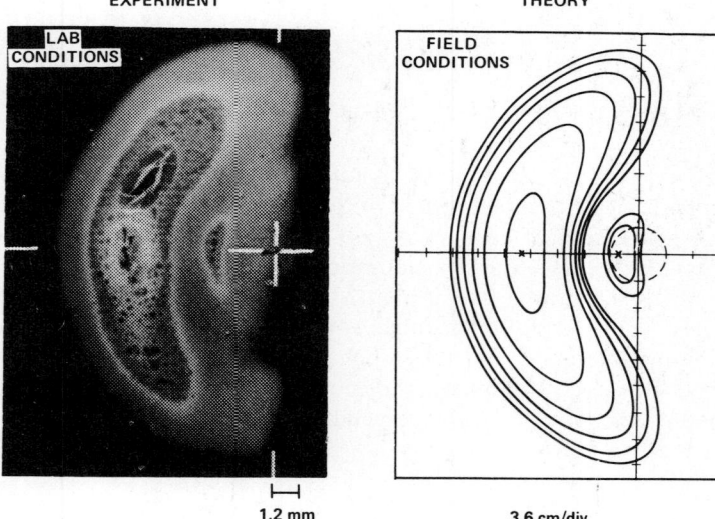

Figure 13-12. Thermal blooming of a high-power CW laser beam dominated by convection. Air flow was from left to right. The circular pattern represents the size and shape of the undistorted beam (from Gebhardt, 1976, with permission).

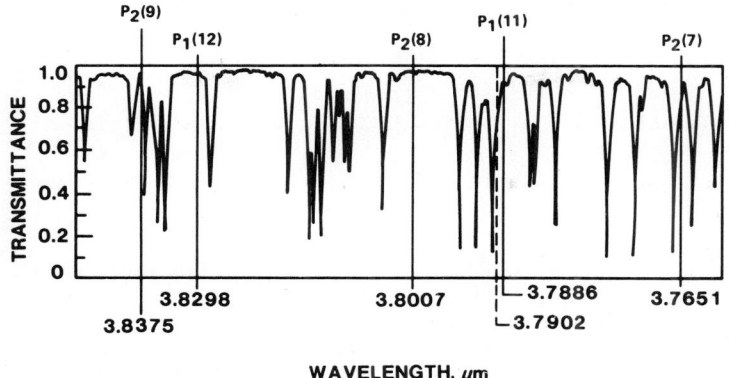

Figure 13-13. Example of narrow atmospheric absorption bands for infrared wavelengths as calculated by McClatchey and Selby, 1972. In this case the spectral band corresponding to the band of DF laser emission is shown from approximately 3.75 to 3.9 μm (from Gebhardt, 1976, with permission).

is typically of concern for beam paths exceeding several km. Absorption varies dramatically in the IR-B and IR-C (Fig. 13-13) and is typically the primary factor contributing toward the attenuation of an infrared laser beam. Atmospheric attenuation (by scattering and absorption) can be expressed mathematically by an exponention function (Eqn. 13-1). But a standard approach for accurately measuring or predicting the attenuation coefficient μ which varies with beam divergence and with meterological conditions is not available. Added to this problem, the effect of scintillation further decreases our predictive ability. Scintillation effects are important for beam paths exceeding several hundred meters. We are left with a statistical approach which prevents us from developing a single "safe" viewing distance if the distances involved exceed 100 m. It is left to the laser safety specialist to be fully aware of the various atmospheric effects as a function of weather, beam path location, and wavelength and recognize the uncertainties in estimating a hazardous viewing distance.

13.8 REVIEW QUESTIONS

1. How does Rayleigh scattering vary with wavelength?

2. Calculate the approximate Rayleigh scattering coefficient at the wavelength of the nitrogen laser (337.1 nm).

3. What causes scintillation of a distant light source?

4. Is scintillation more pronounced at 10.6 μm or at 633 nm?

5. What aerosol parameters influence the value of the Mie scattering coefficient?

6. Which type of scattering is more polarization dependent?

7. Explain how a kidney-shaped beam profile is formed by atmospheric effects upon a high energy CW laser beam.

8. What is the attenuation coefficient for a 15-km visibility range atmosphere for a He-Cd laser operating at 441.6 nm?

9. Along which atmospheric propagation path would a beam experience more scintillation for the same pathlength—a horizontal beam path 2 m above ground or a slant path from atop a 17-story building to a ground-level station?

10. What is the atmospheric attenuation coefficient in dry air for a horizontal beam path at a wavelength of 500 nm between two airplanes operating at 9000 feet above sea level (A.S.L.)?

11. What is the Rayleigh scattering coefficient for the primary line in a low-pressure mercury lamp (254 nm)?

13.9 DEMONSTRATION

A useful demonstration of many of the atmospheric effects discussed in this chapter can be performed with two Class II He-Ne lasers mounted on stable, adjustable tripods. The availability of a Class II He-Cd laser would further enhance the demonstration. Choose a nighttime setting on a warm, cloudless night for best results. Place the first of the two lasers on the roof of a building (at least two stories high) and aim the beam down at a target located 1-1.5 m above the ground about 500 m away. The target location should be chosen away from street lights. Near the base of the building place the second laser and aim its beam at an adjacent area of the same target located 500 m from the building. The ground should be relatively flat below the beam path. To place the beam on the target when a pointing telescope is not available, simply "walk" the beam across the ground on a line between the laser and the target. Use a retroreflective screen or road sign at the target to indicate when the laser beam strikes the target. Care should be taken to choose a reasonably isolated area where few people are likely to be walking so as to avoid unwarranted fears of passersby. The difference in scintillation patterns for a near-earth path and a slant path are evident. The patterns change most during the one hour period following sunset. If a laser beam collimator is available use this with the ground laser, then remove it to show the change in beam wander. Placing a pencil in the beam at 5-10 m from the target (use a white diffuse target board) nicely reveals diffraction patterns around the pencil. Measurements of beam irradiance and output power permit the calculation of an effective divergence. The beam should be observed by all up-range and down-range to permit each participant to visualize the difference between forward scattering and back scattering.

13.10 REFERENCES

Beatrice, E. S. and Frisch, G. D., 1973, Retinal laser damage thresholds as a function of image diameter, *Arch. Environ. Health* **27**:322–326.
Buck, A. L., 1967, Effects of the atmosphere on laser beam propagation, *Appl. Opt.* **6**(4):703–708.
Burch, D. E., Gryvnak, D. A., and Pembrook, J. D., 1971, Investigation of the absorption of infrared radiation by atmospheric gases: water, nitrogen, nitrous oxide, AFCRL-71-0124, *Aeronutronics*, (January 1971).
Buser, R. G. and Rohde, R. S., 1975, Transient thermal blooming of long laser pulses, *Appl. Opt.* **14**:50.
Chernov, L. A., 1967, "Wave Propagation in a Random Medium," Dover Publications, New York.
Clifford, S. F., Ochs, G. R., and Lawrence, N. S., 1974, Saturation of optical scintillation by strong turbulence, *J. Opt. Soc. Am.* **64**(2):148–154.
Dabbert, W. F., 1973, Slant-path scintillation in the planetary boundary layer, *Appl. Opt.* **12**(7):1536–1548.
Dabbert, W. F., and Johnson, W. B., 1971, Atmospheric Effects upon Eye Safety-Part II, Final Report for USAF School of Aerospace Medicine, Stanford Research Inst., Menlo Park, CA, May 1971.
Deitz, P. H., 1969, Probability analysis of ocular damage due to laser radiation through the atmosphere, *Appl. Opt.* **8**(2):371–375.
Deitz, P. H., 1970, Safety considerations in outdoor applications, *Laser Focus* **6**(6):40–43.
DeWolf, D. A., 1968, Saturation of irradiance fluctuations due to turbulent atmosphere, *J. Opt. Soc. Amer.* **58**(4):461–466.
Engstrom, R. W. (ed.), 1974, "RCA Electro-Optics Handbook," (Publication EOH-11), RCA Commercial Engineering, Harrison, NJ.
Elterman, L., 1964, Atmospheric Attenuation Model, 1964 in the Ultraviolet, Visible and Infrared Regions for Altitudes to 50 km, AFCRL-64-740, Hanscom Field, MA (September 1964) (AD 479487).
Eppers, W., 1971, Atmospheric transmission, in "Handbook of Lasers" (R. J. Pressley, ed.) pp 39–154, The Chemical Rubber Co., Cleveland, OH.
Fried, D. L., 1967, Aperture averaging of scintillation, *J. Opt. Soc. Am.* **57**(2):169–174.
Gebhardt, G. and Smith, D. C., 1972, Effects of diffraction of the self-induced thermal distortion of a laser beam in a crosswind, *Appl. Opt.* **11**(2):244–248.
Gebhardt, G., 1976, High power laser propagation, *Appl. Opt.* **15**(6):1479–1493.
Gibbons, M. G., 1959, Experimental study of the effect of field of view on transmission measurements, *J. Opt. Soc. Am.* **49**(7):702–709.
Gilmartin, T. J. and Schultz, F. V., 1969, Laser beam broadening in atmospheric propagation, *Radio Sci.* **4**:983–990.
Gracheva, M. E., and Gurvich, A. S., 1965, Strong fluctuations in the irradiance of light propagated through the atmosphere close to the earth, *Radiofizika* **8**:717–724.
Hill, R. J., and Ochs, G. R., 1978, The calibration of large-aperture optical scintillometers and an optical estimate of inner scale of turbulence, *Appl. Opt.* **17**(22):3608–3612.
Hudson, R. D., Jr., 1969, "Infrared System Engineering," Wiley Interscience, New York.

Kerr, J. R., 1972, Comments on irradiance fluctuations in optical transmission through the atmosphere, *J. Opt. Soc. Am.* **62**(7):916.

Lawrence, R. S., 1972, Irradiance fluctuations in optical transmission through the atmosphere, *J. Opt. Soc. Am.* **62**(5):701.

Livingston, P. M., Deitz, P. H., Alcaraz, E. C., 1970, Light propagation through a turbulent atmosphere: measurements of the optical-filter function, *J. Opt. Soc. Am.* **60**(7):925–935.

McCartney, E. J., 1976, "Optics of the Atmosphere, Scattering by Molecules and Particles," Wiley-Interscience, New York.

McClatchey, R. A. and D'Agati, A. P., 1968, Atmospheric Transmission of Laser Radiation: Computer Code LASER, Air Force Geophysical Laboratory, Hanscom AFB, MA, Report AFGL-TR-78-0029, 31 Jan. 1968.

McClatchey, R. A. and Selby, J. E. A., 1974, Atmospheric Attenuation of Laser Radiation from 0.76 to 31.25 μm. AFCRL-TR-74-0003, Cambridge, MA, January 1974.

Middleton, W. E. K., 1958, "Vision Through the Atmosphere," (rev. printing) University of Toronto Press, Toronto.

Mooradian, G. C., Geller, M., Stotts, L. B., Sephens, D. H., and Krautwald, R. C., 1979, Blue-green pulsed propagation through fog, *Appl. Opt.* **18**(4):429–441.

Ochs, G. R. and Lawrence, R. S., 1971, Measurements of laser beam spread and curvature, *Laser J.* **3**(1):14–17.

Parry, G., and Pusey, P. N., 1979, K distributions in atmospheric propagation of laser light, *J. Opt. Soc. Am.* **69**(5):796–798.

Pearson, J. E., 1975, Comparison of scintillometer and microthermometer measurements of C_N^2. *J. Opt. Soc. Am.* **65**(8):938–941.

Pendorf, R., 1957, Table of the refractive index for standard air and the Rayleigh scattering coefficient for the spectral region between 20 μ and 0.2 μ and their application to atmospheric optics, *J. Opt. Soc. Am.* **47**:176–182.

Plass, G. M., 1966, Mie scattering and absorption cross-sections for absorbing particles, *Appl. Opt.* **5**:149–154.

Poirier, J. L. and Korff, D., 1972, Beam spreading in a turbulent medium, *J. Opt. Soc. Am.* **62**(7):893–897.

Rice, D. K., 1973, Atmospheric attenuation measurements for several highly absorbed CO laser lines, *Appl. Opt.* **12**(7):1401–1403.

Rosenberg, G. V., 1966, "Twilight, A Study in Atmospheric Optics " (translated from Russian by R. B. Rodman), Plenum Press, New York.

Sliney, D. H., 1966, Comments on atmospheric turbulence, *in* "Proceedings of the First Conference on Laser Safety," pp. 86–87, Martin-Marietta, Orlando, FL.

Sliney, D. H., 1970, Evaluating health hazards from military lasers, *J. Amer. Med. Assoc.* **214**(6):1047–1054.

Sliney, D. H., 1976, The safety aspects of atmospheric transmission of lasers, *Ann. N. Y. Acad. Sci.* **267**:366–372.

Spencer, D. J., Denault, G. C., and Takimoto, H. H., 1974, Atmospheric gas absorpton at DF laser wavelengths, *Appl. Opt.* **13**(12):2855–2868.

Strohbehn, J. W. (ed.), 1978, "Laser Beam Propagation in the Atmosphere," Springer-Verlag, New York.

Tartarski, V. I., 1961, "Wave Propagation in a Turbulent Medium," [Institute of Atmospheric Physics, Academy of Science of the USSR] McGraw Hill, New York; Also "Propagation of Waves in a Turbulent Medium," 1967, [translated 1971–NTIS, Springfield, VA].

Traub, W. A. and Stier, M. T., 1975, Theoretical atmospheric transmission in the mid- and far-infrared at four altitudes, *Appl. Opt.* **15**(2):364–377.

Tricker, R. A. R., 1970, "Introduction to Meterological Optics," American Elsevier, New York.

Valley, S. L., 1965, "Handbook of Geophysics and Space Environments," AF Cambridge Laboratories, MacMillan, New York.
Van de Hulst, H. C., 1957, "Light Scattering by Small Particles," John Wiley and Sons, New York.
Weseley, M. L. and Derzko, Z. I., 1975, Atmospheric turbulence parameters from visual resolution, *Appl. Opt.* **14**(4):847–853.
White, K. O., Watkins, W. R., Schleusener, S. A., 1975, Holmium 2.06-μm laser spectral characteristics and absorption by CO_2 gas, *Appl. Opt.* **14**(1):16–18.
Whitman, A. M. and Beran, M. J., 1970, Beam spread of laser light propagating in a random medium, *J. Opt. Soc. Amer.* **60**(12):1595–1602.
Wolf, W. L., 1965, "Handbook of Military Infrared Technology," U.S. Office of Naval Research, Washington, DC.
Yura, H. T., 1971, Atmospheric turbulence induced laser beam spread, *Appl. Opt.* **10**(12):2771–2773.
Yura, H. T., 1974, Temporal frequency spectrum of an optical wave propagating under saturation conditions, *J. Opt. Soc. Am.* **64**(3):357–359.

Chapter 14
Radiometric Measurements Required for Broad-Band Optical Sources

14.1 INTRODUCTION

Although the evaluation of hazards associated with lasers is complex, the evaluation of more conventional, broad-band sources is even more complex, since spectral characteristics and source size must be considered. To evaluate a broad-band optical source, such as an arc lamp, an incandescent lamp, a fluorescent lamp, an array of lamps, or an open-arc process such as those found in industry, it is normally necessary to determine the spectral distribution of optical radiation emitted from the source at the point or points of nearest human access. This accessible emission spectral distribution of interest for a lighting system may differ from that actually being emitted by the lamp alone due to the filtration by any optical elements (e.g., projection optics) in the light path. Secondly, the size, or projected size, of the source must be characterized in the retinal hazard spectral region. Thirdly, it may be necessary to determine the variation of irradiance and radiance with distance. The performance of the necessary measurements is normally not an easy task without sophisticated instruments, as will be shown in this chapter.

14.2 REQUIRED RADIOMETRIC DATA

To evaluate the potential hazards to the eye and skin within the retinal hazard region (400 nm to 1400 nm) it is necessary to obtain spectral radiance, source size, pulse duration and PRF (if pulsed) plus the irradiance and radiance as a function of range. For spectral regions less than 400 nm and greater than 1400 nm (outside of the retinal hazard region) the spectral radiance and source size are not normally required.

14.2.1 Spectral Irradiance

The spectral irradiance E_λ should be measured as completely as possible from 200 nm to at least 1400 nm. Fluorescent lamps and many commonly used arc lamps emit little infrared radiation beyond 1200 nm and the spectral region between 1200 nm and 1400 nm often need not be measured if a suitable instrument is not available. For incandescent lamps, however, it is crucial that the near-infrared (IR-A) radiation be measured. The spectral irradiance E_λ at the nearest point of access is of interest in assessing the potential hazards to both the skin and eye from the ultraviolet component in the spectrum, and the potential hazards to the skin from the entire spectrum. The spectral irradiance in the infrared is also needed to assess the potential hazards to the anterior part of the eye. For wavelengths beyond 1400 nm the spectral irradiance is of marginal interest; although total irradiance in the IR-B and IR-C should be known. For some specialized gas discharges and arc sources as well as specially filtered sources, spectral irradiance data may be required only in one or two spectral regions.

14.2.2 Spectral Radiance

The spectral radiance L_λ is of interest in assessing potential retinal hazards and should be complete from 400 nm to 1400 nm (the retinal hazard region). Again, the actual measurements beyond 1200 nm (or even 1100 nm often can be neglected if the source is an arc or a fluorescent lamp in which the radiant power is heavily concentrated in the visible and near-ultraviolet portion of the spectrum. Likewise the measurements below 300 nm may be neglected if heavy glass filtration is present. However, some quick confirmation measurement check may be necessary at these shorter wavelengths to confirm the efficiency of the filter.

14.2.3 Source Size

The geometrical source size normally specified at half-peak-radiance points plays a major role in *retinal hazard evaluation*. The greatest dimension of the source as seen by a potential viewer is most often used, although a map of the radiance distribution can be even more helpful. This information is only useful, as a general rule, in the 400-nm-to-1400-nm region. The approximate source size for sources not emitting in the retinal hazard region is most useful in calculations of irradiance as a function of distance from the source.

14.2.4 Range Data

For some optical sources, particularly those with projection optics such as searchlights, the variation of radiance and irradiance with range (i.e., viewing distance) must be known in order to determine the hazardous viewing distance. For

Broad-Band Optical Sources

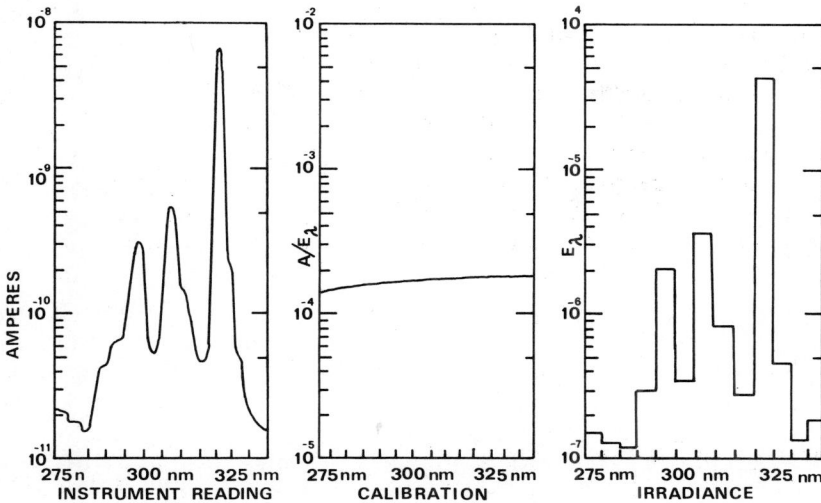

Figure 14-1. Data Reduction for a Spectroradiometer. X-Y chart recording of spectroradiometer detector output (left panel) indicates the instrument bandwidth which must be known along with the spectral calibration curve of the instrument (middle panel), to calculate the line irradiances and continuum spectral irradiance. The line and continuum values are added to achieve the final spectral histogram (right panel).

ultraviolet and far-infrared (IR-B and IR-C) source evaluations, the variations of total irradiance E, or spectrally weighted irradiance with distance also must be known to establish a hazardous viewing distance. Because of the variation in spectral attenuation of the atmosphere, the spectral irradiance E_λ may best be measured also at some distance from the source to ascertain if the spectrum has been altered sufficiently by the atmosphere to warrant further determinations of E_λ at other distances of interest. Normally range data can be readily extrapolated if collimating or focusing optics are not used.

14.3 EVALUATION OF LINE SPECTRAL EMISSION

The spectrum of an arc lamp, a gas discharge lamp, or a fluorescent lamp consists of both line structure and a continuum. Significant errors can be introduced in the representation of the spectrum and in the weighting of the spectrum against biological or safety action spectrum if the fraction of energy in each line is not properly added to the continuum. Figure 14-1 shows a hypothetical spectral recording from the X-Y plotter of a spectroradiometer. If an X-Y recorder were not employed and if spectral points were arbitrarily recorded every 5 nm, most of the line-peak data would be missed. The width of the triangular peak at half maximum is called the bandwidth (or bandpass) of the monochromator. The scan rate of the monochromator must be sufficiently slow to prevent distortion by lag of the X-Y recorder's pen during the recording. Reversing the scan should reveal whether recorder lag or mechanical play in the monochromator or recorder drive exists.

The recommended units for presenting the spectrum in tabulated form should have the measured spectral irradiance in microwatts-per-square-centimeter-per-nanometer [$\mu W/(cm^2 \cdot nm)$] of the continuum at regular intervals (e.g., every 5 nm) with a separate list of the irradiance in microwatts-per-square-centimeter ($\mu W/cm^2$) for each line. This procedure is particularly important in critical spectral regions where biological weighting functions vary rapidly (e.g., 300-320 nm; 395-500 nm). Narrow bandwidth recording (e.g., 1 nm) is also of obvious importance in such transition regions. Some sources with many lines present difficulties, and a broader bandwidth scan may be used to minimize data from the lines outside of the critical spectral regions.

The spectral radiance at each of the significant lines should be separated from the continuum scan. This is accomplished by first drawing an imaginary envelope through the line spectrum to make the continuum spectrum a smooth, continuous line. The region of the triangular-shaped area above the continuum line is then integrated to provide the radiant energy in each line. This calculation is made by taking the peak reading of the triangular-shaped representation $E_{\lambda\,(max)}$ of the spectral line, subtracting the value of the continuum $E_{\lambda(c)}$ at that wavelength, and then multiplying this peak value by the bandwidth (bandpass) of the monochromator $\Delta\lambda_m$ at that wavelength (typically 2 to 5 nm).

$$E_{(line)} = [E_{\lambda\,(max)} - E_{\lambda(c)}]\,\Delta\lambda_m \tag{14-1}$$

This provides the total irradiance or power in each line, and is listed separately from the values of spectral irradiance or spectral power of the continuum. Table 14-1 gives the spectral radiant power distribution of a representative fluorescent lamp found by this procedure.

It is important to realize that the monochromator bandwidth specified by an instrument manufacturer is normally valid only for a central wavelength as the bandwidth varies across the range of the monochromator. The bandwidth is the width of the triangular peak at half of the peak reading when no continuum is present. The bandwidth is determined by the width of the entrance and exit slits of the monochromator (Eqn. 14-1).

The bandwidth of a grating monochromator $\Delta\lambda_m$ is:

$$\begin{aligned}\Delta\lambda_m &= f(\mathcal{R})\,f(W_{s1})\,f(W_{s2}) \cdot f_m \cdot b_\lambda \cdot g_g \\ &= W_{s1}/D \quad \text{for } W_{s1} = W_{s2}\end{aligned} \tag{14-2}$$

where f_m is the focal length of the monochromator, $\mathcal{R}$ the resolution, b_λ the blaze wavelength, D the dispersion, g_g the "grating cut" of the grating, and W_{s1} and W_{s2} the entrance and exit slit widths (Loewen, 1970). For example, a commonly used

Broad-Band Optical Sources

TABLE 14-1. Spectral Radiant Flux Distribution (Watts) from a Fluorescent Lamp

Wavelength (nm)	Power (W)	Wavelength (nm)	Power (W)
380	0.0313	610	0.3956
390	0.0490	620	0.3081
400	0.0708	630	0.2365
410	0.0898	640	0.1774
420	0.1091	650	0.1306
430	0.1329	660	0.0956
440	0.1531	670	0.0718
450	0.1719	680	0.0524
460	0.1867	690	0.0418
470	0.1960	700	0.0304
480	0.1992	710	0.0256
490	0.1988	720	0.0213
500	0.1910	730	0.0265
510	0.1877	740	0.0178
520	0.1972	750	0.0213
530	0.2322	760	0.0198
540	0.3000		
550	0.3851	*Mercury Lines*	
560	0.4902		
570	0.5569	405	0.1897
580	0.5780	436	0.4696
590	0.5415	546	0.2255
600	0.4759	578	0.0769

parameter known as the *throughput* of a monochromator (the F number multiplied by the solid angle field-of-view) is important in choosing a monochromator. The measurement of high intensity sources does not require a high-throughput monochromator. A typical 0.25-m focal length monochromator has a throughput of 0.15 in the visible part of the spectrum (Pierson, 1979).

14.4 SPECTRAL HISTOGRAMS

The spectral distribution of a lamp or arc can be graphically illustrated when the continuum and line structures are recombined in a histogram (Figs. 14-1 and 14-2). The spectral division of the histogram should accurately reflect the spectral resolution of the data. To prepare a histogram from tabulated data (section 14.3) the separate line contributions must be added back to the continuum. Although a spectrum can be represented by a direct, calibrated recording as shown in Fig. 14-3, such an approach makes it difficult if not impossible to read off data for hazard

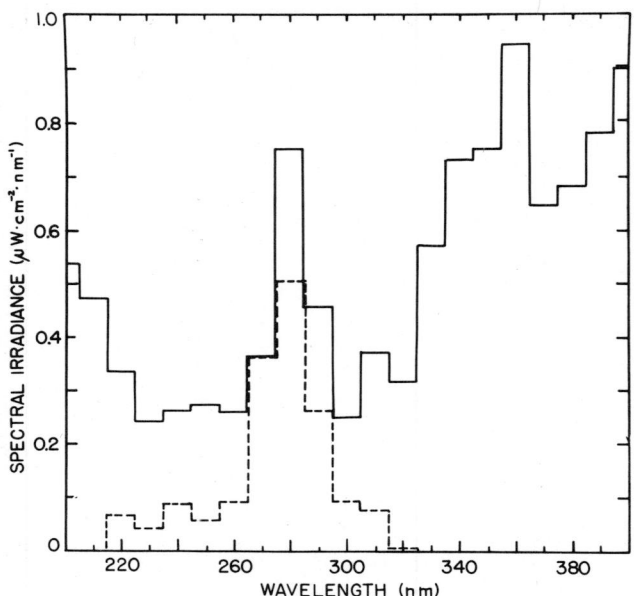

Figure 14-2. Spectral Irradiance of a Welding Arc. The arc's spectral irradiance is the solid line. Dashed line is the final, biologically-weighted spectrum used for hazard analysis.

calculations unless the bandwidth as a function of wavelength is also specified. This type of plot does give a good qualitative presentation, however.

If the spectrum is represented in histogram form in 5 nm intervals, the irradiance of each spectral line is divided by 5 nm and added to the continuum's spectral irradiance value in that 5-nm interval in which the emission line is located. As an example, in the representation of the spectrum of a mercury arc with histogram points at every 5 nm (300 nm, 305 nm, 315 nm, etc.), the 5 nm band centered at 305 nm (that is, from 302.5 nm to 307.5 nm) contains the 303-nm emission line of mercury. Likewise, the band centered at 315 nm contains the 313-nm emission line. Since the band centered at 310 nm contains no emission line of mercury, it alone truly represents the continuum level in this histogram. The histogram points should be separated by a wavelength interval at least as great as $\Delta\lambda_m$.

14.5 BIOLOGICAL WEIGHTING OF SPECTRORADIOMETRIC DATA

Many of the calculations which are useful in hazard analyses require weighting the measured spectrum against a biological action spectrum. There are several, including the erythemal, or photokeratitis action spectrum; the photopic response V_λ of the eye defined by the CIE; and the retinal photochemical injury action

Broad-Band Optical Sources

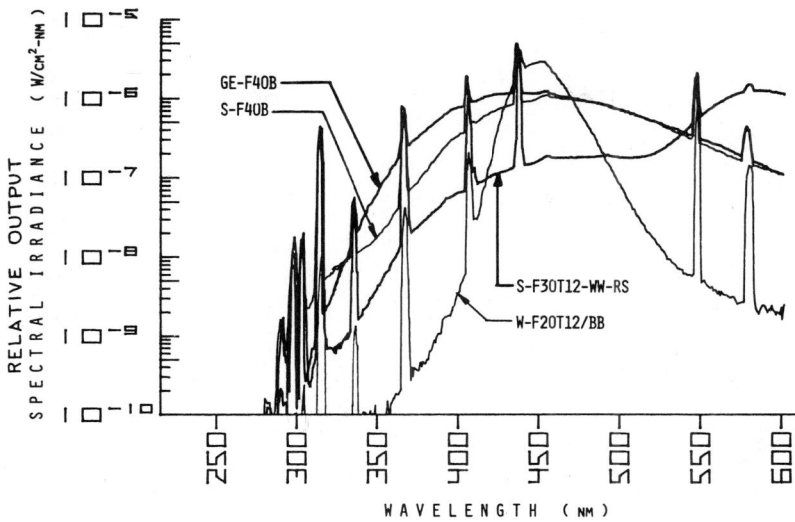

Figure 14-3. Example of a Non-Histogram Plot of Spectral Irradiance. In this case the spectral irradiance of four fluorescent lamps used for phototherapy have been drawn to show the bandwidth of the measuring instrument. The bandwidth of the instrument at a specific peak wavelength is the spectral width at half of that peak (from Coakley, 1976). Note the presence of the lines from the mercury discharge superimposed on the fluorescent continuum.

spectrum B_λ. Little error is normally introduced by using the digitized spectral irradiance values given in the histogram plot produced by this wavelength-by-wavelength band process. However, if the lamp spectrum is changing rapidly at the same location where the biologic weighting spectrum undergoes rapid change, significant errors may be introduced. It is therefore preferable to weight the line values separately for routine evaluation of a single type of lamp. This is most commonly done with mercury-arc lamps, mercury vapor lamps, and fluorescent lamps where the common wavelengths of the mercury emission are encountered at 243.7 nm, 296.7 nm, 302.3 nm, 313.2 nm, 365 nm, 404.7 nm, 435.8 nm, etc. These lines are found in fluorescent lamps as well since a mercury discharge is used to excite the fluorescence. In some cases routine hand-computing or machine-computing routines can be established with the two spectra weighted separately; e.g., continuum spectra plus line spectra (Sliney *et al.*, 1977).

14.6 THE MONOCHROMATOR SLIT FUNCTION, AND STRAY LIGHT

An important part of measuring the spectral distribution of a broad-band lamp source or an arc process is specifying the desired bandwidth, and the intervals at which data will be recorded. One of the most useful approaches is to scan through a

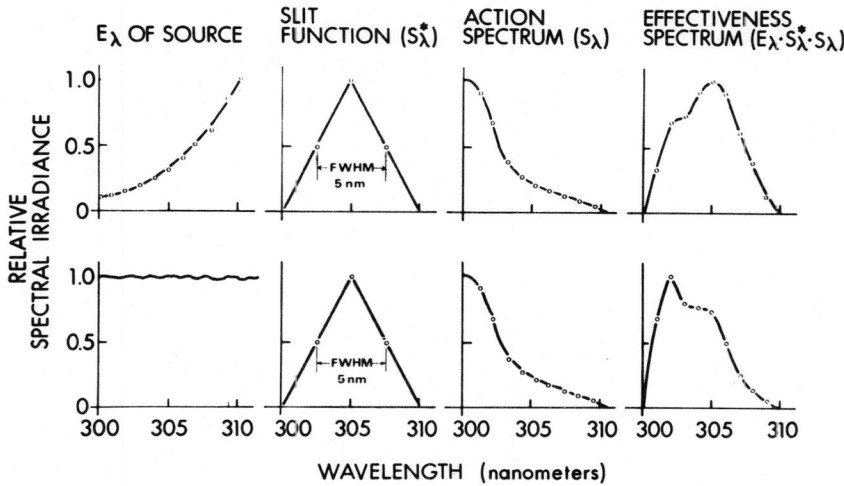

Figure 14-4. Spectral Weighting Errors. The weighting of rapidly changing spectroradiometric data against a rapidly changing action spectrum can result in substantial errors. Such errors are encountered both in the determination of biological action spectra and in the measurement of sources for hazard evaluation. Note the resulting shift in the effective peak wavelength and band being studied.

spectrum and record the detector output in analog fashion on an X-Y recorder, rather than to record digitized data. The reasons for this are straightforward and are not limited to the justifications presented in section 14-4. An X-Y recorder indicates the bandwidth of the monochromator and may quite often indicate which regions of the spectrum will have problems from stray light or extraneous noise. It is also a great deal simpler to make a comparison between successive runs from the same source (especially when the scan direction is reversed) to allow determination of spectral overlay and possible loss of precision in the location of the spectral lines of the source. Any misalignment of the monochromator optics may also be revealed by the shape of the slit function.

The required bandwidth and sampling interval are determined by comparing the so-called "slit function" of the monochromator system with the need for sufficient spectral resolution to permit accurate weighting against action spectra used in hazard analysis. An excellent example of this problem is illustrated by Fig. 14-4. The envelope of the action spectrum used for evaluating ultraviolet radiation hazards changes rapidly between 300 and 310 nm. This function is noted as S_λ in Table 10-1 and is shown as the bold dashed line in Fig. 10-1. If this action spectrum is used

Broad-Band Optical Sources

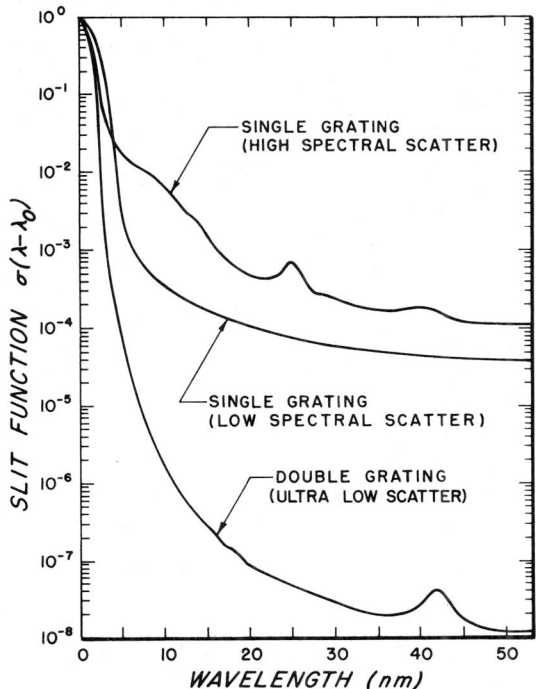

Figure 14-5. Monochromator Slit Function. The slit function of three commercially available monochromators. The upper curves show that significant stray light would be present in measurements of rapidly changing ultraviolet spectra, (e.g., the sun) obtained using those monochromators (courtesy Dr. H. Kostkowski, National Bureau of Standards).

as a weighting function for a source spectrum (such as from the sun) which changes dramatically between 300-310 nm a large error can be produced if the slit width of the instrument is ignored. A 5-nm half bandwidth (S_λ* in Figure 14-4) will allow the midpoint of the action spectrum for the monochromator setting of 305 nm to be shifted substantially. As shown in the lower series of panels this set of conditions will produce an apparent shift of 3 nm. This type of error has caused confusion in some previous biological studies of the action spectrum of UV photokeratitis and UV erythema when monochromator bandwidths of 5 or 10 nm were used.

The considerations above suggest the use of a direct reading UV hazard monitor which has a sharp spectral response similar to the UV envelope safety standard. Alternatively, UV spectral irradiance measurements must be made at intervals of 1 nm or less with a monochromator whose bandwidth is also 1 nm or less. Regrettably, both filter-based and monochromator-based hazard monitors can have intrinsic bandwidth error due to spectral sensitivity shifting with angular movement of a source. Failure to take this effect into account can result in very marked errors for

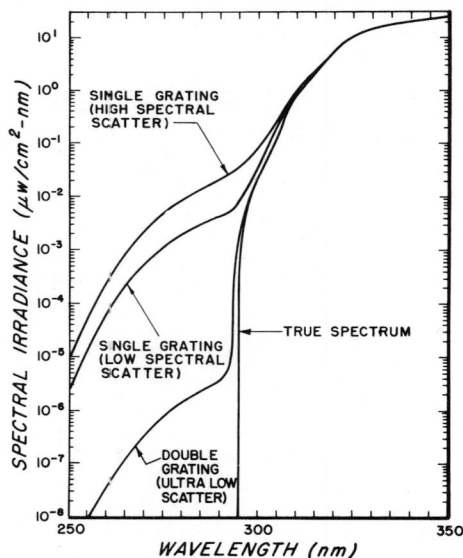

Figure 14-6. Errors Due to Straylight. Sunlight spectral irradiance as obtained with three different types of grating-monochromator spectroradiometric systems is shown. Substantial error is introduced when a grating with significant stray light is used. The problem occurs wherever a rapid change in spectral irradiance is encountered (courtesy, Dr. H. Kostkowski, National Bureau of Standards).

any action spectrum or source spectrum that varies drastically in this spectral region. It should be noted also, that the blue-light retinal hazard function B_λ (Table 10-2) in the 400-500 nm range varies markedly with wavelength. Here again narrow-bandwidth monochromators and small sampling intervals are required.

The slit functions shown in Fig. 14-4 are ideal, theoretical curves for a grating monochromator. However, actual slit functions, when plotted on a semilogarithmic scale, provide an excellent indication of the likelihood of encountering stray light problems originating from scatter from imperfections in the grating and other optical elements, from poor baffling and from re-entry spectra (double diffraction). Fig. 14-5 shows the slit function of three commercially available monochromators: a simple conventionally-ruled single grating instrument; a holographically ruled single grating monochromator, which offers a slight improvement in stray light reduction; and, finally, a double monochromator, which has substantially less stray light.

Figure 14-6 demonstrates how stray light can show up in a spectral irradiance measurement. The rapidly increasing spectral irrradiance of sunlight near 300 nm is poorly characterized by "system #1" which has significant stray light. A telltale plateau (and even increasing values) at shorter wavelength is present. This is shown

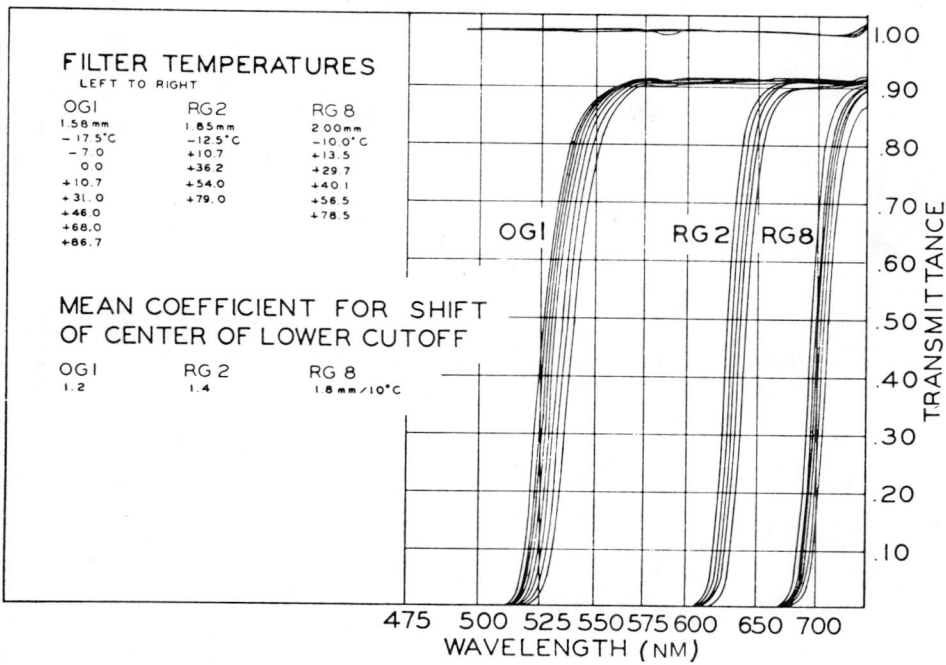

Figure 14-7. Short-Wavelength Cutoff Filters. Spectral transmission curves of short-wavelength cutoff filters vary with temperature. These filters are used for stray-light rejection measurements, and for order sorting with grating monochromators (from Angstrom and Drummond, 1961, with permission).

also in panel C in Fig. 14-1. The double-monochromator curve in Figure 14-6 stops at 5×10^{-17} W/(cm² · nm) because of limited sensitivity. This is low due to the limited throughput characteristic of all double monochromators. Obviously the single-monochromator with a low stray-light figure-of-merit (e.g., a holographic grating) is superior in this evaluation; but the values at wavelengths less than 295 are also high due to stray light.

The presence of stray light can be checked during a measurement by placing a short-wave cut-off filter in front of the monochromator. The filter's cut-off should be at a wavelength just above the wavelength being measured. Hence, a series of filters (Klein, 1979) such as the Schott WG series (Fig. 14-7) are really needed. If the instrument reading is reduced to zero then the reading should be reasonably correct, provided, of course, that there is not significantly more radiation at still shorter wavelengths. If the stray light contribution cannot be reduced to zero, the subtractive technique (section 14.9.1) can be applied to obtain an *estimate* of the spectral irradiance at that wavelength. Obviously all of the facts of monochromator performance must be known and understood before accurate evaluations of broad-band optical sources can be performed.

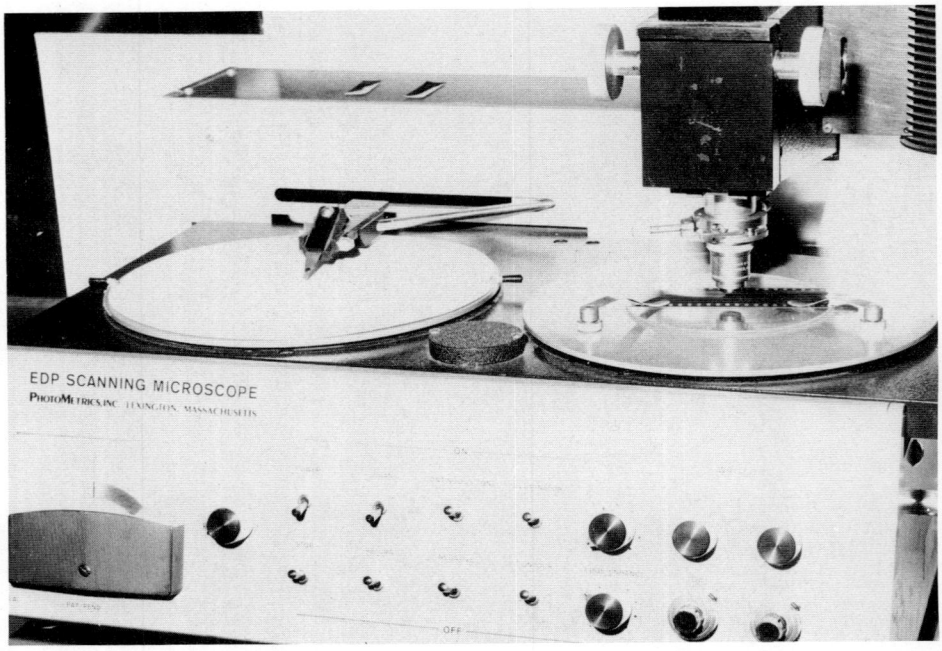

Figure 14-8. Microdensitometer. The source distribution (left disc) can be photographically determined by a scanning microdensitometer provided that the gamma of the film is known and the film density range falls within the linear region of the H-D curve. Iso-density curves of the film image are converted to iso-radiance curves.

Today most spectroradiometers employ grating monochromators, however, it is fair to point out that prism monochrometers typically have had low scattered light. A very superior instrument was employed by Dr. M. Chuchkova of the Institute of Hygiene in Sofia. She performed excellent outdoor environmental field measurements of the ultraviolet solar spectrum in various locales with this spectrograph. The highly portable instrument consisted of a quartz prism and entrance slit which replaced the lens in a 35-mm camera. The data reduction for photographic spectrographs can be very involved, but such an approach provides a permanent record of the actual measurement and a highly portable instrument (Chuchkova and Kurchatova, 1975).

14.7 RADIANCE DISTRIBUTION

The determination of the source size is a serious problem. The most common method is to take photographs of the source at various exposure settings. Enlargements of the photographs, or scanning microdensitometry, is used to reconstruct the

Broad-Band Optical Sources

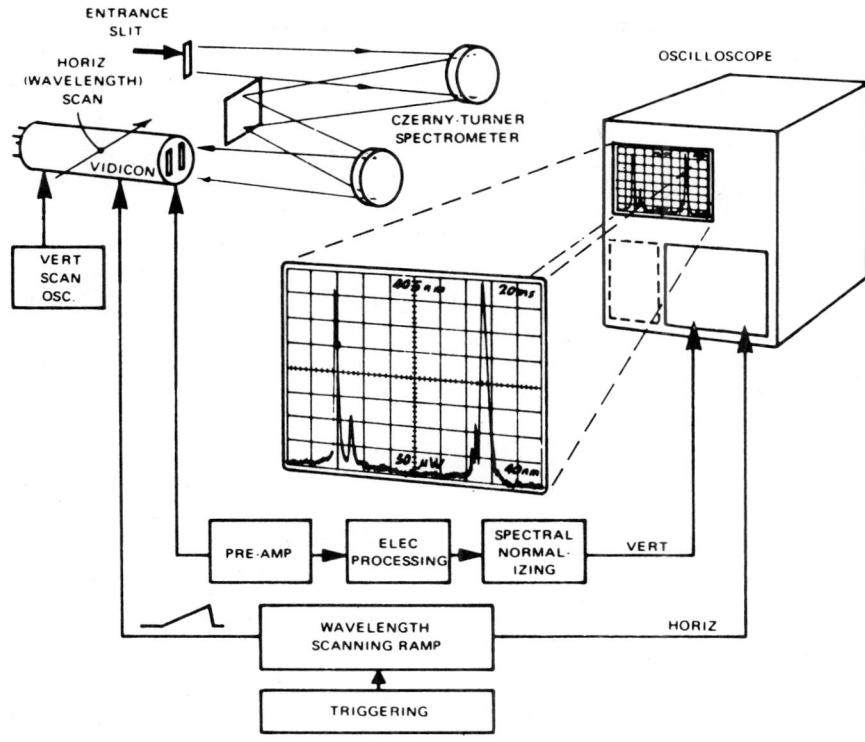

Figure 14-9. A rapid scan spectroradiometer (Textronix, USA). The spectrum from a grating was imaged on a silicon vidicon and an electronic scan of the vidicon was displayed on a cathode ray tube (CRT) (from Pasachoff and Muzyka, 1976).

source distribution to determine the solid angle of the source as seen by the detector. Figure 14-8 (insert) shows a microdensitometer trace of a projected arc source. Of course, the measurements of spectral radiance must be made sufficiently far from the source, (or the source must be masked) to assure that the detector sees only a small solid angle. Figure 23-3 shows a microdensitometry scan of an arc projected by a searchlight reflector. The effective source area was defined where the radiance profiles were at half the peak radiance. Section 12.6.6 considers photographic radiometric techniques in greater detail.

14.8 DIRECT READING INSTRUMENTS

Spectroradiometric measurements are time consuming and awkward, and the interpretation of the data has the same difficulties. Although rapid-scan spectrom-

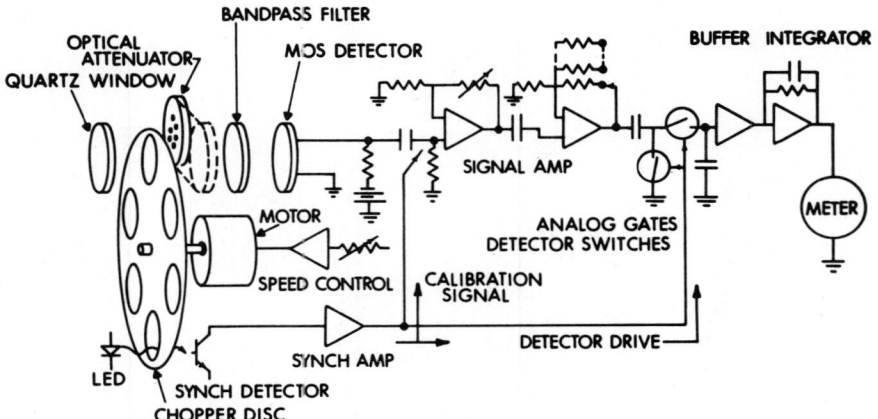

PHOTOTYPE MK I ULTRAVIOLET HAZARD MONITOR FUNCTION DIAGRAM

Figure 14-10. Direct-Reading Ultraviolet Hazard Monitor. The diagram shows the scheme for this instrument which was developed by CBS Laboratories in 1975 for NIOSH (adapted from Roach, 1973).

eters (Fig. 14-9) have shortened the process and permit measurements of some pulsed and time-varying sources, they are, nevertheless, quite complex and expensive and the data reduction remains difficult. It is easy to understand, therefore, that there have been many efforts to develop instruments with spectral responses incorporating the several biologic weighting functions. Because of the great interest in photometry, there are many satisfactory photometers that measure both luminance and illuminance and follow the CIE photopic function V_λ quite well. This is not the case for the other weighting functions. Direct reading UV instruments are a case in point.

14.8.1 The NIOSH UV Meters

To minimize the difficulty in performing ultraviolet safety measurements, a Federal agency in the USA, the National Institute for Occupational Safety and Health (NIOSH) contracted with CBS Laboratories in Stamford, Connecticutt to develop a prototype ultraviolet hazard monitor in 1973 (Roach, 1973). Its design is shown in Fig. 14-10. It made use of a spectrally-weighted UV filter, a silicon diode, and a chopper to reduce noise. This instrument was found to be quite reliable and followed the safety limit curve fairly accurately (Fig. 14-11). Unfortunately, it was never produced commercially since the optical filter was not available in quantity. NIOSH subsequently contracted with another manufacturer to develop a UV instru-

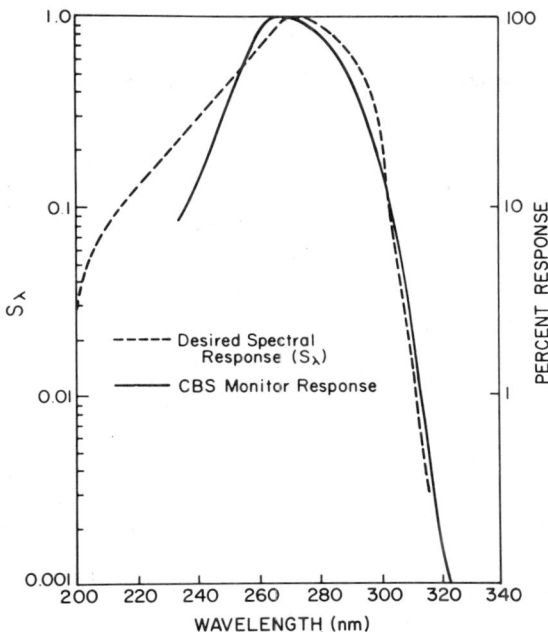

Figure 14-11. Spectral Response of the 1973 CBS UV Monitor. The spectral response of the CBS monitor nearly fitted the desired UV hazard sensitivity curves. This allowed the instrument to be used for direct evaluation of the UV hazard of a light source.

ment of a different design, but this instrument was not very successful either. In 1977 still another Federal agency, the Bureau of Radiological Health (BRH), published a request for quotation for the construction of a similar, but somewhat more versatile UV hazard instrument which employed a solar-blind detector with a dispersive element, an entrance slit and a spectral mask to define the spectral sensitivity function. This instrument, built by Oakwood Electronics, Dayton, Ohio, was successful, but quite expensive (about $10,000 in 1979). In 1977 Acton Laboratories of Acton, Massachusetts began to market a UV filter (Model UVH-1) which followed the UV action curve reasonably well. This filter, in combination with a broad-band UV detector (especially a "solar-blind" CsTe detector) will function reasonably well as a UV hazard monitor.

The principal difficulty in developing an ultraviolet instrument of this nature has been to develop a means for measuring only the UV-B and UV-C radiation with sufficient sensitivity while still rejecting all of the UV-A and visible light. Few instrument designers can believe at first that this design task is as difficult as it really is. They fail to appreciate the critical importance of proper spectral response in the 300

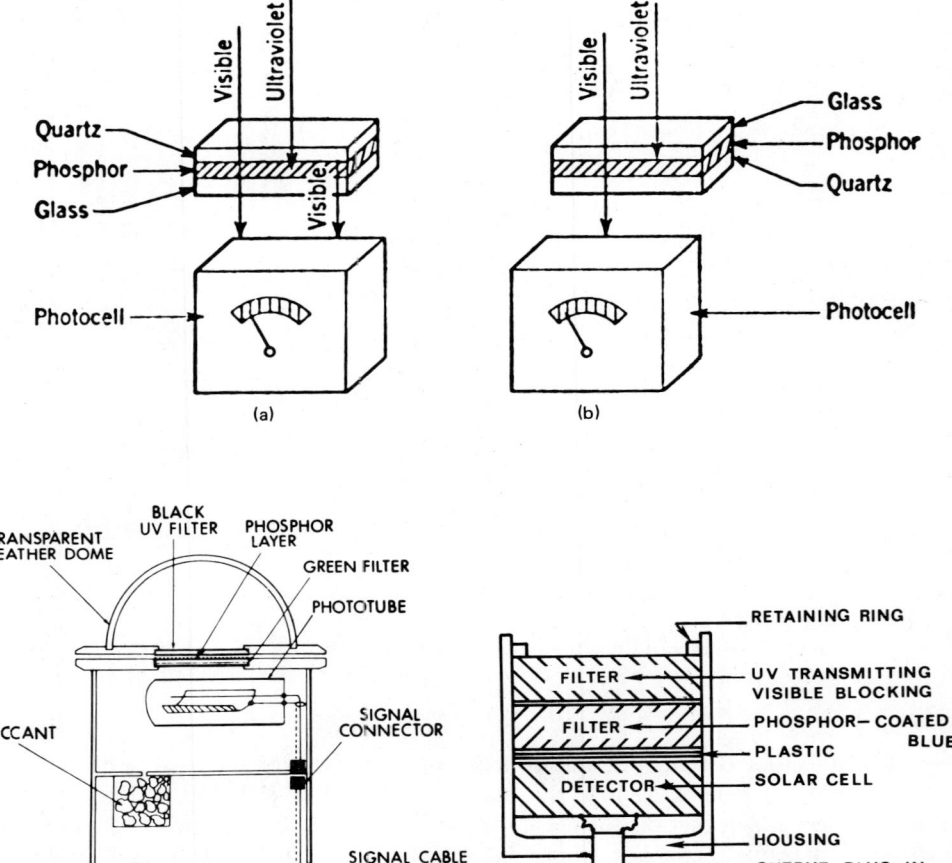

Figure 14-12. Simple Ultraviolet Meters. The Luckiesh–Taylor (a and b) and Robinson–Berger (c and d) direct reading ultraviolet monitors. Both of these instruments make use of the visible fluorescence of materials (e.g., $CaWO_4$) which have excitation spectra somewhat similar to the erythema action spectrum. The Luckiesh–Taylor meter required a shift of the quartz filter (a to b) to allow connection for long wavelength also present (from Koller, 1965 and Berger, 1976).

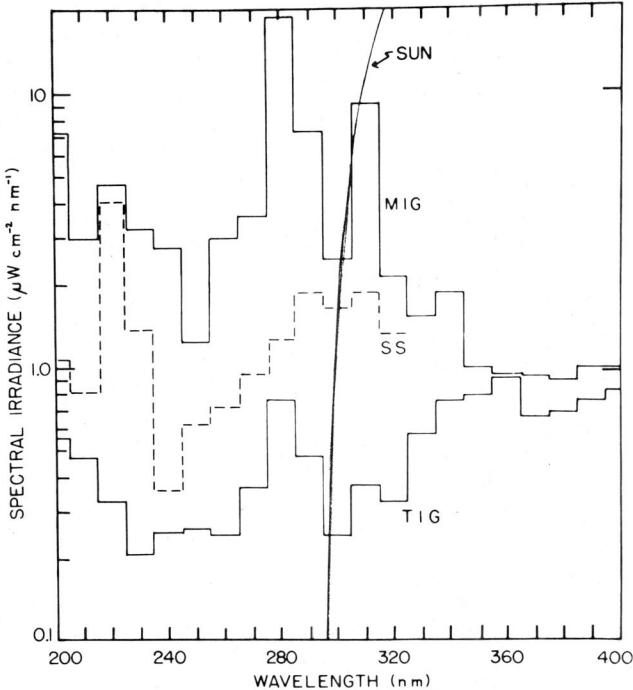

Figure 14-13. Spectral Irradiance of the Sun Compared with Three Types of Welding Arcs. Note the rapid change in the solar spectrum from 300 to 320 nm. Stray-light in the instrumentation obviously introduce far greater errors for measurements of the sun's spectrum in this UV region than in measurements of open arcs (from Sliney, 1972).

to 320 nm band and the need for near total rejection of longer wavelengths. Most ultraviolet sources for which this type of hazard monitor instrument would be used (such as plasma torches, arc lamps and welding arcs) emit far more radiation in the visible and near-ultraviolet (UV-A) regions than in the actinic (UV-B and UV-C) regions. Conventional instruments which were designed to measure actinic ultraviolet radiation would also respond to some degree to the longer wavelength, and therefore could provide an incorrect (larger) spectral irradiance value in the ultraviolet. Efforts to develop ultraviolet photochemical dosimeters for safety purposes have also met the same problem.

A relatively inexpensive instrument for measuring germicidal lamps (254 nm) is the meter shown in Fig. 14-12a. The Robinson-Berger meter with a calcium tungstate ($CaWO_4$) phosphor which has a fluorescence spectrum similar to the erythema action spectrum from 290-315 nm is small and more sophisticated (Fig. 14-12b). It is an improvement over the Luckeish-Taylor meter which used a $ZnSiO_4$ (Willemite) phosphor that required two separate readings with different cover filters.

The measurement of the actinic ultraviolet radiation from the sun at sea level nicely illustrates the UV measurements problem. At noontime in June, the irradiance for wavelengths below 315 nm would be of the order of 0.1 mW/cm^2 vs. 100 mW/cm^2 for the entire spectrum. At noontime in December, the irradiance for wavelengths below 315 nm is of the order of 0.01 mW/cm^2 vs. 80 mW/cm^2 for the entire spectrum (Fig. 14-13). Therefore, to measure the actinic radiation component of the terrestrial solar spectrum, an instrument must be many thousands of times more sensitive to wavelengths below 315 nm than to wavelengths in the visible. The measurement of a welding arc would obviously require less rejection of longer wavelength radiation.

14.8.2 Earlier Direct Reading Instruments

During the 1930's and 1940's Westinghouse Lamp Division marketed an actinic UV measuring instrument which was surprisingly effective in its rejection of unwanted optical radiation. It was termed the "click meter," and made use of a RbTe-phosphor vacuum phototube. The response of this photocathode rapidly decreased from 300 to 320 nm. An electronic integrating circuit produced a click from a speaker each time a capacitor reached a certain charge. Each click corresponded to several μJ/cm^2 and the total number of clicks represented the exposure dose. Unfortunately the techniques for building this phototube have probably been lost with the passage of time. Presputtering of the cathode was critical to assure a pure surface with a sharp cutoff as explained by Rentschler (1930) and his colleagues (1932).

14.8.3 The Outlook

We are not aware of any commercial instrument presently available at a cost below $5,000, which is completely satisfactory for the measurement of actinic ultraviolet radiation (UV-B and UV-C) from most sources. However, many instruments are adequate for the measurement of germicidal ("cold quartz," low pressure-mercury) lamps, which emit very little radiation outside actinic band. The "click" meter and other, more recent, instruments designed for the measurement of irradiance or radiant exposure from germicidal lamps should, therefore, only be used for those lamps. Likewise, ultraviolet meters designed for use with "black light," UV-A sources (normally wavelengths between 320 nm and 400 nm) should only be used to measure such sources in a low ambient or dark environment for best results. The major breakthrough which made the NIOSH instrument (section 14.8.1) practical over a wide range was the ability of an optical coating laboratory to design a very sophisticated filter to limit sensitivity in conformity with the selected biological weighting function.

14.9 PROBLEMS ASSOCIATED WITH MEASUREMENTS

There are two common difficulties encountered in obtaining an accurate radiometric description of a broad-band, extended source. The first problem is to achieve adequate rejection of unwanted wavelengths from the passband of the monochromator (i.e., rejecting "stray light" from other radiometer components). The second most common problem is the proper definition of the actual or effective source size of an arc or a discharge lamp. Several other special problem areas (such as background isolation, wavelength calibration and the proper separation of line and continuous values) are also encountered in specific situations. The most common general source of measurement errors relate to the use of a calibration source that is very different from the source being measured. For example, a spectroradiometer calibrated against a small-size tungsten lamp may provide reproducible but grossly inaccurate measurements of a long tubular fluorescent lamp which has a different geometry and spectrum. Angular field-of-view and spectral sensitivity problems of the instrument may not be revealed during calibration with the small lamp, but introduce substantial errors during the fluorescent lamp measurement.

14.9.1 Stray Light

The problem of rejecting stray light is particularly acute as noted in a previous discussion on the ultraviolet region of the spectrum (section 14.6). The ultraviolet radiation hazard is the most common concern in evaluating lamps. Since the glass envelopes used in lamps or in projection optics normally filter out most of the actinic ultraviolet radiation, lamp evaluation often requires the measurement of ultraviolet spectral irradiance values a million-fold less than the spectral irradiance values in the visible. This requires the use of a high quality monochromator—often a double monochromator—which has excellent stray light rejection. Adequate stray light rejection may require that the monochromator pass less than one part in 10^5 of radiation outside of the desired passband if the source spectrum is not reasonably uniform.

It is difficult to measure ultraviolet radiation from a source rich in visible radiation but weak in actinic ultraviolet radiation. The best example of this challenging type of source would be that of the solar spectrum at sea level. Here the spectral irradiance varies by several orders of magnitude between 295 nm and 325 nm (Figs. 14-6 and 14-13). Reasonable accuracy in this case requires measurement of the spectral irradiance at 1-nm intervals in order to allow use of the proper weighting function for ultraviolet radiation on skin and cornea as discussed previously.

Another problem encountered with all instruments in the ultraviolet is UV radiation damage to optical glass, filters and detector surfaces. Optical materials, particularly plastics, often solarize and increase their absorption or scattering. Photocathodes can be easily damaged by high flux densities.

One method of testing the validity of measurements of actinic radiation is through the use of blocking filters. As an example, if measurements of the spectral irradiance at 300 nm are suspected to contain a significant portion of the stray light from visible or near-ultraviolet radiation, a glass filter (e.g., see Fig. 14-7) which cuts off all radiation below 310 nm may be placed in front of the aperture. Any radiation shorter than 310 nm will be blocked by the filter and should reduce the reading on

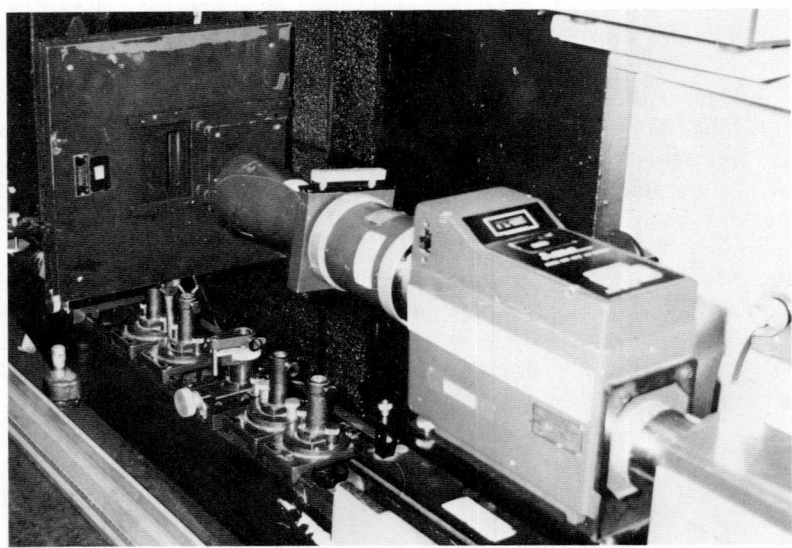

Figure 14-14. Spectroradiometer Calibration. An EG&G 585 commercial instrument is calibrated using a standard of spectral irradiance. Proper calibration protocol, with careful attention to the selection of filters and baffles, is required. The lamp is behind the aperture baffle.

the meter to zero. Any residual non-zero value is the result of stray light. This value can then be subtracted from the original reading to yield the actual 300 nm spectral irradiance. This subtractive technique can also be used with direct-reading UV hazard instruments. The technique is best if the filter does not fluoresce; the filter cutoff is sharp; near the wavelength of measurement the transmission at longer wavelengths is relatively high (e.g., > 90%); and the reading with the filter in place is no greater than 60% of the original reading. It should be remembered that the filter will normally reflect at least 8% of the stray light, and this can be included in the subtractive calculation for greater accuracy.

Stray light can also cause errors in the instrument calibration process in addition to those in the measuring process. A 1000-W tungsten lamp is typically used to calibrate a spectroradiometer (as shown in Fig. 14-14). An examination of the values in Table 14-2 shows that the spectral irradiance values from 250 nm to 400 nm differ by a factor exceeding 100. Hence the spectral calibration function of the spectroradiometer can be in error in the UV-B and UV-C regions if there is inadequate stray light rejection. The measurement of a relatively uniformly varying spectrum at a high irradiance, such as from a welding arc, will have minimal stray light errors (probably undetectable) to place the field measurements in question. But, in fact, the short wavelength measurements could be seriously in error (low) as a result of stray light error introduced during calibration. The instrument user should be wary of any spectroradiometer calibration curve which increases with

TABLE 14-2. Representative Values of Spectral Irradiance for a 1000-W Tungsten-Quartz-Iodide DXW Standard Lamp†

Wavelength (nm)	Spectral Irradiance $\mu W/(cm^2 \cdot nm)$	Wavelength (nm)	Spectral Irradiance $\mu W/(cm^2 \cdot nm)$
250	0.019	480	6.4
255	0.025	490	7.0
260	0.032	500	7.7
265	0.044	510	8.3
270	0.060	520	9.0
275	0.071	530	9.7
280	0.086	540	10.4
285	0.110	550	11.1
290	0.134	560	11.8
295	0.162	570	12.5
300	0.193	580	13.2
305	0.230	590	13.9
310	0.271	600	14.7
315	0.318	610	15.3
320	0.371	620	16.0
325	0.43	630	16.7
330	0.50	640	17.4
335	0.57	650	18.1
340	0.65	660	18.7
345	0.74	670	19.3
350	0.84	680	19.9
360	1.06	690	20.5
370	1.30	700	21.1
380	1.6	710	21.5
390	1.9	720	21.9
400	2.3	730	22.4
410	2.7	740	22.8
420	3.1	750	23.1
430	3.6	760	23.4
440	4.1	770	23.7
450	4.6	780	24.0
460	5.1	790	23.3
470	5.7	800	24.6

† Data for an EG&G Standard DXW lamp at 50 cm.

with shorter wavelengths at wavelengths shorter than 290 nm (Fig. 14-15). Because of this problem a deuterium lamp calibration standard (see Fig. 14-16) has been introduced in recent years. Stray light errors are not limited to the UV. Figure 14-17 illustrates how similar errors can arise in the infrared where a detector's sensitivity (e.g., an S-20 response) rolls off rapidly.

To summarize, errors introduced by stray light can be reduced by adhering to the following steps:

(a) Keep monochromators and input optics in dust-free, smoke-free environments, since stray light is increased by scattering caused by particles on the mirror, grating, filter, or prism surfaces.

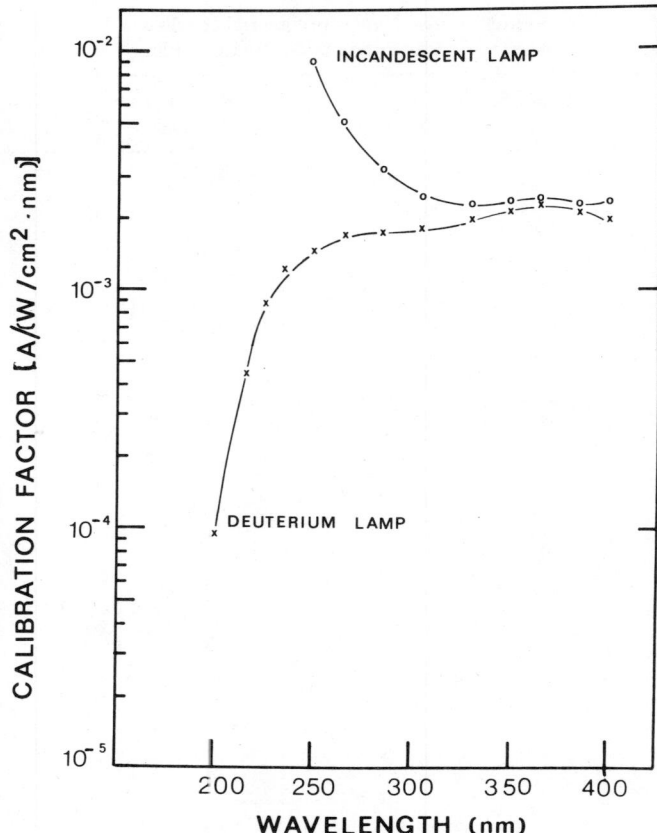

Figure 14-15. Calibration Errors. Calibration curves for a spectroradiometer obtained with a tungsten standard lamp (dashed line) and with a deuterium standard lamp solid line. A serious error in the calibration curve was introduced by straylight from the tungsten lamp. The deuterium-derived calibration curve was accurate.

(b) Use high quality monochromators with low stray light. A double monochromator may be best if the detector is highly sensitive.

(c) Use a series of broad-bandpass filters to reduce second-order radiation and light, and if necessary change filters every 50 to 100 nm. Calibrate the system with these filters in place. Avoid the use of filters which fluoresce.

(d) Check for light leaks throughout the optical path to the detector.

(e) Check for stray light with blocking filters to see if reading is reduced to zero. Table 14-3 provides a list of several useful ultraviolet cutoff filters and their 50% and 0.1% transmission wavelengths.

(f) Be wary of calibration curves that do not follow, at least approximately, the published spectral response of the detector. There will of course be some deviation

Broad-Band Optical Sources

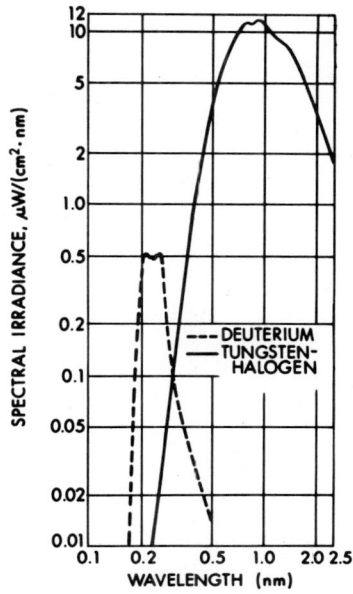

Figure 14-16. Two Calibration Lamps. Comparison of spectral irradiance E_λ from a 150-W tungsten-halogen-quartz lamp and a 30-W Deuterium Lamp. The radiant output of each has been focused to achieve the plotted values at a distance of 20 cm. For calibration the deuterium lamp is typically used only for $\lambda < 300$ nm.

TABLE 14-3. UV Cutoff Filters-Use to Check Stray Light in UV Monochromators and Actinic Ultraviolet Survey Instruments

Filter Type	50%T	0.1%T
WG 280	280	230 nm
WG 295	295	250
WG 305	305	280
WG 320	320	290
WG 335	335	315
WG 345	345	320
WG 360	360	335
GG 375	375	350
GG 385	385	355
GG 395	395	360

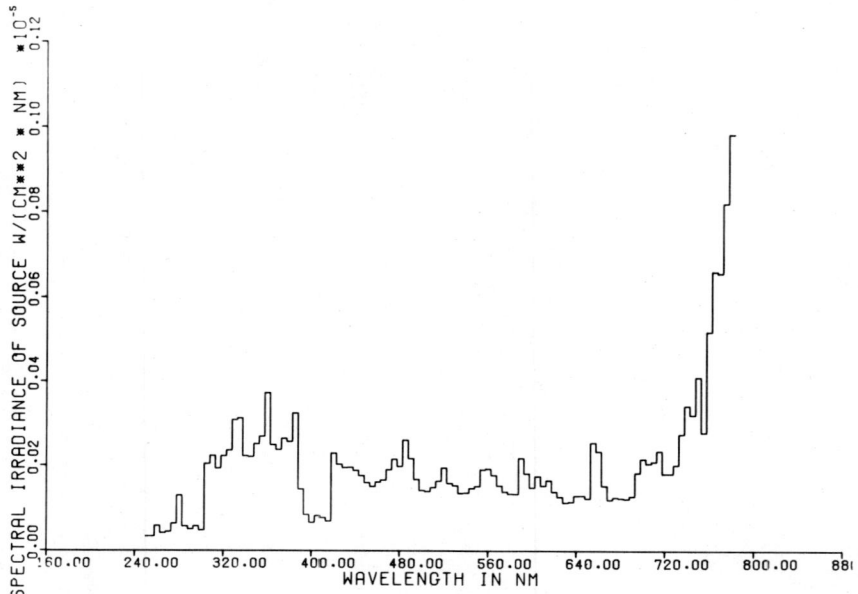

Figure 14-17. Erroneous Spectral Curve in the IR-A. Spectrum near 800 nm shows errors where detector sensitivity falls. Note the steady increase in the "measured" spectral irradiance near 800 nm. Experience with the source spectrum should indicate to the experimentor that this rise is due to either stray light, second-order wavelengths from the monochromator, or background incandescent radiation is superimposed on the entering radiation.

inasmuch as the spectral throughput of the monochromator is never a constant.

(g) Don't be deceived by the "neat appearance" of a computer generated, spectral irradiance curve from an automated spectroradiometer. Check the raw data generated at the detector. Be wary of uniformly increasing spectral irradiance values near the long-wave and short-wave cutoffs of the detector (Fig. 14-17) and discontinuities in the continuum of a spectral printout.

(h) Try to use a calibration source similar to the source to be measured.

14.9.2 Source Size

The source size must be measured in order to apply hazard criteria for extended sources. Even if the radiance can be measured directly, the effective source diameter or length must be determined. For non-uniform radiance distributions, photographic methods are almost always used. Some of the pitfalls associated with photographic radiometry have been reviewed in section 12.6.6. The primary problem area is the definition for the "edge" of the source. The relative source radiance

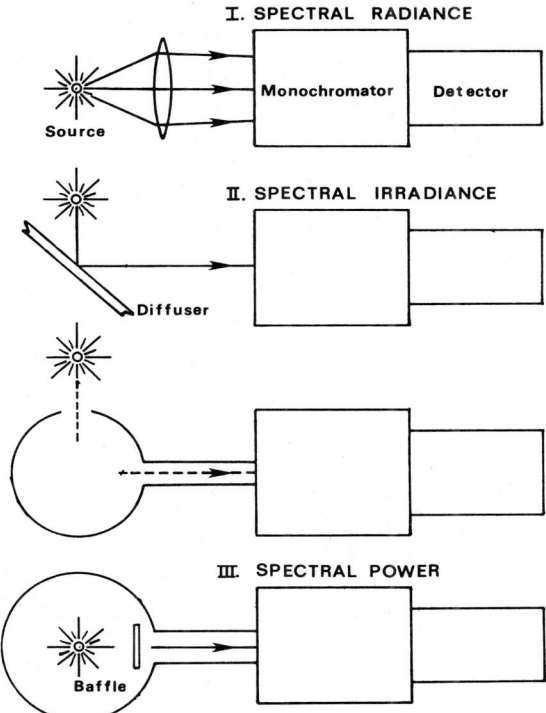

Figure 14-18. Input Optics. The baffles, diffusers and lenses which make up the input optics of a spectroradiometer or radiometer determine the field-of-view, the spatial sensitivity and the angular sensitivity of the instrument. Generally speaking, good input optics reduce throughput.

distribution recorded on photographic film can be reduced to a series of iso-irradiance profiles (Fig. 14-8) using a scanning microdensitometer (Fig. 14-8); but which iso-irradiance line should be considered the edge? If the scanned negative's information is all in the linear portion of the H-D curve the density unit intervals can be directly related to relative radiance by a constant conversion factor. The edge is most often considered to lie at half-peak radiance points defined at the greatest cross-sectional dimension (D in inset to Fig. 14-8).

If the primary purpose of determining source size is for calculating the source's radiance from irradiance measurements at a distance, then a more accurate integration of profile is generally necessary. This is a tedious process with most hand calculation methods, although computer data processing has been used.

If a goniometer mount for a small field-of-view luminance or radiance meter is available a satisfactory estimate of the angular distribution of the beam can be obtained by carefully (slowly) panning across the source; however, this technique is fraught with risk of errors—particularly if the field-of-view is not much smaller than the source size. The field-of-view and angular sensitivity function of the input optics of the radiometer (Fig. 14-18) play a key role in determining the source of errors. The calculated source radiance can be seriously in error even if the source profile is accurate when the radiometer, field-of-view is not matched to the source being analyzed.

14.9.3 Wavelength Measurements

Except for the 300-to-320 nm (and to some extent in the 400-to-550-nm) region a critical measure of wavelength is seldom required. An error in wavelength of 1 nm between 305 and 315 nm can result in a weighted spectral irradiance error of 100% at that wavelength. Monochromator readouts are usually calibrated with low-pressure gas discharge, "pen-ray" lamps. Table 14-4 lists many of the common emission lines used for wavelength calibration checks.

The mercury pen-ray lamp is often used to calibrate simple UV-irradiance meters, since 90% of the low-pressure mercury discharge lamp power is in the 254-nm line. The major problem with this approach is that a stable output occurs only after the lamp (and its housing) has warmed up. With a warm lamp, the infrared output radiant power can be significantly greater than the 254-nm output power. Thus, the infrared must be filtered out with a quartz water filter, etc., then the simple meter is checked against a calibrated thermal (e.g., pyroelectric) radiometer.

14.9.4 Infrared Measurement Problems

The principal problem encountered in the measurement of IR-B and IR-C sources is reradiation from baffles, and heating of detector assemblies. To determine if this is a problem, shields or baffles are temporarily removed, or records are kept of the time history of the measured irradiance after lamp turn-on, since baffle contribution will temporarily increase with time (Fig. 11-20). If pyroelectric detectors and beam chopping techniques are used, then the chopper should be placed near the source to reduce noise from the environment. The choice of an IR-transmitting window can also be important. In general a window having spectral transmission well outside the band of measurement interest is avoided so that unwanted background radiation is reduced. Unfortunately there are only a few windows which have broad, flat transmission bands (Fig. 11-20). If a detector does not have a window, the flattest spectral response is possible, but air currents and degradation of the detector surface can cause other errors.

14.9.5 Spectroradiometric Standards

The preferred calibration method for the radiance levels of interest noted in Table 11-2 is by comparison with a standard lamp. Standard 100-W and 120-W

TABLE 14-4. Commonly Used Wavelength Standards: Gas Discharge Lamps.*

λ (nm)	Lamp	λ (nm)	Lamp	λ (nm)	Lamp
184.91	Hg	430.01	A	696.54	A
194.17	Hg	431.96	Kr	702.41	Ne
226.22	Hg	433.86	A	703.24	Ne
237.83	Hg	435.84	Hg	705.91	Ne
248.20	Hg	436.26	Kr	706.72	A
253.65	Hg	437.61	Kr	717.39	Ne
265.20	Hg	445.39	K	724.52	Ne
280.35	Hg	446.37	K	727.29	A
289.36	Hg	450.24	K	738.40	A
294.51	He	533.08	Ne	743.89	Ne
296.73	Hg	534.11	Ne	748.89	Ne
302.15	Hg	540.06	Ne	750.39	A
312.57	Hg	546.07	Hg	751.46	A
313.17	Hg	556.22	K	753.58	Ne
334.15	Hg	557.03	K	754.41	Ne
336.99	Ne	576.96	Hg	758.74	K
341.79	Ne	579.07	Hg	760.15	K
344.77	Ne	585.25	Ne	763.51	K
346.66	Ne	587.09	K	768.52	K
347.26	Ne	588.19	Ne	769.45	K
352.05	Ne	594.48	Ne	772.38	A
359.35	Ne	597.55	Ne	785.48	K
365.02	Hg	603.00	Ne	794.82	A
365.44	Hg	607.43	Ne	800.62	A
366.33	Hg	609.62	Ne	801.48	A
394.90	A	614.31	Ne	805.95	K
404.44	A	616.36	Ne	810.37	A
404.66	Hg	621.73	Ne	810.44	K
407.78	Hg	626.65	Ne	811.29	K
412.08	He	630.48	Ne	811.53	A
415.86	A	633.44	Ne	819.01	K
416.42	A	638.30	Ne	823.16	Xe
418.19	A	640.23	Ne	826.32	K
419.10	A	650.65	Ne	826.45	A
419.83	A	653.29	Ne	828.01	Xe
420.07	A	659.90	Ne	829.81	K
425.94	A	667.83	Ne	837.76	Ne
427.22	A	671.70	Ne	840.82	A
427.40	Kr	692.95	Ne	842.46	A

* These wavelength values were taken from Ealing Optical Catalog. Wavelengths are given in air (or nitrogen).

tungsten ribbon filament lamps are commercially available calibrated for spectral radiance with an absolute accuracy of 2% to 10%. An estimate of the total response of the radiometer can be made if the spectral characteristics of the window material of the radiometer are known. In addition, 1,000-W tungsten-quartz-halogen lamps are used as standards of spectral irradiance. One approach uses such a lamp to calibrate directly a standard disc calorimeter, a pyroelectric radiometer, or other spectral irradiance (or spectral radiance) instrument. The use of a monochromator always raises the concern of stray light. Calibration errors due to monochromator stray light are particularly common when an incandescent lamp is used to calibrate a spectroradiometer in the UV.

14.10 CALCULATIONS OF BLACKBODY AND TUNGSTEN SOURCES

Many optical radiation sources encountered today are incandescent. Often, by the use of blackbody tables, filter transmission curves, and spectral emissivity data, the need for measurement can be obviated entirely. These curves are discussed in Chapter 22 on Lamp Safety.

14.11 COMPUTER PROGRAM DATA BASE

Table I of Appendix C provides the most useful spectral weighting functions used in the hazard analysis of an arc. Chapter 22 provides a calculation worksheet for evaluating hazards from a broad-band source.

14.12 REVIEW QUESTIONS

1. What is stray light?

2. The spectral irradiance at the 303-nm line of a mercury arc lamp was measured as 57 $\mu W/cm^2 \cdot nm$) at the line peak and the continuum at that point was 7 $\mu W/(cm^2 \cdot nm)$. The bandpass at the monochromator at that wavelength was 2.3 nm. What was the irradiance of the isolated 303 nm line from this arc lamp?

3. What considerations might determine the decision to use spectral measurement intervals of 5 nm versus 50 nm?

4. Could broader spectral intervals be used in measuring an incandescent lamp than used in measuring a fluorescent lamp?

5. A commercial pyroelectric radiometer is available with an optional remote-beam chopper instead of an internal-instrument chopper. Is there any value in such an option?

6. Calculate the error in the measurement of the "effective irradiance" at 303 nm of a line source if the monochromator records this line source as 304 nm.

7. Using a simple ultraviolet UV-C meter, an irradiance of 7 $\mu W/cm^2$ was recorded initially. Then an irradiance of 3.8 $\mu W/cm^2$ was measured with a UV-C blocking filter over the detector. What was the true UV-C irradiance?

8. A spectroradiometer with an S-20 detector records a strong line from a mercury arc lamp at 731 nm. Is this a real line? If not, what is the source?

9. What is the bandpass of a monochromator that has both an entrance and exit slit width of 2 mm and an inverse dispersion of 5 nm/mm.

10. Explain why a radiometer calibration source should be of a type similar to that of the source to be measured.

14.13 REFERENCES

Angstrom, A. K., and Drummond, A. J., 1961, Basic concepts concerning cutoff glass filters used in radiation measurements, *J. Meteorology* **18**(3):360–367.

Bauer, G., 1965, "Measurement of Optical Radiations," Focal Press, New York.

Berger, D. S., 1976, The sunburning ultraviolet meter: design and performance, *Photochem. and Photobiol.* **24**:587–593.

Berger, D., Magnus, I., Rottier, P. B., Sayre, R. M., and Freeman, R. G., 1969, Design and construction of high intensity monochromators, in "The Biologic Effects of Ultraviolet Radiation," (F. Urbach, ed.) Pergamon Press, New York.

Burt, J. E., and Luther, F. M., 1970, Effect of receiver orientation on erythema dose, *Photochem. Photobiol.* **29**:85–91.

Churchkova, M. and Kurchatova, C., 1975, Ultraviolet radiation and photooxidants, (Bulgarian), *Kygiena i Zdraveopazvania* (Sophia) **18**(3):281–286.

Coakley, J. M., 1976, Activities in the control of noncoherent radiation, in "Symposium on Biological Effects and Measurement of Light Sources," (D. G. Hazzard, ed.) pp. 91–105, HEW Publication (FDA)77-8002, U. S. Department of Health, Education and Welfare, Rockville, MD (October 1976).

Eckerle, K. L., 1976, Modification of an NBS Reference Spectrophotometer, NBS Technical Note 913, U. S. Department of Commerce, National Bureau of Standards, Washington, DC (July 1976).

Elenbaas, W., 1972, "Light Sources," Philips Technical Library Series, New York, Crane, Russak and Co., Inc.

Garbuny, M., 1965, "Optical Physics," Academic Press, New York.

Gillham, E. J., 1961, "Radiometric Standards and Measurements," Notes on Applied Science No. 23, National Physical Laboratory, Her Majesty's Stationery Office, London.

Glaser, P. E. and Walker, R. F., 1964, "Thermal Imaging Techniques," Plenum Press, New York.

Jones, O. C. and Preston, J. S., 1969, "Photometric Standards and the Unit of Light," Notes on Applied Science No. 24, National Physical Laboratory, Her Majesty's Stationery Office, London.

Kasha, M., 1948, Transmission filters for the ultraviolet, *J. Opt. Soc. Am.* **38**(11):929–934.

Klein, R. M., 1979, Cut-off filters for the near ultraviolet, *Photochem. Photobiol.* **29**:1053–1054.

Koller, L. R., 1965, "Ultraviolet Radiation," (2nd ed.) John Wiley and Sons, New York.

Loewen, E. G., 1970, "Diffraction Grating Handbook," Bausch and Lomb, Inc., Rochester, New York.

Madden, R. P., 1975, Ultraviolet Transfer Standard Detectors and Evaluation and Calibration of NIOSH UV Hazard Monitor, HEW Publication No. (NIOSH)75 131, NIOSH, Cincinnati, OH, (January 1975).

Martin, D. H. (ed.), 1967, "Spectroscopic Techniques in Far-Infrared, Submillimeter, and Millimeter Wavelengths," North Holland Publishing Co., Amsterdam.

McSparron, D. A., Mohan, K., Raybold, R. C., Saunders, R. D., nd Zalewski, E. F., 1970, Spectroradiometry and Conventional Photometry. An Interlaboratory Comparison, NBS Technical Note 559, National Bureau of Standards, Washington, DC (November 1970).

Nicodemus, F. E., 1972, "Radiometry—Selected Reprints," American Institute of Physics, New York.

Nicodemus, F. E. (ed.), 1977, 1978, 1979, Self Study Manual on Optical Radiation Measurements, NBS Technical Note Series 910, U.S. Department of Commerce, National Bureau of Standards, Washington, DC.

Pasachoff, J. M. and Muzyka, D. F., 1976, Infrared coronal lines, *Vistas in Astronomy* **19**:341–353.

Penning, F. M., 1979, "Electrical Discharges in Gases," Philips Technical Library, The Hague.

Pierson, A. H., 1979, Know your monochromator, *Electro-Optical Sys. Design* **11**(2):31–37.

Piltingsrud, H. V., and Stencil, J. A., 1976, A portable spectroradiometer for use at visible and ultraviolet wavelengths, *Amer. Industr. Hyg. Assn. J.* **37**:(2)90–94.

Rentschler, H. C., Henry, D. E., and Smith, K. O., 1932, Photoelectric emission from different metals, *Rev. Sci. Instr.* **3**:794–798.

Rentschler, H. C., 1930, An ultraviolet meter, *Trans. Amer. Inst. Electr. Engr.* **49**:576–580.

Roach, T., 1973, Final Report on a Method for Field Evaluation of UV Radiation Hazards, prepared by CBS Laboratories for the National Institute for Occupational Safety and Health (NIOSH), Contract No. HSM-99-72-144, NIOSH, Cincinnati, OH.

Saunders, R. D. and Shumaker, J. B., 1977, Optical Radiation Measurements: The NBS Scale of Spectral Irradiance, NBS Technical Note 594–13, U.S. Department of Commerce, National Bureau of Standards, Washington, DC (April 1977).

Saunders, R. D., Ott, W. R., Bridger, J. M., 1978, Spectral irradiance standard for the ultraviolet: The Deuterium Lamp, *Appl. Opt.* **17**:593.

Sliney, D. H., 1972, The merits of an envelope action spectrum for ultraviolet radiation, *Amer. Industr. Hyg. Assn. J.* **33**:644–653.

Sliney, D. H., Bason, F. C., and Freasier, B. C., 1971, Instrumentation and measurement of ultraviolet, visible and infrared radiation, *Am. Ind. Hyg. Assn. J.* **32**:415–431.

Sliney, D. H., Marshall, W. J., Carothers, M. L. and Kaste, R. C., 1977, "Hazard Analysis of Broad-Band Optical Sources," Technical Guide 085, U.S. Army Environmental Hygiene Agency, Aberdeen Proving Ground, MD (available from NTIS as ADA054 802) (December 1977).

Smith, R. A., 1965, Detectors for ultraviolet visible, and infrared radiation, *Appl. Opt.* **4**(6):633–638.

Spears, G. R., 1974, Radiant flux measurements of ultraviolet emitting light sources, *J. Illum. Engr. Soc.*

SPIE, 1979, "Light Measurement in Industry," a meeting held September 12-13, 1978, London, SPIE Proceedings Series, Vol. 146.

Stair, R. 1969, Measurements of natural ultraviolet radiation—historical and general introduction, *in* "The Biologic Effect of Ultraviolet Radiation," (F. Urbach, ed.) pp. 377–390, Pergamon Press, New York.

Stair, R., Schneider, W. E., and Jackson, J. K., 1963, A new standard of spectral irradiance, *Appl. Opt.* **2**:1151.

Vechet, B., 1974, Some problems in the absolute measurements of germicidal ultraviolet radiation: the use of "Pen Ray" lamps as a calibration standard, *Photochem. Photobiol.* **19**:329–335.
Walsh, J. W. T., 1958, "Photometry," 3rd ed., Dover, New York.
Williams, C. S. and Becklund, O. A., 1972, "Optics: A Short Course for Engineers," Wiley Interscience, New York.

Chapter 15
General Hazard Analysis and Controls

15.1 INTRODUCTION

Up to this point, the text has provided the basic information on biological effects, safety standards, and optical radiation measurements. This chapter begins the detailed consideration of hazard analysis and controls for lasers and other optical sources, including general procedures for hazard analysis and broad concepts of control measures. Hence, this chapter should be reviewed prior to study of the following chapters which are devoted to hazards associated with specific groupings or categories of laser equipment and other potentially hazardous optical sources. For the most part, the general hazard analysis and controls presented in this chapter relate to lasers and laser systems.

There are at least three broad areas of concern for any potentially hazardous optical sources: (1) the potential of the source for causing personal injury; (2) the environment in which the laser (or optical source) is used; (3) the individuals who operate and those who are potentially at risk from exposure to the optical radiation emitted by the laser or optical source (Fig. 15-1). For both lasers and lamp systems, it is possible to develop a classification scheme to greatly assist the health and safety professional in evaluating the risk of the optical source in its environment.

In Chapter 9 the laser classification system was examined in detail. It is important to understand that the classification system was developed to aid the user in establishing a safety program for a particular laser device. It was recognized early in the developement of laser safety standards in the United States that such a classification scheme was necessary to relieve the user of the burden of detailed and often complex laser power and energy measurements. The classification system also greatly reduces the need for calculations on the part of the user and even on the part of the health and safety professional. The unique risks and control measures applicable to specific environments depend upon the personnel potentially exposed and vary with each laser application; hence the type of installation could not be made part of

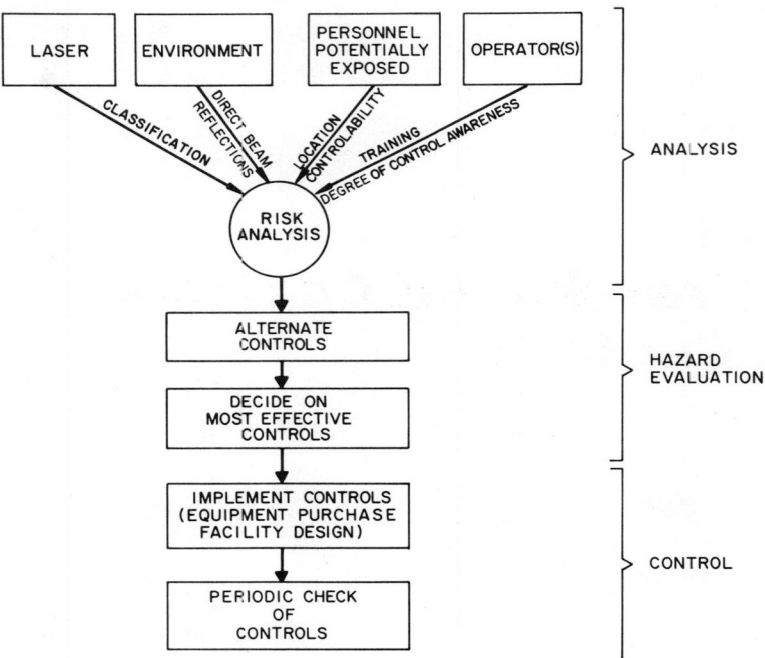

Figure 15-1. Laser Hazard Analysis. General hazard analysis and control by the laser user is shown in a step by step

the laser classification scheme. Fortunately many of the control measures are dependent entirely, or to a great extent, on the laser classification, and considerations of personnel and environment play only a minor role.

Since the control measures required for Class 1 and Class 2 laser systems are minimal or nonexistent for the user, it is the applications of Class 3 and Class 4 lasers that require careful study of the hazards, and the development of detailed control measures. There are several protective methods which can apply to a Class 3 or a Class 4 laser product. The total enclosure of the source is certainly the most desirable control measure. However, since total enclosure with proper interlocks would result in a Class 1 laser product, there must be a reason why a laser system was not originally designed as a Class 1 device. There are a few instances where a specific enclosure must be developed for each application. Where the enclosure approach is feasible, this solution is strongly encouraged.

Where the laser beam is operated unenclosed—either indoors or out-of-doors— the laser safety officer (a health or safety professional or other specially trained individual) encounters the greatest need for resource material and technical data. This data includes the reflective properties of materials found in the environment,

General Hazard Analysis and Controls 473

attenuating properties of filters, windows, or other enclosures, and a working knowledge of several aspects of optical systems. Therefore, this chapter will present several such categories of data.

15.2 THE LASER'S HAZARD POTENTIALS—SYSTEM SAFETY

The laser hazard classification now marked on the label of newly purchased laser systems is the most useful information available to the user that relates to the laser's hazard potential. However, the classification system does have its limits. It was, after all, designed to apply fairly well to most applications, but no such general scheme can ever be perfect. In this section the limitations provided by the classification scheme will be considered along with the risks posed by each laser system even when the classification is known. Chapter 9 provides all the information required to classify a laser system, and provides examples. If the laser system has not already been classified, or if the classification is in doubt, the user is encouraged to follow the procedure given in Section 9.3.3 to determine the appropriate classification. The present chapter will not provide these classification procedures in any detail.

15.2.1 Hazard Classification

The classification of a laser requires that the following output parameters be known: (a) the wavelength or wavelength range; (b) the classification duration (i.e., in the ANSI standard: how long is it possible for a person to be exposed to an applicable AEL); (c) average power output (for CW or repetitively-pulsed lasers); (d) total energy per pulse (or peak power, pulse duration, PRF, and emergent beam radiant exposures) for all pulsed lasers; (e) the laser source radiance or integrated radiance and the maximum viewing angular subtense is required if the source is an extended laser source and is operating in the retinal hazard region (400 to 1400 nm).

If the laser has been modified since manufacture in a way that could affect the hazard classification then the user or the individual performing the modification should go through the procedure of classifying the modified system.

15.2.2 General Concepts of System Safety

Although the Bureau of Radiological Health regulations assure that certain safety features will be incorporated into each type of manufactured laser product, it must be emphasized that these features in themselves do not necessarily ensure optimum system safety, and that user control measures are still the primary means for reducing risks from Class 3 and Class 4 lasers. The possibility of applying further system safety controls in addition to those already imposed by federal regulations should first be considered. Figure 15-2 shows a standard method used by systems designers for detecting potential malfunctions and safety hazards in any piece of equipment, be it an automobile or an electronic device, and for correcting such problem(s).

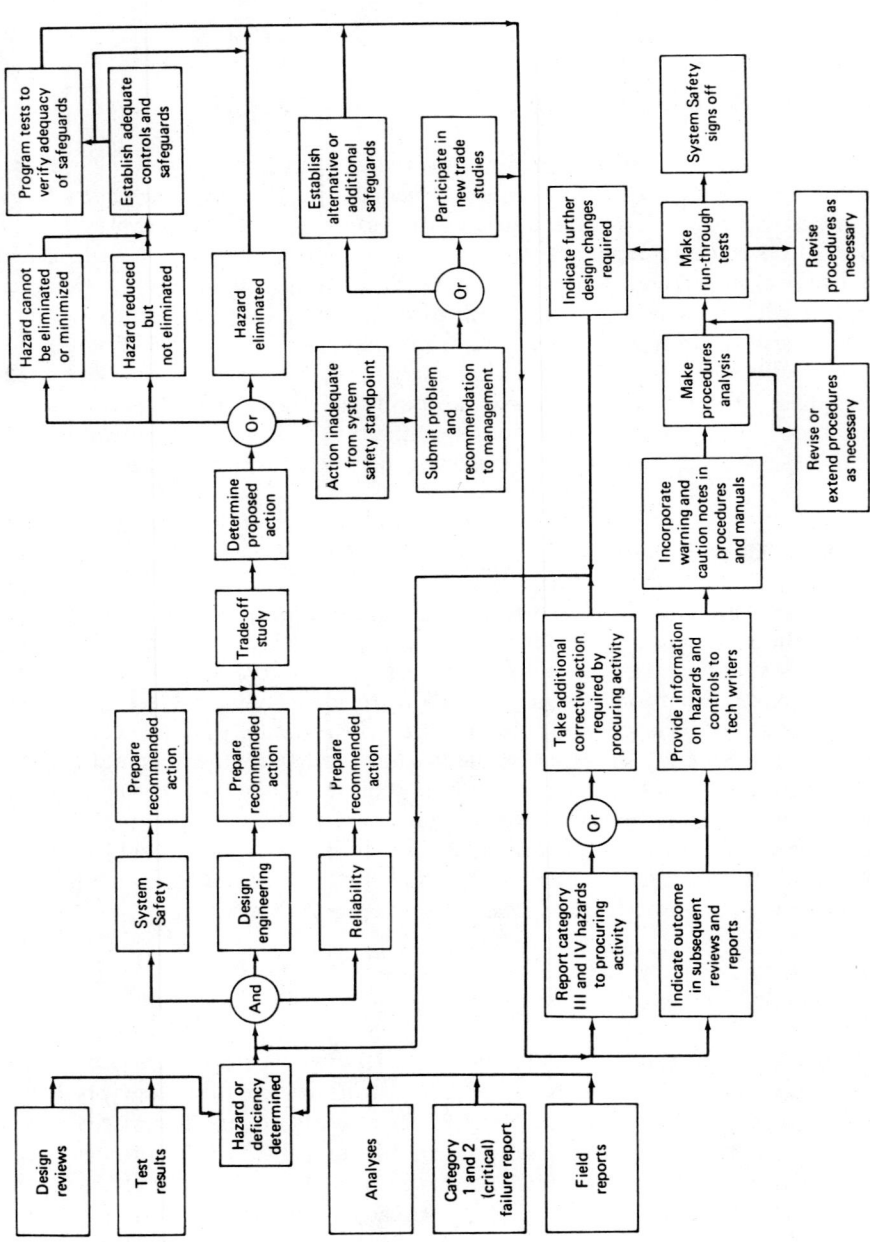

Figure 15-2. Systems Safety Flow Diagram (from Hammer, 1972, with permission).

The careful evaluation of a product's hazard potentials and corrections thereof is termed "system safety." Figure 15-2 is a system safety flow diagram from Hammer (1972). Note that the exercise of system safety requires a judgement of which safety features are economically practical. For instance, an automobile could be designed with highly expensive safety equipment: a collision-avoidance radar, a triple-backup braking system, and many other "desirable" features. The final product would be so expensive to own and operate that only multimillionaires could afford it. Obviously economic trade-offs are a necessity; the "trade-off study" occupies a prominent positon in the upper center portion of the flow diagram (Fig. 15-2). When a hazard cannot be reduced or eliminated, sufficient controls and safeguards should be developed and tested. Hazard control information is then provided to the user in the instructions. Figure 15-2 may be considered as the "brain child" of an enthusiast for management studies. Nevertheless, whether system safety is performed by the sole designer in a small company, or by a panel of experts in a large corporation or government agency, the same thought processes and system safety study take place. Probably the most difficult aspect of system safety is the determination of all of the potential fault conditions. It is practically impossible to anticipate all of the possible things that could happen in the normal use of the product, much less to anticipate those that *could happen* through the misuse of a product. Once a possible fault has been identified the system safety analyst applies a technique known as "fault-tree analysis." This in essence, considers the chain of events which can occur if a particular adverse act or component failure occurs. Clearly, in a multi-component, sophisticated product, a partial or complete component failure should be considered in light of the final resulting hazard. The reliability analyst considers whether or not a system will continue to function, albeit not at maximum performance levels; the system safety analyst considers only those aspects of reliability failure which result in the generation of a risk to life or limb.

One scheme has four categories of hazard resulting from failures (Hammer 1972): Category 1, loss of life or limb; Category 2, loss of property; Category 3, damage to the equipment, and Category 4, only a slight chance of injury or property damage. The various categories of hazards are treated somewhat differently in the flow diagram of Fig. 15-2. Although many potential fault conditions can be explored on paper, or by computer simulation, most large corporations and government agencies perform numerous tests under laboratory and field conditions to determine if unforeseen problems can arise—as they so often do.

15.3 LASER SYSTEM DESIGN

Safe design of laser products is generally oriented toward assuring that the warning mechanisms ("bells and whistles"), beam enclosures, shutters, and filters are appropriate to the level of experience of personnel operating and servicing the equipment. Restricting human access to hazardous optical radiation levels or live current-carrying conductors is achieved by permanent interlocked enclosures.

15.3.1 Interlocks

The Bureau of Radiological Health requires that certain interlocking mechanisms be failsafe (failure-proof). This eliminates the possible use of many all-electronically-activated interlocks, since power loss or circuit failure can prevent the performance of some electrical interlocks and relay contacts can weld shut. Hence, the designer is often faced with the need for a mechanical interlock. Figure 9-2 illustrates two types of mechanical-electrical interlocks for fool-proof electrical switches which are widely employed on various laser systems. A lateral or rotary movement of a hinge or a latch activates the switch which would be in the power circuit for the laser. If the switch contacts welded shut then the panel could not be opened.

No discussion of interlocks is complete without consideration of bypass methods to "cheat" the interlock. An interlock, to be effective, must obviously be designed to require intentional operation to inactivate or bypass the interlock. It is highly desirable that any bypass method which is used in the interlock design include a self-restoring feature to render the interlock effective again when the total system is returned to normal operation. A bypass method is not desirable if the interlock functions to prevent exposure of an operator or serviceman to hazardous exposures within the period of the aversion response. The interlock should be designed and positioned to minimize accidental defeat or bypass. The response time of the interlock must be sufficiently rapid to ensure that hazardous exposure could not occur before system shutdown or similar protective reaction is complete. The interlock and panel should be so designed that even partial opening of the panel to a point where hazardous radiation can be emitted from the opening results in positive activation of the interlock.

Life cycle tests are often required for interlocks, and such tests would typically require at least 10,000 cycles of operation without malfunction. Interlocks which are required to operate in adverse conditions such as high humidity, salt spray, or extremes in temperatures, should be selected so as to function properly in these environments.

15.3.2 Manual Switches

Some system safety standards recommend that if unintentional operation of the switch can result in physical injury, the switch shall operate with a single, straight-line motion. This is based on the assumption that the movement of the hand required to turn off a toggle or push-button switch is more rapid than that for a rotating switch. On the other hand, a cover or protector probably should be used on such a switch to reduce the additional likelihood of unintentional operation. The switch should be readily accessible to the operator in his normal position, yet should be positioned to minimize accidental operation. Operator positive-activated switches (sometimes referred to as positive-action or dead-man switches) are often employed where constant operator alertness is essential for safe operation.

General Hazard Analysis and Controls 477

15.3.3 The Enclosure

A difficult aspect of enclosure design involves possible laser emission or electrical shock hazards following mechanical damage to the enclosure. Damage to a viewing port could allow hazardous optical radiation to pass. A shift in wavelength of the laser could create hazardous conditions if, by such a shift, emission occurs through a sharp-cutoff blocking filter. From a safety standpoint these events are considered highly unlikely, since most lasers will not continue to operate after undergoing severe mechanical shock.

15.3.4 Accidental Laser Firing

Unintentional firing of a pulsed laser can occur in two ways: either by unintentional closure of the firing switch or by capacitor discharge due to extraneous causes. This problem is encountered with small CW lasers, but the possible adverse consequences are clearly of great concern for any Class 4 laser system.

In the early 1960's the complaint was often heard of accidental ruby laser firing due to capacitor discharge without firing-switch closure. The cause could be radio-frequency interference (RFI) or charging circuit transients which triggered flashlamp discharge. These problems are rare now as a result of better power supply circuit design.

Today, a common problem is double pulsing from a q-switched flashlamp-pumped laser. This occurs in a system with a long-pulse lamp flash and a rotating prism system, and from some passive q-switch systems. A second (unnecessary) pulse will increase the hazard distance and can generally only be eliminated by the adjustment or redesign of the pulse-forming network. The two pulses generally follow one another within 0.1 ms.

Desirable control measures to prevent accidental switch closure are switch covers, switch guards, and multiple switches. Of course these controls are only necessary for lasers intended for environments where such accidental firing is possible, and where such firing could create a hazard (e.g., in military lasers). Many Class 4 lasers require positive action such as closure of at least two switches in order to initiate laser action.

15.3.5 Safe Laser Projectors

One question often asked is whether the output laser beam pattern can be altered such that a hazardous output is changed to a relatively safe condition. Obviously a CW laser with an emergent beam diameter of 10 or 20 cm is far less hazardous than a laser of the same power with a 2-mm beam diameter. Although the classification would not change unless the altered output beam diameter exceeded 80 mm (the standard ANSI and BRH measurement aperture for continuous-wave lasers), it is only fair to point out that any expansion of the beam makes an unfocused beam safer since the actual biological effect is not dependent simply upon total power but also upon beam irradiance. Thus, in general, it is more desirable to have a large beam diameter rather than a small beam diameter.† If the beam is propagated over a long distance, however, the larger emergent beam diameter of a highly collimated laser beam will normally result in a higher beam irradiance at points in the far field (downrange) than for the initial, unexpanded beam with normal divergence.

In some instances the demand for laser beams having spatial coherence, or high collimation is not strong. In these cases several methods can be utilized to produce a safe output beam *radiance*. If it is the monochromaticity or pulse characteristic that is of value, as would be the case in a broad-angle beacon, then the laser beam can be directed into a diffuser to give very large solid angle emission. If the diffuser surface is sufficiently large, then the beam radiance may be low enough to place the laser product in Class 1.

The case of a diffused-beam laser system is given as an example. A designer wishes to develop a signal beacon with a total output of 1 joule in a 20-ns pulse at the neodymium:YAG laser wavelength (1064 nm). A hemispherical beam pattern (2π sr) is desired. He realizes that if he directs a laser beam at a white diffuse target and places a diffused plastic hemispherical dome over the beam and diffuser then he can achieve a relatively uniform radiance. How large should the beam diffuser be? Is this diffuser size practical?

From Table 9-2 the BRH limit for a single-pulse 20-ns extended source is 10 $k_1 \cdot k_2 \cdot t^{1/3}$ J/(cm² · sr) = 0.063 J/(cm² · sr). If the diffuser is reasonably Lambertian then the *effective solid angle* into which the 1 J is directed is not 2π sr, but π sr (i.e., $L = H/\pi$). The design requirement is therefore H = 0.063 π J/cm² = 0.2 J/cm² from the surface. The diffuser area A_D required to reduce the surface radiant exposure to 0.2 J/(cm² · sr) is:

$$A_D = (1J) / (0.2 \text{ J/cm}^2) \qquad (15\text{-}1)$$
$$= 5.0 \text{ cm}^2$$

and since:

$$A_D = \pi D_d^2 / 4 \qquad (15\text{-}2)$$
$$D_d = \sqrt{4 A_D / \pi}$$
$$D_d = 2.5 \text{ cm}$$

where D_d is the diameter of the diffuser. Hence, the diameter of the diffuser would not be so large as to make such a beacon system impractical; and obviously the beacon itself is practical. The dome should be of a rugged plastic material rather than glass since dome fracture could cause the laser system to revert to Class 4.

Figure 15-3 shows how diffusing projection optics can be utilized to change a Class 4 or Class 3 laser system into a Class 2, or even a Class 1 laser system, by

---

† For CW lasers having beam diameters of 1 to 10 mm, the actual fire hazard or biological effect upon the skin varies very little for the same beam power.

General Hazard Analysis and Controls

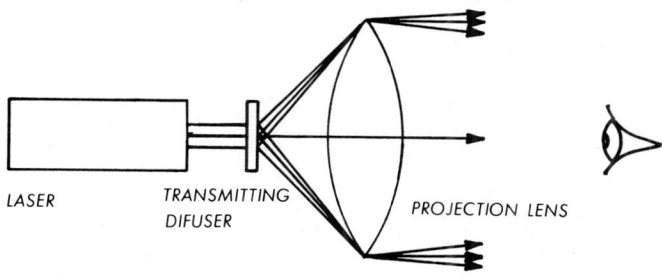

a. TRANSMITTING-DIFFUSER-REFRACTOR OPTICAL PROJECTION SYSTEM

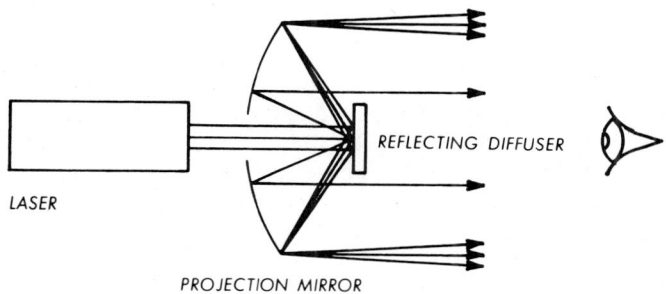

b. REFLECTING-DIFFUSER-CATODIOPTIC OPTICAL PROJECTION SYSTEM

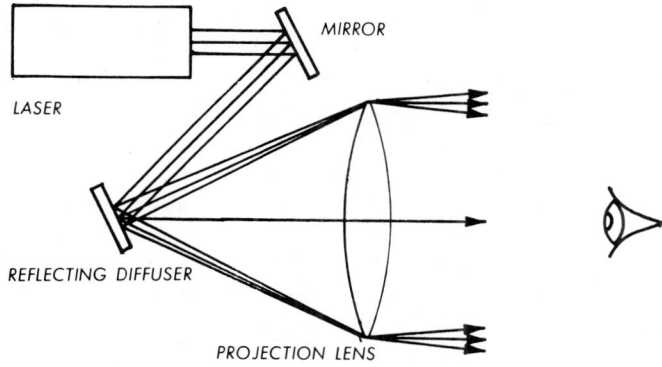

c. REFLECTING-DIFFUSER-REFRACTOR OPTICAL PROJECTION SYSTEM

Figure 15-3. Diffusing Projection Optics. Diffusing projection optics can convert a Class 4 or Class 3 to a Class 1 or Class 2 system by changing the output from point source to an extended source. Three techniques are shown.

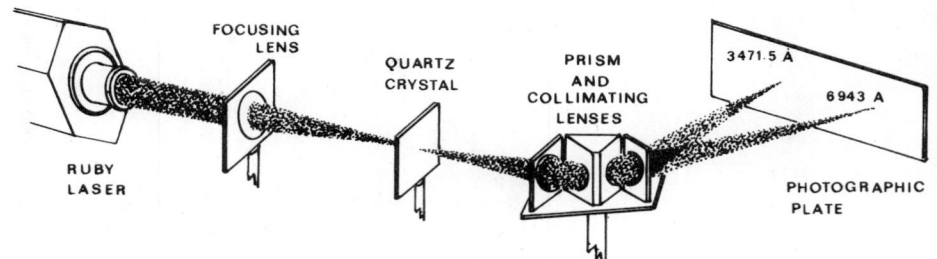

Figure 15-4. Multiple Wavelengths. Production of two laser beams of two different wavelengths: the secondary frequency-doubled beam and the primary beam by SHG. SHG is, in theory, possible at very low conversion efficiencies in any material.

changing the output from intrabeam viewing to an extended source. Unfortunately this is a costly procedure and has limited application. It is only effective if the output of the laser is marginally above the Class 1 limits for a point source, unless very large optical projection elements are incorporated into the design.

15.3.6 Multiple Wavelengths

If non-linear optical components are incorporated into the design of the laser system, increased hazards may be introduced by the production of additional wavelengths, and mode-locked pulses. Figure 15-4 illustrates how a laser beam of sufficient peak irradiance (i.e., a Q-switched pulse) can produce a secondary beam at a wavelength one-half of the initial wavelength through the process of frequency doubling (second-harmonic generation).

The specification of a wavelength or wavelengths by a manufacturer ordinarily refers to the primary output power. That does not preclude the emission of some wavelengths of much lower power which are nevertheless coherent. Occasionally these output wavelengths, overlooked or ignored by most laser designers, are nevertheless of particular concern from the standpoint of laser safety. Fortunately, the threshold power for such secondary laser wavelengths is at least in the milliwatt range and can be detected with some effort. There are additional implications of these secondary wavelengths. For instance, a laser emitting in the infrared may have a more hazardous visible component coaxial with the higher-power infrared beam. Although the far-infrared laser beam is not imaged on the retina, the less powerful visible or near-infrared beam may be at levels which are hazardous. Additionally, the assumption of the emission of a single wavelength leads to the selection of filter glass or plastic windows which may be adequate to attenuate the primary wavelength, but may be insufficient to reduce or eliminate the lower power emission of the secondary wavelength. Fluorescent screens which respond to UV or IR radiation, and image converter viewers may be used to detect unexpected emissions when filters which selectively reject the primary beam are placed over the output beam port. As an example, a frequency-doubled ruby laser operating at 347 nm can be checked by eye for visible or near infrared emission when a UV-absorbing filter is used in front of a fluorescent screen. Ion lasers are particularly noted for producing multiple wavelengths. Argon, krypton, and xenon lasers all emit at a variety of wavelengths. Since most applications require the output to be at one or two wavelengths, the designer usually optimizes the laser output for those wavelengths with a dispersive element (i.e., a prism) in the laser cavity, or resonator mirror coatings with selectively enhanced reflectance for the desired wavelength.

It is difficult to calculate accurately the output power of a laser after use of an electro-optic crystal to produce second harmonic generation (SHG). If an electro-optic crystal is added to the output of a single-mode Gaussian-profile laser of output power Φ and frequency ν (where $\nu = c/\lambda$) incident along the principal axis of an electro-optic crystal of thickness t; is then (Adhav and Orzag, 1974):

$$\Phi_{2\nu} = K_d \cdot \Phi \nu^2 \, t^2 \, K_s^2 \, \sin^2 X \, [\sin(\Delta K \cdot t/2)/\Delta K \cdot t/2]^2 / w_0 \qquad (15\text{-}3)$$

where K_d is the dielectric constant at the fundamental frequency for the SHG crystal, K_s is the coefficient of SHG determined by the non-linear susceptibility of the crystal w_0 is the minimum beam radius (Chapter 12), and X is the angle between the crystal's optic axis and the fundamental beam under phase-matched conditions. ΔK is the wave-vector mismatch parameter due to dispersion resulting from a different index of refraction of the crystal at the fundamental and the SHG wavelengths. Sometimes ΔK is made equal to zero by heating the crystal to a precise temperature. This is known as temperature tuning.

Some of the paramenters of interest for second harmonic generation are given in Table 15-1. It is important to remember that, although electro-optic crystals are used for SHG, it is also possible to produce other wavelengths by parametric amplification. Fortunately, it is unlikely that accidental adjustment of laser components and nonlinear optical crystals would produce parametric oscillations, since lasers that work on this principle are extremely delicate and require constant attention for proper tuning. Obviously the health and safety professional must be aware of the many factors that can contribute to the generation of wavelengths other than the primary specified wavelength, and take appropriate measures to control any unwanted secondary wavelengths at hazardous levels.

15.3.7 Mode Locking

Mode-locked pulses can be produced by using a similar non-linear crystal with a Q-switched pulsed laser (Fig. 2-25). Mode-locking, since it produces sub-nanosecond exposures, presents several problems to the safety specialist. First, there are at present no standards in the U.S.A. for sub-nanosecond exposures and there has always been some controversy as to whether or not self-mode locking actually creates an added hazard inasmuch as the actual average power tends to drop. Conflicting biological data still exists (Chapter 4). The sub-nanosecond exposure limits

TABLE 15.1. Parameters of Interest for Second Harmonic Generation in Crystals.

Material	Formula	Tuning Angle at 1060 nm	Typical Damage Threshold (MW/cm^2)	Typical Efficiency (%) at 1060 nm
ADP	$NH_4H_2PO_4$	41° 09'	100	5
KDP	KH_4PO_4	40° 31'	100	8
RDP	RbH_2PO_4	50° 53'	300	25
ADA	$NH_4H_2AsO_4$	41° 16'	—	—
KDA	KH_2AsO_4	40° 19'	—	—
RDA	RbH_2AsO_4	48° 56'	300	25
CDA	CsH_2AsO_4	83° 30'	300	30
$LiIO_3$	$LiIO_3$	30° 12'	100	8
Li(COOH)	Li(COOH)	81°	200	14
$LiNbO_3$	$LiNbO_3$	10°	50	6
Banana	$Ba_2NaNb_5O_{15}$	90°	5	12

Adapted from Adhav and Orszag (1974), Frequency doubling crystals—unscrambling the acronyms, *Electro-Optical System Design* 6(12):20–24.

proposed in a draft IEC TC76 document in 1979 were to limit the peak irradiance of the EL's to the values always permitted at 1ns (0.5 kW/cm² at the eye for wavelengths between 400 and 700 nm).

Mode-locking which limits the number of longitudinal modes in a laser, was normally achieved through the insertion of an intra-cavity electro-optic modulator which assists the laser to oscillate in the longitudinal mode with the highest gain (and in the associated side-band modes. Passive mode-locking through the use of saturable absorbers is now more common. Single-pulse selection then produces a pulse having a duration of a few ps. In laser cavities that are usually long (e.g., b > 1 m) self mode-locking is not uncommon. There have been some claims, however that almost all HeNe gas lasers self-mode-lock, but the mode locking was difficult to detect because the pulses were not so far apart. If this is so, many of the biological thresholds reported for longer exposures may have been produced using self-mode-locked lasers.

15.3.8 Beam Hotspots

Uncertainties in output irradiance profiles sometimes foul up the hazard analysis. The techniques of laser beam diagnostics discussed in Chapter 12 concentrated on calculations of the axial beam irradiance of a single mode laser beam. However, as illustrated in Fig. 11-1, the irradiance is not easily calculated for the irregular profiles of high-order mode patterns. Sensitive films or detectors with 1-mm apertures to estimate the beam irradiance are the primary methods used to determine diffuse reflection hazards in the retinal hazard region and hazards to the skin and cornea outside of this spectral band. It is useful to remember that the irradiance in a far-field pattern or in the focal spot pattern of a higher-order-mode laser can never exceed that in the single-mode pattern. This is very helpful for outdoor applications and focused beam cases; it is also useful in the analysis of hazards in the near field of a laser. Techniques for analyzing hazardous diffuse reflections will be discussed in greater detail in section 15.5.1.

A value for the maximum output power or energy is necessary for laser classification. An upper limit for the excursion in output power of a laser is difficult to calculate, and therefore maximum output powers are normally estimated by a manufacturer or laser designer based on experience gained during testing identical or similar systems. The maximum output can be affected by changes in the length of the laser cavity, reflectivity of the mirrors, diameter of the discharge tube or laser rod, mirror alignment, and input power or energy. Any changes in these parameters during design or modification of a laser thus require another evaluation of the output. The user who lacks extensive experience in laser design and operating characteristics is encouraged to examine the typical output values from commercially available lasers, in addition to obtaining this data directly from the manufacturer's brochures. Several trade journals publish lists of available commercial lasers and their output characteristics annually in summary product listings [e.g., "Laser Focus Buyer's Guide," (annual in March); "Optical Industry and Systems Directory" (annual); "Electro-Optical System Design's" vendor selection issue (annual in November)].

The output power and energy specifications for a particular type of laser at a specific wavelength with given laser cavity dimensions provides one of the best ideas of laser output, although these specifications are typically minimum rather than maximum values. However, since the advent of the 1976 BRH regulation many manufacturers are listing maximum outputs as well as the minimum design specifications.

Initially the BRH laser hazard classification did not consider the laser application, although an amended regulation was issued in November 1978, which took into account intended viewing conditions as already existed in the ANSI Z-136 standard. This amended BRH regulation included a new Class II-A for CW visible lasers where the intentional viewing duration would be far less than the maximum classification duration of $> 3 \times 10^4$ s. Table 15-2 gives reasonable viewing durations for exposure to CW or repetitively-pulsed laser systems. Clearly, a provision which permits the application to influence the classification obviously requires that the user re-evaluate the classification of the laser if the laser is utilized in an application other than that originally intended.

15.4 THE POPULATION POTENTIALLY AT RISK

15.4.1 Age, Experience, and Frequency of Exposure

The population potentially exposed to laser radiation from any given laser system primarily varies with application. Presumably no one would be exposed to an

TABLE 15-2. Typical Classification Durations for Laser Systems*

Application	Duration (s)
Laser Holographic Display	30,000
Laser Intrusion Detector (GaAs Laser Electric Eye)	100
Laser Alignment Tool intended for intrabeam staring	30,000
Laser Supermarket Point-of-Sales Scanner	1,000
Laser Gun Toy	100
Construction Alignment Laser (no intrabeam viewing intended)	100
Classroom Laser Demonstration Kit	100

* The ANSI Z-136.1 standard and the ACGIH Guide permit the Laser Safety Officer to classify laser systems on the basis of use. The above durations are only representative. Since 1979 manufacturers have been permitted to use a duration of 1,000 s for classification of a laser product not intended for viewing and operating in the visible wavelength region.

unmanned laser system operating in outer space, and considerations of classification are probably not important in such an application. Elsewhere, one or more individuals may be exposed in normal operation during maintenance or during service of a laser. Presumably, laser operators and servicemen would be expected to avoid hazardous exposure based upon their training and experience. On the other hand the mere fact that they work frequently with laser systems increases their probability of exposure.

The type of individuals who may be exposed vary with the location of the laser. Obviously the populations at risk can vary significantly, between those at risk from a laser used in a secondary school as opposed to those at risk from a laser used in a research laboratory or in an underground mine. Potentially hazardous exposure conditions may be most accentuated if the particular laser creates abnormally high levels of curiosity as might occur in a museum exhibition. There is little guidance that can be provided here with regard to the problem of the population at risk. There are so many varied possibilities that it is probably fruitless to attempt to develop generalized guidelines. Nevertheless some observations may be in order. Obviously there will be differences of opinion regarding the expected actions of any particular group under any specific potential exposure condition.

It is often said that safety rules and regulations should be extremely relaxed in a research laboratory so as not to interfere with the pursuit of scientific research. This line of argument continues with the suggestion that research scientists are more careful with a laser simply because they are more aware of the hazards. Are they really? Surveys of research laboratories often produce dismay by the complete lack of understanding of these hazards which some researchers demonstrate even though they have worked with lasers for several years. This ignorance is not limited to laboratory technicians and scientists using the laser as a tool in many diverse fields, but also includes personnel who design and build lasers, or otherwise work in the field of quantum electronics. Over the years the authors have gradually changed their advocacy for relaxed regulations in scientific laboratories, to a position opposing any such relaxation. An examination of serious laser injuries to the eye resulting from accidental exposures indicates that it is the laser specialist who is injured most often and only rarely the curious or the uninitiated. Perhaps in this regard one should remember that "familiarity breeds contempt."

15.4.2 Exposure Duration—Intentional vs. Non-intentional Exposure

It does seem reasonable, however, that system safety precautions and user restrictions should be more severe for the general public or most especially for children. Children have a way of finding new applications (and new hazards) for toys or other objects that come into their possession. A discussion of potential exposure durations indicates that children would not necessarily be sufficiently cautious in limiting their exposure to the laser. On the other hand, the total exposure duration may be limited. At a recent international meeting where exposure durations for classification came under discussion, one representative from the United States suggested that worst-case exposure duration should be assumed for all laser toys (i.e., a maximum time of 3×10^4 s). A delegate from Poland disagreed, pointing out that anyone familiar with children would know that their attention span would never be sufficiently long to warrant a very lengthy classification duration. Of course this is correct, but unfortunately sometimes a greater attention span for toys and games is found in children above the age of 20 or 30. This discussion illustrates the difficulty in coming up with a consensus on what constitutes a reasonable maximum exposure duration for many applications. Table 15-2 lists expected representative durations for classification as judged by the authors.

The aversion response of the eye is a physiologically determined exposure duration that is implicit in present classification schemes. This was explicitly chosen as 0.25 s (250 ms) for both the ANSI Z-136 and the IEC standards, and the BRH performance regulation has this value inherently included. Although the mean duration of the blink reflex is only 150 ms (Geratewold and Strughold, 1956) the inclusion of possible eye movements (and biological variance) suggested the value of 250 ms. This limit of course applies only to visible wavelengths (400 to 700 nm) where the luminous efficiency of radiation is sufficiently great to assure a strong aversion response to bright light sources at levels well below the MPE (see Table 11-3). At wavelengths outside of the visible spectrum a blink reflex is not expected and the aversion response would be considered nonautomatic, unless the corneal irradiance is sufficient to give a general thermal response.

Studies of reaction times for the removal of a hand from a hot surface which would apply to exposure of the skin to relatively high powered CW lasers suggests an aversion response time for the limbs of approximately 0.5 to 3 s and for the whole body of 1 to 7 s. This depends upon the time required for the incident flux to be conducted as thermal energy to sensory nerve endings. This, in turn, depends upon irradiance levels above ambient. Obviously all of these aversion responses are at levels which are of serious concern. Although they are perhaps above levels of long-term chronic exposure they generally are less than 10 s. An aversion response does not reliably limit exposure to the retina from hazardous levels of IR-A radiation. On the other hand it is possible to consider the protective nature of eye movements (Fender, 1965). The normal saccades of the eye would limit the stability of a point image on the retina to a duration seldom exceeding 1 or 2 s, even if the observer concentrates on a point of interest. Therefore unless an individual fixates on a display or a very small area in space for very long periods of time (exceeding 10 seconds), it seems unreasonable to assume that intrabeam retinal exposure to a point laser source would expose the same area of the retina for periods in excess of 10 s.

One physiological fact should be considered, however, in terms of thermal injury to the retina from extended exposure durations. Unlike the photochemical damage mechanism, the thermal injury mechanism is highly dependent upon the area of the retina exposed because of heat flow in the retina (Section 4.7). For a "point-source" exposure the thermal image on the retina could be easily 100 μm in diameter at half-peak-temperature-points under equilibrium conditions. Therefore if the eye movement occurs only to a small extent a large thermal image on the retina would not be substantially affected if the point on the retina being exposed varies only by 25 to 50 μm. This should be kept in mind by designers of oculometers or other devices which may use near-infrared (IR-A) radiation to track eye movements and fixation points. If time-and-motion studies do not appear to provide assurances of a limited exposure duration for a visible (or ultraviolet) laser-type whose exposure limits are additive for exposure exceeding 10 to 100 s, then time-actuated laser power switches may be considered to achieve Class 1 ratings.

15.4.3 Photo-Sensitive Individuals

The possibility exists that a small fraction of the general population will demonstrate abnormal sensitivities to skin or ocular injury from optical radiation. In the work environment it is possible to eliminate the possibility that such individuals will be exposed, but for a consumer product this is essentially impossible. The designer must remember that the exposure limits were based upon normal responses which could be considered excessive for photosensitive individuals. Normally this matter is of concern only for lasers operating at wavelengths shorter than approximately 500 nm where photochemical and photodynamic reactions may exist (Fitzpatrick, 1975).

15.5 ENVIRONMENTAL CONSIDERATIONS - Reflections and the Probability of Exposure

Environmental considerations probably play a greater role in determining the control measures for Class 3 and Class 4 laser systems, and these can only be evaluated by the user. These environmental considerations include the possibility for

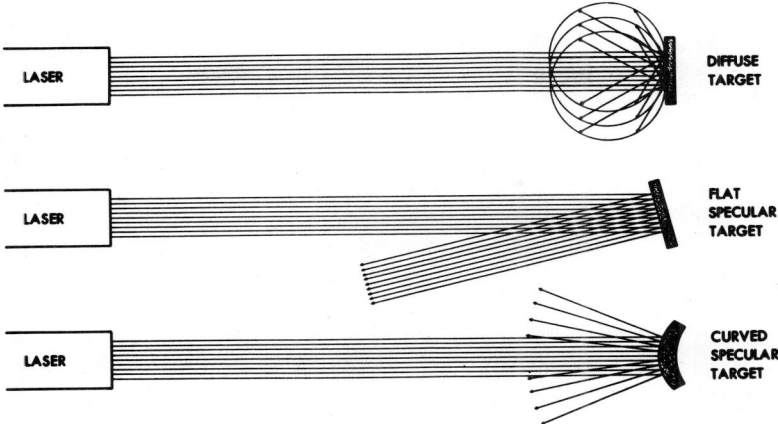

Figure 15-5. Reflections. Three general categories of reflections are illustrated. Diffuse reflections (top) are generally not hazardous (except for Class 4) since the collimated nature of the beam is destroyed. Specular reflection (below) is most dangerous since the beam's collimation or point-source character is retained.

hazardous reflections from both specular and diffuse surfaces, atmospheric effects upon the laser beam in outdoor locations, and building construction techniques.

15.5.1 Reflections

The types of reflections that may be encountered in many environments are shown in Figure 15-5. Diffuse reflections normally greatly reduce the hazards of the primary beam, although for Class 4 visible and near-infrared lasers *hazardous* diffuse reflections are likely. The dividing line between Class 3 and Class 4 visible and IR-A lasers is defined by diffusely reflective hazard conditions. Reflections from flat mirrors produce substantial risks of hazardous exposure at considerable distances from the reflector as can be seen in Figure 15-5. Where random orientation of the reflectors can occur, the hazardous area can be quite large. Curved surface specular reflections on the other hand normally are hazardous only at relatively short distances from the reflector surface. Although specular surfaces are of greatest concern in open laboratory situations, they are not unheard of in outdoor laser applications and in medical applications.

No discussion of reflection hazards is complete without the consideration of the probability of exposure. It must be remembered that the underlying philosophy of the classification system is that the control measures increase with increasing risk of exposure as with increased severity of exposure. Most reported laser accidents occurred when the probability of exposure was very high. At least one was the result of an individual viewing a hazardous diffuse reflection (Curtin and Boyden, 1968), and others occurred when the beam path was greatly enlarged as the result of a reflection from a curved specular surface (e.g., Zweng, 1967). Most recent serious injuries have occurred with neodymium lasers at the essentially invisible wavelengths of 1060 to 1064 nm.

15.5.2 Probability of Exposure

Before specific accident situations can be considered in detail it is useful to perform a few calculations to illustrate the probability of exposure. Consider the random probability of an individual located 100 meters from a single-pulse laser having an output beam diameter of 2 mm and a beam divergence of 1 mrad. If the laser can be randomly oriented in any direction of azimuth, but limited to an elevation angle of ± 10 mrad, it seems reasonable that the likelihood of a single exposure P_{ex} to one person at a distance r = 100 m is the ratio of the area of the pupils of the two eyes divided by the area in space at 100 m to which the laser beam could be pointed. For simplicity first consider that the beam has no chance for vertical movement and the beam can only be placed in one horizontal plane and that the individual's eyes are located in that horizontal plane. Then the probability of exposure to a single eye is:

$$\begin{aligned}
P_{ex} &= (D_L + d_e)/2\pi r & (15\text{-}4)\\
&= (a + r\phi + d_e)/2\pi r & (15\text{-}4a)\\
&= [0.2 \text{ cm} + (10^4 \text{ cm} \cdot 10^{-3} \text{ rad}) + 0.7 \text{ cm}]/2\pi \cdot 10^4 \text{ cm}\\
&= 10.9 \text{ cm}/2\pi \cdot 10^4 \text{ cm}\\
&= 1.7 \times 10^{-4}
\end{aligned}$$

where a is the initial beam diameter, r is the distance, ϕ is the beam divergence, D_L is the beam diameter at r and d_e (taken as 7 mm in this case) is the pupil size of the eye. Obviously the probability is directly dependent upon the size of the pupil, and would be still greater if the laser were observed through an optical collecting instrument such as a telescope. Equation (15-4) can be simplified for the case where the beam diameter is considerably larger than the pupil or emergent beam diameter. This case reduces to:

$$P_{ex} \cong r\phi/2\pi r \qquad (15\text{-}5)$$

Only a slightly different value, 1.6×10^{-4} for P_{ex} would have been calculated with the simplified version. Obviously this is a relatively low probability: 1.6 chances in 10,000 for a single event. Of course the probability increases steadily with time if a number of pulses are emitted by the laser, if the beam or viewer can move.

The next consideration is the probability of exposure in one coordinate in a spherical coordinate system. The probability of the beam being at any given elevation angle is further increased by the ratio of the beam diameter to the vertical range of locations. This is ± 10 mils or a total range of elevation (θ_e) of 20 mils. A 20-mil angle at 100 m give 200 cm. The probability P_{ey} of the beam being directed at a particular elevation so as to intersect this eye is:

$$P_{ey} = \phi/\theta_e \quad (15\text{-}6)$$
$$= 1/20$$
$$= 5 \times 10^{-2}$$

Therefore the total probability of the beam being directed at this particular point in space at 100 m is:

$$P_e = P_{ex} \cdot P_{ey} \quad (15\text{-}7)$$
$$= (1.7 \times 10^{-4})(5 \times 10^{-2})$$
$$= 8.5 \times 10^{-6}$$

Thus, the final probability of exposure to one eye per pulse at 100 m is only one chance in 10^5. The probability that any people will be exposed within this radial distance would increase by the number of people. Nevertheless, it seems obvious why there have been so few laser accidents. The probability of exposure to a collimated beam is relatively low, and, if the beam is rapidly diverged the probability of hazardous exposure at a reasonable distance is also low or negligible.

It is useful to employ the concept of a hazardous volume. In most cases where the laser beam power is far in excess of the exposure limit the calculation of the volume of the hazardous beam space can be simplified by considering the beam as the simple right-angle circular cone. The hazardous volume V_{haz} of the cone is:

$$V_{haz} = 1/3 \cdot r_{haz} \cdot A_L^2 \quad (15\text{-}8)$$

where A_L is the area of the laser beam at a distance r_{haz} (the nominal ocular hazard distance) where the beam radiant exposure or irradiance reaches the exposure limit. For a given output power or energy, a fixed exposure limit, and no atmospheric attenuation, A_L is always constant, and is equal to the output power or energy divided by the intrabeam exposure limit (in W/cm² or J/cm²). With a constant A_L the volume is directly proportional to the hazard distance. Therefore, in theory, if all points in the hazard volume are equally likely to be occupied, then the most hazardous exposure conditions will exist where the beam is at its minimal divergence.

One aspect that has not yet been considered is the state of the individual who may be exposed. The probability of hazardous exposure is modified by the likelihood that an individual's eye is focused to achieve the minimum retinal spot, or that the eye is actually directed back to the laser along the beam path. This event would obviously occur more often in a concentrated setting, e.g., an individual viewing a display system, or observing components in an optical arrangement in the laboratory.

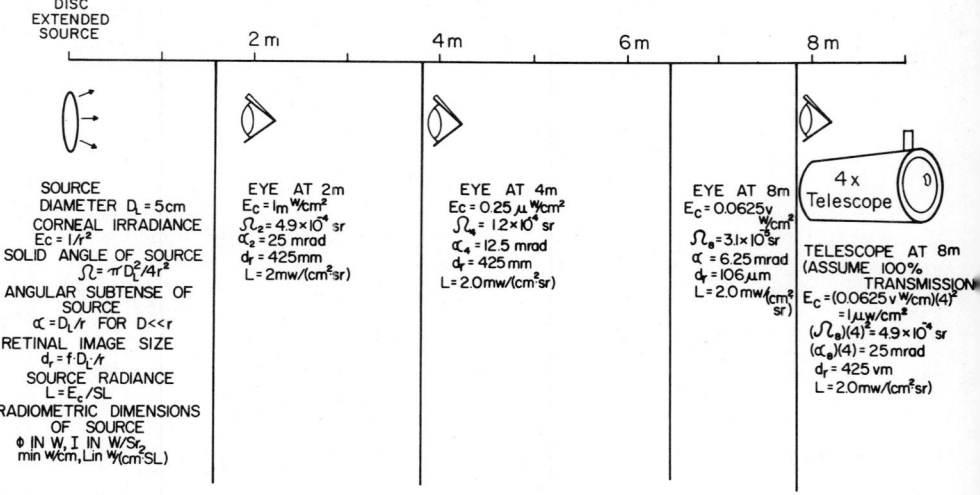

Figure 15-6. Conservation of Radiance. The radiance of an extended source, such as a diffuse reflection does not vary with viewing distance or through the use of ideal collecting optics. Note that although the irradiance decreases as the inverse square of the distance, so also does the solid angle Ω subtended by the source. The retinal image size changes but not the retinal irradiance.

15.5.3 Diffuse Reflection Hazards

In some cases the laser output is sufficiently high so that viewing a diffuse reflection is hazardous. In this instance, as long as the source appears as an extended object to the eye *the same retinal irradiance is achieved regardless of distance.* If this seems strange, consider for instance a glowing source, be it a laser or an electroluminescent panel, 10 cm in diameter. At a distance of 1 m this subtends an angle of approximately 100 mrad; at 10 m it subtends an angle of 10 mrad. Consider next an observer standing 2 m from the source who places an optical detector at his viewing position and measures an irradiance of 1 μW/cm². He then steps backward to a position 4 m from the source, and as one would expect from the inverse square law, measures one-fourth the irradiance or 0.25 μW/cm². The power entering his pupil has therefore been reduced by a factor of 4 unless, of course, his pupil size has changed. But what has happened to his retinal image size? As calculated from Eqn. (4-1); it has decreased in direct proportion to the increase in distance—in this case by a factor of 2 (from 850 μm to 425 μm). The image area (which is proportional to the square of the diameter) of the retinal image is decreased by a factor of 4. Therefore the conclusion is reached that *regardless of the viewing distance the retinal irradiance will remain the same,* although the image size will change directly with the power entering the eye. Figure 15-6 illustrates this by example. If the retinal hazard did not decrease with smaller image sizes, as is the case with thermal injury, it could be concluded that if the radiance of a laser beam reflection from a diffuse surface

General Hazard Analysis and Controls

exceeded the extended source exposure limit, then a hazardous condition would exist regardless of viewing distance until the retinal image reached the limit of 10 to 25 μm, which corresponds to a source angle of approximately 1 mrad.

A truly Lambertian surface, which many real diffuse surfaces approach, produces an irradiance at a given distance which varies as the cosine of the angle from the normal of that surface. As an example, the power entering the eye from an electroluminescent, diffuse Lambertian panel with a viewing angle θ_v = 60° at 2 m, would be reduced by a factor of 2 (cos 60° = 0.5) from that power entering the eye located at 2 m and θ_v = 0°. The retinal image would be foreshortened by this viewing angle—again by the cosine of the angle—such that the image area is reduced by a factor of 2. Hence the resulting retinal irradiance remains constant with viewing angle for a Lambertian light source. Unfortunately not all reflective surfaces are so purely specular as a clear glass mirror or as perfectly diffuse as a magnesium carbonate block. Even a glass mirror will have some surface dust which will produce some diffuse reflections, and magnesium carbonate has some minor departures from a purely Lambertian surface at near-grazing angles of incidence. However, the hazardous reflected intensities are enormously different from these two extreme cases, and even inbetween cases such as a semigloss would not reflect a sufficient percentage of the incident energy with the collimated-beam reflection component to create a hazardous, small image on the retina at realistic viewing distances. This situation is changed in the infrared where the small dust particles do not scatter. A dust covered mirror may be diffuse in the visible and specular in the infrared.

15.5.4 Specular vs. Diffuse Reflections

Figure 17-4 illustrates laboratory or workshop conditions where only the power varies. In panel A of Fig. 17-4 the output of the laser is Class 3 B. In panel B the laser is a Class 4 visible or near-infrared laser. The hazardous zones (shaded areas) are very limited for Class 3 lasers, as diffuse reflections are not hazardous, although specular reflections from curved lens surfaces may be hazardous for a short distance beyond the direct beam path. The hazardous volume in panel B covers most of the room. Not only is the result just derived independent of the viewing distance (for close viewing) but also viewing angle has no effect upon the retinal irradiance from a Lambertian reflective surface.

It should be kept in mind that the difference between the corneal irradiance measured from a diffuse reflector and that from a specular reflector is of interest only if the laser is operating in the retinal hazard region where the direction of the rays plays an important role in image formation at the retina. As a rule of thumb, if an image can be seen from surface reflection, the reflection should be considered specular. If the retinal image from a point source is greatly enlarged, it is very difficult to visualize and is therefore, proportionately safer than one reflected from a more specular surface.

Another facet of surface characteristics relates to the basic definition of a specular surface. As mentioned in section 2.8.1, the specular nature of a surface depends upon the wavelength of incident radiation. A specular surface is one which

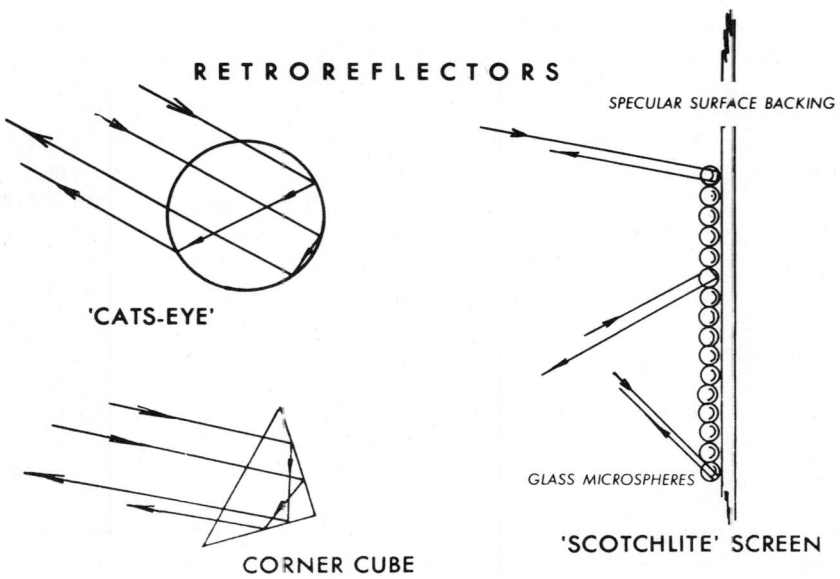

Figure 15-7. Retrodirective Reflection. Three types of retroflectors are illustrated: a corner cube, a cat's eye reflector, and a retrodirective screen. The microspheres in Scoth-Lite retrodirective screen are actually several microns in diameter.

has a surface roughness less than the wavelength of the incident optical radiation. A cast-iron skillet would hardly be considered as a mirror in the visible, and yet at 10.6 μm this surface would be specular, since surface roughness may be of the order of 10 μm or less. The importance of considering the variation of reflection characteristics with wavelength is amply illustrated some years ago by the case of a young physics graduate student who made an adjustment on a CO_2 laser with a flat-bladed screwdriver. The screwdriver slipped into the 10.6-μm beam and was oriented, albeit improbably, just right to direct the beam at one of the young man's eyes—resulting in corneal injury. Had the laser been operating in the visible, most laboratory personnel would avoid using a screwdriver polished to a mirror surface. This avoidance of high specular surfaces in a laser laboratory is natural, but the mirror-like properties of relatively diffuse, brushed or dusty metal surfaces in the infrared are too often overlooked.

Spectral reflectance will also vary with wavelength. The variations in hazard potential as a function of wavelength from spectral reflections are very much less than those from the changes in texture of a diffuse surface. For instance, it is rare to find any surface which has a spectral reflectance at any wavelength exceeding 95%

General Hazard Analysis and Controls

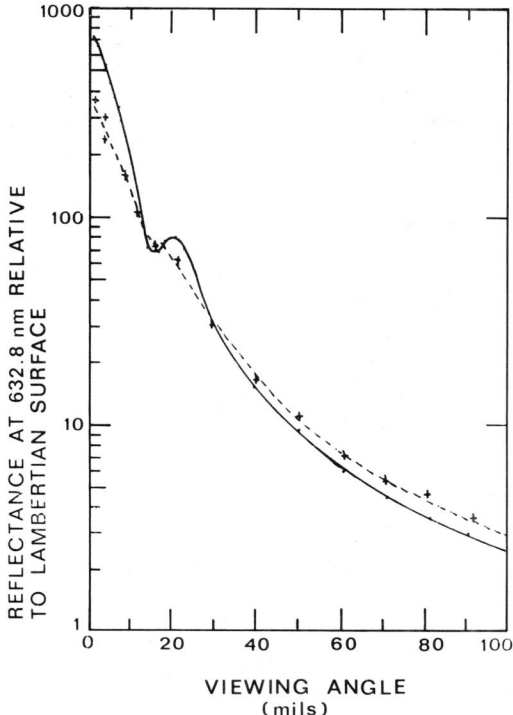

Figure 15-8. Relative reflected irradiance (or radiant intensity) as a function of angle from incident beam found from two types of Scotch-Lite® reflective sheeting.

or less than 4%, a range of 24-fold. On the other hand the variation in the nature of reflections from diffuse to specular for a rough surface with shifting wavelength can increase the irradiance at a distant point by a factor of 1,000,000-fold over that which would exist at other wavelengths for the same incident beam power. For example: a collimated beam of 1 W power incident upon a reflector of 90% spectral reflectance with a beam irradiance of 1 W/cm² would remain at nearly 1 W/cm² at 10 m from a flat mirror surface but would be reduced by Lambert's law (Eq. 2-6) to 0.3 μW/cm² at 10 m—a more than 1,000,000-fold difference in irradiance.

15.5.5 Retroreflection

Some materials exhibit a property known as *retrodirective reflection*. The reflection neither obeys the law of regular reflection applicable to specular reflection, nor does it obey the cosine characteristics of Lambertian reflection. A collimated incident beam may remain collimated and be redirected along the original axis of propagation regardless of the angle of incidence at the retroreflector. Corner cubes

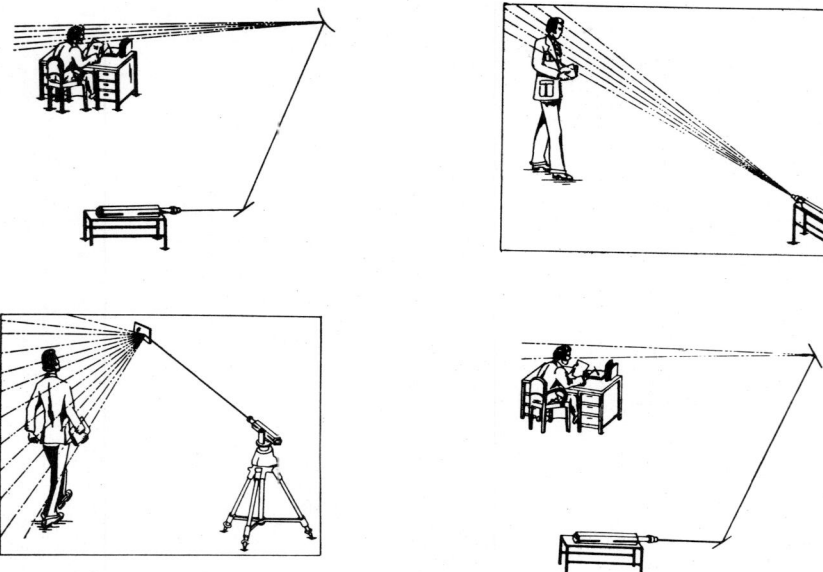

Figure 15-9. Viewing Conditions. Intrabeam exposure from direct or reflected laser radiation is encountered in the laboratory and in other operating environments (drawn by N. P. Krial, USAEHA).

and cat's eye reflectors as illustrated in Fig. 15-7 have such properties. Large arrays of small microspheres embedded on a specular coated surface create a retrodirective screen or sheet material, such as Scotch-Lite (a 3M trademark). Figure 15-8 shows relative reflected irradiance or radiant intensity as a function of angle from an incident helium-neon laser beam as measured from two types of Scotch-Lite reflective sheeting. As shown in Fig. 15-8 it is most useful to describe a retrodirective screen in terms of reflected intensity relative to a perfectly diffuse Lambertian surface. A reflection of an extended source from a retrodirective screen would have a brightness far in excess of the same extended source reflection from a diffuse screen. On the other hand a corner cube retroreflector would give one, or possibly two, slightly displaced point images, and the intrabeam viewing point source exposure limits would apply. Figure 15-9 illustrates four typical viewing conditions encountered in the laboratory and in other operating environments. In each case the individual has entered the hazardous beam or the cone of reflection.

Mirrors, filters and other optical elements are sometimes chosen with the assumption that they either totally transmit or totally attenuate a beam. However, no element is perfect; significant reflection and transmission always occurs when the optical irradiances are of the order of 1,000,000-fold of the exposure limits. The "insignificantly small" fraction of the laser beam power which may actually be transmitted or reflected from an optical component must be considered even though anti-reflection coatings may permit nearly 100% transmission. The fraction of a

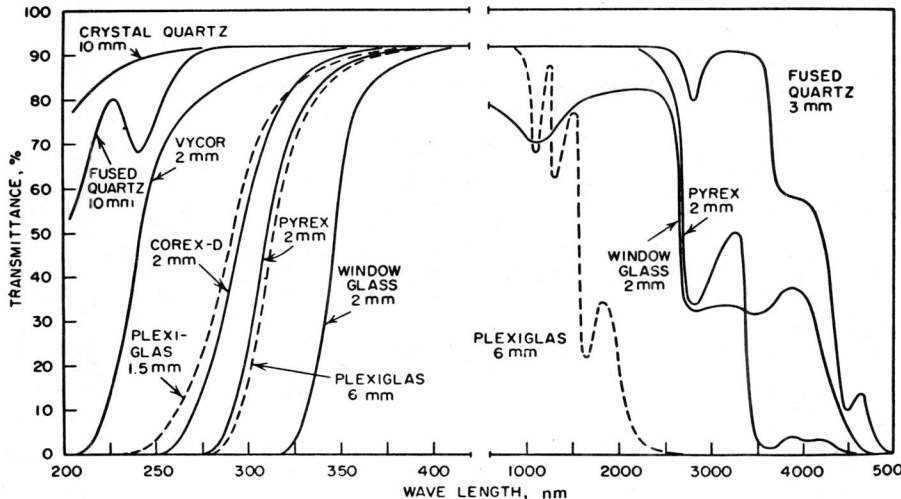

Figure 15-10. Window Materials. Spectral transmission of optical window materials from Withrow and Withrow (1956) with permission.

percent reflection is important here, although insignificant in most applications. A tenth of a percent of a beam which is 1,000,000 times above the exposure limit is still one-thousand times above the exposure limit. Clearly very minimal reflections or transmissions can be of concern in the field of laser safety.

Figure 15-10 illustrates the spectral transmission of many optical window materials which are used as general purpose shields in laboratory environments, or as optical components in actual laser products. Figure 15-11 shows the transmission properties of plastic window materials of the polymethylmethacrylate variety (e.g., Dupont Lucite® or Rohm and Haas Plexiglas®), along with another commonly used polycarbonate plastic (General Electric Lexan®) plastic that is used for shields against flying objects and for lenses in safety goggles.

15.5.6 Calculations of Specular Reflection

As previously noted, specular reflection arises from a mirror-like surface. If the surface is flat the beam characteristics, after the beam has undergone specular reflection, may be considered identical to those of the initial beam. Hence, for tabulation purposes the hazardous distance is the sum of the distances from the laser source to the reflector and from the reflector to the eye. The reflected irradiance is:

$$E = 1.27 \, \Phi \, \rho_\lambda e^{-\mu r} / [a + (r + r_1) \, \phi]^2 \qquad (15\text{-}10)$$

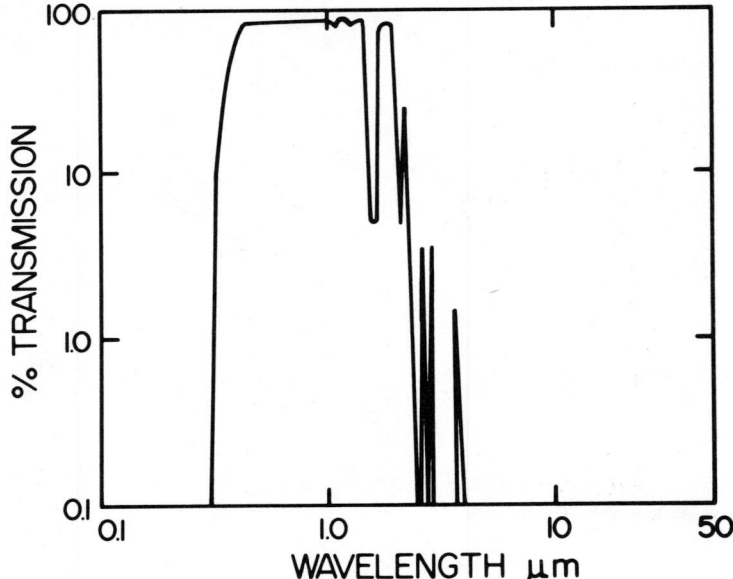

Figure 15-11. Transparent Plastic Windows. The spectral transmission properties of plastic window materials of the polymethylmethacrylate and polycarbonate varieties were determined in the middle-infrared spectral region. High transmission is common in the UV-A, VIS, and IR-A regions; high absorption is characteristic for longer IR wavelengths.

where ρ_λ is spectral reflectance, r is the distance from the laser to the target mirror, r_1 from the target to the point of concern, and other terms are as previously defined (Figure 15-12).

If the surface is not flat the irradiance at the eye for viewing the specular reflection will be less. The corneal irradiance may be calculated for a reflection from a uniformly curved surface. If the radius of curvature of a spherical surface is known and if the beam diameter at the reflector is known the following formula would apply:

$$E_r = \rho_\lambda \cdot E_0 \cdot \cos^2 \theta_r / 4 \, (r_1 + R_1)^2 \qquad (15\text{-}10)$$

where E_0 is the incident irradiance, θ_r is the angle of the reflected ray from the incident beam axis, r_1 is the distance from the reflecting surface, and R_1 is the radius of curvature of the reflecting surface.

Except for finely polished, metallic mirror surfaces, reflecting surfaces normally will reflect only a fraction of the beam, the magnitude of this reflection being

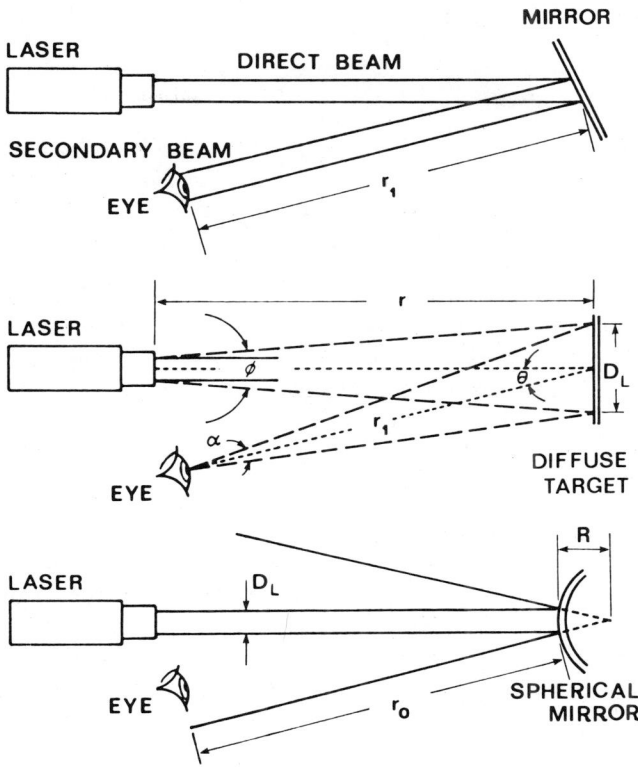

Figure 15-12. Reflection Calculations. The symbols used in describing viewing conditions for diffuse (top) and specular (bottom) reflections.

dependent upon the spectral reflectance and the angle of incidence of the surface. For normal (perpendicular) incidence, typical "transparent" plate glass will reflect approximately 8 percent of the incident beam and "transparent" plastics, approximately 4-percent, but at near-grazing incidence nearly all of the incident radiant energy is reflected. This effect was first noted by Fresnel and is shown graphically in Fig. 2-6. Note that Fresnel reflection is dependent upon polarization, and that light polarized perpendicular to the plane of incidence will always be greater upon reflection than that light initially polarized parallel to the plane of incidence. The plane of incidence is the plane defined by a line perpendicular to the surface of the reflector and the incident ray. The polarization of the beam is defined by the electric vector. The curve for Fig. 2-6 shows a polarizing (or Brewster's) angle of 57° for glass with an index of refraction of 1.5. On the other hand, water, with a 2-percent reflectance at normal incidence and an index of refraction of 1.33, would have the polarizing angle at 53° instead of the 57° shown for glass.

The coefficient of specular Fresnel reflection is:

$$\rho_\lambda = p_\| \cdot \tan^2(\theta - \theta')/\tan^2(\theta - \theta') + p_\perp \cdot \sin^2(\theta - \theta')/\sin^2(\theta - \theta') \tag{15-11}$$

where $p_\|$ and $p_\perp$ are the fraction of the total incident beam energy which are polarized in the plane, parallel ($\|$) to the plane of incidence and perpendicular ($\perp$) to the plane of incidence, respectively; θ is the angle of incidence; θ' is the arc sin (sin θ/n) i.e., the angle of the refracted ray; and n is the index of refraction. For an unpolarized beam $p_\|$ and $p_\perp$ are both 0.5.

The practical significance of the variation of the Fresnel reflection as a function of angle is illustrated in Fig. 21-7 where a collimated beam has struck a plate glass window. The hazard envelopes for the perpendicularly-polarized light occupy the greater area as would be expected from the higher specular reflectance coefficients.

15.5.7 Diffuse Reflection

In the actual determination of the radiance of diffuse reflection the radiance exposure limit (or integrated radiance exposure limit) for pulsed exposures can be directly related to the incident irradiance or radiant exposure for a Lambertian surface having a spectral reflectance of known value. Table 15-3 provides a list of permissible laser beam radiant exposures incident upon a diffuse reflecting surface in joules-per-square-centimeter. This table is based upon the following equation:

$$L_p = \rho_\lambda H_i/\pi \tag{15-12}$$

where L_p is the reflected integrated radiance, ρ_λ is the spectral reflectance and H_i is the incident radiant exposure. Because pupil size plays a role in adjusting retinal irradiance, these permissible radiant exposures could be raised by a factor of 3 for conditions of relatively bright ambient lighting as the exposure limits are based on a 7-mm (dark adapted state) pupil. Caution should be used here as not all pupils will constrict the same. Such adjustments for pupil sizes are not permitted for intrabeam exposure because there is little variation of peak retinal irradiance with increased pupil size for a point image. This is discussed in section 4.5.2 in connection with the eye's Strehl ratio.

As noted here, the reflection from a flat diffuse surface generally obeys Lambert's law, at least at small angles from the normal where the greatest reflected radiant intensity exists. Table 15-3 is based upon the assumption that the incident radiant exposure is measured through a 1-mm aperture in the plane of the surface at or at least parallel to it. For oblique incidence, the beam's radiant exposure may be increased as the reciprocal of the cosine of the angle of incidence.

This discussion assumes that the size of the beam is sufficiently large to produce an "extended source" subtending an angle α (Fig. 15-12) as seen by the viewer. If the size of the reflection subtends an angle less than α_{min}, the maximum allowable radiant exposure to produce a hazardous integrated radiance would be greater. In this instance the irradiance in the reflected beam arriving at the eye would again

General Hazard Analysis and Controls

TABLE 15-3. Maximum Allowable Radiant Exitance from a Diffuse Surface Reflection As Measured at the Reflecting Surface

Duration of Exposure (seconds)	Threshold Limit Value at Cornea ($J \cdot cm^{-2} sr^{-1}$) See Figure 8-6 for graphic presentation of this column	Limiting Angle, a_{min} (See Table 8-4)	Permissible Laser Beam Radiant Exposure Incident on the Diffuse Reflecting Surfaces ($J \cdot cm^{-2}$) Values in Columns 4, 5, 6 = Values in Column $2 \times \frac{\pi}{\rho}$		
			Reflectance (ρ) = 100%	Reflectance (ρ) = 50%	Reflectance (ρ) = 10%
1	2	3	4	5	6
10^{-3}	1.0×10^{-2}	8.0	3.1×10^{-2}	6.3×10^{-2}	3.1×10^{-1}
10^{-8}	2.2×10^{-2}	5.4	6.8×10^{-2}	1.4×10^{-1}	6.8×10^{-1}
10^{-7}	4.6×10^{-2}	3.7	1.5×10^{-1}	2.9×10^{-1}	1.5
10^{-5}	1.0×10^{-1}	2.5	3.1×10^{-1}	6.3×10^{-1}	3.1
10^{-5}	2.2×10^{-1}	1.7	6.8×10^{-1}	1.4	6.8
10^{-6}	4.6×10^{-1}	2.2	1.5	2.9	15
10^{-3}	1.0	3.6	3.1	6.3	31
10^{-2}	2.2	5.7	6.8	14	68
10^{-1}	4.6	9.2	15	29	150
1	10	15	31	63	310
10	20	24	68	140	680

NOTE: The actual radiant exitance (the light reflected from a diffuse surface) may be calculated by multiplying the radiant exposure or irradiance of the beam impinging upon the surface by the reflectance (a property of the material). These values may be approximately tripled for conditions of bright ambient light. From ACGIH (1976).

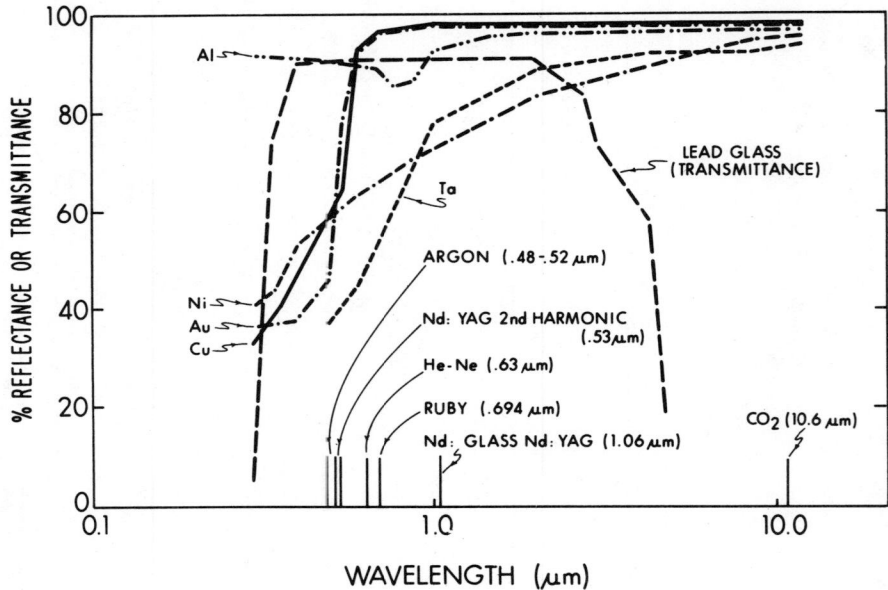

Figure 15-13. Metallic Spectral Reflectance. The spectral specular reflectance of a number of metallic surfaces used as mirrors is shown (adapted from a figure in the catalog of the Corion Corporation).

be calculated by Lambert's Law (Eq. 2-6). At wavelengths outside of the retinal hazard region the concept of a permissible surface radiance does not apply, and Lambert's Law must be used to calculate the irradiance or radiant exposure from the reflected surface at the point of interest.

The maximum incident radiant exposure for a diffuse surface can also be considered an upper safe limit for reflections from arrays of small reflectors such as raindrops and water droplets on a surface. As a general rule, laser irradiances or radiant exposures in a beam which are safe to view by diffuse reflection will not create hazardous reflections from water droplets, natural foliage, fog, and dry snow at viewing distances greater than 1 m.

15.5.8 REFLECTANCE

The spectral reflectance coefficient, a unitless radiometric quantity, is the ratio of the total reflected power to the total incident radiant power at a given wavelength. It is normally expressed for either diffuse or specular conditions, but may apply to both. It can be specified in a variety of ways (Nicodemus, 1977) when the surface is not clearly specular or diffuse, but rather glossy or semi-glossy. For the present an attempt will be made to distinguish between the two.

General Hazard Analysis and Controls 501

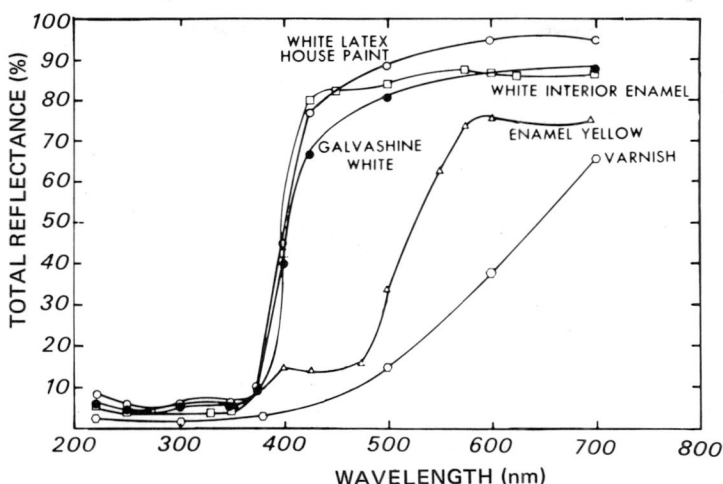

Figure 15-14. Spectral Reflectance of House Paints. The spectral reflectance of five representative paints are shown from 200 nm to 800 nm. Note the low reflectance in the UV-B and UV-C range. The data were compiled by Ulrich and Johnson (1976) for the American Welding Society (AWS).

The specular spectral reflectance coefficients of a number of metals used in mirror surfaces are shown in Fig. 15-13. It should be noted that for infrared wavelengths all these values generally exceed 90 percent, and only in the ultraviolet are most values (except aluminum) relatively low.

A useful collection of spectral diffuse reflectance coefficients for a variety of materials are given in Figs. 15-14 to 18. A large book of spectral reflectance values for different materials could be compiled, but its utility to the laser safety specialist would be minimal. The approximate values as shown in Figs. 15-18 are sufficient. As previously mentioned, the maximum variation in spectral reflectance is only 24-fold (except for laboratory standards), and the influence of such a small change upon safety conditions is normally inconsequential. It need be considered carefully only for reflections from a laser system which is on the borderline between Class 3 and Class 4 in the retinal hazard region.

15.6 OPTICALLY AIDED VIEWING

Nearly all laser workers know that viewing a laser source with a telescope substantially increases the hazard. This increase in hazard is most dramatic for intrabeam viewing of a collimated source. An increase in power entering the eye is

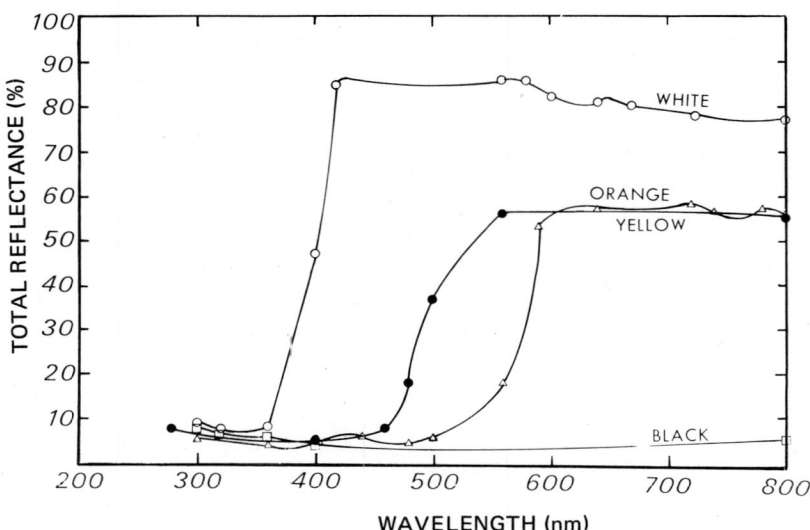

Figure 15-15. Spectral Reflectance of Paints on Metals. The spectral reflectance of paints on metals is low in the UV and high beyond 2 μm. Source: Martin-Marietta (1964).

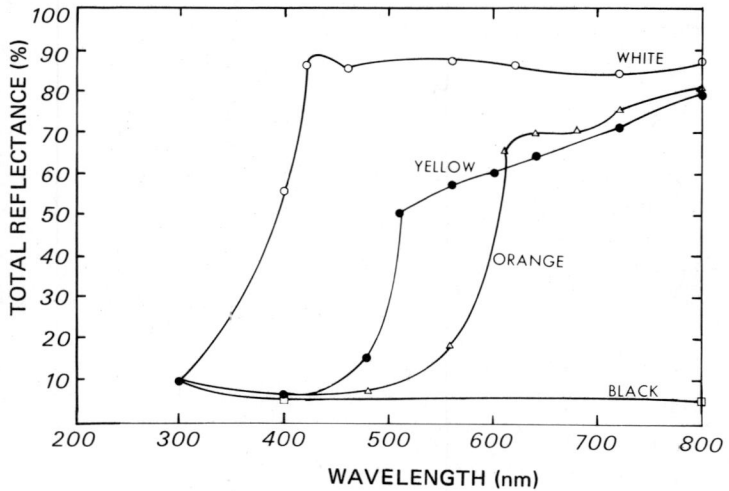

Figure 15-16. Spectral Reflectance of Paints on Wood. There is little or no difference in the diffuse spectral reflectance of paints on wood or on metals between 200 nm and 800 nm.

General Hazard Analysis and Controls 503

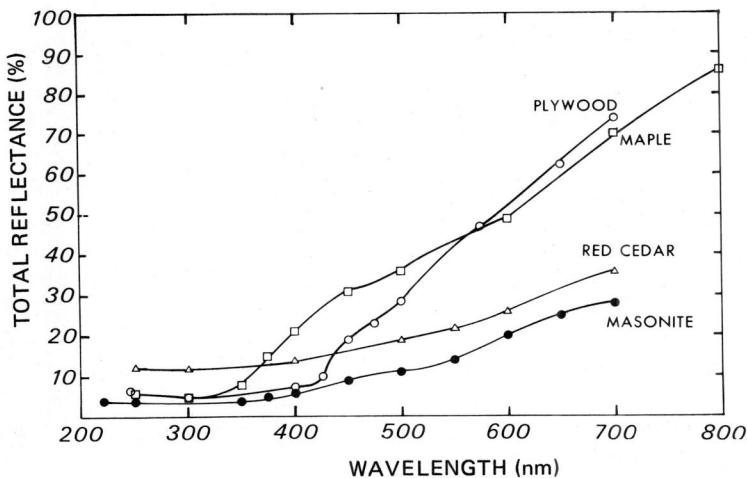

Figure 15-17. Spectral Reflectance of Building Materials (Woods). The reflectance data of maple and red cedar came from Thomas (1973) and the data for plywood and masonite were obtained by Ulrich and Johnson (1976) for the AWS. Again, note the low UV reflectance values.

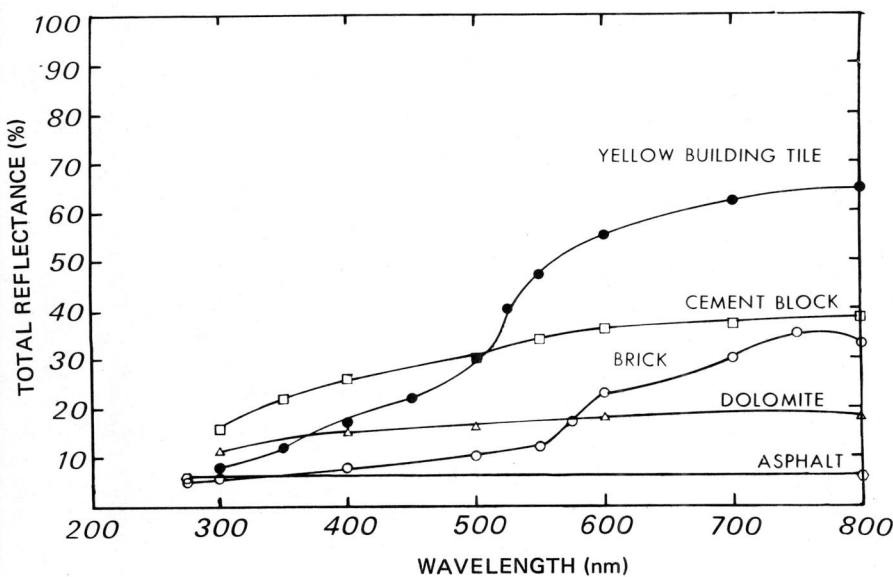

Figure 15-18. Spectral Reflectance of Building Materials (Non-Wood). These reflectance data are representative. Source: Thomas (1973).

possible because the diameter of the objective D_0 of the telescope or binocular is much larger than the eye's pupil d_e. The actual increase in hazard G depends upon whether the eye's pupil is larger or smaller than the exit pupil D_e of the optical system and the spectral transmittance τ_λ of the optical system at the laser wavelength(s).

When a bright object larger than a point source is viewed through a well-designed optical system, the radiant power reaching the retina (Visible and IR-A) is theoretically increased by the square of the instrument's magnifying power. However, since there is a commensurate increase in the area of the retinal image the retinal irradiance remains unchanged, except for a slight reduction due to the reflective loss and the absorption of light in the optical system. If, however, a distant star or a collimated laser beam is viewed directly the retinal image will be formed as if from a true point source, and this retinal image may remain diffraction-limited with an interposed optical system. Thus, the retinal image size remains the same, while the radiant power reaching the retina is increased by as much as the square of the magnifying power of the optical system with a commensurate increase in the retinal irradiance. There is a borderline condition—usually close to the laser (near field)—where the retinal image formed by viewing through an optical system may actually be larger than the diffraction-limited image. Nevertheless, the collimated beam laser would behave nearly as a point source and a reduction of the retinal irradiance should really not be assumed.

A consideration of the effects of optical viewing of any light source allows an application of the law of conservation of radiance, no optical system can increase the true radiance (brightness) of a source. The source radiance for a laser can be extremely large, and may only be defined if the "point source" is resolved by an extremely high resolution optical system. For this reason the assumption that a collimated laser beam is a point source, and that the retinal irradiance will increase by as much as the square of the magnifying power is not unreasonable.

The increase (or gain) in retinal irradiance for optically-aided viewing, called ratio G, is also dependent upon how well the optical system is matched to the eye. The exit pupil D_e of the optical instrument is defined by the objective diameter D_0 divided by the magnifying power P of the instrument:

$$d_e = D_0/P \qquad (15\text{-}13)$$

The exit pupil may be visualized (and measured) by aiming the instrument at the sky or other very large, uniformly bright surface. A piece of white paper behind the eyepiece as it is moved away will pass through a point where the emerging light rays form a sharply defined circle. This is the instrument's exit pupil. For example, the exit pupil of a 7 × 50 binocular is 50 mm/7 = 7.1 mm. Instruments with large exit pupils are employed for nighttime use or when eye motion relative to the eyepiece is common (e.g., at sea or in a vehicle).

The exit pupil must be larger than the pupil size in order for the rule-of-thumb of G equal to P^2 to apply. The following equations apply for the more general case. For intrabeam viewing of a point source:

$$G = D_0^2/d_e^2 \quad \text{for } d_e \geqslant D_e \qquad (15\text{-}14)$$

General Hazard Analysis and Controls

and

$$G = D_0^2/D_e^2 = P^2 \text{ for } d_e \leq D_e \quad (15\text{-}15)$$

where d_e is the pupil diameter for the human eye and D_e is equal to the exit pupil of the optical instrument. All dimensions must be consistent. For viewing of an extended source such as a diffuse reflection where the object subtends an angle greater than 1 mrad following magnification, the following formula would apply:

$$G = D_0^2/P^2 \cdot d_e^2 \leq 1 \text{ for } d_e \geq D_e \quad (15\text{-}16)$$

and

$$G = D_0^2/P^2 D_e^2 = 1 \text{ for } d_e \leq D_e \quad (15\text{-}17)$$

As noted earlier, the ratio G is affected by the actual optical transmission τ of the instrument. Normally this value is relatively insignificant for wavelengths between 450 and 750 nm if the system has coated optics (anti-reflection coatings). If this is not the case then the factor τ of the instrument should be used. It appears in the numerators of all of the previous equations [(15-14) through (15-17)]. As an example, if an individual were to view a laser flash from a diffuse reflector through a pair of 10X50 binoculars (P = 10; D_0 = 50 mm) then the increase in retinal irradiance for a daylight pupil of 3 mm would be calculated as follows:

Since D_e equals 5 mm from Eq. (15-13), and $D_e > d_e$, then using Eq. (15-17):

$$G = (50 \text{ mm})^2 / (10^2) \cdot (5 \text{ mm})^2$$
$$= 2500/(100)(25)$$
$$= 1$$

On the other hand, if the pupil of the eye d_e were dilated (dark adaptation) such that it would be larger than the exit pupil of the instrument D_0 (5 mm) then Eq. (15-16) would apply and:

$$G = (50 \text{ mm})^2 / (10^2) \cdot (7 \text{ mm})^2$$
$$= 2500/(100)(49)$$
$$= 0.51$$

If the corneal exposure is of interest, equation (15-15) also provides the ratio of corneal (exit-pupil) irradiance to objective irradiance. Corneal exposure is generally of interest for wavelengths outside of the retinal hazard region but within the optical glass transmission range, namely 320-400 nm, and 1400-5000 nm. If the irradiance at the front of a 10X optical instrument were 1 $\mu W/cm^2$, then the irradiance at the cornea would be 100 $\mu W/cm^2$, a factor of 100 over the case where the optical instrument is not used. As another example, if an individual chose to view a specular reflection of a laser beam with a pair of 7X50 binoculars, the corneal irradiance would be increased by the square of the magnifying power and the retinal irradiance by Eq. (15-15).

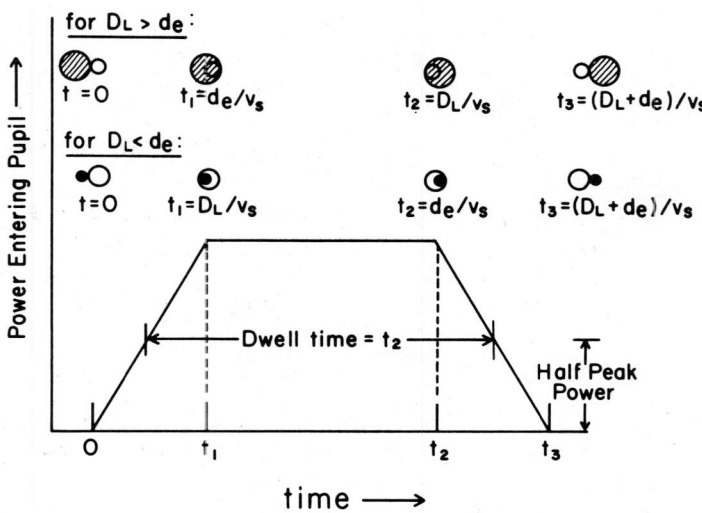

Figure 15-19. Pulsed Exposure from a Laser Scan. The temporal profile for laser beam power entering the eye for a scanning laser beam passing over the pupil is shown in the lower portion of the figure. The diagrams above illustrate the relative position of the laser beam (shaded) and the eye's pupil at each point.

15.7 SCANNING LASER BEAM

15.7.1 Linear Scans

There are a number of applications where a continuous-wave laser beam of divergence ϕ is scanned over a total scan angle θ_t. As the beam passes the pupil of the eye, or any other spot, there is a dwell time t over a given spot. If, as a first-order approximation, the beam is assumed to have a rectangular profile, Fig. 15-19 would represent the total beam power entering the eye as a function of time. More sophisticated calculations with a Gaussian beam profile would make only a slight change. The duration t of the exposure is obviously dependent on the angular speed of the beam (θ_t/s) in rad/s and the ratio of the pupil size d_e to the beam diameter D_L at the range r, the location of the viewer. The eye's scan rate s is the number of scans over the eye per second. The following formulas (Eq. 15-18 and 15-19) will apply equally as well to skin exposure for a large beam scanning past the entire body (substitute body width for d_e) but the beam passing over a pupillary aperture d_e is a far more likely situation. The pulse duration depends upon whether the beam diameter ($a + r\phi$) is greater or smaller than d_e:

General Hazard Analysis and Controls

$$t = (a + r\phi)/r \cdot s\theta_t \quad \text{for } d_e \leq (a + r\phi) \tag{15-18}$$

or

$$t = d_e/r \cdot s \cdot \theta_t \quad \text{for } d_e \geq (a + r\phi) \tag{15-19}$$

Since the radiant exposure at range r is the product of the exposure duration t and the beam irradiance at range r, the formula for beam irradiance downrange (Eq. 12-4) may be multiplied by the preceding expressions of t:

$$H = [1.27 \, \Phi \, e^{\mu r}/(a + r\phi)^2] [d_e/r \cdot s \cdot \theta_t] \quad \text{for } d_e > [a + r\phi] \tag{15-20}$$

or

$$H = 1.27 \, \Phi \, e^{\mu r}/(a + r\phi)(r \cdot s \cdot \theta_t) \quad \text{for } d_e \leq (a + r\phi) \tag{15-21}$$

If each scan passes across the eye, then the pulse repetition frequency (F) is equal to s. If the scan has a stationary pattern without overlap, then the PRF of the train of pulses entering the viewer's eye would be S/n, where n is the number of lines per frame and S is the total number of scans of the beam per second then S/n should be used for s in the equations above. Other conditions for scanning lasers can obviously be calculated by a simple geometrical analysis of the problem, and the same general approach as given for a linear scan will apply.

15.7.2 Lissajous Scans

Some scans are effectively Lissajous patterns, and two sine functions of w_x and w_y refer to the sinusiodal scan rates in the x and y coordinates. The following formulas apply to the scan pattern as a function of scan time t_s and describe the beam position in x,y coordinates in a plane normal to the beam:

$$x = A_x \sin(w_x t_s) \tag{15-22}$$

and

$$y = A_y \sin(w_y t_s) \tag{15-23}$$

were A_x and A_y are the amplitudes of the beam deflection calculated as:

$$A_x = \theta_t (x)/2r \tag{15-24}$$

$$A_y = \theta_t (y)/2r \tag{15-25}$$

and w_w and w_y are the angular frequencies of oscillation defined as $2\pi f_x$ and $2\pi f_y$. In order to derive more convenient formulas for beam velocity, two more related factors are defined:

$$\text{The Lissajous factor} = \Lambda = w_x/w_y = f_y/f_x, \tag{15-26}$$

$$\text{and The Pattern Aspect Ratio} = u = A_x/A_y \cdot \Lambda \tag{15-27}$$

The beam velocity v_s across the pupil at a distance r is of primary interest:

$$v_s = \sqrt{v_x^2 + v_y^2} \qquad (15\text{-}28)$$

where
$$v_x = dx/dt = \Lambda \cdot w_x \cdot u \cdot A_y \cdot \cos(w_x \cdot t) \qquad (15\text{-}29)$$

and
$$v_y = dy/dt = \Lambda \cdot w_x \cdot \cos(a \cdot w_x \cdot t) \qquad (15\text{-}30)$$

Combining equations (15-28) (15-29) and (15-30) gives:

$$v_s = w_x \cdot \Lambda \cdot A_y \sqrt{u^2 \cos^2(w_x \cdot t) + \cos^2(\Lambda w_x \cdot t)} \qquad (15\text{-}31)$$

From Eq. (15-31) it is clear that v is not a constant for a Lissajous scan pattern as it was for the linear scan. Also the beam's dwell time at the pupil is not a single value as for the linear scan [Eq. (15-18) and (15-19)]. The only reasonable approach is to plot Eq. (15-31) for a given scan, and study the eye exposure for minimal and maximal v_s (min) and v_s (max)]. v_s (max) can be calculated by noting that v_s (max) will occur when $(w_x t) = 0$ and $\cos(w_x t) = 1$:

$$v_s(\max) = w_x \cdot \Lambda \cdot A_y \sqrt{u^2 + 1} \qquad (15\text{-}32)$$

But v_s (min) will occur at the edge of the scan pattern other than near the center as v_s (max). For this reason, v_s (min) is not readily calculated without a plot. The "pulse duration" or beam dwell time at the eye is:

$$t = d_e/v_s \qquad \text{for } D_L \geqslant d_e \qquad (15\text{-}33)$$

$$t = D_L/v_s \qquad \text{for } D_L \leqslant d_e \qquad (15\text{-}34)$$

as shown in Fig. 15-19.

For some scanning laser applications the eye may not be focused at the beam scanning mirror, in which case the retinal image will be a line and not a point. The line image length d_r' is dependent on the distance of the eye from the scanner and pupil size d_e. This will be considered in greater detail in Chapter 20.

15.8 LASER ACCIDENTS

To this date, retinal injuries with loss of sight from visible and near-infrared laser systems have been the most catastrophic of all effects from laser radiation. Although the relatively high-powered far infrared laser such as the CW CO_2 laser, have caused numerous burns to the hands, and clothes, these are considered inconsequential in comparison to the serious retinal injuries. One mail survey conducted several years ago appeared to indicate that there have been at least 100 injuries to the eye from laser radiation in the U.S.A. Only a few, and those the earlier more dramatic cases, have been reported in the medical literature. As the novelty of laser eye injury diminished, editors of ophthalmic journals no longer saw the value of publishing case reports. A few of these earlier cases will be briefly discussed to provide a general background for accidents. The vast majority of the serious eye injuries occurred from exposure to Class 4 laser systems. Although there are a few cases in the literature of retinal injury following prolonged viewing (staring) into the beam of a small helium-neon laser, these cases are generally considered sufficiently controversial that they will be neglected in the following discussion.

Curtin and Boyden (1968) reported on a young college student who, apparently desiring to view directly and "safely" a ruby laser beam without eye protection, decided to use the reflection off of a chalk block. Little did he realize that the reflection from a Class 4 high-power ruby laser, even from a diffuse surface, was hazardous, and he ended up with a retinal injury in the eye which he had used to observe the reflection.

Other cases involved laser reflections from specular surfaces, either soft drink bottles and other curved specular surfaces in the beam path, or from secondary beams produced at Brewster-angle windows and similar optical elements within the laser optical system (Anon, 65; Anon, 72; Armstrong, 1970; Blancard, 1965; Henkes and Zuidema, 1975; Jacobson and McLean, 1965; Rathkey, 1965; Pecker, 1977; and Zweng, 1967). All of these cases could have been prevented had the individuals working in the laser laboratory worn eye protection. The authors are aware of other unpublished cases, which are repetitions of the events in the case studies in the literature where the individual felt that he could get by without eye protection. A laser worker who once forgets to wear eye protection and is exposed, but not injured, often assumes that there is no need to wear the goggles. He does not appreciate the risk associated with the probabilistic event of the eye being in the beam path. The probabilities discussed earlier in this chapter amply illustrate the low chance of a single event causing an injury. It is for this reason that there have been so few accidents. The greatest share of accidents in recent years since the advent of great interest in laser safety have been with neodymium-YAG lasers—normally repetitively-pulsed—where the probability of injury is low, but not vanishingly small, and where the beam is invisible. In one instance a laser technician even reported after his injury that he had been wearing safety goggles and that the beam had been seen through a gap between the goggle and his nose (Anon, 1977). Since his retinal injury was a central scotoma, this would mean that he would have had to have been staring through the crack in his goggles, an unlikely, if not impossible, event.

In investigating an accident one must remember two things. The individual who has received an injury is often embarrassed to admit that he did not follow proper practices, and may tend to emphasize, if not invent, the accidental nature of the event. Secondly, any attempt to measure accurately the reconstructed exposure dose is normally hopeless unless the beam is so large, and of relatively uniform irradiance in the general region of the accident, that there would be little variation in exposure dose as the result of head movement.

One individual in 1963, attempting to show that laser safety predictions and calculations were completely inaccurate, voluntarily (and without the knowledge of supervisors) went down range 500 meters from a ruby laser rangefinder looked into the beam, and saw a brilliant red flash. An ophthalmoscopic examination did not reveal any sign of a retinal lesion and there was no visual field loss. Until a rabbit was placed at the same location downrange and received serious retinal hemorrhage from such an exposure, the "volunteer" was not convinced that he had merely been slightly off-axis of the beam and had simply seen the brilliant flash characteristic of the small-angle forward scatter from the beam. Obviously, had he been near the center of the beam and received the full beam irradiance he would have had a very serious retinal injury. Thus, even "eye witness" exposures can be misleading.

Although an accident case rarely provides any significant biological data, the estimates of retinal exposure from a number of cases appear to substantiate the retinal injury thresholds reported in primates as a result of laboratory studies. In any discussion of probabilities of exposure special note must be taken of those conditions where an individual would have a relaxed normal eye which would focus a collimated beam to the minimal retinal image, and would be using central-foveal vision to look at the laser source. This could occur out-of-doors where the person would be in the beam path looking back towards the laser. This could occur in a military laser environment, in surveying, or alignment over considerable distances. On the other hand, a laboratory exposure with a collimated beam would have a considerable factor of safety in the image would probably not be focused and considerably greater energy into the eye would be required to cause injury. However, if the reflection were from a curved surface, with the eye focused near the center of curvature for that surface, then there would be a nearly minimal image at the retina. In the period of 1965-1969 it was not uncommon for ill-informed salesman of He-Ne lasers to look directly into a 3-mW He-Ne laser held up to their eyes to "prove that the laser product was safe." Of course they received no retinal injuries because their eyes were not relaxed or focused at infinity.

Finally the subject of laser accidents should not be left without noting that the severity of injuries are by far the greatest with very short pulses, such as Q-switched or mode-locked trains of laser pulses, where retinal hemorrhaging can occur. A retinal hemorrhage greatly increases the possibility of loss of vision. Exposure within the blink reflex to a 0.1 to 0.5-W CW visible laser would not normally result in an injury over a very large area of the retina. Although a permanent scotoma (blind spot) would probably develop, this type of visual loss would not be serious. Catastrophic loss of vision would probably only occur from hazardous exposure to a very short laser pulse at levels exceeding 25 to 100 times the MPE (Gibbons and Allen, 1978).

15.9 GENERAL CONTROL MEASURES

15.9.1 Engineering Controls, Personnel Protection and Administrative Control

In a manner similar to laser hazard analysis, control measures may be broken down into three groups: the laser, the environment, and the personnel who may be exposed. Normally as a variation of this theme, these three general types of control measures are considered:

1. Engineering controls (e.g., enclosures, interlocks, beam stops);
2. Personnel protection (e.g., eyewear, gloves); and
3. Administration controls (e.g., signs, warning lights, bells, whistles, and safe operating procedures.

The three groups were mentioned in order of effectiveness, and unfortunately, in order of highest-to-lowest cost (in general).

Effective engineering controls at the laser itself generally mean placing the entire laser system within an opaque enclosure, as is done in most industrial lasers used today. This approach is always the most desirable. In some applications it is possible to reduce the laser's output irradiance below exposure limits without interfering with the operation. This approach may become more widespread in many applications as advances in detector technology make lower beam power adequate. This is particularly true of the less hazardous infrared wavelengths which are now limited by detector technology. Beam shutters, key controls, and cover interlocks (all engineering controls), and warning labels (administrative) are examples of other controls that work directly on the laser.

Environmental (engineering) controls may differ widely, depending upon whether the laser is used in an indoor or out-of-door environment. Back-stops and shields to exclude the beam from occupied areas are commonly used both in and outdoors. Well illuminated laboratories and limited-access rooms are also important environmental controls. The prevention of unsafe acts by personnel may be achieved by the use of physical barriers (engineering controls) and/or by the application of administrative controls, procedures, training and education, and through careful supervision.

Control measures which apply directly to the potentially exposed individual are the prevention of unsafe acts by personnel through administration procedures and the use of protective eyewear. This latter is a major control that should be mandatory when any risk of exposure of the eye to hazardous levels exists. However, such situations should be avoided by the use of other control measures if possible. The advantages and limitations of protective eyewear are discussed in detail in Chapter 16.

Most control measures fall into the category of common sense procedures aimed at limiting the laser exposure, thus reducing the probabilistic risk of exposure. General control measures were broken down as a function of laser hazard classification in Chapter 1. It is recommended that these controls be reviewed as listed in that chapter. It should be evident by now that most of the classification differences between Class 3 and Class 4 lasers relate only to degree of control, since the principal and substantial difference between a Class 3 and Class 4 laser is in probabilistic risk and severity of exposure. Table 15-4 summarizes some of the most commonly used control measures.

15.9.2 Control Measures for Very High Power Lasers

It has sometimes been suggested that there be a separate class for super high-powered lasers which operate at levels far in excess of the lower limits of Class 4.

TABLE 15-4. General Control Measures

I   **Engineering Control Measures**
- Protective Housing and Service Panel Requirements
- Interlocks on the Protective Housing
- Door Interlocks and Remote Conrol Connector
- Beam Attenuator or Beam Shutter
- Key Switch or Padlock over Aperture Cover
- Filtered Viewing Optics and Windows
- Emission Delay (BRH)
- Warning Lights, Emission Indicators (audible or visible)
- Enclosed Area or Room
- Beam Enclosure
- Remote Firing and/or Monitoring

II   **Personal Protective Equipment**
- Eyewear
- Clothing
- Gloves

III   **Administrative and Procedural Controls**
- Laser Safety Officer
- Standard Operating Procedures (SOP's)
- Limitations on Use by Class
- Education and Training
- Maintenance and Servicing Manuals
- Marking of Protective Devices
- Warning Signs and Labels
- Entry Limitations for Visitors, etc.

This would include the multi-kilowatt, CW infrared lasers used for industrial welding of large structures. When this suggestion is considered carefully, it becomes evident that it is based on the assumption that the probability of hazardous reflection and/or the severity of reflection injury is far greater with such higher powered lasers. In fact, the truth may be just the opposite. A very high-powered infrared laser beam incident on a metal surface almost immediately alters the surface and the specular nature is lost. Hence, such specular reflections do not normally occur from a metal surface, unless its thermal conductive ability is so high, or the beam irradiance is so near the threshold for surface ablation that the metal surface remains intact (or unablated) for a substantial duration following initiation of the exposure. The reflected beam from a 100-W CO_2 laser beam incident upon a metal surface is probably more hazardous than from a 1,000 W system as it would not cause surface ablation, and therefore is a specular reflection hazard. From this it appears that one general set of guidelines for control measures can be applied to all Class 4 laser systems. Most are potential fire hazards; all are nearly so. Some lasers operating in the visible and IR-A present diffuse reflection eye hazards, and most Class 4 lasers operating in the ultraviolet can produce injury of the skin or eye within a fraction of second for direct-beam exposure.

15.9.3 The Choice of Control Measures

Hazard control guidelines are not mutually exclusive. Following one or two guidelines may reduce the risk sufficiently so that the other recommended control measures of the particular class are no longer essential. As an example, if the beam path of a Class 4 laser is enclosed then it would hardly be necessary to remove all glass objects, or other specular surfaces, near the beam path but outside the enclosure, nor would it seem necessary to wear eye protection. However, the eyewear should be available when the enclosure is being modified or during initial alignment.

In performing hazard analyses it is useful to use the techniques for beam location that are discussed in Chapter 17. Once the hazardous locations are determined then attempts should be made to design enclosures, baffles, and beam stops to reduce risk of exposure.

15.9.4 Class 4 Laser Controls

Because of the greater risk associated with exposure to Class 4 high-risk lasers, the safety precautions associated with these laser installations indoors generally include the installation of door interlocks to prevent exposure to unauthorized or transient personnel entering the laboratory, the use of baffles to terminate the primary and any secondary beams, and the use of safety eyewear by personnel within the interlocked facility. A requirement for all Class 4 laser systems is that they be manufactured with remote control connectors which allow deactivation of the laser by door interlocks or other remote switches. In general, personnel permitted to enter a high-power laser facility should be familiar with hazard control measures, and the restricted entry often used at indoor, high power laser facilities will assist in this aim. Because of the electrical hazards associated with pulsed discharge laser systems, the accidental release of a stored charge or spurious firing should be avoided by design of a fail-safe firing circuit. The safety controls for some Class 4 laser systems require an alarm system such as a muted sound, or a flashing light which can be seen through the proper laser protective filters. Count-down procedures have been used for pulsed lasers in order to assure that personnel required to wear eye protection have them properly adjusted during laser activation.

At one time it was recommended the ambient light levels be high enough to constrict the pupil. However, since a constricted pupil provides only a small factor of safety, the requirement for good illumination which remains in present safety standards is related to good general visibility as the wearing of eye protection limits visual capabilities. Light-colored, matte surfaces in the room help to achieve minimum glare, and thus promote visibility.

Very high energy laser systems should generally be operated by remote control with television monitoring, or filter windows where feasible. Such an approach can eliminate the need for the physical presence of personnel in the laser room. This approach is reasonable in the few research facilities where both explosions and multiple specular reflections are possible. An equally attractive alternative is to enclose the associated beam and target area within a light-tight or filter box which lowers transmission at the laser wavelength to a safe level.

Since many Class 4 laser systems present fire hazards, in particular high-powered CW sources, a sufficient thickness of back stops such as fire brick, asbestos, or earthen materials should be available, or a water cooled beam stop should be used, or the beam should be diverged prior to striking the back stop. Other specific guidelines are provided in Chapter 17.

The operations of Class 4 visible or near infrared (IR-A) laser systems out-of-doors for optical ranging (LIDAR), or similar uses, should be avoided in rainy, snowy, or foggy conditions or if there is substantial dust in the air, unless eye protection can be provided for all personnel within the immediate vicinity of the beam.

15.9.5 Precautions for Class 3 Medium Risk Laser Systems

Since Class 3 lasers are generally hazardous only for direct exposure, most specific control measures are designed to reduce greatly the probability of viewing either the direct beam or reflections from flat specular surfaces. The general precautions are directed at the operator of the system so that he will avoid aiming the beam at specular surfaces.

15.9.5.1 Indoor Operations

The laser should be operated indoors in a well-controlled facility. The laser's primary and secondary beam shall be terminated, where feasible, at the end of the usable beam path. The beam stop material should have a diffuse reflectance at the laser wavelength to make beam visibility optimum, but glare and potentially hazardous reflections should be minimized. It is particularly important to remove specularly reflectant surfaces, particularly flat ones in and near the beam path. Optical elements are often specular but must remain in the beam. However, chrome-surfaced instruments and similar surfaces should be kept away from the beam path unless protective eyewear will be routinely worn. Eye protection should be required if intrabeam viewing is even slightly possible. Eye protection should always be required for Class 4 systems but should be optional for Class 3 systems if the arrangement is relatively stable, and the likelihood of direct intrabeam viewing is extremely remote.

15.9.5.2 Authorized Operators

It is particularly important that the operator of an outdoor Class 3 or Class 4 laser

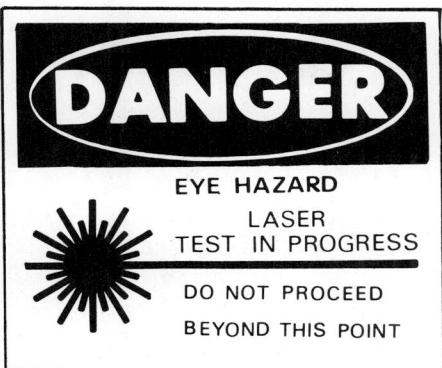 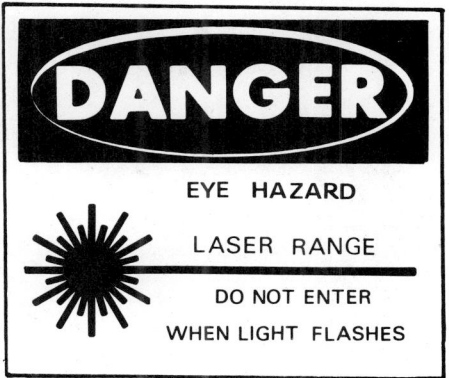

Figure 15-20. Warning Signs. The standard warning signs recommended by the ANSI Standard Z-136.1 for indicating controlled laser areas both indoors and outdoors allow flexibility in wording. The DANGER logo would apply to operations with Class 3B and Class 4 lasers.

system be appropriately trained to install, adjust, and operate such equipment. Some local authorities require that proof of qualification of the laser equipment operator be available. In the State of New York a Laser Operator's permit is needed for out-of-doors operation of a mobile laser, and operators must take a test to prove their knowledge of laser safety in this regard.

15.9.5.3 Outdoor Operations

Where lasers are operated that have an output power well above those used for alignment, the area should be posted with standard laser warning placards. When the laser is not being operated, or if it is not necessary that it be continuously operated, beam shutters should be used to terminate the beam at the laser, or the laser power should be turned off. These efforts will minimize accidental exposures. Direct intrabeam viewing of a laser for alignment purposes should be minimized, unless there is no chance that personnel can be exposed to levels in excess of the exposure limit. The laser should be terminated at the end of its usable beam path unless the beam is directed into the airspace. If the laser is directed into airspace, precautions must be taken to assure that personnel in elevated positions or aircraft are not exposed to hazardous levels. The local FAA offices in the United States should be consulted for appropriate precautions (ANSI, 1976). When the laser is not actually being operated or supervised it should be stored or located where unauthorized personnel cannot gain access to the unit. Placement of the laser beam path at or near eye level should be minimized to reduce the risk of accidental exposure.

Standard warning signs, which can be used at the entrance of laser facilities or near laser outdoor applications, are illustrated in Figs. 15-20 and 15-21. It should be

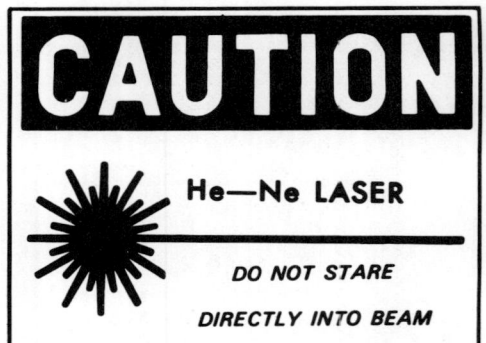 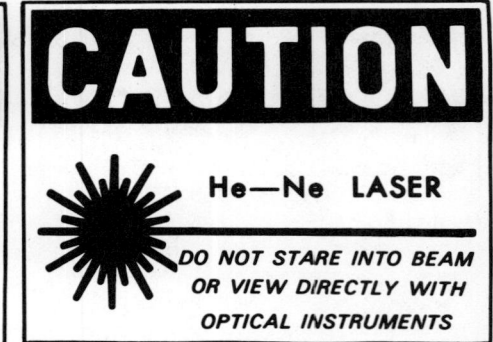

Figure 15-21. Warning Signs. The CAUTION warning sign would be used for Class 3A (left) or Class 2 laser operations both indoors or outdoors where concern would exist about people being surprised from a bright light exposure. Such signs are rarely used, and many feel such signs are unnecessary.

noted that there are two general logotypes used in the United States and another is recommended in the draft of the international IEC standard.

15.9.5.4 Ancillary Hazard Controls

It is important to consider that additional hazards beyond those due to the optical radiation hazards may exist in the use of high-risk Class 4 laser (and in a few cases of medium-risk Class 3 laser) systems, especially electrical hazards (Chapter 27). These industrial hazards normally include the vaporized target materials, or the gases or dyes used in laser systems. Ultraviolet radiation may also be emitted as a secondary byproduct in an optically-pumped or gas discharge laser system, and hazards may also exist from explosions at capacitor banks or gas storage tanks. Significant levels of X-radiation are possible from high-voltage (over 30-kV) power supply tubes in some systems. These additional hazards and their controls are discussed in detail in Chapter 26.

15.10 CONCLUSIONS

In summary, the ability to analyze potential hazards from any laser system is enhanced by a broad knowledge of optics, laser technology in general, and the imaging process of the human eye. In the preceding chapters a background of the basic information necessary to perform a hazard analysis has been presented. This chapter showed that the hazard analysis depends upon at least three aspects—the laser

General Hazard Analysis and Controls 517

system and its potential hazards, the type of personnel who may be exposed, and, finally, the reflective materials and other optically important materials in the environment which can influence the hazard analysis. Normally, once a hazard is recognized, the control measures are obvious. The next several chapters will give the detailed hazard control measures for specific laser applications. The hazard analysis and control measures for Class 1 and 2 laser systems are largely left up to the manufacturer. The control measures developed by the user are most important for Class 3 and 4 systems.

15.11 REVIEW QUESTIONS

1. There is little need for safety inspections in research laboratories since the scientific personnel using such lasers are aware of the hazards and can be relied upon to take appropriate control measures. True or False?

2. A laser beam (wavelength 694.3 nm) is incident upon a dull, diffuse surface with a spectral reflectance of 0.32. The beam energy is 1 Joule and the beam diameter is 0.8 cm. What is the reflected radiance? Is this reflection hazardous for the pulse duration of 1 ms?

3. Estimate the probability of ocular exposure from a direct beam entering the eye of an individual located 10 m from a laser that accidentally falls from its mount if it can land directed at any possible postion. The laser beam will fire once as the device strikes the ground. The individual is standing 10 m away and is looking at the laser. The beam divergence is 4 mrad, the emergent beam diameter is 1 mm, and the output peak power is 1 mW. The individual has a 4-mm pupil and both eyes are unprotected.

4. A laser beam is directed at a flat glass plate 100 m away. The beam is horizontal and the glass plate is vertical. The entire beam strikes the glass window and the emergent beam divergence is 0.5 mrad and the emergent beam diameter is 2 cm. What is the probability that an individual 100 m from the target whose eye is on the plane of the incident and reflected laser beam and who is looking at the target would receive an exposure to the collimated reflected beam?

5. Should eye protection be used around a high-power laser operated outdoors in the rain? Need eye protection be worn 10 m away from a Class 3 laser beam to protect against reflections from the rain or fog or snow?

6. Why is it important to install door interlocks in a Class 4 laser facility, but not a Class 3 facility?

7. Why is a hazardous diffuse reflection considered a more likely risk than a hazardous reflection from a flat mirror surface within a laboratory environment for a Class 4 laser operating at 530 nm?

8. Are special laser operator permits required for lasers used out-of-doors? Give at least one example if this is so.

9. Which hazardous reflection has the greatest hazard volume for a 1 J ruby laser (694.3 nm), 10 ns pulse, 1 cm emergent beam diameter, 1 mrad divergence: (a) a diffuse reflection from a 90% diffuse white magnesium carbonate block; (b) a flat glass beam splitter oriented at 10° from the normal of the beam path; (c) a reflection from a curved lens surface which creates a specularly-reflected beam having a divergence of 24 mrad.

10. A laser beam is incident upon 1-mm thick plain glass window with an index of refraction of 1.5 for normal incidence. The specularly reflected beam will have an energy: (a) 1% of the initial beam; (b) 4% of the initial beam; (c) 8% of the initial beam; (d) 17% of the initial beam.

15.12 GENERAL REFERENCES

Adhav, R. S., and Orszag, M., 1974, Frequency doubling crystals—unscrambling the acronyms, *Electro-Optical Sys. Design* **6**(12):20–24.

American National Standards Institute, 1976, "Safe Use of Laser," Standard Z-136.1, ANSI, New York (under revision, 1979).

American Conference of Governmental Industrial Hygienists, 1976, "A Guide for Control of Laser Hazards," ACGIH, Cincinnati, OH.

Charschan, S. S., 1977, Avoiding eye damage, *Laser Focus* **13**(12):8 (December 1977).

Fender, D. H., 1964, Control mechanisms of the eye, *Sci. Am.* **211**(1):24–33.

Fitzpatrick, T. B., Pathak, M. A., Harber, L. C., Seiji, M. and Kukita, A., 1974, "Sunlight and Man, Normal and Abnormal Photobiologic Responses," University of Tokyo Press, Tokyo.

Gibbons, W. D., and Allen, R. G., 1978, Retinal damage from suprathreshold Q-switch laser exposure, *Health Phys.* **35**(3):461–469.

Girard, A., Chin, S. L., and Delisle, C., 1979, Penetration depth of 10.6-μm radiation in plexiglas, *Appl. Opt.* **18**:1295–1296.

Goldman, L., Rockwell, R. J., Jr., and Hornby, P., 1971, Laser laboratory design and personel protection from high energy lasers, *in* "Handbook of Laboratory Safety," (N. C. Steere, ed.) 2nd edition, pp. 381–389, The Chemical Rubber Company, Cleveland, OH.

Gray, D. E. (coordinating ed.), 1972, "American Institute of Physics Handbook," McGraw-Hill, New York.

Green, A. E. S., (ed.), 1966, "The Middle Ultraviolet: Its Science and Technology," John Wiley and Sons, New York.

Hammer, W., 1972, "Handbook of System and Product Safety," Prentice-Hall, Englewood Cliffs, New Jersey.

International Electrotechnical Commission, 1979, "Radiation Safety of Laser Products and Equipment Classification, Requirements and User's Guide," Technical Committee, TC-76 Laser Equipments Draft Standard, IEC, Geneva.

Koller, L. R., 1965, "Ultraviolet Radiation," 2nd edition, John Wiley and Sons, Inc., New York.

Laser Institute of America, 1976, "Laser Safety Guide," LIA, Cincinnati, OH.

Lowenstein, E. V., Smith, D. R., and Morgan, R. L., 1973, Optical constants of far-infrared materials 2: Crystalline solids, *Appl. Opt.* **12**(2):398–406.

Lytle, J. D., Wilkerson, G. W., and Jaramillo, J. G., 1979, Wideband optical transmission properties of seven thermoplastics, *Appl. Opt.* **18**(11):1842–1846.

Martin-Marietta, 1964, "Night Reconnaissance Subsystem," Final Technical Document Report, Martin-Marietta Corp., Orlando, Contract AF33(657)-12490 (November 1964).

Nicodemus, F. E. (ed.), 1976-1978, "Self-study Manual on Optical Radiation Measurements," NBS Technical Notes 910 series, National Bureau of Standards, Optical Physics Division, U.S. Government Printing Office, Washington, DC.

Pert, G. J., 1978, Laser satellite ranging as a hazard to overflying aircraft, *Opt. and Laser Tech.* **10**(2):77–79.

Peters, G. A., 1975, Systematic Safety, *Natl. Safety News* **112**(3):83–90.

Sliney, D. H., Marshall, W. J., Del Valle, P. F., Franks, J. K., Lyon, T. L., and Krial, N. P., 1976, "Laser Hazard Classification Guide," National Institute for Occupational Safety and Health, NEW Publication No. (NIOSH) 76-183, Government Printing Office, Washington, DC (July 1976).

Sliney, D. H., and Palmisano, W. A., 1968, The evaluation of laser hazards, *Am. Industr. Hyg. Assn. J.* **129**:425–431.

Sliney, D. H., 1969, Evaluating hazards and controlling them, *Laser Focus* **39**:42–46 (August 1969).

Smith, D. R., and Lowenstein, E. V., 1975, Optical constants of far infrared materials 3:Plastics, *Appl. Opt.* **14**(6):1335–1341.

State of New York, 1969, Code Rule 50, Lasers, Albany, New York.

Thomas, W., Jr. (ed.), 1973, "SPSE Handbook of Photographic Science and Engineering," John Wiley and Sons, New York.

Ullrich, O. A., and Johnson, G., 1976, "Spectral Measurements of Paints," Report of AWS, Battelle Columbus Laboratories, Columbus, OH.

Withrow, R. B., and Withrow, A. P., 1956, Generation, control, and measurement of visible and near-visible radiant energy, in "Radiation Biology," (A. Hollaender, ed.) Vol. III, pp. 125–258, McGraw-Hill, New York.

U.S. Department of the Army, 1975, Control of Hazards to Health from Laser Radiation, TB-MED 279, Department of the Army, Washington, DC.

15.13 SOME LASER ACCIDENT REFERENCES

Anonymous, 1972, Accidental laser exposure. Health and Safety Information, Issue No. 322, U. S. Atomic Energy Commission, Washington, DC (December 15, 1972) [25-ps Nd exposure, 1064 nm].

Anonymous, 1965, More light on lasers, *Electronics* **38**(11) [Dr. D. Rounds reports of laser injury to lens muscle].

Anonymous, 1977, ILS employee regains central vision lost for a month after laser accident, *Laser Focus* **13**(12):21–22 (December 1977).

Armstrong, C. E., 1970, Eye injuries in some modern radiation environments, *J. Amer. Opt. Assn.* **41**(1):55–62 [2-mW HeNe reflected exposure for 1-2 seconds, 632.8 nm].

Blancard, P., Sorato, M., Blonk, K., Iris, L., and Liotet, S. A., 1965, Propos d'une photocoagulation maculaire par laser, accidentalle, *Ann. Oculist* **198**:263–264 [100-ns ruby, 0.1 J, 694.3 nm].

Charschan, S. S., 1977, Avoiding eye damage, *Laser Focus* **13**(12):8 (December 1977).

Curtin, T. L., and Boyden, D. G., 1968, Reflected laser beam causing accidental burn of retina, *A. J. Ophthal.* **65**(2):188–189 [diffuse reflection of 30-J, 1 ms ruby, 694.3 nm].

Decker, C. D., 1977, Accident victim's view, *Laser Focus* **13**(8):6 (August 1977) [10-ns, 6-mJ Nd exposure at 1064 nm].

Henkes, H. E. and Cuidema, H., 1975, Accidental laser coagulation of the central fovea, *Opthalmologica* **171**:15–25 [20-ns, 3-mJ/cm^2 ruby-pumped dye laser exposure, 800 nm].

Jacobson, H. J. and McLean, J. M., 1965, Accidental laser retinal burns, *Arch. Ophthal.* **74**:882 [two cases; 0.2-J, 35-ns; ruby 694.3 nm].

Rathkey, A. S., 1965, Accidental laser burns of the macula, *Arch. Ophthal.* **74**:346–348 [0.8-ms ruby laser reflection, 694.3 nm].

Zweng, H. C., 1967, Accidental Q-switched laser lesion of human macula, *Arch. Ophthal.* **78**:597–599 [1 to 3-mJ exposure to 10-ns Raman and Brillouin scattered radiation from a ruby laser pulse at 650, 694.3 and 746 nm].

Chapter 16
Eye and Skin Protection

16.1 INTRODUCTION

From a safety standpoint the most desirable laser hazard control measure is complete enclosure of the laser or laser system; however, this may not always be practical and laser eye protection generally offers the best alternative. Although most industrial laser applications do not require the use of eye protection, this is not usually true for laser applications in the research laboratory. Eye protection provides the simplest solution to the laser safety problem for a constantly changing experimental arrangement. Several factors play a role in determining whether eyewear is necessary and, when so, which eyewear is proper for a specific situation. At least three output parameters of the laser must be known: maximum exposure duration, wavelength, and output power (or output irradiance, radiant exposure, or energy) as well as the applicable safe corneal radiant exposure. In addition, some knowledge of such environmental factors as ambient lighting and the nature of the laser operation may also be required.

Laser eye protection generally consists of a filter (often composed of several individual filter plates) which selectively attenuate at specific laser wavelengths, but elsewhere transmit as much visible radiation as possible (Schreibeis, 1968; Scherr, et al., 1969; Sliney, 1974; Straub, 1965, 1970; Swope, 1969, 1970; Swope et al., 1965). Eyewear is available in several designs—spectacles, coverall types with opaque side shields, and coverall types with somewhat transparent filter side shields (Fig. 16-1). Active electronic imaging devices have also served an additional role as eye protection. Although this chapter is devoted primarily to laser eye protection, we shall also discuss sunglasses, sunscreens and protective garments.

16.2 APPLICATIONS

In the indoor shop or in the laboratory environment, eye protection is tradi-

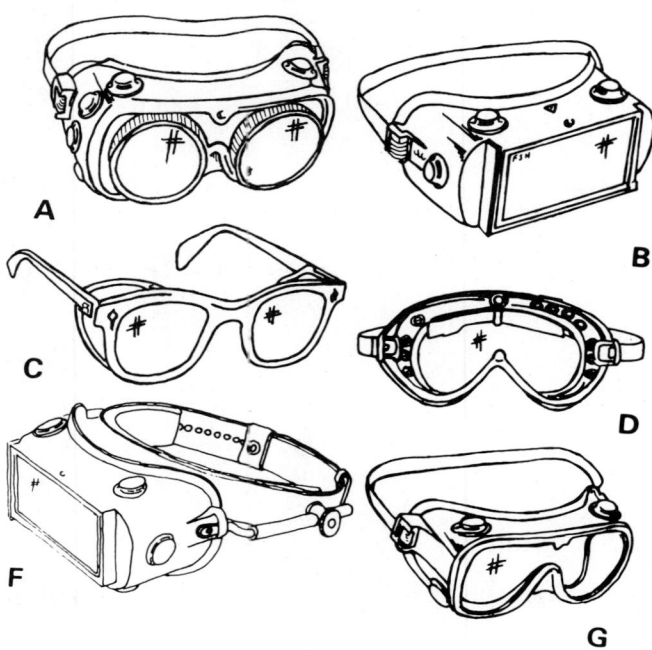

Figure 16-1. Protective Eyewear Designs. Six common types are shown: (A) Goggles with separate glass lenses; (B) Coverall-type with hard rubber or soft vinyl frames, glass and/or plastic flat filter plates; (C) Spectacles with side shields; (D) Plastic wrap-around lens in ski-type frames; (F) Headrest coverall-type goggles; and (G) Full-view soft vinyl goggles.

tionally required for unenclosed high-risk Class 4 lasers. However, where viewing the beam is essential, as in many holographic applications and optical alignment procedures, other precautions must be taken to prevent ocular exposure to levels above the exposure limits.

Several laser applications exist in which a potentially hazardous laser beam is propagated in the outdoor environment. Many applications for construction, atmospheric research, air pollution monitoring, and military use fall into this category. For these, individuals are normally prevented from entering the beam path or the laser is shielded from occupied areas, and eye protection is therefore not used. However, eye protection is extensively utilized where individuals must be "downrange" within the beam path. This is usual in some atmospheric laser beam propagation studies, laser communication experiments, and in tests of rangefinders and similar military lasers (Sliney, 1970). If a laser is directed at a specular target, eye protection is required for all within the hazardous envelope (see Chapter 19, Fig. 19-7).

Eye and Skin Protection

Before deciding that laser protective eyewear offers the best solution for controlling potential hazards, disadvantages of such eyewear force consideration of alternative controls. Most goggles are somewhat uncomfortable to wear for extended periods of time; lens surfaces fog in some environments; at best, peripheral vision is reduced and many goggles provide only "tunnel" vision; and visual acuity is always impaired and color vision is seriously compromised, often to such a degree that warning lights of certain colors are not visible. This reduction of vision by protective eyewear can introduce increased risks in many occupations, e.g., aircraft pilots, electricians or operators of hazardous mechanical equipment. Moreover, an individual wearing eyewear in the vicinity of a laser beam path introduces an additional risk of exposing any unprotected bystanders to specular reflection from the polished protective filter surface. Likewise, an individual wearing safety goggles who increases a laser's output power by a large factor to permit himself to see the beam path sufficiently for alignment purposes will at the same time increase by the same factor the hazard to any unprotected bystanders.

16.3 LASER VIEWING ENHANCEMENT GOGGLES

Several manufacturers offer goggles designed to selectively transmit, rather than attenuate, at a specific laser wavelength. Such goggles have been designed for use with He-Ne lasers used in daylight in the construction industry. The goggles permit workers to readily locate a He-Ne beam at much lower irradiances than would otherwise be possible. Hence, a lower power laser may be used, and potentially hazardous conditions at the laser may be reduced or eliminated. When a 0.5-mW laser can be utilized instead of a 2-mW device, most hazard control measures may be dropped. Obviously, such goggles must be clearly marked, as they *do not* offer eye protection.

16.4 PARAMETERS OF LASER EYE PROTECTION

Several physical parameters are necessary to provide an adequate description of specific eyewear: the protective wavelength or wavelength range; the filter's optical density; visual transmittance; damage threshold (i.e., maximum irradiance); and filter curvature.

16.4.1 Wavelength

The laser wavelength(s) for which the type of eyeshields were designed should be specified. Commercial protective eyewear is designed to greatly reduce or essentially prevent particular wavelength(s) from reaching the eye. It is emphasized that many lasers emit more than one wavelength and that *each* wavelength must be considered. It is seldom adequate to merely mark that the goggle will protect against radiation from a particular type of laser based upon a design to protect against the wavelength corresponding to the greatest output power. For instance, a He-Ne laser may emit 100 mW at 632.8 nm and only 10 mW at 1150 nm, but safety goggles which absorb at the 632.8-nm wavelength may absorb little or nothing at the 1150-nm wavelength. Hence the wavelength range of use should be specified.

16.4.2 Optical Density

Optical density is a parameter for specifying the attenuation afforded by a given thickness of a filter. Since laser beam irradiances may be a factor of a thousand or a million above safe exposure levels, *percent-transmission* notation can be unwieldy. For instance, goggles with a transmission of 0.000001 percent can be described as having an optical density of 8.0. Optical density D_λ is a logarithmic notation and is described by the following expression:

$$D_\lambda = \log_{10}[E_0/E] \qquad (16\text{-}1)$$

or

$$= \log_{10} \tau_\lambda$$

where E_0 is the irradiance of the incident beam, E is the irradiance of the transmitted beam of wavelength λ, and τ_λ is the transmittance of the filter at the specified wavelength. Thus a filter attenuating a beam by a factor of 1,000 or 10^3 has an optical density of 3, and one attenuating a beam by 1,000,000 or 10^6 has an optical density of 6. The required optical density is determined by the maximum laser beam irradiance to which the wearer could be exposed. The optical density of two highly absorbing filters when stacked is nearly (but not exactly if glued) the sum of the two individual optical densities.

The total transmittance of an absorbing optical filter is the product of the internal transmittance of the absorbing medium (which is dependent upon the filter thickness) and the transmission losses due to Fresnel reflection at the filter surfaces. Hence, two stacked filters bonded with optical cement will have slightly less density (~ 0.04) than if separated.

The spectral transmittance of a thin glass or plastic filter sample (molded or ground to useful thickness) is generally measured with a high quality spectrometer to provide no less than one percent transmittance within the wavelength band of interest. The optical density for the material of a given thickness t_2 at a given wavelength may then be calculated from the spectral transmittance τ_λ, of the sample of thickness t_1 if the Fresnel reflection component is adequately accounted for (Ditchburn, 1963). The total spectral transmittance τ_λ is the product of the internal transmittance τ_i (dependent upon thickness) and the loss by reflection ρ_1 (dependent only upon index of refraction) for a beam incident perpendicular to the filter surface.

$$\tau_\lambda = \rho_1 \cdot \tau_i = 2n/(n^2 + 1) \cdot \tau_\lambda \qquad (16\text{-}2)$$

The density D_i due to internal transmission is dependent upon thickness t:

$$D_i = -\log_{10} \tau_i = \log_{10} \rho_1 - \log_{10} \tau \quad (16\text{-}3)$$
and
$$D_i(t_1)/D_i(t_2) = t_1/t_2 \quad (16\text{-}4)$$

For example, if a 2-mm thick Schott BG-18 filter (Schott, 1977) has a density due to internal attenuation of 1.96 (2.00 total density at 694.3 nm), then a 5-mm BG-18 filter would have a density of 9.8 due to internal attenuation, plus 0.04 due to reflection, hence 9.84 at 694.3 nm. Table 16-1 provides useful comparison values of percent transmittance and optical density for quick reference.

16.4.3 Visual Transmittance of Eyewear

Since the object of laser protective eyewear is to filter out the laser wavelengths while transmitting as much of the visible light as possible, visible (or luminous) transmittance should be noted. A low visible transmittance (usually measured in percent) creates problems of eye fatigue and may require an increase in ambient lighting in indoor environments. However, adequate optical density at the laser wavelengths should not be sacrificed for improved visible transmittance. For nighttime viewing conditions, the effective visual transmittance will be different since the spectral response of the eye is different. Figure 3-12 shows the CIE "standard observer's" scotopic (night vision) and photopic (day vision) responses of the eye (Commission International de L'Eclairage 1970). These are mathematical functions that attempt to show approximately the two types of spectral sensitivities of human vision; these are probably the extremes of actual viewing conditions encountered with laser eye protection. Certain colored filters would therefore affect daylight vision differently than night vision. For example, blue-green filter lenses such as BG-18 have scotopic transmission values than red or orange lenses of the same photopic transmission values.

16.4.4 Laser Filter Damage Threshold (Maximum Irradiance)

At very high beam irradiances filter materials which absorb the laser radiation are crazed, cracked, melted or otherwise damaged. Thus it becomes necessary to consider a damage threshold for the filter. Damage thresholds from Q-switched and mode-locked pulsed laser radiation fall between 10 and 100 J/cm^2 for absorbing glass, and 1 to 100 J/cm^2 for plastics and dielectric coatings.

Irradiances from *CW lasers* which would cause filter damage are in excess of those which would present a serious skin hazard or fire hazard and therefore would normally not need to be considered; i.e., personnel would not normally be permitted in the area of such lasers. Studies by BRH (Envall, 1975) confirm that damage occurs to both filter and frame material from 5- and 10-W CW lasers. In fact, in several cases plastic frames and vent caps had lower damage threshold than the filter (Fig. 16-2).

Pulsed lasers damage eye protection in a different manner. Figure 16-3 shows

TABLE 16-1. Optical Density vs Transmission Table

Percent	Density	Percent	Density	Percent	Density	Percent	Density	Percent	Density
100.00	0.00	33.11	0.48	10.96	0.96	3.631	1.44	1.20	1.92
92.72	0.01	32.36	0.49	10.72	0.97	3.548	1.45	1.17	1.93
95.50	0.02	31.62	0.50	10.47	0.98	3.467	1.46	1.15	1.94
93.33	0.03	30.90	0.51	10.23	0.99	3.388	1.47	1.12	1.95
91.20	0.04	30.20	0.52	10.00	1.00	3.311	1.48	1.10	1.96
89.13	0.05	29.51	0.53	9.772	1.01	3.236	1.49	1.07	1.97
87.10	0.06	28.84	0.54	9.550	1.02	3.162	1.50	1.05	1.98
85.11	0.07	28.18	0.55	9.333	1.03	3.090	1.51	1.02	1.99
83.18	0.08	27.54	0.56	9.120	1.04	3.020	1.52	1.00	2.00
81.28	0.09	26.92	0.54	8.913	1.05	2.951	1.53	0.89	2.05
79.43	0.10	26.30	0.58	8.710	1.06	2.884	1.54	0.79	2.10
77.62	0.11	25.70	0.59	8.511	1.07	2.818	1.55	0.71	2.15
75.86	0.12	25.12	0.60	8.318	1.08	2.754	1.56	0.63	2.20
74.13	0.13	24.55	0.61	8.128	1.09	2.692	1.57	0.56	2.25
72.44	0.14	23.99	0.62	7.943	1.10	2.630	1.58	0.50	2.30
70.79	0.15	23.44	0.63	7.762	1.11	2.570	1.59	0.45	2.35
69.18	0.16	22.91	0.64	7.586	1.12	2.512	1.60	0.40	2.40
67.61	0.17	22.39	0.65	7.413	1.13	2.455	1.61	0.36	2.45
66.07	0.18	21.88	0.66	7.244	1.14	2.399	1.62	0.32	2.50
64.57	0.19	21.38	0.67	7.079	1.15	2.344	1.63	0.28	2.55
63.10	0.20	20.89	0.68	6.918	1.16	2.291	1.64	0.25	2.60

61.66	0.21	20.42	0.69	6.761	1.17	2.239	1.65	0.22	2.65
60.26	0.22	19.95	0.70	6.607	1.18	2.188	1.66	0.20	2.70
58.88	0.23	19.50	0.71	6.457	1.19	2.138	1.67	0.18	2.75
57.54	0.24	19.05	0.72	6.310	1.20	2.090	1.68	0.16	2.80
56.23	0.25	18.62	0.73	6.166	1.21	2.040	1.69	0.14	2.85
54.95	0.26	18.20	0.74	6.026	1.22	2.000	1.70	0.13	2.90
53.70	0.27	17.78	0.75	5.888	1.23	1.950	1.71	0.11	2.95
52.48	0.28	17.38	0.76	5.754	1.24	1.910	1.72	0.10	3.00
51.29	0.29	16.98	0.77	5.623	1.25	1.860	1.73	0.09	3.04
50.12	0.30	16.60	0.78	5.495	1.26	1.820	1.74	0.08	3.10
48.98	0.31	16.22	0.79	5.370	1.27	1.780	1.75	0.07	3.15
47.86	0.32	15.85	0.80	5.248	1.28	1.740	1.76	0.06	3.20
46.77	0.33	15.49	0.81	5.129	1.29	1.700	1.77	0.04	3.40
45.71	0.34	15.14	0.82	5.012	1.30	1.660	1.78	0.025	3.60
44.67	0.35	14.79	0.83	4.898	1.31	1.620	1.79	0.016	3.80
43.65	0.36	14.45	0.84	4.786	1.32	1.580	1.80	0.010	4.00
42.66	0.37	14.13	0.85	4.677	1.33	1.550	1.81	0.006	4.25
41.69	0.38	13.80	0.86	4.571	1.34	1.510	1.82	0.003	4.50
40.74	0.39	13.49	0.87	4.467	1.35	1.480	1.83	0.0018	4.75
39.81	0.40	13.18	0.88	4.365	1.36	1.450	1.84	0.0010	5.00
38.90	0.41	12.88	0.89	4.266	1.37	1.420	1.85	0.0006	5.25
38.02	0.42	12.59	0.90	4.169	1.38	1.380	1.86	0.0003	5.50
37.15	0.43	12.30	0.91	4.074	1.39	1.350	1.87	0.00018	5.75
36.31	0.44	12.02	0.92	3.981	1.40	1.320	1.88	0.00010	6.00
35.48	0.45	11.75	0.93	3.890	1.41	1.290	1.89	0.00001	7.00
34.67	0.46	11.48	0.94	3.802	1.42	1.260	1.90	0.000001	8.00
33.88	0.47	11.22	0.95	3.715	1.43	1.230	1.91	0.0000001	9.00

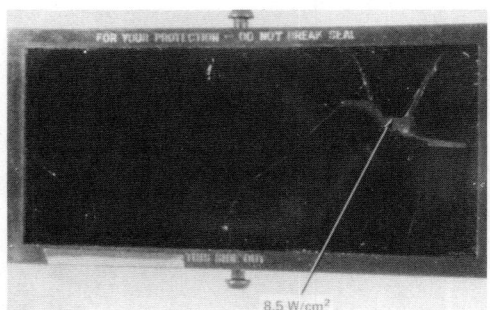
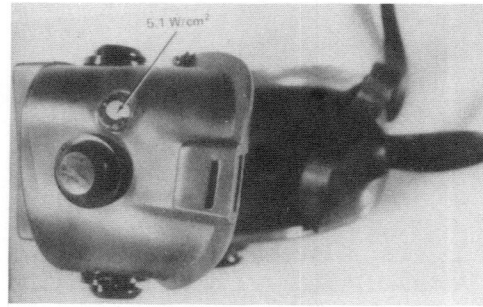

Figure 16-2. Damaged Glass Plate and Plastic Frames from CW Lasers. The upper panel shows the result of a 10-W Nd:YAG laser incident upon a glass filter plate. It shattered immediately whereas plastic filters burned through only after 15-s exposure. Bottom panel shows burn-through of frame material after ~ 16-s exposure to the same beam (from Envall et al., 1975).

examples of damage to laser filters from intense pulsed laser beams. Generally, only surface effects are noted, and little change in optical density results. Plastic materials melt superficially, glass surfaces craze, and dielectric coatings vaporize. These effects contrast with the more serious fracturing of glass and complete burn-through of plastic filters (Fig. 16-2) that occur from CW laser irradiation.

16.4.5 Filter Curvature

As potentially hazardous specular reflections can exist to significant distances from flat lens surfaces, curved filter lenses are far more desirable than flat ones. If curved protective filters are required for personnel in a laser target area, then personnel in the vicinity of the laser and elsewhere would not also require eye protection. Also, the use of the standard 6-diopter curvature on spectacle lenses reduces prismatic distortion. But some curved glass filters which are manufactured by thermal shaping rather than by lens grinding have noticeable edge distortion.

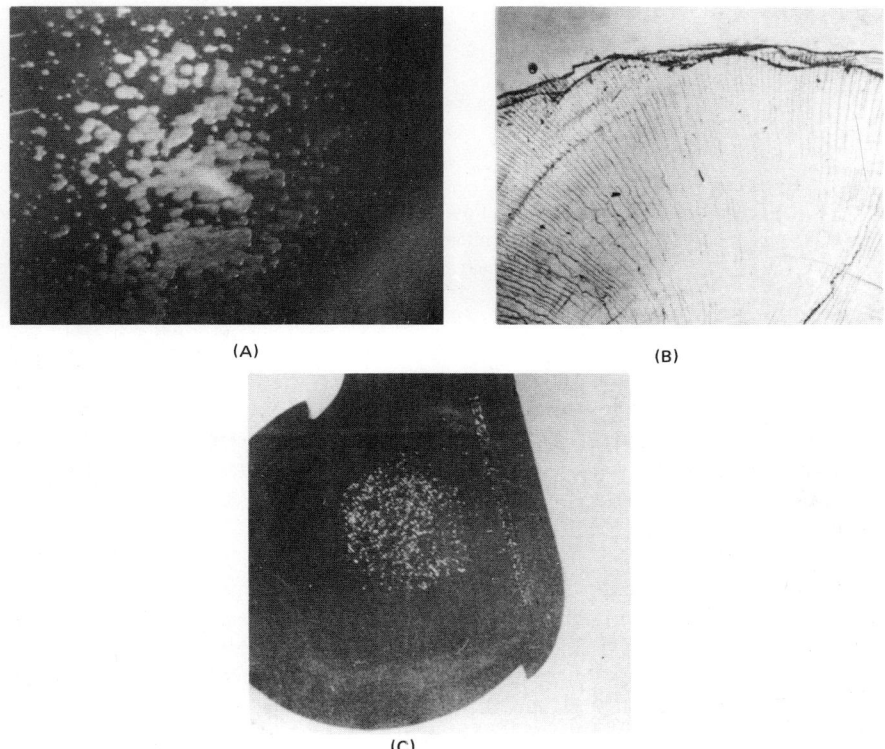

Figure 16-3. Surface Damage of Protective Filters by Laser Irradiation. (A) Photomicrograph showing holes formed in a dielectric coating of filter plate from a Q-switched laser beam radiant exposure of 1-10 J·cm^{-2}. (B) Photomicrograph of an absorbing glass filter (BG-18) illustrating concoidal fractures after exposure to a 2-J Q-switched laser beam focused to a 2- to 3-mm spot. (C) Surface damage in a plastic filter caused by a radiant exposure of approximately 30 J·cm^{-2} delivered in a 2-ms pulse.

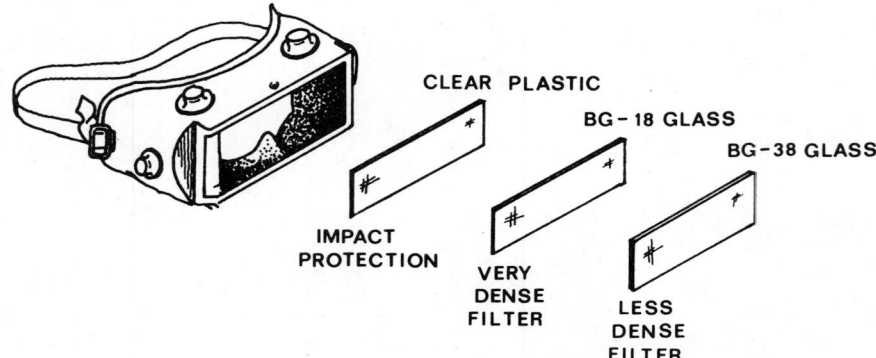

Figure 16-4. Design of Laser Goggle for High-Power, Q-Switched Lasers. First glass plate has lower absorption coefficient than second glass plate so as not to shatter as readily as the second and to protect the second plate, and a clear plastic sheet protects the eye from glass breakage (after Swope, 1969 and 1970).

16.5 METHODS OF CONSTRUCTION

There are basically two effects which are utilized in passive goggles to filter out specific laser wavelengths: selective absorption by colored glass or plastic, or selective reflection from dielectric coatings on glass. Combinations of each are also possible. Each method has its advantages.

The simplest method of fabrication is to use colored glass absorbing filters. These are generally the most effective in resisting damage from wear and from very intense laser sources. The inorganic colorants in glass are quite stable. Unfortunately, many absorbing glass filters such as phosphate glasses cannot be chemically hardened to provide impact resistance by normal methods. However, sufficient impact protection can be provided by clear plastic sheets placed over the glass filter if this is considered an important feature (Fig. 16-4). A more serious drawback is the lack of absorbing-type filters which have a sharp transmission "cut-off" or "notch" near the laser wavelengths in the visible.

Dichroic reflective coatings can often be used with advantage as they can be designed with a relatively sharp spectral "cut-off;" that is, they can selectively reflect a given wavelength while transmitting most of the rest of the visible. However, this spectral attenuation factor is angular dependent. At off-normal incidence, the attenuation factor is reduced. Hence, these dichroic coatings are generally used in conjunction with absorbing filters, or in small field-of-view (narrow-acceptance-angle) optical instruments. If used with an absorbing filter substrate, the increased pathlengths of off-normal rays through the substrate results in increased attenuation factors which compensate for the reduced coating attenuation at those angles of incidence.

Absorbing plastic filter materials have many advantages: greater impact resistance, lighter weight, and ease of molding into curved shapes. The disadvantages are that they are more readily scratched, quality control appears to be more difficult, surfaces are often damaged by chemical solvents, and the organic dyes used as absorbers are more readily affected by heat and ultraviolet radiation. Also, they may saturate or bleach under Q-switched or mode-locked pulsed laser irradiation. Many of these problems have been solved for the plastic laser eye protection that is now commercially available. The major difficulty is that some plastics will become denser with age and the visual transmittance will be reduced. There are even some unusual cases where the laser protection characteristics degrade with time in an ultraviolet rich, humid environment.

16.6 SELECTING APPROPRIATE EYEWEAR STEP–BY–STEP

16.6.1 Step 1

Determine wavelength(s) of laser output. If more than one wavelength is emitted, it is useful to know the relative output powers at each wavelength.

16.6.2 Step 2

Determine required optical density. Table 16-2 lists required optical densities (or alternatively, attenuation factors) for various laser beam irradiances E_i or radiant exposures H_i which could be incident upon safety eyewear. Some margin for error is built into Table 16-2. The exact minimal density D_{min} for a given wavelength can be calculated as:

$$D_{min} = \log_{10} [E_i/E_{EL}] \qquad (16\text{-}5)$$
$$= \log_{10} [H_i/H_{EL}]$$

To determine the maximum incident beam irradiance (or radiant exposure) that is relevant for Table 16-2 or Eq. (16-5) follow the following rules:

(a) If the emergent beam is not focused down to a smaller spot, and the beam is greater than 7 mm in diameter, the emergent beam radiant exposure/irradiance may be considered the maximum that could reach the unprotected eye, and is thus used in Table 16-2 or Eq. (16-5).

(b) If the emergent beam is *focused* after emerging from the laser system or if the emergent beam diameter is *small* (less than 7 mm in diameter), one should assume that all of the beam energy/power could enter the eye. In this case divide the laser output energy/power by the maximum area of the 7-mm pupil (approximately 0.4 cm²). This "equivalent" radiant exposure or irradiance may be used in Eq. (16-5) or in Table 16-2. Alternatively the output energy/power is also listed in the table for direct application.

(c) If the observer is in a fixed position and cannot receive the maximum output radiant exposure/irradiance, then a measured or calculated value may be used (e.g., "downrange" from the laser and within the beam).

TABLE 16-2. Simplified Method for Selecting Laser Eye Protection for Intrabeam Viewing for Wavelengths Between 200 and 1400 nm

Q-Switched Lasers (1 ns to 0.1 ms)	Non-Q-Switched Lasers (0.4 ms to 10 ms)		Continuous Lasers Momentary (0.25 s to 10 s)		Continuous Lasers Long-Term Staring Greater than 3 hrs		Attenuation	
Maximum Output Energy (J) / Maximum Beam Radiant Exposure ($J \cdot cm^{-2}$)	Maximum Laser Output Energy (J)	Maximum Beam Radiant Exposure ($J \cdot cm^{-2}$)	Maximum Power Output (W)	Maximum Beam Irradiance ($W \cdot cm^{-2}$)	Maximum Power Output (W)	Maximum Beam Irradiance ($W \cdot cm^{-2}$)	Attenuation Factor	OD
10 / 20	100	200	NR†	NR	NR	NR	100,000,000	8
1.0 / 2	10	20	NR	NR	NR	NR	10,000,000	7
10^{-1} / 2×10^{-1}	1.0	2	NR	NR	1.0	2	1,000,000	6
10^{-2} / 2×10^{-2}	10^{-1}	2×10^{-1}	100*	200*	10^{-1}	2×10^{-1}	100,000	5
10^{-3} / 2×10^{-3}	10^{-2}	2×10^{-2}	10	20	10^{-2}	2×10^{-2}	10,000	4
10^{-4} / 2×10^{-4}	10^{-3}	2×10^{-3}	1.0	2	10^{-3}	2×10^{-3}	1,000	3
10^{-5} / 2×10^{-5}	10^{-4}	2×10^{-4}	10^{-1}	2×10^{-1}	10^{-4}	2×10^{-4}	100	2
10^{-6} / 2×10^{-6}	10^{-5}	2×10^{-5}	10^{-2}	2×10^{-2}	10^{-5}	2×10^{-5}	10	1

* Only where exposure is considered extremely remote.
† NR = not recommended.

(d) In general, having an optical density in excess of one density unit above the minimum requirement is not desirable since the visual transmittance may be sacrificed. This general guideline often must be disregarded if the eyewear is designed for several wavelengths. Additionally, it may be necessary to view reflections from the laser beam of a CW laser for positional alignment; e.g., a 1-W argon laser could be safely operated by a worker using goggles with only a density of 3.5 to 4, which would permit momentary viewing of the direct beam, although intentional direct viewing would not be advisable with these goggles. If continuous intrabeam viewing were anticipated, then greater densities corresponding to EL's for the duration of viewing (E_{EL} or H_{EL}) should be worn.

16.6.3 Selecting the Most Suitable Eye Protector

Once the minimal density is determined, the user must fabricate his own eyewear (which should not be attempted without experience) or purchase a commercially available protector. Salient features of a variety of such protectors are presented in Table 16-3. Depending upon the application, one should consider the best model having the proper density. Advantages of one model must be weighted against the disadvantages of another. One should strive for a protector having:

(a) high photopic visual transmittance;

(b) high scoptopic visual transmittance if the protector is to be used in the dark;

(c) high resistance to fogging (particularly important if use outdoors or in hot environments is envisioned);

(d) good peripheral vision (important for work in hazardous areas, and essential for aviators)

(e) adequate resistance of filter, side shield frame and vent ports (important if working with Class 4 systems—particularly CW where beam irradiances are likely to exceed 1 W/cm^2 for beam powers exceeding one watt).

(f) availability of optical correction (use coverall goggles for prescription laser safety spectacles)

(g) resistance to degradation by UV and harsh environments (important largely for outdoor applications)

(h) comfort (the goggles are of little value if a worker stops wearing them).

TABLE 16-3. Standard Laser Eye Protection. Optical Densities (OD) at Common Wavelengths (nm)

	320	325	332	337.1	347.1	441.6	457.9	488	514.5	530	611.8	632.8	647.1	694.3	840	905	1060	1184	1152	TRANSMITTANCE
AMERICAN OPTICAL																				
580*& 586*+	>2	>2	>2	>2	>2	<1	<1	<1	<1	<1	1	2	2	3	4	3	2	2	1	10
581* & 587*+	>2	>2	>2	>2	>2	<1	<1	<1	<1	<1	3	4	4	6	13	14	11	10	8	46
584	>2	>2	>2	>2	>2	<1	<1	<1	<1	<1	<1	1	3	8	21	22	17	16	13	35
585**	>2	>2	>2	>2	>2	<1	<1	<1	<1	<1	1	3	3	7	17	17	13.8	13	11	33
588						17	16	13	9	7	<1	2.5	<1	<1	<1					24
598						17	13	13	9	6	<1	<1	<1	<1	<1					33
599						14	11	11	8	8	<1	<1	<1	<1						25
698	>2	>2	>2	>2	>2	12	11	10	8	6.4	<1	<1	<1	<4	<10	11	8.5	8	6	5
OMNITECH																				
182+						<1	<1	<1	<1	<1	2	4	4	2						22.5
GLENDALE																				
NH	>16	15	15	16	16	<1	<1	<1	<1	<1	<1	<1	<1	<1	<1	<1	<1	<1	<1	70
HN	>10	>10	>10	>10	>10	<1	<1	<1	<1	<1	<1	6	5	2	<1	<1	<1	<1	<1	17
A	20	20	21	19	18	1	1	1	1	<1	<1	<1	<1	<1	<1	<1	<1	<1	<1	45
R	10	8	9	9	9	14	14	15	11	5	3	4	1	1	<1	<1	<1	<1	<1	19
NDGA~	>20	25	25	24	23	7	6	6	6	<1	<1	<1	<1	3	<1	<1	10	10	<1	45
NDGA,R&NN	25	25	25	25	25	<1	<1	<1	<1	<1	<1	<1	<1	6	14	16	16	10	<1	20
NDGA,db ND,A,N	25	25	25	25	25	14	12	11	7	4	<1	<1	<1	<1	30	30	30	2	<1	48
HADRON																				
1+	>10	7	5	2	2	<1	<1	<1	<1	<1	3	4	7	>10	>10	>10	>10	>10	>10	25
2	10	10	10	10	10	10	>10	>10	>10	>10	<1	<1	<1	<1	<1	<1	<1	<1	<1	1.5
3															>1	>2	>3	>3	>3	
5	>10	>10	>10	>10	>10	>10	>10	>10	>10	>10	8	4	>1	>1	>1	>1	>1	>1	>1	17.6
FRED REED OPTICAL *																				
FR6-PL-BG18-GBS-C	>5	5	2	1.7	1.4	<1	<1	<1	<1	<1	<1	1.5	2.2	5	>5	>5	>5	>5	>5	35
FR6-PL-KG3-GBS-C	<1	<1	<1	<1	<1	<1	<1	<1	<1	<1	<1	<1	<1	<1	>2	3	4	>5	<1	76
RG610	>5	>5	>5	>5	>5	>5	>5	>5	>5	>5	<1	<1	<1	<1	<1	<1	<1	<1	<1	
RG630	>5	>5	>5	>5	>5	>5	>5	>5	>5	>5	4	<1	<1	<1	<1	<1	<1	<1	<1	
RG665	>5	>5	>5	>5	>5	>5	>5	>5	>5	>5	>5	>5	>5	<1	<1	<1	<1	<1	<1	
GG9	>5	>5	>5	>5	>5	4	2	2	4	<1	<1	<1	<1	<1	<1	<1	<1	<1	<1	
OG530	>5	>5	>5	>5	>5	>5	>5	>5	>5	<1	<1	<1	<1	<1	<1	<1	<1	<1	<1	
OG550	>5	>5	>5	>5	>5	>5	>5	>5	>5	<1	<1	<1	<1	<1	<1	<1	<1	<1	<1	
OG570	>5	>5	>5	>5	>5	>5	>5	>5	>5	<1	<1	<1	<1	<1	<1	<1	<1	<1	<1	
OG590	>5	>5	>5	>5	>5	>5	>5	>5	>5	2	<1	<1	<1	<1	<1	<1	<1	<1	<1	
FISH SCHURMAN																				
1060-9	>1	>1	>1	>1	>1	>1	>1	>1	>1	>1	>1	>1	>1	>1	2	5	9	9	9	64
2800-4 •	>1	>1	>1	>1	>1	>1	>1	>1	>1	>1	>1	>1	>1	>1	1	1	2	2	2	78
633-5						>10	>10	>10	7				5	>10			>30			
515-7	>10	>10	>10	>10	>10	>10	>10	7				5								
PHASE-R																				
blue	5	>5	5	5	5	<.5	<.5	>1	>2	>3	>5	>5	5	1						
red								>4	>4	4	2	1	<1							
EALING																				
	(Helium Neon)							10	7			5	10				30			
25-2437																	9	9	9	
25-2460															5		4	4	4	
25-2478																				
25-2486																				
25-2494																				
QUANTRAD CORP																				
Yag	>2	>1																		
Xenon	>5	>5	>5	>5	>5	>5	>5	>5	>5	>5			2		>5	>5	>5	>5	>5	

Eye and Skin Protection

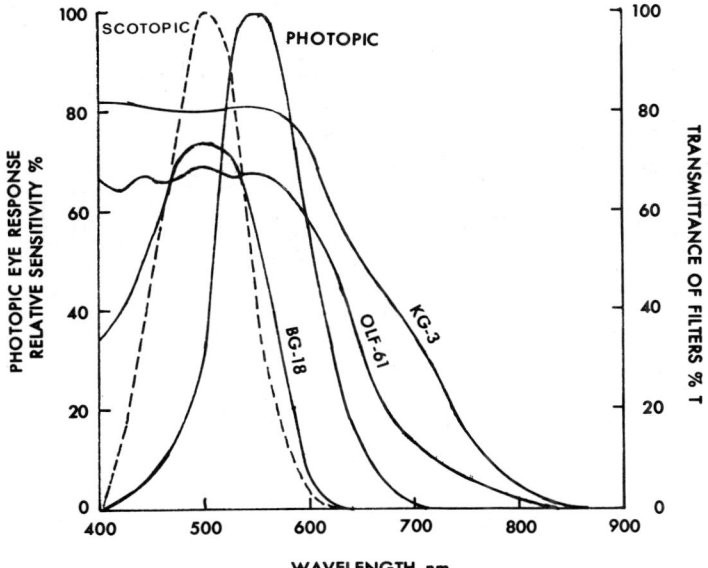

Figure 16-5. Filter Spectral Transmission Curves and Visual Transmission. Three types of IR-A laser protective filter materials are shown which provide adequate protection from neodymium lasers. Only BG-18 glass provides substantial protection at the 694.3-nm ruby wavelength but that interferes far more with photopic vision.

16.7 COMMERCIAL SOURCES OF LASER EYE PROTECTION

A variety of commercially available eye protection exists. Table 16-3 presents the optical densities at principal UV-A visible, and IR-A laser wavelengths and for actinic ultraviolet radiation (200 to 320 nm) for a large group of such products. The authors made every effort to collect the available data from all present American manufacturers of laser eye protection. If any data were overlooked the authors would appreciate knowing for use in future editions of this book.

16.8 EYE PROTECTION FOR INFRARED LASERS

Optical radiation at wavelengths greater than 1.4 μm is absorbed in the anterior portion of the eye and does not usually reach the retina. The same EL values have been used in protection standards for both the eye and skin. If is therefore necessary to consider also the need for skin protection at these IR-B and IR-C wavelengths. Protection of the eye is nonetheless of paramount importance, since an injury to the eye (specifically the corneal stroma in most instances) can result in nearly total or

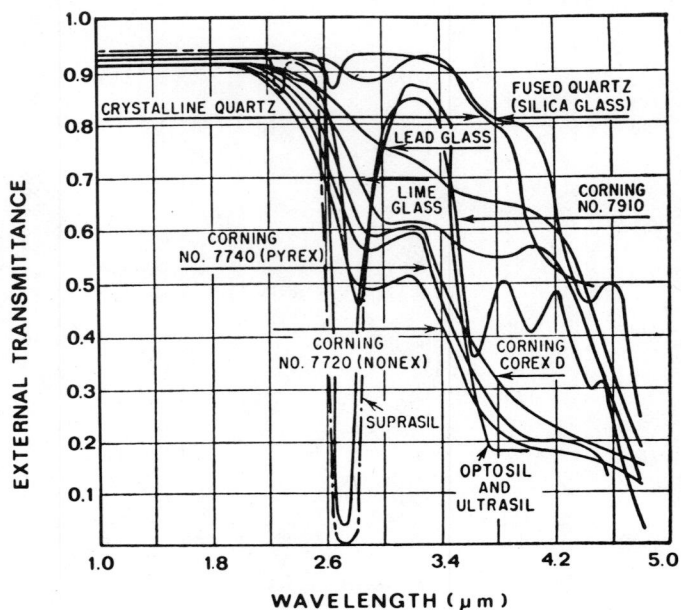

Figure 16-6. IR Spectral Transmission of Glass. The IR-B and IR-C spectral transmission of a variety of glass materials is shown. Adapted from Figure 6c83 of the American Institute of Physics Handbook (1973); data from GE and Amersil quartz catalogs.

partial blindness, whereas a skin burn from a comparable laser exposure would heal without much disability. Eye protectors for IR-A have already been discussed in the context of protecting against retinal hazards. Figure 16-5 summarizes the most common IR-A filter materials.

Most optical materials which are transparent in the visible spectrum (transparent plastics, glass and quartz) are essentially opaque at wavelengths greater than 5 μm (Figure 16-10). All of these materials can, therefore, be used for eye protection for CO_2 (10.6 μm) laser radiation and most are adequate for the CO laser (wavelengths of 4.8 to 6 μm). Plastic goggles, despite the fact that they may burn, are preferred for protection where there is a low-probability of exposure to reflection from CO_2 lasers having an output power less than 100 W. Quartz (e.g., AO Model 300) or heat-resistant glass (e.g., Hadron Type 112-4) goggles worn in conjunction with face shields and skin protection have been used when very high-power CO_2 laser beams cannot be enclosed.

Eye protection between 1.2 and 4 μm has become a problem at those wavelengths where polymethylmethacrylate (Lucite ®, Plexiglas ®, and Perspex ®) and lime glass do not have aborption bands (Figures 16- 6, 16-10, and 16-11). Possibly the best all-purpose filter for wavelengths greater than 1.4 μm is a water cell which indeed is the common IR filter used in the radiometry laboratory. Because of weight and other design problems the H_2O filter has not been considered a practical eye protection method except in a laboratory window. Although water goggles have been made (Spencer and Bixler, 1972), more practical, lightweight goggles may be fabricated by using 3 to 5-mm Schott KG-3 glass filters which provide an optical density of 3 to 5 at the DF laser wavelengths (3.8 to 4.2 μm) and at the HF wavelengths (2.6 to 3.3 μm). Fred Reed Optical Company manufactures safety spectacles with KG-3 glass. American Optical Company has also made an infrared protective filter glass (Type OLF 51) but did not incorporate it into commercially available safety glasses. Most inexpensive clear plastic visitor goggles are made of polymethylmethacrylate which transmits in some of the HF band between 2.5 μm and 2.8 μm, but are reasonably opaque at longer wavelengths.

16.9 TESTING LASER EYE PROTECTION

Eye protection should be checked periodically for integrity. The measurement of eye-protection-filter optical densities in excess of 3 or 4 without destruction of the filter is very difficult (Bauer et al., 1968). Because of this problem, the requirement that the optical density of protective eyewear be periodically checked, as originally proposed for many laser hazard control guidelines, has been deleted.

16.9.1 Routine User Tests

The user should periodically check for the integrity of the filter, frame, vent ports, etc. Hold the goggle up to a luminaire and look for light leaks. A crack or pinhole in a colored filter will show up as white light (if using a white light source). Visually inspect coatings for obvious scratches or blotches. Look for evidence of cracking, pitting or crazing. Minor scratches in a filter will not seriously degrade its protective performance (albeit, it can degrade its visual performance). Remember that the OD of an absorbing filter is proportional to thickness. Hence a 0.1-mm deep scratch in a 3-mm filter plate (OD 8) will only reduce the OD by (0.1/3 = 3.3%) or from 8 to 7.73 in theory. In practice, the diffraction effects caused by the scratch would probably distort the retinal image sufficiently to more than compensate for the increased filter transmission. If the filter is plastic and appears to have become lighter from use outdoors or in indoor, high-UV environments, the filter should be tested for OD or discarded. Check to see that side shields fit snugly and hinges are properly functioning. When the reliability of an eye protector is in doubt, discard it (unless OD testing is much less than the cost of the eyewear). Testing of OD is complex and relatively costly as will become apparent in the next paragraph.

16.9.2 Testing Optical Density

The actual measurement of filter optical densities between 3 and 10, and perhaps greater densities, can be performed with special techniques using either a

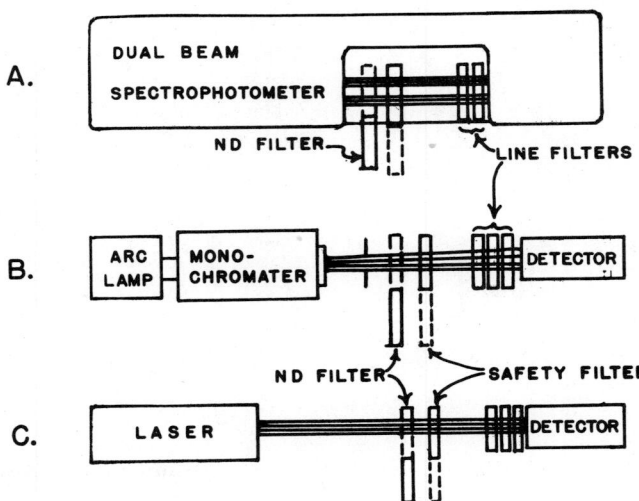

Figure 16-7. Measuring Optical Density of Filters. Three methods used for direct measurement of laser filter transmission are shown; several other variations of combinations of filters, light sources and monochromators are possible. In all arrangements, one or more neutral density filters calibrated at the wavelength of interest are inserted in place of the protection filter until the transmission comparison is within 1 OD unit. This procedure is necessary to reduce errors for detector nonlinearity. Laser line filters are continuously added in series until the addition of filters (to reduce unwanted light of other wavelengths) results in the same measured OD for the protection filter (from Sliney, 1974, with permission).

spectrophotometer or a laser. As noted previously, spectrophotometers found in most chemical laboratories are limited to measurements of densities of 2.7 to 3 when sharp wavelength-cutoff filters are measured. This limitation arises from errors introduced by "stray light" passing through the monochromator (Cook and Jankow, 1972). Stray light arises principally from dust and microscopic imperfections in the prisms or diffraction gratings. These imperfections scatter light of wavelengths other than the one wavelength of interest into the exit slit of the monochromator. Obviously, this stray light can be greatly reduced by placing monochromators in tandem or by using narrow-band filters in conjunction with a monochromator (see Fig. 16-7). However, further measurement problems arise after one achieves a relatively pure monochromatic beam if the detector does not have sufficient sensitivity. Unless a laser is used as the light source, the bandwidth (related to slit width) of the monochromator may be so increased as to achieve a measurable signal at the detector that a broad-band attenuation factor is measured for the protective filter—a very serious shortcoming for filters having a rapidly changing optical density with changing wavelength. The stray-light problem does not arise when measuring the transmittance of a welding filter (or any neutral filter) with a spectrophotometer. A calibrated neutral density filter is added to the reference beam path in order to change the transmission measurement range in the sample path. The limit to the measurement range is then determined by the sensitivity of the instrument tested in 1971 at the U.S. Army Environmental Hygiene Agency. Using a CW light source and monochromator the filter had an OD = 6 at 694.3 nm, but when tested with an irradiance of 10 mW/cm^2 from a ruby Q-switched laser (694.3 nm) the measured OD = 1.3. Without the laser testing procedure this defect in the filter material would never have been detected. The reversible bleaching characteristic was also found in plastic filters in some commercially available goggles (no longer manufactured), but the changes were not of importance since the goggles still met minimal density specifications. For example, densities were reduced from values of 14 and 16 down to 8 and 10.

The greatest concern has been with goggles having specified optical densities at, or only slightly above, the density required for protection. The normally required densities do not exceed 8. Goggles having densities less than 8 are usually designed for use at either the helium-neon, neodymium or ruby laser wavelengths. Therefore, if a more comprehensive goggle testing program were initiated, the goggles which should receive first attention are those having a density less than 8 for the ruby and helium-neon lasers. Sliney and his associates have periodically checked the optical density of various types of commercial eye protection. In general, the goggles met or exceeded specifications given by the manufacturer (Table 16-3). However, in some rare instances protective filters were shown to have densities less than specified. One type of glass filter was low by 0.2 density units. In another case, the lower density of a plastic filter still exceeded 8 and was therefore not of real concern. In a third case, the density of a blue plastic filter was significantly less than a specified density of 6 and a product recall was initiated by the manufacturer.

16.9.3 Environmental Tests

At present, almost all evidence indicates that the optical density of commercially available eyewear does not decrease with use although some plastics "age" by becoming slightly more dense after considerable exposure to solar radiation (or age on the shelf simply with time). One exception to this general rule was a commercially available plastic filter designed to protect against argon laser lines. In studies performed at the USAF School of Aerospace Medicine (for BRH) it was noted that this filter bleached under a combination of ultraviolet radiation and high humidity. Although the manufacturer had not detected such changes from earlier solarization tests, his tests were not performed in high-humidity environmental chambers.

16.9.4 Tests of Translucent Side Shields or Frames

Occasionally it is desirable to have some limited vision through side shields. This is possible by using filter side shields or diffusing transparent side shields. Testing the color filter side shield would require the same methods as 16.9.2. To test diffusion side shields requires the measurement of transmitted radiance. Total transmitted power would be measured, and a photograph of the diffused laser spot on the side shield is used to determine the new diffuse source area. Typical values would be OD-5 to 6 equivalent.

For example, a clear plastic side shield is diffused by abrasion. A beam irradiance of 10 mW/cm² in an 11-mm beam diameter is incident on the exterior side of the side-shield. The transmitted projected radiance is 1.2 mW/(cm²·sr), and is the same at both 0° and ±40° on the opposite side, hence the surface is reasonably diffuse. Visual observation confirms that the projected spot seen on the exit side is uniformly bright. Now the "effective optical density" D_{eff} is converted from a diffusion attenuation factor C_D of:

$$C_D = L(trans)/E_i \quad (16\text{-}6)$$
$$= [1.2 \text{ mW}/(\text{cm}^2 \cdot \text{sr})]/[10 \text{ mW}/\text{cm}^2]$$
$$= [0.12 \text{ W}/(\text{cm}^2 \cdot \text{sr})]/[\text{W}/\text{cm}^2]$$

The exposure duration of $t = 0.25$ s (momentary viewing) has $\alpha_{min} = 12$ mrad. The largest value of $\alpha_{min} = 24$ mrad (for exposures where $t \geq 10$ s). At the greatest reasonable exposure duration the dual visible EL's at $t = 10$ s are 1 mW/(cm²·sr) and 2.2 W/(cm²·sr). Therefore with the $C_D = 1.2$ W/(cm²·sr)/W/cm² the D_{eff} is:

$$D_{eff} = \log_{10}[L_{EL}(\text{extended})/C_D \cdot E_{EL}] \quad (16\text{-}7)$$
$$= \log_{10}\{[2.2 \text{ W}/(\text{cm}^2 \cdot \text{sr})]/[(0.12 \text{ W}/(\text{cm}^2 \cdot \text{sr})/(\text{W}/\text{cm}^2)][(10^{-3} \text{ W}/\text{cm}^2)]\}$$
$$= \log_{10}[1.83 \times 10^4]$$
$$= 4.26$$

Now, to illustrate the importance of making this calculation at an exposure duration where α_{min} is large let us calculate D_{eff} at 10 μs where α_{min} is a very small value. We can express C_D in joules instead of watts. Using a visible wavelength:

$$D_{eff} = \log_{10}\{[0.22 \text{ J}/(\text{cm}^2 \cdot \text{sr})]/[(0.12 \text{ J}/(\text{cm}^2 \cdot \text{sr})/(\text{W}/\text{cm}^2) \cdot (5 \times 10^{-7} \text{ J}/\text{cm}^2)]\}$$
$$= \log_{10}[3.67 \times 10^6] \quad (16\text{-}8)$$
$$= 6.56$$

16.10 MARKING OF EYE PROTECTORS

The optical density at appropriate laser wavelengths should be marked indelibly on the eye protection. This will assist in eliminating the mistaken use of goggles designed for one laser with another laser—a mistake that could result in ocular injury. Less technical marking (e.g., "use only with ruby laser") may also be desirable in some limited applications where non-technical persons must wear the eye protector. A manufacturer or model number should also be on the filter or frame. Literature supplied with the goggle should provide data on visual transmittance and limitations of the product such as available estimates of damage thresholds for several exposure conditions.

16.11 EYE PROTECTION FOR PUMP LAMPS AND TUNABLE WAVELENGTH LASERS

Occasionally eye protection is necessary for work around unenclosed arc lamps used as optical pumping sources for both pulsed or CW lasers. Eye protection developed for welding is quite suitable for this purpose. Likewise, welding goggles may provide the only temporary solution to some viewing requirements such as for dye lasers that may be scanned over most of the visible spectrum.

Eye protection filters for welders were developed empirically based more upon available materials than upon the knowledge of ocular protection requirements. The first organized study of glass filter materials was due to Sir William Crookes (1914) in England. Optical transmission characteristics are now standardized as "shades" and specified for particular applications (Coblentz and Stair, 1930; Stair, 1948; ANSI, 1959). Although maximum transmittances for ultraviolet and infrared radiation are specified for each shade, the mean photopic visual transmittance τ_v or visual optical density D_v has traditionally defined the shade number S#:

$$S\# = 7/3\, D_v + 1 \cong -\ln \tau_v + 1 \qquad (16\text{-}9a)$$

or
$$D_v = 3/7\, (S\# - 1) \qquad (16\text{-}9b)$$

where
$$D_v = -\log_{10} \tau_v \qquad (16\text{-}10)$$

For instance, a filter with a photopic visual attenuation factor of 1000 (i.e., $D_v = 3$) has a shade number of 8. Electric arcs typically have luminances of the order of 10^4 to 10^5 cd/cm² and filter densities ranging from 4 to 5 corresponding to shades 10 to 13 are required for comfortable viewing (Sliney and Freasier, 1973). Likewise, a shade of at least 13 is required to comfortably view the sun which has a luminance of approximately 10^5 cd/cm². These densities are well in excess of those necessary to prevent retinal burns, but are required to reduce the luminance to 1 cd/cm² or less for viewing comfort. The user of the eye protection should therefore be permitted to choose the shade most desirable to him for his particular operation. It can be stated that actinic ultraviolet radiation from quartz-enclosed arcs is effectively eliminated in all standard welding filters. Chapter 24 (Welding Arcs and Open-Arc Processes) describes welding filters in greater detail.

16.12 POLARIZING FILTERS

At first thought, the use of polarizing spectacles is appealing as eye protection for multiple laser wavelength use, since many laser beams are highly polarized. Unfortunately, optical densities above 2 can scarcely be achieved with polarizing spectacles, and a tilt of the head would render even that protection almost non-existent. Nevertheless, in many laboratory arrangements, such filters are often used in a rotatable mount at the laser exit port as a means of reducing the laser output to a reasonably safe level for alignment purposes. Rotatable, cross-polarizers have occasionally been mounted in eyewear and in viewing optics to serve as variable density filters for work with variable luminance light sources. However, this technique is used rarely since commercially available polarizing sheet material is effective only within a limited band of wavelengths. That is, while densities up to at least 2 may exist in the visible spectrum, much higher (and in a few instances, potentially hazardous) levels of near-infrared radiation could pass almost unattenuated through the filters. The increased IR-A transmission of such a filter is not as hazardous at might at first be expected (Ham et al., 1973).

16.13 DYNAMIC EYE PROTECTION DEVICES

Numerous dynamic systems have been studied as eye protection against pulsed optical sources such as the nuclear fireball. The ideal dynamic filter would be nearly transparent except when activated by a hazardous light source, at which time it would rapidly become nearly opaque for the duration of the light flash. These systems usually consist of photodetector-actuated shutters (which may be mechanical, electro-optic, or magneto-optic) or photoreactive filters (such as photochromic materials). They are all generally rather cumbersome when compared with typical laser safety goggles or welder's goggles. Batteries are required to power the first category of such devices. However, dynamic filters may offer the only practical solution for eye protection against unexpected white-light (broad-band) pulsed sources.

The dynamic filter approach has not been employed in the development of laser eye protection since sharp-cutoff filters have been available which strongly attenuate most laser wavelengths and still transmit sufficient light for vision. In addition, present-day dynamic filter devices are not capable of achieving significant optical densities within 10 μs, which is far greater than the duration of a typical Q-switched laser pulse ($\cong$ 20 ns), although such a fast response is theoretically possible (Fox, 1961; Thursby et al., 1971; Williams and Duggar, 1965; Cook and Jankow, 1972; Spencer and Bixler, 1972; Harris and Cutchen, 1972). Figure 16-8 shows an active PLZT filter. Note that an electronic power source and an optical detector are required to activate the filter.

An active welding helmet with a Motorola filter that has a 0.15-ms closure duration and another with a liquid crystal filter having a closure duration of 0.2 s are available from some welding safety suppliers. Liquid crystal sheets with cross polarizers have also been used in the laboratory to achieve a density of 3 within 150 μs. An electric current is used to break up a polarized pattern in the crystal. Such helmets are sometimes useful in working with arc lamps and searchlights where the arc source is repeatedly turned off and on and shields or enclosures are not practical or are ineffective.

16.14 IMAGE CONVERTER TUBES

Image converter viewers designed as night-vision viewing devices to view near-

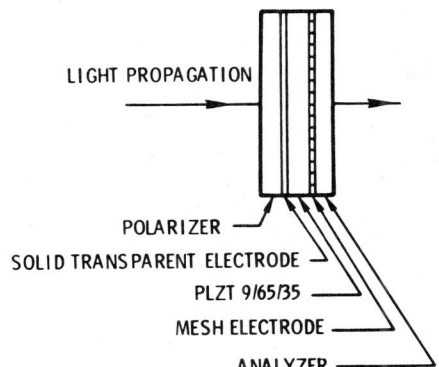

Figure 16-8. PLZT Active Filter. Light is transmitted or attenuated depending upon the polarization of the PLZT ceramic layer (courtesy Sandia Laboratories).

infrared radiation can serve as laser protective eyewear. Although the image converter tubes may be damaged by direct laser irradiation, these devices provide equivalent optical densities of at least 8 for all wavelengths. Their disadvantage is bulkiness and a monochromatic presentation with some loss of resolution of the objects being observed.

Infrared image-converter tubes and image-intensifier tubes are utilized in many military surveillance systems and are now available for scientific applications. Night vision goggles have also been used as prosthetic appliances for the partially blind. These devices may be subjected to laser or other high intensity optical irradiation during use which would otherwise expose the operator's eye to hazardous irradiation. However, the physical construction of these tubes provide eye protection in a unique way since the optical path consists of nearly opaque components which afford viewing by electronic optical amplification. Studies were conducted at the Army Environmental Hygiene Agency by T. L. Lyon and D. H. Sliney to determine the degree of protection that these viewing devices provide for an observer under various conditions.

Image converter systems can be divided into two categories: "active" and "passive." Most older night vision equipment was employed as part of an "active" system consisting of an infrared source to irradiate the selected scene which was then viewed through an infrared image converter tube. These systems normally consisted of an S-1 photocathode screen (peak sensitivity in the near-infrared) and a P-20 phosphor screen (peak luminance in the green), but the overall optical gain was low. However, the newer, passive systems use available lighting with a high-gain, image-amplifier tube to view an area. These systems typically consist of an S-20 (extended range) photocathode screen with a P-20 phosphor screen. Figure 16-9 illustrates the approximate geometrics of four groups of these devices. The maximum luminance (brightness) produced by a P-20 phosphor tube when the tube is

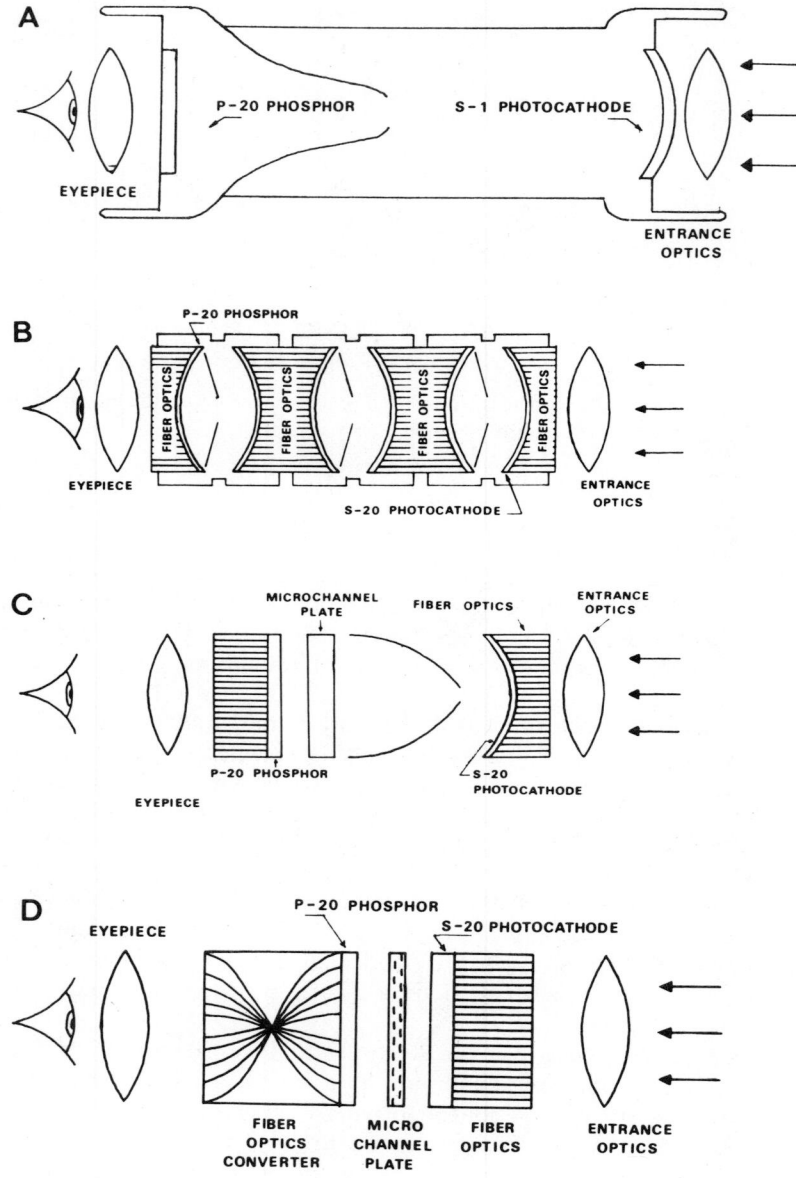

Figure 16-9. Geometries of Four Image Converter Tubes (A) Simple image converter; (B) Three-stage image amplified; (C) Advanced single-stage amplifier; with micro-channel plate; and (D) Amplifier with fibre optic twist for an upright image.

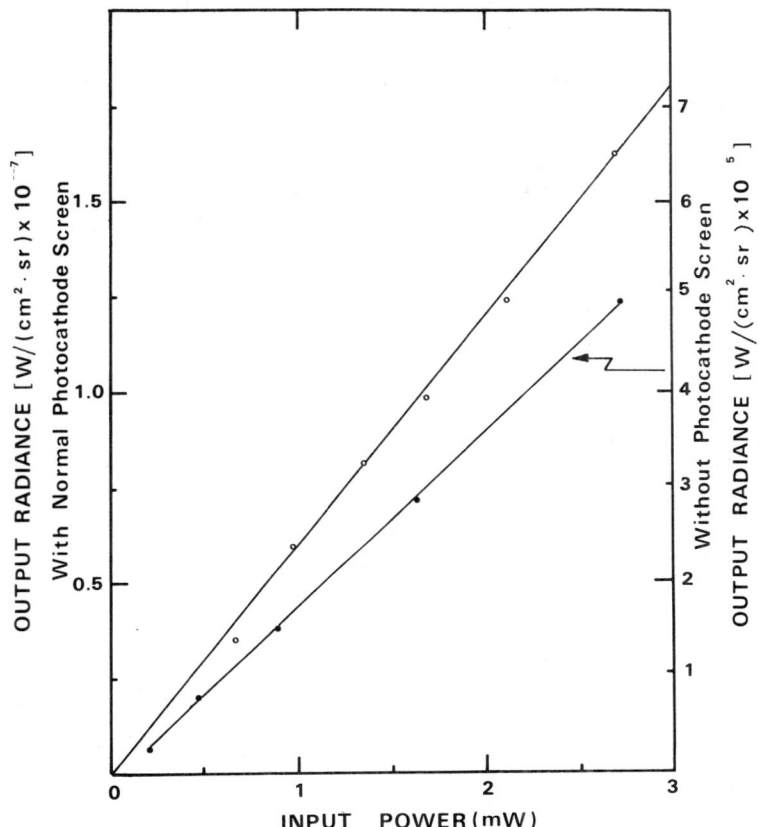

Figure 16-10. Transmission Measurements of Image Converter Tubes. The relevant measure of transmission for safety purposes is to measure the radiance of the diffused transmitted laser radiation.

operated in a normal manner is approximately 80 cd/m² (i.e., 80 nits = 0.008 cd/cm²).

Night-vision devices have a low transmittance (see Fig. 16-10) of the incident light due to absorption by the photocathode and phosphor screens, scattering due to internal components and their geometries, and refraction losses due to the lenses. Not only is the potential hazard from intrabeam viewing reduced due to the low transmittance, but also the highly collimated light from the laser is diffused by the device to produce a larger source size at the phosphor screen (see Fig. 16-11). The result is that instead of a laser beam being focused to a small spot ($\sim$ 10 to 20 μm) on the retina, a much larger image size is formed, thus substantially reducing the

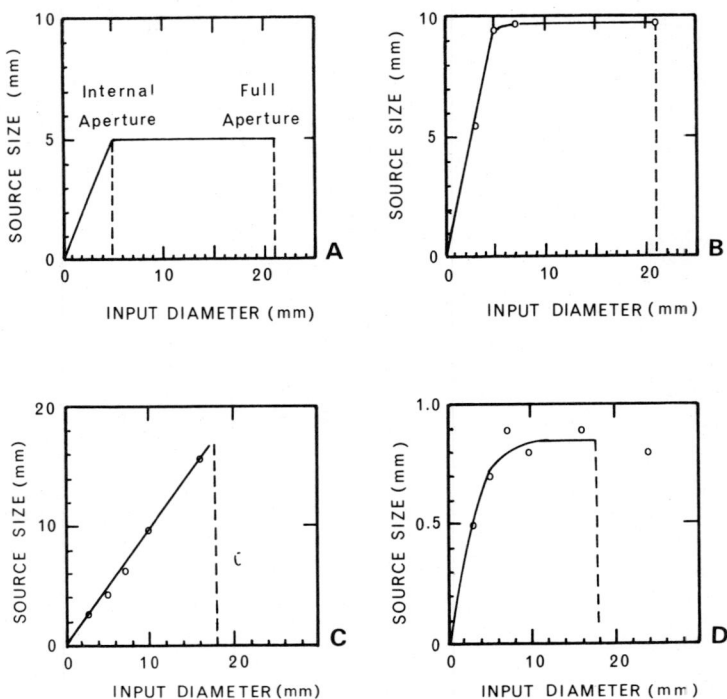

Figure 16-11. Diffused Image of a Laser Source. The source size of transmitted laser radiation at a photosphor screen surface is shown for four types of image converter and image intensifier tubes. Instead of viewing a point source the viewer sees an extended source.

retinal irradiance and hence the potential hazard. It is possible to determine an effective optical density for a point source such as a laser based upon measurements of the tube's actual transmission and the increase in projected source size (i.e., using an approach similar to that in Eq. 16-6 and 16-7).

The source radiance is the most important parameter used in evaluating the potential hazard of an extended source in the retinal hazard region of the spectrum (400-1400 nm) since it is directly related to retinal irradiance. Many laser systems encountered in the laboratory would contain either a Q-switched ruby laser operating at 694.3 nm or a neodymium laser at 1064 nm or at 530 nm with a pulse duration of approximately 20 ns. The exposure limits are 0.027 J/(cm² · sr) for the visible laser wavelengths and 0.14 J/(cm² · sr) for the 1064-nm neodymium wavelength under the above conditions. The power-to-radiance conversion factor can be computed for the converter tube; for example this factor was computed for two tubes at the ruby and neodymium wavelengths using Fig. 16-10 and Fig. 16-11. The results

TABLE 16-4. Power-to-Radiance Conversion Factor C_D from Direct Transmission of Optical Radiation at Ruby and Neodymium Wavelengths

Night Vision Device	Wavelength	Power-to-Radiance Conversion Factor ($[W/(cm^2 \cdot sr)]/W$)	Effective Optical Density (D_λ)
System using 6929 tube	694.3 nm	4.2×10^{-5}	---
	1064 nm	3.5×10^{-3}	---
System using 6929 tube with photocathode screen removed	694.3 nm	3.2×10^{-2}	4.6
	1064 nm	1.0	3.1
System using second generation tube with fiber optic converter	694.3 nm	6.0×10^{-4}	6.5
	1064 nm	8.8×10^{-2}	4.2

of these computations appear in Table 16-4. From this table it is possible to compute the incident radiant energy (within the input limiting aperture of systems using these two tubes) that would be required to exceed the exposure limits at these wavelengths. The results indicate that reflections from most laboratory laser systems do not have sufficient radiant exposure (greater than 1 J/cm^2) for the transmitted radiance through present image converters to exceed the EL's. These devices provide adequate protection to personnel from intrabeam viewing of many lasers even if the photocathode screen is removed. Some other devices are also available that have still lower transmittance with increased diffusion of the laser beam due to their internal geometries and hence provide greater protection from intrabeam viewing. Intrabeam viewing of radiation from a searchlight or arc source through a night-vision device reduces transmitted fraction of the incident radiation to an unmeasurable level and therefore provides the observer with adequate eye protection. Under normal operating conditions the phosphor luminance of these devices are less than 80 cd/m^2. This is a level at which adverse effects normally do not exist. However, the dark-adapted eye may lose much of its dark adaptation at 80 cd/m^2. Operational limitation secondary to loss of dark adaptation therefore must be considered.

16.15 EYE PROTECTION FILTERS FOR SOLAR RADIATION

From the optical hazards discussed in previous chapters it is evident that direct viewing of the sun, either because of insufficient knowledge of the hazard or because of interest in a solar eclipse, requires protection against several different portions of

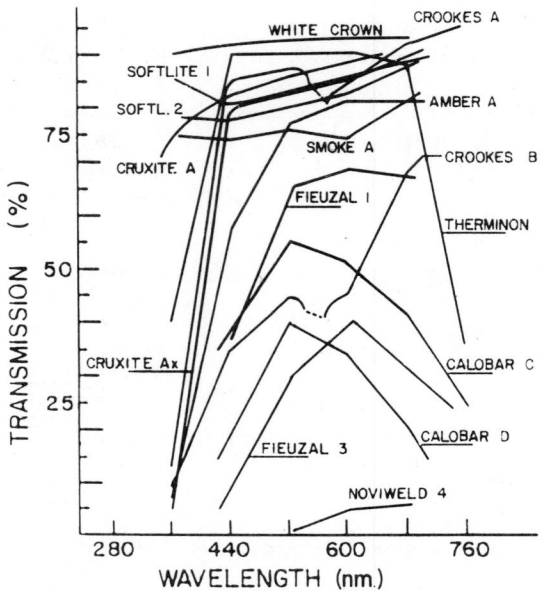

Figure 16-12. Filters for Sunglasses and Industrial Spectacles. The spectral transmission of commonly used tinted glass lenses is provided for comparison (from Borish, 1970, with permission).

the spectrum. Protection against ultraviolet radiation may be accomplished by choosing a yellowish or reddish filter which attenuates UV. Protection against intense visible rays should be weighted to filter more of the blue light than the rest of the visible spectrum. It is generally found that a shade 12 or 13 welder's filter is quite adequate to protect against both the ultraviolet radiation and the visible radiation. Protecting against the IR, however, is more complicated.

One should be warned against the use of darkened colored slides since these slides (usually made by developing unexposed color film) use organic dyes which transmit in the near-infrared (IR-A) spectral band. In fact, it is very uncommon to find any type of organic dyes that absorb in the near-infrared. Although the near-infrared is not considered as dangerous to the retina as once thought, unnecessary exposure should be limited. Crossed polarizing filters have often been suggested for looking at such bright sources. Unfortunately most polarizing materials used in sunglasses do transmit in the IR-A region. The study of Ham, Mueller, Williams, and Geeraets (1973) is particularly relevant to the question of viewing the sun through such filters. Probably the best solution for observing a solar eclipse, or any arc process, is to view indirectly an image with a pinhole camera as shown in Fig. 6-15.

The spectral transmittance of commonly used ophthalmic glass tinted lenses is provided in Fig. 16-12 (Borish, 1970). However, Hedblom (1961), Anderson and Gebel (1977) have shown that some commercially available plastic, non-prescription

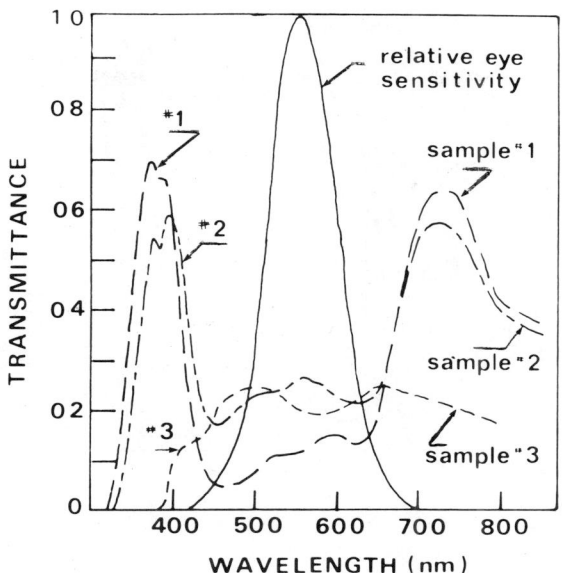

Figure 16-13. Non-Prescription Sunglasses. Spectral transmission of three commercial, non-prescription sunglasses measured by Anderson and Gebel (1977), with permission.

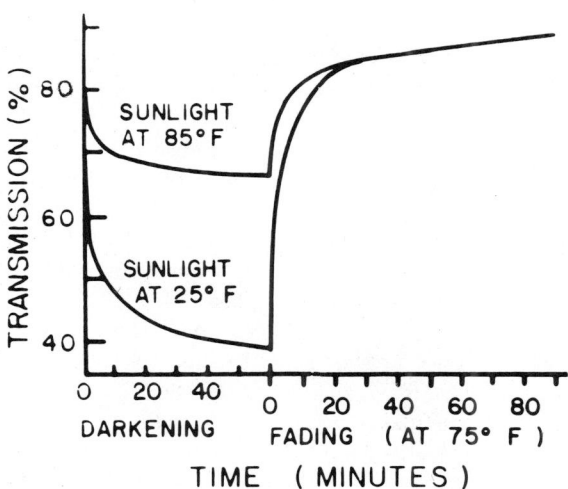

Figure 16-14. Photochromic Glass. The speed of response and change in density are too small to be of any value for eye safety applications (from Borish, 1970, with permission).

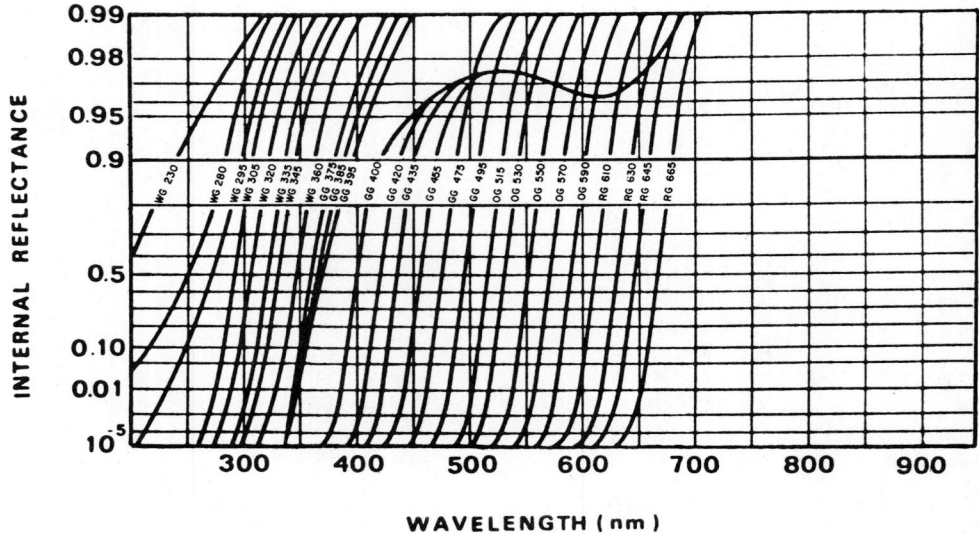

Figure 16-15. Short-Wavelength Blocking Filters. The spectral transmission curves of Schott cut-off filters (1-mm thickness) are at left while the curves for Blue cut-off filters (3-mm) are shown at right (from Schott Color Filter Glass Catalog).

"sunglasses" absorb ultraviolet radiation poorly (Fig. 16-13), which is, of course, very undesirable.

Photochromic glass filters darken when exposed to ultraviolet radiation. This Gebel (1977) have shown that some commercially available plastic, non-prescription "sunglasses" absorb ultraviolet radiation poorly (Fig. 16-13), which is, of course, very undesirable.

Photochromic glass filters darken when exposed to ultraviolet radiation. This characteristic has been employed for use in both prescription and non-prescription sunglasses. Unfortunately the speed of response of this effect and the total change in density would appear to be useful for comfort only and not for any useful degree of eye protection from intense optical sources. Figure 16-14 illustrates the speed of darkening and lightening of a photochromic glass.

Yellow filter lenses have been used to protect the eye and to reduce haze in certain industrial and outdoor applications. In the U.S., American Optical Noviol ® (a safety lens) and Hazemaster ® (an impact resistant lens) yellow lenses are probably the most common. The glass ("Helios" or "Striking Yellow" from Schott Glass Company or PPG 1397) is a sharp cut-off, cadmium-sulfide colored glass that generally will have a 50%-transmission point between 485 nm and 495 nm for a 2-mm thickness which corresponds to an optical density of about 5 at 300 nm, 3 to 360 nm, and 2.4 at 440 nm. This type of filter lens is an adequate alternative for a shade 2 welding goggle lens worn under a welding helmet by electric-arc welders since it substantially reduces hazardous blue light as well as market laser safety spectacles for UV and blue-light lasers which have Schott sharp-cut-off lenses. The spectral transmission curves of some of the common Schott filter materials used in such applications are provided in Figure 16-15. Plastic UV contrast goggles (Ultraviolet Products, Inc.) filter out UV-A but still transmit most blue-light wavelengths. These goggles were developed not as eye protection (although they can be used to protect the eyes), but to filter out UV-A used to generate fluorescence in several non-destructive testing procedures. Argon laser eye protectors (see Table 16-3) are also suitable to eliminate UV-A and blue light.

16.16 PROPER FIT

The potential hazards resulting from light leaks around a goggle are often debated. If large gaps existed (as with no side-shields) direct irradiation of the eye could result, although central macular exposure would be unlikely if not impossible. Side exposure would probably be most hazardous for UV exposure. One laser accident a victim who sustained a central scotoma claimed (according to a news note in Anonymous, *Laser Focus*, 1977) that he was wearing laser safety goggles when exposed and that the beam entered through an opening near his nose. How someone could receive a central scotoma in such a manner is baffling. The most obvious explanation would be that he did not wear his eyewear, was injured, and then concocted the story of wearing goggles. If eyewear fits tightly it becomes more uncomfortable and fogs more readily. The authors are therefore not convinced that loosely fitting eye protection should be considered a shortcoming. A "universal" nose bridge and contour goggle frame is probably impossible. It is normally desirable, therefore, to make use of more than one size or style within a laboratory to assure the best fit for a variety of employees. Still another area of concern that should be addressed when selecting goggles is illustrated in Fig. 16-16. Flat filter plates in oversize goggles may present the greatest chance for serious retinal injury as shown in that figure.

16.17 SKIN PROTECTIVE AGENTS FOR ULTRAVIOLET RADIATION (SUNSCREENS)

A number of topical screening agents have been developed which provide nearly total or in some cases partial filtration of ultraviolet radiation. Since actinic UV-B and UV-C radiation are the most hazardous, and since the skin's senses are not sensitive to this radiation, efforts to develop topical agents have normally concentrated on filtering out primarily this more actinic radiation. These have generally been developed as "sunscreens" because of the large market for such products. These agents include para-aminobenzoic acids (PABA) and its esters, salicylates and cyanamates. These materials are placed in solution with substances that have good *substantivity*.

Substantivity is the term used by dermatologists to indicate that the solution has an affinity for absorption into the skin and retention by that tissue. In some

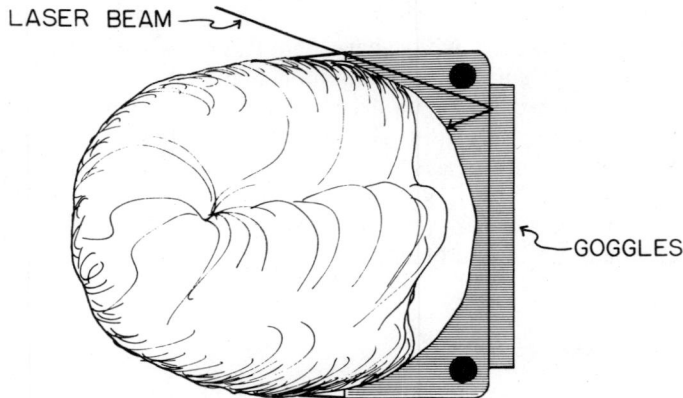

Figure 16-16. Reflection Hazard. The potential hazard to the eye from a specular reflection from a laser beam entering from behind the viewer.

cases it is believed that substantivity is enhanced by chemical reactions between the solution and the stratum corneum. Many of the standard sunscreens provide an attenuation factor (for UV-B) of approximately 10 when applied in a normal manner, which suggests that the duration for achieving a minimum erythema while sunbathing would be increased ten-fold. Rather than a half hour exposure at noontime, The sunscreen would permit an exposure of well more than five hours before sunburn would result in a lightly pigmented sunbather. The Food and Drug Administration has worked out a grading index, The Sun Protection Factor System, for judging the protection afforded by sunscreens. An application of a sunscreen material that increases the permissible exposure time by two would have a sunscreen Protection Factor of two.

The standard commercial sunscreens permit a much greater fraction of UV-A to be transmitted to the skin than UV-B. UV-A, although much less efficient than UV-B, does contribute to solar erythema. Because of the fact that many specialists believe that exposure to UV-A is more conducive to producing both an immediate and a delayed tanning reaction at a range of exposure levels below an erythema threshold, most sunscreens deliberately transmit UV-A*. Other, more highly absorbent materials are used by dermatologists to protect highly photosensitive individuals from excessive UV and UV-visible exposures. Such materials may be used as protective creams in certain industrial or research environments where for some reason clothing or protective face masks may not be appropriate. Several excellent reviews of sunscreen formulations have been prepared and are referenced at the end of this chapter (Parrish, 1971; Fitzpatrick, 1974). The reader must be careful to remember that agents designed for protection against solar UV-B may not provide much protection from industrial sources which emit in the UV-C or UV-A.

---

* In fact several European lamp companies market a very high intensity UV-A lamp for rapid tanning.

16.18 DESIGN SPECIFICATIONS FOR LASER PROTECTIVE EYEWEAR

Although no design specification standards exist in the United States expressly for laser eye protection, such standards do exist for welding protection and safety spectacles, specifically ANSI standard Z-87. During the writing of this book the International Standards Organization (ISO) Technical Committee 94, Subcommittee 6, Working Group 3, (Chairman, E. Sutter, PKB, West Germany) was drafting a standard on "Filters and Eye Protectors Against Laser Radiation." Although the standard was then only in draft form, several of the proposed requirements of this standard are considered desirable goals for any protective filter design. The following draft proposals are of particular interest:

1. Spectral transmittance measurements would be at an angle of incidence of 0° for absorptive laser filters and between angles of 0° to 30° for filters with interference layers. The minimum optical density at any of these angles would be considered the protective density. Protective filtration requirements were most rigid for the spectral region between 200 nm to 1400 nm and the standard specified ocular exposure limits which were based on earlier German safety standards.

2. With reference to a CIE standard of illuminance (a tungsten source) the visual transmittance (photopic) would be required to be greater than 0.15 if at all possible.*

3. The filter could not melt, break or show other indications of damage upon repeated exposures of the maximum recommended exposure for up to 10 exposures, and reversible bleaching (induced transmission) would of course not be permitted.

4. The quality of the lens would have to meet the following standards. For filters, the refractive errors would be restricted depending upon the quality desired. Two classifications of quality would be permitted. For the highest quality class, Class 1, the spherical error would be limited to ±0.06 diopter, the astigmatic error to 0.06 diopter and the prismatic error to 0.12 cm/m within a circular area in the filter 52 mm in diameter centered about the pupillary axis. The specifications would be slightly relaxed for quality Class 2 to 0.12 diopter spherical error, 0.12 diopter astigmatic error and 0.25 cm/m prismatic efficiency. The scattered light of the filters could not exceed 1 $cd/m^2/lx$. The quality of the material would be of good optical quality with no blisters, streaks, inclusions, cloudiness, pits, mold impressions, draw lines or other production defects notable within the central zone of the filters except for a marginal zone of 5 mm; that is, within a 52-mm diameter zone (if one plate, two areas spaced 66 mm apart). Furthermore, induced emission from fluorescence, or conceivably even from stimulated emission, would be restricted such that any induced emission would be limited to safe levels of corneal irradiance. [Fluorescence is normally striking only for ultraviolet lasers. The ISO would also recommend tests to assure stability under ultraviolet radiation (solarization tests) and recommend tests of thermal stability to show that all of the optical specifications are met over a wide range of temperatures and humidity.]

---

* In the design of sunglasses it is customary to limit filtration to a minimum of 15% transmittance to avoid disability glare resulting from reflections off of the inside surface of the lens. However, with side shields in eye protection, this type of limit is not nearly as important or critical.

5. The eye protection filters and frame would be flame-resistant or self-extinguishing [since the laser exposure that would result in a flame would probably be limited to 3 seconds due to head movements, such a requirement should limit burn-through to at least 3 seconds].

6. The laser filters would be resistant to impact and meet certain requirements of contemporary safety spectacles (i.e., the filter materials must withstand standard ball-dropping tests). The eye protection should be so manufactured that separation of stacked filters cannot readily occur. Frame and side shield materials should provide equivalent or superior protection against laser radiation as the filter, and resist exposure from "lateral penetration of laser light;" and holes in the frames would be prohibited. Whether such a requirement would prohibit venting is not completely clear.

7. The eye protection would be required to be marked with the wavelength, protective density, manufacturer's symbol and refractive quality classification. A protective code was also proposed by the ISO draft.

In addition to the recommendations of the ISO, the authors of this manual would suggest that the filter materials withstand damage from expected environmental contaminants such as chemicals, insecticides, insect repellants, high humidity, mildew, and sunlight, which may be encountered in certain environments, and the manufacturer should supply additional information available to him as regards the filter transmission curves or tables and data on filter damage thresholds or frame damage thresholds.

16.19 PROTECTIVE SHIELDS AND PROTECTIVE GARMENTS

16.19.1 Window Ports

To this point only the eyewear use of filter materials has been discussed. Of course the same color filter glass materials may be used in viewing ports or windows. Figures 15-10, 15-11 and 16-6 provide spectral transmittance values for many commonly available large-sheet filter materials that may be used for these applications to filter either ultraviolet or infrared radiation, or both. It should be noted, however, that the formulations of some commercial trade-name products vary. For instance, polymethylmethacrylate (e.g., DuPont Lucite® or Rohm and Haas Plexiglas®) are available in a variety of colors and with and without UV absorbers added. The important characteristic of polymethylmethacrylate is that it is a good absorber of all IR-C wavelengths. For example the absorption coefficient is 40 cm^{-1} at 3.8 μm and 178 cm^{-1} at 10 μm.

In selecting a color glass filter for eye protection one normally must use a thicker filter than is used in many other applications. For this reason, optical companies may provide data for only one thickness and extrapolation is required. A novel approach to this problem is that of the Schott Glass Company. Figure 16-17 shows the Schott catalog's spectral transmission curve for type BG-18 and type BG-38 glass. A colored plastic overlay is provided with the catalog to permit an immediate shift of the ordinate lines by the cue circle on the left. In the figure

Eye and Skin Protection

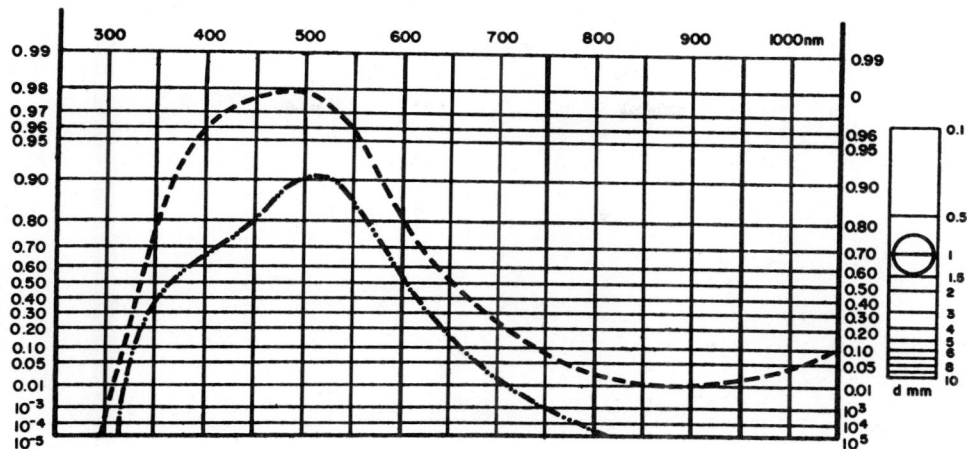

Figure 16-17. Two IR-A Filters. Spectral transmission curve of the Schott type BG-18 filter glass (1 mm) and BG-38 from the Schott Filter Glass catalog. Note the logarithmic ordinate to permit the use of a shifting overlay scale for varying filter thickness.

shown the cue circle is aligned with the thickness d of 1 mm. Shifting the overlay downward from 2 to 10 mm is possible to permit direct readings for thicker glass samples. Another sliding scale of τ_λ for a variety of colored glasses has been prepared by Dobrowolski and colleagues (1977) at NRC in Canada and is a very useful reference to have available.

16.19.2 Area Shields and Large Windows

In choosing a general area shield for far infrared lasers ($\lambda > 3$ μm) one could use glass, but the thermal expansion coefficients of most glass will often cause the shield to shatter upon impact with a Class IV laser beam. Hence, polymethylmethacrylate (e.g., Lucite or Plexiglas) or polycarbonates (e.g., Lexan) are used. These materials all burn upon impact with IR-C laser beams at sufficient irradiances. Typical threshold values are provided in Figure 16-18. Polyethylene transmits some IR-C. For example, polyethylene wrap (Handi-Wrap® and Glad Wrap®) transmit 10.6-μm radiation at a substantial value and Saran Wrap® and Stretch and Seal® absorb at 10.6 μm.

Thermal screens are commonly used in heavy industry around foundary facilities and steel mills; for example in glass windows of offices, in cool-off rooms and in cabs for overhead crane operators. Normally an EC (electrically conductive) coating has been employed. Some recent use has been made of solar film or "sun control" films which are metalized (aluminum vapor coated) polyester film with an adhesive backing to permit application to glass by the user. The film is typically 25-30 μm

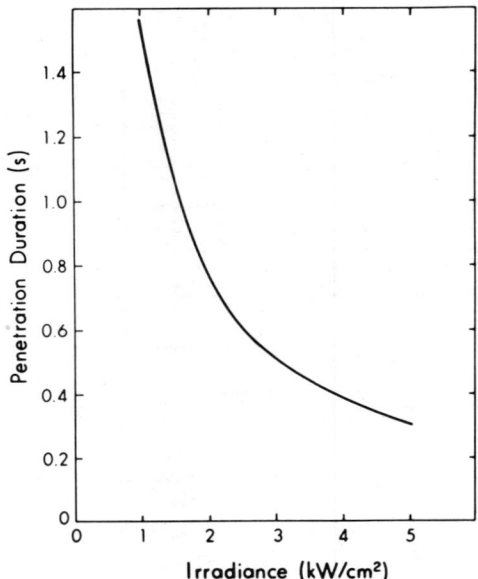

Figure 16-18. Damage to Plastics. Damage thresholds for polymethylmethacrylate (Lucite® or Plexiglas®) of 5-mm thickness.

thick. Such polyester coatings also offer limited shatter resistance. Thicker coatings have been used for shatter resistance applications alone. The lifetime of these types of coatings has yet to be tested under harsh industrial applications. Figure 16-19 shows the spectral transmittance of three commercially available "sun control" films. Plastic *laser safety* films for direct application to windows have also been manufactured by Glendale Optical in the U.S.A., but again, the effects of harsh industrial environments could affect such plastic films.

16.19.3 Protective Garments

Aluminized fabrics were greatly improved during the NASA manned space program (Stoll and Chiantra, 1971). Such fabrics when used in thermal protective garments have been shown to offer equivalent or superior reflective and mechanical properties to those of conventional aluminized asbestos garments (Wren *et al.*, 1977). Aluminized rayon (basket weave) and certain aluminized cotton were shown to have the least transmission of infrared radiation. The aluminized basket-weave rayon offered the best molten-metal splash protection, followed by cottons, fiberglass, asbestos, other rayons and wool. The selection of an aluminized suit should

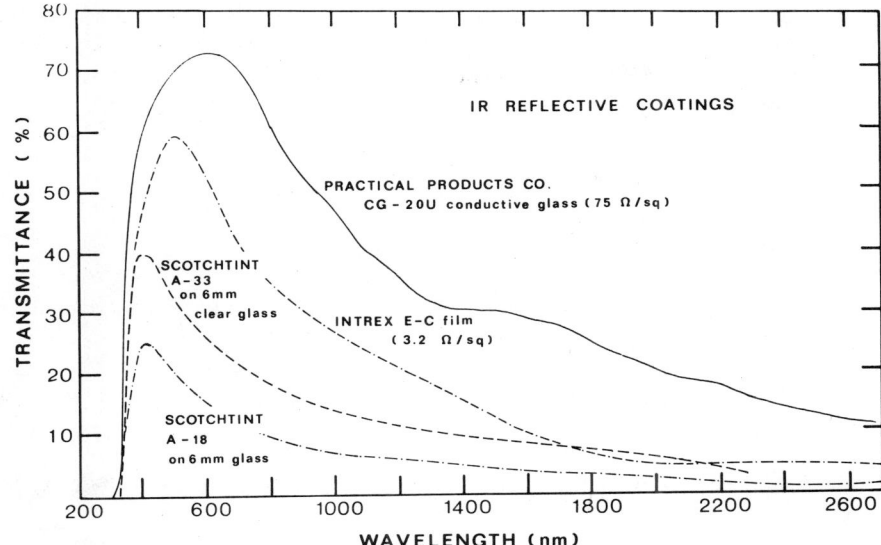

Figure 16-19. Sun Control Films. The spectral transmittance curves of three types of 3-M sun-control films are shown.

include considerations of the abrasion resistance of the aluminized coating, design of seams, the insulation layers behind the fabric (the more the better), looseness (loose garments are desirable) and whether the protection should be against metal splashes as well as optical radiation. The study of Wren *et al.* (1977) is a useful source of information in this regard.

16.20 FUTURE DEVELOPMENTS

It is difficult to predict future developments in laser technology. In the future, more laser systems will be commercially available in the infrared, and improvements may be expected in infrared detectors. It appears reasonable that present laser applications which require unenclosed lasers (e.g., laser distance measurement equipment) but do not require a visible beam (as do alignment lasers) may best be realized by using an infrared laser operating in the relatively "eye-safe" region beyond 1.4 μm.

The Federal codes tend to encourage the manufacturing of enclosed laser systems, and lasers which require the use of eye protection will probably be limited to the research environment.

It is technologically feasible that new filter materials could be developed which have narrower absorption bands in the vicinity of a laser wavelength. Such a development would be more likely to be in a plastic material rather than in a glass. Interference filter coatings sealed between layers of absorbing plastic now show promise. However, unless a much greater demand arises for laser protective eyewear it is unlikely that much development effort will be directed toward these areas.

16.21 REVIEW QUESTIONS

1. What are the advantages and disadvantages of using welding protective filters for laser protection?

2. What optical density is required for safety goggles being used with a 1.2-W argon CW laser?

3. What should be specified for protection when working with a 1200-W CO_2-N_2 laser operating at 10.6 μm?

4. What optical density is required for protection against a ruby laser (694 nm) having a 20-ns, 100-mJ pulse output with a 6-mm emergent beam with a 1-mrad divergence at a range of 0, 100 m, and 1 km for the unaided eye? For a 10 × 50 binocular at 1 km?

5. What eye protection would be recommended for a laboratory worker who uses a 1-mW He-Ne CW laser?

6. Using only the facts that a factor of two change in transmission (or attenuation) corresponds to a density change of 0.3, and a factor of 10 corresponds to a density change of 10, give the optical density for the following attenuation factors (use no calculators or log tables):

    (a) 1.25×10^4 (d) 4×10^3
    (b) 5×10^6 (e) 8×10^5
    (c) 1×10^7 (f) 2.5×10^6

7. A durable, scratch-resistant dichroic coating is developed which has a $D_\lambda = 4.0$ at 694.3 nm at normal incidence. It is used successfully as a safety filter in a telescope, but it should not be used for safety spectacles. Why?

8. A commercial laser safety goggle (Glendale LGB) has a specified density of 4 at 530 nm for "doubled neodymium." A laboratory worker, desiring added protection takes two goggles, removes the filter from one and inserts it along with the other goggle to achieve his goal. The specified luminous transmittance of a single filter is 48%. Estimate the luminous transmittance of the two filters together.

9. What is PLZT?

10. What is the optical density of a 5-mm thickness of BG-18 glass at 650 nm?

16.22 REFERENCES

American National Standards Institute, 1959, Safety Code for Head, Eye, and Respiratory Protection, ANSI Z-2.1, American National Standards Institute, New York.

Anderson, W. J., and Gebel, R. K. H., 1977, Ultraviolet windows in commercial sunglasses, *Appl. Opt.* **16**(2):515–517.

Bauer, G., Hubner, H. J., and Sutter, E., 1968, Measurement of light scattered by eye protection filters, *Appl. Opt.* **7**:325–329.

Borish, I. M., 1970, "Clinical Refraction," 3rd Ed., Professional Press, Chicago.

British Standards Institution (BSI), 1952, Green Protective Spectacles and Screens for Steelworks Operatives, British Standard Specification B.S. 1729:1952, London, British Standards House.

British Standards Institution (BSI), 1967, Industrial Eye-Protectors, British Standard Specification BS 2092:1967, London, British Standards House.

Coblentz, W. W. and Stair, R., 1930, Correlation of the Shade Numbers and Densities of Eye-Protective Glasses, NBS, Circular 471, National Bureau of Standards, Washington, DC (November, 1930).

Commission Internationale de L'Eclairage, 1970, "International Lighting Vocabulary," 3rd ed., p. 51, Bureau Central de la CIE, Paris.

Cook, R. B. and Jankow, R., 1972, Effects of stray light in spectroscopy, *J. Chem. Educ.* **49**:405–408.

Crookes, Sir Wm., 1914, The preparation of eye-preserving glass for spectacles, *Phil. Trans., Roy. Phil. Soc.* **A204**:1–25.

Dahling, R. F., Shapiro, S. I., Berry, C. Z., and Schreiber, M. M., 1970, A method of evaluating sun screen protection from long-wave ultraviolet, *J. Invest. Derm.* **55**:164–169.

Ditchburn, R. W., 1963, "Light," 2nd ed., Chapter 15, John Wiley and Sons, New York.

Dobrowolski, J. A., Marsh, G. E., Charbonneau, D. G., Eng, J., and Josephy, P. D., 1977, Colored filter glasses: an intercomparison of glasses made by different manufacturers, *Appl. Opt.* **16**:1491–1511.

Envall, K. R., Coakley, J. M., Peterson, R. W., and Landry, R. J., 1975, Preliminary evaluation of commercially available laser protective eyewear, US Dept. of Health, Education and Welfare, Bureau of Radiological Health, DHEW Publication (FDA) 75-8026:32 (March, 1975).

Fitzpatrick, T. B., Pathak, M. A., and Parrish, J. A., 1974, Protection of the human skin against the effects of sunburn ultraviolet (290-320 nm) *in* "Sunlight and Man: Normal and Abnormal Photobiological Responses," (M. A. Pathak, L. C. Harbour, M. Seiji, A. Kita, editors; T. B. Fitzpatrick, consulting ed.) pp. 751–765, University of Tokyo Press, Tokyo.

Fox, R. E., 1961, Development of Photoreactive Materials for Eye-Protective Devices, Report No. 61-67, USAF School of Aerospace Medicine, Brooks Air Force Base, Texas (AD 261608).

Haertling, G. H., and Land, C. E., 1972, Recent improvements in the optical and electrooptic properties of PLZT Ceramics, *Ferroelectrics* **3**:269–280.

Ham, W. T., Mueller, H. A., Williams, R. C., and Geeraets, W. J., 1973, Ocular hazard from viewing the sun unprotected and through various windows and filters, *Appl. Opt.* **12**(9):2122–2129.

Harris, J. O., Jr., and Cutchen, J. T., 1972, Electrooptic Variable Density Optical Filter, Sandia Laboratories, Albuquerque, New Mexico.

Hedblom, E. E., 1961, Snowscape eye protection, *Arch. Environ. Health* **2**:685–704.
Holst, G. C., 1973, Proper selection and testing of laser protective materials, *Am. J. Opt.* **50**:477–483.
Kahn, G. and Wilcox, G., 1969, Comparison of *in vitro* and *in vivo* sun screen testing methods, *J. Soc. Cosmetic Chem.* **20**:807–824.
La Marre, D. A., 1977, Development of Criteria and Test Methods for Eye and Face Protective Devices, Publication DHEW (NIOSH) No. 78-110, NIOSH, Cincinnati, OH, August 1977.
Novikov, N. P., and Kholodilou, A. A., 1971, Destruction of thermoplastics by powerful heat fluxes, *Mekhanika Polmerov* **1**:122–130.
Parrish, J. A., Pathak, M. A., and Fitzpatrick, T. B., 1971, Protection of skin from germicidal ultraviolet radiation in the operating room by topical chemicals, *New Eng. J. Med.* **284**:1257–1258.
Scherr, A. E., Tucker, R. J., and Greenwood, R. A., 1969, New plastics absorb at laser wavelengths, *Laser Focus* **5**:46–48.
Schott Glass Co., 1969, "Color Filter Glass," p. 19, Schott and Gen., Mainz, West Germany.
Schreibeis, W. J., 1968, Laser eye protection goggles, based on manufacturer's information, *Amer. Indus. Hyg. Assn. J.* **29**:504.
Sliney, D. H., 1970, Evaluating health hazards from military lasers, *J. Am. Med. Assn.* **214**:1047–1054.
Sliney, D. H., 1974, Laser protective eyewear, *in* "Laser Applications in Medicine and Biology," (M. L. Wolbarsht, ed.), Vol. 2, pp. 223–240, Plenum Press, New York.
Sliney, D. H. and Freasier, B. C., 1973, The evaluation of optical radiation hazards, *Appl. Opt.* **12**:1–24.
Spencer, D. J., and Bixler, H. A., 1972, IR laser radiation eye protector, *Rev. Sci. Instr.* **43**:1545–1546.
Stair, R., 1948, Spectral-transmissive Properties and Use of Eye-Protective Glasses, NBS Circular 471, National Bureau of Standards, Washington, DC (October 8, 1948).
Stoll, A. M., and Chianta, M. A., 1971, Heat transfer through fabrics as related to thermal injury, *Trans. N. Y. Acad. Sci.* **33**:649–670.
Straub, H. W., 1965, Protection of the human eye from laser radiation, *Ann. N. Y. Acad. Sci.* **122**:773–776.
Straub, H. W., 1970, Laser eye protection in the U.S.A., Die Berufsgenossenschaft Zeitschrift fur Unfallversicherung und Betriebssicherheit **3**:83–87.
Swope, C. H., 1969, The eye–protection, *Arch. Envir. Health* **18**:428–433.
Swope, C. H., 1970, Design considerations for laser eye protection, *Arch. Envir. Health* **20**:184–187.
Thursby, W. R., Richey, E. O., Bartholomew, R. V., and Ebbers, R. W., 1971, Evaluation of Photochromic Goggle System for Nuclear Flash Protection, SAM-TR-71-20, USAF School of Aerospace Medicine, Brooks Air Force Base, Texas (AD 726544).
Williams, D. W., and Duggar, B. C., 1965, Review of Research on Flash Blindness, Chorioretinal Burns, Countermeasures and Related Topics, DASA-1576 rev., Defense Atomic Support Agency, Washington, DC (AD).
Williams, D. R., 1970, Some comments on the properties of absorptive lenses, *J. Am. Opt. Assn.* **41**(1):82–91.
Withrow, R. B., and Withrow, A. P., 1956, Generation, control and measurement of visible and near-visible radiant energy, *in* "Radiation Biology," (A. Hollaender, ed.) Vol. III, pp. 125–128, McGraw-Hill, New York.

Wren, J. E., Scott, W. D., and Bates, C. E., 1977, Thermal and mechanical properties of aluminized fabrics for use in ferrous metal handling operations, *Am. Industr. Hyg. Assn. J.* **38**(11): 603–612.

Chapter 17
Laser Safety in Research Laboratories and Medical Facilities

17.1 INTRODUCTION

The laser was considered little more than a fascinating laboratory device for at least six years following its initial development. All of the original laser safety guidelines and early standards were based solely on laboratory experience. Today, despite the wide use of lasers in industry, the potential for hazardous exposure to laser radiation is probably still greatest for the research worker who is experimenting with new laser devices and new laser applications. This is due to the need for flexibility in the arrangement of laser components and ancillary system components while studying new techniques. Also unenclosed, high-power laser beams will most likely be encountered in the research laboratory.

In the research and engineering laboratories more than in any other laser environment, administrative safety measures are relied upon instead of engineering control measures. Here, likewise, protective clothing and protective eyewear have found their greatest usage. By contrast, the use of medium-power and high-power lasers in most industrial production lines would rely on the use of engineering control measures to prevent exposure to any workers in the vicinity of the equipment. For maximum flexibility, few scientists and engineers consider the installation of permanent beam enclosures and similar fixtures, since optical beam-path layouts can change daily, if not hourly. Under these conditions the workers normally wear eye protection despite the associated reduction in visual capability, and possible discomfort.

Of course, laser devices are used in commercial instruments in some laboratories; for example, laser particle sizing equipment, interferometers, and Raman spectrometers. These products, like other complete laser systems, normally include sufficient engineering controls that the user has few if any worries. Other unenclosed lasers, originally used as tools in research, are finding their way into most chemical physics laboratories for basic studies in photophysics and photochemistry, e.g., high resolution spectroscopy and coherent Raman spectroscopy. This chapter is primarily concerned with the use of experimental lasers and prototype lasers in applications where sufficient experience has not accumulated to establish conventional engineering control measures.

17.2 HAZARD EVALUATION OF NEW LASERS

When a new laser is being designed and developed, there is often a very real lack of knowledge of the laser output characteristics, and hazard classification of the laser may be very difficult. Several principal and secondary wavelengths of the experimental device are theoretically possible and all may or may not be known. In these cases, the hazard evaluation presents quite a challenge. Fortunately there are only a few research laboratories where situations of this type are likely to be encountered. In most instances all principal wavelengths are known and the theoretical limit of output power can be predicted sufficiently closely to permit a conservative determination of the hazard classification. The most conservative approach is to consider a laser to be in Class 4 until its output has been completely defined by appropriate beam measurements. However, although desirable, it may not be possible to define completely all output characteristics.

In the construction of a breadboard-type laser the potential hazards of the optical pumping system should be considered first. This includes checking the safety of any associated electrical systems, or the potential hazards of toxic chemicals used in either optical pumping or the laser medium itself.

Before the laser is initially operated, the relative strengths of all emitted wavelengths must be determined so the proper optical filter materials can be chosen if eyewear or protective screens are to be used. Multi-wavelength and tunable-wavelength lasers will present the most serious hazard control problems. Some examples are liquid dye lasers, and lasers employing either frequency-doubled, second-harmonic generation, or parametric oscillators which operate in the ultraviolet, visible, and near-infrared portions of the optical spectrum. Tunability in the IR-B and IR-C spectral regions is of little significance since the permissible exposures do not vary with wavelength. For safety the most important aspect of tunability is the consideration of the suitability of the available eye protection.

17.3 PUMP LAMPS AND GAS DISCHARGE TUBES

In most cases laser radiation presents the chief problem; however, it may not be the only optical hazard. In a prototype gas laser a check must be made on the electronic discharge tube to ascertain that it is made of quartz or a similar material which will allow actinic ultraviolet radiation to be emitted, as this can result in acute photokeratitis, conjunctivitis, and skin burns (Figure 17-1). Ultraviolet radiation is also emitted from xenon flashlamps to varying degrees depending upon the envelope material and gas pressure. For this reason, most experimental designers now use heat-resistant glass discharge tubes which are opaque in the UV-B and UV-C spec-

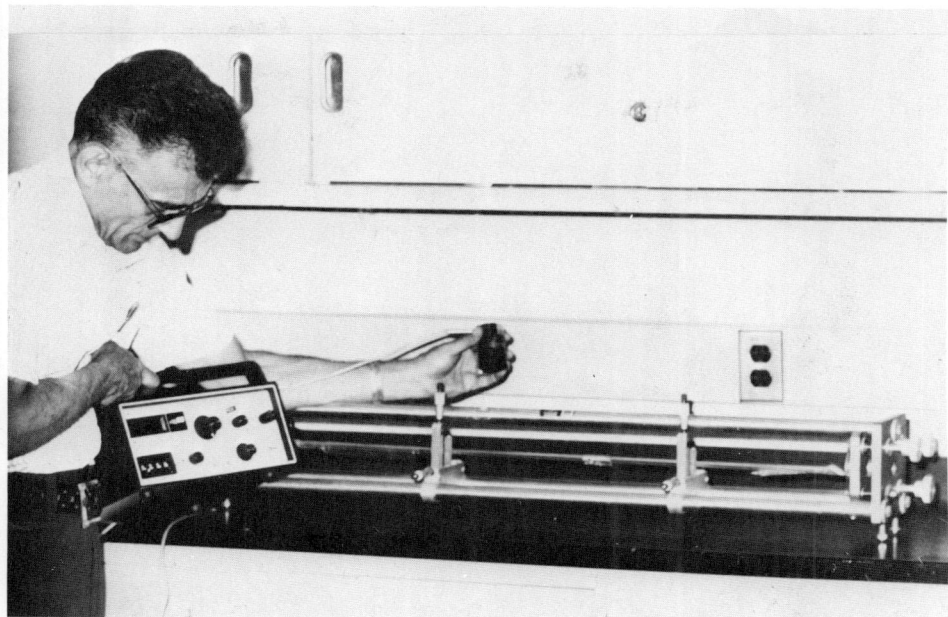

Figure 17-1. Ultraviolet Hazards. An early gas laser with a quartz discharge tube. A laboratory technician checks for the presence of ultraviolet radiation by using a simple meter or a fluorescent paper.

trum. The same examination should be given to the end windows (mirrors) since they may also transmit ultraviolet radiation if constructed of quartz or other ultraviolet window materials.

It is desirable to consider at least a temporary enclosure or shield around the lamps in optically-pumped systems. These lamps are often brighter than the permissible radiance limits, and are always annoying. Preparations for the explosion potential of flashlamps and capacitor banks must be considered. Although this type of explosion is rare in properly engineered production laser systems, it has not been uncommon in the research laboratory in experimental laser systems. Therefore, flashlamp enclosures should be sufficiently rugged to withstand an explosion (Fig. 17-2). The enclosure should be designed to rupture only enough to allow reduction of pressure while still containing any shattered elements. In the early 60's, one commercial model research ruby laser used very high-pressure xenon flashlamps which frequently exploded. However, the housing was always partially torn, and flying fragments were minimized. Thus, despite several reported explosions of this model, no one was ever injured. Experience has now made these accidents rare or nonexistent.

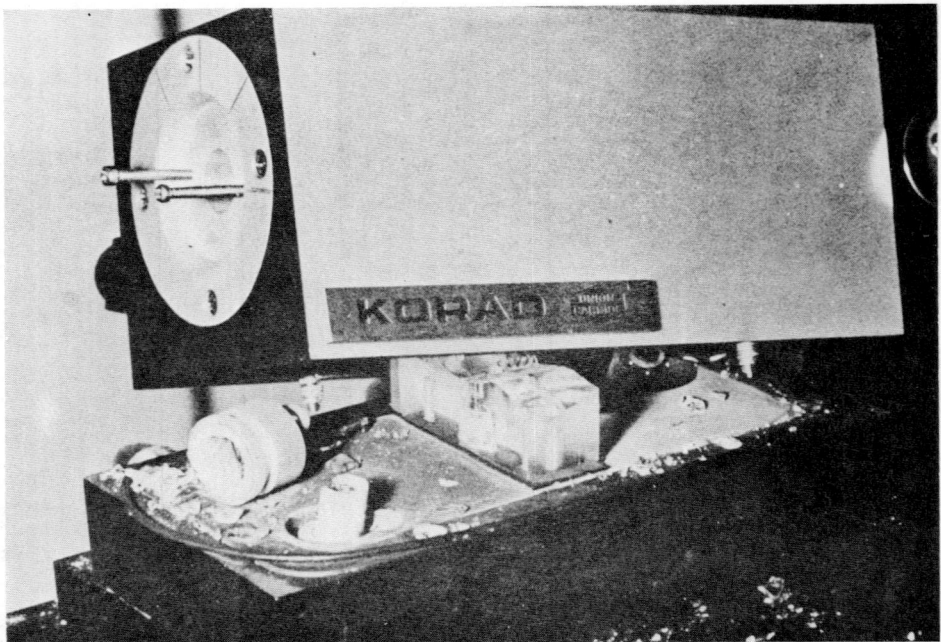

Figure 17-2. Lamp Explosion Hazards. Ruptured casings of an early research laser following flashlamp explosion. This photograph was kindly provided by D. A. McSparron.

17.4 BEAM PATHS

Many lasers used in experiments in research laboratories are very high-powered (Class 4) devices. It is desirable for such lasers to be operated within an enclosed area. There is, however, often the need for experimenters to remain in the laboratory with the unenclosed laser beam. It is therefore very important that these individuals are aware of the beam path, not only of the primary beam, but any secondary beams as well. Prior to the initial operation of such lasers, and at each subsequent increase of output power, the operator should carefully check the alignment of all optical elements in the train, and consider the likelihood for generation of any hazardous secondary beams. At least two personnel should be present during such laser operations.

One must realize that when the beam power is 1,000,000 times above permissible exposure levels at the eye, the secondary beam transmitted through a mirror coating and through its substrate (from behind a "100%" reflective mirror) may be hazardous. More specifically, many mirrors which employ metallic coatings on a

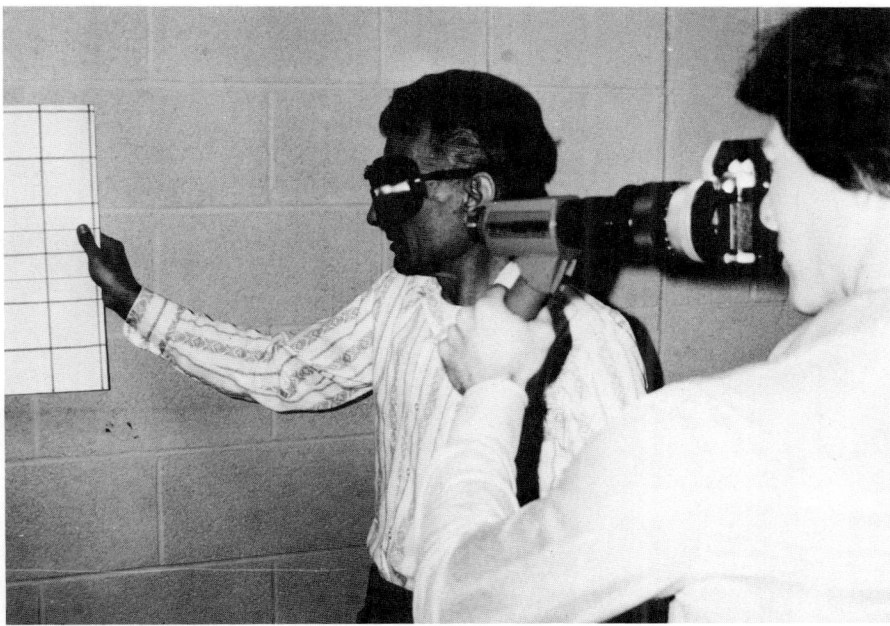

Figure 17-3. Viewing Infrared Laser Beams. Use of infrared image converter for detection of CW GaAs or neodymium beam reflections.

glass substrate may transmit a measurable fraction of the incident power. Only an opaque backing to the mirror, such as a solid metal mirror mount will block this secondary beam. A transmission of even 0.1% of the initial beam power would result in a secondary beam 1,000 times above the permissible exposure limits. After considering the location of the most obvious secondary beam paths, it is then desirable to carefully look for other secondary and even tertiary beams. If as much as 0.5% of the total beam power is unaccounted for after measuring the principal secondary beams of a high-powered laser, then a very careful analysis of potential beam paths may be required before a worker can be confident that eye protection is not required. On the other hand, for a Class 3 laser, eye protection might be required only during realignment or changes in the beam path.

For visible CW lasers, it is generally wise to darken the room and look for any secondary beams incident upon the surrounding walls. If the beam's wavelength is in the far infrared, a pyroelectric vidicon may be used, or the walls and ceiling may be simply examined for burn spots created by the high-power beam. Figure 17-3 shows the use of an infrared image converter to search for CW neodymium laser beam reflections. This is highly desirable, as most recent accidental retinal injuries have resulted from "invisible" neodymium laser exposures.

The typical beam path is normally a few centimeters above a laboratory bench

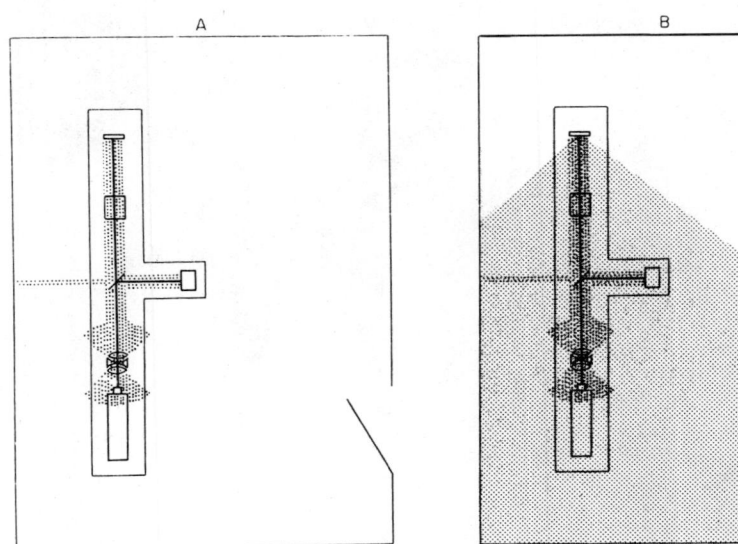

Figure 17-4. Hazardous Reflections. Potentially hazardous (shaded) areas in a laser laboratory are vastly different for a pulsed laser that produces only hazardous specular reflections (A), rather than hazardous diffuse reflections as well (B).

top. Therefore it may be approximately at eye level for a person seated at a desk. The area where any individual might be sitting should be examined most carefully. Perhaps because of the design of most optical-bench hardware, laser holographic arrangements and other similar optical layouts normally have beams limited to a horizontal plane. This horizontal beam plane should also not be located at the eye level of a standing individual, because of the greater probability of movement placing the experimenter unknowingly in a hazardous position. Secondary beams are also emitted quite frequently from some open laser resonators into a vertical plane above the laser (e.g., from Brewster end-windows). At least two laser laboratory personnel have received eye injuries from "invisible," neodymium laser beams reflected in a vertical plane from a Brewster window.

17.5 DIFFUSE REFLECTIONS AND BEAM TRAPS

In all fields of safety—automotive safety, fire safety, electrical safety, etc.—the major aim is to reduce the probability of injury. One can seldom achieve "total, absolute safety" or "fool-proof" safety. This is particularly true in the laser laboratory or in medical applications of the laser. As noted in Chapter 15, the likelihood

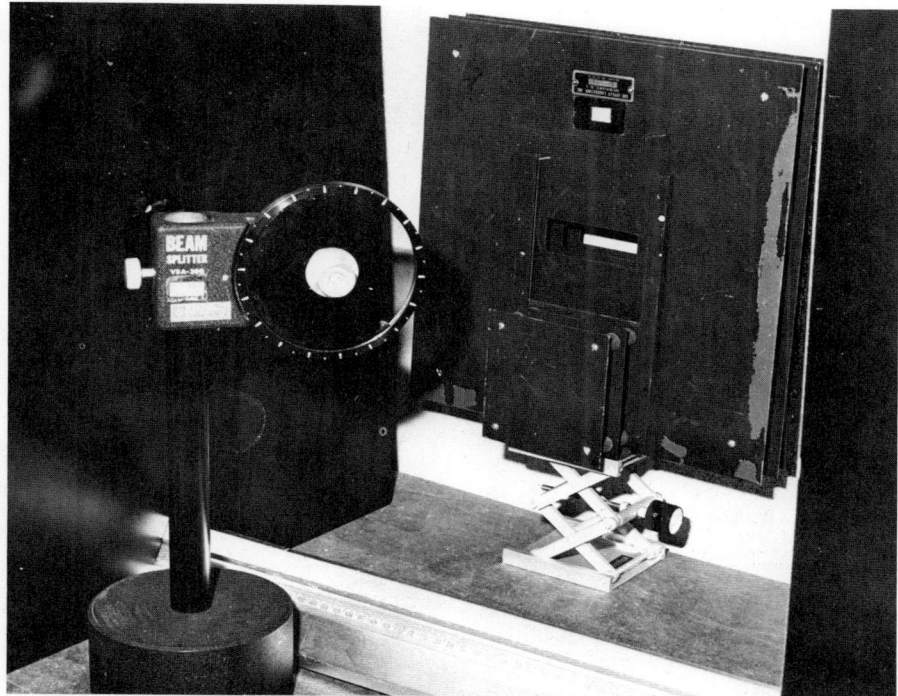

Figure 17-5. Beam Dump. Variable reflectance beam splitters are often used to direct the unused fraction of a beam into a beam trap.

of a highly collimated pencil beam of light randomly entering a person's eye is quite small. This explains why, overall, there have been so few eye injuries amongst laboratory laser workers. The shaded area of Figure 17-4A illustrates the dangerous zones for intrabeam viewing for a Class 3 laser. If the output radiant exposure of a pulsed laser is increased so that the laser is considered Class 4 then the probability of eye injury anywhere within the shaded zone in Figure 17-4B is now likely. It is for this reason that control measures must be more stringent with the pulsed Class 4 laser.

If high-powered (Class 4) lasers are used with low reflectance surfaces and beam traps as backstops, the normally accessible laser radiation levels are often reduced to Class 3 levels, and the probability of hazardous exposure is greatly reduced. Figure 17-4 provided an explanation of the need for eye protection whenever hazardous diffuse reflections are possible from visible and near-infrared lasers; this is one situation where eye protection should not be optional. Figure 17-5 provides examples of a beam splitter/beam trap combination; Figure 17-6 illustrates the design of typical beam traps. One type of beam trap which is not shown makes use of metallic, aircraft honeycomb which is spray painted black.

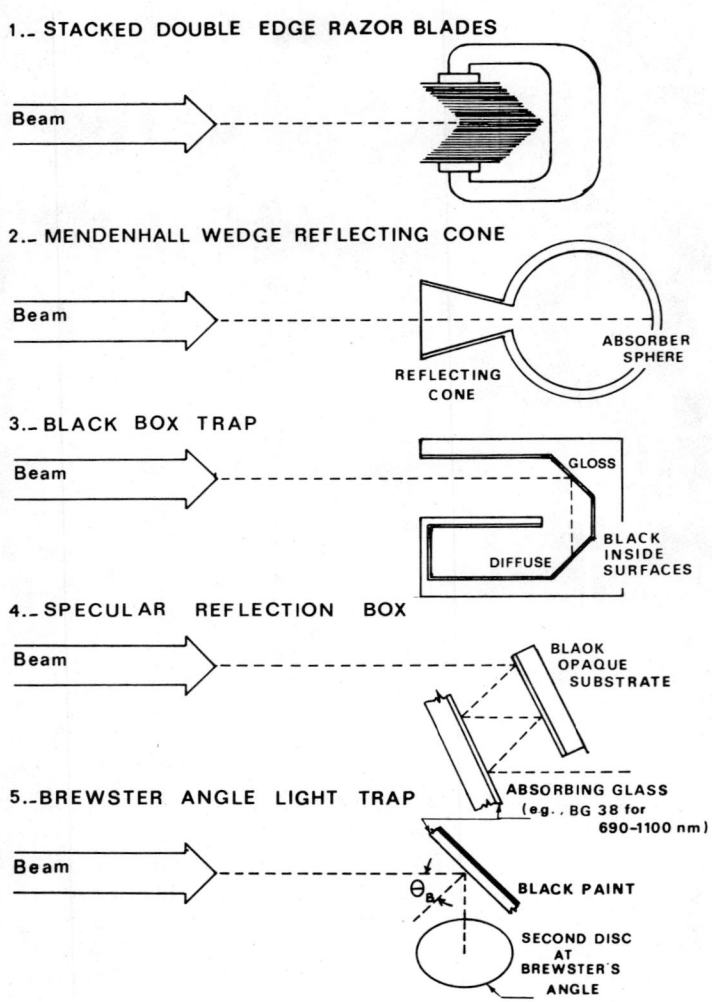

Figure 17-6. Beam Traps. In each of the five types of laser beam traps the concept is to minimize the reflected energy leaving the trap without placing too great a thermal burden on the absorbing surfaces.

17.6 CONTROL MEASURES FOR OPEN BEAM PATHS

As previously mentioned in Chapter 16, it is most conventional for research laboratories to rely heavily upon protective eyewear rather than beam enclosures. This is necessary so that the optical elements of the laser system can be adjusted along all parts of the beam path(s). Several general safety procedures have been employed with great success when working with such experiments. The output power of a laser is first optimized by directing the exit beam into a calorimeter or other radiometric instrument. Usually such an instrument can be placed directly at the output port of the laser to give, effectively, an enclosed optical pathway. Once the laser output has been optimized, then some variable output device can be installed as close to the beam output as possible.

For CW laser power outputs below 1 W, polarizing materials can be rotated in front of a normally polarized laser beam to serve as variable attenuators. In addition, variable reflectance beam splitters can also be used to direct the unused portion of the beam into a beam trap (Fig. 17-6). A variable attenuator is useful whenever the output power of the laser cannot be adequately reduced by lowering the electrical input power. In essence the safety filters are placed over the laser instead of the eyes. By this technique the CW laser can normally be reduced to comparatively safe levels of the beam without the need for eye protection. Also, it is seldom necessary to view the laser beam path once the experimental setup has been aligned.

A common complaint of research workers who use argon lasers is that the only commercially available eye protection filters have such enormous optical densities as to make the beam not only safe, but also, invisible. In many of these instances an attenuator on the output beam to reduce the level to approximately 1 mW would be particularly useful. An alternative method for viewing the location of such a laser beam is the use of a fluorescent card whose longer-wavelength fluorescence can be seen through the eye protection. Image converter monoculars or goggles are often used for looking at near-infrared or ultraviolet laser radiation. Studies performed at the U.S. Army Environmental Hygiene Agency show that modern image converter tubes (Fig. 16-10) transmit only a small fraction of the incident optical radiation and are, therefore, suitable as laser eye protection (see section 16.14). They are effective over a very broad-band spectrum in attenuating incident laser radiation to a permissible level. The disadvantages of image converter systems—or for that matter, of closed-circuit TV systems—are: some loss of detail; usually a monochrome presentation; and a limited field-of-view. Also, image converter tubes and closed-circuit TV cameras are not highly resistant to damage by laser radiation. In fact, they will not resist levels much below those which are hazardous to the eye. Therefore, one would not normally employ such devices without protective filters on the camera or converter tube unless hazardous direct exposure is very unlikely. Such TV and image-converter approaches are becoming more common when working with some tunable dye lasers because of wide tuning ranges. On the other hand, the use of a single dye does not always require such an approach since each dye has a limited spectral range as shown in Figure 17-7.

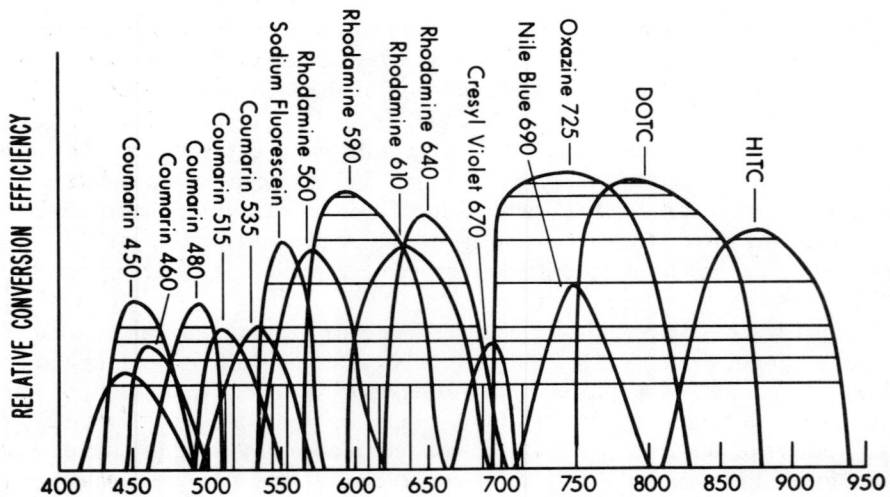

Figure 17-7. Laser Dyes. A variety of laser dyes permit a tunable laser range from the violet to the IR-A. The relative spectral conversion efficiency is shown.

17.7 CONTROLLED ENTRY

For open beam Class 4 laser operations (and also in a few cases for Class 3 installations) it is generally advisable to allow laboratory entry only to those persons actually engaged in setting up or conducting the laser experiment. The laboratory is then termed a *controlled area* (ANSI Z-136.1, 1976). Presumably the laboratory personnel have been instructed in basic laser safety procedures, and are familiar with both the experimental arrangement, and any dangerous conditions. At one time, such a restriction was imposed to limit the number of individuals requiring eye examinations. However, the laboratory manager is generally receptive to a limited entry policy as it will also keep away the curious.

Restrictions on entry are generally administrative, and enforced through the use of signs, special door latches, and interlocks (Fig. 17-8). The safety guidelines have always recommended safety latches or door interlocks for Class 4 laser installations along with opaque window covers. Most manufacturers of early Class 4 laser systems provided a power supply relay connector to connect with a door switch interlock to disable the power supply when the door was opened. The installation at the time of manufacture of such remote connectors has been required in the U.S.A. since August 1976 by Federal regulation. If control of a high-power CW laser can be

Research Laboratories and Medical Facilities 573

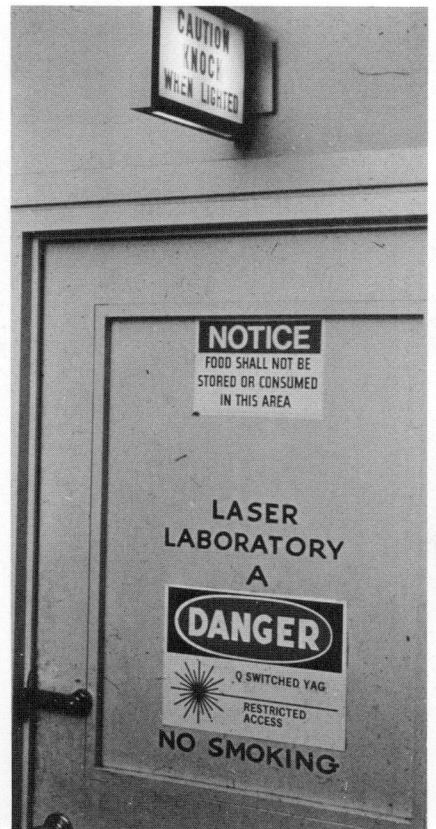 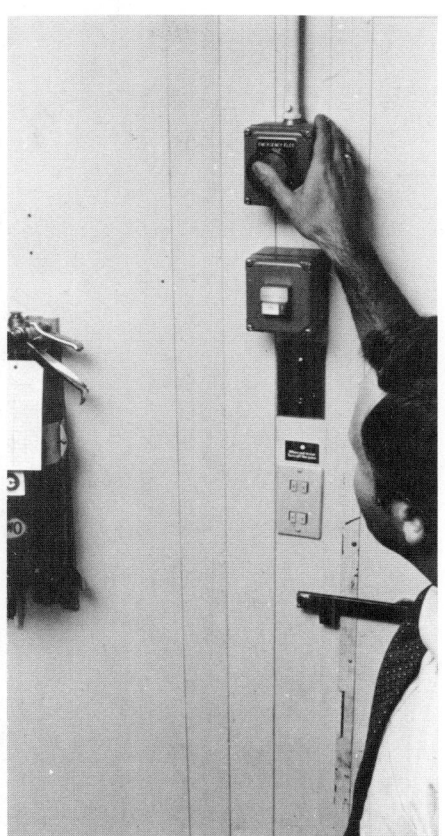

Figure 17-8. Laser Facility Entrance. Warning signs, lights, door interlocks, and emergency shutdown switches are employed with Class 4 lasers.

lost in case of an accident, then "panic buttons" (control-disconnect switches) should be located at several accessible locations within the laboratory—at least at the point of egress from the laboratory. The idea here is to permit rapid shutdown in case of fire or "runaway" operation. These types of precautions are most important for CW lasers with output powers exceeding 100 W.

17.8 STANDARD OPERATING PROCEDURES

Because of the attendant risks in a Class 4 laser laboratory, it is advisable for the research personnel to draft a standard operating procedure (SOP). This effort

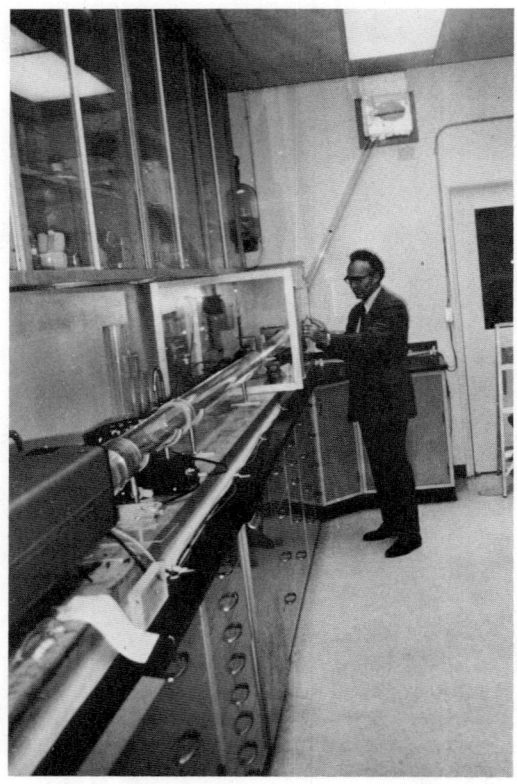

Figure 17-9. Beam Enclosures. Temporary beam enclosures around beam path of a high-power CO_2 laser. Note the use of glass pipe.

serves several goals. The laboratory personnel themselves are forced to consider safety and generally will follow their own self-imposed rules more readily than those imposed by a central safety office. Secondly, they may well be more familiar with some of the potential hazards than would be the central health and safety office, although, a review of the SOP by that office should hopefully uncover any points overlooked by the laboratory personnel.

17.9 TEMPORARY BEAM ENCLOSURES

It is often desirable, when working with high-power lasers, to fabricate temporary shields or beam enclosures which are mounted on flexible stands and placed around the beam path (Fig. 17-9). Telescoping tubes and tube supports have been considered quite useful in this regard. Small portable shields made of glass or trans-

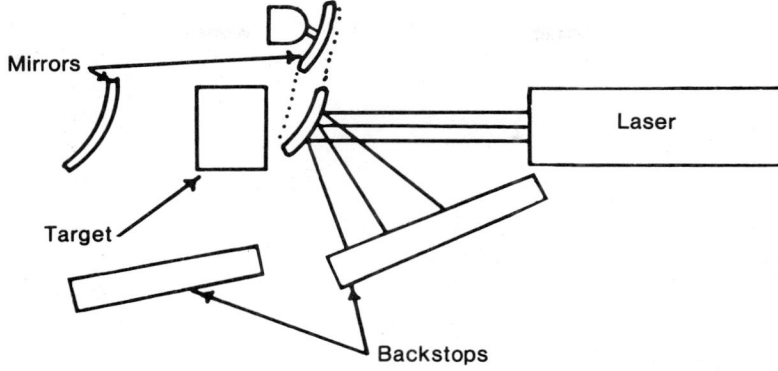

Figure 17-10. Beam Shutter. A shutter for high-power laser beam must be able to dissipate the high beam power. In this instance the beam irradiance is reduced.

parent plastic are frequently used to prevent skin injury from far-infrared, or high-powered, lasers. Such shields are particularly important if the laser beam is invisible. By trial and error most investigators have been able to develop similar fixtures suited to their particular laboratory activities since they only minimally impede the experimental progress and flexibility. Glass pipe, of the type used in the chemical industry, is a relatively inexpensive beam enclosure. Transparent shields permit a view of the optical path, yet prevent insertion of either the hand or reflective objects. Such enclosures may also reduce the problems of dust collecting or UV degraded organic material upon optical surfaces. A safety specialist can often more readily "sell" his idea of enclosures to a laboratory worker if he points out the other advantages of such enclosures.

17.10 VERY HIGH POWER CW LASERS

Laboratory controls for very high-power CW lasers (> 500 W) vary only slightly from those required for the smaller Class 4 systems. The added difficulty for the higher power systems stems from the limits of protective materials. It is difficult to terminate a very high power beam unless the beam is spread out. Figure 17-10 illustrates how a convex reflector and beamstop can be shifted into the beam when necessary. The convex mirror causes the reflected beam irradiance to drop below a fire-hazard irradiance within a short distance. A fire-resistant backstop then terminates the beam.

17.11 ASSOCIATED HAZARDS

The research laboratory laser usage can be accompanied by many potential hazards not directly related to the laser radiation itself. In general, these ancillary hazards have been minimized or eliminated from any industrial applications. Improvised cryogenic fluid connections, exposed electrical connectors, and other unsafe conditions, which would never be permitted in an industrial or field environment, are often present in a research laboratory. Class 4 High Risk lasers generally present a fire hazard and an appropriate class of laboratory fire extinguishers should be present at a readily accessible location.

The ancillary hazards are always of concern. To date most of the severe injuries, and all of the four deaths associated with laser usage, were in laboratory environments, and resulted from these ancillary hazards. The deaths were all from electrocution. Chapter 27 discusses the electrical hazards and Chapter 26 considers the other ancillary hazards.

17.12 SAFETY ASPECTS OF LASERS IN MEDICINE

Many of the safety problems encountered in the laser laboratory are also common in the clinical setting. Although clinical studies of laser applications in medicine have seldom included the collection of minimal biological threshold data, clinical experience has produced most of the evidence to support the extrapolation of animal tissue reaction thresholds to human-tissue thresholds. This is particularly true in the case of skin exposure levels. Studies directed toward a better understanding of tissue damage mechanisms often have direct impact on both clinical applications and the setting of permissible exposure levels.

The application of specific laser laboratory precautions to the clinical use of lasers is difficult. Problems can arise because the object of the medical laser application may well be to coagulate or destroy tissue, whereas the aim of the safety rules is to minimize or prevent exposure to hazardous levels of laser radiation. Clearly all laser safety standards must contain a clause to exclude irrelevant restrictions on the medical exposure of humans to laser radiation. The primary reliance for safety in these types of applications must rest on the properly trained medical personnel who administer treatment, especially since such lasers are generally Class 4. In the USA, the BRH has set rules which exclude the requirement for a medical laser exit port to be marked with a warning label, but the incorporation of power meters and other features (USDHEW, 1979) are required. When first proposed the BRH regulations were met with objections by some medical research groups. The following is extracted from the Federal regulation:

1040.11 Specific Purpose Laser Products

(a) Medical laser products. Each medical laser product shall comply with all of the applicable requirements of 1040.10 for laser products of its class. In addition, the manufacturer shall:

(1) Incorporate in each Class III or IV medical laser product a means for the measurement of the level of that laser radiation intended for irradiation of the human body with an error in measurement of no more than ±20 percent when calibrated in accordance with paragraph (a) (2) of this section. Indication of the measurement shall be in International System Units.

(2) Supply with each Class III or IV medical laser product instructions specifying a procedure and schedule for calibration of the measurement system required by paragraph (a) (1) of this section.

(3) Affix to each medical laser product, in close proximity to each aperture through which is emitted accessible laser radiation in excess of the accessible emission limits of Class I, a label bearing the wording: "Laser aperture."

Probably the best engineering design feature for Class 4 medical laser products is to employ short-focal-length projection optics in the beam delivery port. Although not always feasible, this feature often dramatically reduces the probability of very hazardous exposure of personnel in the vicinity of the laser device. Positive-action exposure switches, beam shutters and key-lock master switches are all features that provide some additional safety. It seems reasonable that diagnostic medical laser devices should be limited to Class 1 or Class 2 systems unless actual patient exposure is truly below the EL.

17.12.1 Laser Surgical Facilities

Although extensive surgical facilities for experimental laser applications were built in the 1960's (Goldman and Rockwell, 1971; Riggle *et al.*, 1971; and Gamaleya, 1977) such elaborate facilities now are uncommon because of the development of modular laser surgical systems with delivery systems which do not require restriction to a specific room. Three types of lasers are most often used in various surgical procedures: the argon laser at 488 and 514.5 nm; the neodymium laser at 1064 nm; and the CO_2 laser at 10.6 μm. Each type of laser has a different penetration depth into tissue and therefore has advantages as well as disadvantages in comparison with the other two.

The CO_2 laser, because of higher power available in early models and because of very high attenuation in tissue, was used early as a surgical knife for a number of specialized procedures (Steller *et al.*, 1971), and is the only common type of surgical laser which operates outside of the retinal hazard region. Hence, CO_2 laser reflections from specular metal surfaces such as surgical instruments and stainless steel operating room fixtures are not as serious a problem as reflections from a laser of similar power emitting within the retinal hazard region.

Argon (1-10 W) lasers and CW neodymium-YAG lasers (10-50 W) were used more extensively later—particularly with fiber optic light guides for use in endoscopy (Auth *et al.*, 1976). Figure 17-11 illustrates such a delivery system with characteristics output irradiance and radiance patterns. When incoherent optical fiber bundles are used in a delivery system, the laser beam is no longer characterized as a point source (Gulacsik *et al.*, 1979). In the design of the fiber optic endoscope the first concern was protection of the surgeon's eye as he viewed the optical cautery action of the laser through the fiber optic guide. The reflections back through the laser catheter were of the order of 2 mW for a flashback (as a specular reflection) returning through the endoscope per watt of power at the distal element of the fiber optic delivery system for the neodymium-YAG systems, and less than 1 mW/W for neodymium-YAG systems, and less than 1 mW/W for the argon laser. They used a

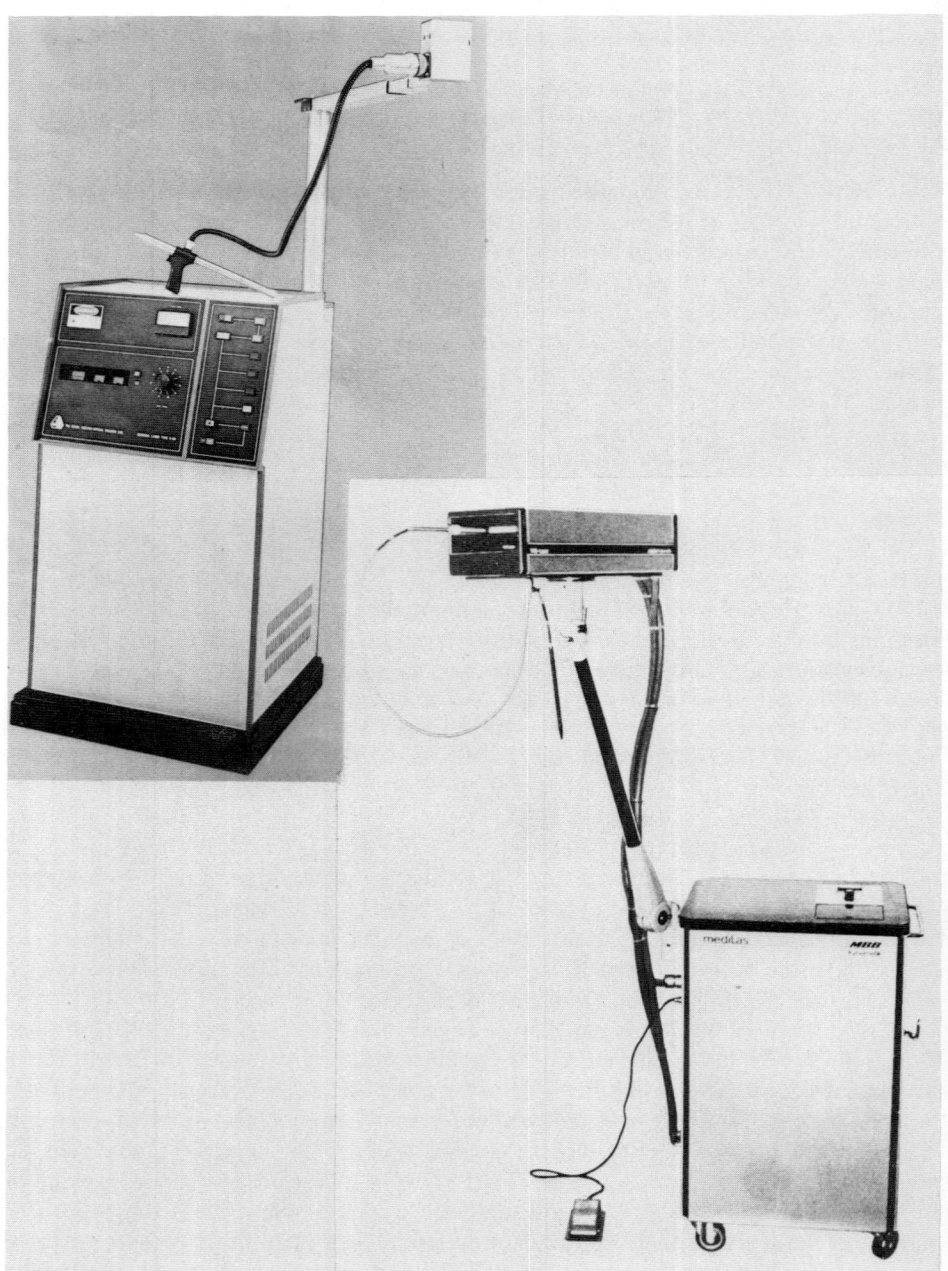

Figure 17-11. Surgical Lasers. A CO_2 surgical laser with positive action foot pedal (courtesy Sharplan, Inc., Tel Aviv, Israel) is seen at the top and a CW Nd-YAG Coagulator is shown in the lower panel (courtesy of Messerschmidt-Bolkow-Blohm GmbH, Munich, Germany).

A quartz glass target represents the worst-case specular reflection condition, i.e., the mucosal membrane of the intestine. Thus, minimal filtration would be required to protect the surgeon's eye from injury during momentary viewing. However, eye protection of the order of density 3 to 4 would be required at the argon wavelength to provide protection as well as comfortable viewing during extended exposures. A protective factor density 1.5 to 2.0 would be required for use with a neodymium laser. Diffuse reflection values were always considerably less than specular reflection values in terms of corneal irradiance. Hence, the operator's viewing of a diffuse reflection was reasonably safe with these devices.

Because of the deeper penetration of the 1064 nm radiation as compared to the blue and green lines of the argon laser, higher power levels (on the order of 50 W) are typical of neodymium-YAG laser coagulators and endoscopic coagulators, whereas argon and CO_2 laser systems could be limited to possibly 10 W and certainly 15 W distal power for coagulation. CO_2 surgical lasers used for vaporizing tissue are 25 W or greater.

Both the neodymium-YAG and CW argon laser systems used for endoscopy typically make use of fiber optic delivery systems to permit maximum flexibility for the surgeon. Recently, optical fiber materials have been developed for the 10.6 μm wavelength of the CO_2 laser. Various types of beam focusing heads are attached to the end of the fiber optics cable. Obviously the connection of the fiber optics cable to the laser output should be constructed so that if the cable is removed, a spring-loaded shutter or similar device assures that no laser radiation escapes from the housing.

Laser surgical instruments are most often operated by a footswitch to allow the surgeon freedom for his hands. The footswitch should be operated only after throwing a master control switch. An emergency shutdown switch should also be located at a point of ready access.

Quite often surgeons have available a fire-resistant target such as alumina, silicon, or silicon-carbide firebrick to focus a hand-held laser "scalpel." This inanimate target assists in developing a "feel" for the equipment and gives a visible adjustment of the beam's focal spot. Metallic surfaces are unacceptable for this purpose.

Eye protection for all personnel at the laser wavelength(s) is almost always required for surgical laser operations. Surgeons using CO_2 laser devices should be reminded that materials which do not appear specular mirror-like to the eye may be specular at the 10.6 μm wavelength, e.g., brushed metal surfaces and enamel-metal surfaces. The beam should not be directed near any such surface, particularly if flat. Surgical implements which have convex surfaces to diverge the beam should be used in or near the beam path. If this is not possible, the concave surfaces of instruments should be tested by first directing the beam under controlled conditions at the concave surfaces to determine the extent of the hazardous recollimation of the laser beam by the concave surface.

To obtain a better understanding of the reflective hazards associated with the use of any of these surgical lasers, consider for example, the specular reflection from a relatively flat metal surface for a beam with the following characteristics. A 50 W beam, whose initial beam diameter is 5 mm, is focused to a 0.1-mm spot by a 50-mm focal length lens. A focal beam focussed on a flat specular surface will diverge the same as the convergence of the focused rays. The change in beam diameter for the beam traversing the 50-mm focal length is:

$$\Delta D_L = 5 \text{ mm} - 0.1 \text{ mm}$$
$$= 4.9 \text{ mm}$$

Hence the divergence of the beam will be:

$$\phi = \Delta D/r \tag{17-1}$$
$$= 4.9 \text{ mm}/50 \text{ mm}$$
$$= 0.098 \text{ rad}$$
$$= 98 \text{ mrad}$$

Obviously this divergence is quite substantial compared to a collimated beam. However there is still as much as 50 W in the reflected beam. The irradiance in the reflected beam at a distance r_1 from the reflector can be calculated using formula (12-4) by setting the initial beam diameter (a) equal to the focal spot diameter of 0.1 mm:

$$E = 1.27 \, \Phi \, / \, (a + r_1 \phi)^2$$

At a distance of 30 cm of (r_1) the irradiance is:

$$E = 1.27 \, (50) \, / \, [(0.01) + (30)(0.098)]^2$$
$$= 7.3 \text{ W/cm}^2$$

At a viewing distance r_1 of 100 cm:

$$E = 1.27 \, (50) \, / \, [0.1 + (100)(0.098)]^2$$
$$= 661 \text{ mW/cm}^2$$

From Tables 8-1 and 8-3, and Figure 8-4, the exposure duration for an allowable CO_2 laser irradiation at 661 mW/cm² is less than 1 ms. From this, skin protection as well as eye protection must be considered when using such high powers around relatively flat specular surfaces. However, considerable experience with laser surgical equipment has shown that eyewear only (but not face shields and heavy protective clothing) is required.

The previous calculation shows that the shorter the focal length of the lens, the more strongly converging the focused laser beam rays will be, and therefore the more rapidly diverging will be the rays from a flat specular surface. Hence from a safety standpoint a short focal-length lens is more desirable than a long.

To summarize, the procedures that reduce the chance for personnel injury from laser radiation and which are generally followed by laser surgeons include:

- (a) draping the area of the surgical incision with wet towels rather than dry towels to avoid towel combustion;

- (b) the use of focusing guides which not only assist the surgeon in keeping the focal spot on the tissue, but also reduce the chance of hazardous specular reflection because of their geometry;

- (c) exclusion of combustible anesthetic gases from laser surgical procudures (Snow et al., 1974);

- (d) a positive action switch, either a hand trigger squeeze switch or foot switch, to ensure rapid shut-off in case of emergency;

- (e) prohibition of misuse by unauthorized personnel with a key switch. Of course, since the BRH regulation of 1976 such a key-switch master control is required in the United States.

17.12.2 Laser Retinal Photocoagulators

Many of the precautions that are relevant to higher power surgical lasers apply also to the much lower power (but still, Class 4) laser photocoagulators for ophthalmic work. Originally, the first photocoagulators as developed by Meyer-Schwickerath (1960) in the 1950's in Germany consisted of a high-power, high-radiance, xenon-arc lamp with a direct ophthalmoscope delivery system. Following the development of the ruby laser it was sometimes used to replace the xenon lamps (for review see Wolbarsht and Landers, 1979). A long-pulse 0.2-ms to 0.8 s ruby laser was the first available and was used most often for retinal reattachment surgery. Then the treatment of proliferative diabetic retinopathy and other vascular retinal diseases made the argon laser photocoagulator by far the most popular type (L'Esperance, 1969). The delivery systems in commercial instruments differ, but the most common consist of a slit lamp—biomicroscope which can be adjusted to deliver a variable cone (but usually of a minimal divergence) of radiation to the retina. The power delivery normally exceeds 0.2 W and may typically range upward to 1.5 W, placing the system into Class 4. Although the total power delivered is less than previously discussed in regard to multi-watt argon surgical lasers, the power is still sufficient to present potential eye hazards. Unfortunately, because of the low divergence of the beam the irradiance does not decrease rapidly with distance. Figure 17-12 gives a diagram of a typical argon laser photocoagulator.

The return laser reflection from the eyeball is quite modest for a ruby laser. A collimated beam would provide the sharpest cone of back reflection. As the beam strikes the curved corneal surface, a 2% normal reflection is encountered [calculated by Eq. 16-2, using a refractive index of 1.3 for the cornea]. For a reflection from a

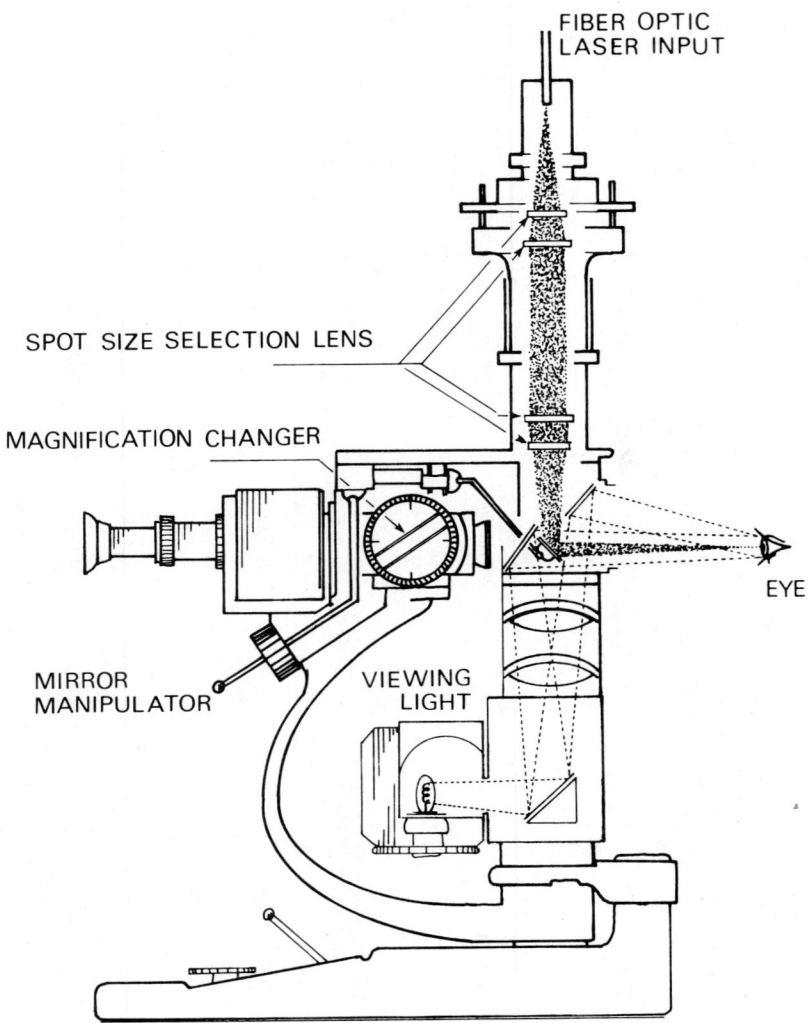

Figure 17-12. Ophthalmic Laser Photocoagulator. The specular reflection of the therapy beam from the cornea (or flat-faced contact lens) is generally terminated by the instrument.

curved specular surface the irradiance E as a function of distance from the reflecting surface r_1 can be determined from Eq. (15-10). A reflection at a distance r_1 of 30 cm may be of the order of 12 mW/cm² for a 1-W beam with a beam diameter of 3 mm. However, because of the design of the delivery system, this reflection is terminated by the ophthalmoscopic delivery system itself. Some argon laser photocoagula-

figures a contact lens to be placed on the patient's eye. Further, the reflections from the flat front surface from the Goldmann or gonial contact lens introduces a real hazard (Jenkins, 1979). Reflections of the alignment beam are not hazardous, but those from the direct beam may be Class 4. All direct beam reflections from the contact lens should be considered hazardous, although an antireflection coating will limit the hazardous range to 1.6 m. Thus all personnel except the ophthalmologist and the patient should wear the proper eye protection.

The ophthalmologist is protected from direct argon laser irradiation during the operation of the therapy beam by a filter in the viewing optics. This filter is not in place when the aiming beam (Class 2) is operating as the ophthalmologist must see the spot on the retina. The reflection of the aiming beam off contact lens is often several microwatts if the contact lens is not anti-reflection coated. The reflection seen by the ophthalmologist is dazzling, but is not hazardous even in the context of the number of possible exposures in a day. As mentioned above, a more serious problem is the occasional reflection of the treatment beam off the contact lens to an observer (e.g., a resident in training or attendant nurse). Such an observer should wear laser eye protection.

With the early ruby laser systems it was not uncommon for an ophthalmologist to direct the beam at a wall or at the ceiling to see if a red flash resulted, indicating that there were no glass surfaces such as picture frames or lighting fixtures which would create a specular reflection. Because of the higher reliability (and CW operating characteristics) of the argon laser, such checkouts are seldom necessary now.

17.13 LASER DIAGNOSTIC EQUIPMENT IN MEDICINE

Although the laser's unique characteristics make it useful in numerous diagnostic investigations, they are, as yet, only at the research level; few devices have made their way to commercial production, and most of these have been failures.

One of the most interesting applications has been the utilization of the speckle characteristics of coherent radiation to determine directly refractive errors. The laser furnishes the means to distinguish between defects in the optical system and defects in the neuronal system in an objective fashion. The speckle pattern image at the retina is formed when laser light is reflected from a rough diffuse surface and passes through the eye's pupil, or any other aperture. Any lens system produces conjugate interference patterns. If the source moves laterally very slightly, the conjugate images in the focal plane at the retina will also move very slightly. The direction of movement indicates whether the image plane is in front of or behind the focal plane. Using this property of laser light, small variations from proper focus can be translated into changes in movement easily detectable by the human visual system. Both spherical and cylindrical corrections can be made to about one-eighth diopter in this way. For comparison, usual spectacle lenses are considered satisfactory if prescribed within one-quarter of a diopter. The important feature of this method is that it depends only on proper focus, on the retina, neural factors in the visual pathway do not contribute. Thus, if the lenses have been fitted in this fashion, any residual lack of adequate performance by the visual system can be blamed on the neural components. Although speckle pattern refractometers have been produced, they are not in widespread use. The laser power involved is very low, only a 1 mW laser source is really required if the ambient illumination is low.

Occasionally the optical system is deranged sufficiently to prevent proper refraction, but some assessment of visual function is still desired. For example, prior to a cataract operation, the ophthalmic surgeon may desire to know if the retina has sufficient function to justify this surgery. The artificial production of interference patterns on the retina has been used in this manner (Green, 1970), and retinal irradiance levels for such procedures are not hazardous.

Holography has also been used to assist in diagnosis. It provides the possibility of documenting the structure of many parts of the eye simultaneously and it also allows precise computation of intraocular distances (Vaughan et al., 1974). The retinal irradiances to produce a holograph however approach very closely hazardous levels (Hochheimer, 1974; Rosen, 1973). Blood flow has also been measured in retinal vasculature through the use of Doppler laser tonometry (Riva et al., 1979). For all of the diagnostic techniques other than holography, the retina is always exposed to a very low irradiance, well within the comfort range, and therefore well below hazardous levels. It is only when the output of the laser system is focussed on the retina that there is any concern for hazard.

Many ophthalmic laboratories now have automatic lens refractometers which make use of a Class 2 He-Ne laser which is enclosed within a system. Using the laser it is possible to fully automate the technique of measuring the optical properties of spectacle lenses, including sphere, cylinder, axis, prism and optical center. These instruments are capable of measuring optical prescriptions to the nearest one-eighth diopter. The lens in a pair of spectacles is placed over a lens cone on a lens holder and the beam directed upward through the lens. Emitted radiation is typically of the order of 0.9 mW. The operator would normally never be able to place his eye in the beam. Only if a mirror were placed within the beam where the lens would normally be located would the beam be directed outward to other personnel in the laboratory. Then, since the power would be less than 1 mW, the beam would not be hazardous if viewed within the blink reflex.

Laser cell sorting has also been developed for laboratory use (Mullaney et al., 1974), but such systems are usually totally enclosed Class 1 systems. Holographic reconstruction has also been used to visualize ultrasonic images for diagnostic radiology. In these instances the helium-neon or argon laser beam is greatly expanded to produce an interference pattern over a large surface of water. Again, however, this is a rather uncommon technique and because of the beam irradiances used there is no great hazard. No doubt there will be many other future applications of lasers for diagnostic tools but only very low beam irradiances would be involved.

Low-power Class 2 helium-neon lasers have been used to position patients for radiation therapy treatment as shown in Fig. 17-13. However, despite the very low Class 2 or even Class 1 beam irradiance levels involved in these applications, needless exposure of the patient's eyes as shown in that figure should not be permitted. Originally two or three Class 2 (0.04-0.1 mW output) He-Ne lasers would be employed to provide a cross-over point on a patient in the center of a therapy field. Later, scanning He-Ne lasers (Class 2) were used to provide crossed lines, instead of single

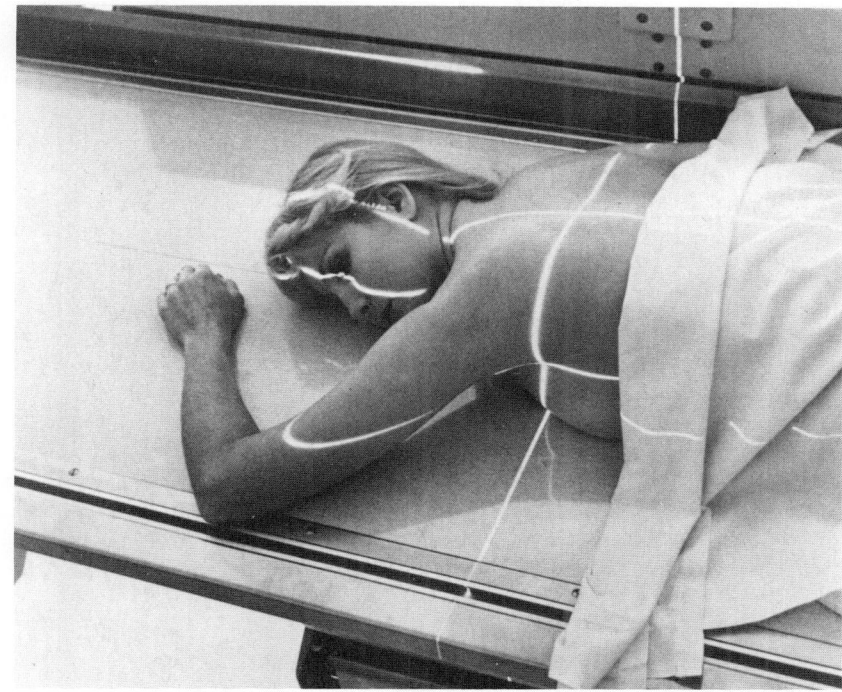

Figure 17-13. Teletherapy Alignment Laser. A scanning He-Ne laser (Class II) is used for patient positioning. By using low ambient light levels, beam irradiance at the patient is less than 0.1 mW/cm^2 (courtesy of Gammex, Inc., Glendale, Wisconsin).

beam points, on the patient. In either case the patient's eye would be exposed to Class 1 or lower Class 2 levels. The retinal image would be a point (or line) image if the eye were relaxed. However, no hazard could exist unless the patient were to overcome his aversion response, and intentionally stare into the beam.

17.14 LASER SURVEYS

Corporate or governmental health and safety personnel are often required to survey laser installations. This task is the most difficult for experimental laser arrangements. Figures 17-14 and 17-15 illustrate two useful survey forms—one centered about the laser and the other centered about its operation. The forms are designed to be used with a machine records program, and in actual practice each box could have its own code number.

LASER EQUIPMENT SURVEY FORM

LASER DATA

1. Manufacturers ☐☐☐☐☐☐☐☐☐☐☐☐☐☐☐☐☐☐☐☐☐☐☐☐
2. Model Number ☐☐☐☐☐☐☐☐☐☐
3. Serial Number ☐☐☐☐☐☐☐☐☐☐
4. Output Power (W) ☐☐☐☐☐☐
5. Output Energy (J) ☐☐☐☐☐☐
6. Wavelength(s) (nm) ☐☐☐☐☐☐☐ or (μm) ☐☐☐☐☐☐☐
7. Emergent Beam Diameter (cm) ☐☐☐☐☐☐
8. Emergent Beam Divergence (mrad) ☐☐☐☐☐☐
9. Emergent Beam Irradiance (W/cm^2) ☐☐☐☐☐☐
10. Emergent Beam Radiant Exposure (J/cm^2) ☐☐☐☐☐☐
11. Classification ☐☐☐☐☐☐☐☐☐☐
12. Hazardous Range (cm) ☐☐☐☐☐☐
13. Labels: ☐ Caution ☐ Danger ☐ 21CFR1040 ☐ Emission Port
14. Safety Features: Beam Port Shutter ☐ Filter ☐ Polarizer ☐
15. Electrical Safety Features: ☐ Indicator Light ☐ Cabinet Interlock ☐ Remote Control Connector ☐ Exposed Current Carrying Points
16. Location: Bldg ☐☐☐☐ Room ☐☐☐☐ Installation ☐☐☐☐☐☐☐ ☐ Fixed ☐ Mobile ☐ Accessory Use ☐ Collimator ☐ Diverging Lens ☐ Beam Scanner

Figure 17-14. Laser Equipment Survey Form. This form could be improved by adding the output duration and recycle time if a pulsed laser is being studied.

CLASS III AND CLASS IV
LASER INSTALLATION SURVEY FORM

A. PERSONNEL

No. Workers ____ In Medical Surveillance Program ____

B. SYSTEM CONTROLS

☐ Beam Attenuator   ☐ Beam Shutter   ☐ Door Interlocks

C. INSTALLATION/ENGINEERING CONTROLS

☐ Beam Path Not Easily Accessible ____
   (Not at eye level while standing or sitting)
☐ Rigid Mounting ____
☐ Changing Beam Path ____
☐ Multiple Wavelength Use ____
☐ Scanning Beam   ☐ Diffuse Reflection Hazard
☐ Unused Secondary Beams Terminated ____
☐ Beam Enclosure ____
☐ Ventilation ☐ General ☐ Local Exhaust ☐ Hood at Target
☐ Second Laser Beam Port ☐ Capped
☐ Beam Backstop ☐ Fire Resistant ☐ Diffuse ☐ Low Reflectivity

Laboratory: ☐ Overcrowded ☐ Multiple Operations at One Time
☐ Windows Closed or Covered
☐ Communication Problem For All Potentially Exposed ____
☐ Significant Skin/Fire Hazard ☐ Beam Collimator

Safety Equipment Available: ☐ Eye Protection – Model ____ OD ____
☐ Fire Extinguisher λ ____

D. ADMINISTRATIVE CONTROLS

☐ SOP ☐ Posted ☐ Resuscitation Chart Posted ☐ Warning Lights
☐ Audible Alarm ☐ Warning Signs ☐ Viewing Restrictions
☐ Visitor Restrictions ☐ Personnel Training ☐ Completed Safety Course

E. SECONDARY ASSOCIATED HAZARDS

☐ Flashlamp Exposed ☐ UV ☐ Fumes ☐ Toxic Dyes ☐ Explosion
☐ Biological Materials: ____
☐ Solid Conducting Grounding Rod   ☐ Cryogenic Liquids

Figure 17-15. Laser Installation Survey Form.

Most of the form is completed at the time of the survey. Some values, such as beam irradiance and hazardous distance, may be looked up or calculated at a later time. If the laser is not a commercial product "line 1" in Fig. 17-14 becomes "IN HOUSE," and the box marked 21CFR1040 is checked if the BRH label is intact. This box further serves to indicate whether the laser was manufactured after August 1, 1976, when the Federal Laser Performance Standard became effective. Man of the checks on the second page of the form serve to remind the experienced surveyor of potential problem areas. In actual use, a third page is provided for writing additional comments and recommendations.

17.15 REVIEW QUESTIONS

1. A Class 4 laser installation should normally possess a door interlock or similar means to preclude laboratory entry during laser operation. True or False? A Class 3 installation?

2. A research technician complains bitterly that the eye protection he must wear when working with a 2-W argon laser does not permit him to see the beam. He contends that he could burn his hand in the 2-mm beam. The only commercially available protective lenses have an optical density of 13 at 514.5 nm and 17 at 488 nm. What can you recommend?

3. A laboratory manager comes to you as the safety director to ask if you would help him justify the purchase of a closed-circuit TV system since he is working with a 15-mW He-Ne laser. What would be your response?

4. A laser worker testing gas discharge laser tubes comes to you and complains to you that she awoke at 2 a.m. with a feeling of sand in her eyes. She is puzzled and wonders if it could result from working with lasers. What do you think?

5. A laboratory worker insists that he must maintain a versatile "breadboard" power supply without covering exposed current-carrying conductors. He only needs it for two more days. What do you recommend?

6. A laboratory technician requests that he be issued a fire extinguisher for use in his laboratory. He has a 2-W argon-krypton ion laser. Should he have a fire extinguisher?

7. Does the probability of hazardous retinal exposures (a) barely increase; (b) significantly increase; (c) remain the same or (d) decrease when an open Class 4 ruby laser replaces an open Class 3 ruby laser?

8. What is the reflected beam power from a 1 W argon laser beam incident upon an uncoated glass contact lens?

9. Using Figure 17-10 suggest hazard controls.

10. How can a Class 4 laser be aligned without the use of eye protection?

17.16 REFERENCES

American National Standards Institute, 1976, The Safe Use of Lasers, Standard Z-136.1.
Auth, D. C., Lam, V. T. Y., Mohr, R. W., Silverstein, F. E., and Rubin, C. E., 1976, A high-power gastric photocoagulator for fiberoptic endoscopy, *IEEE Trans.* BME-23(2):129–135.
Baily, N. A., 1972, Further developments in the use of holographic methods for the storage of roentgenographic images, *Invest. Radio.* 7:118–123.
Burch, J. M. and Gates, J. W. C., 1967, Lasers: practical control and protection in experimental laboratories, *Ann. Occ. Hyg.* 10 (Laser Safety Suppl.):65–73.
Elterman, P. B., 1977, Brewster angle light trap, *Appl. Opt.* 16(9):2352.
Floriam, H. J., 1975, Laser and the eye—occupational protection for physicians, *Hefte Unfallheilkd.* 121:514–519 (German).
Gamaleya, N. F., 1977, Laser biomedical research in the USSR, *in* "Laser Applications in Medicine and Biology," (M. L. Wolbarsht, ed.) Vol. 3, pp. 1–173, Plenum Press, New York.
Goldman, J. R. and Meyer, R., 1965, Transmission of laser beams through various transparent rods for biomedical applications, *Nature* 205:892–894.
Goldman, L., 1967, Laser laboratory design, *in* "CRC Handbook of Laboratory Safety," pp. 294–301, Chemical Rubber Co., Cleveland, OH.
Goldman, L. and Hornby, P., 1965, The design of a medical laser laboratory, *Arch. Environ. Health* 10:493–497.
Goldman, L. and Rockwell, R. J., 1971, "Lasers in Medicine," Gordon and Breach, New York.
Goldman, Hornby, P., and Rockwell, R. J., 1967, Investigative studies with quartz rods for high energy laser transmission, *Med. Res. Eng.* 6:12–17.
Goldman, L., Rockwell, R. J., Jr., Fidler, J. P., Altemeier, W. A., and Siler, V. E., 1969, Investigative laser surgery: safety aspects, *Biomed. Eng.* 4:415–418.
Goldman, L., Rockwell, R. J., Jr., Fox, S. H., and Fidler, J., 1974, Optical aspects of laser surgical instrumentation, *Opt. Eng.* 12(5):176–179.
Green, D. G., 1970, Testing the vision of cataract patients by means of laser-generated interference fringes, *Science* 168:1240–1242.
Gulacsik, C., Auth, D. C., and Silverstein, F. E., 1979, Opthalmic hazards associated with laser endoscopy, *Appl. Opt.* 18(11):1816–1823.
Harding, D. C., and Baker, D. W., 1968, Laser schlieren optical system for analyzing ultrasonic fields, *Biomed. Sci. Instr.* 4:223–230.
Hillenkamp, F., Hutzler, P. and Kinder, J., 1976, Coherent and quasi-coherent optical methods in biology and medicine, *Ann. N. Y. Acad. Sci.* 267:216–221.
Hochheimer, B., 1974, Lasers in ophthalmology, *in* "Laser Applications in Medicine and Biology," (M. L. Wolbarsht, ed.) Vol. 2, pp. 41–75, Plenum Press, New York.
Ingelstam, E. and Ragnarsson, S. I., 1972, Eye refraction examined by aid of speckle pattern produced by coherent light, *Vis. Res.* 12:411–420.
Jenkins, D. L., 1979, Non-ionizing radiation protection, Special Study No. 25-42-0310-79, Hazard Evaluation of the Coherent Model 900 Photocoagulator Laser System, January-February 1979. U.S. Army Environmental Hygiene Agency, Aberdeen Proving Ground, MD (NTIS No. ADA068713).
Kaplan, Z., Sharon, U., and Ger, R., 1974, The carbon-dioxide laser in clinical surgery, *in* "Laser Applications in Medicine and Biology," (M. L. Wolbarsht, ed.) Vol. 2, pp. 295–307, Plenum Press, New York.

Krasnov, M.M., 1974, Q-switched laser goniopuncture, *Arch. Ophth.* **92**(1):37–41.
L'Esperance, F. A., Jr.,1969, Photocoagulation delivery systems for continuous-wave lasers, *Brit. J. Ophthal.* **53**:310–322.
Marich, K. W., Orenberg, J. B., Treytl, W. J. and Glick, D., 1972, Health hazards in the use of the laser microprobe for toxic and infective samples, *Am. Ind. Hyg. Assn. J.* **33**(7):488–491.
Meyer-Schwickerath, G., 1960, "Light Coagulation," Mosby, St. Louis.
McSparron, D. A., Douglas, C. A., and Badger, H. L., 1966, Radiometric methods for measuring laser output, Tech. Note 418, National Bureau of Standards, Rockeville, MD.
Mohon, N. and Rodemann, A., 1973, Laser speckle for determining ametropia and accommodation response of the eye, *Appl. Opt.* **12**(4):783–787.
Mullaney, P. F., Steinkamp, J. A., Crissman, H. A., Cram, L. S., and Holm. D. M., 1974, Laser flow microspectrophotometers for rapid analysis and sorting of individual mammalian cells, *in* "Laser Applications in Medicine and Biology," (M. L. Wolbarsht, ed.) Vol. 2, pp. 151–204, Plenum Press, New York.
Rentzepis, P. M., 1970, Ultrafast processes, *Science* **169**:239–247.
Riggle, G. C., Hoyle, R. C., and Ketcham, A. S., 1971, Laser effects on normal and tumor tissue, *in* "Laser Applications in Medicine and Biology," (M. L. Wolbarsht, ed.) Vol. 1, pp. 35–65 Plenum Press, New York.
Riva, C. E., Feke, G. T., Eberli, B., and Benary, V., 1979, Bidirectional LDV system for absolute measurement of blood speed in retinal vessels, *Appl. Opt.* **18**(13):2301–2306.
Riva, C. E., Timberlake, G. T. and Feke, G. T., 1979, Laser Doppler technique for measurement of eye movement, *Appl. Opt.* **18**(14):2486–2490.
Rosen, A. N., 1973, Fundus holography through a wide-angle contact lens, *Invest. Ophthal.* **12** (10):786–788.
Sliney, D. H., 1969, Evaluating hazards and controlling them, *Laser Focus* **5**:39–42.
Solon, L. R., 1963, Occupational safety with laser beams, *Arch. Environ. Health* **6**:414–416.
Snow, J. C., Kripke, B. J., Strong, M. S., Jako, G. J., Meyer, M. R., and Vaughan, C. W., 1974. Anesthesia for carbon dioxide laser microsurgery on the larynx and trachea, *Anesth. Analg.* **53** 507–512.
Stellar, S., Polanyi, T. G., and Bredemeier, H. C., 1974, Lasers in surgery, *in* "Laser Applications in Medicine and Biology," (M. L. Wolbarsht, ed.) Vol. 2, pp. 241–293, Plenum Press, New York.
U. S. Department of Health, Education and Welfare, 1979, Title 21, Code of Federal Regulations Part 1040, Light Emitting Products.
Vaughn, K., Laing, R., and Wiggens, R., 1974, Holography of the eye: A critical review, *in* "Laser Applications in Medicine and Biology," (M. L. Wolbarsht, ed.) Vol. 2, pp. 77–132, Plenum Press, New York.
Wilkening, G. M., 1970, A commentary on laser-induced biological effects and protective measures, *Ann. N. Y. Acad. Sci.* **168**(3):621–626.
Winburn, D. C., 1976, Safety considerations in the laser research program at the Los Alamos Scientific Laboratory, *Ann. N. Y. Acad. Sci.* **267**:135–151.
Wolbarsht, M. L., and Landers, M. B., III, 1979, Lasers in ophthalmology: the path from theory to application, *Appl. Opt.* **18**:1518–1526.
Zweng, H. C., 1971, Lasers in ophthalmology, *in* "Laser Applications in Medicine and Biology," (M. L. Wolbarsht, ed.) Vol. 1, pp. 239–254, Plenum Press, New York.

Chapter 18
Safety with Lasers Used in Construction

18.1 INTRODUCTION

From 1964 to 1968 there were several attempts to place a helium-neon laser on a surveyor's transit tripod and to use it for aligning various equipment used in heavy construction. The photograph of Figure 18-1 shows an early application of such a laser mounted on a transit as used for aligning a dredge in the construction of the Bay Area Rapid Transit tunnel under the San Francisco Bay. In this application the dredge operator knew he was in a position when he could stare directly into the vertically fanned-shaped beam. Since 1968 the variety of applications for alignment, leveling, and surveying has greatly increased. During this period experience with the control of the associated eye hazards has shown that such applications can be made relatively safe. None of the lasers used for these purposes in construction presents a skin hazard. They are normally helium-neon lasers whose output power is not more than 5 mW.

The first alignment lasers were designed for use in the laboratory and then placed on tripods for outdoor use as an afterthought. Not surprisingly their reliability was poor, but their great advantage for providing a straight and easily seen red-light reference line for tunneling, dredging, and surveying spurred further development. Since that time several manufacturers have designed completely ruggedized, waterproofed laser systems especially for these applications and the equipment no longer appears to be slightly modified from a laboratory instrument. Figures 18-2 and 18-3 show two types of common laser systems. Figure 18-2 shows a laser designed for utility contractors to use for aligning sewer pipes. Figure 18-3 shows a scanning laser product which emits a beam that rotates on a horizontal plane for more rapid installation of suspended ceilings; the workmen adjust the ceiling suspension wires by noting the location of the scanning laser beam as it is reflected from the side walls and from special targets located on the ceiling suspension structures. The output powers of the present helium-neon lasers used in these applications were

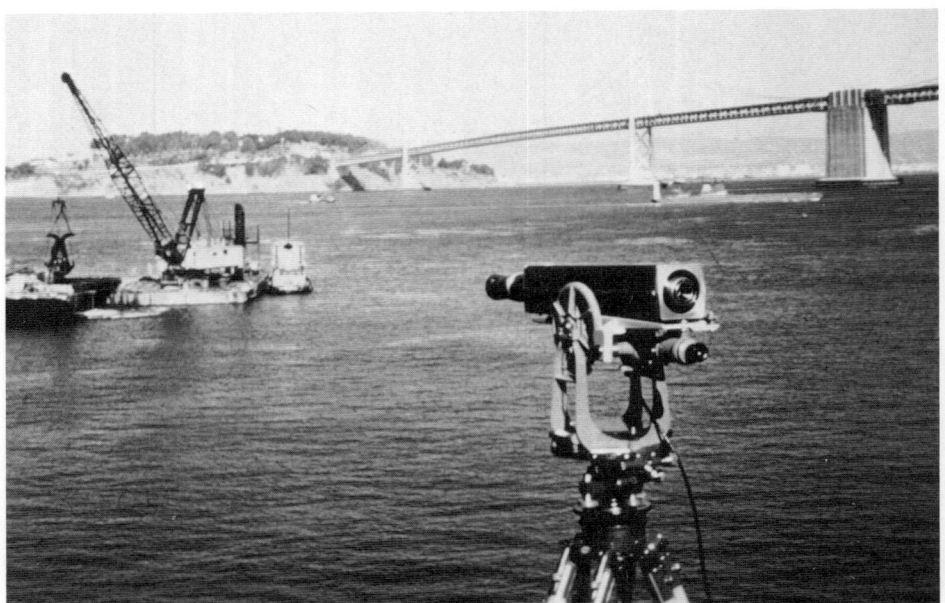

Figure 18-1. Early Alignment Laser. An early prototype alignment laser used for visual alignment of a dredging barge in construction of the Bay Area Rapid Transit tunnel under the San Francisco Bay (courtesy Spectra Physics).

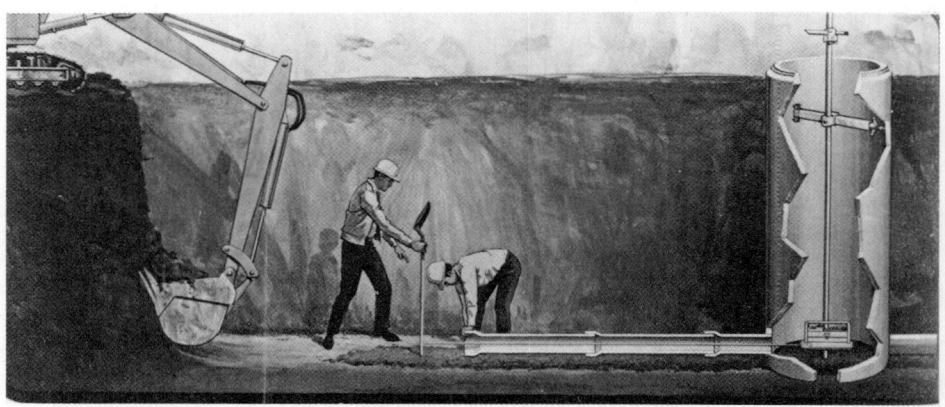

Figure 18-2. Sewer Pipe Alignment. Probably the greatest application of HeNe alignment lasers has been for sewer pipe installation. The reference beam is normally below ground but may in some instances be at or above ground level. Note that direct eye exposure in this scenario is next to impossible (courtesy Blount and George).

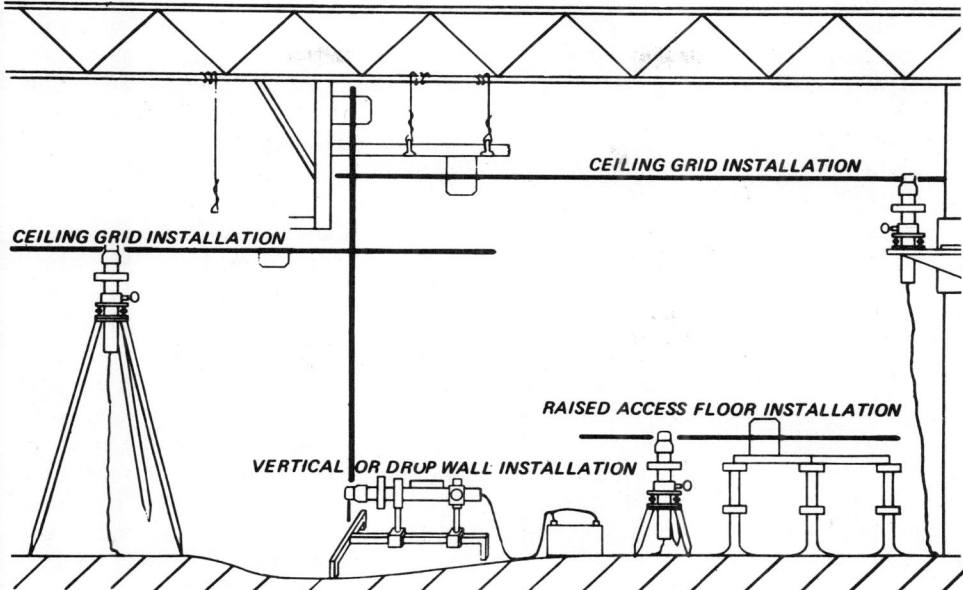

Figure 18-3. Ceiling Alignment. A rotating beam from an alignment laser is used for installing suspended ceilings. The rotating beam forms a reference plane that intercepts target cards that attach to ceiling supports (courtesy Spectra-Physics).

shaped by the typical requirement, to have the reflected beam from an alignment target visible in daylight. To achieve this, approximately 5 mW in a 1-cm diameter beam are needed. These lasers are therefore normally Class 3 lasers which may present a hazard even from momentary direct viewing, unless the beam diameter is sufficiently large that no more than 1 mW enters the eye's pupil. Reflection from these lasers are seldom hazardous even from flat specular surfaces unless the specular reflectance is far greater than from ordinary plate glass. Only mirrors are likely to have such characteristics.

18.2 PROTECTION STANDARDS FOR CONSTRUCTION LASERS

During the 1970's the manufacturers and users of construction laser products played a significant role in the development of the national concensus standard of the American National Standards Institute (ANSI). This special interest group was particularly concerned about safety standards because the greatest number of lasers that had been manufactured to that date (more than 100,000) were small helium-neon lasers with an output of 0.5 - 5 mW for their use. A great deal of attention was paid, therefore, to this type of laser during the development of both the ocular exposure limits, the classification scheme, and safety procedures.

Many of these laser users and manufacturers felt very strongly that no significant hazard existed from ocular exposure to helium-neon lasers having an output power of less than 5 mW. They sincerely felt that the permissible exposure limit should be 5 mW for a momentary exposure. This would place all of their lasers in a relatively safe category, making the lasers easier to market and relieve the manufacturer and the user from complying with the future governmental regulations which were then just on the horizon. The basis for their position was that no one had adequately documented an eye injury as the result of working with these devices. Furthermore, they pointed to the biological research data (Lappin, 1971; Ham et al., 1970; Davis and Mautner, 1969) which showed that the ED-50 "threshold" for retinal burns from the helium-neon laser emitting at 632.8 nm was typically of the order of 7 to 10 mW in the rhesus monkey eye for an exposure duration of 0.1 to 2 s. They considered the rabbit threshold data of 2.5 mW obtained by Blabla and John (1966) for a 0.65 s exposure as not being relative to the human eye and generally overlooked one data point in the Ham report which showed a retinal injury at 1.9 mW. They had been told that the rhesus monkey eye should be more vulnerable to injury from this type of laser exposure than the human eye because of the greater pigmentation of the rhesus monkey retina compared to a human retina. Since the thresholds for this type of exposure were close to their proposed exposure limit of 5 mW, a great deal of debate ensued. The proponents of the 5-mW limit argued that the biologic data supported their position. In Great Britain the exposure level for momentary viewing was set at 5 mW in 1972 by the British Standards Institute, although they have since lowered this value.

Most health and safety personnel and experts on eye injury on the ANSI Z-136 committee argued for more conservative exposure limits at values between 0.1 and 1 mW for this momentary exposure. The argument for a momentary (0.18– 0.25 s) limit relied on the concept of an aversion response which would normally cause a viewer to blink and turn away when he or she looked, unexpectedly, into the beam. Some pointed out that an individual could overcome his natural aversion to bright light. There was, therefore, concern about setting a momentary exposure limit; some conservative members questioned whether one could even make the distinction which was later made between a Class 3 and a Class 2 laser based on the aversion response. The users and manufacturers of this type of laser eventually won part of the argument by pointing out the very low incidence, if any, of injuries from these types of lasers.

One of the problems that fueled the controversy was that the "threshold" generally reported in the biomedical literature was actually not the lowest limit at which injury occurred. The data for "threshold" were normally expressed as "ED-50" exposure data (explained in Chapters 4 and 7, particularly Chapter 7). Some thresholds of injury in individual animals were well below the value of 7-10 mW often noted in the literature. One single data point that created much discussion was the previously mentioned individual point of 1.9 mW reported by Ham and his colleagues in 1970 for a 1-second exposure of the retina of a rhesus monkey.

The proponents of the 5-mW safety limit went on to question the applicability of the experimental data in the rhesus monkey to the real world and quite

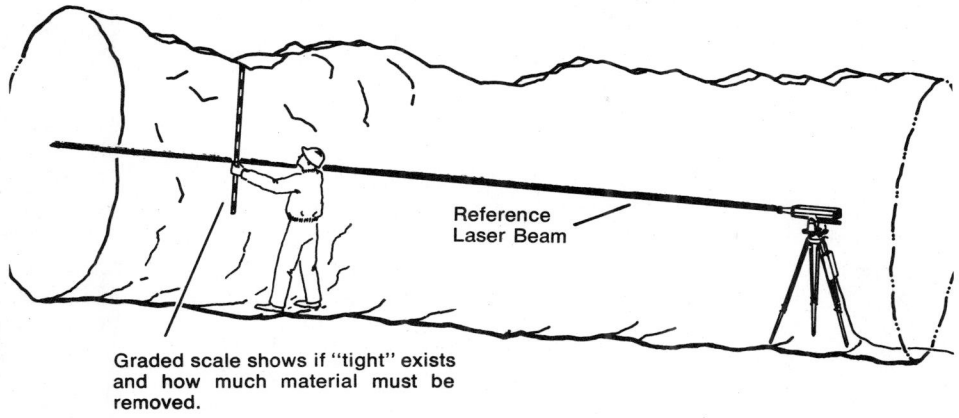

Figure 18-4. Tunnel Laser. A HeNe laser is often used in tunnel construction. Normally the beam is placed above eye level (courtesy Spectra-Physics).

reasonably asked whether the retinal image of the laser in the eye of an individual standing at a construction site could ever be as stable as the image placed in the eye of an anesthetized experimental animal. Surprisingly, the image in the human eye may be more stable if he were staring in the direction of the laser; the human eye has a remarkable ability by muscular movements to stabilize an image (Fender, 1964). The eye of the anesthetized monkey, on the other hand, may tend to slightly wander during an experimental exposure; and more importantly, the accommodation (focusing) will not be consistently adjusted for the optimal "point" image as it would be for the man standing at the construction site. The tentative conclusion was that the experimental threshold data could not be considered conservative, and the final limit for momentary viewing (a 0.25-s exposure) of the helium-neon laser was set at a power of 1 mW into the eye, or 2.5 mW/cm^2 when expressed as an irradiance. That exposure limit will probably remain the concern of many because of its great impact upon the practical application of the versatile helium-neon laser.

The constriction of the pupil in daylight would tend to allow a greater safety margin, although probably no greater than 4 for the outdoor construction applications as opposed to the use of this type of laser for tunneling or indoor applications. This factor is not accounted for in present safety standards since some individuals naturally have enlarged pupils, as well as others who are on medication. Fortunately, lasers designed strictly for construction applications in a lowered ambient illumination normally have lower outputs, and helium-neon lasers used in tunneling and mining (Fig. 18-4) normally do not exceed 1 mW in total output power.

18.3 HAZARD CLASSIFICATION

Following this brief review of the controversies associated with setting one of the applicable ocular exposure limits, it is appropriate to turn to the operational safety rules for construction laser devices. The rules depend upon the hazard classification.

18.3.1 Class 1 Systems

Only a few applications can make use of safe, Class 1 lasers. The Class 1 lasers are normally gallium-arsenide lasers designed to be used in laser distance-measuring equipment and of course are safe to stare into for long periods of time without risk. Of course, no safety procedures are required for using this type of laser. The GaAs laser diodes are also used in intrusion detection devices for security in and around construction sites at night or on weekends.

18.3.2 Class 2 Systems

The Class 2 low-risk lasers, which are not considered hazardous to view momentarily, are used in tunneling and in certain other applications where the 2-5 mW power is not considered essential. The only safety requirement here is that a cautionary label must be located on the laser housing. Nevertheless, it is generally good practice to try to terminate these beams within the controlled construction area. Even if the beam is below 1 mW in total power, a passerby outside of the construction site who might accidentally walk through the beam could be sufficiently surprised by the bright, unexpected light to be seriously concerned about his vision and could bring a complaint against the construction contractor. Construction contractors often realize this potential problem and generally try to follow practices that would keep the beam from being seen by onlookers despite the lack of a legal safety requirement.

18.3.3 Class 3 Systems

The Class 3 medium-risk lasers would include the 1-2 mW lasers that could be hazardous even for momentary intrabeam (direct) viewing. The earlier lasers normally had beam diameters of less than 1 cm and many would be considered Class 3B by present standards. After the promulgation of the BRH standard for product performance in 1976, some manufacturers began to discontinue or modify certain Class 3B construction lasers. If the output irradiances were to be kept below 2.5 mW/cm^2, and the power were below 5 mW, then the system would be Class 3A. This means that the only significant risk to personnel would be if the 1-5 mW beam were collected by an optical instrument. Hence the required BRH label on these devices gave a cautionary warning against viewing the beam directly with optical instruments. One might ask whether any real chance of such viewing could occur. Actually, surveyor transits and other optical instruments are not completely uncommon in some construction sites and workers should be cautioned about the added risk of using their optical instruments in or near a laser beam path.

Because the use of any Class 3B helium-neon laser presents a significantly greater risk to the general public if misused, it is fortunate that the added hazard control restrictions for these devices have tended to encourage the use of lower power Class 2 or Class 3A lasers and the development of visual enhancement target screens for use with survey and alignment lasers. In any case the U. S. Federal Government has taken positive steps to prohibit the manufacture and use of (U. S. Department of Labor, 1977) surveying, alignment and leveling lasers with an output power above 5 mW (BRH Regulation 1976:21CFR1040.11(b)) in the visible (400-700 nm) and above Class 1 for other wavelength regions.

§ 1040.11

(b) *Surveying, leveling, and alignment laser products.* Each surveying, leveling, or alignment laser product shall comply with all of the applicable requirements of § 1040.10 for a Class I, Class II, or Class III laser product and, in addition:

(1) Shall not permit human access to laser radiation in the wavelength range of greater than 400 nm but less than or equal to 710 nm with a radiant power that exceeds 5.0×10^{-3} W for any emission duration greater than 3.8×10^{-4} second; and,

(2) Shall not permit human access to laser radiation in excess of the accessible emission limits of Class I for any other combination of emission duration and wavelength range.

At least two variances to 1040.11 were granted. One variance (No. 77004) for an output power of 8 mW (exceeding the 5 mW limitation unless measured in an 80-mm aperture having a 20 sr[sic] field of view at a distance of 20 cm). The variance was granted for the Coherent Radiation Model 81-11L laser linemaker [see Federal Register, 42(242):63470-1, December 16, 1977]. A greater output was required to make the 120°-fan-shaped beam visible in sawmills and steel mills. Another variance from the 5-mW limit was issued in March 1977 to RCA Corporation for the RCA RangePole.

The only OSHA standards that applied to laser use are in the OSHA Safety and Health Regulations for Construction—Part 1926. These regulations were drafted in 1970 and first issued in 1971—two years before the first ANSI standard. The exposure limits are therefore more conservative, but at present have not created any major controversy as they are generally readily complied with. The following paragraphs are from 29CFR1926.54, "Nonionizing Radiation" (U.S. Department of Labor, 1977):

§ 1926.54 Nonionizing radiation.

(a) Only qualified and trained employees shall be assigned to install, adjust and operate laser equipment.

(b)   Proof of qualification of the laser equipment operator shall be available and in possession of the operator at all times.

(c)   Employees, when working in areas in which a potential exposure to direct or reflected laser light greater than 0.005 watts (5 milliwatts) exists, shall be provided with antilaser eye protection devices as specified in Subpart E of this part.

(d)   Areas in which lasers are used shall be posted with standard laser warning placards.

(e)   Beam shutters or caps shall be utilized, or the laser turned off, when laser transmission is not actually required. When the laser is left unattended for a substantial period of time, such as during lunch hour, overnight, or at change of shifts, the laser shall be turned off.

(f)   Only mechanical or electronic means shall be used as a detector for guiding the internal alignment of the laser.

(g)   The laser beam shall not be directed at employees.

(h)   When it is raining or snowing, or when there is dust or fog in the air, the operation of laser systems shall be prohibited where practicable; in any event, employees shall be kept out of range of the area of source and target during such weather conditions.

(i)   Laser equipment shall bear a label to indicate maximum output.

(j)   Employees shall not be exposed to light intensities above:
   (1)   Direct staring: 1 micro-watt per square centimeter;
   (2)   Incidental observing: 1 milliwatt per square centimeter;
   (3)   Diffused reflected light: 2½ watts per square centimeter.

(k)   Laser unit in operation should be set up above the heads of the employees, when possible.

18.4   DISTANCE MEASUREMENT LASER SYSTEMS

Up to this point only those lasers have been considered which are used for alignment and leveling. Another application of the helium-neon laser has been in distance measurement and in surveying. Originally this application was limited to large-scale geodetic surveys but smaller units have found their way into general survey in the past few years. Output powers of approximately 5 mW appear to be required for distances of more than 1 mile (1.8 km). Figures 18-5 and 18-6 show two types of lasers used for surveying. In general the opeator of the laser aims the distance meter at a distant reference point where a retroflector (Fig. 18-7) is located. The retroreflector returns some of the beam power to the distance measuring instrument and the operator can see this reflection through his optical telescope.

The first question that must be answered is whether the operator is exposed to a hazardous level when viewing a retroreflection through the telescope. It has been shown adequately that the beam diameter at the distance is so large where reflectors are used, that far less than 1 mW is ever returned to the opeator. Likewise because of the displacement of the beam output optics from the input optics in most of these devices, it is nearly impossible for a nearby retroreflection to find its way back into the input optics. In theory it is sometimes possible for a beam to leave the instrument, be displaced by reflection from a retroreflector and enter the viewing optics. This possibility is quite remote.

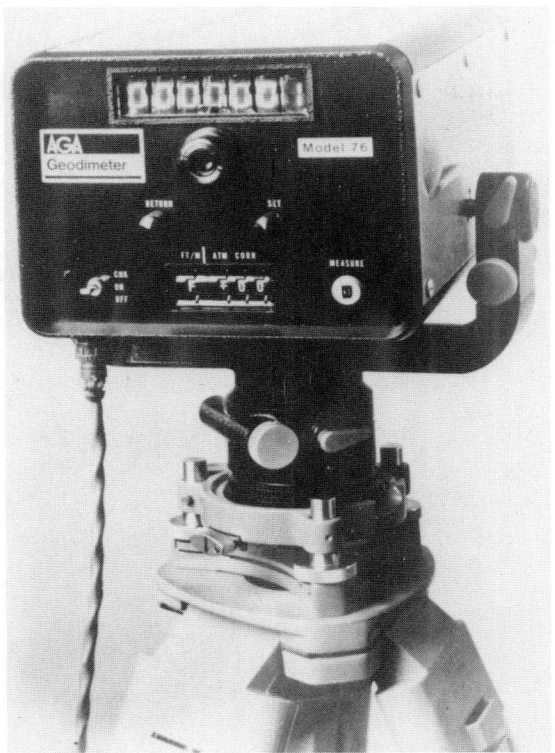

Figure 18-5. Geodetic Survey Laser. This HeNe laser is used for measuring distance by a multiple modulation of the beam. This is used for geodetic work over long distances (courtesy AGA of Seacaucus, New Jersey).

The laser beam for distance measurement must be modulated since the basis of the measuring technique is the comparison of typically three superimposed frequencies which may be of the order of 10 MHz. The phase separations of the received three frequencies indicates the precise distance if an approximate distance is known. The same general principle is applied in the gallium-arsenide laser distance measuring devices which operate to a maximum distance of approximately 1,000 meters. These Gallium-arsenide lasers may be either Class 1 or Class 3. It is not normally hazardous to view the direct beam by the unaided eye. The only hazard that exists would be viewing the direct beam by an optical collecting instrument. The BRH regulation 21CFR1040.11 now requires a Class 1 GaAs laser for these applications.

The use of the survey and distance measuring helium-neon lasers normally requires that the beam be well above well-trafficked areas for two reasons—to attain a long distance line of sight and to operate above the severe atmospheric turbulence

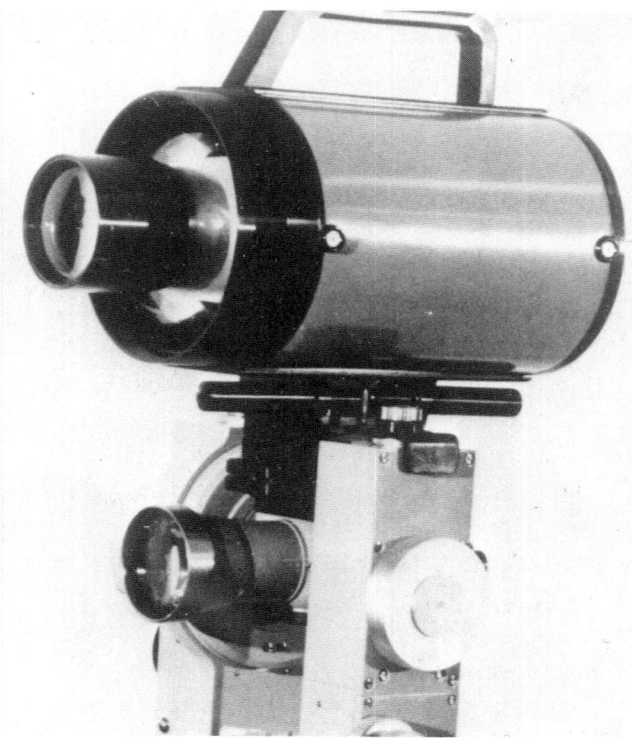

Figure 18-6. Land Survey Laser. A GaAs laser can be used for land surveying over short distances (courtesy Keuffel and Esser, Morristown, N.J.).

in the near ground layer [0 to 6 meters (20 feet)] that causes major errors in the distance measurement (see Sec. 13.3.5 for additional discussion).

18.5 CONTROL MEASURES FOR VISIBLE CLASS 3 CW LASERS USED FOR SURVEYING ALIGNMENT AND LEVELING

Although it is desirable to utilize Class 2 laser systems for construction applications, some applications in high ambient illumination require output powers of approximately 2 mW but in no case should the laser output exceed 5 mW from a visible laser with a circular beam. Adherence to the following rules will minimize the hazards in all matters relating to construction lasers:

Rule #1. Only qualified trained employees should be assigned to install, adjust or operate the laser equipment.

Rule #2. Proof of qualification of the laser equipment operator should be available and in possession of the opeator at all times. An operator card is often provided by a representative of the manufacturer following the completion by the

Safety with Construction Lasers   601

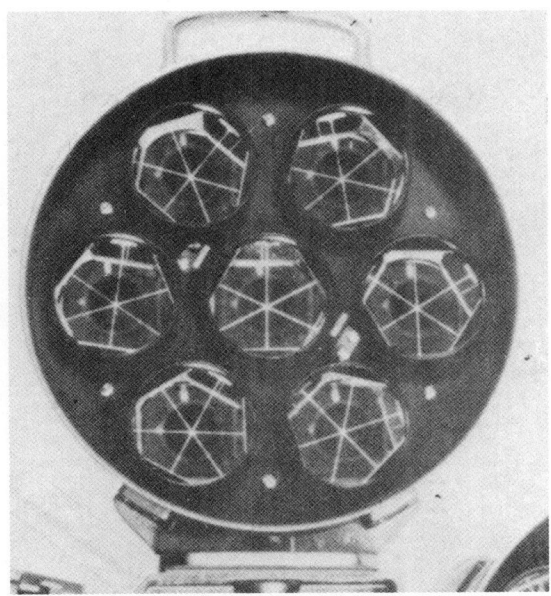

Figure 18-7. A Corner-cube Retroreflector. Corner cube retroreflectors used for enhancing the return laser beam for distance measurement.

operator of a minimum of one hour of training on the safe use of laser equipment. In some states, such as New York, it is required that such opeators have a "mobile laser" operator's permit. To obtain such a permit requires the operator to attend a three-day course on laser safety, or to have had a certain number of years of experiance operating the laser, or to have a college degree and a certain period of experience.

Rule #3. Areas in which Class 3B lasers are used should be posted with standard laser warning placards.

Rule #4. When the laser is not required for substantial periods of time, such as during lunch period, overnight, or at the change of shifts, beam shutters or caps should be utilized, or the laser should be turned off.

Rule #5. Mechanical or electronic means should be used for detecting and for guiding the alignment of the laser where feasible. Several newer types of lasers employ automatic alignment and leveling, as shown in Figure 18-8.

Rule #6. Precautions shall be taken to ensure that persons do not look directly into the beam unless the beam irradiance is below the applicable exposure limit at that observing location. Figure 18-9 shows the use of translucent, diffusing targets in sewer pipes precludes intra-beam viewing.

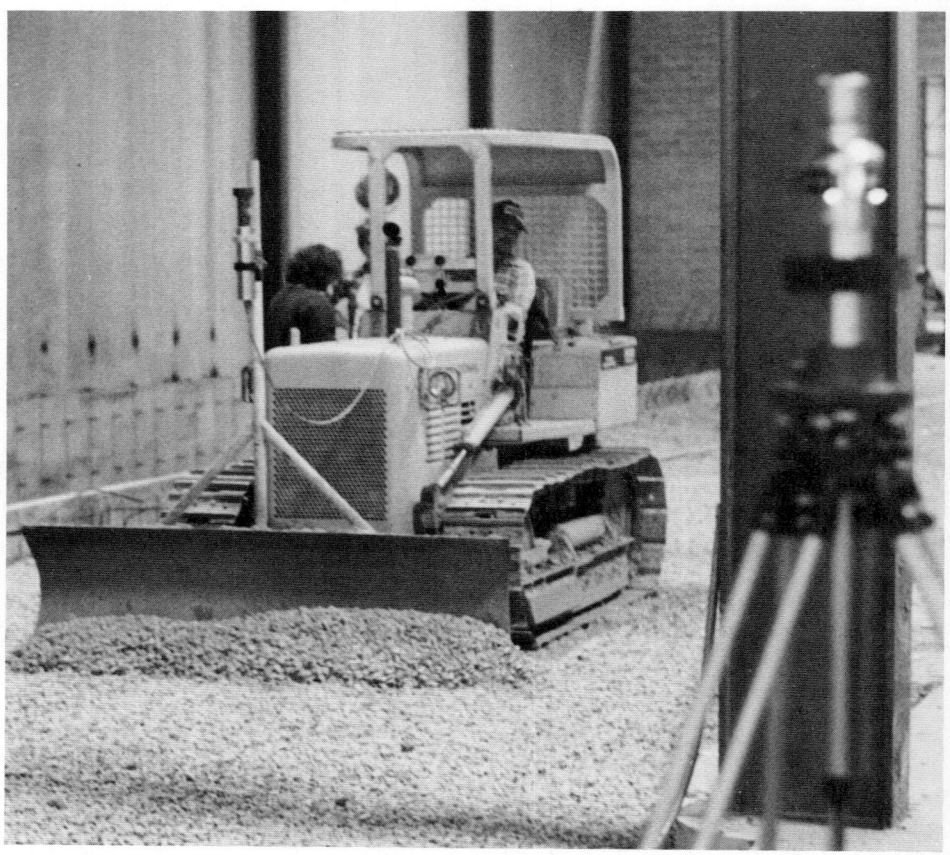

Figure 18-8. A Laser Sensor. A sensor which detects a rotating He-Ne laser beam is mounted above a bulldozer blade to permit accurate grading. The sensor moves up and down automatically to indicate the plane of the scanning laser beam. The dozer operator then adjusts the blade to maintain proper grading. Photograph courtesy of Laser Alignment, Inc., Grand Rapids, Michigan.

Rule #7. The laser beam should be terminated at the end of its useful beam path and should in all cases be terminated if the beam hazard extends beyond the controlled area of the construction site. The hazardous distance is defined as the point where the beam irradiance is $2.5 \text{ mW} \cdot \text{cm}^{-2}$.

Rule #8. Laser equipment should bear a label to indicate the maximum output and the nominal ocular hazard distance beyond which the laser beam irradiance is not expected to exceed $2.5 \text{ mW} \cdot \text{cm}^{-2}$.

Safety with Construction Lasers 603

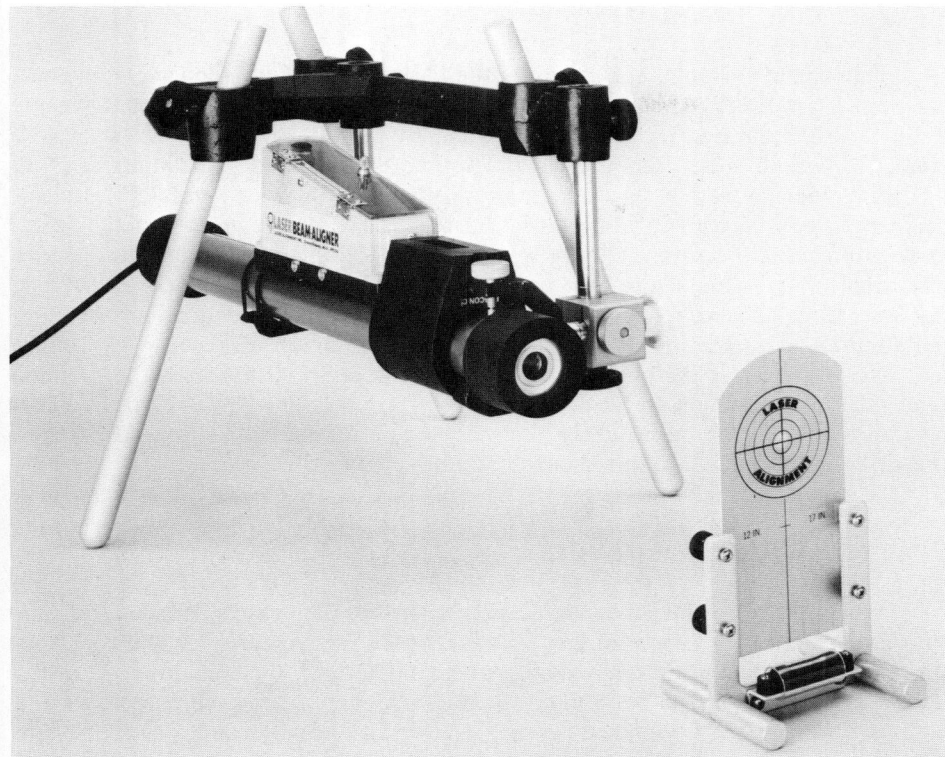

Figure 18-9. Translucent Alignment Target. Translucent plastic alignment targets are used in laying sewer pipe. Generally, a reticle of concentric circles is painted on the target to permit rapid centering. The plastic screen is mounted in a jig designed for the size of pipe and quick placement in the pipe opening. Photograph courtesy of Laser Alignment, Inc., Grand Rapids, Michigan.

Rule #9. When the laser is not being used it should be stored in a location where unauthorized personnel cannot gain access to it.

Rule #10. Placement of the laser beam path at or near eye level should be avoided whenever feasible. In sewer pipe alignment if the beam is in the ground it is normally well below eye level.

Rule #11. Precautions should be taken to ensure that the laser is not pointed at mirror-like (specular) surfaces.

Rule #12. Use the lowest power laser suitable for the particular construction task. Higher powers than required merely introduce additional hazards. The visibility of a laser beam may be enhanced by the appropriate eyewear filter (see section 16.3). Also, a modulated beam (4 to 10 hz) may be more easily identified over long distances.

18.6 WEIGHING THE RISKS

This chapter should not close on the subject of helium-neon surveying and alignment lasers leaving the erroneous impression that these devices present serious public health hazards. The present low accident rate experienced with at least a hundred thousand such lasers used in the United States is proof that the hazard is not serious. What must be remembered is that the probability of an accidental intrabeam exposure is very low, and that, to date, these devices have been treated by most users with adequate caution. It is then to everyone's best interest that this attitude of caution be maintained, and that the respect for these devices is not lost. There is only one sure method to accomplish this objective: assure adequately informed operators. The construction industry notes that the use of lasers for sewer pipe alignment actually reduces the overall hazards. This reduction results from the reduced period that the workmen are in deep ditches subject to the serious risk of cave-ins. Apparently cave-ins are more likely as time passes after excavation since the trench walls dry out and earth movement becomes more likely.

18.7 TYPICAL LASER PRODUCTS

Table 18-1 provides the characteristic output parameters, and hazard and caution distances of a variety of laser products used for alignment in the construction industry. The output parameters are manufacturer specifications or actual measured values obtained by Sliney and his associates. Table 18-2 provides the details on a variety of presently available laser distance measuring systems. The "hazard distance" applied to momentary viewing (i.e., 0.25 s, where the EL = 2.5 mW/cm^2). The "caution distance" is that distance where the beam irradiance falls below the long-term staring exposure limit (i.e., the EL for $t > 10^4$ s).

18.8 REVIEW QUESTIONS

1. Helium-Neon lasers have been used for long-distance measurement and Gallium-Arsenide lasers for shorter-distance measurement because of the tighter divergence characteristics of the He-Ne laser. T or F?

2. Calculate the hazard distance and caution distances of a laser geodimeter having a beam output power of 7 mW, wavelength 632.8 nm, output beam diameter of 1.2 cm and a beam divergence of 0.2 mrad.

3. What is the value of having a key switch master control on a 2.5-mW alignment laser used for aligning ceilings?

4. A laser emits 7 mW in a 360° horizontal beam plane. The beam is a fan and does not rotate. The vertical divergence is 1 mrad. Can this laser be Class 2 or Class 3A? Could it meet the requirements of 21CFR1040.11(b)?

Safety with Construction Lasers

TABLE 18.1 Typical He-Ne Laser Alignment Systems

Manufacturer	Model	Emergent Beam Diameter (cm)	Emergent Beam Divergence (mrad)*	Average Emergent Beam Radiant Power (mW)	Emergent Beam Irradiance Averaged over 7-mm Aperture (mW/cm^2)	Hazard Distance (m)	Caution Distance (km)
Allied	930, 930-30	1.0	0.1	2.0	5.2	<100	1.2
Blout & George	AGL-S-352	0.7	0.1	1.9	4.9	<100	1.2
	AGL-TCL	1.0	0.1	2.3	5.8	<100	1.3
	AGL-LTL	—	0.1	1.6	4.1	<100	1.1
	AGL-LTL-11A	0.7	0.1	3.5	9.1	<140	1.6
Coherent Radiation	Gradomat I to IV	0.7	0.1	1.9	4.9	28	1.2
Construction Laser Systems	Accubeam IIA	1.0	0.8	1.7	2.2	0	140
	Accubeam IV & V	0.8	0.8	1.2	2.6	1	0.1
	Accusweep 710 and 711	1.1	0.8	1.1	2.3	0	0.1
	Tru-Square TS-40	0.6	0.8	2.1	5.4		0.16
Keufel & Esser	740130	4.0	0.1	2.5	0.4	0	1.4
	712600	1.0	0.1	0.7	1.8	0	0.73
	712605	1.1	0.1	0.7	1.4	0	0.73
Laser Alignment	1278	0.8	0.1	2.4	6.3	<100	1.3
	1348	0.6	0.1	2.4	5.4	<100	1.2
	2100	0.5	0.1	2.3	6.0	<100	1.3
	2300	0.6	0.1	2.5	6.5	<100	1.4
	2400	0.6	0.1	2.1	5.4	<100	1.2
	2500	0.6	0.1	2.3	5.8	<100	1.3
	2600	0.6	0.1	2.4	6.1	<100	1.3
Spectra-Physics	611	3.3	0.06	5.0	1.2	0	1.9
	655	—	—	2.2	5.7	<100	1.5
	833 Tunnel Laser	—	0.1	2.2	5.7	<100	1.3
	840 Rotolite	—	0.1	4.0	10	<100	1.7
	842 Rotolite	0.3	0.1	4.0	10	<100	1.7
	855 Dial-A-Grade	0.6	0.1	2.4	6.2	<100	1.3
	944 Laser Level SL	0.7	0.12	3.0	5.4	30	1.0
Trice V Developments	Plan-O-Lite Model A	0.2 by 17	1.0 by 6280	3.5	1.0	0	

*Most alignment lasers are adjusted to have a minimal spot at approximately 100 m and are therefore "focused." It is difficult to place an accurate effective divergence for any of these laser products, although most that have been measured at distances greater than 100 m approach 0.1 mrad.

TABLE 18-2. Commercial Laser Distance Measuring Systems

Manufacturer	Model	Wavelength (nm)	Emergent Beam Diameter (cm)	Emergent Beam* Divergence (mr)	Average Emergent Beam Radiant Power (mW)	Emergent Beam† Irradiance (mW/cm²)	Hazard# Distance (m)	Caution# Distance (km)
AGA	Model 4L, He-Ne	632.8	1.2	0.1	1.3	1.1	10	3.5
AGA	Model 4LA, He-Ne	632.8	0.72	0.07	6.8	16.5	300	9
AGA	Model 8, He-Ne	632.8	0.84	0.1	4.1	7.3		
AGA	Model 76, He-Ne	632.8	1.2	1.3	0.9	0.92	0	
Cubic Industrial	Cubitape DM6, GaAs	910	4.0	1.8	8.8			
Cubic Industrial	Cubitape DM60, GaAs	910	4.0	1.8	0.0088	0.00045	0	0
Hewlett-Packard	Model 3800, GaAs	910	3.3	4.0	0.0024	0.00012	0	0
Hewlett-Packard	Model 3805, GaAs	910	2.9	4.8	0.0023	0.00012	0	0
Keufel & Esser	LSE Rangemaster, He-Ne	632.8	0.54	0.064	4	2.3	0	0
Keufel & Esser	LSE Ranger I, He-Ne	632.8	1.2		3.0	5.3		2.5
Keufel & Esser	LSE Ranger II, He-Ne	632.8	1.2		3.0	5.3		4
Keufel & Esser	LSE Ranger III, He-Ne	632.8	1.2	0.08	1.3	1.4	0	1.0
Keufel & Esser	LSE Ranger IV, He-Ne	915	1.4	0.07	2.2	1.5	0	1.6
Keufel & Esser	LSE Microranger, GaAs	915	2.8	4	210	0.035	0	0
Spectra-Physics	Geodolite 3A, He-Ne	632.8		1	24	12		
Spectra-Physics	Geodolite 3G, He-Ne	632.8	0.72	0.1 to 1.5	6	12	40	1.3
Spectra-Physics	LT3, He-Ne	632.8			7	10	50	7
Spectra-Physics	Model 611, He-Ne	632.8	3.3	0.06	1.0			
Plessy Group	Tellurometer, MA 100, GaAs	910		4.2			0	
Wild-Heenbrugg	Distomat DI-10, GaAlAs	875	3.5	4.2	0.08	0.009	0	0

†Average over 7-mm aperture.
*Defined at 1/e points.
#Without intrabeam viewing with optics.

5. What is the basis of the 1-mW limit for Class 2 lasers?

6. What is the upper limit in power permitted by the OSHA construction laser safety standard?

7. What would be the applicable irradiance limit for calculating a caution distance for a wavelength of 442 nm? for 632.8 nm?

8. What is the exposure limit used to calculate a hazard distance for a CW visible laser beam operating at 442 nm? at 632.8 nm?

9. Does a rotating-beam visible laser alignment system have to have a scan-failure interlock?

10. What is the OSHA requirement for eye protection with construction lasers? What is the practical effect of this role?

18.9 REFERENCES

American National Standards Institute, 1976, The Safe Use of Lasers, Standard Z-136.1, (with proposed revision 1979).

Blabla, J., and John, J., 1966, The saturation effect in retina measured by means of He-Ne laser, *Am. J. Ophth.* **62**:659–663.

British Standards Institute, 1972, Protection of personnel against hazards from laser radiation BS4803, British Standards Institution, London.

Bureau of Radiological Health, 1979, Title 21, Code of Federal Regulations (CRF), 1979 ed., Part 1040, "Performance Standards for Light-Emitting Products."

Davis, T. P., and Mautner, W. J., 1969, Helium-Neon laser effect on the eye, Report C106-59223, EG&G Inc., Santa Monica Division, Los Angeles, CA (April 1969).

Fender, D. H., 1964, Control mechanisms of the eye, *Sci. Am.* **211**(1):24–33.

Ham, W. T., Jr., Geeraets, W. J., Mueller, H. A., Williams, R. C., Clarke, A. M., and Cleary, S. F., 1970, Retinal burn thresholds for the helium-neon laser in the rhesus monkey, *Arch. Ophth.* **84**:797–809.

Lappin, P. W., 1970, Ocular damage thresholds for the helium-neon laser, *Arch. Environ. Health* (Chicago) **20**:177–183.

Sliney, D. H., 1968, The amazing laser, Trans. of the 56th National Safety Congress, Chicago, *National Safety Council* **8**:38–44.

Sliney, D. H., 1974, Lasers in construction, *Natl. Safety Cong. Trans.* **8**:19–21.

Sliney, D. H., 1971, Laser distance measuring equipment used by US Army Topographic Command, US Army Environmental Hygiene Agency Special Study No. 42-073-71 (February-April 1971) (AD 729346).

U.S. Department of Labor (OSHA), 1977, Title 29, Code of Federal Regulations (CFR), 1977 ed., Part 1910, "Occupational Safety and Health Standards."

Chapter 19
Safety with Lasers Used in Manufacturing

19.1 INTRODUCTION

The first industrial applications of the laser were in the field of material processing. Pulsed ruby lasers were used for drilling small holes in the diamond dies used for pulling thin wire at the Western Electric Company as early as 1965 (Charschan, 1972). Since then many more industrial production line applications have evolved. The laser is now used for microwelding, microdrilling, scribing ceramic materials, surface treating, high-speed marking, precision wire stripping, resistor trimming, and integrated circuit manufacture. These types of industrial material processing laser systems now generally make use of a CO_2 laser or a neodymium YAG laser, operating CW or repetitively pulsed. Dependent upon whether the material is to be drilled or welded, a short or longer pulse duration will be employed. The highest CW powers are available from CO_2 lasers; therefore, CO_2 lasers are used for the heavy-duty applications. In any event, all of these laser applications present similar hazards. These include viewing the heated material, or exposure to the airborne contaminates produced in this material processing. The amount of toxic material produced by very small units is normally not significant enough to warrant local ventilation. However, in larger units, where significant amounts of material are released, local exhaust ventilation is often needed. Chapter 26 considers these ancillary hazards of laser material processing. The present chapter concentrates on the hazards from the laser radiation itself.

For most equipment now used on production lines, either the manufacturer or the user of the laser system normally encloses the target area to prevent direct viewing of the laser beam impact on the material. In research laboratories, no such precautions are formally required, and it is not uncommon to find a laser welder or driller apparatus without an enclosure.

Lasers such as He-Ne and Argon CW are used for nondestructive testing and

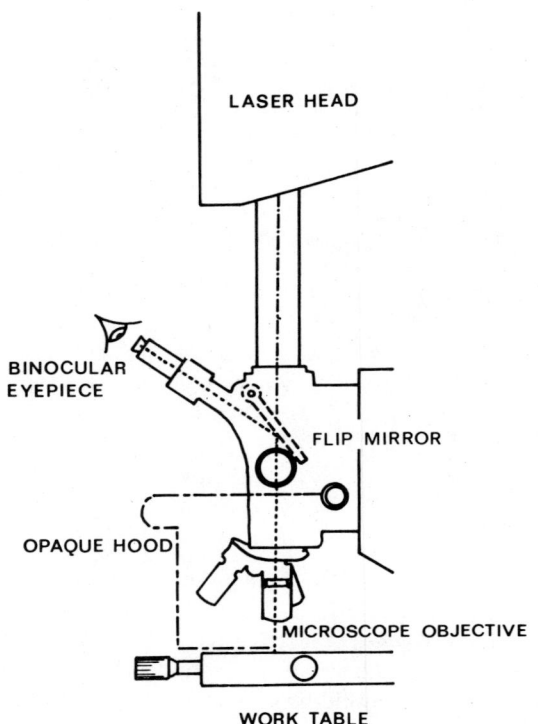

Figure 19-1. Viewing Optics. Fail-safe procedure for assuring that target reflections do not reach the operator's eye. The use of a flip mirror which blocked direct eye exposure was often used in early ruby laser microdrilling systems.

measurement. Some, but not all, non-destructive testing techniques make use of holography. The hazards associated with these applications are for the most part somewhat different than for material processing applications.

19.2 NEODYMIUM:YAG LASER MATERIAL PROCESSING

The most commonly used laser for small scale material processing (e.g., in the electronics industry) is the neodymium:YAG laser which operates at 1064 nm. Output energy typically ranges from 50 to 500 mJ per pulse for pulsed lasers and from 10 W to 100 W for CW lasers. Because the 1064-nm wavelength is in the retinal hazard region, relatively low-power reflections can be a serious hazard if they are from a specular (glass or polished metal) surface.

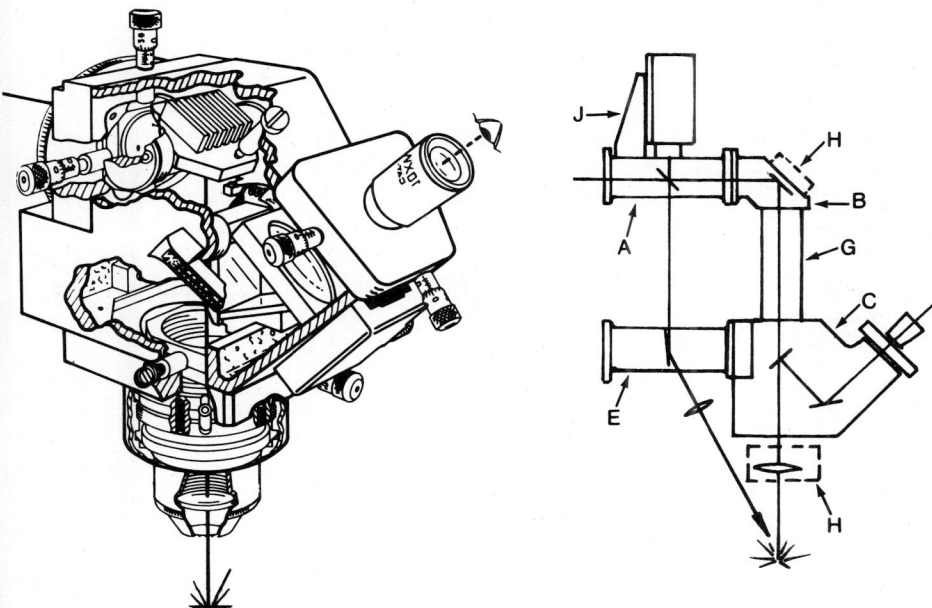

Figure 19-2. Two Types of Commercial Viewer Configurations with Flip Mirrors. Target enclosures are not shown. The left panel shows a system used with a Nd:YAG laser and the right panel shows a viewer which also includes a closed circuit TV (CCTV) as well as conventional optics for on- or off-axis viewing the water cooled lens. Courtesy of Optimation, Londonderry, New Hampshire.

19.2.1 Viewing Optics

In microdrilling and microwelding apparatus the laser beam is usually focused by a microscope objective. The microscope's viewing optics are used to position the target material. Although some very early laser microwelding and microdrilling equipment did not incorporate safety shutters, it is now almost universal that a fail-safe viewing system be utilized. A typical example is shown in Figure 19-1. The target area can only be observed when mirror M-1 is in position. In the viewing position the direct laser beam is blocked to ensure that no laser radiation is transmitted through M-1 to be reflected back through the viewing optics into the operator's eye. An electrical shutter or similar device would not alone to considered sufficiently fail-safe for this application.

Some manufacturers of microwelding and microdrilling equipment have found that closed circuit TV displays compare favorably in cost to the optical components in a direct view microscope. Also, some users prefer this indirect approach as the target may be seen during laser impact. Of course the camera tube must be protected from reflected laser radiation. Indeed, the usual eye protective filters are often used for this purpose. Figure 19-2 shows the design of two Optimation laser control viewers; the unit shown in the right-hand panel was designed for use with CO_2 far-infrared radiation as well. The CO_2 laser wavelength requires the use of reflecting optics and a far-IR lens such as zinc selenide (ZnSe) germanium (Ge), Cadmium telluride (CdTe), or gallium-arsenide (GaAs) since glass is opaque at that wavelength.

An alternative to a shutter is the incorporation of eye protective filters into the viewing optics. This removes the necessity for any fail-safe shutter system in the viewing optics. The neodymium laser has an advantage in this respect as its wavelength is sufficiently outside of the normal visible spectrum for protective filters (e.g., Schott KG-3) to combine ample visibility with high attenuation at the laser wavelength. Figure 16-5 provides spectral transmittance curves for filters used with neodymium lasers.

19.2.2 Enclosures

Once the hazard has been minimized for the direct beam path, the possibility that a bystander, or even the operator himself, may view the target directly during laser irradiation is lessened. Many different approaches have been followed in eliminating or reducing this hazard because of the myriad of applications. In some operations enclosures are installed around the work place. The time required to open the enclosure, insert the material, and close the enclosure can become significant with a repeat of this process for each operation. This time may not be considered a serious drawback because of the long duration of the entire manufacturing procedure. On the other hand, high volume production lines may make automatic-feed modifications economical.

The safe design requirements of most industrial production lines requires the use of a total beam enclosure. This eliminates the need for eye protection, enclosed rooms, medical surveillance of personnel, and any controversies concerning alleged exposures. Recent federal regulations encourage strongly, or even in some cases require, enclosure of the entire operation to the point that the accessible radiation does not exceed the permissible exposure limits. The definitions of accessibility become very important for these applications. For instance, a shield around the work piece which does not completely touch the base may be satisfactory in practice, if it can be shown that hazardous radiation levels are not scattered and reflected through this opening. This may be exceedingly difficult to prove, since the range of materials that might be placed in the laser system have such different reflectance characteristics that some radiation may leak through those small openings. According to the Federal performance standard, the permissible size of the opening would be quite small to preclude accessibility. Effectively, the opening should bar a straight line probe of any diameter and 1-m long in the BRH standard openings larger than 5 cm in diameter (simulating a small hand) were not to be allowed in a proposed (1977) OSHA standard. Interlocks should be required on the equipment to disable the laser or at least otherwise ensure that the beam will not exit from the system if the protective enclosure is out of position.

Safety with Lasers Used in Manufacturing

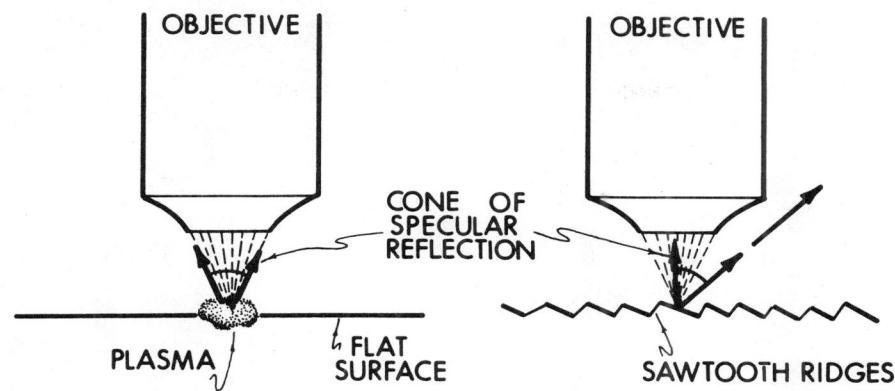

Figure 19-3. Target Reflections. The reflections which are not terminated by the objective assembly are almost always diffuse in nature (A) unless from a machined ruled surface (B); but even then, plasma formation would cause diffuse reflections.

19.2.3 Reflections

Studies conducted at the U.S. Army Environmental Hygiene Agency show that ruby and neodymium laser beam irradiances capable of causing surface ablation in any material are orders of magnitude above safe exposure limits for specular (mirror-like) reflections and are even almost always about the safe viewing levels for diffuse reflections. This is to say, any unprotected view of a laser target, close enough to appear as an extended source, is hazardous for wavelengths in the retinal hazard region (400–1400 nm). As previously noted, laser microwelders and microdrillers, during their exploratory development, were operated with the target area open for the greatest flexibility. The question arises as to why observers did not receive retinal burns when looking at these target areas during laser exposure. The answer is that the beam was focused to a very small spot (10–100 μm); the specular reflection was terminated by the objective assembly (left panel of Figure 19-3); the diffuse reflection was effectively a point source for anyone viewing the target from the side; and the operator viewed through protective filters in the microscope viewing optics if he or she viewed the target at all. An extended analysis of the situation follows.

The major hazard to the bystander is the diffuse reflection. This reflection irradiance decreases inversely as the square of the distance from the target. The specular components of the reflection are normally directed in a cone upward toward the beam focusing optics and terminated by the optical housing unless the target has very unusual surfaces as shown in Figure 19-3 (right panel). For a Q-switched laser drilling unit the hazardous viewing distance r_{haz} is estimated with the following

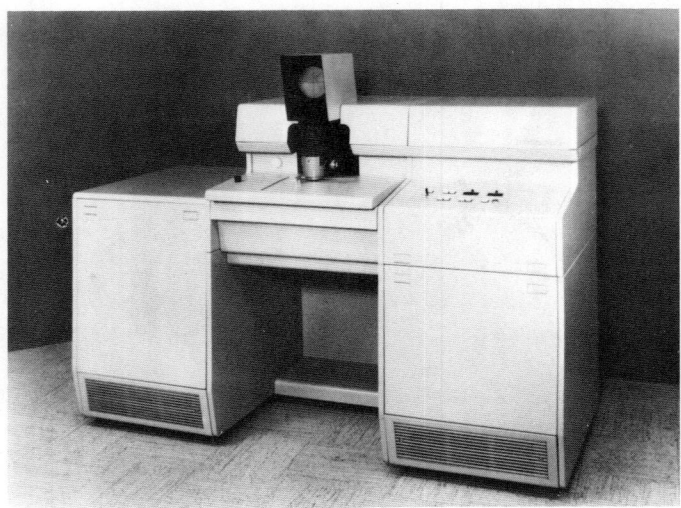

Figure 19-4. Enclosed Laser System. Laser micromachining device with interlocked cover over target (courtesy of Quantronix).

formula derived from Lambert's Law (Eq. 2-6):

$$r_{haz} = \sqrt{Q \cdot \rho_\lambda \cdot \cos\theta / \pi H_{EL}} \qquad (19\text{-}1)$$

where θ is the smallest angle from the beam axis for viewing the target, ρ_λ is the diffuse reflectance of the target, H_{EL} is the permissible exposure limit (e.g., H_{EL} is 3×10^{-6} J/cm² for a single, 200-μs pulse from a ruby laser, and H_{EL} is 1.5×10^{-5} J/cm² for a single 200-μs neodymium laser pulse). From Eq. 19-1 it can be calculated that a 1-joule ruby laser beam incident upon a target with a 20% diffuse reflectance will produce a hazardous reflection at a 60° angle from the vertical for a distance of 1.03 m. Actual measurements of the reflected levels in this case would typically be below this because of self absorption by the plume formed by target ablation. However, a consideration of a possible target surface with its multi-angled specular elements (Fig. 19-3, right panel) shows the need for shielding to prevent reflections if total safety is to be assured. Figure 19-4 shows a Class 1 production laser system with interlocked enclosure.

19.3 HIGH-POWER CO_2 LASER CUTTING AND WELDING EQUIPMENT (1 kW to 20 kW)

The engineering safeguards appropriate for low energy lasers discussed in the previous section are also applicable in many cases to the very high-powered laser

Safety with Lasers Used in Manufacturing

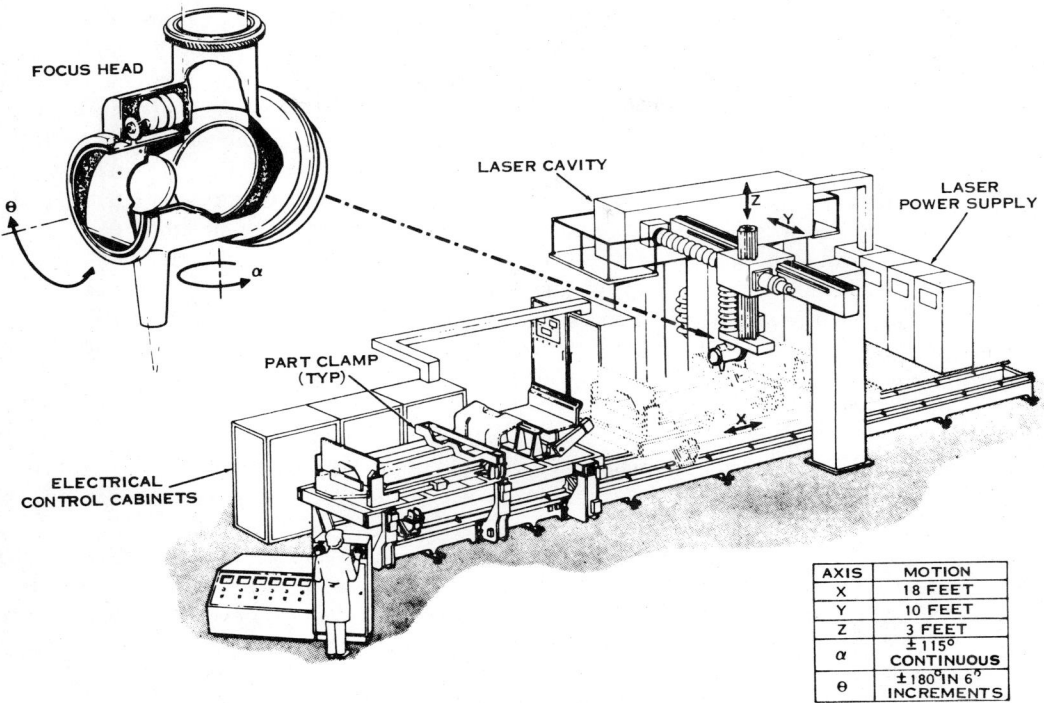

Figure 19-5. High-power experimental CO_2 laser (3 kW CW) system which welds automatically (from Hoag *et al.*, 1974).

systems used in certain material processing systems. Very high power CO_2 laser systems have entered the commercial market for production welding. These systems most often use dynamic flow CO_2 lasers, and typically have an output power of between 2 kW and 20 kW. This is sufficient for the rapid automated welding of various metal structures including batteries and automotive bodies, and also for cutting aluminum. In most of the production applications, safety policy requires total enclosure of the operation such as the one shown in Fig. 19-5. Both local opaque enclosures of steel or aluminum, and small, room-like enclosures of polymethylmethacrylate (e.g., Lucite or Plexiglas) or similar transparent materials which are opaque to far-infrared laser radiation are found. Plate glass shields would be less suitable since glass would shatter upon beam impact rather than burn.

High speed laser welding or cutting of metals forms many of the same metal oxides and other fumes as conventional welding operations. In addition to the general ventilation which is sufficient for conventional welding, local exhaust ventilation may be required to remove the potentially hazardous metal fumes and metal oxides. The laser process may, after all, be much faster than the conventional arc process, hence the greater potential volume of fumes. Plastic enclosures can normally not withstand long-term exposure to irradiances greater than 1 W/cm^2 without gradual surface deterioration. However, in most applications such high irradiances are seldom reached at the surface of the enclosure. While metal enclosures can withstand higher reflected irradiances, such surfaces are specular and may increase the hazard zone by reflections. Interlocks are generally considered essential to assure that the laser will not operate when entry is possible into the enclosure.

With the higher power systems, misalignment of the beam delivery optics can produce the most serious problems. The reduced output power from misalignment can prevent ablation of the metal target surface and thereby create hazardous specular reflections. This should be noted by all developmental and service personnel, as malfunction or reduction in power, in this case, almost uniquely, increases the hazard.

The semiconducting materials such as Ge, GaAs, ZnSe, and CdTe which are used in focusing lenses can be damaged by "thermal runaway" which at first causes beam distortion, and finally a loss of power. Ignition of some of these optical materials produces hazardous airborne contaminants (e.g., from ZnSe). Thermal runaway can be caused by the use of a poorly designed lens system, by operating the laser above the power rating of the lens and by contaminants on the exterior lens surface. A high-volume gas flow shield is generally used to prevent fumes from the target from reaching the lens surface. Unfortunately, the gas flow rate required to be totally effective may produce splatter from the melted target, hence the flow rate must be carefully controlled to provide the needed protection of the lens surface without serious spattering. Specht (1977) recommends the use of automatic gas flow interlocks and flow gages rather than pressure gages to alleviate this problem. The surface of the workpiece is often tilted to limit back reflections into the lens. While protecting the lens from specular reflections this approach does send the reflected beam elsewhere—where it should be terminated safely. It is obvious that poorly trained operators or service personnel could create hazardous situations by improperly cleaning lenses, improper placement of clamps and cooling hoses, misalignment of optical and mechanical parts, and by not setting the proper focus.

CO_2 lasers have also been used for high speed marking of wooden crates. In these cases the lasers are used often in a relatively open assembly line without complete enclosure, although some baffling is used so that the beam path is not readily accessible. It is easy enough to imagine how a laser container marking system could be set up so that wooden crates could go down a conveyor belt, stop in front of a large open aperture and the beam could scribe on the wood without real concern about hazardous reflections. Only a specular, metallic surface, such as crating metal bands or nail heads would produce hazardous specular reflections. However, if the aperture port is sufficiently close to the crate, and if a shield around the open aperture extended for sufficient distance to terminate the specular reflections, then this could be considered an essentially safe operation. The metal surfaces would have to be at off angles from the scribing port to produce reflected secondary beams out in the open. Obviously baffles and shields could be set up in such a way as to effectively eliminate any chance of hazardous reflections to personnel in the general area.

CO_2 lasers have been used in high speed assembly lines to punch holes in non-metallic surfaces such as plastics or rubber materials, e.g., puncturing holes in rubber nipples for baby bottles. In such instances the beam is chopped or repetitively pulsed such that a focused beam drills a hole only at the precise instant that the object is underneath the beam objective. Hazardous reflections would not be expected unless metal surfaces were within the conveyor area. Transparent plastic baffles placed around the entrance into the laser device would effectively shield most individuals from hazardous exposure to the far infrared. Similar levels of power have been used to burn off paint surfaces on bottle caps and other containers in rapidly moving bottle works. In all cases the individual exposures are not sufficient to produce hazardous reflections at reasonable distances. Such devices are, nevertheless, normally Class 4 and the user must design some general arrangement of shields and baffles to attenuate potentially hazardous reflections near the scribing area. Somewhat similar applications involve the use of CO_2 lasers for cutting fabric for wearing apparel in production tailoring. In these instances the beam or the fabric table moves to permit computerized cutting along predetermined paths. The beam path is open for 1-10 cm above the table, and unless metal objects were placed on top of the cutting board (e.g., a pair of conventional scissors or other small tools) hazardous reflections would not be a problem. Administrative controls and barriers are used to keep people from getting onto the table during operation, and the beam path is seldom within arm's reach.

19.4 LASERS IN THE PRINTING INDUSTRY

Lasers have been employed in a variety of applications in the printing industry. He-Ne lasers have been extensively used in scanning-beam optical readers of copy, and higher power lasers have been used in the preparation of printing plates (i.e., "laser plate making"). In these applications the lasers have typically been enclosed and the products have been classified as Class I. In some cases the users of the equipment have been unaware that a laser was being used in the system.

He-Ne laser beams used in the "reader" applications scan the "paste-up" copy in order to digitize copy in much the same manner as the facsimile process. The laser beam can be used as an optical character reader to read the printed material which may then be introduced into a computer for playback in a CRT display for computer editing. The copy to be scanned is either placed on a rotating drum below a static laser beam or is on a flat bed below a scanning laser beam. In either case, in commercial systems the laser exposure area is interlocked and not accessible during operation.

The lasers actually used to manufacture printing plates depend upon which of the several processes used. Both letterpress or offset plates have been manufactured. Letterpress plates were traditionally composed of lead to form raised letters which transferred the ink from rollers to paper. Offset plates have traditionally been manufactured by photographic and photoresist methods and do not have raised letters. The letters are treated with an ink-retentive material that picks up the ink from the rollers and transfers it to the paper. This latter type of plate was the first candidate for laser employment.

At least one manufacturer has produced CO_2 laser systems to make a raised-letter type of plate—the flexographic plate used in printing wallpaper and fabrics. Figure 19.6 (lower panel) illustrates this process. Since the CO_2 laser actually burned away plastic materials, the engraving head had to be enclosed for fume extraction. The Laser Technique process (Doxey, 1977) started with a flexographic cylinder with a plastic or hard-rubber coating covered by a thin copper layer. The copper was etched to produce a mask for the laser exposure. A 240-W CO_2 laser beam was reflected from the remaining copper negative image but burned away the exposed plastic or rubber, thus creating a raised printing cylinder. In a commercial product of this nature both the reading laser and the engraving laser exposure sites are enclosed.

A more common type of laser printing plate process uses an Ar laser to expose a photographic negative. An example of this process is the EOCOM system shown in the top panel of Figure 19.6. The photographic negative is then employed in a conventional plate maker where an intense ultraviolet source (e.g., a carbon arc or mercury arc lamp) exposes the photo-offset plate. Once reliable UV lasers are available that operate in the proper wavelength region, the intermediate step of producing a negative could be dropped.

Another process (LogEtronic, Inc.) makes use of an infrared neodymium-YAG laser beam to thermally treat an ink-retentive material on a bare metal plate to produce a photo-offset type of plate. In this system, as in the others, the entire laser exposure site is totally enclosed. With all of these systems, the principal hazards would relate to laser servicing with the enclosure opened and to the potentially hazardous airborne contaminants produced in some of the processes.

19.5 ANCILLARY HAZARDS

The ancillary hazards of high power lasers are covered in detail in Chapter 27. The following material is placed here to alert the reader to those problems particular to materials processing.

19.5.1 Noise Hazards

Micromachining systems would not be expected to present a noise hazard. However, some recent, multi-kilowatt laser systems for high volume production lines deserve attention in this regard. For hearing conservation measures see section 27.7. Hazardous noise levels generally exist only in the immediate vicinity of the laser or target where personnel are usually excluded for other safety reasons.

19.5.2 Airborne Contaminants

Many of the materials required for laser operation as well as the byproducts produced by the laser during operations, or by beam interaction with the target in

Safety with Lasers Used in Manufacturing

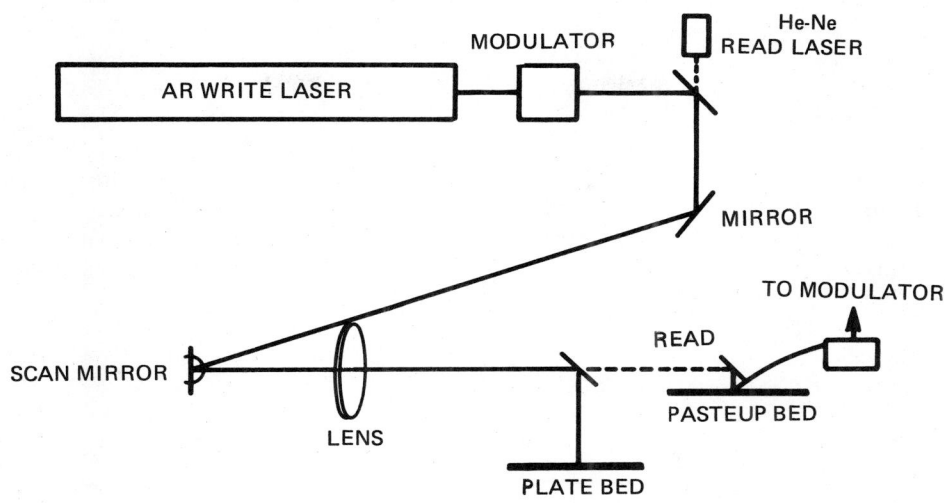

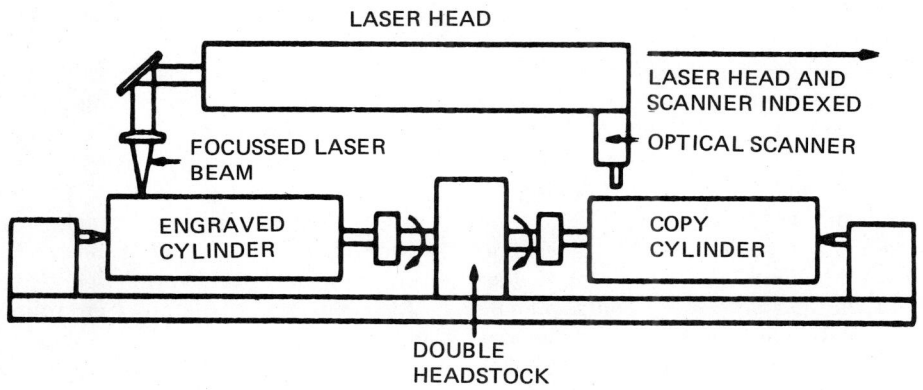

Figure 19-6. Lasers Used in Platemaking. Top photo employs Class 4 Argon laser for rapid scan exposure of photo-offset plates. Digitized signal from pasteup can be sent to satellite printing plants (courtesy EOCOM, Irvine, CA). Bottom photo shows a 240-W Class 4 CO_2 laser system engraving letter press cylinder plates. A metallic (copper) mask or controlled beam output is used to produce the image (from Doxey, 1977, with permission).

materials processing are potentially hazardous. Exposure of operating personnel to those hazardous materials should be kept below established safe concentrations. This can be accomplished by local or dilution ventilation, isolation, shielding, the use of personal protective devices, and other engineering or administrative controls. Airborne contaminants are normally captured near the point of evolution before they have a chance to be distributed throughout the room. Local exhaust systems should be designed to provide a capture velocity of 100 to 150 linear feet per minute in the direction of the exhaust inlet at the point of contaminant evolution. The exhaust inlet should be designed to ensure contaminant capture. For this purpose, total enclosure is optimal but not always attainable. Thus, efforts should be made to enclose as much of the contaminant source as is practical. The location of the exhaust inlet should be selected to take advantage of the natural movement of the contaminant. The material, however, should not be allowed to pass through an individual's breathing zone enroute to the exhaust inlet.

19.6 NONDESTRUCTIVE TESTING

A variety of lasers are used for nondestructive testing in manufacturing. One of the best methods of nondestructive testing involves double exposure laser holographic interferometry to produce an interferogram of a surface placed under stress during one of the exposures and released from stress during the other. A hologram is recorded of an object and the second holographic exposure is made of the object being strained while in its same position. The light from the strained object passes directly through the hologram and interferes with the constructed wave of the unstrained object in some applications of holographic strain interferometry. Pulsed ruby lasers have been used for this as well as frequency-doubled neodymium-YAG (532 nm) lasers where very short pulsed exposure is desirable, as in testing a vibrating engine. An argon laser and sometimes even a helium-neon laser have also been used in some twin exposure holographic interferogram systems such as the one shown in Fig. 19-7. Often such techniques are used to sample only a small lot of products and such equipment is generally not found on the production line. When such equipment is found in a particular laboratory or test cell it is often operated in the open, and procedural controls analogous to an open laser laboratory are followed. In other instances, such as the tire analyzer shown in Fig. 19-7, the device is made into a Class 1 product by enclosing the entire holographic exposure process. Since holograms normally must be taken in total darkness the enclosure serves a dual purpose. Although high power Class 4 lasers are generally required for producing a holographic exposure on film the viewing of the hologram may be through the use of a Class 2 or a Class 3 helium-neon laser. In this case, off-axis holographic viewing, such as shown in Fig. 20-2, is obviously to be desired.

Class 2 lasers are also employed in precise machine tool alignment and as non-contact laser micrometers. For example, one company (Techmet Co.) produces a scanning He-Ne laser micrometer which uses a 0.2-mW beam to continuously measure wire diameter. In this system it would be impossible to place one's head in the beam although the beam is accessible in an opening.

Safety with Lasers Used in Manufacturing 621

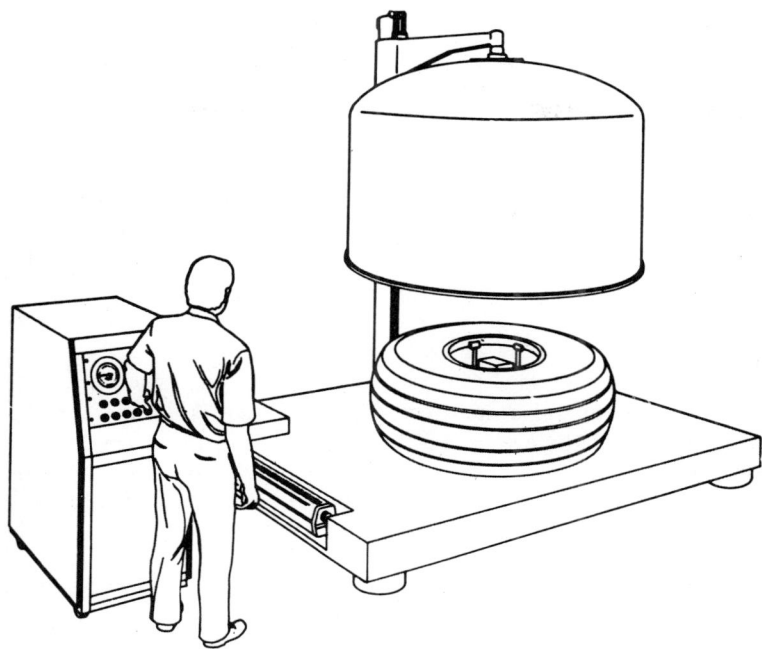

Figure 19-7. Nondestructive Testing. This NRC Tire Inspector 4 is used to locate structural defects by using a double-exposure hologram technique. The laser operates only when the cover is down (courtesy of Newport Research Corporation, CA).

19.7 REVIEW QUESTIONS

1. A laser scribing system has an access panel for items moving on a conveyor belt into the laser enclosure which is a heavy rubber flap. The flap touches the conveyor belt and 2-cm high object pass through the flexible door. Would this type of enclosure meet the accessibility criteria for Class 1 systems under BRH? Suppose the rubber flaps were replaced by rigid baffles such that no straight line access to the laser was possible and the flexible line distance was 35 cm; that is, items on the conveyor belt did not pass through any opening and closing doors but merely through an aperture in the housing and were moved to the left through a narrow corridor into another enclosure after undergoing two right-angle turns in their passage into the exposure chamber. Would this entrance arrangement complete the BRH requirements?

2. A 0.4-J neodymium-YAG laser with a 20-ns pulse width is used in a microdrilling operation where there is insufficient enclosure of the target. An individual views the target from an angle of 45° at a distance of 1 m. If the reflectance of the plasma is 8%, what will be the radiant exposure at the

individual's eye? Will it exceed the permissible exposure for a single pulse case?

3. A double-pulsed (30-ns) ruby system is used in nondestructive testing of large aircraft structures. The output energy per pulse is 5 J; the two pulses are 2 µs apart; the emergent beam diameter is 0.4 cm; the divergence is 0.3 rad and the surface being exposed is 2 m away. Some flat polished surfaces on the target are exposed and could redirect the beam back at the operator's eye. The operator is 3 m from the reflection. What will be the exposure at the operator's eye? What optical density for safety goggles would you recommend for this operator?

4. A CO_2 TEA laser is used to scribe bottle caps. The irradiance at the cap is 1 kW/cm² and the pulse duration is 200 ns. What is the radiant exposure at the bottle cap? If there were 100% reflection, and the beam divergence from the 1-cm diameter illuminated area was 5 mrad, what would be the radiant exposure at 1 m from the bottle cap? Would this exceed permissible exposure limits for a single pulse; for 100 pulses per second?

5. Sketch a production line facility where a laser scriber could operate for scribing wooden and cardboard containers. The area of the scribe must be at least 40 × 40 cm. Show how to design baffles to permit varying size containers varying in width on the conveyor belt between 20 cm and 80 cm.

6. A 10-kW CO_2 laser is used to replace a conventional plasma arc welding operation. General exhaust ventilation has been adequate to rid the area of potentially hazardous metal fumes and oxides produced in the conventional welding process. Could you therefore assume that no such improvement in ventilation would be required after the installation of the laser welding unit? What information would you need to know to make this determination?

7. A TEA laser produces an impact noise of 120 dBA every 4 s. Is this noise level hazardous?

8. A 2-cm diameter objective lens with focal length of 4 cm is used to focus a neodymium-YAG CW laser beam on a target surface. The surface does not ablate, and faces a 45° angle to the beam. What would be the irradiance at a viewing distance of 1 m from the target if the beam power was 1 W, and the specular reflection factor (reflectance) was 0.8?

9. What sort of reflections would you expect for a laser beam incident upon plasma? What optical density at 1064 nm would be required in the viewing optics of a 1-W CW YAG scribing system? Assume maximum back reflection through the microscopic objective back to the viewing microscope eyepiece. Calculate the same for a 0.4-J ruby laser system (694.3 nm) operating at 20 ns.

10. Are there any BRH special use restrictions on laser material processing applications?

19.8 REFERENCES

American Conference of Governmental Industrial Hygienists, 1976, A Guide for Control of Laser Hazards, ACGIH, Cincinnati.
American National Standards Institute, 1976, The Safe Use of Lasers, Standard Z-136.1 (1976), ANSI, New York (in revision, 1979).
Charschan, S. S. (ed.), 1972, "Lasers in Industry," Rheinhold-Van Nostrand, New York.
Doxey, B. C., 1977, How a laser system engraves cylinders for printing by the flexographic process, *Laser Focus* 12(7):66–68 (July 1977).
Duley, W. W., 1976, "CO_2 Lasers, Effects and Applications," Academic Press, New York.
Herreman, G. O., 1977, Manufacturing accuracy and the laser interferometer, Tech. Paper MR77-966, Society of Manufacturing Engineers, Dearborn, Michigan.
Herreman, G. O., Berry, F., Dowdy, C., 1977, The laser interferometer and programmable calculator as an inspection and metrology tool, *in* Effective Utilization of Optics in Quality Assurance, *Proc. SPIE* 129:37–48.
Hoag, E., Pease, H., Staal, J., and Zar, J., 1974, Performance Characteristics of a 10 kW Industrial CO_2 Laser System, Research Report 396, AVCO Everett Research Laboratory, Everett, MA, (February 1974).
Iceland, W. F., 1977, Design and development of equipment for laser wire stripping, Tech. Paper MR77-978, Society of Manufacturing Engineers, Dearborn, Michigan.
Kashuba, V. A., 1976, Problems of industrial hygiene in the use of neodymium lasers in the production of watches, *Gig. Sanit.* 8:28–32 (in Russian).
Locke, E. V., 1974, Multi-Kilawatt Industrial CO_2 Lasers, Tech. Paper MR74-952, Society of Manufacturing Engineers, Dearborn, Michigan.
Ready, J. F., 1978, Coupling of CO_2 laser energy into ionized blowoff material, *Opt. Let.* 2(5): 130–132.
Ready, J. F., 1978, "Industrial Applications of Lasers," Academic Press, Inc., New York.
Rockwell, R. J., Wilson, R. M., Jander, S., and Dreffner, R., 1976, Occupational Hazards of Laser Material Processing, College of Medicine of the University of Cincinnati, Report 0859 for Grant No. R01 OH 00371, National Institute of Occupational Safety and Health, Cincinnati, OH (May 1976).
Scherman, G. H., and Frazier, G. F., 1978, Transmissive optics for high power CO_2 lasers: practical considerations, *Opt. Eng.* 17(3):225–231.
Schwarz, H. J., and Hora, H., 1972, "Laser Interaction and Related Phenomena," Vol. 2, Plenum Press, New York.
Sliney, D. H., 1975, Health hazards from laser material processing, Tech. Paper MR75-581, Society of Manufacturing Engineers, Dearborn, Michigan.
Sliney, D. H., Bason, F. C., and Freasier, B. C., 1971, The measurement of ultraviolet, visible, and infrared radiation, *Am. Industr. Hyg. Assn. J.* 32:415–431.
Specht, W. A., 1977, Laser safety hazards—problems solvable, Tech. Paper MR77-983, Society of Manufacturing Engineers, Dearborn, Michigan.
Weiner, M. J., 1976, Product marking with Nd:YAG and CO_2 lasers, Tech. Paper MR76-853, Society of Manufacturing Engineers, Dearborn, Michigan.

Chapter 20
Laser Safety with Consumer and Office Products

20.1 INTRODUCTION

The primary impetus to early laser legislation in the 1960's was the concern of some legislators that the general public might be exposed to hazardous laser beams. The legislation was directed toward controlling potential misuse of lasers. Some legislators had visions of "laser guns" in the public sector.

This concern with public exposure also was probably a major factor in the drafting of the Laser Product Performance Standard (21CFR1040) of the Bureau of Radiological Health. Many of the provisions of the BRH Laser Product Performance Standard clearly related to that agency's experience with general commercial products such as color television sets and microwave ovens. A number of safety provisions of 21CFR1040 pertained to leakage radiation and accessibility to the radiation sources, enclosure interlocks, etc. The provisions were similar to those found in the microwave oven standard and the X-ray leakage standard for color television sets. Unfortunately, some laser users felt that many of those well-intentioned provisions created significant problems and increased costs for laboratory and industrial lasers where the same degree of control was perhaps not as essential. Today, most of the BRH performance requirements are no longer questioned.

This chapter will consider the means of assuring that exposure of the general public to laser equipment is not hazardous. At the time of the writing of this book the principal public applications of the laser were in the fields of "laser art," laser exhibitions, and point-of-sale laser scanning devices used at checkout counters in supermarkets. On the near horizon were laser applications in home entertainment electronic systems, such as video disc recorders.

20.2 LASER DISPLAYS AND LASER ART

In the first 20 years of the laser's existence there have been a number of

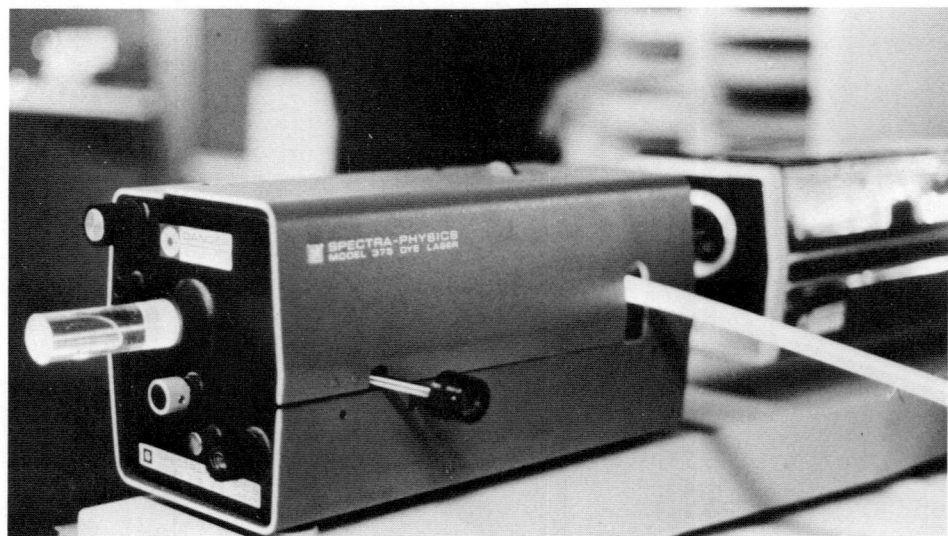

Figure 20-1. Laser Output Diffuser. The photograph shows an argon-laser-pumped dye laser at an exhibition. A solid plastic rod diffuser at the output port reduces the beam to a safe diffuse source. The beam paths of the pump laser are enclosed by plastic covers.

attempts to employ the laser with its monochromatic brilliance as an artistic tool, either as a supplementary element in multi-media artistic work or as a primary element in an artistic work with light. Some of these exhibitions have been indoors and employed small lasers; others have employed a variety of high-powered argon and krypton lasers for displays outdoors in the general environment and inside auditoriums or planetariums. The principal safety effort in all of these laser art applications was to contain the laser beams within an inaccessible space. For instance, beams would be kept above the heads of the crowd or directed directly upward into the clouds, or shielded behind a window in a museum exhibit.

20.2.1 Lasers in Science Exhibits

The procedures for protecting the public in a museum exhibit or a technical exhibition are obvious. The use of plastic or glass beam enclosures, opaque beam stops, and beam paths which do not permit secondary beams to go out into the viewing area are the obvious solutions. An example of one such approach is shown in Figure 20-1, which illustrates a small Lucite® or Plexiglas® cylindrical tube with a wide diffuser at the end. This has been used by a number of CW-visible laser manufacturers as a beam stop when displaying the laser output of their equipment. In these instances, as long as the beam power is well below 0.5 W the existence of a safe diffuse reflection is almost definitely assured and a colorful display is achieved.

Numerous attempts with rotating mirrors and oscillating mirrors to create a dynamic display of laser beams have been presented at art and science museums. In many cases the approach was to try to maintain the beams in a single plane which was inaccessible to the public. The beams were made visible by the Tyndall scattering of smoke or dust in the air of an exhibit hall.

20.2.2 Holographic Displays

The first holograms required on-axis (intrabeam) viewing (Fig. 20-2, top). However, since the development of off-axis holograms, intrabeam viewing is not necessary (Fig. 20-2, bottom). Therefore, holographic displays should be designed so that a viewer cannot directly view the illuminating source either directly or by specular reflection. A transparent shield (e.g., a display case) should exist between the viewer and the hologram. There should be no concern over viewing of the holographic display itself. If the hologram is comfortable to view, the radiance of the extended source hologram will be far below extended source criteria for 8-hr continuous viewing [$2 \text{ mW}/(\text{cm}^2 \cdot \text{sr})$] —even in the blue end of the spectrum. Indeed, if the radiance of the hologram were hazardous, the illuminating beam irradiance for such a condition would probably damage the hologram. Measurements performed by one of the authors (Sliney) suggest a typical ratio of radiance-to-incident-beam-irradiance factor of 0.03 to 0.05 sr^{-1}. For example, an incident beam irradiance of 50 $\mu\text{W}/\text{cm}^2$ on a transmission hologram would create areas of maximum radiance in the holographic image of approximately 2 $\mu\text{W}/\text{cm}^2 \cdot \text{sr}$).

20.2.3 Sound and Light Shows

A number of rock music groups found that the laser added significantly to the total sensory impact of their concerts. They would often apply high-power 5 to 10 W argon and krypton lasers with versatile scanning mechanisms to create abstract, colorful patterns on the ceiling or walls behind them. In some instances the audience has been illuminated by direct scanning laser beams. Public health officials were very concerned about the potential hazards of such exposure conditions. The scanning beams were created by a variety of means, e.g., by the initial beam passing through an array of spinning gratings to produce a rotating fan of diffracted orders. The use of such lasers during a rock concert would typically be limited to a few 90-s "on" periods during a concert. In some instances there would be efforts toward protective procedures by placing beam stops and minimum elevation stops in front of the laser beam. This would assure that the beam plane would not reach the performers or audience. Similar attempts were made with laser scanning equipment in planetariums.

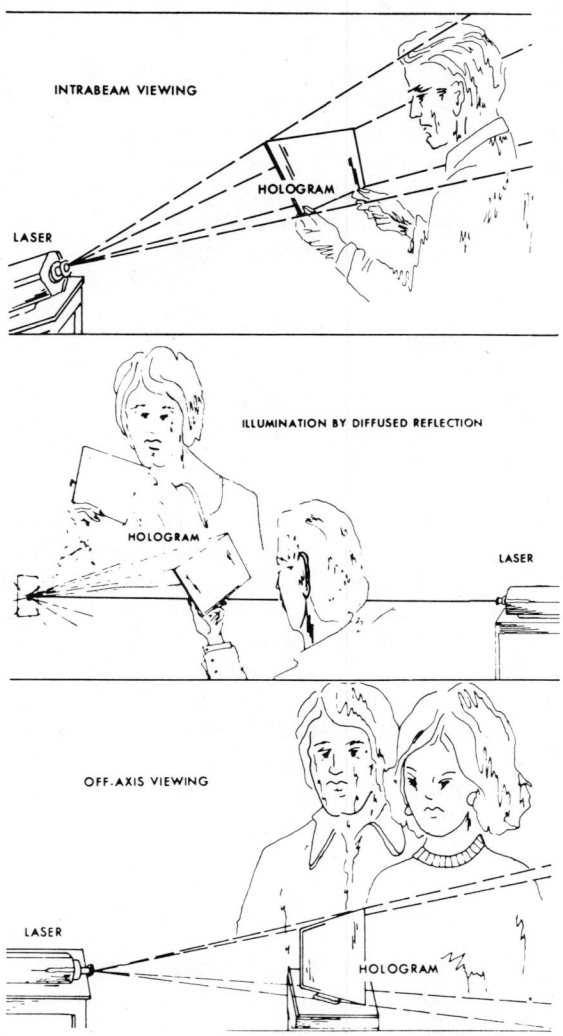

Figure 20-2. Holographic Viewing. Intrabeam viewing was characteristic of the first holograms (upper diagram). Diffuse viewing is helpful when each individual of a large group has a hologram. Off-axis viewing with the eye restricted from the direct beam is encouraged, as shown in the lower illustration.

Several organizations have toured the country presenting a laser show with accompanying music in large planetariums. In these cases 0.5-W to 5-W argon and krypton laser beams were used to create abstract patterns on the ceiling in synchrony with the music. Although some of these lasers were Class 4, the beam paths and reflective surfaces were sufficiently distant that no hazardous diffuse reflection would exist at the level of the viewing audience. For such shows it becomes necessary to demonstrate that, if one of the laser beam scanners should fail, the radiance of the stationary beam would not be hazardous. Although in excess of permissible exposure limits for very close viewing distances (less than 10 to 50 cm from the target), the stationary beams' diffuse reflection would not be hazardous when point-source criteria were used at the nearest audience viewing distance. Hence the diffuse reflection from the planetarium dome from any of the laser beams employed would be completely safe.

As an example, consider a 1-W argon laser beam at 488 nm. The minimal spot on the diffuse dome is a = 3 mm. The dome reflectance ρ_λ at 488 nm is 0.8. Using Eq. (2-6), the reflected irradiance E at $\theta = 0°$ (worst case) at a distance r_1 would be:

$$E = \rho \Phi \cos \theta / \pi r_1^2 \qquad (20\text{-}1)$$
$$= (0.8)(1\text{ W})(1.0)/(3.14) r_1^2$$
$$= 0.25/r_1^2$$

Hence the distance to the 2.5 mW/cm² level is:

$$r_1 = \sqrt{(0.25/E)}$$
$$= \sqrt{(0.25/2.5 \times 10^{-3})}$$
$$= 10 \text{ cm}$$

The radiance L at the diffuse dome is:

$$L = E_o/\pi \qquad (20\text{-}2)$$
$$= 1.27 \, \Phi/\pi a^2$$
$$= (1.27)(1\text{ W})/(3.14)(0.09 \text{ cm}^2)$$
$$= 4.5 \text{ W}/(\text{cm}^2 \cdot \text{sr})$$

Under these viewing conditions the source is so small that a momentary viewing (0.25-s) hazard would exist at only a very short distance (10 cm). Even very long-term (assume 1000 s = 16 minutes) viewing conditions are limited to a short distance from the dome:

$$E_{EL} = 10 \text{ mJ/cm}^2/1000 \text{ s}$$
$$= 10 \, \mu\text{W/cm}^2$$

$$r = \sqrt{(0.25/E)}$$
$$= \sqrt{(0.25/10^{-5})}$$

$$r = 1.57 \times 10^2 \text{ cm}$$
$$= 1.6 \text{ m}$$

Skin exposure to any of the four beams would be safe even if the beam were accessible to the outstretched hands of the curious. In these applications the hazard would only exist if an individual could place his or her eye into the direct beam or if a flat mirror surface were placed into the beam after the beam left the central enclosure. This secondary beam directed into the eye of an individual could be hazardous. Either engineering or administrative control measures should be used to preclude human access to the emergent beams in this application; and the engineering controls are, by far, more preferable.

The following obvious control measures could be implemented whenever the general public would be in the planetarium and the laser operating:

1. During actual operation, the public access to the beam paths could be prevented by one or more of the following four procedures:

   (a) Place an usher in front of the laser projection system and not allow seating near the projection system, especially in front of it (administrative control).

   (b) Place a barrier (e.g., fence) around the laser enclosure to preclude anyone from placing a mirror into the beam (engineering control).

   (c) Extend the accessible sides of the enclosure sufficiently high to preclude human access to the beams (engineering control).

   (d) Raise the entire system at least one meter above the tallest individuals to preclude human access to the beams (engineering control). This control measure is also highly desirable. However, it may limit the total scan coverage over the entire screen or planetarium dome.

2. In all cases only an experienced operator should operate this type of system. The master control key should not remain in the system power supply when an operator is not present. The enclosure panels should not be removed if the laser is operating when other than trained service personnel are present. These concepts were embodied in standards developed on this subject by BRH and ANSI.

3. The access panels to the laser and laser scanning system enclosure should not be removed if the laser were operating, or if untrained personnel (general public) were present within the planetarium.

These kinetic laser light and sound shows generally attempt to have the widest variety of wavelengths. For this reason krypton, as well as argon lasers have been typically employed. As a general rule, the various wavelengths from these ion lasers are divided by directing the beam into a prism or grating. The useful krypton laser lines would generally be in the blue (476.2 nm and 482.5 nm), in the green (520.8 nm and 530.9 nm), in the yellow (568 nm) and in the red (647.1 nm). In some instances these krypton laser beams would be added to the primary 488-nm blue line and 514.5-nm green line of the argon laser. In many indoor light shows only a 1-W krypton laser is employed. The beams may be further separated and exit from one or several beam ports in an enclosure. The enclosure shields the public from both the laser and the variety of optical parts, lenses, prisms, static mirrors, vibrating mirrors, flexible mirrors, rotating mirrors, etc., that are used for the scanning and spreading of the beam. Normally a control console would be located adjacent to this beam shaping enclosure. Measurements made by Sliney have shown that some of these systems used in auditorium displays often have had beams reduced in power to as low as 5-10 mW after the laser beams had been separated in wavelength and directed through many beam-shaping objects. However, such low-power beams could only be used in totally dark planetarium environments.

Much higher power beams are typically used in rock concert shows or outdoor laser art shows. The saving feature of diffuse reflection viewing is that visible CW laser beams of any power would burn any diffuse reflecting surface before hazardous reflections could occur at any reasonable viewing distance (>2 or 3 m). Viewing scattered light from raindrops, snow, sleet, fog and aerosol particulates is likewise safe at such distances from any CW visible laser beam.

20.2.4 Regulations and Standards for Laser Light Shows

A review of the BRH performance standard for laser products reveals that only Class I or Class II laser products may be manufactured and sold as "demonstration laser products" (see paragraph 9.3.11). The Bureau of Radiological Health in a policy statement dated November 28, 1977, interpreted 21CFR1040.10 and 21CFR1040.11 to apply to groups putting on laser shows to the public. The statement explained that musical groups themselves would be construed as manufacturers of a laser product if they assembled their own light show for use in their own performances, even if the act of "manufacture" was simply a rededication of a general-purpose laser product to use in a light show without the addition of any components. Subsequently, BRH issued an interim enforcement policy on February 21, 1978 which provided lengthy light show guidelines. It indicated to light show "manufacturers" using Class III and IV Laser Systems, that BRH would take no enforcement action against a "manufacturer" if three conditions were fulfilled. First, he must provide BRH with documentation that the show would be conducted safely in accordance with BRH guidelines. Secondly, BRH must be allowed to inspect the products and operational shows. Thirdly, the "manufacturer" must certify his product(s) and provide an initial report on his products along with an application for a variance from the performance standard (for those aspects of the product which the manufacturer deems appropriate) prior to the introduction of the laser light show(s) into commerce.

The guidelines of BRH were as follows:

1. Laser radiation outside of the visible range (400 nm to 710 nm) must not exceed Class I limits.

2. The levels of laser and collateral radiation may not exceed Class I limits where the audience is seated or standing.
3. Operators, performers and employees must be able to perform their duties without having to view laser and collateral radiation exceeding the Class I limits and without having to be exposed to such radiation exceeding the Class II limits.
4. All scanners including mirror balls must incorporate scanning safeguards if scan failure could cause exposure exceeding the limits of criterion 2 or 3.
5. Class III and IV levels of laser radiation must be at least 6 m vertically above or 2.5 m horizontally from any standing surface or position where the audience may be *if the show is NOT under the continuous control of an operator* (Figure 20-3).
6. Class III and IV levels of laser radiation must be at least 3 m vertically above or 2.5 m horizontally from any standing surface or position where the audience may be *if the show is under the continuous control of an operator* (Figure 20-4).
7. There must be an accessible control and a designated person to terminate laser radiation under unsafe conditions.
8. Levels of laser radiation above the Class II limit must be the lowest possible to achieve the desired effects.
9. Other criteria may be included to suit the requirements of a particular show. This may include maintenance of a checkout log, contacting the Federal Aviation Administration (FAA) for outdoor shows, having additional safety equipment, or certification of operators.
10. Measurements for the determination of levels are to be made in accordance with the laser standard.

Except for criterion #6, these requirements have not created a serious problem for the light show industry (Taylor, 1979). Physical dimensions of the show hall often made strict compliance difficult or impossible. In specific variance applications, BRH has reduced the 3-m requirement where Class III levels were not greatly over 1 mW. Since most of the laser shows incorporate scanning laser beams, a defining measurement aperture of 7 mm rather than 80 mm has applied to beam measurements and therefore the exposure measurements have more nearly reflected an assessment of user EL's or MPE's rather than product performance AEL's. Exposure limits for the eye obviously should not be exceeded. Subsequent to the BRH publication of light show safety criterion, the ANSI Z-136 Committee developed recommendations that could be framed in the context of a user standard rather than in terms of product performance.

If the reader is planning a laser light show, it would be advisable to contact the BRH Division of Compliance, Rockville, MD, for the latest information on BRH requirements in this area.

In the 1979 ANSI Z-136.1 revision document, a set of controls for laser light shows were introduced. These control measures closely followed the BRH criteria just ennumerated (Rockwell et al., 1979). The dividing line between supervised and unsupervised light shows was shifted from the limits of Class II (BRH) to the upper

Consumer and Office Products 633

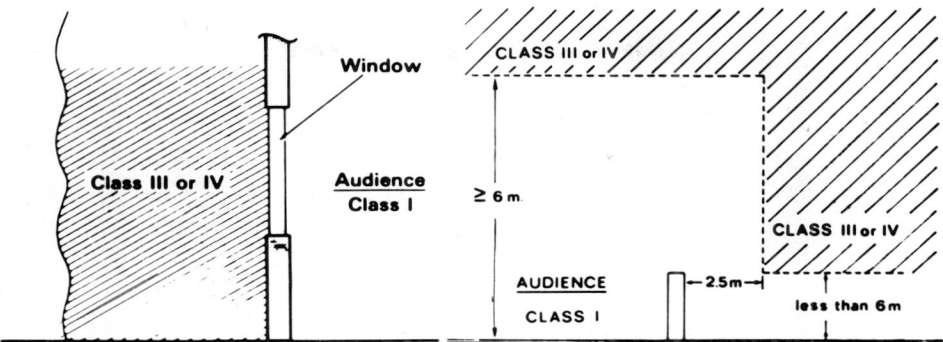

Figure 20-3. Unsupervised Laser Light Show. The BRH requires that any Class III or Class IV laser radiation be at least 6 m vertically and 2.5 m horizontally from a standing surface. This normally means that a visible laser beam having a CW power exceeding 1 mW must be far above the heads and well beyond the reach of a standing audience. A physical barrier of transparent glass or plastic can be used as a shield in lieu of the required distances as shown on the right. The drawings are from Smith and Dennis (1979).

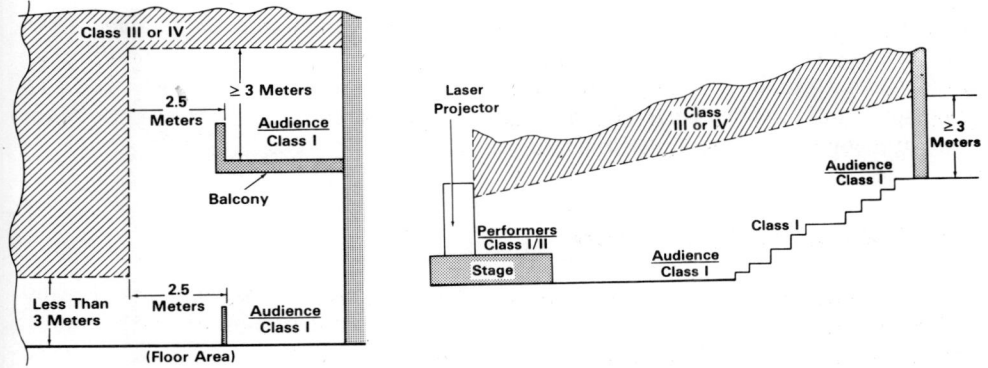

Figure 20-4. Supervised Laser Light Show. With an operator present, Class III and Class IV laser radiation levels must be at least 3 m above any surface and 2.5 m horizontally from any surface upon which an audience may stand. The drawings are from Smith and Dennis (1979).

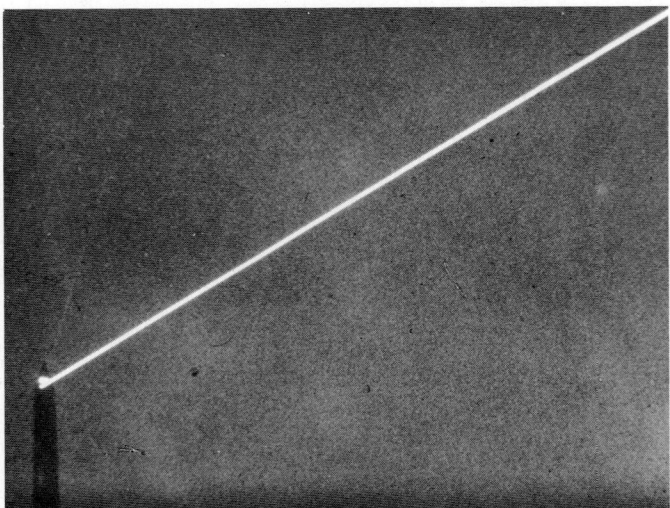

Figure 20-5. Outdoor Laser Art Show. Scanning laser beams from argon lasers leave the windows of the Washington Monument during the Bicentennial Fourth of July Laser Display presented by artist Richard Lefrak. The beam paths were limited to positive elevation angles and airspace was monitored to assure that the beams did not intercept aircraft. Photo by Les Henig, courtesy of Richard Lefrak.

limit of Class 3a (ANSI). The distances of 3 m, 2.5 m and 6 m, were retained; however, the Laser Safety Officer (LSO) could relax these distances if equivalent protection were afforded. The key point in the ANSI proposal was that the permitted exposure limits applicable to the viewers would be based on the relevant MPE's for the total combined operational time during any 8-hour period.

20.2.5 Laser Beams in the Airspace

Outdoor laser beam shows typically would employ horizontally-to-vertically directed beams where the public could note the scattering of light off of the atmosphere. In some cases these beams were directed through scanning optical systems. These were controlled by computers to write on the walls of buildings or clouds. Figure 20-5 shows one such situation where a high-power argon laser beam leaves the window of the Washington Monument during a Fourth-of-July celebration. In this latter case the beam was directed horizontally, or slightly above horizontal, to assure that the beam did not strike the ground. In these instances, provided that the beam does not strike uncontrolled areas of tall buildings, the principal concern is assuring that aircraft do not fly through a beam at hazardous levels. It has generally been considered adequate that the laser beam irradiance be below 2.5 mW/cm^2 (visible laser wavelengths). This assures that no airborne personnel are exposed to levels above Class 2 momentary viewing limits. The possibility that a 2.5-mW/cm² exposure from a laser would dazzle a pilot is discounted, as typical pilots and FAA personnel note that the FAA never has had regulations against dazzle from searchlights which can be of comparable magnitude in brightness. In almost all instances the expected exposures would be far less than the 2.5 mW/cm² (0.25 s) permissible exposure.

In general, outdoor laser exhibitions are permissible if the beam is limited to horizontal or vertical paths above accessible ground areas, (above 10 m) with adequate precautions to assure that personnel in aircraft are not exposed to hazardour levels. Laser beams employed in a city area with high buildings must be directed with some care. Not only are exposures to personnel in tall buildings possible, but, in addition, firemen and utility repairmen on ladders or in "cherry pickers," could be exposed. It is generally advisable that there be operating personnel present at all times to watch the beam path for any unexpected conditions which could expose personnel. As a secondary precaution, the fire department and utility companies could be made aware of any such hazards, particularly if the beam were more permanent and an operator not present. Weather conditions, such as rain, snow, sleet or fog would not create an additional hazard from any 5-W argon or krypton laser beam used in such exhibitions. The hazardous reflections would extend only 10 to 20 cm from the beam.

20.2.6 The Speckle Pattern and Laser Displays

Until 1976 there were no suggestions that the speckle pattern in itself could present a potential hazard. Studies by Zwick and Jenkins (1978) revealed that monkeys exposed to a large-field (a ganzfeld) blue light speckle pattern for long periods while sitting in a diffuse sphere developed abnormal color and spatial vision responses. These adverse changes did not occur in the monkeys exposed in the same chamber to uniform diffused light from the same laser wavelength with the speckle pattern eliminated. The changes occurred at levels *below* the EL for long-term ($>10^4$ s) exposure, which is 2 mW/(cm² · sr). It is unlikely that anyone would consent to viewing large-field speckle patterns with, or without, image information (patterns) present for such an extended period. Most people complain of annoyance from viewing the speckle pattern in a hologram or other laser visual display for even a short time. For this reason, much effort has been expended in reducing or eliminating speckle. At this time, no definitive conclusions can be made regarding the hazards to humans from speckle. We do know that detectable adverse changes in vision have not been noted in scientists and technicians working with holograms for extended periods of time.

20.2.7 Raster Scanned Laser Displays

Most laser display systems which project images upon a viewing screen are front-or rear-projection scanning systems. A three-color scanning beam in an audito-

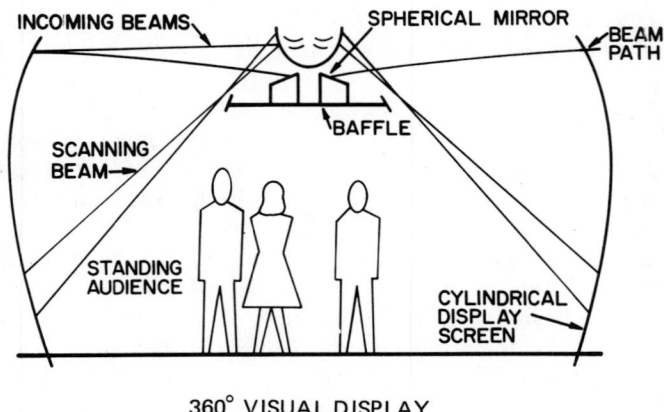

Figure 20-6. Scanned Laser Visual Display. The drawing depicts a large, walk-in cylindrical laser projection system. Twelve Ar lasers are located above and the beam scanned in six raster displays below. The audience is well below the beam paths at heights where the beam would be hazardous.

rium would have to meet access requirements such as that shown in Figure 20-4 with the beam direction reversed. The beam paths can normally be kept above the audience's accessible space. The major question that arises regarding hazards from such a system is: Is the screen safe to view if the beams stop? Determining the actual ocular exposures can be very complex.

An example prepared by Mr. Wesley J. Marshall of USAEHA illustrates these points very well. A large walk-in cylindrical screen system for a few seated observers is shown in Fig. 20-6. Twelve identical 3-W Ar/Kr laser beams are used to cover a $90° \times 360°$ area on the inside of a very large, walk-in cylindrically-shaped screen in the proposed system. The actual transmitted power could be either 0.25 W or 0.5 W per beam. Each laser covers a $30°$ horizontal $\times$ $90°$ vertical sector of the screen with 300 equally spaced vertical lines at 60 Hz. The scan immediately following would interlace the first scan. Therefore, a complete scan would take 1/30 s. The output of each laser should be between 3 and 5 W yielding an output through the optics of between 0.25 and 0.5 W. The only hazard from a single laser need be considered in the direct viewing mode, since multiple beam laser exposure would not normally be additive for intrabeam viewing. The beam leaves the laser projector more than 3 m above a standing surface, but a person standing near the screen could look in a scanning beam.

(a) Intrabeam Viewing Condition

A 30° horizontal sector would contain 0.52 rad with 300 lines, 1 line would cover every 1.74 mrad. At an arbitrary distance from the laser r, the number of lines N entering an individual's eyes while looking toward the scanning laser beam, with a 0.7 cm pupil size would be:

$$N = (0.7 \text{ cm})/[r\,(1.74 \times 10^{-3} \text{ rad})] \quad \text{every } 1/60 \text{ s} \qquad (20\text{-}3)$$

On the average he would receive in 1 s a number of pulses equal to:

$$N = 24{,}064/r \text{ (cm)} \qquad (\text{for } r > 2 \text{ cm}) \qquad (20\text{-}4)$$

However, an individual standing directly on one of the 300 vertical scanning lines or one of the interlaced lines at any distance from the laser projector would receive at least one pulse every frame (1/30 s). The above approximation (Eq. 20-4) therefore must be modified to a step function. In the worst possible location for exposure, the number of pulses exposing the eye could be represented by the following step functions:

$$\begin{aligned}
N &= 30 & &\text{for } r > 8 \text{ m} \\
N &= 60 & &\text{for } 4 \text{ m} < r < 8 \text{ m} \\
N &= 120 & &\text{for } 2 \text{ m} < r < 4 \text{ m, etc.}
\end{aligned} \qquad (20\text{-}5)$$

A 90° vertical sector would contain 1.57 rad. For one vertical sweep of the laser beam, the distance traveled s of the beam is a function of the distance r from the laser scanning projector:

$$s = 1.57\,r \qquad (20\text{-}6)$$

where r is expressed in cm.

Since the pupillary diameter is small compared to this arc length, the duration that the beam could enter a person's eye would be:

$$\begin{aligned}
t &= (0.7/1.57\,r)\,(1/300)\,(1/60) \qquad &(20\text{-}7)\\
&= 2.48 \times 10^{-5}\,r
\end{aligned}$$

The radiant exposure per pulse H from the scanning system for an individual located a distance r (cm) from the laser projector is equal to:

$$\begin{aligned}
H &= (0.25)\,(2.48 \times 10^{-5})/[(0.385)\,(r)] \qquad &(20\text{-}8)\\
&= 1.61 \times 10^{-5}/r
\end{aligned}$$

for a 0.25-W output. For the 0.5-W output this value is doubled.

The exposure limit (EL) for a multiple-pulse laser system, with a pulse width of less than 10 μs, is the product of the single-pulse EL and the repetitive pulse correction factor C_P. The single pulse EL for visible lasers with a pulse width of less than 18 μs is 5×10^{-7} J/cm². Pulse durations are shorter than 10 μs at distances greater than 2.5 cm from the laser projector. The EL for all reasonable distances is given by:

$$\text{EL } (r > 2 \text{ cm}) = (5 \times 10^{-7}) C_P \text{ J/cm}^2 \qquad (20\text{-}9)$$

where C_P is given in Figure 8-11 as a function of the pulse rate frequency F. C_P may be approximated by the following functions:

$$C_P = \begin{cases} 1/\sqrt{F} & \text{for } F = 1 \text{ to } 100 \\ 0.3317\, F^{-0.265} & \text{for } F = 100 \text{ to } 500 \\ 0.133\, F^{-0.116} & \text{for } F = 500 \text{ to } 1000 \\ 0.06 & \text{for } F > 1000 \end{cases} \qquad (20\text{-}10)$$

The biological effect, however, is not simply a function of the number of pulses received in 1 s, but rather the intrapulse spacing between pulses. The intrapulse spacing for two adjacent lines would be 1/300 of 1/60 of 1 s or 56 μs, corresponding to 18,000 pulses per second (pps). The C_P value then would always be 0.06 for an individual close to the laser scanner. At 4 m from the scanner, however, the distance between two adjacent lines is greater than the nominal pupillary diameter (0.7 cm). The maximum pulse rate at distances exceeding 4 m is then 60 pps. The corresponding EL for 60 pps is 6.4×10^{-8} J/cm². At 8 m from the laser projector, only one pulse per frame (1/30 s) could be received. The corresponding protection standard for 30 pps is 0.1×10^{-8} J/cm². At distances between 2 m and 4 m, two pulses every 1/60 s could be received, which would cut the EL for 60 pps in half. If it is assumed that the two closely spaced pulses add linearly, the EL would be 3.2×10^{-8} J/cm².

Graphical means are convenient for determining at what distance the radiant exposure value exceeds the EL. Both the radiant exposure-per-pulse and the multiple pulse protection standard have been plotted as a function of distance in Fig. 20-7. For a 0.25-W output, the multiple-pulse protection standard is exceeded at distances less than 4 m from the laser scanner. For a 0.5-W output, this EL is exceeded within 5 m.

For very long intrabeam viewing (several hours), the EL (1.0 μW/cm²) is sometimes more restrictive. Figure 20-7 also shows the 8-hr viewing criterion as a function of range calculated on a per pulse basis. These levels are exceeded within 8 m for a 0.25-W output or within 9.5 m for a 0.5-W output.

EL's for several minutes viewing time may be exceeded at the hazard distance based on multiple pulses. For the 0.25-W output, 3.5 minutes is the recommended maximal viewing time at 4 m. For the 0.5-W output, 4.3 minutes is the recommended viewing time at 5 m. For other power levels, the permissible viewing time (t > 10 s) may be computed by the formula:

$$t \text{ (s)} = (0.01 \text{ J/cm}^2)/E_{\text{avg}} \text{ (W/cm}^2) \qquad (20\text{-}11)$$

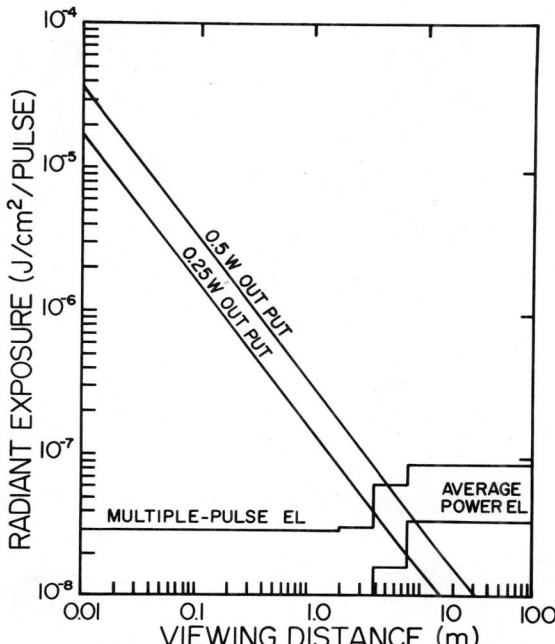

Figure 20-7. Graphical Determination of Hazardous Viewing Distances. Exposure limits for multiple-pulse viewing of the scanned laser display are plotted as a function of distance in accordance with Eq. 20-5. The hazardous viewing distances are the points where the calculated beam irradiances intercept the exposure limits. Redrawn from a plot kindly provided by Mr. Wesley J. Marshall.

Clearly the viewers must be kept out of the projection beam for short times.

(b) Diffuse Reflection

The luminance (and radiance) of the raster scan is safe (quite low) and comfortable to look at. For example, a 0.5-W beam covering a 6 m² screen area A would produce an average radiance of:

$$L = \Phi \cdot \rho / \pi A = (0.5)(2)/(3.14)(60{,}000 \text{ cm}^2) \quad (20\text{-}12)$$
$$= 5.3 \ \mu W/(cm^2 \cdot sr)$$

which is nearly 400 times below the 8-hour viewing EL. But the diffuse reflection hazard for a static laser beam of this type must be calculated. Using formula 2.6 in Chapter 2, the reflectivity should be replaced by the gain of the screen (G) which

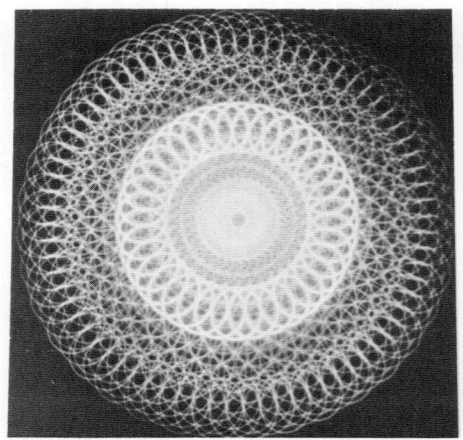
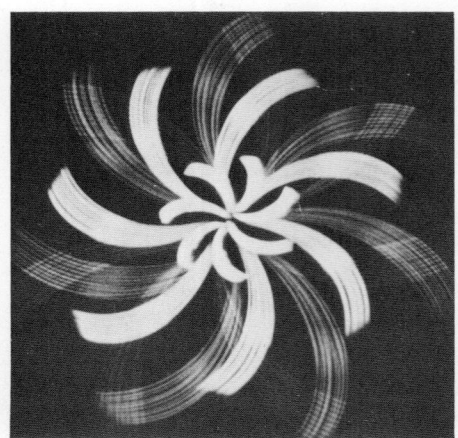
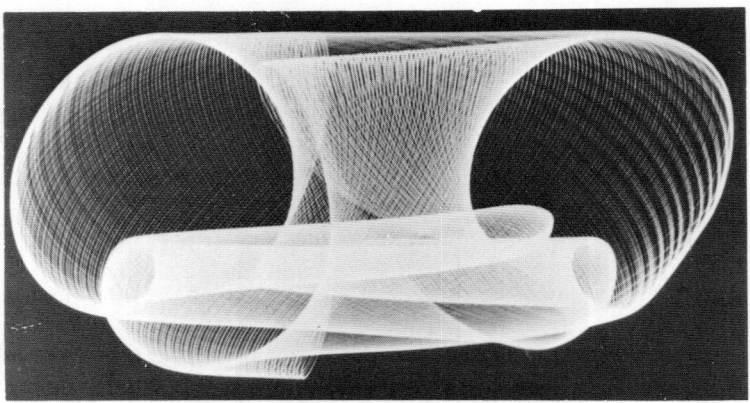

Figure 20-8. Laser Art Scan Patterns. These scan patterns from laser beams illustrate some of the intricate artistic effects created for "Laserium" laser art shows. Unfortunately the brilliant colors cannot also be shown (Photographs courtesy of Laser Images, Inc., Van Nuys, CA).

may be as great as 3 for this example. Then the hazardous distance $r_{1\,(haz)}$ for staring at the static beam for 100 s (EL = 0.1 mW/cm^2) would be:

$$r_{1\ haz} = \sqrt{\Phi G/(\pi E)} \qquad (20\text{-}13)$$
$$r_{1\ haz}\,(0.25\ \text{W}) = \sqrt{0.25\,(3)/\pi\,(10^{-4})} = 49\ \text{cm}$$
$$r_{1\ haz}\,(0.5\ \text{W}) = \sqrt{0.50\,(3)/\pi\,(10^{-4})} = 69\ \text{cm}$$

It is very unlikely that any person would be so close or stare at a static beam spot, but scanning-failure cut-off switches are clearly advisable. If only to prevent intrabeam exposure. For strongly retroreflective screens the gain G is not a simple function but can vary dramatically with small viewing angles as was shown in Figure 15-8. Figure 15-7 showed how the retroreflective screen works. Normally the viewing angle θ_v is considered to be the angle between the laser beam path and the viewer's line-of-sight. This is not the angular subtense α of the source.

20.2.8 Demonstration Lasers in the Classroom

Many secondary schools and universities make use of HeNe lasers to demonstrate principles of optics. Thousands of He-Ne lasers having output powers ranging from 0.4 mW to 4 mW have been specifically sold for this purpose. Some of these lasers have been sold in teaching kits with optical accessories. Since August 1976 the BRH regulation 21CFR1040.11 has limited sale of such demonstration laser products to Class I or Class II. For most demonstrations a 0.8-mW Class II laser beam is sufficiently bright to illustrate most optical effects in a dimly lit classroom. Some secondary school science teachers had argued that this beam power would be insufficient for some multiple-beam demonstrations and opposed this limit in public hearings. Since BRH only regulates the manufacture, sale, and advertisement of such products, some teachers simply purchase a 3-to-5-mW laser sold for other purposes (e.g., a "research" laser or an alignment laser). Many Class 4 scientific laboratory lasers are "demonstrated" in universities, however these lasers were not designed and sold expressly for "demonstration."

Teachers should instruct pupils not to stare into the direct laser beam prior to turning on the laser. Some He-Ne lasers, particularly near the end of their lifetime, emit intermittently or have an extensive delay in emission after turn-on. These malfunctions have led to intra-beam eye exposures to the uninitiated who foolishly stared down the bore of the laser tube and then were exposed. Events such as these appear to underscore the need to limit the radiant power to 1 mW *in any one beam* of a laser light demonstration.

The Bureau of Radiological Health has published a book on safe laser light demonstrations (Van Pelt, *et al.*, 1970a and 1970b) that provides useful information for secondary school teachers. Additionally the annual catalog of Metrologic Instruments, Inc. of Bellmawr, New Jersey, includes a 40-page "Laser Handbook" with 101 demonstrations possible with small He-Ne lasers and other useful information.

20.3 LASER POINT-OF-SALE TERMINALS

During the 1970's a number of American corporations introduced laser scanners in point-of-sale (POS) checkout equipment. These scanning laser beams were used to illuminate the international standard product code (Fig. 20-9 inset) which is now located on most merchandise packaging. Figure 20-9 illustrates one such laser point-of-sale installation as employed in a supermarket. Most systems use a nominal 1-mW He-Ne laser with a scanner. The scanning patterns of different laser scanners varies with manufacturer. Some have Lissajous patterns at the beam exit window, others have rectangular or linear criss-cross patterns (see Section 15.7). All employ

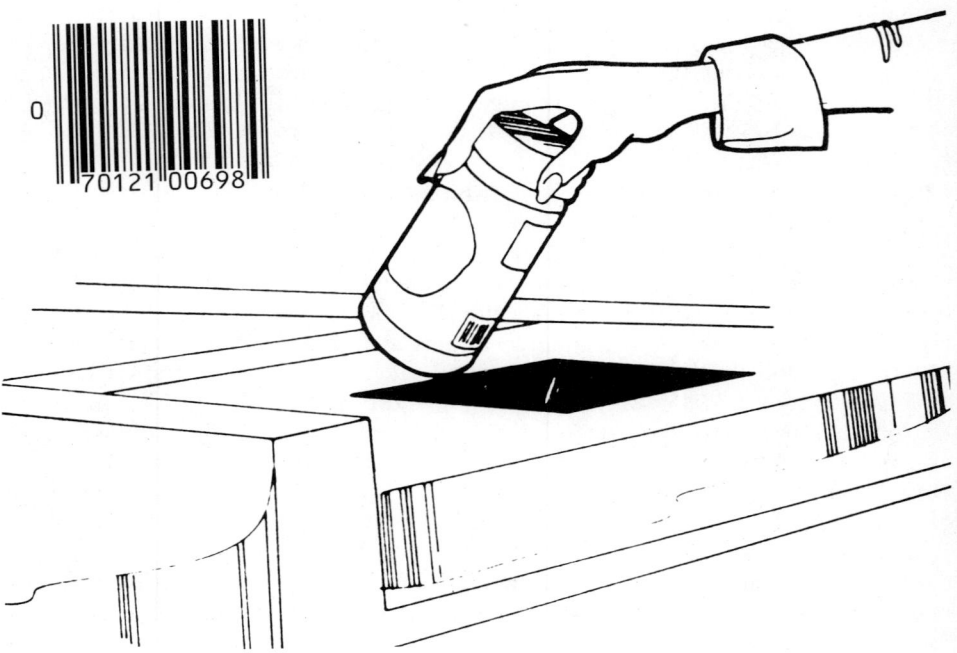

Figure 20-9. Laser Point-of-Sale Terminal for a Supermarket. The laser beam exits a window in the counter and scans the universal product code (inset). Scratches in the window deteriorate the system's performance and the window must be replaced periodically unless it is recessed.

some means to reduce operator exposure and all were designed to be Class I laser products, in accordance with the Bureau of Radiological Health Laser Product Performance Standard. The primary safety control designed into this equipment is a positive means to assure that the laser beam does not emerge from the output window if the scanning motor fails, since in this case the exposures could approach 1 mW if directed into a static 7-mm pupil. A further requirement was that a static 7-mm pupil at any given point (such as the crossover point on a criss-cross pattern) could not be exposed to levels in excess of 0.39 μW in any 8-hr exposure limit. To limit the total emission duration, the scanning beam is usually on only when an object is located within the scan area as determined by an electric eye detector on the counter.

The writing of an "air-tight" performance standard for this equipment was a very difficult matter. After the publication of the initial standard in 1976, there was a debate between manufacturers and the Bureau of Radiological Health as to the desirability, and need, for certain requirements in measurement of the beam, and the practicality of assuming that an operator could really be exposed continually or even as much as 4-8 hours for any one day. It was also questionable that an apparent line source should be treated the same as a static point source. As a result of this interchange of ideas, BRH modified the performance standard in late 1978. A new BRH classification (Class IIa) was born. POS scanners would be considered Class IIa if the measured laser output did not exceed the Class I limit for 1,000 s (i.e., 3.9 μW measured through a 7-mm aperture). To the user by all outward appearances, the Class IIa product appears as a Class I product. This relaxation also eliminated the need in some models for an electronic accumulator (sometimes referred to as a "gas tank") to assure that the Class I accumulated limit of 3.9 mJ was not exceeded.

The repetitive pulse correction of ANSI Z-136.1 and the draft IEC standard places many POS scanners into Class 2. Since the BRH performance standard does not distinguish between CW and repetitively pulsed exposures, the BRH limits for Class IIa are seldom exceeded. In any case no one ever stares into the scanner source constantly, and such concerns are academic.

An accurate hazard analysis of a POS laser scanner can become quite involved. The fundamental scan equations were presented for simple scan patterns in Section 15.7 (pp. 506–508). The retinal image is not always equivalent to a static point source. Depending upon the arrangement of the scanners, there may or may not be a point or an array of points in space where the eye can focus upon an apparent point source. Generally there will be such a point behind the laser, but it would be nearly impossible to accommodate to that point in normal store lighting. The POS operator (checkout clerk) could not stare into the window for any length of time and would not accommodate on the point image during the course of passing merchandise across the window. The operator would be exposed to levels far below worst-case conditions. What would a passerby or curiosity seeker see? Most likely he would see a line source by imaging on one of the scanners. The retinal image width d_r would be minimal ($\sim$ 20 μm). The retinal image length d_r' is, curiously enough, a function of pupil size d_e and is also determined by the viewing distance z from the laser beam's waist and the distance l_s of the beam waist from the last scanning mirror:

$$d_r' = d_e \cdot l_s \cdot f / z (l_s + z) \qquad (20\text{-}14)$$

where f is the eye's focal length.

The retinal exposure dose H_r is simply the energy-per-pulse divided by the image area ($d_r \cdot d_r'$). The average retinal irradiance E_r is the average power entering the eye divided by the image area. Since both the energy entering the eye and d_r' are directly proportional to d_e for cases where the beam diameter is much less than d_e (common condition), the retinal irradiance is constant for different pupil sizes. This illustrates that a Class 2 laser could hardly be considered a hazard in this application. Unfortunately the measurement requirements for classification do not take into account the range of focus of the eye, variation in retinal image area and the nature of the scan pattern which truly affect a more accurate hazard analysis. Measurements of actual POS systems revealed typical source radiances of 1 to 10 W/(cm$^2 \cdot$sr) or 180 to 1800 cd/cm^2 at 633 nm which are comparable to ordinary tungsten filaments. Since the lasers are normally HeNe (633 nm) there should be no serious blue-light retinal injury hazard. Fortunately blue-light (HeCd) lasers have not been employed for POS systems. One may therefore conclude that present day Class I or Class IIa POS HeNe laser systems operate at levels with a very large margin of safety.

20.4 LASERS IN OFFICE MACHINES

Lasers have been employed for high speed printers, for facsimile recorders, and for recording data (as in holographic storage of data) on a photosensitive recording medium and for readout from the same medium. In almost all instances, practical, commercial systems have been made as Class I products. Hazards associated with servicing (Section 9.3.8 and Fig. 9-6) were minimal as these embedded lasers were typically Class 2 or only slightly above Class 2 limits. HeNe, Ar and HeCd lasers have generally been used, although at least one desktop printer makes use of an 810-nm laser diode to sensitize a CdS drum. The blue (441.6 nm) and UV-A (325-nm) wavelengths of the HeCd laser have been considered ideal for most photochemical reactions since photographic emulsion sensitivity and the sensitivity of photochromic and photoresist reactions are enhanced for shorter wavelengths. Some high-speed systems in the printing industry use high-power Ar lasers (see Section 19.4).

The control measure most desirable for servicing is a service-mode filter which can be manually (or preferably, automatically) inserted into the beam path as close to the laser beam exit as is feasible. The filter should reduce the beam power below 1 mW (UV-A and visible, 320 nm to 700 nm) to permit reasonably safe viewing of the beam path by visible reflection or by fluorescence from a calibration card. In many such products most components can be replaced without the need for laser operation while the cabinet (protective housing) is open. Lasers in optical computers, copy machines recorders, photo-offset platemakers, color printing, map makers, and video recorders all fall into this category.

One example of a well engineered Class I office machine product is the Xerox Model 200 Telecopier Fascimile System. This system incorporates a Class 2 embedded HeNe laser, which operates in both the recording and the printing modes. However, the total system was designed to be a Class I product. The operator cleans the platen glass, replinishes dry ink and paper (maintainence), and adjusts print density. Operator access to the laser area is only needed when the platen is cleaned, and the laser itself is shut off by redundant interlocks during this task. When the opeator opens the automatic document feeder cover to clean the platen, three interlocks preclude laser exposure: one inserts a laser output filter, a second shuts off the machine's electrical power, and a third is a mechanically actuated shutter which is pulled over the beam path when the feeder cover is raised.

During service of the Model 200, one interlock assures that the power is shut off when the outer covers are removed. This interlock is on the rear panel, and side panels cannot be removed until the rear panel is off. Once these service panels are removed, the optical cavity area is still shielded by other panels. The first interlock may be overridden by the serviceman. If the shields are removed, a laser caution label becomes visible to the serviceman (Edmunds, 1979).

Interlocks used in such commercial products must, of course, undergo extensive life testing. Interlock reliability is not only necessary for safety, but to preclude

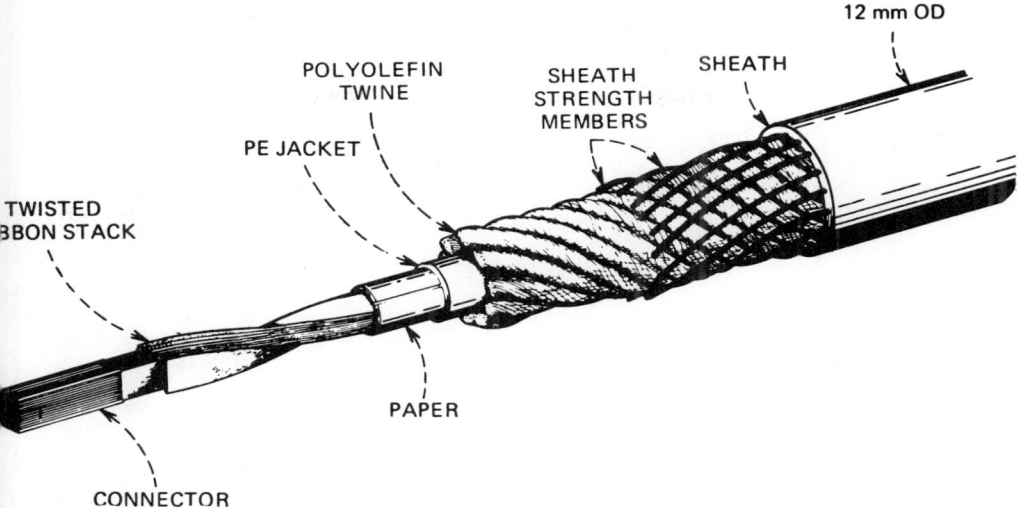

Figure 20-10. Fiber-Optic Cable. A rugged fiber-optic cable carrying at least 144 optical fiber channels is shown. The principal safety questions relate to servicing and the adequacy of connectors. From Buckler and Miller (1978) with permission.

removal of these safety features by frustrated users and servicemen if repeated machine failure were traced to faulty interlocks.

20.5 LASER OPTICAL FIBER TRANSMISSION SYSTEMS

The late 1970's showed an explosion of activity in the development of practical optical communications using IR-A diode lasers and light emitting diodes (LED's). Both glass and plastic optical fibers were under study, although glass fibers had a clear lead. During much of this development there appeared to be little concern with regard to laser hazards. After all, the entire system would always be enclosed and surely would present no hazard. However, by 1978 it was recognized that some optical cables carrying 100 or more separate fibers could carry a total power exceeding 0.1 W. An example of a rugged cable having 144 separate optical fiber units is shown in Figure 20-10. Concern now developed regarding the safety of cable service personnel and bystanders who might look into such a cable.

An optical fiber transmission line alters the beam pattern of the initial laser beam. The degree of alteration depends upon both the quality of the initial beam and the quality of the optical fiber. An important parameter in this regard is the numerical aperture. The numerical aperture NA depends upon the index of refraction of the cladding n_{cl} and of the core n_{co}:

$$NA = \sin(\theta/2) \tag{20-15}$$

$$= \sqrt{n^2_{co} - n^2_{cl}} \tag{20-16}$$

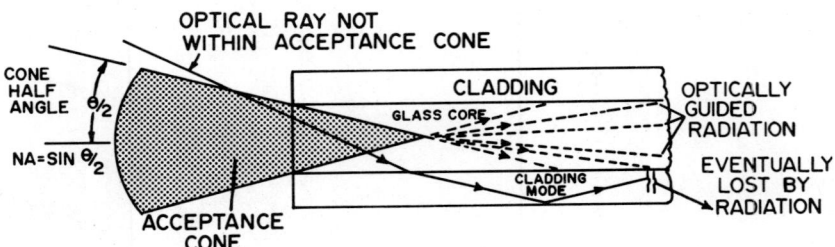

Figure 20-11. Optical Fiber Characteristics. The numerical aperture of an optical fiber is one of the principal parameters required when estimating the spread of a beam after it leaves the end of a fiber. Adapted from Hickey and Kuhfeld (1979).

The f-number of the fiber is the reciprocal of the NA. Figure 20-11 shows the field-of-view as defined by the numerical aperture of a single optical fiber. The numerical aperture also determines the beam spread of the emerging beam—often a significant angle exceeding 100 mrad (i.e., several degrees). Thus, the eye would have to be placed very near to an open cable to encounter a real hazard.

The optical communication signal typically consists of trains of modulated 850 to 910-nm pulses (Fig. 20-12), and the appropriate EL must be determined when assessing the intrabeam eye hazard. The ANSI Z-136.1 standard, proposed IEC standard, and the ACGIH TLV's all require the use of correction factor C_p for sub-microsecond pulses. For communications the pulse widths are typically less than 100 ns, and the PRF always greatly exceeds 11 kHz. The following sample calculations demonstrate that for pulse trains exceeding 11 kHz, the limiting EL criterion will be the average power rather than the energy/pulse. The limit per pulse at 905 nm is 1.25 C_p $\mu J/cm^2$ and C_p is 0.06 for F > 1 kHz; hence EL = 75 nJ/cm^2 per pulse. But at an F of 11 kHz this corresponds to an average irradiance of 0.83 mW/cm^2. This exceeds the irradiance limit of 0.8 mW/cm^2 that applied to purely CW sources for exposures greater than 1000 s. Regrettably, this EL is based upon extrapolation as retinal injury studies for lengthy GaAs laser exposures do not exist.

Although the spread beam from an optical fiber or an array of fibers is not a point source, the source itself is almost always smaller than α_{min} (21 mrad) at the near point for human vision (10 to 20 cm). For example a 0.1-mm (100-μm) source diameter viewed at 10 cm is only 1 mrad. Even a large array of fibers 1 mm across would subtend only 10 mrad at 10 cm. For small, local cable systems an average output power of 3 mW at λ = 905 nm from a cable having NA = 0.1 (ϕ = 12° = 200 mrad) might be characteristic. In this instance the approximate irradiance at r = 10 cm from the cable end is:

$$E = \frac{1.27 \, \Phi}{(\phi r)^2} = \frac{1.27 \, (3 \text{ mW})}{[(0.2)(10 \text{ cm})]^2} = 0.95 \text{ mW/cm}^2 \qquad (20\text{-}17)$$

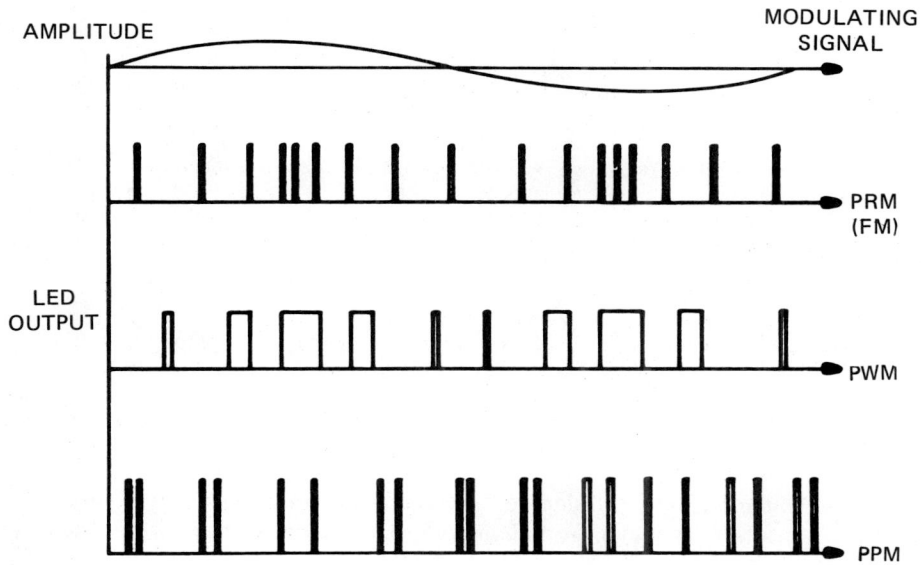

Figure 20-12. Pulse Trains Used in Optical Communications. The communication signal (top) modulates a train of optical pulses in one of several ways, such as the three shown above: pulse rate modulation (PRM), pulse width modulation (PWM), and pulse position modulation (PPM) or pulse interval modulation. Drawing courtesy of Irwin Math Associates.

which slightly exceeds the EL for very lengthy exposures. At 20 cm, E is 0.24 mW/cm^2 which is below the previously derived 8-hour limit of 0.8 mW/cm^2. Many small data links have a maximum power of only 0.1 mW and are in practice not hazardous, but the output beam should be measured to confirm this in any given installation. Most present systems use GaAlAs (850 nm) or GaAs (905 nm) but future systems are expected to operate at 1.15–1.3 µm (e.g., InGaAsP diode lasers) where transmission loss and pulse spreading (due to dispersion) are minimal in glass.

Efforts to establish safe fiber-optic communication installations have centered on safe connectors. Revised, 1979-vintage safety standards (IEC, ANSI) require that fiber-optic connectors be so designed that disconnection can only be accomplished using a tool (e.g., a screw driver). The following extract from the 1979 ANSI Z-136.1 revision distinguishes between open, accessible cable connections and those connections in a secured junction closet:

4.4.4 Laser Optical Fiber Transmission Systems. Laser transmission systems which employ optical cables shall be considered enclosed systems with the optical cable forming part of the enclosure. If a disconnection of a connector results in accessible radiation being reduced to below the applicable MPE by engineering controls connection or disconnection may take place in an uncontrolled area and no other control measures are required. When the system provides access to laser radiation above the applicable MPE via a connector, the conditions given in 4.4.4.1 or 4.4.4.2 shall apply.

4.4.4.1 Connection or Disconnection during operation shall take place in a laser controlled area described, as appropriate, in 4.2.12 through 4.2.12.2.

4.4.4.2 Connection or Disconnection during maintenance, modification or service shall take place in a temporary laser controlled area described in 4.2.14. When the connection or disconnection is made by means of a connector other than one within a secured enclosure, such a connector shall only be disconnectable by the use of a tool.

When the connection or disconnection is made within a secured enclosure, no tool for connector disconnect shall be required, but a warning sign appropriate to the class of laser or laser system shall be visible when the enclosure is open.

Note: In all instances where radiation above the MPE levels can be accessed by disconnection of a connector, the connector shall bear a label or tag with the words "Hazardous Laser Radiation When Disconnected."

A secondary safety problem of some concern in some fiber experiments is injury of the skin and eye from handling glass fibers. During work where glass fragments can be generated, safety glasses should be worn.

20.6 LASER CANE FOR THE BLIND

Under the sponsorship of the Prosthetic and Sensory Aids Service of the U.S. Veterans Administration, Bionic Instruments Inc., Bala Cynwyd, PA, developed a laser cane (Typhlocane) for the blind during the 1960's to serve as a mobility aid. The hazard analysis of this device is illustrative of the difficulties in assessing the potential hazards of a small, portable, diode laser transmitter. The goal of the laser cane was to retain the proven physical and psychological advantages of the conventional long cane, yet add protection of head and shoulders, as well as early warning of objects and major breaks in the terrain, such as steps or edges of platforms.

20.6.1 General Characteristics

The 1969-vintage Bionic Model C-4 Laser Typhlocane weighed 1-1/3 pounds and employed three gallium-arsenide (Ga-As) infrared-emitting laser diodes, with associated detectors, logic circuits and power supply self-contained. A diagram of the unit is shown in Figure 20-13.

In normal use the cane simultaneously emitted three collimated beams which were directed upward, straight ahead, and downward. A low-pitched tone was heard if the reflection from the downward beam ceased. The user's index finger was vibrated if the forward-looking detector was reflected from an object straight ahead. A high-pitched tone was heard if the upward-looking detector received a reflection from an obstacle, such as a tree, a branch or an awning. The cane would normally be rotated about, rhythmically sweeping the three laser beams.

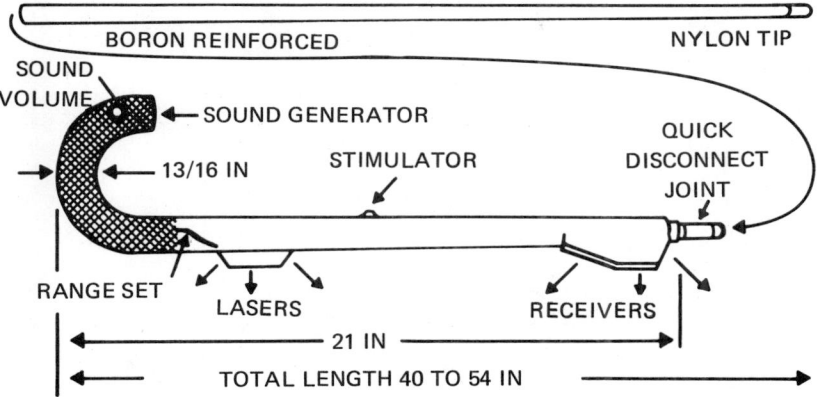

Figure 20-13. Laser Cane. The laser cane in this drawing is separated into two parts, the electronic section and the staff. Drawing courtesy of Bionic Instruments, Inc., Bala Cynwyd, PA.

The emergent beam of each laser was collimated by a single positive lens of 13.6 mm focal length. The beam emitted from one prototype Typhlocane was measured in 1969 with a spectroradiometer to obtain the relative spectral irradiance. The peak spectral irradiance occurred at approximately 902 nm with a spectral width at half-power points of 15 nm. The total average power measured within the beam of each laser was 30 μW. The PRF of the lasers was 40 Hz, with a pulse duration of approximately 100 ns, hence the peak power of each pulse would be 7.5 W. Actual oscilloscope traces of single pulses provided a nominal value of 5 W.

20.6.2 Beam Divergence

The beam divergence of a laser-diode projector is theoretically determined by the length of the active area of the emitting junction, the intrinsic beam divergence in the plane perpendicular to the junction plane, and the focal length of the collimating lens. The length of the junction of the General Electric Type H1D1 diode was 200 μm and the focal length of the lens was 13.6 mm; therefore, the divergence in the plane of the junction was: (0.2 mm) / (13.6 mm) or 14.7 mrad. The divergence in the other plane would be less than 1 mrad.

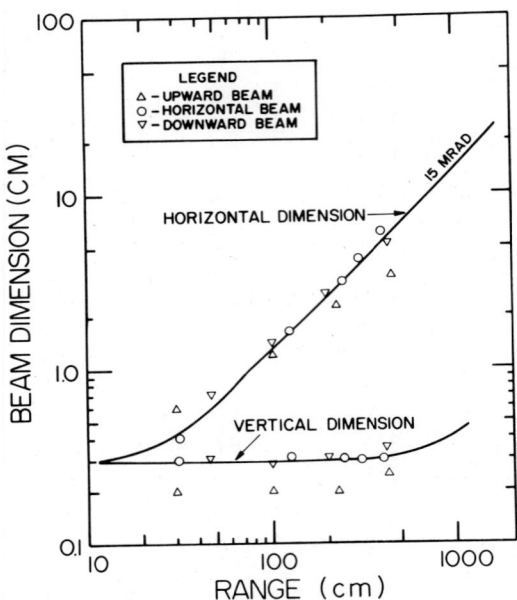

Figure 20-14. Laser Cane Beam Dimensions. The beam width across the narrowest dimension is shown in the lower curve. The beam heights (broadest dimension) are shown in the upper curve with individual data points for the three beams. The measurements were made in 1969 using an infrared image converter and grid paper. Newer canes have different characteristics.

The beam profiles of three beams from one cane, as measured at several distances out to a range of 3 m, gave divergences of 6 mrad, 14 mrad, and 19 mrad for the upward, downward and forward-looking beams, respectively. The 14 and 19 mrad beams were just as expected; however, the 6 mrad beam was somewhat surprising at first. Apparently, the laser source was defective, or partially occluded. The narrower dimensions of the beam profiles indicated a divergence of less than 1 mrad.

The diameter of the beam emerging from the collimating optics was estimated to be 3 mm. This value was obtained by viewing the emergent beam pattern on a mm grid through the use of an infrared image converter. The beam pattern was likewise defined for selected distances out to 3 m. A summary of the beam profile data is presented in Figure 20-14.

20.6.3 Beam Irradiance

The beam irradiance was calculated from the beam divergence and the 30 μW average power value. The resulting calculated emergent beam irradiance was 3.8×10^{-4} W/cm^2; the emergent beam irradiance measured through a 7-mm aperture was

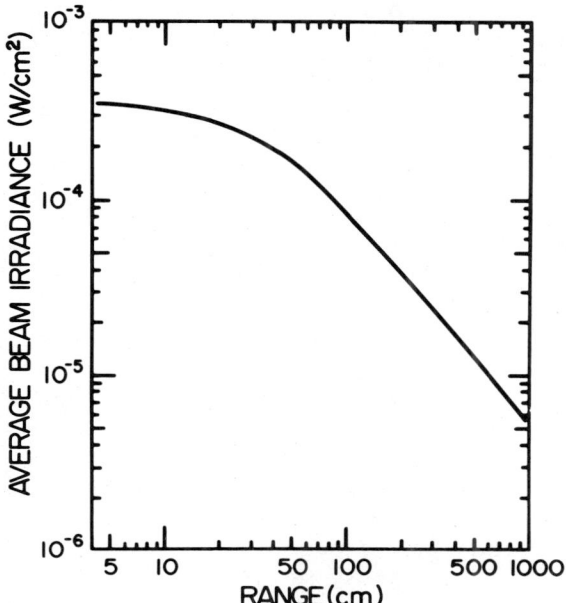

Figure 20-15. Beam Irradiance of an Early Laser Cane. The average beam irradiance for the 30-μW elliptical beam was calculated using Eq. 12-8 on p. 388 and is plotted above.

only 7.8×10^{-5} W/cm^2. The beam irradiance at a given distance from the laser is determined by the beam divergence (Figure 20-14) and is given in Figure 20-15.

20.6.4 Projected Radiance

The projected radiance of the source is determined approximately by the beam irradiance measured at a given point, divided by the solid angle subtended by the apparent size of the source viewed from that point. It is convenient to choose a point at a distance of 25 cm, (the typical "near point" of the adult eye) where the magnifying power, P, of the collimating lens is:

$$P = (25/f) + 1 \qquad (20\text{-}18)$$

where f is the focal length of the lens in cm. As f is 1.36 cm, the magnifying power is 19.4 X or approximately 20 X. Hence, the apparent length of the source is 4 mm. Likewise, the apparent width is approximately 0.2 mm, which is also the width predicted by diffraction theory for a 5-mm diameter lens. The solid angle, Ω, in steradians (sr), subtended by this source is calculated by Figure 2-32, where r is the viewing distance, 25 cm; and A_s is the projected area of the source of 25 cm, 0.8 mm². By this, Ω is 1.3×10^{-5} sr, which in turn leads to an approximate effective radiance of 30 W/(cm²·sr).

20.6.5 Hazard Analysis

Within a viewing distance of approximately 50 cm, it is possible for the entire laser beam to enter the eye. If the normal eye were relaxed, the image upon the retina would be approximately 20 μm by 250 μm, or 5×10^{-5} cm². These retinal image dimensions were obtained by assuming a minimum line spread function of 20 μm (Section 4.5.3) and an image length, s, determined by ϕf, with ϕ the greater divergence ~ 15 mrad, and f the effective focal length of the eye, 1.7 cm.

It is therefore possible to estimate a worst-case retinal irradiance of 30 μW/5 × 10⁻⁵ cm² or 0.6 W/cm². Likewise, the estimated retinal exposure dose per pulse is 7×10^{-7} J/5×10^{-5} cm² or 14 mJ/cm². For a PRF of 40 Hz the exposure dose for such image sizes can be expected to be slightly additive. This exposure dose is below the reported retinal injury levels for pulse durations less than 1 μs, but little data really exists for repetitive-pulse exposures to line sources. It is more relevant to examine the exposure limits. The exposure from one sector of the line source within an angle of α_{min} must not exceed the intrabeam EL.

Since the maximal projected source length is 15 mrad, this angle is less than α_{min} for a CW, 905-nm source. But it is greater than α_{min} for a 100-ns pulse, which is only 3.7 mrad, or 25% of the line source. The EL for such a 905-nm source is the lesser of the single-pulse and CW criteria. Specifically, the 40 Hz single-pulse EL at 905 nm is:

$$H = 5 \, C_p \cdot C_A \cdot \mu J/cm^2 \qquad (20\text{-}19)$$
$$= 0.2 \, \mu J/cm^2$$

and

$$E_{avg} = (0.2 \, \mu J/cm^2)(40 \, Hz) = 8 \, \mu W/cm^2$$

which is well below the "pure-CW" criterion of:

$$E = 320 \cdot C_A \cdot \mu W/cm^2 \qquad \text{for} \quad t \geqslant 1000 \, s \qquad (20\text{-}20)$$
$$= 0.8 \, mW/cm^2$$

Hence the permissible long-term viewing distance for this prototype based upon the pulse limit criterion and from Figure 20-15 was 750 cm. If the objective of the cane could be met with a higher PRF and the same average power it would have been Class 1 by the ANSI standard. It is interesting to note that the present Typhlocane uses a different laser diode which operates at a higher PRF of 80 Hz.

20.7 REVIEW QUESTIONS

1. What is a hologram? How should a hologram be safely viewed?

2. What is the safe radiance and the equivalent safe luminance for long-term (>10^4 s) viewing of extended-source laser displays at each of the following three wavelengths: 441.6 nm; 514.5 nm; 632.8 nm?

3. What is the limiting angle (α_{min}) for long-term (>10 s) viewing of extended visible light laser display sources?

4. Calculate the hazardous viewing distance for a 0.5-W krypton CW laser beam at 647.1 nm striking a 99% reflectance diffuse white surface if the beam diameter is 2 mm. Assume viewing duration of 0.25 s and 10^4 s.

5. What is the beam irradiance at an aircraft illuminated by a 2-W visible CW laser beam which has an emergent beam diameter of 8 mm, and a divergence of 0.3 mrad, if the airplane intercepts the beam at an altitude of 20,000 ft above ground level (a.g.l.) and at a ground distance of 1 km from the laser? At a ground distance of 1 km and at an elevation of 3,300 ft a.g.l.?

6. How does one prevent public exposure in a planetarium during a laser sound and light show? Who requires a variance from the BRH regulation?

7. An artist wishes to make use of total internal reflection of a laser beam in water (n = 1.33) to keep a laser beam from exiting a water tank. Calculate the angle of incidence with an air interface to which the beam must be limited.

8. What type of fiber optic cable connections were recommended in the 1979 ANSI Z-136 and IEC proposals?

9. What is the numerical aperture of a glass fiber (index of refraction of 1.56) which has a plastic cladding (index of refraction of 1.36)? A GaAs laser with a beam spread of 40° × 20° is coupled to one end of the fiber. What is the approximate beam spread at the other end?

10. A toy gun has a GaAlAs (850-nm) laser diode which emits an average power of 20 μW with 200-ns pulses at 1 kHz PRF. What is the hazard classification?

20.8 REFERENCES

Abel, L. A., Dell'Osso, L. F., Daroff, R. B., and Parker, L., 1979, Saccades in extremes of lateral gaze, *Invest. Ophthal. Vis. Sci.* **18**(3):324–327.
American National Standards Institute, 1976, The Safe Use of Lasers, Standard Z-136.1, ANSI, New York (with proposed 1979 revision).
Anonymous, 1979a, Philips shows a 'compact' audiodisk with digital playback by a diode laser, *Laser Focus* **15**(7):38–41 (July 1979).
Anonymous, 1979b, IBM introduces an intelligent copier with a laser and two microprocessors, *Laser Focus* **15**(5):24 (May 1979).
Anonymous, 1969, Laser systems, recent legislation, lasers and risks, *Illinois Med. J.* **135**:85–86.
Beiser, L., 1978, Augimented laser scan equations, *Appl. Opt.* **8**(17):1161.

Buckler, M. J., 1978, Optical crosstalk evaluation for two end-to-end lightguide system installations, *Bell Sys. Tech. J.* **57**(6):1759–1769.
Commission Internationale de L'Eclairage, 1970, (International Commission on Illumination), "International Lighting Vocabulary," 3rd Ed., Publ. CIE No. 17 (E-1.1), CIE, Paris.
Charlton, D., and Reitz, P. R., 1979, Making fiber measurements, *Laser Focus* **15**(9):52–64 (September 1979).
Edmunds, H. D., 1979, Interlocks, *Proc. SPIE* **144**:33–37.
Garbor, D., 1972, Holography 1948–1971, *Science* **177**:299–313.
Goldman, L., 1970, Laser light, a new visual art and a new occupational hazard, *Arch. Envir. Health* **20**:145.
Goodson, J. E., 1979, Dynamics of an image viewed through a rotating mirror, *J. Opt. Soc. Am.* **69**(5):771–775.
Hecht, J., 1977, Light shows and safety, *Laser Focus* **13**(7):6 (July 1977).
Hickey, J., and Kuhfeld, R., 1979, Fiber optics—looking better all the time, *Instr. Contr. Syst.* **52**(3):17–26 (March 1979).
Hopkins, R. E., and Buzawa, M. J., 1979, Optics for laser scanning, *Opt. Eng.* **15**(2):90–94.
Jacobs, I., 1978, Atlanta fiber system experiment: overview, *Bell Syst. Tech. J.* **57**(6):1717–1721.
Kiesling, G. A., 1979, Assuring an efficient effort for complying with the BRH laser standard, *Proc. SPIE* **144**:74–79.
Makous, W. L. and Gould, J. C., 1968, Vision and Lasers, the effects of lasers on the human visual system, with some implications for the design of laser displays, IBM Research Report RC-1702, IBM Watson Research Center, Yorktown Heights, NH (October 28, 1966) and IBM *J. Res. Div.* **12**:257.
Malina, F. J. (Ed.), 1978, "Kinetic Art: Theory and Practice," Dover Publications, New York.
North, J. C., 1978, Handling optical cables: safety aspects; comments, *Appl. Opt.* **17**(13):1987.
Parker, G. S., 1970, The current status of state regulation on laser radiation, *Laser J.* **2**(3):17–20.
Rockwell, R. J., Jr., Sliney, D. H., and Smith, J. F., 1979, Laser safety, part III: controls for safe operation, *Electro-Opt. Syst. Design* **11**(5):34–46 (May 1979).
Royston, D. D., 1979, Special measurement problems, *Proc. SPIE* **144**:46–53.
Runge, P. K., and Cheng, S. S., 1978, Demountable single-fiber optic connectors and their measurement on location, *Bell Syst. Tech. J.* **57**(6):1771–1790.
Smith, L. D., and Dennis, J. E., 1979, Laser light show safety criteria, *Proc. SPIE* **144**:106–110.
Solon, L. R., and Sims, S. D., 1970, Fundamental physiological optics of laser beams, *Med. Res. Eng.* **9**(3):10–25.
Stroke, G. W., 1969, "An Introduction to Coherent Optics and Holography," Academic Press, New York.
Takeda, Y., and Tsunoda, Y., 1978, Use of heterostructure diode lasers in video disk systems, *Appl. Opt.* **17**(6):863–867.
Taylor, S. L., 1979, The impact of the Federal Laser Performance Standard on planetarium laser light shows, *Proc. SPIE* **144**:101–106.
Timmerman, C. C., 1977, Handling optical cables: safety aspects, *Appl. Opt.* **16**(9):2380–2382.
U.S. Department of Health, Education and Welfare, Food and Drug Administration, 1978, Approval of Variance for Laserium Projector, *Federal Register* **43**(168):38626–38628 (August 29, 1978).
Van Pelt, W. F., Stewart, H. F., and Peterson, R. W., 1970a, A safety oriented laser manual for science teachers. Electronic Product Radiation and the Health Physicist BRH/DEP 70-26, 385–389, U.S. Department of Health, Education, and Welfare, Bureau of Radiological Health, Rockville, MD (October 1970).
Van Pelt, W. F., Stewart, H. F., Peterson, R. W., Roberts, A. M., and Worst, 1970b, Laser Fundamentals and Experiments, Report BRH/SWRHL 70-1, Bureau of Radiological Health, Rockville, MD, (May 1970).
Zwick, H., and Jenkins, D., 1978, Effects of coherent light on retinal receptor processes of pseudemys, *Invest. Ophthal. Vis. Sci.* **17**(Suppl):172.

Chapter 21
Laser Hazards in Outdoor Applications: Military and Lidar

21.1 INTRODUCTION

The use of lasers in the tactical military environment on the ground and sea, and by aircraft present eye hazards to personnel in aircraft and surface personnel. Many similar hazards are presented by the use of high-power laser satellite trackers and by LIDAR (Laser Radar). Methods have been developed for applying ocular exposure limits to the solution of practical field safety problems. Laser pointing accuracy, and the extent of backstops and the presence of hazardous specular reflections from flat glass and standing areas of water strongly influence safe laser operations. Many of the hazard controls used for military lasers apply to civilian outdoor laser usage such as LIDAR and open communication links.

Many medium-power laser systems are being used in tactical military ground and airborne applications. Those include rangefinding, target designation (Figure 21-1), ordinance guidance, and, during periods of darkness, night vision illuminators for covert detection, identification and surveillance. Several papers in the open literature have described hazard evaluation for ground based and airborne military lasers, and laser range controls (Freasier, 1969; Sliney, 1970; Sliney and Yacovissi, 1975).

The military services have documents promulgating safety control procedures (U.S. Department of the Army, 1975; U.S. Department of the Air Force, 1973) and follow permissible laser exposure limits (Table 21-1) which follow the ANSI Z-136.1 limits. It is the purpose of this chapter to review the factors useful in evaluating and controlling the operational hazards for both ground and airborne laser systems used out-of-doors.

21.2 OCULAR EXPOSURE CONDITIONS

Personnel can receive hazardous retinal exposure by intrabeam viewing of

Table 21-1. Some Protection Standards Applicable to Some Representative Military Lasers from the 1976 ANSI Standard Z-136.1

Type of Laser Exposure	Example for PRF (Hz)	Wavelength (nm)	Exposure Duration	Exposure Limit for Intrabeam Viewing by the Eye [$J/(cm^2 \cdot pulse)$]	Exposure Limit for a Diffuse Reflection: Surface Radiant Exposure ($\rho = 90\%$) [$J/(cm^2 \cdot pulse)$]	Exposure Limit for the Skin [$J/(cm^2 \cdot pulse)$]
Single-Pulse Ruby Laser Rangefinder	Single Pulse	694.3	1 ns to 18 μs	5×10^{-7}	$28\ t^{1/3}$	0.02
Repetitively Pulsed Ruby Laser Rangefinder or Designator	10	694.3	1 ns to 18 μs	1.6×10^{-7}	$9\ t^{1/3}$	0.02
	20	694.3	1 ns to 18 μs	1.1×10^{-7}	$6.2\ t^{1/3}$	0.02
Single-Pulse Neodymium: YAG Laser Rangefinder	Single Pulse	1064	1 ns to 50 μs	5×10^{-6}	$141\ t^{1/3}$	0.1
Repetitively Pulsed Neodymium:YAG Rangefinder or Designator	10	1064	1 ns to 50 μs	1.6×10^{-6}	$45\ t^{1/3}$	0.1
	20	1064	1 ns to 50 μs	1.1×10^{-6}	$31\ t^{1/3}$	0.1

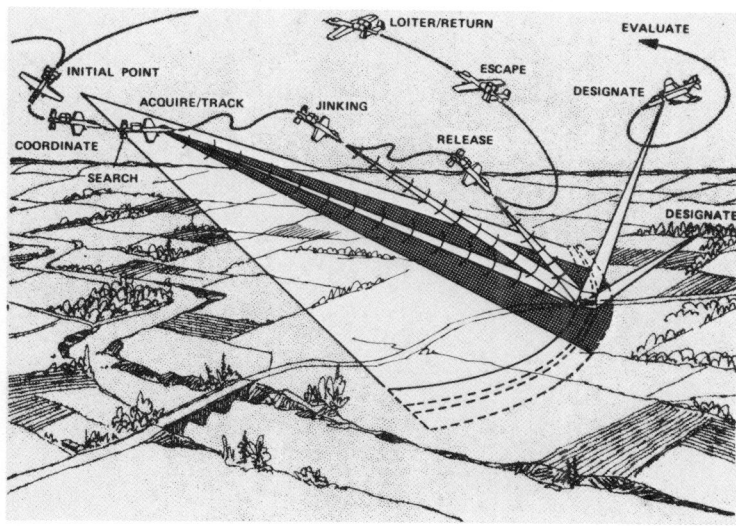

Figure 21-1. Target Designator. An airborne laser target designation beam from the aircraft in the upper righthand corner (or from the ground laser) points out a target for a bombing by the aircraft to the left (Reprinted from *Laser Focus,* June 1977, with permission).

most laser rangefinders and laser target designator lasers (Figure 21-2), and in a few situations, by viewing the diffuse reflection of such a laser beam. Many of the present day laser rangefinder systems have nominal intrabeam ocular hazard distances (NOHD's) between 1 and 10 km. In many field situations it is not feasible to exclude all personnel from the vicinity of the laser. Therefore, the hazardous areas must be carefully defined, and safety precautions followed to minimize the potential for accidental ocular injury.

21.3 LASER HAZARD ANALYSIS AND CONTROLS

In contrast to the control of laboratory lasers, the control of field military lasers must rely on the determination of hazardous zones of occupancy. The safety guidelines for field lasers have centered on limiting personnel access to laser areas, limiting laser operation in occupied areas, and limiting the exposure of personnel to laser radiation. The performance of personnel hazard evaluation of the laser device in accordance with appropriate safety standards is necessary to establish the hazardous zones. Adequate controls for personnel protection must be established without unduly restricting the operation of the system. The unjudicious application of unnecessary controls can have serious consequences. The following sections will consider those factors which should be included in such an evaluation.

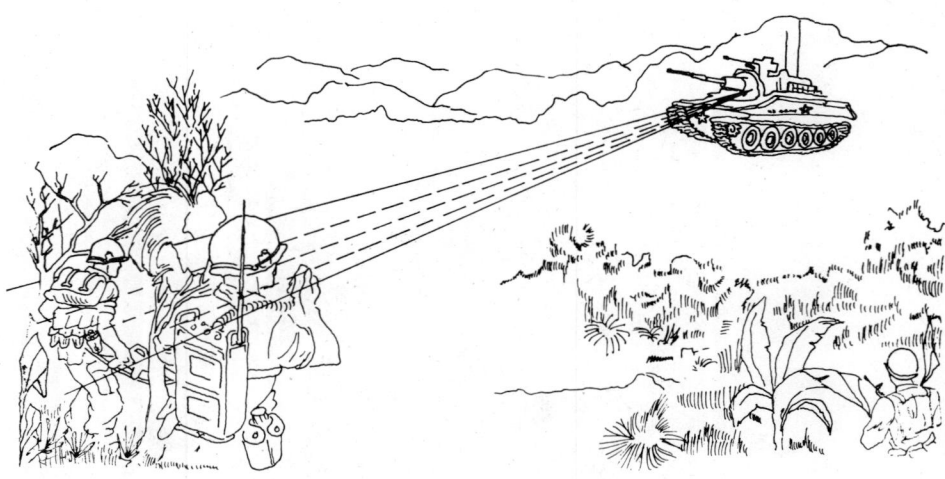

INTRABEAM VIEWING

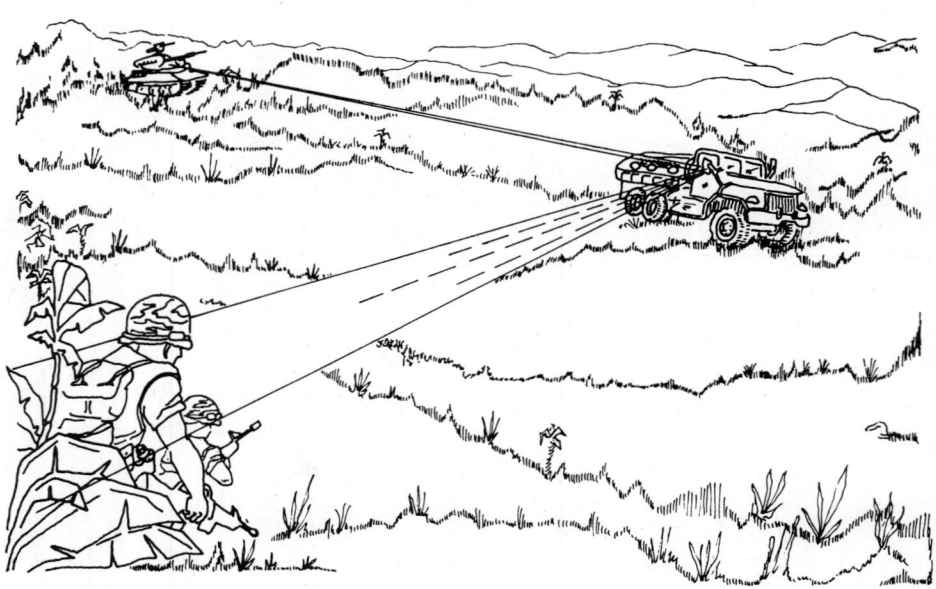

INTRABEAM VIEWING OF SPECULAR REFLECTION

Figure 21-2. Intrabeam Viewing. Intrabeam viewing of a military tank laser rangefinder can occur when a soldier is located within the direct beam (top) or within a specularly reflected beam from a flat glass surface (bottom).

21.4 DIRECT BEAM EXPOSURE

Laser exposure limits for the direct beam are specified in terms of the corneal irradiance or corneal radiant exposure. It is therefore essential that some estimate of the beam irradiance E or radiant exposure H as a function of distance be known. The values of H at different ranges r is used in evaluating reflection hazards, optical viewing hazards and eye protection requirements. The beam irradiance, $E(W/cm^2)$, or radiant exposure, $H(J/cm^2)$, can be calculated at a distance r by using the following equations developed in Chapter 12 (Eq. 12-6 and 12-7) for a circular beam:

$$H = 1.27\, Q\, e^{-\mu r}/(a + r\cdot\phi)^2 \quad \text{or} \quad E = 1.27\, \Phi\, e^{-\mu r}/(a + r\cdot\phi)^2 \qquad (21\text{-}1)$$

where Q is radiant energy (expressed in Joules); Φ is radiant power (expressed in Watts); r is range (in centimeters); μ is the atmospheric attenuation coefficient (typically 5×10^{-7} to 5×10^{-6} cm^{-1}); a is the emergent beam diameter (in cm) at 1/e-peak-irradiance points; and ϕ is the beam divergence (in radians) at 1/e-peak-irradiance points. These parameters are often available from the system specifications, but they should be supported by direct measurements. For hazard analysis purposes, it is desirable to use the divergence value obtained at the 1/e-peak-irradiance points to calculate the maximum axial beam irradiance or radiant exposure, rather than the average beam irradiance (or radiant exposure) which would be calculated using the $1/e^2$ divergence points often specified by the manufacturer. The $1/e^2$ points also correspond approximately to the cone angle which includes 90% of the beam power or energy. Figure 13-10 presents the theoretical and measured values of the radiant-exposure-per-pulse for a typical neodymium (Nd) laser rangefinder. Beyond a range of a few hundred meters, the focusing and defocusing of small parts of the beam due to localized atmospheric turbulence will result in a highly irregular beam profile (Chapter 13). Figure 13-6 illustrates this scintillation effect upon the beam of a ruby laser at 500 and 1500 meters. It is believed that the spreading of the beam by the atmosphere will largely counteract the adverse effects of "hotspots" which, previously, were thought to considerably extend the hazardous range beyond that calculated for a nonturbulent medium. As turbulence is greatest for near-ground laser beam paths, scintillation is far less noticeable for air-to-ground, or ground-to-air paths.

The beam irradiance or radiant exposure as a function of range will first determine whether hazardous exposure conditions exist in the target area from the laser. Precautionary controls can then be determined, and a decision made as to whether personnel should be restricted from the target area, or be required to wear laser eye protectors. Restrictive minimum altitudes or slant ranges of operation for airborne lasers and controlled beam paths and buffer zones around the target area can be established as required.

21.5 REFLECTED BEAM EXPOSURE

Reflections of the laser beam can result in exposure to personnel outside of the controlled areas of the immediate beam path and the target as shown in Figure

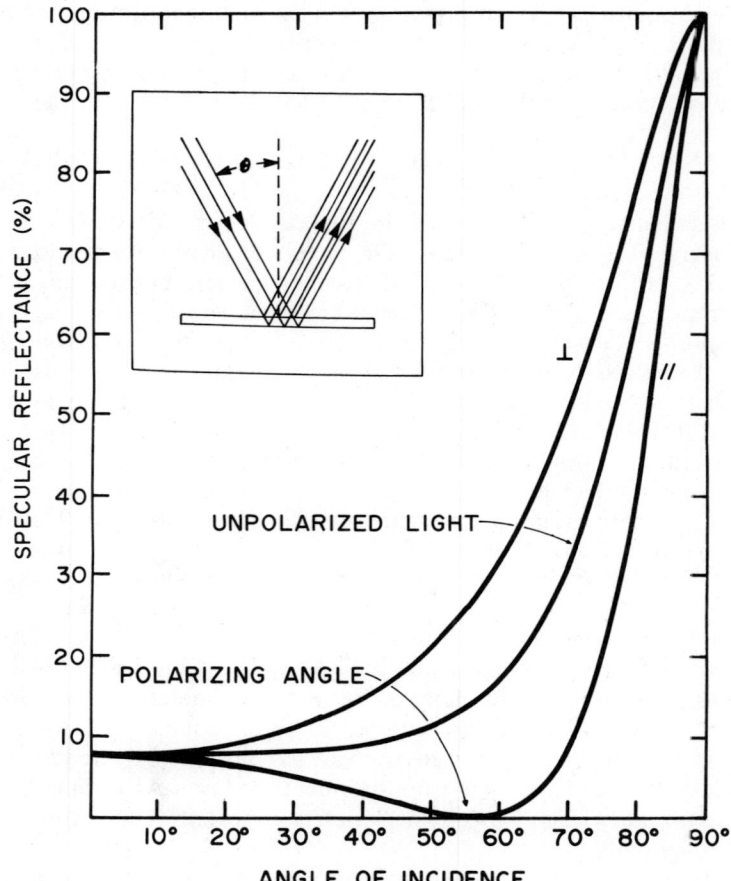

Figure 21-3. Fresnel Reflection. Specular reflectance from two surfaces of a glass plate ($n = 1.5$). Note that a beam whose electric vector is oriented parallel (||) to the plane of incidence is not reflected at Brewster's angle (i.e., the polarizing angle). Inset shows beam incident upon glass for specular reflection. Employing a vertically polarized beam for airborne lasers and a horizontally polarized beam for ground-located lasers minimizes hazardous specular reflections since most glass surfaces are oriented vertically and water surfaces are oriented horizontally.

21-2 (bottom). The reflections can be considered as two general types: specular and diffuse.

21.5.1 Diffuse Reflections

Normally, diffuse reflections down-range (away from the laser) will not be of concern since the laser energy can no longer be readily focused to a concentrated spot. In some cases, the laser's radiant exposure at the output port is capable of producing a radiance level of diffuse reflection that is unsafe to view. Such a reflection would be hazardous at all viewing angles and not just within the localized and collimated secondary beam. Laser exposure standards give the value either of the radiant exitance at a diffuse surface, or the time-integrated surface radiance capable of producing a hazardous diffuse reflection. Lasers capable of exceeding these levels are normally classified as Class 4 "high risk" laser systems. In these instances, all objects should be excluded from the beam path until the beam's radiant exposure has decreased to a value that will not produce a hazardous diffuse reflection. For airborne lasers in flight, hazardous diffuse reflections will not be of concern. However, during maintenance and testing of some aircraft lasers, or for some ground lasers, hazardous diffuse reflections can be very significant. If they exist, stringent control procedures will be required within approximately 1 to 10 m of the laser.

21.5.2 Specular Reflections

Specular reflections from flat surfaces are of greatest concern since the reflection will maintain the collimated beam characteristics. Hence, hazardous levels are possible out to considerable distances. Most targets encountered in field situations are reasonably diffuse. Most natural surfaces which have some form of specular reflection (e.g., water droplets, glossy leaves, etc.) have a small enough radius of curvature that hazardous reflected levels exist only near the reflector. Flat mirrors will reflect almost all of the incident beam energy, other flat reflective surfaces will reflect a part of the beam depending on the angle of incidence and the inherent reflectivity of the surface. Figure 21-3 illustrates that approximately 8-percent of the beam incident on clear glass (4% per surface) is reflected at normal (perpendicular) incidence, but at large angles (θ approaching 90°) most of the incident beam will be reflected. From a water surface, approximately 2-percent of a beam incident at 0-20° is reflected.

For hazard evaluation, still ponds of water, glass surfaces on target vehicles, and windows in target structures are the principal specularly-reflecting surfaces of importance. When the reflecting surface lies in a vertical plane, the reflected beam from an airborne laser will be terminated in the ground zone around the target, and thus could be of concern only to ground personnel in the immediate area of the target. On the other hand, vertical glass surfaces present the primary source of hazardous reflections from ground lasers. Noting this, it has been suggested that the polarization of ground based and airborne lasers be different: that the polarization be adjusted to minimize hazardous reflections.

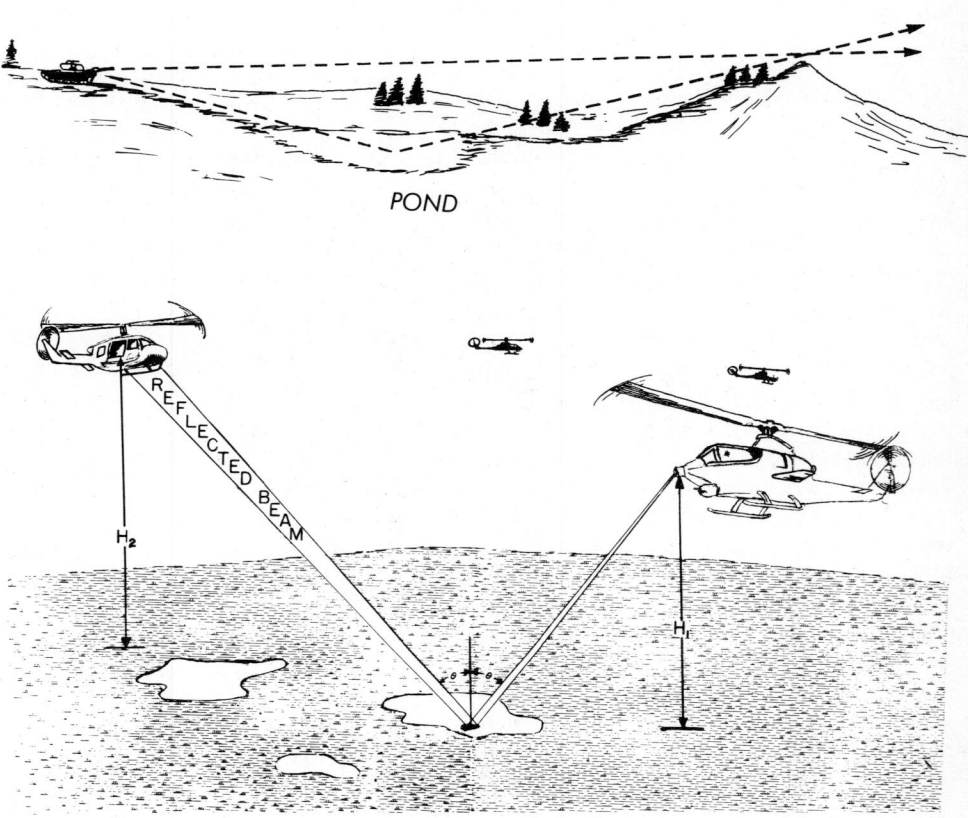

Figure 21-4. Specular Reflections from Water. Upper panel shows reflected beam from a ground laser; lower panel shows reflected beam from laser redirected upward from still water. The altitudes H_1 and H_2 are R_1 and R_2 in Equation (21-2).

21.5.2.1 Standing Water

In situations where laser equipped aircraft would be operating along with other aircraft over swamps or areas of *standing* water, the reflection hazard to personnel in other aircraft should be considered. Since the water surface in this case is always horizontal, the path of the reflected beam would continue along the same azimuth as the primary beam but angled upwards so that the angle of incidence would equal the angle of reflection (Figure 21-4), thus defining a hazardous plane. Equation 21-2 can be used to predict the reflected beam radiant exposure at an altitude equal to the sum of the altitudes of the two aircraft.

$$H = \frac{1.27 \, Q \cdot e^{-\mu(R_1 + R_2)/\cos\theta}}{\left[a + \left(\dfrac{R_1 + R_2}{\cos\theta}\right)\phi\right]} \left[\frac{p_\| \tan^2(\theta - \theta')}{\tan^2(\theta + \theta')} + \frac{p_\perp \sin^2(\theta - \theta')}{\sin^2(\theta + \theta')}\right]$$

(21-2)

where Q is the output energy in joules; R_1 is the altitude in cm of the aircraft firing the laser; R_2 is the altitude of any other aircraft on the azimuth of the laser beam in cm; θ is the angle the laser beam makes with a line perpendicular to the water surface (angle or incidence); θ' is the angle of the refracted laser beam in water [Arcsin (sin θ/n)]; n is the index of refraction (1.33 for water), $p_\perp$ is that fraction of the laser beam polarized perpendicularly to the plane of incidence (horizontal polarization); $p_\|$ is that fraction of the laser beam polarized parallel to the plane of incidence (vertical polarization) and ϕ is the beam divergence in radians. Figure 21-5 is a plot of the reflected beam radiant exposure for a Neodymium laser rangefinder as a function of the incident angle using Equation 21-2. The polarization of the beam for a worst-case and best-case reflection is illustrated.

21.5.2.2 Snow

Studies of reflections from snow indicate that snow is a nearly perfect diffuser. Since most tactical lasers are not a diffuse reflection hazard, no hazard will result from reflections of the laser beam incident upon snow.

21.5.2.3 Ice

Reflections from naturally occurring ice surfaces indicate a relatively strong specular component in the reflection, but despite the strength of this specular component, the reflection is insufficiently collimated to be of much concern. No truly collimated reflections are observed from ice. At close distances, patterns as shown in Figure 21-6 are observed with narrow bright areas superimposed over a diffuse reflection. Few lasers would produce hazardous reflections at distances greater than 100 meters from the reflecting surface.

21.5.2.4 Water-Covered Ice

Reflections from ice covered with a thin layer of water resemble reflections from water alone. These reflections are hazardous since the laser beam retains its collimation. Reflections at near-grazing angles provide the most reflection and hence the greatest hazard. This effect is also illustrated in Figure 21-6.

21.5.2.5 Glass Windows and View Blocks

Reflections from truck windows and from glass view blocks of armored

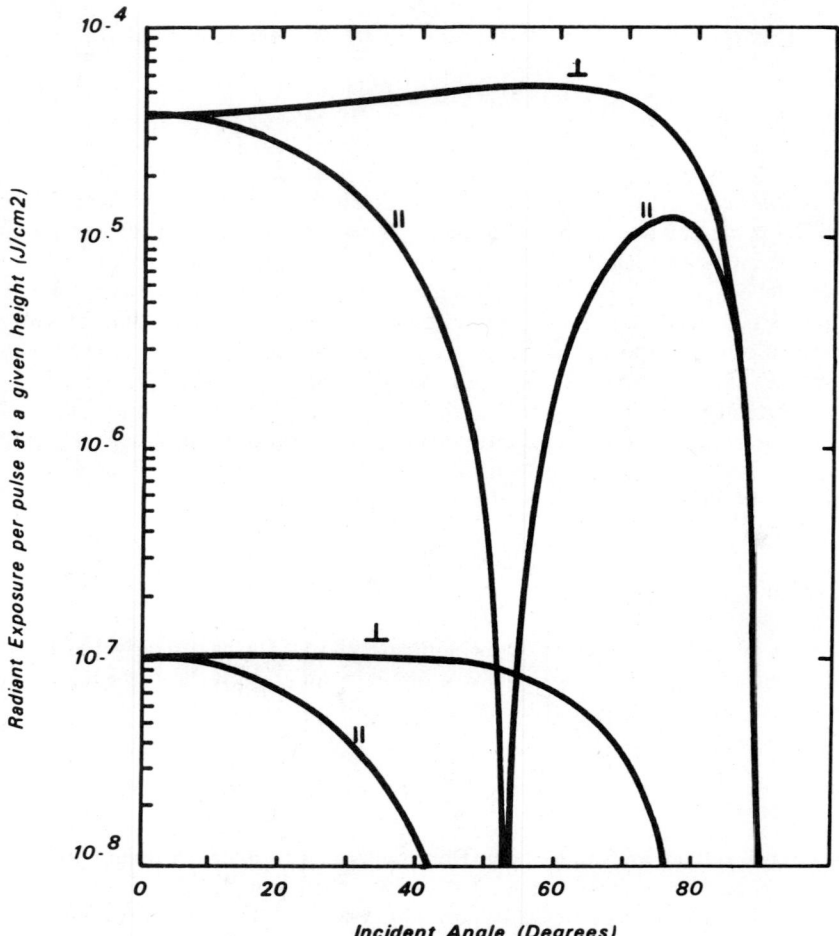

Figure 21-5. Specularly Reflected Levels. Reflected beam radiant exposure resulting from a typical laser rangefinder beam incident upon still water for a value of $R_1 + R_2 = 35$ m (upper curves) and for $R_1 + R_2 = 1000$ m (bottom curves).

vehicles produce a well-collimated beam, much as reflections from water; however, the pattern of optical radiation is altered slightly due to reflections from both the front and rear surfaces. Figure 21-7 shows the ground hazard envelopes for such reflections.

21.6 SCANNING LASERS

Some airborne laser devices used as illuminators, or as obstacle avoidance

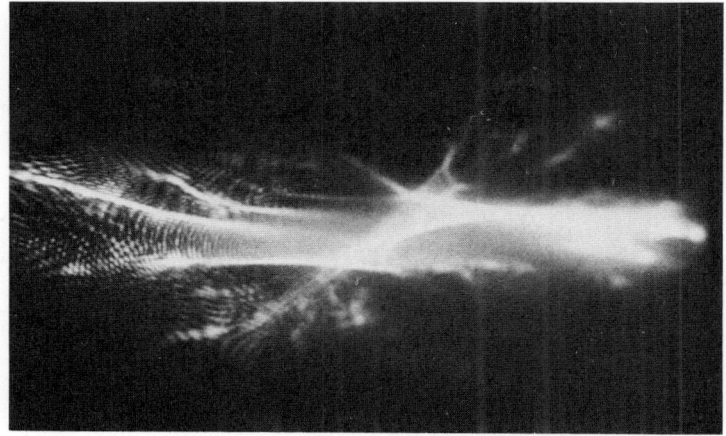

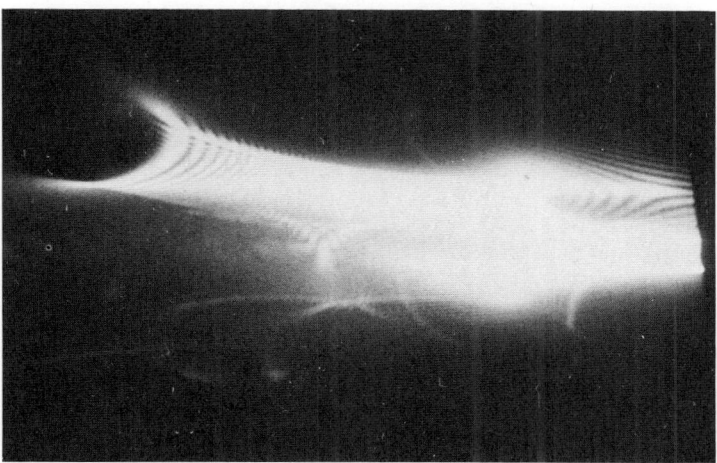

Figure 21-6. Reflections from Ice. Samples of the types of laser reflections observed from ice imaged on a card placed 0.5 to 1.0 m from the ice surface. The upper panel shows the reflection from ice alone, whereas the lower panel shows the reflection from melting ice where the water creates a collimated reflection in a small central white spot.

optical radar, may employ a scanning beam. The raster scanning beam in a surveillance laser generally has a pattern that will expose for at least one brief exposure per frame an individual on the ground looking up at the aircraft. This single exposure to

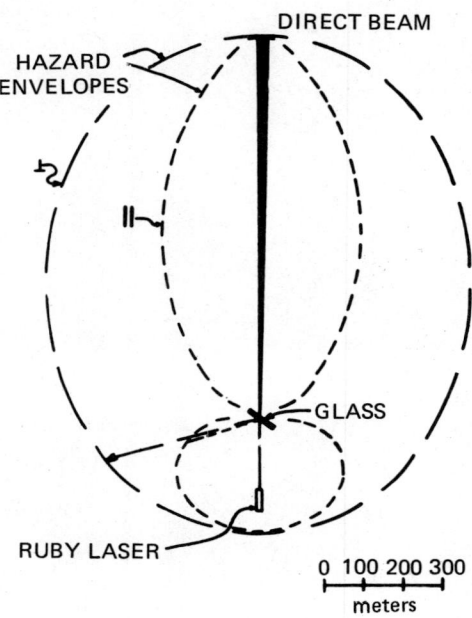

Figure 21-7. Hazard Envelopes. Ground hazard envelopes for a laser beam incident upon a vertical glass surface at 250 m is shown. Note the strong dependence upon polarization.

the retina is generally of a short duration t (in seconds). It depends upon the beam path to ground (approximately the altitude of the aircraft) r (in cm), the scan rate S (in scans per second), the pupil diameter d_e (in cm), and the sweep angle of each scan θ (in radians):

$$t = \frac{(a + r\phi)}{rS\theta} \quad \text{for} \quad d_e \leq (a + r\phi) \quad (21\text{-}3)$$

or

$$t = \frac{d_e}{rS\theta} \quad \text{for} \quad d_e \geq (a + r\phi) \quad (21\text{-}4)$$

The radiant exposure H (J/cm²) is simply the CW beam irradiance at the distance r multiplied by the exposure duration t. H is determined by the emitted CW laser power (in watts); the initial beam diameter a (in cm), the atmospheric attenuation factor μ (in cm^{-1}), (Figure 13-2), and the beam divergence ϕ (in cm):

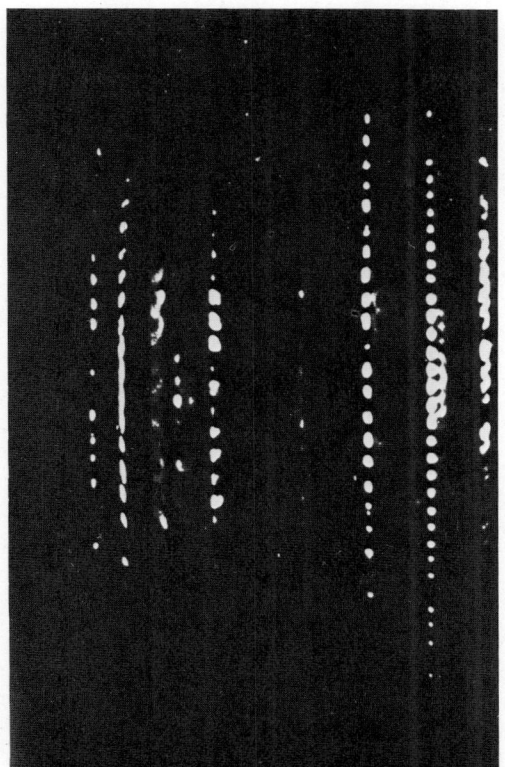

Figure 21-8. Laser Diode Array. This intrabeam photograph of a GaAs illuminator shows the diode rows created by an optical integrator. Hundreds of liquid-nitrogen-cooled laser diodes produced several watts of optical power.

$$H = \frac{1.27\, \Phi\, e^{-\mu r}}{(a + r\phi)^2} \cdot \frac{d_e}{rS\theta} \quad \text{for } d_e > (a + r\phi) \quad (21\text{-}5)$$

or

$$H = \frac{1.27\, \Phi\, e^{-\mu r}}{(a + r\phi)\,(rS\theta)} \quad \text{for } d_e < (a + r\phi) \quad (21\text{-}6)$$

Most airborne laser scanning systems have a relatively short hazardous range of 100 m or less since the duration of a single exposure is of the order one μs, and only a few pulsed exposures are possible during one flyover by the aircraft.

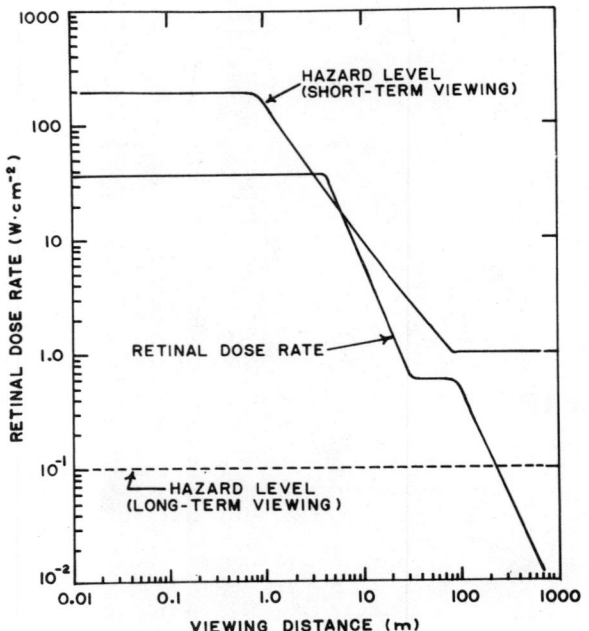

Figure 21-9. Retinal Hazard. Absorbed retinal irradiance is a function of viewing range for the infrared illuminator of Figure 21-8. The source was a liquid-nitrogen cooled GaAs array having a total average radiant power of 4.5 W. Solid line hazard level is USAEHA image-size dependent limit shown in Figure 10-3 (p. 337) and dashed line was early retinal limit for chronic exposure (from Sliney and Freasier, 1973).

21.7 EXTENDED SOURCES

Gallium-arsenide-diode arrays used as near-infrared illuminators do not normally present an intrabeam single-point image to the retina at distances in which the source can be resolved into a geometrical image (Figure 21-8). Applying intrabeam point-source laser retinal exposure standards to these lasers may be too conservative. A more valid criterion is based on the radiance of the source. Generally, photographic methods are employed to determine the effective source size of the various elements of the array at different intrabeam viewing distances. At close distances the individual source elements may be resolved. The radiance of each element can be determined, and the appropriate permissible exposure level applied. At greater ranges, the retinal image of the individual elements will tend to coalesce and the radiance of the entire source can be calculated (this occurred at $r > 30$ m in Figure 21-9). The radiance may be defined as the ratio of the irradiance at a given range divided by the solid angle subtended by the effective source size. The curious outcome of this hazard evaluation (Fig. 21-9) was that the array was hazardous at 4 to 6 m but not hazardous closer to the source. Biological experiments using animal subjects later confirmed this. Significant retinal temperature rises only occurred when the diode images coalesced. The potential for injury from extended sources will depend on the viewing duration. For example, the sun with a radiance of approximately 1300 W/(cm^2·sr) is safe for momentary (~0.25 second) viewing but definitely unsafe for long-term viewing. Of course the principal hazard of lengthy viewing of the sun is due primarily to blue light, even prolonged viewing of a near-infrared source is more dangerous than momentary viewing.

For near-infrared sources such as gallium-arsenide laser arrays and infrared searchlights, consideration must be given to the reduced visual response. The near-infrared wavelengths (700-1400 nm) are transmitted through the clear structures of the eye in various degrees depending on the wavelength, and "focus" on the retina. Since there is little visual sensation in this region, the normal protective mechanisms of the blink reflex and the natural aversion to bright light are ineffective for personnel protection. Consequently, uninformed personnel can, in many cases, view these infrared sources with comfort, unaware of the hazard.

21.8 OPTICAL VIEWING INSTRUMENTS

Intrabeam viewing of a collimated laser beam or a specularly reflected beam through a telescope or binoculars can increase the retinal irradiance considerably. Although the retinal image size will not be appreciably affected by the magnification of the optical system (i.e., it will remain essentially a diffraction-limited image), the greater light collecting power of the instrument will increase the retinal irradiance by a factor as great as the instrument's magnifying power squared.

The viewing of a large diffuse reflection (or intrabeam viewing of an extended source) through optical instruments will produce a retinal irradiance essentially the same as when viewed with the unaided eye. The retinal irradiance is actually reduced due to transmission losses in the instrument. Although the amount of light energy entering the eye is increased, it will be distributed over a proportionally increased retinal image area. The image area will increase proportionally to the square of the instrument's magnifying power. The power entering the eye will increase as the square of the objective diameter, but the increase cannot exceed a factor of the magnifying power squared. The potential for retinal injury for a given retinal irradiance is a strong function of the retinal image size. For example, the potential for a retinal injury from the sun is greater when the sun is viewed through binoculars. This increased hazard is due to the larger retinal image size. Thus at locations where a light source is considered safe to view by the unaided eye, it may not be safe when viewed through optical devices. Generally, the hazardous range will be extended by a factor approaching (but no greater than) the magnifying power of the instrument when one views either an extended source or a point source.

If the objective is not fully illuminated, then the simple rule-of-thumb hazard increase of the square of the magnifying power G does not apply. An alternative formula to Equation 21-1 has been developed by Marshall (1980) which permits one to calculate that fraction of a Gaussian beam energy entering an aperture (objective D_o) that can then be averaged over a 7-mm aperture for safety calculations:

$$H = 2.6\, Q\, e^{-\mu r} [1 - e^{-D_o^2/(a + r\phi)^2}] \qquad (21\text{-}7)$$

Equations 15-14 through 15-17 can be used in the hazard analysis of optically aided viewing. It is customary to assume a worst-case maximum objective diameter of 80 mm when calculating extended hazard distances. An exception to this rule would develop if large tracking telescopes were in use, e.g., at a missile range.

The use of optical instruments to observe the target during laser exposure should not be permitted unless all specular target surfaces have been removed, or appropriate protective filters are used. The use of manually operated cameras to photograph the laser beam, or its reflection from the target, should not be performed without approval of the Laser Range Safety Officer. He must analyze whether the camera viewfinder magnifies the view.

21.9 LASER RANGE CONTROLS

During system development and operator training programs, laser safety procedures should be established and applied to all personnel connected with laser ground and/or flight operations. The personnel hazard evaluation of the particular device will provide guidelines on which to base the necessary controls. A standard operating procedure (SOP) should be enforced to control personnel movement in the vicinity of the laser or the laser beam path, and to assure that personnel exposure is limited to established, permissible levels (see Section 17.8).

The underlying concept of range safety is to prevent intrabeam viewing by unprotected personnel. This is best accomplished by locating target areas where no lines-of-sight exist between lasers and uncontrolled, potentially occupied areas, and by removing flat-glass surfaces from targets. Recommended target areas are those without flat specular surfaces. Examples of flat specular surfaces are: windows in vehicle buildings, vision blocks, searchlight cover glass, plastic sheets, and mirrors. Glossy foliage, raindrops, and other natural objects are not hazardous targets. If target areas have no flat specular surfaces, then range control measures can be limited to the control of the beam path between the laser and backstop.

21.9.1 Hazardous Range (NOHD)

The nominal ocular hazard distance (NOHD) for direct intrabeam viewing of a typical ruby military LRF is 7-10 km or 1-4 km for a Nd LRF. The NOHD for a military laser designator (LD) will normally be still greater. At the NOHD an unprotected individual may stand in the beam and be exposed repeatedly without fear of injury, provided only that he does not look at the laser with binoculars or telescopes. When viewing the collimated beam with a telescope, the hazardous range is

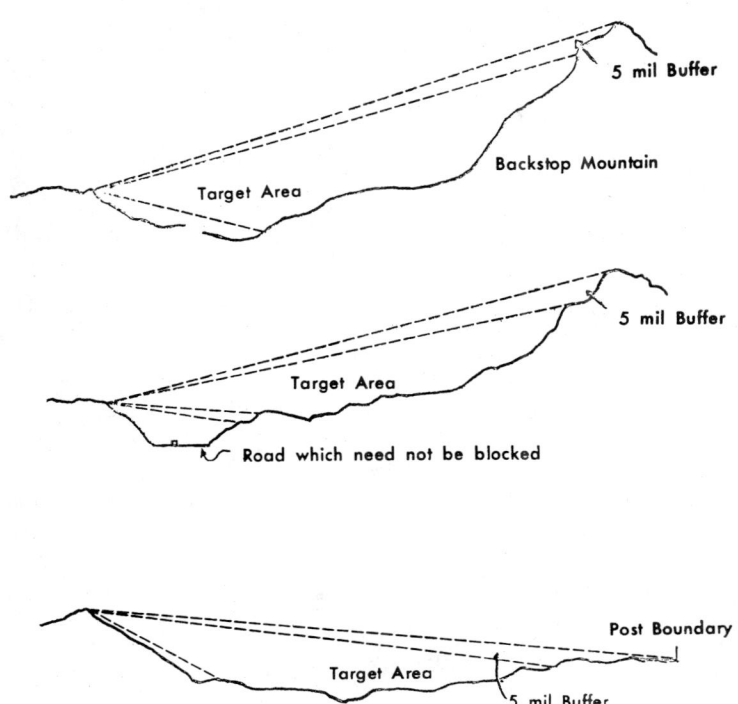

Figure 21-10. Backstops. Backstops such as a dense tree line or hill should terminate the beam. Without the use of such backstops there can be little assurance that persons at a great distance with telescopes will not be at risk, unless the NOHD is relatively small (e.g., less than 1 km).

greatly increased (Section 21.8). For instance, a 10-km NOHD would typically be increased to 80 km for an individual looking back at the laser from within the beam with 13X optics. In almost all cases it is not possible to control such sizable areas of real estate. The solution to this problem is to use a backstop to ensure that a clear line-of-sight does not exist between the LRF and potential observers behind the target.

21.9.1.1 Caution Range

Beyond the normal occular hazard distance (NOHD) or hazard range for momentary viewing is the caution range in which a laser may still be hazardous for prolonged viewing or staring. The lower limit has the general criterion of 1 $\mu W/cm^2$

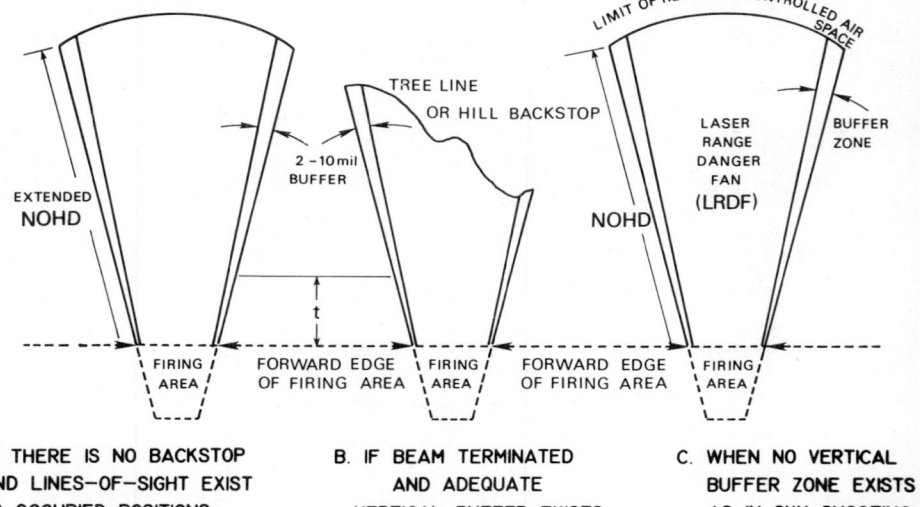

Figure 21-11. Laser range safety fans are used in the U.S. Army for a ground LRF. As can be seen, a backstop normally establishes the NOHD. The theoretical NOHD is used only for control of airspace.

as formulated for prolonged exposure to CW lasers and is modified (usually upwards) as a function of wavelength and other characteristics of the laser output. Personnel in this area should be advised to use care and avoid staring at any bright, or unfamiliar lights either with the naked eye or through optical aids.

21.9.2 Backstops

Backstops are opaque structures or terrain such as a dense tree line, a windowless building, or hill that completely obstructs any view beyond it, and would therefore completely terminate the laser beam that may miss the target. In most cases the hazard distance of the LD or LRF is the distance to the backstop. This hazard distance must be controlled. Defining hazardous range areas when establishing a laser range is somewhat different from the procedures used with direct-fire weapons. The terrain profile plays a very important role since the laser presents only a line-of-sight hazard. Figure 21-10 illustrates the concepts of backstops and Figure 21-11 illustrates types of range safety fans used with a LRF by the U.S. Army.

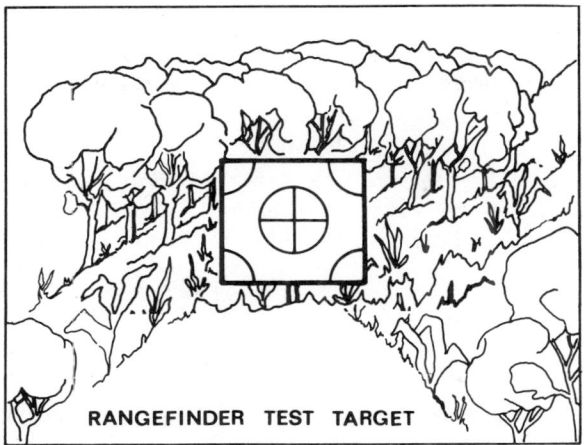

Figure 21-12. Example of one type of LRF boresight test target. The reticle cross-hairs of the LRF are aimed at each corner of the target. The target is set well in front of a substantial backstop.

21.9.3 Buffer Zones

The extent of horizontal and vertical buffer zones around the target of a military laser, as viewed from the firing area depends upon the aiming accuracy of the laser. Appropriate buffer zones for some military fire-control lasers are:

Laser in a stationary tank – 2 mils
Laser on tripod, moving tank, or aircraft with stabilizing optics–5 mils
Hand-held laser in an aircraft, or in a moving vehicle without stabilizing optics–10 mils minimum.

These buffer zones presume that the LRF or LD is in proper boresight with the aiming optics. Where this is not confirmed a boresight test target should be used at medium range (200 to 400 m) in front of a very substantial backstop. Figure 21-12 shows a very practical type of alignment target which is ranged upon at each corner of a square. There will be a range return from each corner only if the laser is in proper boresight provided that the target is at the proper distance for its size.

21.9.4 Laser Range Safety Fan (LRSF)

The downrange distance consumed by these laser range safety fans vary for all ground-based lasers. The lateral extent of the LRSF is controlled by target placement. The lateral extent would include the leftmost target plus the appropriate buffer zone and the rightmost target plus the appropriate buffer zone.

21.9.4.1 Hazardous Diffuse Reflection Area

This area extends from the laser firing point to a distance where the beam irradiance is safe to view by a diffuse reflection—a distance typically less than 10 m downrange. All surfaces potentially within the beam path should be removed in LRSF Area T.

21.9.4.2 Hazardous Area

This area extends from the laser to the NOHD. The NOHD is usually the distance to the backstop. On ranges with no backstop (e.g., desert flats) this area could in theory extend out to extremely long ranges (e.g., to the "Extended NOHD" where the beam is safe to view with 80-mm optics. This occurs, however, only where there are lines-of-sight from the laser to uncontrolled ground positions. Firing at targets on the horizon (no vertical buffer zone) is permitted as long as airspace is controlled to the NOHD downrange. In this case, the controlled area on the ground extends downrange only to the backstop, and to the NOHD—typically 10 to 20 km in the airspace. The controlled surface area extends to the skyline as seen from the firing on the ground.

21.9.5 Airborne Laser Controls

For many airborne laser systems, the procedures normally followed for direct-fire aerial gunnery ranges can also be applied to laser ranges. The designation of a single individual such as a gunnery sergeant as a Laser Range Safety Officer (LRSO) to insure implementation of safe operating procedures and proper administrative controls is desirable.

Airborne fire-control laser systems may typically have an operational slant range of 1-20 km, and the target area may be an area of potential ocular hazard to personnel. The nomogram in Figure 12-2 (page 390) can be used to provide an estimate of the distance at which the beam radiant exposure equals the permissible exposure level for typical neodymium and ruby laser rangefinders. A buffer zone should be established around the target area based on the aiming accuracy and reliability of the system, the slant range, the aircraft altitude, and ground constraints. A 5-mil buffer zone on each flank would be a reasonable value in many cases. The ground width of these lateral buffer zones would simply be equal to: $(5 \times 10^{-3})(r)$, where r is the beam path to ground. On the other hand, the calculation of the fore and aft buffer zones requires more complex trigonometric functions. Figure 21-13 gives the ground length of the foreward buffer zone which can be very large for low altitudes if the ground is level. For example, using Figure 21-13, one can determine

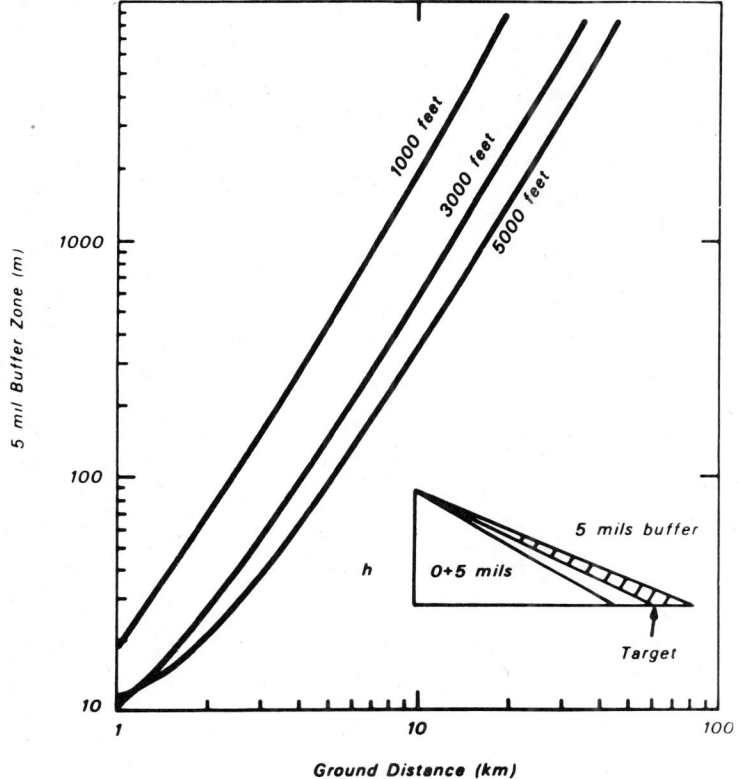

Figure 21-13. The ground width of a 5-mil forward buffer zone vs. ground distance of the aircraft from the target.

that the aircraft located 10 km from the target and at 1,000 feet (3 m) elevation a.g.l. will require a 2,100 m forward buffer zone if there is no hill behind the target. Of course, the beam should be terminated at the ground within a controlled range area. For shallow slant angles, the beam should be terminated against a natural terrain feature, such as a very dense tree line, or hill, or a ridge. Figure 21-14 shows how the length of the aft buffer zone varies with aircraft elevation and beam slant path.

By far the greatest concern about airborne laser safety relates to pointing reliability. Unlike a ground laser operator, the airborne laser operator can normally direct his laser beam in almost any direction and because of this large field-of-view, potential targets can occupy enormous areas on the earth's surface. Therefore the operator's responsibility for directing the beam only at approved targets and assuring proper laser system performance is greater than his ground-based counterpart. Since the laser pointing optics of many modern airborne laser devices rely not upon mechanical linkages, but upon electronically controlled gimbal mirrors, the use of several

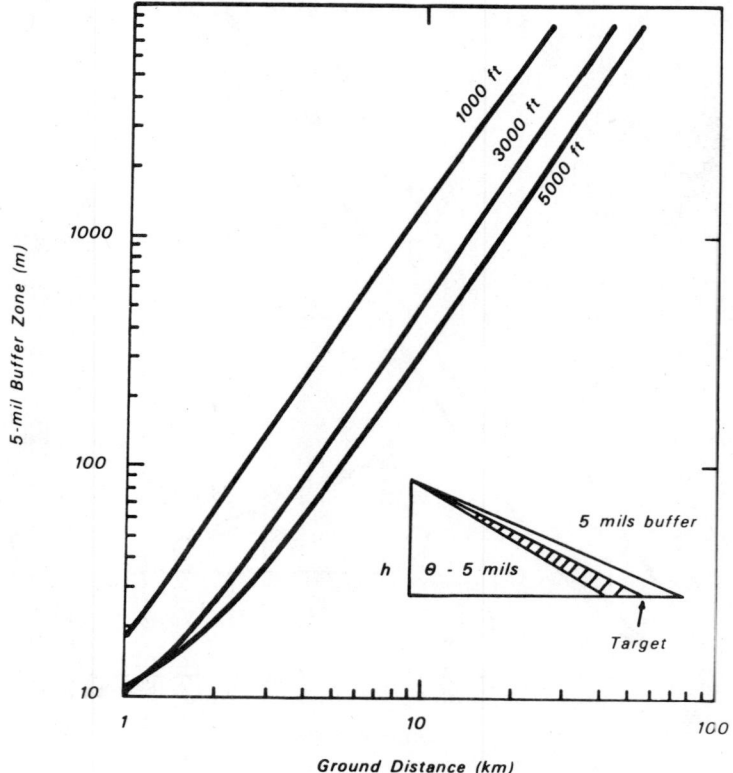

Figure 21-14. The ground width of a 5-mil aft buffer zone vs. ground distance of the aircraft from the target.

types of system safety features are paramount to reduce accidental misfiring and misdirection of the beam:

  (a) Protected master control switch (ground as well as airborne);
  (b) Automatic laser inhibit switch which disables the laser when tracking instability (e.g., "break-track") occurs;
  (c) Automatic laser inhibit switch which turns off the laser at the maximum traverse angle;
  (d) Positive action ("dead-man" type) laser firing switch (ground as well as airborne);
  (e) "Safe" stow-lock position for the laser when the aircraft is on the ground or when not flying over authorized range areas.

Some system safety features required in the BRH Federal Laser Performance standard need not be applied if they interfere with the mission; tactical military lasers are covered in a 1976 Department of Defense Exemption.

21.9.6 Eye Protection

Eye protectors should be worn by personnel required to be in the target area during laser operation. It is unnecessary for persons outside the target area to wear them provided that the target is nonspecular. The eye protection filter(s) should be curved (preferably 6 diopters if spectacle type) to prevent collimated specular reflections if the laser beam strikes the filter. As can be seen from the reflection pattern in the lowest panel of Figure 15-5 on page 487, the reflection from curved lens surfaces will rapidly diverge. This greatly limits the hazards from specular reflection in the target area to less than 30 m from the lens. The eyewear should be marked with the optical density at the specified wavelength so that eyewear designed for another laser system operating at a different wavelength will not be inadvertently used. Alternative, simple wording relating the eyewear to specific lasers rather than these technical specifications is often advisable when non-technical personnel must wear the eye protectors. Communication with personnel in the target area must be maintained to insure that protective eyewear is worn during laser operations. If communication is broken, laser operation should cease. Eye protectors for aviators should be avoided unless intentional lasing upon the aircraft is expected, since eye protection will reduce visual performance.

21.9.7 Limitations on Targets

Precautions should be taken to avoid targets which can produce specular reflections. If such targets are required or cannot be avoided, personnel in the range area who could be exposed to hazardous specular reflections should be equipped with eye protectors or the specular surfaces oriented to direct reflected beams into the ground. If areas of standing water exist in the target area, the laser should not be fired if other aircraft or elevated ground positions are located along the same azimuth as the laser target and the sum of the altitudes is less than the safe value determined by Equation 21-2, unless aircrews are provided with eye protectors.

21.9.8 Laser Maintenance Tests

Adequate control measures must be observed when the laser is operated on the ground during hanger or maintenance-shop testing. The direct beam can be extremely hazardous to personnel. If the laser output is capable of producing hazardous diffuse reflections, then all objects must be removed from the beam path, the beam enclosed, or all personnel within line-of-sight in the facility should wear laser protective eyewear. Firing of the laser into a light-tight box designed to contain

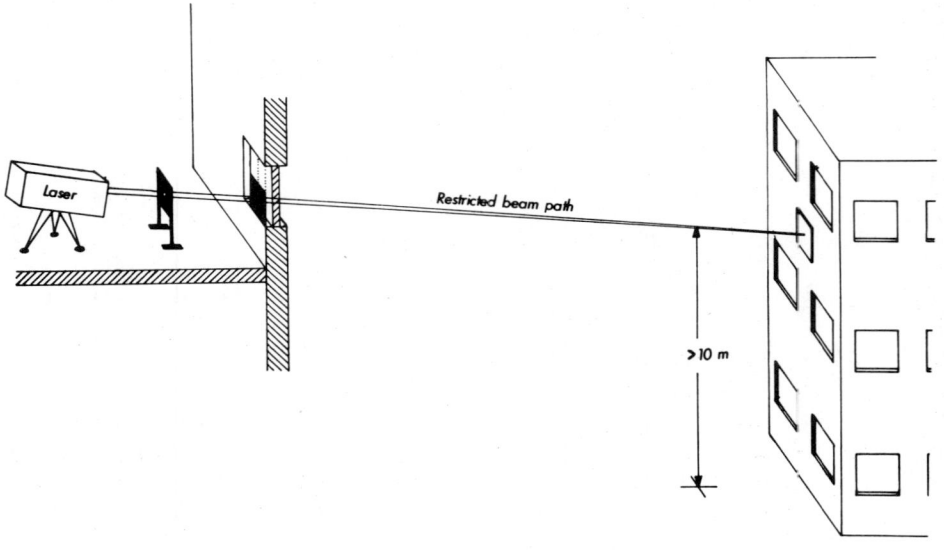

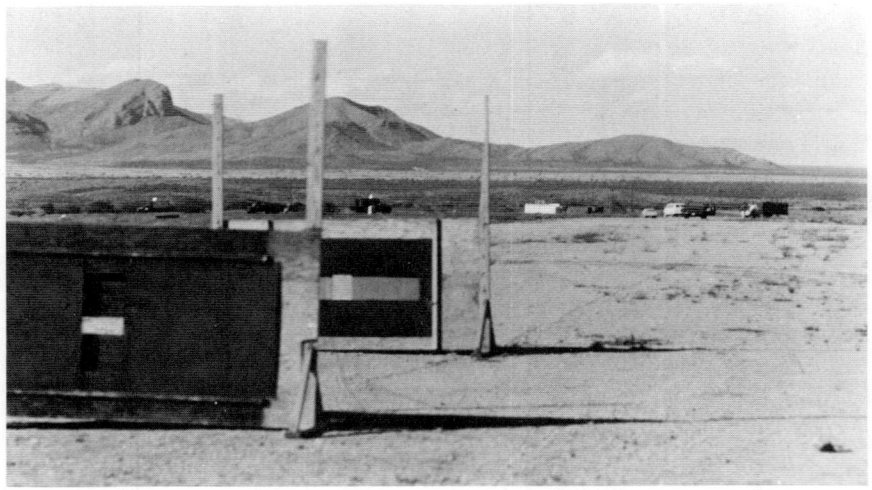

Figure 21-15. Laser Beam Baffles. Laser beam baffles to assure proper beam pointing for maintenance checkout. The top panel shows the concept in a factory area. The bottom panel shows the same scheme at a desert range.

all of the laser output is a desirable control for laboratory or maintenance testing. Assuring that the beam always hits a test target in a controlled outdoor test range, as shown in Figure 21-15, should be a required safety procedure when beam alignment is uncertain.

21.9.9 Medical Surveillance

Employees who routinely perform maintenance on military lasers or whose occupation or assignment may result in a significant risk of exposure to optical radiation in excess of the exposure limits have typically been included in an occupational vision program, which normally has included an ophthalmologic examination before assignment and at termination of assignment, and a simple vision test at periodic intervals during assignment. In many instances the periodic and termination examinations are no longer required. Employees who are suspected of receiving an accidental exposure in excess of the applicable exposure levels, and persons complaining of other visual disturbances such as persistent after-images should be examined. Hazard control measures for most laser operations should be adequate to preclude the need for all such examinations. Chapter 26 explores this subject in greater detail.

21.10 OPERATIONAL USE OF LASER SYSTEMS

The safe operational use of all tactical laser equipment will depend upon the operator's training and judgment. Fortunately, for combat situations there is a low probability of injury to personnel by reflections from unintentional viewing. Nevertheless, it is important that a hazard evaluation be performed on laser devices and the hazard zones delineated. This is especially true where the laser rangefinders, designators, and night vision illuminators are used in surveillance, and for acquiring targets of opportunity. The use of unfiltered optical viewing instruments, which may increase the hazard, make it difficult to assess situations other than the controlled field environment. For example, when an aircraft is ranging upon or illuminating ships at sea, it is to be expected that watchstanders will be viewing the aircraft through optical viewing devices. Because of the possibility of individuals with binoculars being located beyond a hazardous range developed for the unaided viewer, no single safe range for safety control purposes appears practical for laser equipment operating in the retinal hazard region (400–1400 nm). Air-crew eye protection is often not required, but is available as plastic visors or glass spectacles.

21.11 VIEWING PROBABILITY

A LRF operates by sending out a single pulse and measuring the elapsed time to and from the target. Each laser beam pulse lasts for only 10 to 20 ns. That time is so short that compared with one second, one second compares with about a year-and-a-half. Light traveling at 186,000 miles per second travels only six meters (20 feet) in 20 ns. Obviously, within such a short pulse, there is no chance to react.

There have been few accidents with military field lasers. The reason that so few laser accidents have occurred is two-fold. Early laser users, such as test engineers, have been cautious; and a laser safety program has been established in the Army since 1962. Perhaps most important, however, is the very low chance of the extremely compact laser beam entering a person's eye downrange. Indeed, in making

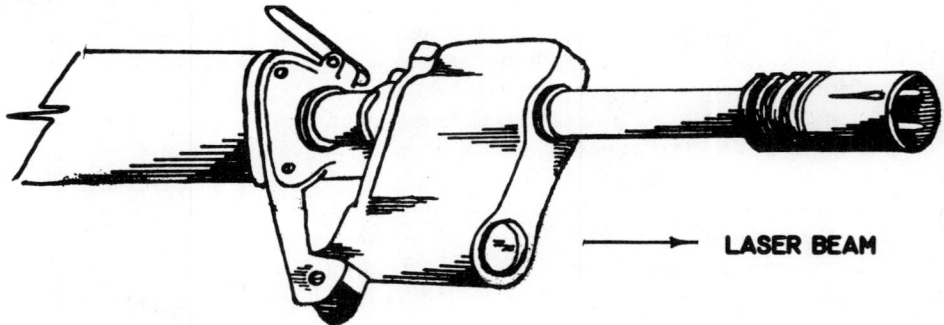

Figure 21-16. A small GaAs laser transmitter mounted on the muzzle of a rifle used to simulate direct weapon fire. Laser detectors are located at the target.

laser beam measurements downrange it is often very difficult to place a detector into the center of the beam on purpose. Of course, eye protection is always worn when performing such measurements.

21.12 TRAINING MODE

It is possible for training purposes to filter or otherwise reduce the output energy of some lasers for the purpose of shortening the hazardous distance, but unless the output is filtered down by a factor of 500,000 times, the laser beam will be hazardous at some distance in front of the laser, and the use of sighting optics will increase that distance. However, some tests have been conducted which show that a LRF will function with a safe-output filter which converts the laser to a Class 1 system if corner-cube retroreflectors are used at the target.

A corner-cube retroreflector is a glass prism which reflects a laser beam back precisely towards the laser, regardless of its orientation to the beam. Figure 15-7 (page 492) shows how it works. Reflective screens and bicycle reflectors work in a similar manner but are not nearly as efficient as a corner-cube. Military training agencies in the USA are now studying whether this approach for total LRF training safety is practical, feasible, and economically justified.

Range safety control measures can also be simplified if the extended NOHD (NOHD for 80-mm-objective optics) is reduced to 1,500 m or less. In some instances, a safety filter which does not reduce the output energy to Class 1 may nonetheless permit ranging on nearby targets while reducing this extended NOHD to a controllable distance.

Small, Class 1, GaAs lasers such as the unit shown in Figure 21-16 have been used extensively to simulate direct fire weapons. For the most part, such lasers are

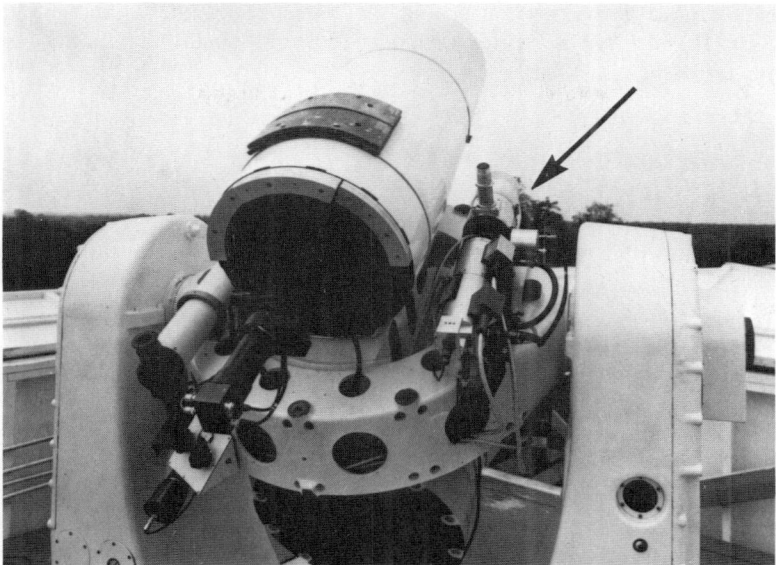

Figure 21-17. An early laser satellite tracker that used a ruby laser (arrow) and large telescope collecting optics. The laser was boresighted with receiving and aiming optics by firing at the water tower.

not a direct viewing hazard. Class II HeNe lasers have also been used in this fashion. The generally accepted rule of not looking into the bore of a gun should be fostered with all of these devices, regardless of hazard.

21.13 CONCLUSIONS ABOUT MILITARY LASER SAFETY

Methods have been developed for applying laser radiation exposure limits for the eye to the solution of practical field problems of controlling laser hazards from tactical lasers. The underlying concepts of laser range safety are termination of the beam and removal of flat specular surfaces. In many cases the terrain, rather than protection standards, defines the hazardous ranges of laser systems. In the end, it appears that the continuation of an almost perfect record for laser safety by the armed forces rests on each individual laser operator.

21.14 LASER AIMING DEVICES

HeNe lasers have been employed on special police rifles to assist policemen when aiming at a terrorist, a sniper or a criminal holding a hostage. Some criminals have been known to give up when seeing the red spot on them. Such lasers are generally Class III and BRH has issued variances to permit such "alignment" lasers to exceed the criteria of Class IIIa.

21.15 OPEN-AIR COMMUNICATION LINKS

The practical approach to follow in establishing a fixed ground-to-ground laser communication link requires several steps. First, assure the termination of the entire beam. Second, design the receiving optics so that a collimated specular reflection is not created. Third, locate the beam above traffic, but below navigable air space if possible (see Figure 21-15, top). None of the aforementioned steps require a careful study of atmospheric effects. Except for some GaAs laser transmitters, the laser beam will probably be hazardous. Admittedly, the beam irradiance of a far-infrared laser beam may be below the personnel exposure limit of $0.1 \text{ W} \cdot \text{cm}^{-2}$, but the entire beam could be reflected (or refracted by glass lenses for wavelengths less than 4 μm) to create a hazardous hot spot.

Today, open-air laser communications are far less common than fiber optic laser communication links. The hazards associated with FO communication systems are discussed in Section 20-5.

21.16 LIDAR

LIDAR (from Light Detection and Ranging) has been used on a limited scale for scientific studies. In this grouping could be included laser cloud-height ceilometers, remote atmospheric probes moon ranger, and satellite trackers, such as the NASA unit shown in Figure 21-17. Wavelengths from the UV to the far IR have been employed. In almost all cases, the beam may be directed into many elevation and azimuth angles.

Safety controls center on assuring that the beam is normally not directed at occupied areas on the ground or at non-target aircraft. To prevent ground exposure, almost all units employ beam elevation lower limit switches or mechanical stops. Mechanical stops are of course preferable to electrical switches because of their higher reliability. Azimuth switches or sector blanking techniques are also employed where high buildings or air traffic corridors are within potential lines-of-sight. It is, of course, possible in some remote locations (e.g., above military reservations) to restrict airspace, but even so, LIDAR operators must be concerned with the beam intercepting a non-target aircraft within the NOHD. In some instances when microwave radar was available, it has been slaved to the laser such that the laser beam would be inhibited when an aircraft intercepted the much broader radar beam. It is more conventional, however, to make use of ground spotters to visually search the sky for aircraft. Reflections of a laser beam from fog, rain or clouds would not be hazardous to the ground spotters, even if they were to use binoculars.

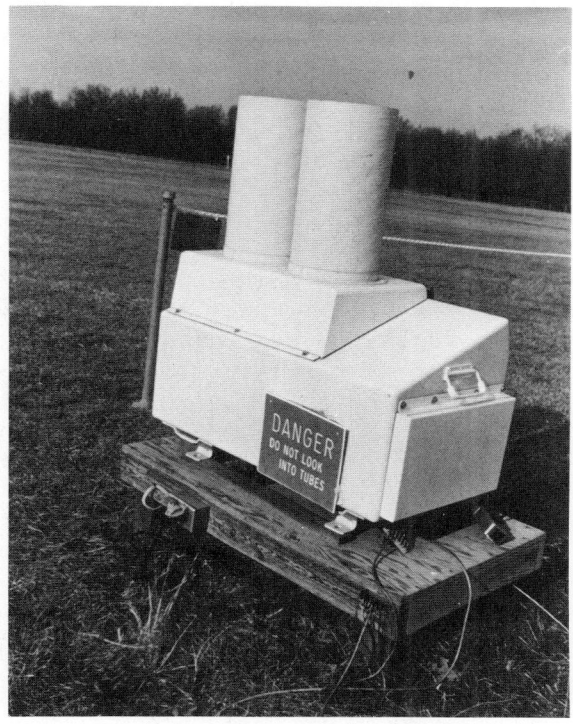

Figure 21-18. Laser Cloud Ceilometer. This prototype GaAs cloud ceilometer developed for the Weather Service has one tube enclosing the vertical beam and one tube around the receiving optics. This unit was designed as a Class IIIb instrument; however, the beam is so enlarged for collimation that E_0 is below the exposure limit. Since the beam is vertical, and since a hood prevents an individual from staring into it, there is virtually no hazard.

A specialized application of LIDAR is the determination of cloud ceiling, i.e., as in a cloud *ceilometer*. Ceilometers are often found at airports—generally within a fenced-in area not too far from a runway. Some early ceilometers for meteorlogical research had ruby (694.3 nm) or frequency-doubled neodymium (532 nm) lasers. GaAs laser systems (910 nm) with lower radiant power levels are more common today. Figure 21-18 illustrates such a GaAs system developed for the Weather Service as a Class 3b system. Most GaAs laser ceilometers studied by the authors were Class 3 systems, but were not hazardous for intrabeam viewing because of the large emergent beam size and low beam irradiance. The hood further diminished the possibility of prolonged staring. Intrabeam viewing of the vertical beam with optical instruments could theoretically be hazardous, but in practice such a condition is virtually inconceivable. The GaAs laser ceilometers have been designed to replace older types which used incandescent-lamp projectors. The latter presented a similar theoretical retinal hazard only through intrabeam viewing with optical instruments.

21.17 ENVIRONMENTAL IMPACT

It is not uncommon for laser operations out-of-doors to be considered in Environmental Impact Statements (EIS) that must be prepared to meet certain Federal Regulations in the USA. For example, the flight of birds through static CW laser beams should not be hazardous. Concern has in the past been expressed by wildlife conservationists that Class 3 and Class 4 lasers could be hazardous to wildlife. Obviously, deer, rabbits, eagles, falcons and other wildlife would not read laser range warning signs or observe FAA restricted airspace. However, only if such wildlife were within the direct beam of very short-pulse military lasers used for fire control, would eye injury even be possible. And then, such injury could only occur if the animal were well within the NOHD, a range easily seen by the operator. Hence, precaution by the laser operator not to fire at wildlife would preclude any adverse environmental impact.

The control measures required to eliminate exposure to unprotected personnel also protect wildlife. The susceptibility of wildlife depends upon the presence of foveae. Not all vertebrates display a fovea, but this structure has been identified in some mammals (mostly primates, some carnivores, and the horse), in birds, various reptiles, frogs, and some species of fish (Prince, 1956). It has been postulated that the fovea in birds may function in the detection of polarized light, and is therefore indirectly involved in navigation (Kreithen and Keeton, 1974). Also some birds and reptiles display two foveae in each eye. Animals without a fovea have little potential risk of incapacitation due to laser eye injury, whereas those with two foveae might be at greater risk than a human. The only animals that would be greatly affected by laser induced eye injury, would be those whose activity is dominated by visual input. These would be squirrels, primates, and birds. However, these animals would only be affected if they happened to be staring directly at the laser as it emitted its light. The falcon with its telephoto system might be susceptible to laser eye injury in the near field at a slightly greater distance than for humans.

Another structure in the avian eye that would be susceptible to additional injury is the pecten. The pecten arises from the junction of the retina and the optic nerve, and extends into the interior of the eye. Because the avian retina is avascular and the pecten consists almost exclusively of capillaries, the pecten is believed to be a nutritional device (Walls, 1942), i.e., it is an analog to the retinal circulation. The pecten also has some pigmented cells which may be involved in the regulation of intraocular pressure. Strong pigmentation in these cells would in theory decrease the threshold for injury from laser impingement because of increased light absorption; however, the pecten is not at the focal plane of the image laser. The pecten has also been suggested as a shield against solar retinal injury as it absorbs the direct rays of the sun.

The nocturnal habits of many animals are an additional consideration in assessing the potential laser hazard. Night tests may find more animals moving about the range than during the daytime. Some of them are attracted to light and might stare directly down the laser beam if it were to catch their attention by directly hitting their eyes. However, when passing through clear air (i.e., with limited airborne particulates, such as dust, smoke, or vapor), the laser beam undergoes less scattering, and is difficult to see if it is not directed into the eye. Therefore, animals will not be attracted to the beam path. Many lasers emit infrared which is not readily visible to the animal and would not catch its attention. Studies of color receptors in animals reveal that red (and IR-A) vision is not significantly extended in wavelength over that of humans.

Certain nocturnal animals have a special layer of tissue behind the retina, the tapetum lucidum, which improves vision in dim illumination by reflecting the incident light so that it traverses the visual receptors twice, thus increasing apparent visual brightness. This structure is what causes the cat's eyes to shine at night when illuminated by a spotlight. Because of this reflection, less laser light would be absorbed by the pigment below, thus increasing the threshold for laser eye damage.

Some animals have rather large eyes to gather as much light as possible, and a lens set far back from the cornea to place the optical center near the retina so that light transmitted through the system is concentrated into a small image of the maximum possible brightness. The increased amount of light entering the eye would decrease the damage threshold, and theoretically the smaller image size on the retina also might decrease the threshold for laser damage. This combination in addition to the effect of the tapetum would probably balance each other so that the resulting threshold to laser eye damage would be similar to that for man. Whatever the case, the pigmentation and final minimal image could not be so different from the rhesus monkey such that the human exposure limits would not apply to animals as well. In the past, some animals, such as the owl, were thought to have more superior night vision than man. However, research has shown that their night vision is actually similar to man's, and that their nocturnal activity is mostly dependent on auditory input (Martin, 1978). Bats would also not be significantly affected by laser eye injury due to their heavy reliance on auditory senses. It is important to realize that spherical aberrations and diffraction effects preclude an image much smaller than the 10-20 μm retinal image in man. Furthermore, since there is a 10-fold difference between safe exposure levels for man and thresholds for noticeable retinal injury, no animal would be at risk at distances greater than the nominal ocular hazard distance (NOHD) set for man.

21.18 EXAMPLES

Example 21-1. Gallium Arsenide Array Illuminator

A number of infrared projector systems have been developed that make use of GaAs injection lasers. Such systems, used in military night-vision systems, normally have had a total optical power output of 0.5–20 W. As an example, consider the following system:

    Output power Φ :   4.5 W

    Beam spread: 6° × 2°

    Number of diodes: 240

    Pulse width: 1.4 μsec

    PRF: 10 kHz

    Wavelength: 855 nm (liquid nitrogen-cooled GaAs)

Irradiance measurements and infrared photographs of the source were taken at several distances within the beam. Because of the relatively large beam spread, the near field of the projector system only extended to a distance of 2 m, and photographs of the projected source radiance distribution (Fig. 21-8) beyond this distance did not vary. The use of trapezoidal-prism optical integrators to provide a uniform rectangular irradiance distribution added to the complexity of evaluating the array. Figure 21-8 is a photograph of the projected source that shows the 240 diodes and two additional rows for each primary row of diodes, which are the first reflections produced by the optical integrator. Other, secondary and tertiary, reflections are produced by the optical integrator but were ignored in the calculations because of their small contribution to the total irradiance. From the photographs and irradiance measurements, it was determined that the radiance of each of the 480 source elements was approximately 1000 W/(cm$^2 \cdot$sr); the average radiance of each row was approximately 400 W/(cm$^2 \cdot$sr); and the average radiance of the entire array was approximately 15 W/(cm$^2 \cdot$sr) The retinal hazard criterion for a CW source at 850 nm was once obtained by using Equation 4-4 (page 123) to calculate the radiance, which corresponded to a "safe" retinal absorbed irradiance of 0.1 W/cm^2, i.e., 2.6 W/(cm$^2 \cdot$sr), since R_λ = 0.5 at 850 nm (see page 339).

One may wish to relate this criterion to present day laser safety criteria (Table 8-2, page 263) for diffuse reflections or extended sources of laser radiation. This criteria is 1.3 W/(cm$^2 \cdot$sr) for the wavelength of 850 nm and for exposures greater than 1000 s. Assuming that the retinal injury mechanism of interest is strictly thermal, the array may be treated as a CW source, since the high PRF (10 kHz) does not permit thermal relaxation within the retina. The thermal relaxation time of significant areas of retinal tissue is approximately 0.1 sec, whereas the duration between pulses is approximately 100 μsec. Unfortunately there is very little biologic data available to substantiate this approach, and the application of a safety factor of as much as 100 may be advisable in such a hazard analysis until biologic investigations into the effects of high-repetition-rate lasers provide injury thresholds upon which to base hazard criteria.

Determining the Caution Range

Since the radiance of the illuminator was greater than 1.3 W/(cm$^2 \cdot$sr), the *caution distance* (Section 21.9.1.1) applicable for long-term viewing (staring) must be determined by the CW laser criterion (Table 8-1) of 0.64 mW/cm^2. In the present case this irradiance occurrs at 14 m.

Determining the Hazardous Range (NOHD)

As previously discussed (Section 21.9.1), the *hazardous range* for short-term (momentary) viewing depends upon the source radiance and the retinal image size. As the viewer moves away from the source, fewer distinct source elements are seen. The relative position of the retinal image of each element becomes closer to neighboring elements and they coalesce. The retinal irradiance E_r of any element may be calculated from the element's radiance L using Equation 4-4 (page 123). However, formula 4-4 is strictly valid only for extended sources subtending an angle greater than 3.1 mrad, which corresponds to a retinal image disk diameter of approximately 50 μm. For elements that have smaller geometrical images on the retina, the limiting effects of diffraction and other phenomena must be taken into account. Using the work of Gubisch (1967) the reduction in the retinal irradiance for small images could be calculated, and the resulting irradiance of adjacent, coalesced elements could be determined. The retinal irradiance of two adjacent elements is essentially uniform when their image edges as predicted by geometrical optics were within 5 μm of each other for a 7-mm pupil. It has been determined from the work of Mainster and collaborators (1970) that a significant overlap of retinal thermal profiles occurred when the image edges were within 100 μm of each other.

Using the above criteria, the maximum permissible retinal irradiance was plotted in Figure 21-9. When the separation of retinal image edges of the various elements in the laser array was 100 μm, the critical area increased to the next largest element size and the corresponding maximum permissible retinal irradiance decreased, hence the changes in slope of this curve with increasing range. Likewise the curves of retinal irradiance, which are also plotted in Figure 21-9, demonstrate these changes in critical areas. The hazardous range for intrabeam viewing of the illuminator was 6 m.

Hazard Control Measures

Positive control measures were taken to prohibit individuals from entering the beam path within 6 m. Individuals were instructed not to *stare* into the source if within 6-14 m. By earlier 1969 criteria the caution distance was 220 m.

Example 21-2. Calculate the NOHD for a laser rangefinder which has the following specifications:

Q = 100 mJ
a = 4 cm
λ = 1064 nm
ϕ' = 0.5 mrad (at $1/e^2$ –points)
τ = 13 ns

Step 1. Determine EL. From Table 8-1 the EL for a 1064-nm pulse of 1 ns–100 μs is 5×10^{-6} J/cm².

Step 2. Rearrange Equation 21-7 to solve for r (NOHD) by ignoring the atmospheric attenuation.
$$\text{NOHD}(r) = (1/\phi) \, [(\sqrt{1.27 \, Q/H_{EL}}) - a]$$

Step 3. Convert ϕ' to ϕ:
$\phi = 0.707 \, \phi' = (0.707)(5 \times 10^{-4} \text{ rad})$
$= 3.5 \times 10^{-4}$ rad

Step 4. Solve for NOHD(r).
NOHD(r) = 4.6 km

Step 5. If greater accuracy is desired, apply a conservative value of the atmospheric attenuation coefficient μ at a shorter range r until a value of the true NOHD is obtained. This can be best accomplished by using a programmed calculator and solving Equation 21-1. If we use $\mu = 6 \times 10^{-7}$ cm^{-1} from Figure 13-1 and r = 4 km, then the NOHD is reduced to 4.0 km.

Example 21-3. CO Laser Atmospheric Probe

Output Parameters:

λ = 4.9–5.0 μm
Φ = 200 W
a' = 1.4 cm
ϕ' = 2 mrad (specified at 1/e^2 points of axial peak beam irradiance).

Background: The exposure limit for t > 10 s is E = 100 mW/cm^2. Since the wavelength is greater than 4.8 μm we may assume that glass optics will not transmit, hence telescopes and binoculars in the beam beyond the NOHD would not increase the risk to the observer. Calculating the NOHD:

Step 1. Convert a and ϕ to values defined at 1/e points:

$a = a'/\sqrt{2} = 1.4$ cm$/1.414 = 1.0$ cm

$\phi = \phi'/\sqrt{2} = 2$ mrad$/1.414 = 1.4$ mrad

Step 2. Determine atmospheric attenuation coefficient μ. Since this laser operates in the spectral region of sharp molecular absorption bands, μ depends dramatically on the precise wavelength(s) of the laser. Hence one can only assume that the μ could be exceedingly small for safety calculations and neglect it.

Step 3.

$$\begin{aligned}
\text{NOHD} &= (1/\phi)\ [(\sqrt{1.27\ \Phi/E}\ ) - a] \\
&= (1/1.4 \times 10^{-3})\ [(\sqrt{(1.27)(200)/(0.1)}\ ) - 1] \\
&= (714)\ [\sqrt{2540}\ ) - 1] \\
&= (714)\ [49.4] = 3.53 \times 10^4\ \text{cm} \\
&= 350\ \text{m}
\end{aligned}$$

Example 21-4: Multiwavelength LIDAR

Laser #1   Ruby, λ = 694.3 nm, Q = 0.5 J, a = 2 cm
τ = 30 ns, F = 1 Hz, ϕ = 0.5 mrad
Laser #2   Carbon-Dioxide, λ = 2.5 to 11 μm, Q = 0.7 J,
a = 2.5 cm, τ = 20 ns, F = 1 Hz, ϕ = 1.2 mrad.

Step 1. Applicable exposure limits:
Single pulse criteria (λ=694.3 nm) – 5 $\times$ 10^{-7} J/cm^2
(λ=2–11 μm) – 10^{-2} J/cm^2

Step 2. NOHD Calculation

Laser #1 – NOHD = $(1/5 \times 10^{-4})[(1.27 \times 0.5/5 \times 10^{-7})^{1/2} - 2]$
= 2.25 $\times$ 10^6 cm = 22 km

or by Figure 13-1 the NOHD = 13 km if μ = 10^{-6} cm^{-1} (Haze)

Laser #2—NOHD=$(1/1.2 \times 10^{-3})[(1.27 \times 0.7/0.01)^{1/2} - 2.5]$
$= 5.8 \times 10^3$ cm $= 580$ m

Step 3. Eye Protection Calculations

Laser #1: OD $= \log_{10}[(1.27 \times 0.5)/(2)^2/5 \times 10^{-7}]$
$= \log_{10}[3.2 \times 10^5] = 5.5$

Laser #2: OD $= \log_{10}[(1.27 \times 0.7)/(2.5)^2/10^{-2}]$
$= \log_{10}[14.2] = 1.2$

NOTE: Since almost all materials such as glass and plastics absorb strongly beyond 4.5 µm, any safety eyewear designed for protection at 694.3 nm will also protect at 10.6 µm.

21.19 REVIEW QUESTIONS

1. Fire control lasers are used to stop forest fires. True or False.

2. Which of the following characteristics do not influence the hazard of a laser rangefinder?
    a. Beam polarization
    b. Output Energy
    c. Beam pointing accuracy
    d. Range readout accuracy
    e. Wavelength
    f. Weight
    g. Beam Divergence
    h. Emergent Beam Diameter

3. Calculate the NOHD for the unaided eye and for viewing through an 80-mm aperture for a laser rangefinder with the following specifications: $\phi = 1$ mrad, $\lambda = 850$ nm, $\tau = 20$ ns, $a = 2$ cm, $\mu = 0.1$ km^{-1}.

4. Is there a hazard when viewing a diffuse reflection from a nearby smoke cloud when the beam radiant exposure at 570 nm is 4.4 J/cm² for a 10-ns pulse.

5. An airborne scanning laser beam has a beam power of 4 W at 10.6 µm; $\phi = 2$ mrad, and the beam scans a full angle of 14° at a rate of 20 scans per second by a rotating polygonal mirror (i.e., no return beam). What is the NOHD? What is the ocular exposure duration for an eye located at the NOHD for a 7-mm pupil?

6. A military training rifle uses a laser diode firing simulator. At each pull of the trigger the laser sends out a 5-pulse code of 100-ns pulses in 40 µs, 1-W peak

power at 850 nm, one pull per second maximum. The emergent beam diameter is 1 cm. What is the laser's class?

7. The laser diode transmitter of problem 6 above is redesigned to be used in a machine gun. All of the output parameters remain the same except that the pulse train is repeated at 300 "rounds-per-minute." What is the hazard classification?

8. A lunar sounding ruby laser emits 5 J at 694.3 nm. The beam divergence is 0.01 mrad and the emergent beam diameter is 26 cm. What is the NOHD? Is there a hazard when viewing a reflection from a white cloud at 400 m above ground level through the 400X aiming telescope?

9. How high should a backstop at 8 km be to permit a 2-mil buffer zone above a 3-meter target? For a 5-mil buffer zone?

10. What is $R_1 + R_2$ for a water reflection for a Nd:YAG airborne LRF with Q = 0.1 J, ϕ = 1 mrad, τ = 20 ns and a = 2 cm?

21.20 REFERENCES

Crescitelli, F., 1977, "The Visual System in Vertebrates," Handbook of Sensory Physiology, Vol. VII/5, pp 549–737, Springer-Verlag, Berlin.

Dunsky, I. L., Fife, W. A., and Richey, E. O., 1973, Determination of revised Air Force permissible exposure levels for laser radiation, Am. Indust. Hyg. Assn. J. 34(6):235–240.

Fox, R., Lehmkuhle, S. W., and Westendorf, D. H., 1976, Falcon visual acuity, Science 192(4236): 263–265.

Fite, K. V., and Wessels, S. R., 1975, A comparative study of deep avian foveas, Brain Behavior and Evolution 12:97–115.

Freasier, B. C., 1970, Army laser range controls, in "Electronic Product Radiation and the Health Physicist," pp. 365–372, DEP 70-26, USBRH, Rockville, MD.

Gardner, C. S., 1979, Technique for remotely measuring surface pressure from a satellite using a multicolor laser ranging system, Appl. Opt. 18(18):3184–3189.

Gubisch, R. W., 1967, Optical performance of the human eye, J. Opt. Soc. Am. 57:407–415.

Kreithen, M. L., and Keeton, W. T., 1974, Detection of polarized light by the homing pigeon, Columbia livia, J. Comp. Physiol. 89:83–92.

Mainster, M. A., White, T. J., Tips, J. H., and Wilson, P. W., 1970, Retinal-temperature increases produced by intense light sources, J. Opt. Soc. Am. 60:264–270.

Marshall, W. J., 1980, Hazard analysis of Gaussian shaped laser beams, Am. Industr. Hyg. Assn. J. (in press).

Martin, G., 1978, Through an owl's eye, New Scientist 75:72–74.

Nicholson, A. N. (Ed.), 1975, Laser hazards and safety in the military environment, AGARD Lecture Series, No. 79, North Atlantic Treaty Organization (NATO) Advisory Group for Aerospace Research and Development, NTIS, Springfield, VA.

Prince, J. H., 1956, "Comparative Anatomy of the Eye," Thomas, Springifled.

Robson, J. G., and Enroth-Cugell, C., 1977, Light distribution in the cat's retinal image, Vis. Res. 18:169–173.

Shlaer, R., 1972, An eagle's eye: quality of the retinal image, Science 176:920–922.

Sliney, D. H., and Freasier, B. C., 1973, Evaluation of optical radiation hazards, Appl. Opt. 12: 1–24.

Sliney, D. H., 1976, The safety aspects of atmospheric transmission of lasers, *Ann. NY Acad. Sci.* **267**:366–372.
Sliney, D. H., 1970, Evaluating health hazards from military lasers, *J. Am. Med. Assn.* **214**(6): 1047–1054.
Sliney, D. H., and Yacovissi, R., 1975, Control of health hazards from airborne lasers, *Aviat. Space Environ. Med.* **46**(5):691–696.
Snyder, A. W., and Miller, W. H., 1978, Telephoto lens system of falconiform eyes, *Nature* **275** (5676):127–129.
U.S. Deparment of the Army, 1978, Policies and procedures for firing ammunition training, target practice, and combat, AR 385–63 (22 February 1978).
U.S. Department of the Air Force, 1973, Laser Health Hazards Control, AF Manual 161–32 (Washington, D.C.).
U.S. Department of the Army, 1975, Control of Hazards to Health from Laser Radiation, TB MED 279, Washington, D.C., 54 pp. (May 1975).
U.S. Deparment of the Army, 1974, Control of Health Hazards from Lasers and other High Intensity Light Sources, Army Regulation 40–46 (February 1974).
U.S. Department of the Army and U.S. Department of the Navy, 1978, Policies and Procedures for Firing Ammunition for Training, Target Practice, and Combat, Army Regulation 385–63 MCOP 3570.1, Chapter 20, "Lasers" (February 22, 1978).
U.S. Department of the Army and U.S. Department of the Navy, 1969, Control of Hazards to Health from Laser Radiation, TB Med 279 and NAVMED P-5052–35, Washington, D.C., 9 pp. (superceded by ANSI Z-136.1–1976 and 1975 Edition of TB Med 279).
Walls, G. L., 1942, The vertebrate eye and its adaptive radiation, Cranbrook Inst. Sci., Bull. No. 19, Bloomfield Hills, Mich.

Chapter 22
Lamps and Lighting Systems

22.1 INTRODUCTION

It may seem strange that the subject of lamp safety has been relegated to nearly the end of this book. After all, lamps and lighting systems have been around far longer than the laser. On the other hand, despite the short history of the laser, safety standards for the use of lasers and for the manufacture of lasers were developed within 10-15 years after the invention of such devices. This was not really true in the case of the electric lamp. Indeed, at the time of publication of this book, there were essentially no standards devoted to lamp safety. There are several reasons for this. First of all, lamps were developed and produced in large quantities and became commonplace in an era when product standards and, certainly, safety standards were rare if not totally unknown. Furthermore, there was no public fear of hazards from lamps such as was associated with the development of laser devices. Finally, the evaluation and control of lamp hazards is a far more complicated subject than similar tasks for a single-wavelength laser system. The required radiometric measurements are quite involved, for they do not deal with the simple optics of a point source, but rather with an extended source which may or may not be altered by a projection system that is almost always involved. Also, the wavelength distribution of the lamp may be altered by ancillary optical elements, diffusers, lenses, and the like.

In this chapter the evaluation and control of hazards associated with specific types and uses of lamps and visual displays will be discussed. When lamps are used in illumination systems which have collimating optics, such as projection systems, the hazard evaluation procedure is more complex. This subject is discussed in detail in Chapter 23.

22.2 LIGHTING TERMINOLOGY

Prior to a detailed discussion of lamps it is useful to review a few of the principal terms used by lighting engineers. The general photometric and radiometric terms were introduced in Chapter 2. It would be useful to review the photometric terms in Table 2-3 (page 56) prior to reading this chapter. Other specific terms described below will then be more understandable.

Two useful terms relate to a lamp's light output efficiency. These terms, *luminous efficacy* and *luminous efficiency*, are often used loosely in an interchangeable fashion. Indeed, *luminous efficacy* has two meanings. There has also been some past disagreements over definitions used by the IES of North America and those used by her sister societies in other countries. For this text we shall try to abide by the International Lighting Vocabulary, (CIE, 1970) and in general, these terms are also in accordance with the IES vocabulary.

A lamp's *luminous flux (power)* output is measured in *lumens*, its *radiant power (flux)* output in *Watts*; but then its electrical input power is also measured in Watts. Hence one must be careful not to confuse an attempt to describe a lamp's effectiveness in 1m/W-electrical with its 1m/W-radiated.

Luminous efficacy (of radiation) K is defined as the quotient of luminous flux Φ_v by the corresponding radiant flux Φ_e:

$$K = \Phi_v/\Phi_e \qquad (22\text{-}1)$$

Luminous efficiency has in the past often referred to K, but this term now correctly only refers to a more abstract concept that is not frequently used. The luminous efficiency V(*) of a broad-band source is the ratio of its luminous efficacy K to that of a source at the peak of the luminosity curve K_m; that is, the ratio of the radiant flux weighted according to V(λ)—the spectral luminous efficiency function—to the corresponding radiant flux:

$$V(*) = \int \Phi_{e,\lambda} \cdot V(\lambda) \cdot d\lambda \;\Big/\; \int \Phi_{e,\lambda} \cdot d\lambda \qquad (22\text{-}2)$$
$$= K/K_m$$

Remember that K_m = 683 1m/W at 550 nm. Another more commonly used term is the *radiant efficiency* η_e of a source, which is the ratio of the radiant flux emitted to the power consumed. On the other hand, the analogous photometric term is termed the luminous efficacy η_v (of a source), which is the quotient of luminous flux (power) emitted to the electrical power consumed (in 1m/W).

Many lamps are rated in terms of candlepower, or more correctly, the *luminous intensity* I_v in candelas (cd). The value of this unit is that the illumination at a distance from the lamp (in the far-field) can be easily calculated. The illuminance E_v at a range r from the lamp is:

$$E_v = I_v / r^2 \qquad (22\text{-}3)$$

For example a PAR-56 headlamp may emit approximately 80,000 cd in the tight central beam. At a distance of 10 m from the lamp, the illuminance is:

$$E_v = 80{,}000 / (10)^2$$
$$= 800 \text{ lm/m}^2 = 800 \text{ lx}$$

Radiometric characteristics of lamps which are of interest to the health or safety specialist are generally not provided by lamp companies. For example, the spectra of lamps are often presented relative to the photometric unit, the lumen, e.g., $\mu W/(nm \cdot lm)$, or simply as relative spectra. The luminance of a lamp is generally not provided, and almost certainly not the radiance. Nevertheless, with a relative spectrum and a measurement of the luminance of a lamp, it is possible to calculate the radiance and spectral radiance of the lamp which are important in any hazard evaluation. When lamp companies specify ultraviolet emissions from a lamp, they often provide data in terms of $\mu W/lm$, or $\mu W/cm^2$-per-footcandle. This is not really surprising since lamp companies sell lamps for lighting and photometric units are used almost exclusively for that purpose. In fact, if one becomes used to these strange units, most hazard evaluations can be performed with a simple light meter. This should become more evident later in this chapter and in Chapter 23.

22.3 TYPES OF LAMPS AND LIGHT SOURCES

The general characteristics of lamps and pertinent technical characteristics of interest to the health and safety specialist will be reviewed in this section. There are several methods for cataloging lamps and light sources. From the standpoint of potential hazards it is convenient to use the following categories:

a. incandescent filament lamps and incandescent heating sources
b. low pressure discharge lamps
c. fluorescent lamps
d. high intensity discharge lamps
e. short arc lamps
f. carbon arcs
g. electroluminescent lamps and light-emitting diodes

There are other light sources such as radioactive-phosphor combinations, radioactive phosphorescent panels, and gas lamps which are never sufficiently bright to be of concern, and therefore will not be discussed. Figure 22-1 is a summary of the hazards of different types of lamps.

22.3.1 Incandescent Sources

Incandescent sources and blackbody sources were introduced in sections 2.11 to 2.13. Because solid-body incandescent materials such as iron and tungsten used in filament lamps, (or nickel, chromium and iron in heating elements) seldom exceed

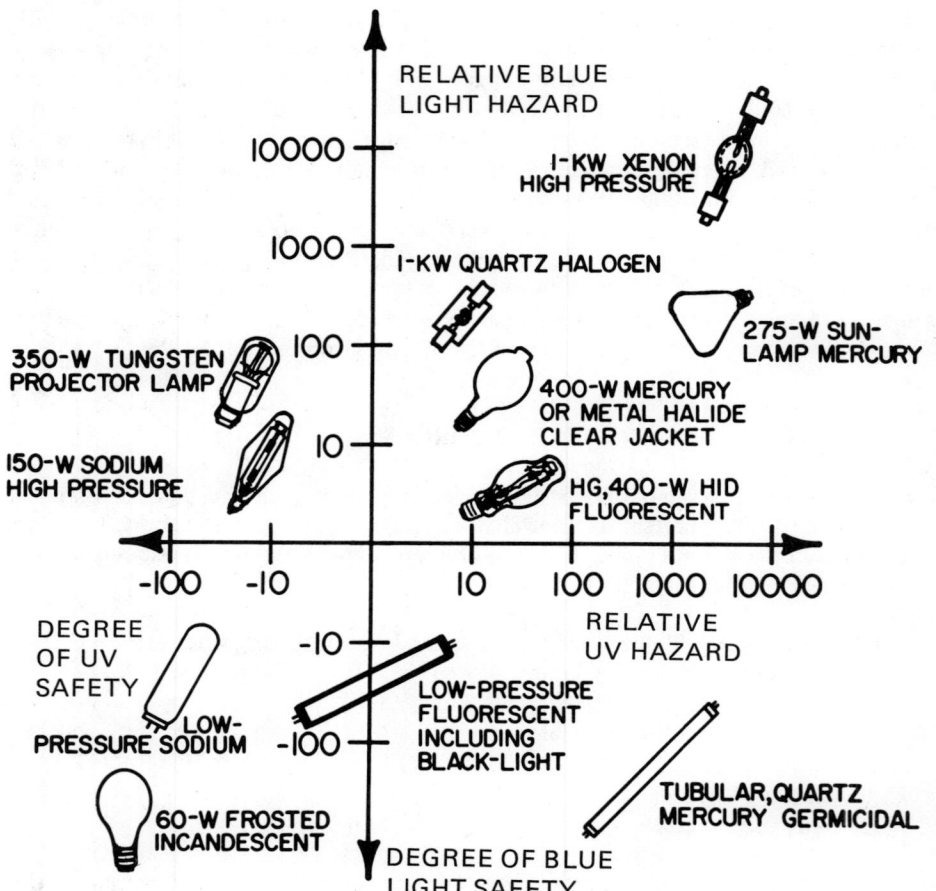

Figure 22-1. The Relative UV and IR Hazards of Different Types of Lamps. The type of envelope, voltage and current ratings obviously influence the exact degree of hazard.

blackbody temperatures of 3000 K, their spectral distributions peak in the red end of the spectrum with a relatively small fraction of blue and ultraviolet radiation. Since, as explained in Chapters 4 and 14, the shorter wavelength bands of the optical spectrum create the biggest problems from a hazard standpoint, incandescent light sources, as a general rule, present less problems from a safety standpoint than any other type of light source. The incandescent lamp was the first to be developed and utilized on a broad scale. This was probably fortunate because incandescent sources were extensively used long before there was an understanding of the blue-light hazard to the retina.

The first incandescent lamps in the nineteenth century were carbon, iron, osmium, or tantanum filament lamps. However, in spite of its low ductility tungsten has replaced all these filament materials because of its low vapor pressure, high melting point (3655 K), and strength. Today tungsten is typically alloyed with metals such as thorium and rhenium.

Although tungsten is a selective radiator, its spectrum still rather closely approximates a "graybody." The emissivity of tungsten varies with temperature as is shown in Figure 2-13 (page 33). The maximum theoretical luminous efficacy of tungsten wire at its melting point (3655 K) is approximately 53 lumens per watt. This luminous efficacy is not realized in practical lamps which are operated at lower filament temperatures—typically 2800 K to 3200 K—to obtain reasonable lifetimes for the filament. The theoretical limit for the luminance of an incandescent source is the luminance of a true blackbody at that temperature. The luminance of a blackbody as a function of temperature is given in Figure 22-2.

Lamp manufacturers and particularly the photographic industry often refer to an incandescent lamp's *color temperature*. This is useful in color applications where the approximate spectral distribution is important. It is important to understand, however, that the color temperature of the source is not necessarily the actual temperature of the filament or other source material. Color temperature, as used for a selective radiator (or graybody), is the actual temperature of a blackbody which has the closest possible approximation to a color match with the output spectrum of the selective radiator. Color temperature is of interest to the health and safety specialist since it gives a clue to the spectral distribution of the lamp and the luminous efficacy. The luminous efficacy η_v of most incandescent lamps varies from approximately 8 lumens-per-electrical-Watt at 2500 K to 14 lumens-per-electrical-Watt at 2800 K, 20 lumens-per-electrical-Watt at 3000 K and 27 lumens-per-electrical-Watt at 3200 K. Vacuum lamps operate typically between 2400 K to 2600 K; gas filled lamps operate at approximately 2700 K to 3050 K; and photoflood lamps operate between 3400 K and 3450 K. Figure 22-3 provides a plot of the luminous efficacy of radiation K as a function of blackbody temperature for a theoretical blackbody. The luminous efficacy of a true blackbody at a given temperature is obviously higher than the values for tungsten. The luminous efficacy and spectral distribution play key roles in hazard evaluation.

Color temperature is sometimes used with non-incandescent sources but with less than perfect success. Any attempt to estimate the spectral distribution of a non-incandescent source from the color temperature will generally result in a substantial error. Sometimes the phrase "correlated color temperature" is used to describe the output of a non-incandescent source.

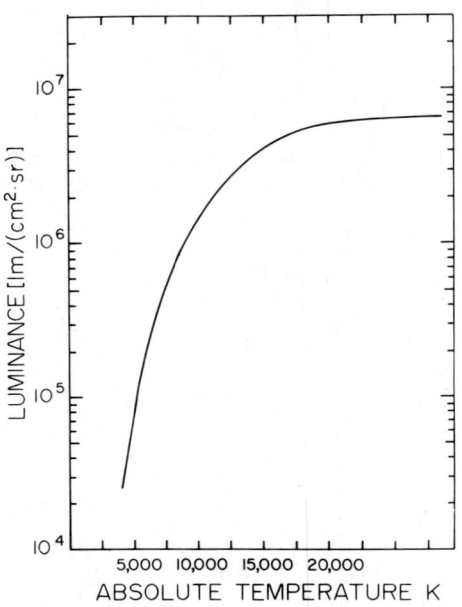

Figure 22-2. Luminance of Blackbody Sources. The theoretical luminance for a perfect blackbody is provided from 4000 to 30,000 K (courtesy of J. K. Franks, USAEHA).

Since the color temperature does describe the relative spectral distribution of an incandescent source, it can be used in calculating an estimate of the relative absorbed exposure at the retina for a given radiance or luminance of that type of source. Figure 22-3 also gives the function R, the relative retinal hazard factor of Sliney and Freasier (1973), which is that fraction of corneal optical power which is actually absorbed in the retina and choroid, and contributes to temperature elevation of the retina. The close similarity of the two functions is not surprising.

Tungsten lamp filaments, bulb structures and envelopes vary considerably. All components can contribute to the potential safety hazards from discomfort glare (this is discussed in detail in Section 4.5.11, page 141). Filaments may be single-strand, coiled, or coiled-coiled (a coil within a coil) as shown in Fig. 22-4. These three different types of filaments can then be arranged in a variety of complex structures.

The envelope of a lamp bulb is normally "soft" lead glass or lime glass for low wattages, and a "hard" glass—a high silica glass, or quartz—for high temperature applications. Except for the quartz-envelope lamps there are no measurable levels of actinic UV-B or UV-C radiation emitted from incandescent lamps. Even the ultra-

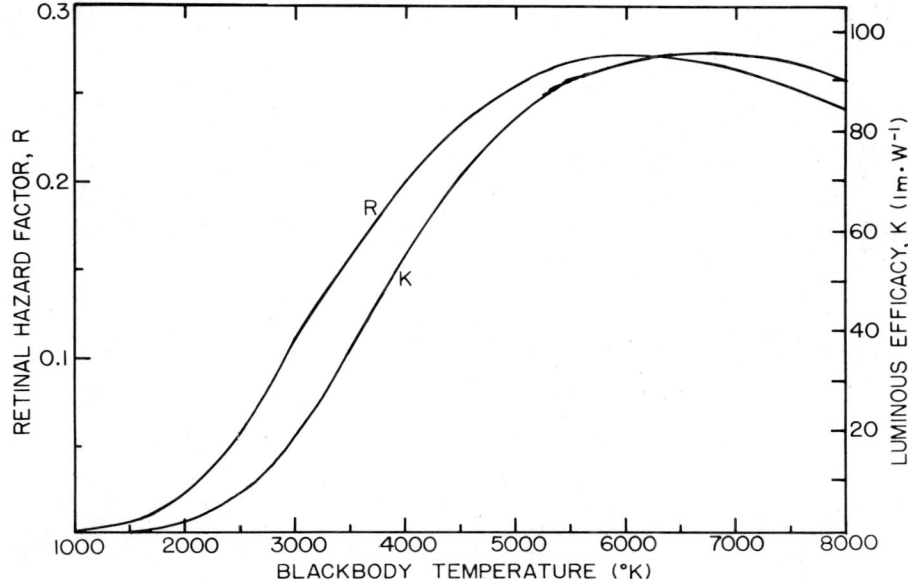

Figure 22-3. Luminous Efficacy K and Retinal Hazard Factor R for Theoretical Blackbodies. The retinal hazard factor is the ratio of absorbed power at the retina to power incident upon the cornea.

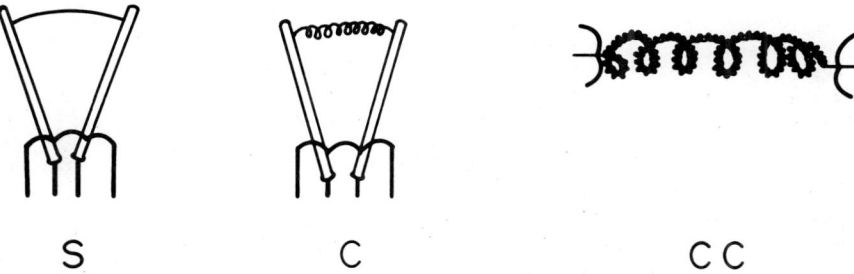

Figure 22-4. Types of Incandescent Filaments. Filaments are arranged upon support structures within the bulb in a variety of ways. The filament itself may be either straight (S), coiled (c), or coiled coil (cc).

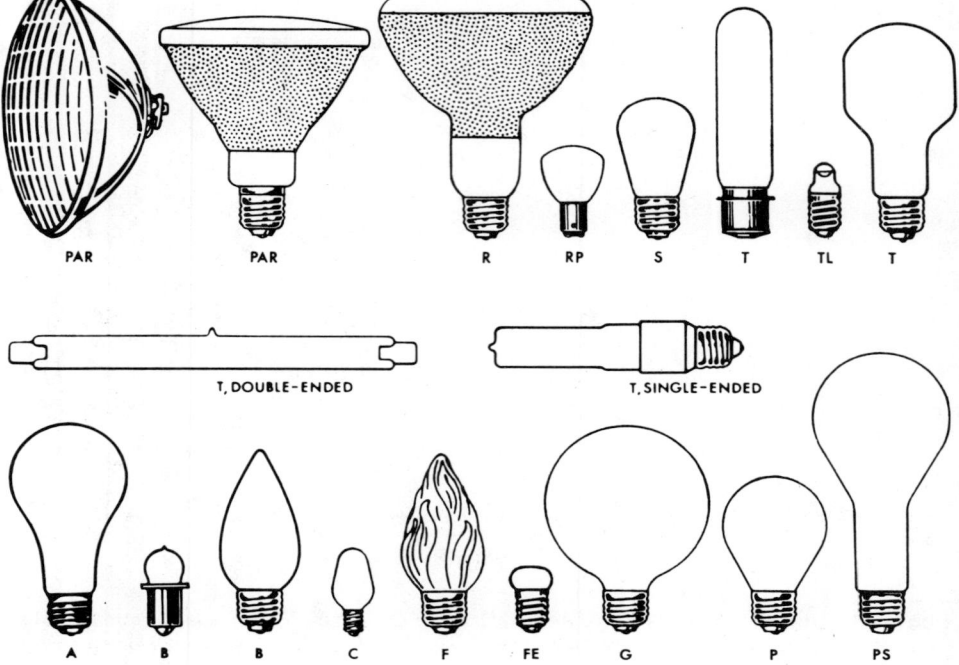

Figure 22-5. Incandescent Lamp Bulb Shapes. A variety of lamp bulb shapes—some with internal reflectors (PAR and R) and Fresnel lenses (PAR)—are encountered in general use. The codes used by the Illuminating Engineering Society (IES) are shown below each type. The relative sizes are not to scale. PAR stands for parabolic aluminized reflector, P for pear shaped, G for globular, C for cone shaped, S for straight side, F for flame shape, and T for tubular.

violet irradiance levels from a quartz-envelope tungsten lamp are relatively low except from the tungsten halogen types. Occasional cases of photokeratitis, conjunctivitis and erythema (sunburn) have accompanied prolonged use of these quartz-envelope halogen lamps. These lamps have been used often as photofloods and exposures of subjects for several hours can result in discomfort or damage.

Many lamp bulbs are frosted. That is, the inside of the glass shell is washed with hydrofluoric acid during manufacture in order to diffuse the source, and reduce the perceived brightness of the filament. The greatest glare and highest retinal irradiances are possible only with clear envelopes. Figure 22-5 provides an indication of the wide variety of bulb shapes encountered in the United States with their IES designations. For example, a sealed beam reflective automobile headlight is of the PAR category; a typical automobile headlight designation might be PAR-56. Some lamps make use of colored glass bulbs which absorb some of the output radiant energy in order to produce a specific color at the expense of a reduction in the total output of radiation.

Most modern incandescent lamps are filled with gas to increase the lifetime of the filament. The fill gasses are generally a mixture of argon and nitrogen, with a high percentage of argon for low voltage lamps, and a very high percentage of nitrogen for high-voltage projection lamps. Occasionally krypton is added for still greater lifetime. The high heat conductivity of hydrogen is utilized in signal lamps where a rapid on-off cycle must be maintained for quick flashing. None of these gasses appreciably influence the spectral quality of the incandescent source. However, in one category of lamps—the tungsten-halogen type which has become increasingly common in the last twenty years, the emission is modified by the gas. Generally iodine vapor is used, hence the common term "tungsten iodine" lamps. The halogen gas plays a regenerative role by combining with vaporized tungsten to form a tungsten halide which then breaks down near the filament, thereby permitting the vaporized tungsten to redeposit back on the filament. In order for this tungsten-halogen cycle to operate, the envelope must be maintained at a high temperature, at least 250° C, and for this reason the envelope is of quartz. As mentioned above, the UV-B emitted by this lamp can be a substantial hazard for long exposure durations. The high temperature of the lamp can cause skin burns or ignite materials upon touch. Therefore, these lamps should be used in protective fixtures where feasible.

One highly specialized type of incandescent lamp is the radio-frequency (RF) lamp which is used in certain laboratory instruments and in motion picture printers. A small ceramic disc (typically 8-mm diameter) is heated to more than 3000 K. Its color temperature can vary between 3100 and 3700 K and luminance is of the order of 1000 to 5000 cd/cm^2.

In the evaluation of the hazard of any lamp or the measurement of radiometric or photometric quantities, the question is often raised of the relevance of those measurements to the emission conditions earlier in the lamp's life or in the future for the same or similar lamps. Tungsten lamps can be reasonably well categorized in this regard. The lifetime specified by lamp manufacturers is generally the 50% survivability time. In other words, a lamp rated for a 2000-hour lifetime has a 50/50 chance of reaching that age. By 2800 hours (140% lifetime), almost all of the lamps will have ceased operation. The lumen and radiometric output of incandescent lamps depends upon the fill gas and type of filament, among other things. Lamps used in current-regulated or series circuits suffer little appreciative change during their lifetime with a reduction in lumen output as little as 10%. Tungsten-halogen lamps will have still less reduction. Indeed, the greatest depreciation to be expected is 20%. Thus, radiometric measurement performed on a lighting bulb near the end of its life would at worst case be only 20% low, or 80% of what would be measured with a new one. On the other hand, lamps with current regulators may show an extremely small, less than 5%, *increase* in lumen output during the first quarter of the lamp's lifetime.

The relative spectral radiant distributions from a variety of incandescent sources is shown in Fig. 22-6. It is noteworthy that not even the photoflood lamp operating at 3360 K color temperature has a peak in the visible portion of the electromagnetic spectrum. By far the greatest fraction of energy in all incandescent lamps is emitted as infrared radiation. Therefore, a radiometric measurement of an incandescent lamp with a broad-band detector (such as a disc calorimeter or a

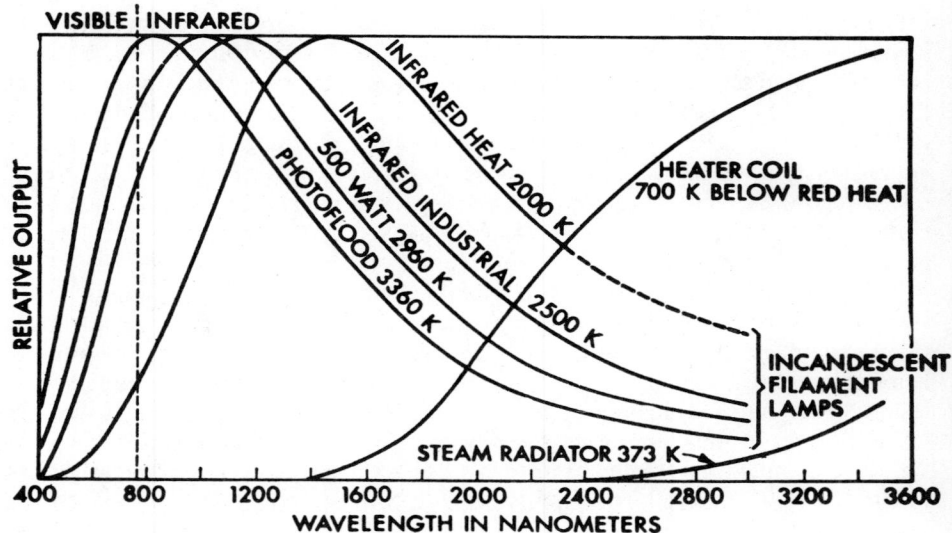

Figure 22-6. Relative Spectral Distribution of Incandescent Sources in the Visible, IR-A and IR-B. Notice the shift in peak wavelength with temperature. The curves are all normalized to peak at the top line (from the IES Lighting Handbook, with permission).

thermopile without a window) would show a far greater radiant output or irradiance than would be found with a limited-band radiometer such as a 450-to-900-nm detector radiometer. Since most of the radiant output is outside of the retinal hazard region, a reasonable estimate of the relative hazard can be made from simple photometric measurements, and a knowledge of the color temperature. The high stability of incandescent lamps has led to their use as radiometric and spectro-radiometric standards. Coiled-coiled tungsten-filament, quartz-halogen lamps are now the most common type of standard for spectral irradiance (Fig. 14-6 and Table 14-2) and tungsten ribbon filament lamps are used as standards of spectral radiance. Ribbon filaments are utilized to provide a very uniform spot of uniform radiance where a filament must be imaged on an area.

Since incandescent lamps are so efficient in producing infrared radiation, there are a variety of applications in the form of infrared lamps and incandescent-wire heating elements in space heaters, electric ovens, toasters, and industrial heating and drying applications. The hazard evaluation of such equipment will be discussed in greater detail in section 22.5.2.

The infrared radiation emitted by some lamps is sometimes a liability in pure lighting applications as it may give an unwanted temperature rise in the illuminated area. In many instances, proper design of the lamp can reduce this problem. For instance, PAR projector lamps include built-in dichroic reflectors built so that visible radiation is reflected toward the target being illuminated, and the infrared radiation is transmitted through the reflector and dissipated. Hence a certain color temperature of an incandescent lamp does not always ensure that certain fraction of infrared radiation will be in the beam. The use of various glass envelopes, lenses and such in projection systems will further alter the luminous intensity and the spectrum, as will be discussed in detail in Chapter 23.

22.3.2 Low-Pressure Gaseous Discharge Lamps

The most common types of low-pressure gaseous discharge lamps are those often referred to as "neon" sign lamps. This is a survival of the time when the first low-pressure gas discharge tubular lamps; filled with neon gas, were used in advertising signs which glowed red. However, the variety of colors now available in "neon" signs are really the result of electric discharges in other gasses, such as argon (blue) and krypton (yellow). Lighting engineers call these *"luminous tube signs."* Often fluorescent phosphors are combined to coat the interior of the glass tubing to achieve a shift in color. Standard tubing varies from 9 to 15 mm outside diameter. This glass tubing is sufficiently thick to attenuate any ultraviolet actinic UV-B radiation which could be of concern from a safety standpoint. A high starting voltage is required to start low-pressure lamps. In order to maintain the discharge at the optimum efficiency the gas temperature has to be relatively high. Hence, specialized power supplies are required. Once the gas has reached a critical temperature, the resistance of the gas is sufficiently low that discharge can be maintained with a lower voltage to give the optimum luminous output. Again, quartz envelopes will transmit the ultraviolet B and ultraviolet C gaseous discharge, whereas heat resistant glass tubing will not.

There are two other types of low-pressure gaseous discharge lamps which are of interest: mercury and sodium lamps. *Low-pressure mercury lamps* are commonly encountered in germicidal applications. Low-pressure sodium lamps were at one time relatively common for certain specialized illumination applications as the sodium doublet emission (at 589 nm and 589.6 nm) is near the peak of the photopic response of the eye (550 nm) and gives a high luminous efficacy of radiation K. The nearly monochromatic emission, however, often poses visual problems. Besides these two general types of lamps, other low-pressure lamps are sometimes encountered in laboratories when they are used for special purposes such as spectroscope calibration. Some of these spectroscopic lamp calibration sources are listed in Table 14-4 (page 465). Aside from the low-pressure mercury lamps none of these lamps pose any special hazards beyond the typical hazard of operating at a temperature sufficient to cause contact skin burns.

22.3.3 Fluorescent Lamps

One of the most common lamps in use today is the fluorescent lamp. It is a close cousin to the low-pressure discharge lamp since the only addition is that of a fluorescent phosphor. The usual fluorescent lamp consists of a low-pressure mercury discharge lamp which emits almost 90% of its energy at 253.7 nm, as shown in Fig. 2-14 (p. 35). These high energy UV-C photons can excite a large variety of phosphors very efficiently. The available phosphors have peak emissions ranging from the UV-B (FS sunlamp) through the UV-A (BL blacklight) to the visible (daylight, white, warm white, cool white, etc.). The mercury gas is normally maintained at approximately 0.008 Torr and the operating temperature is typically 40°C (104°F). Fluorescent lamps use two types of cathodes: cold and hot. Cold cathodes are used when a rapid start is unnecessary. Hot cathode electrodes have a tungsten filament structure which operates at approximately 1100°C. The hot cathode has a drop of only 10-12 volts, as opposed to the cold cathode drop of over 50 volts. The low cathode drop in the hot cathode lamp gives it greater luminous efficiency, and therefore most fluorescent lamps today are of the hot cathode type.

Most common tubes have one or two-pin bases at either end, with the identifying label printed near one end. For example, in T12F40CW, the initial letter refers to the shape (tubular) and the next number is the tube diameter in eighths of an inch (3.2-mm steps). Thus T12 refers to a tubular (T) lamp 12/8 or 1½" (3.8 cm) in diameter. The next figure is the power of the lamp in watts, and finally the phosphor is specified. Thus, the remainder is translated as: F, fluorescent; 40, 40 watts; CW, cool white. It is this latter type of notation that is stamped on the lamp. Lighting engineers often talk about a "T8" or "T12" lamp.

The luminous efficacy of a fluorescent lamp increases with length. An 80-inch tube is 40% more efficient than a 15-inch one. Furthermore, lamp efficiency is affected by the ambient temperature. For instance, the luminous output can be reduced to less than 5% of the rated output at sub-zero temperatures; therefore outdoor fluorescent lamps are often placed in heated enclosures. However, if the temperature is held constant, fluorescent light output may vary as little as 20% over the lamp's lifetime, although near the end there is often a rapid decrease in radiant output and luminous output. Fluorescent lamp lifetime is greatly dependent upon how frequently the lamp is started and how long the lamp is operated (Kaufman and Christensen, 1972).

A problem that was sometimes encountered in the early fluorescent tubes was flicker (Eastman and Campbell, 1952). The 60-Hz AC low-pressure mercury discharge will vary considerably due to the 60-Hz or 120-Hz oscillation in the voltage applied to the lamp. If the phosphor operated purely by fluorescence, this flicker would be translated to the luminous output. However, most phosphors have sufficient phosphorescence to smooth somewhat the luminous output. Nevertheless, rapidly moving objects illuminated by fluorescent lamps will sometimes show a slight stroboscopic flicker. This flicker can most readily be seen in a stationary fluorescent lamp by viewing the end of the lamp by the peripheral retina which is more sensitive to flicker. Some special applications may have circuits which operate the bulb above 60 Hz as this reduces the flicker, and also can increase the luminous efficacy by 10%.

In performing any radiometric measurements of fluorescent lamps it is important to document the ballast used. The ballast has a marked influence on the output of the lamp, and a laboratory measurement of a bulb with one type of ballast may not necessarily reflect the performance of the bulb in another fixture ouside the laboratory. Another characteristic measurement problem relates to geometry. A lamp that is 1 m long will subtend a large angle at close distances. Since many instruments have neither a large field of view or a cosine-corrected response, a segment of a lamp is often measured.

The output of a fluorescent bulb is a function of the type of ballast. Most modern fluorescent tubes are designed to operate with rapid start ballast and one of the major differences between the ballasts is the "sound rating." Some ballasts, however, are more efficient than others in terms of light output as a function of electrical power.

The importance of the ballast can be illustrated by an example from a phototherapy application. During our evaluation of some bilirubin phototherapy lamps (Westinghouse 20-Watt, F20 T12/BB, special blue) it became evident that the outputs of different fixtures with the same bulbs had wide variations. Two types of ballasts were found in the various fixtures in use at the Duke University Medical Center: a preheat starter type (Advance No. L-220 F 118 Volts 60 Hz), and a rapid start (Advance type RL-2SP20, 120 Volts, 60 Hz, 0.55 amps). For our test program two standard bulbs and standard starters (where required) were used in each fixture. The difference between the preheat and rapid-start type was quite marked. The light output was approximately 20% higher from the preheat-start ballast than the rapid-start, 121 mW/(cm$^2 \cdot$nm) versus 100 mW/(cm$^2 \cdot$nm) at 456 nm at the treatment distance. It is interesting to note that one manufactor suggested that a rapid-start ballast should be used in this application. Since output was the major consideration in phototherapy and the bulbs were replaced when their output had decreased by 20%, it seemed reasonable to select the ballast to maximize the current rating, which is roughly proportional to light output. On this basis, we are now testing some preheat 25-W ballasts which appear to give a 50% increase in light output over the rapid-start type. Obviously our program was not an exhaustive test of all types of ballasts. However, it indicates that care should be exercised in the selection of the type of ballast where light output (as well as lamp life) is an important factor. Ballasts must be circulated as well as lamps in any fluorescent lamp measurement intercomparison.

22.3.4 High Intensity Discharge (HID) Lamps

The most common high intensity discharge (HID) lamps are mercury, high-pressure sodium, and metal-halide lamps. The Illuminating Engineering Society defines HID lamps as those with a thermal loading on the bulb wall of 3 W/cm^2 or greater (Kaufman and Christensen, 1972). Gas pressures are typically 2-4 atmospheres. These lamps often present potential hazards and require evaluation. High intensity mercury discharge lamps are sometimes operated with fluorescent phosphors in the outer envelope.

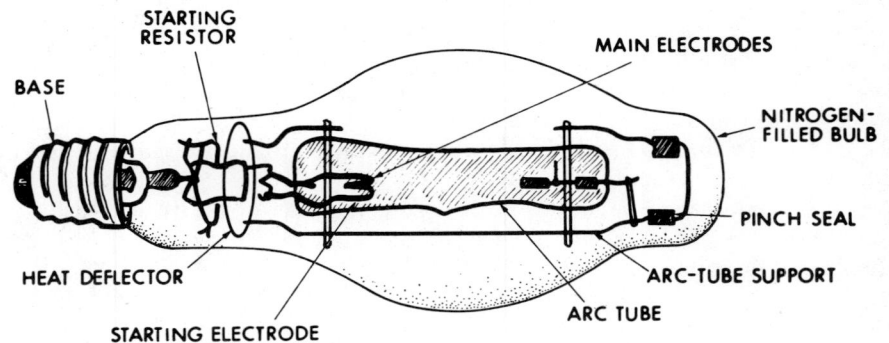

Figure 22-7. Mercury HID Lamp. This cutaway drawing shows a cutaway drawing of the construction of a Hg-HID lamp. The inner envelope is of quartz; the outer envelope of borosilicate glass (adapted from Kaufman and Christensen, 1972).

22.3.4.1 Mercury Lamps

A small amount of argon gas is introduced into the inner tube (Fig. 22-7) to facilitate starting and is responsible for the first arc. As this arc heats up the mercury is vaporized and the high pressure mercury discharge then sustains the light output. This process usually takes a few minutes. Most mercury HID lamps employ two envelopes. The inner envelope or arc tube is generally of quartz. The outer envelope is typically constructed of hard borosilicate glass. Nitrogen is typically used to file the interstitial space. The outer envelope shields the arc tube from ambient changes in temperature and drafts and also plays an important role in filtering out UV-B and UV-C radiation. These lamps are usually of the 400-W size and are used most often in highway or industrial applications.

Mercury lamps with only a quartz envelope, often as large as 3000 W, are employed in photochemical applications such as photoresist and ultraviolet ink and paint "drying," and similar ultraviolet curing applications. The spectral output of a mercury lamp is strongly dependent upon the vapor pressure and the discharge current, as was illustrated in Figure 2-14 on page 35. Not only does a continuum appear in a high-pressure mercury discharge, but also the five principal visible emission lines (405, 436, 546, 557, and 559 nm) have much of the output radiant power. This spectrum is unlike that of the low-pressure mercury lamp where the largest fraction of radiant power is in the 254-nm line. These mercury lamps have a typical luminous efficacy ranging from 30-65 lm/W (electrical) and a very bluish or bluish-green emission. A phosphor coating is employed inside of the outer envelope of a HID fluorescent lamp. This makes use of the substantial fraction of energy emitted by the mercury discharge in the ultraviolet. Figure 22-8 provides a characteristic spectral radiance spectrum of a 400-W HID fluorescent lamp. The luminous output

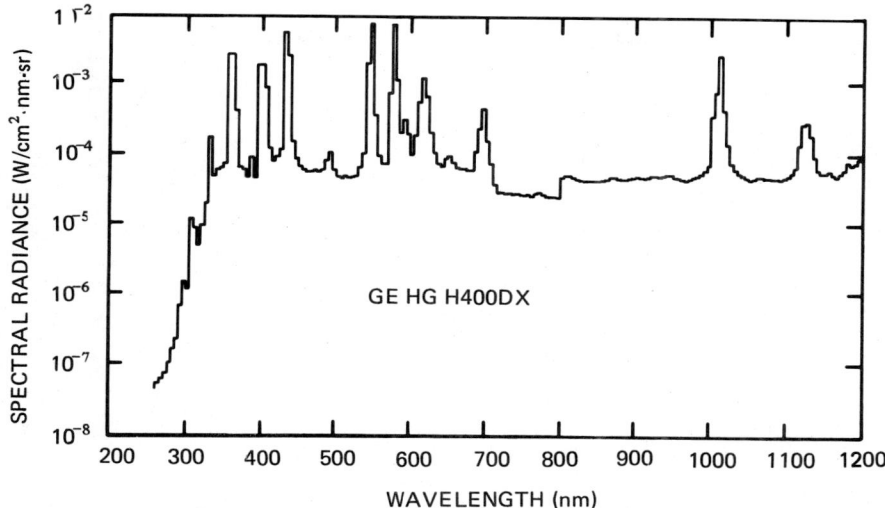

Figure 22-8. Spectral Radiance of a 400-W Hg-HID Lamp. The spectral radiance of a lamp is required for retinal hazard analysis. One can calculate the spectral irradiance at a distance if the bulb size is known.

of a 400-W mercury lamp typically decreases by only 10% for 8000 hours of operation.

22.3.4.2 High-Pressure Sodium Lamps

High pressure sodium lamps are becoming much more common in roadway lighting in this era of increased energy conservation. Like the high pressure mercury lamp, this lamp also is constructed with two envelopes. Figure 22-9 shows a cutaway structural diagram of a typical high pressure sodium lamp. The inner envelope is a polycrystalline allumina which resists deterioration by the highly reactive sodium vapor. This material is nearly 90% transmitting in the visible, but is translucent. The translucence therefore increases the apparent source size of the discharge. The trade names for two of the most common versions of this lamp in the United States are Lucalox® (trademark of the General Electric Corporation) and Lumalux® (trademark of GTE Sylvania). Like the mercury HID lamp the high-pressure sodium lamp includes another gas, in this case xenon, to aid in starting. There is also a small amount of mercury which would contribute to ultraviolet emission if the polycrystalline allumina transmitted much UV-B or UV-C.

The spectrum of a high-pressure sodium lamp is markedly different from that

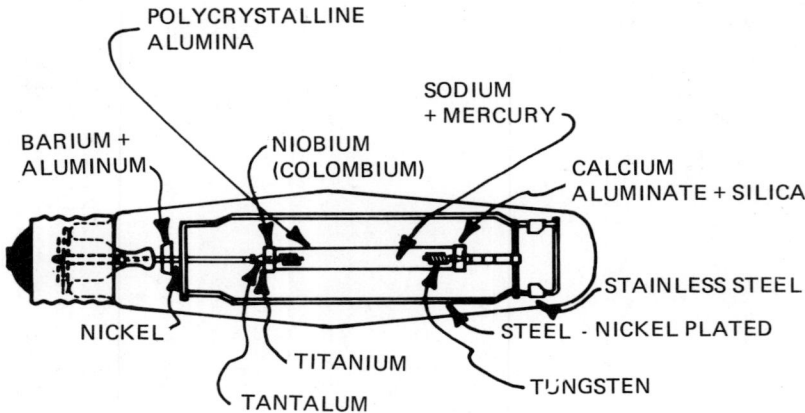

Figure 22-9. High-Pressure Sodium Lamp. This cross-sectional diagram shows the construction of a typical Na high-pressure lamp (adapted from Kaufman and Christensen, 1972).

of a low-pressure sodium lamp as shown in Fig. 22-10. This figure also provides an excellent illustration of self-absorption in a gas discharge. In the low-pressure sodium discharge almost all of the energy is limited to the sodium D-lines (doublet at 589 nm and 589.6 nm), but at higher sodium pressures (approximately 200 Torr) this doublet is self absorbed by the gas and reradiated as a continuum on either side of the doublet. In the high-pressure discharge spectrum there is actually a "dark" region at 589 nm. Therefore the appearance of the emitted light is more of a golden color than the intense yellow appearance of the low-pressure sodium discharge lamp. Since the outer lamp envelope is not diffuse, the luminance and even the blue-light radiance is greater than for the HID lamp.

A special lamp starter is required to produce a high-frequency, high-voltage pulse to start the sodium low-pressure lamp. The lamp requires approximately 15 minutes warm-up for it to emit at an optimum luminous efficacy. By contrast, the warm-up time for a 400-W mercury lamp is only 4-5 minutes.

22.3.4.3 Metal Halide Lamps

The metal halide lamps appear very much like mercury lamps with a phosphor coating. Generally these lamps contain mercury as well as a mixture of metal halides such as sodium, thalium, and indium iodides; sodium and scandium iodides; or dysprosium and thalium iodides. The spectral distribution of such a lamp is illustrated in Fig. 22-11. Certain of these lamps are used where it is important to have

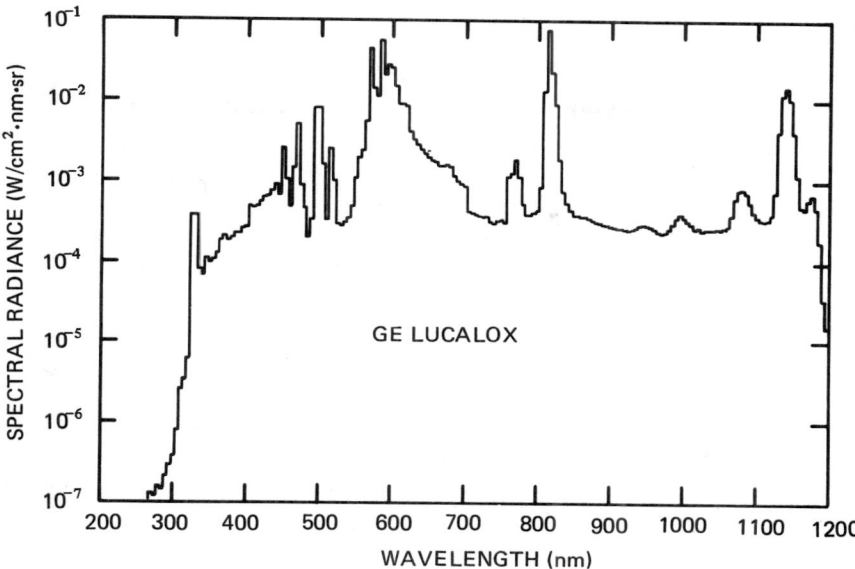

Figure 22-10. Spectral Radiance of a High-Pressure Sodium Lamp. The electrical power consumption for this lamp (GE Lucalox) was 150 W.

nearly monochromatic emission in certain lines. For instance the sodium halide emits principally at the 589-nm line (yellow); thalium at 535 nm (green); and indium at 435 nm (blue). Certain color balances can be attained by appropriate combinations of the radiating elements. A lead halide emits a strong near-UV discharge. Some metal halide lamps also employ phosphors in the outer envelope's inner surface, much like the mercury HID phosphor coated lamps. Metal halide lamps typically have smaller arc tubes than their mercury cousins of the same wattage. This can be used to tell them apart.

22.3.5 Short-Arc Lamps

Short, compact-arc (0.3 to 10 mm gap) lamps are the brightest continuous lamp sources available, and are typically used for searchlights and solar simulators. The short-arc lamps are generally direct current (dc) and specialized starting circuits and high-current, low-voltage power supplies are required. Xenon, mercury-xenon, and mercury are the most common. All of the short-arc lamp types employ quartz envelopes and therefore emit sufficient actinic UV-B and UV-C radiation to present serious eye and skin hazards for direct exposure. The quartz envelopes are exceedingly hot and would cause burns of the skin if touched momentarily. In addition, the high-pressure lamps present an explosion hazard if not handled very carefully. Specialized polycarbonate plastic, or metal enclosures are designed for installation of

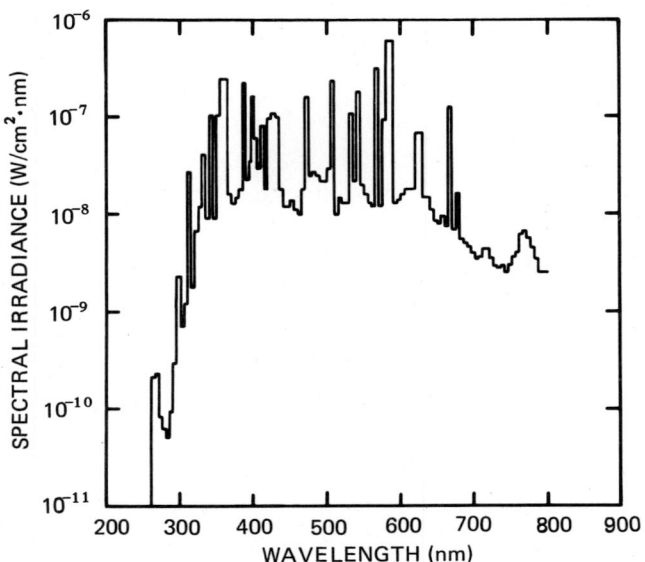

Figure 22-11. Spectrum of a Metal Halide Lamp. A representative spectrum of a 400-W clear jacket Sylvania Metalarc® lamp is shown. Note the dominant line spectra.

these lamps into a fixture. For searchlights it is almost universal to employ a glass ultraviolet-absorbing glass faceplate over the source to filter out the ultraviolet radiation, and to guard the lamp. Ozone is often produced around the quartz envelope and this must be exhausted to the outside of a laboratory or maintenance shop.

Figure 22-12 shows a drawing of the design of a typical short-arc lamp. The cathode is often a curved surface which the anode has a sharp point which creates a roughly triangular shaped discharge. The *xenon short-arc lamp* is chosen for solar simulators or when good color rendering is important, as its arc emission approximates daylight very closely The arc radiance exceeds 1 kW/(cm² · sr). It has a color temperature of approximately 6000 K and a continuous spectrum in the visible. Indeed it is almost the only arc lamp without pronounced lines in the visible. Strong emission lines are found only in the IR-A region between 800 nm and 1000 nm, but a few weaker emission lines appear in the blue between 400 and 490 nm. Figure 22-13 shows a typical 1-kW xenon-arc spectrum. The luminous efficacy of the lamp can be 35 to 50 lumens per electrical watt with the radiated luminous efficacy about 100 lumens per watt for 3-5 kW lamps. Small laboratory xenon short-arc lamps are made with electrical inputs as low as 30 W while large experimental searchlight lamps have been made to 30 kW. Above 10 kW, liquid cooling of the electrodes is usually required. The typical searchlight and solar-simulator applications are 1 kW to 5 kW.

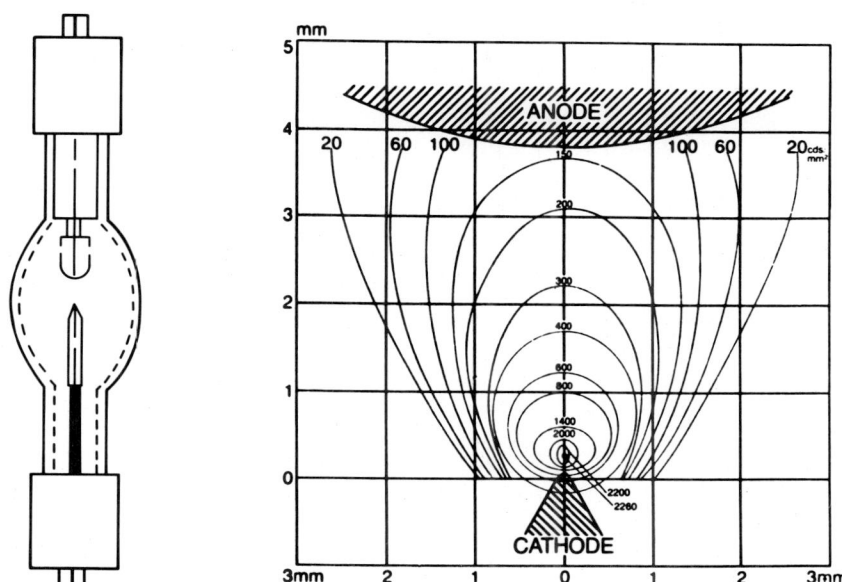

Figure 22-12. The Short-Arc Lamp. The cross section of a short-arc lamp is shown at left. The anode is typically dome shaped as shown and the cathode cone shaped. An iso-luminace plot of a xenon-arc lamp is shown at right.

High-pressure, *mercury short-arc lamps* are used where very intense ultraviolet sources are required, such as in solarization test chambers and in the photochemical industry. For such applications, mercury short-arc or even high-intensity-discharge (HID) lamps are almost always enclosed in a sealed processing chamber, as in photo-etching units and machines that employ ultraviolet curing of inks and plastics. This is necessary because of the extremely high emissions of ultraviolet radiation.

The spectrum of a mercury xenon lamp is useful where high UV and white light are both demanded. Again, the characteristic emission lines of mercury are superimposed on a continuum which peaks at 240 nm. Luminances of mercury-xenon arcs range upwards to 1000–7500 cd per square millimeter (cd/mm^2), which corresponds to radiances of the order of 1000 to 7000 $W/(cm^2 \cdot sr)$.

22.3.6 Carbon-Arc Sources

Carbon-arc sources were once widely used, but they now most often have

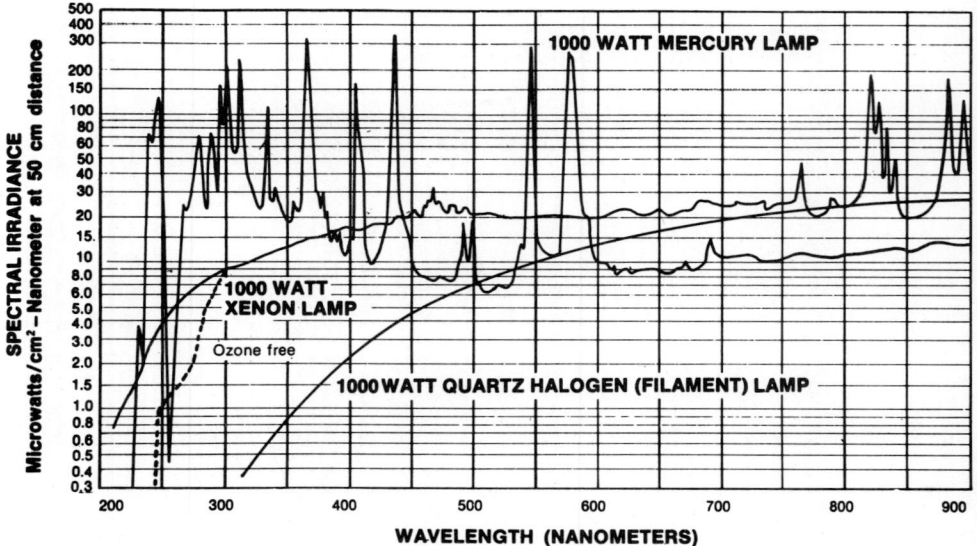

Figure 22-13. Spectra of Three 1-kW Lamps. The spectral irradiance of a quartz halogen lamp is compared to two types of short-arc lamps: A 1000-W Xe, and e 1000-W Hg lamp (courtesy of the Oriel Corporation of America, Stamford, CN).

been replaced in motion-picture projectors, spotlights, searchlights, and in many laboratory situations by short-arc lamps. Nevertheless, they are still sometimes encountered. The arc is open, as in a welding arc and must be vented. The carbon arc produces a rich spectrum in the UV-B and UV-C as well as in the visible. There are three general types of carbon arcs: *low-intensity, flame,* and *high-intensity*.

The actual light source in the *low-intensity arc* is the white-hot tip of the positive electrode carbon. The temperature at this point is very nearly the vaporization sublimation point of carbon, about 3700° C (about 3400 K). Although the arc-stream center is almost 6000° C, the low current density gives the arc proper only a small total emission, and the carbon tip itself is the chief radiator (Kaufman and Christensen, 1972). Hence, the positive electrode is placed at the focus of reflectors and concentrators.

In contrast to a low intensity arc, a flame arc uses electrodes which are made with other materials compounded with the carbon and the luminous of the arc is comparably uniform. The flame consists of vaporized carbon along with a very hot combination of other vaporized materials. The materials are chosen to alter the

the spectrum for specific applications. The vaporized materials, besides the various oxides of carbon, include iron (to increase UV emission), some rare earths, calcium, and strontium compounds, all of which have a high luminosity when heated to a high temperature. These compounds are made into a composite electrode along with the carbon. The spectral emission from the flame consists of the characteristic line spectra of the elements in the composite electrode and the band spectra of the compounds formed in the flame and will vary with electrode manufacturer. The flame arcs used in the graphic arts industry are designed to have a peak emission in the UV-A and blue portion of the spectrum. It would be of little value to present representative spectra of carbon arcs since they vary so greatly due to the flame materials. Indeed, it might even mislead the reader into trying to (incorrectly) apply a given spectrum to a different carbon arc. As the actual concentration of the luminous flame materials is not as high as in either a low intensity or high intensity carbon arc, the brightness of the flame arc is even less than that of a low intensity carbon arc. For searchlights, the large arc area is suitable only for broad-beam applications. Although the arc is not highly concentrated, it can have a high luminous efficacy—80 lumens per input electrical watt.

A *high-intensity carbon arc* has compound electrodes like the flame arc. However, the current density is much greater and the anode bright spot encompasses the entire carbon anode tip causing a rapid evaporation of flame material from the core of the anode, creating a crater. The most brilliant point of the arc exists near the crater. There is a greater continuum superimposed on the characteristic line and band spectrum in the high-intensity carbon arc. The luminance of the high-intensity carbon arc may be 55,000 to 150,000 cd/cm^2 at the crater and the color temperature may be as great as 6500 K. These values contrast with the luminances of low-intensity arcs of 150 to 180 cd/cm^2 with their color temperatures of 3600 to 3800 K. High-intensity arcs may have an input electrical power ranging from 2 to 30 kW, whereas flame arcs generally have an electrical input power of 1 to 4 kW. A high-intensity arc often has an offset cathode carbon to permit the flame to get outward from the anode and a rotating anode to permit uniform ablation of the positive carbon.

The peak luminance of a carbon arc or other open-arc process is often difficult to specify without sampling an extremely small central bright spot of the plasma. The spectrum can vary widely in the flame arc and the high intensity arc depending upon the flame materials compounded with the carbon electrodes. Certain compounds, such as iron, will cause a strong ultraviolet emission. In some carbon arc lamp systems, an air jet is used to stabilize and control the position of the flame relative to the positive electrode and to aid in the exhaust of combustion products.

During the early years of the motion picture industry when open carbon-arc reflector floodlights and spotlights were used, it was not uncommon to hear of cases of erythema and photokeratitis among the actors. Likewise, accidents which resulted in skin and eye burns from ultraviolet radiation among workers in graphic arts reproduction facilities were also not uncommon. However, with the advent of other arc lamps, and greater ease of control of UV-B and UV-C radiation, these problems are now rarely encountered.

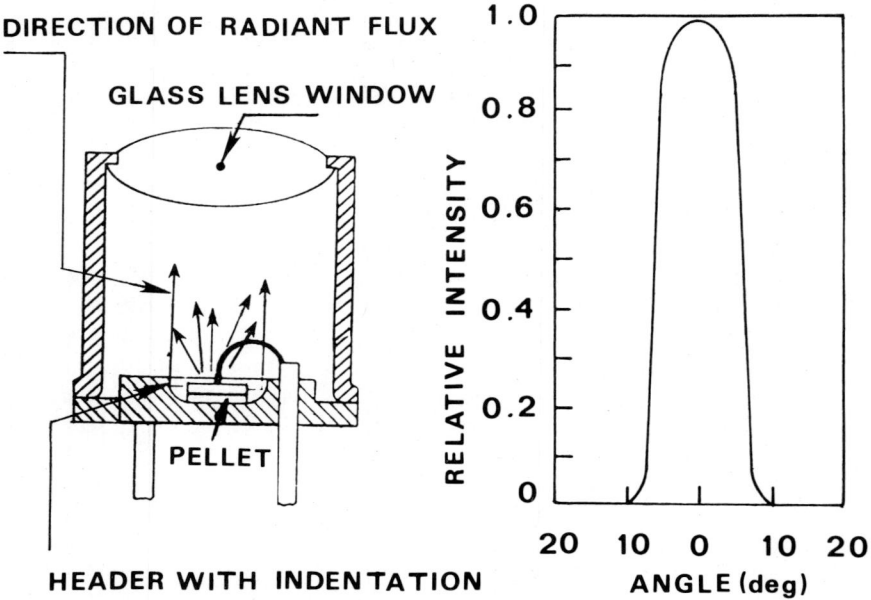

Figure 22-14. Light Emitting Diode (LED). Light emitting diodes come in a variety of configurations, one of the most common employs a built-in collimating lens as shown at left. Otherwise the diode emission would be hemispherical. The beam profile (right) of a collimated beam is shown at left (courtesy of Texas Instruments and RCA Corps.).

22.3.7 Electroluminescent Lamps, Radioactive Sources, and Light-Emitting Diodes

These are a variety of different types of relatively low luminance light sources used in panel indicators, as emergency night lights, and for readouts. They are seldom of concern from an ocular hazard standpoint because of their relatively low radiance and luminance.

At one time, *radium light sources* and radium dials on watches were common. However, with recognition of the hazards associated with the ionizing radiation emitted from these sources, the radium phosphor compounds have almost disappeared. The most common radioactive light sources today are tritiated phosphors which are safely sealed in glass beads to control the ionizing radiation hazards. The illuminance of such sources is generally below 7×10^{-4} cd/cm² (2 ftL) which is far less than any retinal hazard levels, nor are the ultraviolet radiation levels sufficient to be of concern either.

There are many so-called *electroluminescent lamps*. These are solid-state devices with a phosphor embedded in the dielectric between the transparent parallel plates of a capacitor. A variety of phosphors are used to produce different colors. These lamps are typically used as night lights, panel light switch plates, and instrument panels. Again, their luminance is quite low, varying from 0.0007 to 0.007 cd/cm^2 (2 to 20 ftL) with the most common sources under 0.0035 cd/cm^2.

Another type of fluorescent light source in use today is the *chemical light source*. The fluorescence is produced by a chemical reaction similar to that in fireflies. Typically, two chemical liquids are kept separated within a plastic tube, with one in a glass vial. When the glass vial is broken, the two chemicals mix, producing a reaction which emits light of a greenish color very much like that of a firefly. The luminance of these sources may be of the order of 0.0035 cd/cm^2 (10 ftL).

The *light-emitting diode* (LED) is the only type of light source discussed in this section ever to be of concern from an eye hazard standpoint. Light emitting diodes are similar to semiconductor lasers except that Fabry-Perot faces are not cut in the crystal. The total radiant power emission from a LED may be greater than that of a diode laser but the luminance and radiance are always less. Quite often the fan of radiation produced at the PN semiconductor junction is somewhat collimated by a glass lens which is placed immediately above it as shown in Fig. 22-14. Some characteristic spectral emissions of light emitting diodes are shown in Fig. 22-15. Near-infrared gallium-arsenide light emitting diodes are commonly used in communication, intrusion detection and instrument control devices. Gallium-phosphide and silicon-carbide LED's are used in calculator displays, and whenever visible emission is desired. The chip size is typically on the order of 0.25 to 0.1 mm. LED's generally require a voltage of 1 to 3 V with a continuous current of 1 to 100 mA. The visible LED's emit around 0.01 cd whereas the infrared LED's tend to be more efficient, emitting up to 10 to 30 mW. A gallium-arsenide source emitting at 900 nm is basically no different from the hazard standpoint than a gallium-arsenide laser diode of the same projected source size. At one time some manufacturers sold GaAs laser diodes as LED's. One can always check for laser emission by checking the spectral width of the emission—the laser emission being in a far narrower band.

22.3.8 Flashlamps and Flashbulbs

There are a variety of electrical flashlamps and chemical flashlamps that are used in photographic and specialized applications where a short pulse of optical radiation of less than 10 msec is required. Figure 22-16 shows the spectra of two characteristic xenon flashlamps used for photographic purposes with two types of current densities. Figure 22-17 shows the spectra of representative photographic flashbulbs and flashcubes which have a magnesium wire electrically or chemically ignited. These sources generally have a color temperature of 6000° K for the xenon lamps, and 3200° K for the destructible flashbulbs. Both sources emit both ultraviolet and visible radiation. Where quartz envelopes are used in xenon flashtubes the UV-B radiation can be of significant concern unless the arc tube is enclosed in another glass envelope. The chemical flashbulb is an *incandescent* or "combination"

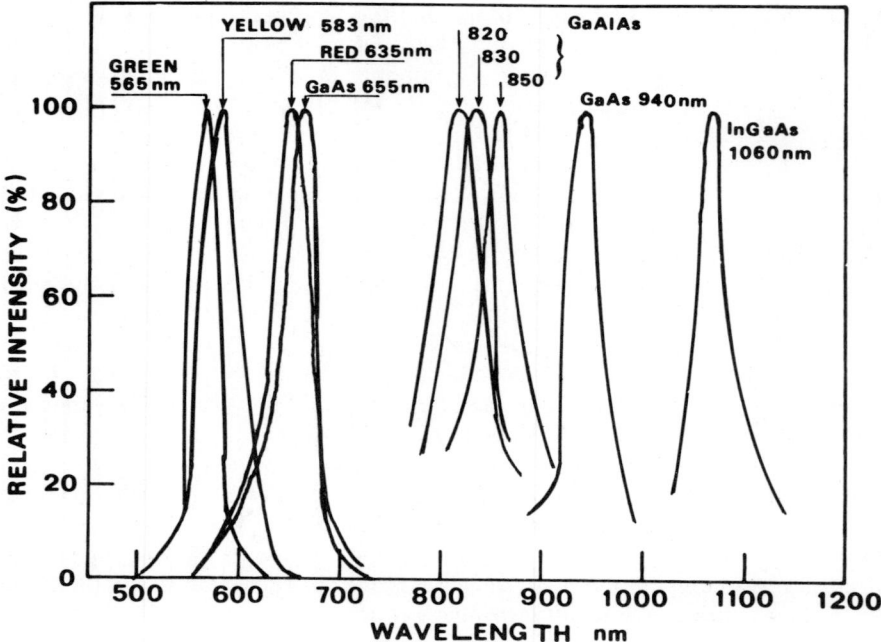

Figure 22-15. Spectral Characteristics of LED's. A variety of LED spectral emissions are available depending upon the choice of semiconductors. The spectral bandwidths are much broader than those of laser diodes. This spectral data is based upon information from RCA and Texas Instruments data sheets.

source of zirconium or aluminum and may have a color temperature of 5500 K only through the use of a blue filter.

22.4 HAZARD EVALUATION OF A LAMP SOURCE

22.4.1 Preliminary Evaluation

Prior to exhaustive measurements and safety calculations, it may be worthwhile to determine the need for a comprehensive hazard evaluation. Many categories of lamps can be excluded from all or several of the evaluations. Table 22-1 provides a list of common light sources and a few useful parameters for retinal hazard evaluation. Table 22.2 lists all the relevant hazard evaluation parameters for several specific lamps; this data may permit direct comparison or extrapolation to the source of interest.

Lamps and Lighting Systems

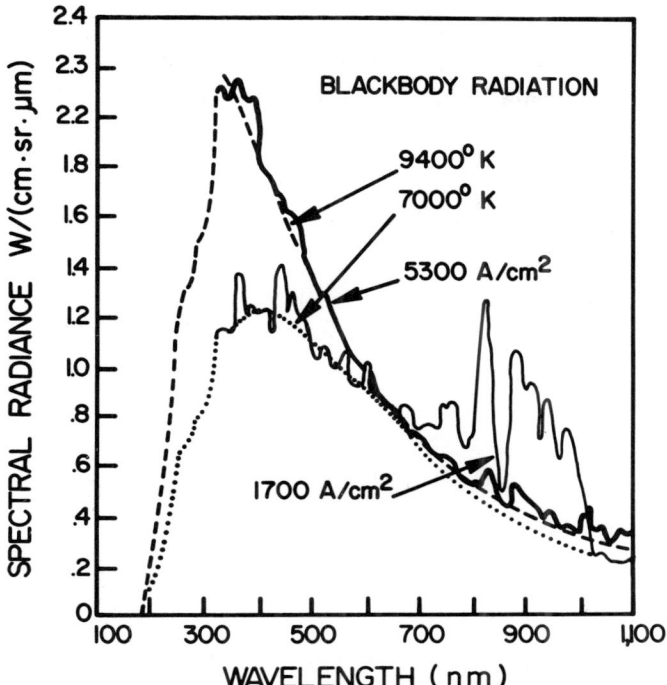

Figure 22-16. Xenon-Arc Flashlamp Spectra. The spectral radiance of an EG&G Type FZ-47A xenon flashtube is shown for two current densities. Flashtubes used in photography are normally designed to operate a current density sufficient to provide a daylight color temperature of 6500 K. Note how the visible spectra output dominates the spectrum as compared to a CW Xe lamp.

- *STEP 1 — Categorize the Lamp.* Certain hazards are not possible with all types of lamps. The grouping from Section 22.3 is particularly useful in this regard:

    a. Incandescent lamps and incandescent heating sources
    b. Low-pressure discharge lamps
    c. Fluorescent lamps
    d. High-intensity discharge (HID) lamps
    e. Short-arc (compact arc) lamps
    f. Carbon arcs
    g. Solid-state sources (LED's, etc.).

- *STEP 2 — Determine the Source Envelope.* Any glass between the actual source of radiation (e.g., the arc or tungsten filament) and the point of access can greatly influence the potential hazard. Soft glass of any reasonable thickness will greatly attenuate UV-B and UV-C radiation.

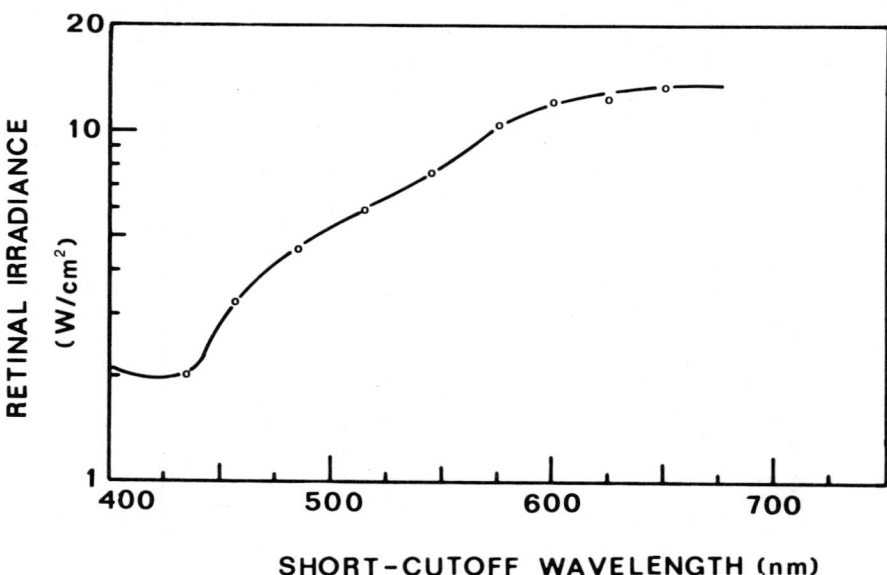

Figure 22-18. Retinal Injury Thresholds for a Filtered Xenon-Arc Spectrum. The 100-s retinal injury thresholds reported by Ham *et al.* (1979) for a 500 μm image in the rhesus monkey are plotted against the short-wavelength cut-off of the spectrum. For a full-spectrum exposure, the threshold was 2 W/cm^2 since blue light was present. For a flat spectrum with the wavelengths below 550 nm eliminated, the threshold jumped to 8 W/cm^2.

a. *Incandescent lamps*, other than quartz-halide lamps, normally have a sufficiently thick glass envelope to completely preclude a UV hazard. The blue-light hazard is also not theoretically possible at blackbody temperatures below 2000 K.

b. *Low-Pressure Discharge Lamps.* Low-pressure discharge lamps normally do not present a retinal hazard because of the relatively low radiance. Only those lamps with quartz envelopes can transmit sufficient UV-B and UV-C to be of concern. Of the common low-pressure lamps only mercury lamps can create a severe UV hazard. Many may be quite hot to the touch.

c. *Fluorescent Lamps.* Low-pressure tubular lamps in almost all cases have a thin glass envelope, but often present a *theoretical* UV hazard at the surface. They are certainly never a retinal thermal injury hazard and seldom a blue-light hazard.

d. *HID Lamps.* These lamps may present both blue-light and retinal thermal hazards, and possible UV hazards. Since most lamp envelopes are glass, there is little UV-B leakage. Nevertheless, the UV-B leakage may be of concern at very close distances. Quartz-mercury HID lamps require a UV hazard evaluation.

Lamps and Lighting Systems

TABLE 22-1. Approximate Characteristics of Typical Optical Radiation Sources

Source	K (0.25–1.4 μm)* [lm/W]	L_e [W/(cm²·sr)]	L_v(cd·cm²)	L_V (fL)
Sirius (star)	150	10^4	1.5×10^6	4×10^9
Nuclear fireball (~7000 K)	110	4×10^3	4×10^5	1×10^9
High pressure xenon short-arc lamps				
1 kW	70	3×10^2	2×10^4	6×10^7
2.5 kW	80	9×10^2	7×10^4	2×10^8
10 kW	90	1×10^3	10^5	3×10^8
20 kW	100	3×10^3	3×10^5	9×10^8
30 kW	120	4×10^3	5×10^5	1.5×10^9
Xenon long-arc lamp (20 kW)	70	2	2×10^2	6×10^5
High intensity mercury short-arc lamp	100	10^3	10^5	3×10^8
Electric welding arcs				
Stainless steel (115 A × 220 V)	140	10^2	10^4	4×10^7
Aluminum-TIG (80 A × 18 V)	60	6×10^2	4×10^3	10^7
Aluminum-MIG (100 A × 18 V)	80	10^2	8×10^3	2×10^7
Tungsten filament (500 W)	80	12	10^3	
Frosted tungsten filament lamps				
500 W	50	0.7	34	10^5
100 W	35	0.5	17	5×10^4
40 W	25	0.2	5	1.5×10^4
Sodium arc lamp	100	50	5×10^3	1.5×10^7
Sodium arc-transluscent tube (400 W)	266	2.8	750	2×10^5
Oxyacetylene torch	100–250	10^{-2} to 4×10^{-3}	10	3×10^4
Fluorescent lamps (40 W)	300	2×10^{-3}	0.7	2×10^5
Fluroescent HID lamp (HG 400 DX)	266	0.23	60	1.8×10^5
Candle flame	90	0.01	1	3×10^3
Bright sky (clear)	100	3×10^{-3}	0.3	10^3
General earth terrain	100–200	10^{-3} to 10^{-2}	0.1–1	3×10^2 to 3×10^3
Tungsten iodide lamp (1000 W)	100	25	3×10^3	10^7
Lightning bolt	120	8×10^4	10^7	3×10^{10}
6500 K blackbody	110	3×10^3	3×10^5	10^9
High intensity carbon arc	145	7×10^2	10^5	3×10^8
Electronic photoflash	100–200	0.5 to 1.5×10^3	1–3 $\times 10^5$	3-10 $\times 10^8$
Sun (at zenith)	130	1.3×10^3	1.7×10^5	5×10^8
Flashlight (3 V)	30	1–3	30–90	9×10^4 to 3×10^5
Snow field at noon	120	0.025	3	9×10^3

* The luminous efficacy of radiation K is correctly defined only if based upon total irradiance. The values in Table 22-1 are based upon the irradiance measured between 0.4 μm and 1.4 μm (the retinal hazard spectral region). The actual value of K is normally at least 30% less than K (0.25–1.4 μm).

TABLE 22-2. Optical Radiation Hazard Data for Representative Bare Lamps*

Type of Lamp Source	Apparent Source Size A_s (cm²)	Radiance (200-1400 nm) L_e [W/(cm²·sr)]	Blue-Light Radiance L_B [W/(cm²·sr)]	Luminous Efficacy of Radiation K (lm/W)	Luminance L_v (cd/cm²)	Retinal Hazard Factor R	Retinal Hazard Factor $\overline{R}$	Ultraviolet† E_{eff} (μW/cm²)	Ultraviolet† t_{max} (min)
Incandescent: Quartz-Tungsten Halide, DXW; 1-kW	0.69	58	0.95	45	2,6000	0.25	1.02	2.1	24
HID Fluorescent: GE, HG400DX; 400-W	45	0.23	0.048	266	60	0.46	2.5	1.1	46
High Pressure Sodium: GE Lucalox; 150-W	2.3	2.8	0.084	266	750	0.54	1.02	0.008	Safe
Low-Pressure Fluorescent:									
—Cool White, GE, F40CW	—	0.0027	0.0006	290	0.8	0.63	2.5	0.14	360
—Blacklight, Westinghouse, F40BL	—	0.0015	0.0001	26	0.04	0.07	1.0	0.12	420
—Royal White, Sylvania, F403K	—	0.0026	0.0005	270	0.7	0.57	2.3	0.14	360
Sunlamp: Sylvania Type RSM, 275-W	4.8	15	2.3	170	2,600	0.3	1.85	510	0.1
Xenon Short-Arc Lamp: Hanovia 976C1	0.36	980	109	110	110,000	0.36	1.5	680	0.07
Medium-Pressure, Clear-Jacket Mercury: 400-W Sylvania	2.6	2.1	0.42	160	340	0.32	2.5	1.0	50
Medium-Pressure, Clear-Jacket Metal Hallide, Sylvania 400-W Metalarc	2.2	4.1	0.60	220	880	0.62	4.6	1.2	42

* These values can vary considerably from lamp to lamp and are only provided as a relative indication of these parameters.
† Ultraviolet effective irradiance values are for a distance of 50 cm. The effective irradiance varies greatly from lamp to lamp as a function of the thickness of the glass envelope.

Lamps and Lighting Systems

e. *Short-arc Lamps.* Of all the electric lamp categories, this group will require the most extensive hazard evaluation. All potential hazards may be present (UV-B/c, UV-A, Blue light, retinal thermal injury, and skin thermal injury). Because of the high temperature of the arc, a quartz envelope (which transmits UV-B and C) is characteristic.
f. *Carbon arcs.* Since there is often no glass lens or filter plate between the open arc and a point of access, the carbon arc, like the short-arc lamp may present every potential injury.
g. *Solid-State Lamps.* Aside from LED's at very close viewing distances, there should be no concern, regardless of envelope. Only a retinal thermal hazard is possible with presently available green, red and infrared LED's—and then only in very rare circumstances where highly efficient collimators are employed, need there be any concern.

- *STEP 3 − Obtain All Available Manufacturer's Radiometric and Photometric Data and Lamp Divisions.* Any radiometric or photometric specification may be of value either for calculation or for direct intercomparison with measurements. Spectral data is most useful. The dimensions of the emitting area of the lamp will be required for retinal hazard evaluation.

- *STEP 4 − Compare Lamp Specifications with Those of Previously Evaluated Lamps.* In this regard Table 22-2 will often be of value.

- *STEP 5 − Perform Detailed Spectroradiometric Measurements when Necessary.* Where feasible, complementary measurements of luminance, illuminance, total irradiance should be performed. The pulse duration must be measured for a pulsed source. These will provide confirmation of the spectroradiometric measurements.

- *STEP 6 − Determine the Source Dimensions.* A photograph and microdensitometer scan of the negative may be necessary for a non-uniform source. Calculate the maximum angular subtense α of the source at the point of human access or at 15 cm from the source whichever is closer.

- *STEP 7 − Apply the Exposure Limits of Chapter 10 to Determine the Degree of Hazard.*

22.4.2 Required Data

To evaluate a broad band optical source it is necessary to first determine the spectral distribution of the optical radiation at the location of interest. The spectral distribution of the *accessible* emission may differ from that of the source due to the filtration by a glass window, or other optical elements used in projection systems. The spectral irradiance E_λ at the nearest point of human access or accessible viewing should include all parts of the spectrum from 200 nm to at least 1400 nm when significant levels exist. Incandescent lamps typically emit little ultraviolet radiation and the spectrum is predictable (Section 22.4.5) and with experience one can often justify elimination of measurements below 250–300 nm. Other lamps, such as fluorescent lamps, generally have little infrared radiation beyond 1200 nm and this region can, therefore, be neglected. This is important to note, since many radiometric instruments with photomultiplier tubes or silicon photodetectors do not have spectral sensitivity beyond 1100–1200 nm. Likewise, if it is known that UV-C is definitely not present due to a glass enclosure, the spectral region below 300 nm (and certainly below 250 nm) can be ignored. The spectral irradiance at the nearest point of access must be measured to assess potential ultraviolet hazards to the skin and the eye from the ultraviolet, and from the rest of the spectrum also.

The spectral radiance L_λ should be complete within the retinal hazard region, i.e., from 400 nm to 1400 nm to assess potential hazards to the retina. Again, the actual measurements beyond 1200 nm can generally be neglected for most sources. The measurement techniques and the required spectral intervals have been discussed in Chapter 14.

Lamp manufacturers often do not have readily usable spectral irradiance and spectral radiance tables (or curves) for each lamp. Published data or quality control data may present a spectrum over all or most of the bands of interest. However, the available spectrum may be in spectral power Φ_λ or in normalized or specialized units such as $\mu W/(nm \cdot lm)$. In these instances the measurements of luminance or illuminance at accessible points may provide the necessary keys to calculate all of the aforementioned data. For example, you are provided with a spectral power table for an exposed lamp and you measure a lamp luminance of 100 cd/cm² and an illuminance at the accessible point of greatest illumination of 5 lm/cm². You also take a photograph of the lamp source. Using either a machine-computing or hand-computing routine it is possible to total the spectral power and to calculate a weighted sum of the spectrum against B_λ, R_λ, and V_λ, or against V_λ alone.

The specified spectral power Φ_λ, when weighted against the CIE photopic function V_λ, provides the luminous power Φ_v:

$$\Phi_v = \Sigma V_\lambda \cdot \Phi_{e,\lambda} \cdot \Delta\lambda \qquad (22\text{-}4)$$

and the total radiant power Φ_e is the sum of the spectral power across the spectrum:

$$\Phi_e = \Sigma \Phi_{e,\lambda} \cdot \Delta\lambda \qquad (22\text{-}5)$$

The luminous efficacy of radiation K is Φ_v/Φ_e (Eqn. 22-1). For this example, assume it is 100 lm/W. One can now calculate the total irradiance E_e across the specified spectrum:

$$\begin{aligned} E_e &= E_v/K \qquad (22\text{-}6)\\ &= (5 \text{ lm/cm}^2) / (100 \text{ lm/W})\\ &= 50 \text{ mW/cm}^2 \end{aligned}$$

and the radiance L_e across the weighted spectrum:

$$L_e = L_v/K \qquad (22\text{-}7)$$
$$= (100 \text{ cd/cm}^2) / (100 \text{ lm/W})$$
$$= 1 \text{ W/(cm}^2 \cdot \text{sr})$$

The spectral irradiance E_λ and spectral radiance L_λ are directly proportional to E_e and L_e respectively:

$$E_\lambda = \Phi_\lambda \cdot E_v/\Phi_v \qquad (22\text{-}8)$$

and:

$$L_\lambda = \Phi_\lambda \cdot L_v/\Phi_v \qquad (22\text{-}9)$$

22.4.3 Hazard Evaluation Using the Proposed Army/ACGIH Criteria

As previously explained, aside from arc sources, the retinal thermal injury criteria will not be required. Generally the retinal thermal hazard criteria will only apply to projection sources. The blue-light hazard weighting should be applied to all light sources which are discomforting to stare at. The UV criteria apply generally to open-arc or quartz-envelope lamps:

- *STEP 1 — UV Hazard.* Weight the spectral irradiance E_λ against S_λ (generally for arc sources or quartz-envelope lamps). Use Eqn. 10-1 on page 332. Calculate the maximum permissible exposure time using Eqn. 10-2 on page 332.

- *STEP 2 — Blue-Light Hazard.* Weight *spectral irradiance* E_λ against B_λ if the source appears to be nearly a point source at the closest point of access and determine the maximum viewing duration. Use equations 10-6 and 10-7 on page 340. Otherwise, weight the *spectral radiance* L_λ against B_λ to determine this viewing duration using Eqn. 10-8 on page 340.

- *STEP 3 — Retinal Thermal Hazard.* For pulsed sources or exceedingly high-brightness CW sources, use Eqn. 10-3 on page 340 to calculate whether a retinal hazard exists. If the lamp has been filtered to eliminate visible light, use Eqn. 10-9 on page 341. Sources of possible concern would be cesium and rubidium halide lamps and filtered xenon lamps.

- *STEP 4 — Practical Use Considerations.* Probably the greatest difficulty encountered in any hazard analysis of a lamp is determining the actual, realistic exposure conditions—both typical and worst-case. For example, essentially all fluorescent lamps emit UV-B radiation exceeding an E_{eff} of 0.1 μW/cm² at the lamp surface. But at a realistic exposure distance of 100 cm, even for lengthy exposures, there would not be a hazard (Spears, 1974). When the UV exposure limits were first promulgated, knowledgeable lighting engineers thought that the limits were far too conservative. They argued that even if an individual were placed immediately beneath a bank of ordinary fluorescent lamps for eight hours, there would be no erythema of exposed skin. Such a test was run with a volunteer and he did receive erythema. That experience amply illustrated the difficulty of performing a fair assessment of worst-case exposure conditions. Other illustrations of this problem are evident by examining Table 22-2. Note that the permissible direct-viewing (staring) times for two common lamps used in high-bay industrial areas and in street lighting are less than 30 minutes. It is difficult to conceive of anyone staring at such high-luminance sources. One to ten seconds would probably be a reasonable estimate for the greatest duration someone might really stare into such a source.

Returning to the lamp example given in Section 22.4.2, it would be illustrative to calculate a blue-light-hazard viewing duration. Again from the manufacturer's spectrum, it is clearly possible to calculate the absolute blue-light-weighted radiance L_B. If the B_λ function weighted against the manufacturer's spectral power distribution:

$$L_B = (\Sigma \Phi_\lambda \cdot B_\lambda \cdot \Delta\lambda)(L_v/\Phi_v) \tag{22-10}$$

were to result in a value (for this example) of 0.04 W/(cm²·sr). Then from Eqn. 10-8 (page 340), the permissible viewing duration t_{max} would be:

$$\begin{aligned} t_{max} &= 100 \text{ J/(cm}^2 \cdot \text{sr)} / 0.04 \text{ W/(cm}^2 \cdot \text{sr)} \\ &= 2500 \text{ s} \\ &= 52 \text{ min} \end{aligned}$$

In most instances the calculation of t_{max} is purely an academic exercise. Any source exceeding the long-term, blue-light exposure limit will in fact be discomforting to view. A substantial after-image would result even for a 10-s viewing period.

Another fair criticism of the presently proposed blue-light hazard limits is that it may overestimate the hazard of sources which have L_B values exceeding 1 W/(cm²·sr). This overestimate results from the great difficulty of drafting a set of hazard criteria with an action spectrum changing with exposure duration. A set of experimental retinal lesion thresholds reported by Ham et al. (1979) illustrate this problem. They inserted short-wavelength blocking filters with successively longer cutoff wavelengths. As would be expected, the 100-s retinal exposures which included blue light were lowest, as illustrated in Figure 22-18. Hence a yellow filter over any xenon-arc source would obviously reduce the risk of retinal injury. Further experiments of this type with 1000-s and 10,000-s exposure durations would be highly desirable to establish the validity of weighting the spectrum of a light source with the B_λ function.

22.4.4 The Sliney-Freasier Method for Retinal Hazard Evaluation

The Army/ACGIH hazard criteria (Section 10.5) for retinal injury are a simplification of an earlier, more rigorous, method of analysis published by Sliney and Freasier (1973). Occasionally there is an interest in calculating the retinal irradiance for direct comparison with retinal-injury thresholds (e.g., those in Figure 4-18).

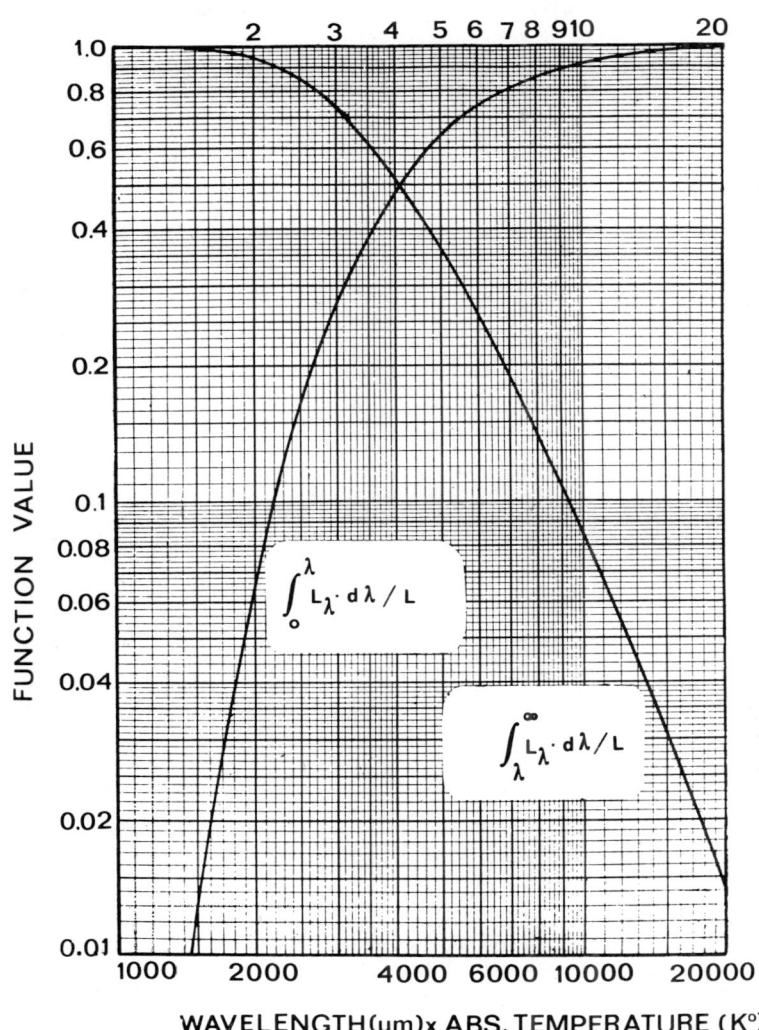

Figure 22-19. Blackbody Radiance Calculation Curves. Through the use of Equations 2-16 and 2-18 with the above two functions, it is possible to calculate the theoretical radiance of a blackbody within any given spectral band from λ_1 to λ_2. The fraction of the total radiance within the band is found by subtracting the two function values from 1.0. Adapted from Engstrom (1974).

TABLE 22-3. Maximum Permissible Absorbed Retinal Irradiances (W·cm^{-2}) as a Function of Retinal Image Size

Length (μm)	Width of Rectangular Images (μm)											Circular Image Diameter (μm) in First Column
	25	50	75	100	150	200	250	500	750	1000	1500	2000	
25	109	56	36	26	16	12	9.2	4.2	2.7	1.9	1.2	0.88	150
50	56	50	35	26	16	12	9.2	4.2	2.7	1.9	1.2	0.88	62
75	36	35	32	25	16	12	9.2	4.2	2.7	1.9	1.2	0.88	38
100	26	26	25	23	16	12	9.2	4.2	2.7	1.9	1.2	0.88	26
150	16	16	16	16	14	11	9.0	4.2	2.7	1.9	1.2	0.88	17
200	12	12	12	12	11	10	8.7	4.2	2.7	1.9	1.2	0.88	12
250	9.2	9.2	9.2	9.2	9.0	8.7	8.1	4.2	2.7	1.9	1.2	0.88	8.0
500	4.2	4.2	4.2	4.2	4.2	4.2	4.2	3.7	2.6	1.9	1.2	0.88	4.2
750	2.7	2.7	2.7	2.7	2.7	2.7	2.7	2.6	2.3	1.8	1.2	0.88	2.7
1000	1.9	1.9	1.9	1.9	1.9	1.9	1.9	1.9	1.8	1.7	1.2	0.88	2.0
1500	1.2	1.2	1.2	1.2	1.2	1.2	1.2	1.2	1.2	1.2	1.1	0.84	1.3
2000	0.88	0.88	0.88	0.88	0.88	0.88	0.88	0.88	0.88	0.88	0.84	0.77	1.0

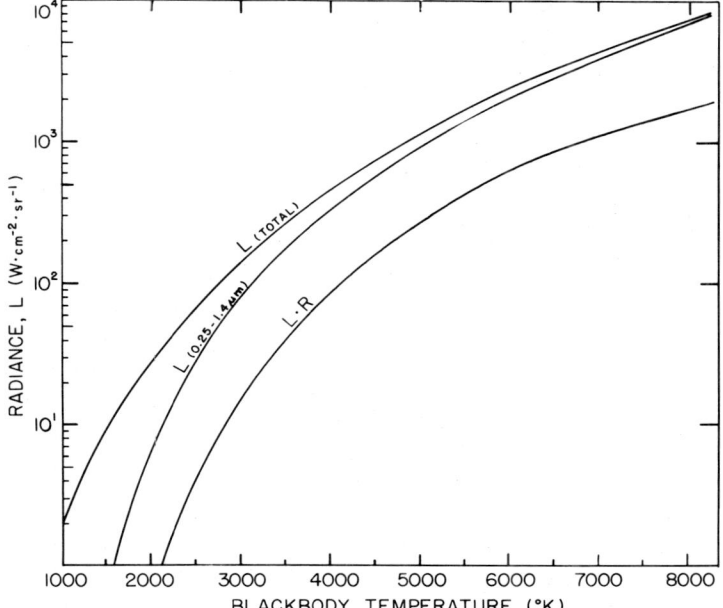

Figure 22-20. Radiance of theoretical Blackbody Sources. The lower curve shows the radiance multiplied by the hazard factor R which is the T·A value of equation 22-11 (from Sliney and Freasier, 1973).

Table 22-3 lists the maximum recommended retinal exposure limits for circular images (right-most column) and rectangular images. These limits assume momentary (0.2 to 1-s) viewing. These absorbed irradiance E_r values must be calculated with equation 4-4 modified to include a retinal absorption term:

$$E_r \text{ (absorbed)} = (0.27)(TA) \cdot L_e \cdot d_e^2 \qquad (22\text{-}11)$$

where (TA) is the spectral retinal absorption plotted in the uppermost curve of Figure 4-12 on page 121. The radiance L_e is computed from 200-250 to 1400 nm and d_e is the pupil diameter in cm. No further reduction in the limits are made for retinal image sizes in excess of 2 mm. The experimental evidence (although limited) suggests that the thresholds of injury at these larger images do not continue to decrease for larger image sizes. This is probably explained by the influence of choroidal blood flow in cooling the retina. The only shortcoming of the Sliney-Freasier method is that more recent retinal injury data suggests that even momentary exposure to blue light may not be purely thermal as can be seen in Figure 4-21

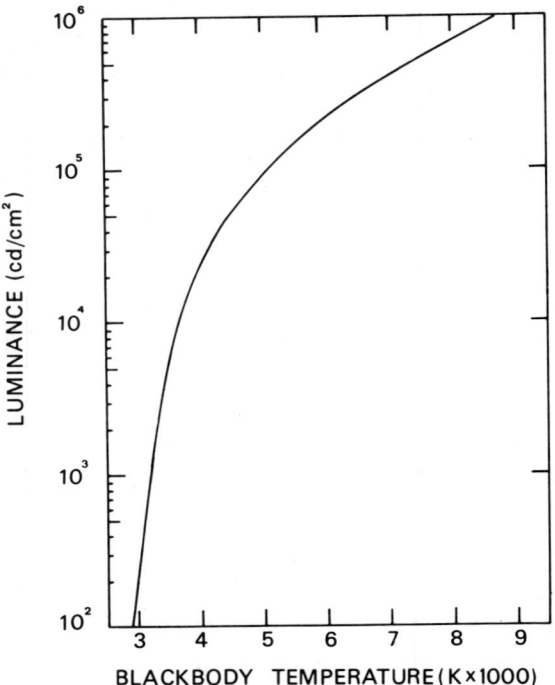

Figure 22-21. Luminance of Blackbody Sources. The theoretical luminance for a perfect blackbody is provided from 2800 to 9000 K.

on page 136 (441.6-nm data). For this reason, the ACGIH R_λ function has increased values between 400 nm and 500 nm (see also Appendix B).

22.4.5 Evaluating Blackbody Sources

Incandescent lamps, heating coils and molten metals can often be evaluated through the use of Planck's Equation for the spectral radiant exitance of a blackbody (Eqn. 2-21 on page 37). Figure 2-16 on page 37 shows the spectral radiance for several representative blackbodies. Figure 22-19 provides two blackbody functions which are very useful in the evaluation of incandescent sources and hot bodies. The functions permit one to calculate the fraction of radiance below a cutoff wavelength (lower-left curve) and that fraction above that wavelength (lower-right curve). The functions would apply to irradiance and radiant exitance as well. The curves are tabulated in the American Institute of Physics Handbook and other reference works.

To illustrate the value of Figure 22-19 one may calculate the fraction of radiant power in a 5000-K incandescent graybody source (i.e., the emissivity is constant) between 400 nm and 1400 nm. The two wavelengths in μm multiplied by the

Lamps and Lighting Systems

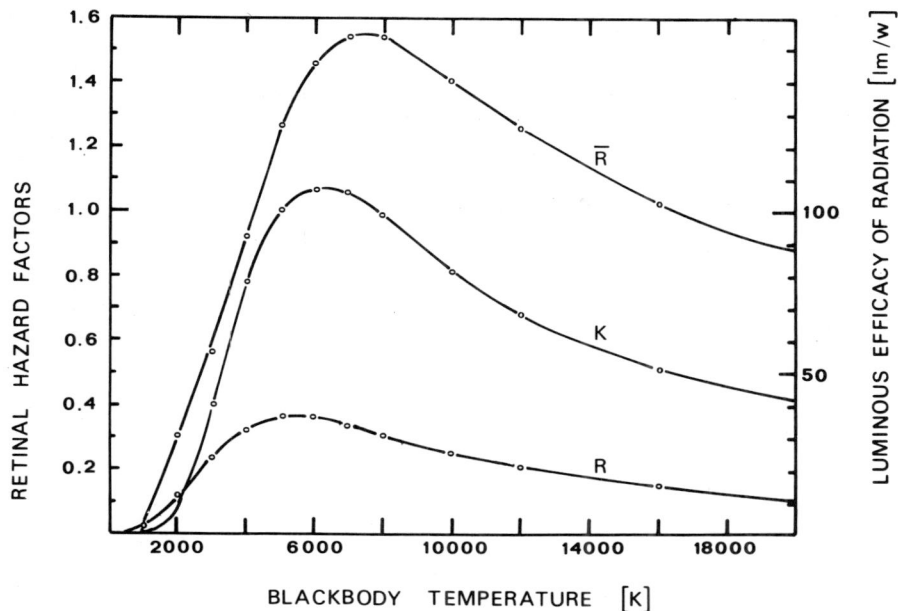

Figure 22-22. Luminous Efficacy of Blackbodies. The values of the luminous efficacy of radiation K, the ACGIH retinal hazard factor $\overline{R}$, and the other retinal hazard factor R (i.e., TA of Eqn. 22-11) display a similar dependence as a function of blackbody temperature (updated from Sliney and Freasier, 1973).

temperature give 2000 and 7500 for the short-wavelength and long-wavelength cutoffs respectively. The function values from the graph are 0.065 and 0.165 for the fraction of short wavelength and fraction of long-wavelength radiation to be subtracted from the total power. Hence the radiant power in the 400–1400-nm band is (1.00−0.065−0.165) or 0.77 of the total power. Since the two curves are complementary, one could have used just one curve for this calculation—with some loss of accuracy.

The spectral distribution of most incandescent sources approximate blackbodies within the accuracy of interest to hazard analysis. For this reason, it is convenient to plot the pertinent radiometric and photometric parameters of blackbodies. The absorbed retinal irradiance for blackbody radiators can be a theoretical guide for those using the Sliney–Freasier method. Figures 22-20 through 22-25 present the pertinent characteristics of blackbody radiators. The retinal absorbed irradiance values (Figure 22-23) are considered maximum since they were calculated using uppermost TA curve in Figure 4-12 (page 121) by means of Eqn. 4-4 (page 123).

As an example, the total radiance of a typical, general service 100-W tungsten lamp with a color temperature of approximately 2900°K and an emissivity of approximately 0.45 in the visible spectrum is obtained from Figures 22-20 and 2-13

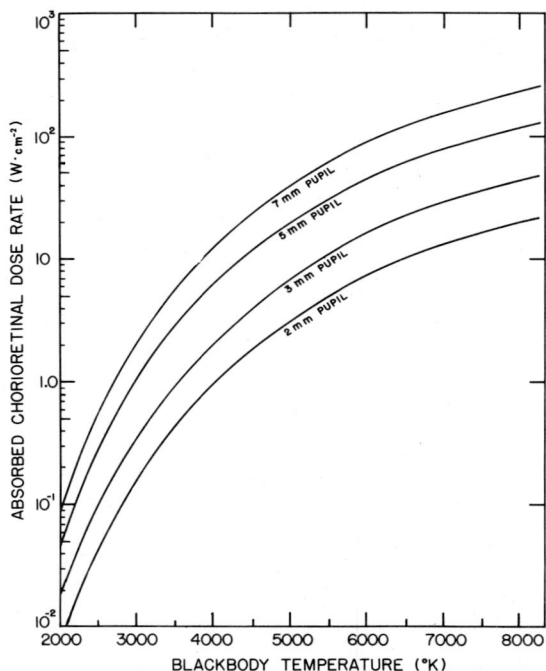

Figure 22-23. Absorbed Chorioretinal Irradiance for Blackbodies. From Eqn. 22-11, the above four curves were calculated to illustrate the dependence of retinal irradiance upon pupil size (from Sliney and Freasier, 1973).

(page 33). L is 130 W/(cm²·sr) for this temperature; and this theoretical radiance, when multiplied by the emissivity of 0.45, results in an actual radiance of 58 W/(cm²·sr). A source size and viewing distance would have to be given to apply the Army/ACGIH criteria. Using Figure 22-22 the luminous efficacy is approximately 18 lm/W and the retinal hazard factor R is approximately 0.1. Since the retinal hazard factor R as defined above by Sliney and Freasier (1973) is approximately 50% of that which would be calculated using the R in Table 10-2 (page 339), it is assumed that the R for this particular source weighted against the spectrum would be 0.2. From Figure 22-23 the absorbed chorioretinal dose rate for an observer with a 3-mm pupil is about 0.3 × 0.45 W/cm² or approximately 0.14 W/cm².

From Lambert's Law, using the weighted ultraviolet radiant exitance W_{eff} from Figure 22-25, one can estimate the effective UV irradiance E_{eff} at a distance r from a Lambertion incandescent source. The projected area of the source A_s and ϵ, the emissivity of the source must be known:

Lamps and Lighting Systems

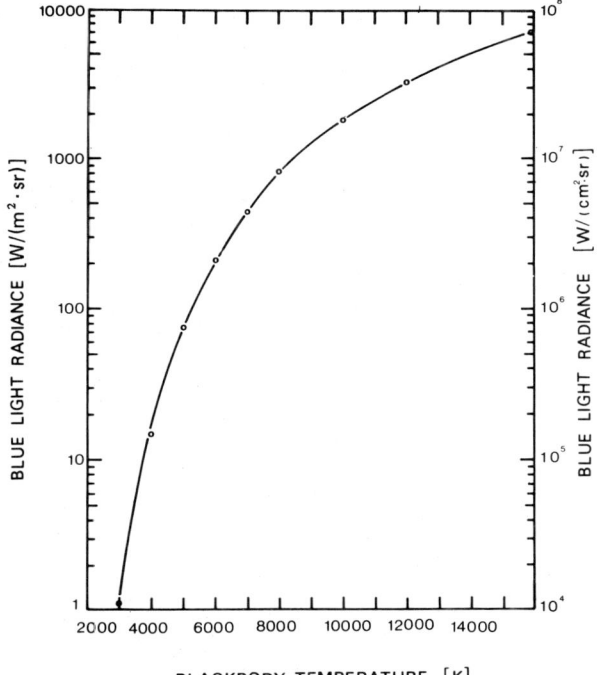

Figure 22-24. Blue-Light Radiance of Blackbody Sources. The blue-light radiance of blackbody sources follows a curve much like that for luminance.

$$E_{eff} = \epsilon \cdot W_{eff} \cdot A_s / \pi \cdot r^2 \qquad (22\text{-}12)$$

For example, a coiled-coil tungsten-halogen lamp (quartz envelope) has a coil which has an outside diameter of 3 mm and a length of 2.3 cm. From a distance of 50 cm, an area of 3 mm by 2.3 cm, or 0.69 cm², appears to be filled with the source. It is this apparent area, not the actual surface area, of the coiled coil that must be used for A_s. From Figure 2-13 on page 33, ϵ is about 0.4. If the color temperature is 3200 K, we can estimate the real temperature to be only marginally less for a 3200-K blackbody. From Figure 22-25, W_{eff} is about 0.066 W/cm², and:

$$\begin{aligned} E_{eff} &= (0.4)(0.066)(0.69) / (3.14)(50)^2 \\ &= 2.3 \times 10^{-6} \text{ W/cm}^2 \end{aligned}$$

This compares with the value of 2.1 μW/cm² given in Table 22-2 for a DXW lamp which operates at 3200 K. Obviously, we have neglected the transmission of the envelope which is probably about 0.9 for 250 nm to 320 nm.

Blackbody calculations are also useful for evaluation of the upper limits of ultraviolet, visible and infrared radiation emitted from arcs and hot plasmas. The

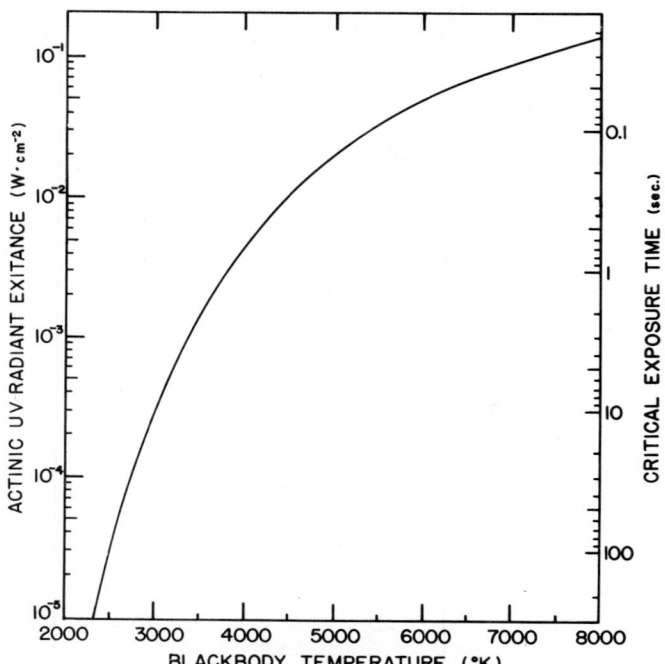

Figure 22-25. Actinic UV Radiant Exitance of Blackbody Sources. Since the E_{eff} of ultraviolet radiation will vary as a function of distance and source size the weighted radiant exitance is provided along with the permissible exposure time at the surface of the source. One can calculate E_{eff} at a distance by Eqn. 22-12 (from Sliney and Freasier, 1973).

emissivity of an open-air arc is generally quite small (0.01 to 0.04). If the emissivity and the arc temperature are known, then reasonably good estimates of several useful radiometric quantities may be calculated. Figure 22-26 presents the ultraviolet spectral radiance of a variety of ultraviolet. One could use the values in Figure 22-16 and calculate the spectral irradiance at a distance r from one of the sources by using a modified version of equation 22-12:

$$E_\lambda = \epsilon \, L_\lambda \cdot A_s/r^2 \qquad (22\text{-}13)$$

Equation 22-13 can also be used to estimate the total irradiance at a distance from a hot source. For example, many electrical resistance heaters operate at approximately 1450° F (1060 K). A red-hot, 2 cm × 30 cm bar of steel with a temperature of 1000° K and an estimated emissivity of 0.2 would have a total radiance of 0.73 W/(cm² · sr) as calculated by equation 2-25. Almost all of the radiant power would be in the infrared. Since area of the source is 60 cm², at a distance of 100 cm from this bar, the total irradiance would be:

Lamps and Lighting Systems

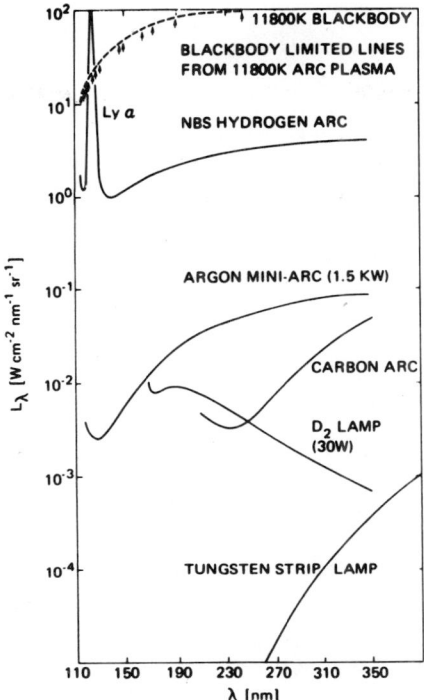

Figure 22-26. UV Spectral Radiance of Very Intense Sources. The ultraviolet spectral irradiance of UV sources at a distance can be calculated using Eqn. 22-13 (from Bridges and Ott, 1977, with permission).

$$E = \epsilon \cdot L \cdot A_s/r^2 \quad (22\text{-}14)$$
$$= (0.2)(0.73)(60)/(100)^2$$
$$= 1.6 \times 10^{-3} \text{ W/cm}^2$$
$$= 1.6 \text{ mW/cm}^2$$

With a very large radiating area, as would be found in a steel mill or foundry, one can imagine the large radiant heat loads on workers.

22.5 PROTECTION AND CONTROL MEASURES FOR BROAD–BAND OPTICAL SOURCES

Protective procedures, engineering controls and safety equipment used with non-laser optical sources often differ markedly from those used for protection against laser radiation hazards. This is not particularly surprising since almost all non-laser sources are broad-band and are far less bright than most lasers.

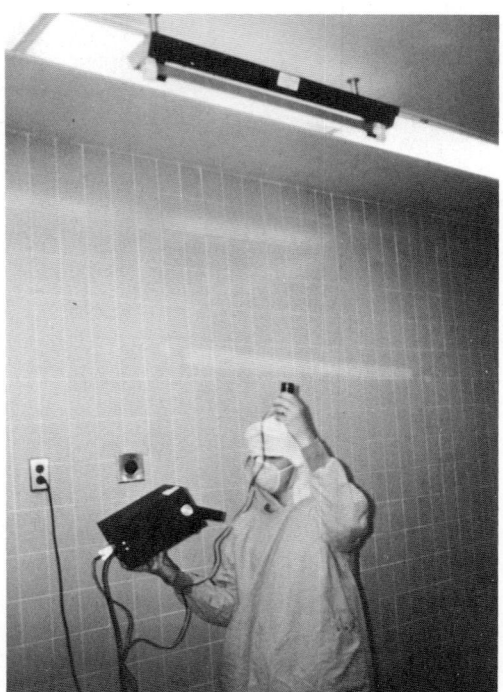

Figure 22-27. Germicidal Lamp in an Operating Room. A technician measures the effective ultraviolet irradiance from an overhead quartz-mercury-discharge lamp.

22.5.1 Control Measures for Ultraviolet Sources—Germicidal Lamps

The most common ultraviolet lamps—low pressure mercury ("quartz lamps")—are used for germicidal control in hospital hallways, intensive-care wards, operating room suites, and biological laboratory hoods. In some cases these lamps have been installed in fixtures to insure that the exposure of personnel is indirect. However, these fixtures have not generally been very effective. Therefore direct skin and eye exposure often occurs from exposed lamps. The selection of certain oil base paints instead of water base paints near these indirect fixtures in hallways has apparently resulted in increased UV reflection, and erythema of passers-by have resulted. Figures 15-14 through 15-18 (pp. 501–503) provide some representative reflectance values for several types of painted and non-painted surfaces.

Effective germicidal action in a room or in a laboratory hood requires such high actinic ultraviolet levels that personnel in the area must always be protected. Obviously, the glass shields in front of laboratory hoods filter out most ultraviolet radiation. However, in an operating room with quartz-mercury-discharge lamps mounted in the ceiling as shown in Fig. 22-27, protective clothing should be worn.

Lamps and Lighting Systems

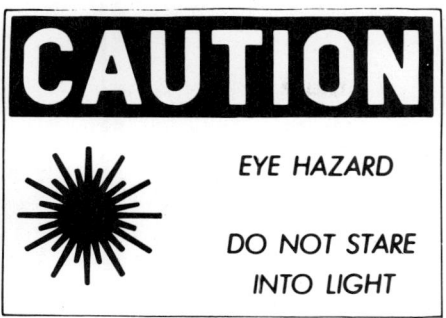
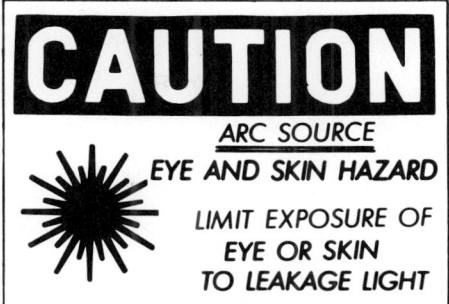
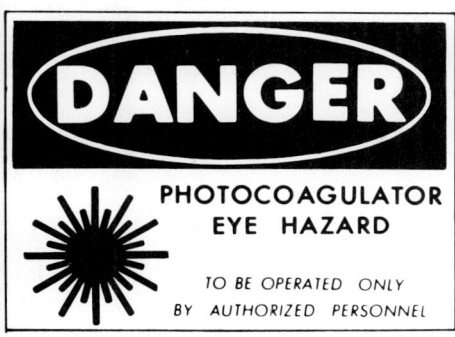
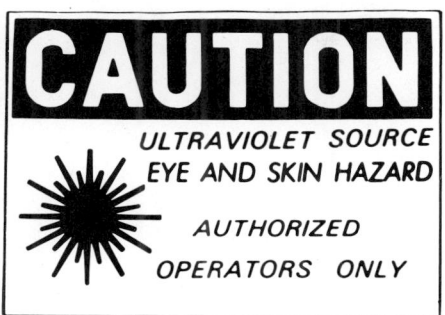

Figure 22-28. Warning Labels. Warning labels such as these are useful on equipment with high intensity lamps. The sunburst symbol for high-intensity light is distinguished from the laser symbol by the lack of an elongated bar going to the right which symbolizes the directionality of laser light.

Figure 22-27 also shows a man underneath a lamp fitted with a gown, face shield, and gloves to protect his skin and eyes. However, the patient is generally not protected in the area of the operation and some effects on internal tissue may occur during long-duration operations.

Some companies which sell quartz-mercury lamps also sell protective goggles or face shields, although almost any plastic face shield or goggles will be almost as effective. Most transparent plastics such as polymethylmethacrylate and polycarbonates transmit a significant fraction of UV-B, but fortunately UV absorbers are normally added to deter ageing. If question is raised of the adequacy of such protection, the spectral transmission of the material should be checked in the 300-320 nm spectral band. Any measurable transmission in this spectral band detected by a conventional spectrophotometer is considered unacceptable. Indeed a 0-100% graphical printout should show an ultraviolet cutoff in the 330-nm region, or at longer wavelength if appropriate UV absorbers have been added to the plastic.

When germicidal lamps are used in air-flow ducts, toilets, and laboratory pass-

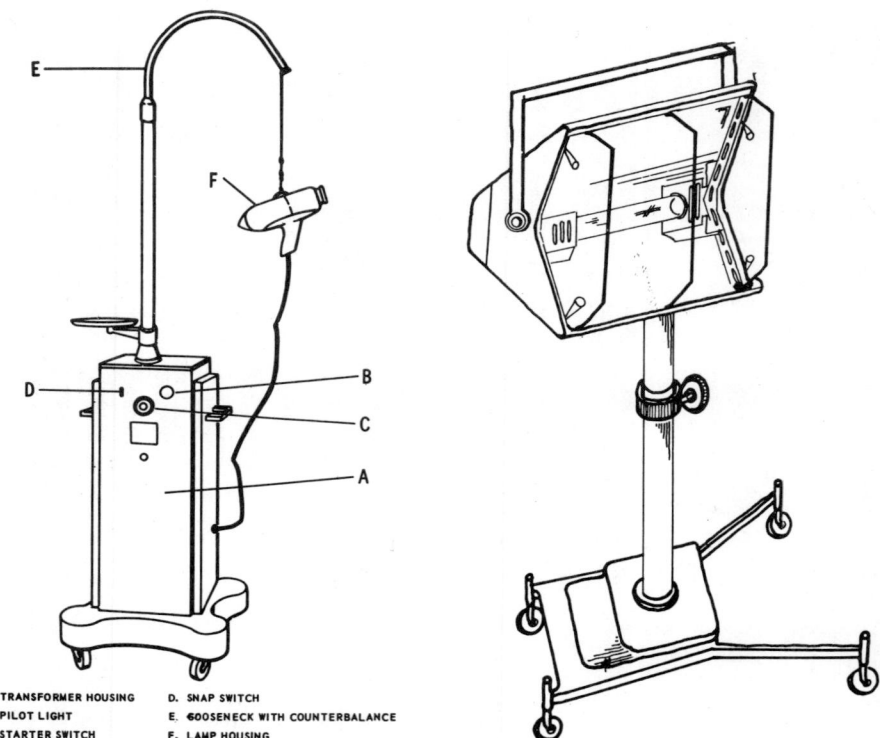

A. TRANSFORMER HOUSING	D. SNAP SWITCH
B. PILOT LIGHT	E. GOOSENECK WITH COUNTERBALANCE
C. STARTER SWITCH	F. LAMP HOUSING

Figure 22-29. UV Lamp Systems Used for Skin Testing and Treatment. The Hanovia Aero-Kromayer UV spot lamp (left) is used for patch testing and emits an intense, highly localized UV spot on the skin. The Burdick Model 800, 410-W ultraviolet therapy lamp (right) is used to treat larger areas of skin.

boxes, interlocks should be installed to ensure that an intruder is not injured. There have been a number of cases reported of an individual developing erythema of the back while sitting on a toilet where germicidal lamps failed to shut off when the toilet seat was lowered to the horizontal position. Any windows of hoods or pass-boxes should be constructed of ordinary plate glass (lime glass) which filters out wavelengths below 320 nm. Special warning labels, such as the one shown in Fig. 22-28 can be useful in assuring that users of ultraviolet equipment are adequately informed.

22.5.2. Phototherapy Lamps and Sunlamps

Dermatologists often make use of ultraviolet lamps for special phototherapy treatment. These lamps are usually vertically arranged in treatment booths as shown in Fig. 5-9 on page 180, and typically have several tubular UV fluorescent sunlamps and UV fluorescent "black lights." Normally only one set of lamps is used for any

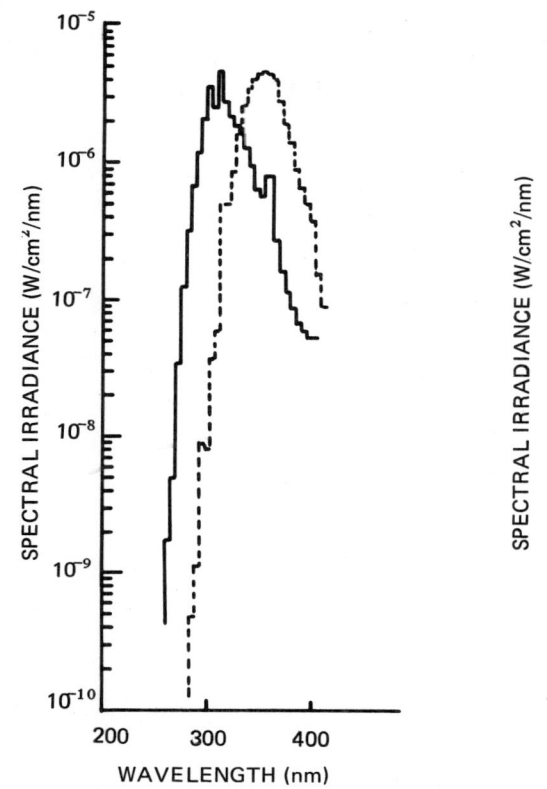
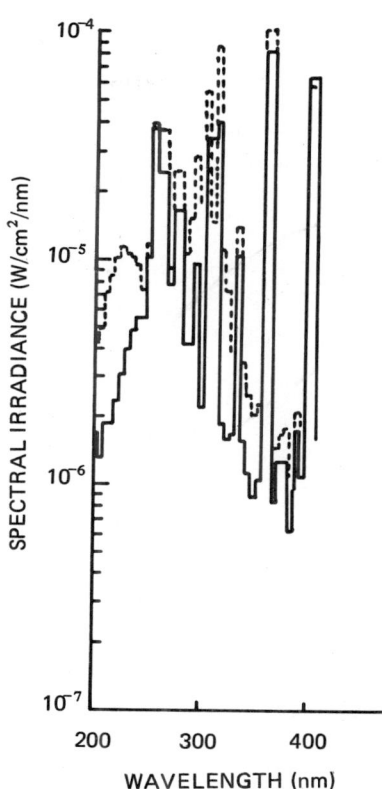

Figure 22-30. Spectral Irradiance of Skin Treatment Lamps. The spectra on the left are for a point 40 cm from a bank of fluorescent lamps mounted in a treatment box. Tubular UV-A, Type F 40-BL lamps (dashed line) were alternately placed as closely as possible with Type FS40 sunlamps (solid line). The spectra on the right are for the sources in the equipment shown in Figure 22-29. The dashed-line spectral irradiance is at a distance of 16 cm from the quartz window tip of the Aero-Kromayer gun. The solid line is the spectral irradiance at 28 cm from the edge of the standard treatment cone of the Burdick Model 800 Therapy Unit.

one treatment. For example UV-A lamps are used for treating psoriasis patients with 8–methoxypsoralen. Dermatologists are well aware of the hazards of excessive exposure and normally employ timing switches to limit exposure. The protective enclosures, or booths, are often open at the top for ventilation but the levels of actinic ultraviolet radiation reflected off a normal ceiling are generally below the 8-hr hazard limits for personnel standing outside the booth. The Committee on Photobiology (1979) of the Illuminating Engineering Society issued a detailed set of precautions for the construction of light boxes.

A variety of high-pressure and medium-pressure, mercury, quartz lamps

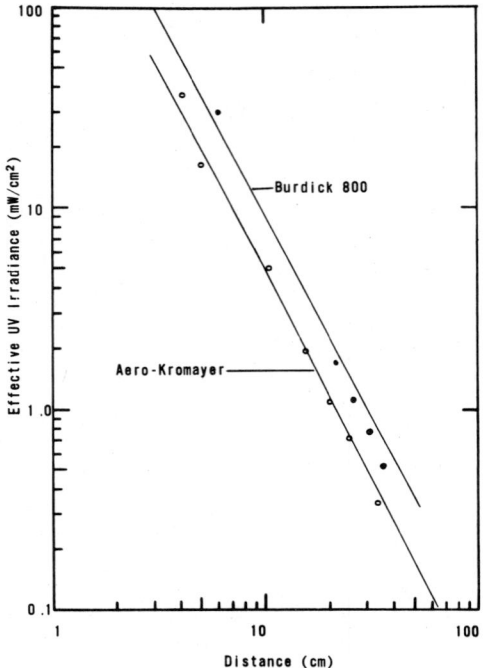

Figure 22-31. Effective UV Irradiance from Two Dermatology Lamp Systems. The effective UV irradiance for the two systems follows the inverse square law if the zero reference point is 5 cm behind the cone edge of the 4.5-cm diameter cone on the Burdick unit and 4 cm behind the applicator tip window on the Aero-Kromayer unit. The light skin minimal erythemal dose (MED) is typically 25 mJ/cm² which contrasts to the ACGIH occupational TLV of 3 mJ/cm².

(sometimes referred to as "hot quartz" lamps) are used for localized skin treatment. Figure 22-29 shows the design of two common UV delivery devices. The left panel shows a hand-held Aero-Kromayer device and the right panel is a drawing of a larger, general UV source—the Burdick Model 800. Figures 22-30 and 22-31 provide the spectral irradiance and E_{eff} for these two sources.

The following sample operational procedure for a dermatology clinic illustrates the control measures applicable to such a medical facility:

OPERATION OF UV LAMPS

Serious and painful ultraviolet induced eye and skin irritation may result to unprotected personnel if these units were improperly used. The following precautions reduce needless occupational exposure:

   a.   *Only authorized personnel familiar with the potential hazards and control measures shall use the unit.*

b. The unit shall be used in a designated area with limited access which affords added protection to passers-by. Operation from within a closed well-ventilated room or draped area reduces the risk of exposure.

c. Operator protective measures include the usage of dark glasses with side shields, long sleeved shirts, gloves and long pants. Although these devices may not completely eliminate the ultraviolet radiation, they lessen the risk of a severe burn.

d. Avoid needless exposure even when skin or eyes are covered.

e. Never look directly at the lamp. Cover eyes and skin of patients which do not require exposure. Avoid an overdose. Time carefully. Know the erythemic reaction of the patient. Avoid needless exposure to patients.

22.5.3 "Black Light" Lamps

The so-called "black light" or UV-A lamp often referred to as a "Wood's Lamp" is used with fluorescent powders in many nondestructive testing application, for special effects in entertainment, or in medical facilities. These lamps are normally not considered hazardous since the UV-A radiance at the lamp surface is only 1-5 mW/cm^2 and the skin or eye would not normally be exposed to levels exceeding 1 mW/cm^2. Problems with such lamps arise normally in two instances. One situation occurs when the lamp envelope insufficiently filters out the actinic UV lines of the mercury spectrum (297, 303, and 313 nm). The second situation occurs when photosensitive individuals use these lamps. In industry it is not uncommon for a worker who has been working with black lights for many years to suddenly have a skin reaction. Investigation normally reveals that the workers has been taking some medication, such as tetracycline, which photosensitizes his skin to UV-A radiation and sunlight. Protective creams or temporary removal from the job site are the most common cures for this situation. Photosensitive individuals should not be assigned to work with UV-B sources when pre-employment medical screening reveals such a problem. Tables 5-4 and 5-5 (pp. 177–179) provide useful lists of photosensitizers. In a few instances actinic ultraviolet UV-B and UV-C radiation from lamps used in UV-A illumination systems has leaked out of cooling louvers or cracks in an instrument housing causing skin reactions or conjunctivitis and photokeratitis which at first were thought to be due to UV-A radiation.

There are a variety of small portable "blacklight" units used for fluorescence studies. Some of these have a "shortwave" (UV-C and UV-B) mode as well as a "longwave" (UV-A) mode. The spectral irradiance values for four such lamps are given in Figures 22-32 through 22-36. The measurement distance for each spectral histogram plot was 15 cm from the lamp surface. The effective UV irradiance for each mode of operation is provided in the upper part of each figure. The measurements were performed on representative units by J. K. Franks of USAEHA and should only be considered indicative of the output characteristics of other units of the same model.

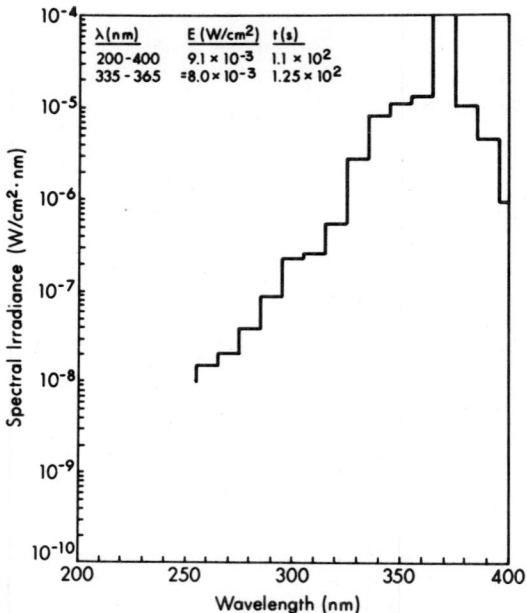

Figure 22-32. Lamp Spectrum. Absolute spectral irradiance of Blak-Ray Model B-100 made by Ultraviolet Products, Inc., lamp is H44GS-108.

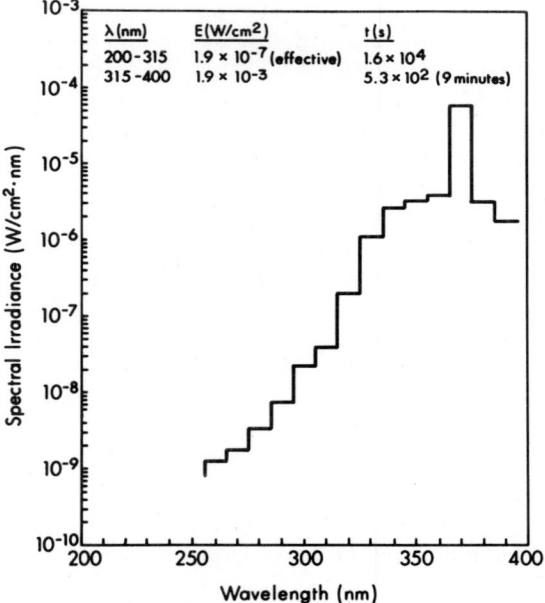

Figure 22-33. Lamp Spectrum. Absolute spectral irradiance of the B-100 Spectroline manufactured by Blacklight Eastern Corporation.

Lamps and Lighting Systems

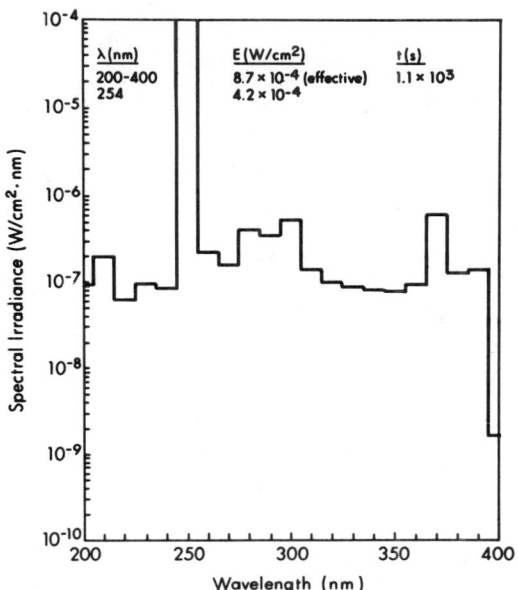

Figure 22-34. Lamp Spectrum. Absolute spectral irradiance of the mineral light Model R52. This fixture is manufactured by Ultraviolet Products, Inc.: spectrum emitted by shortwave side.

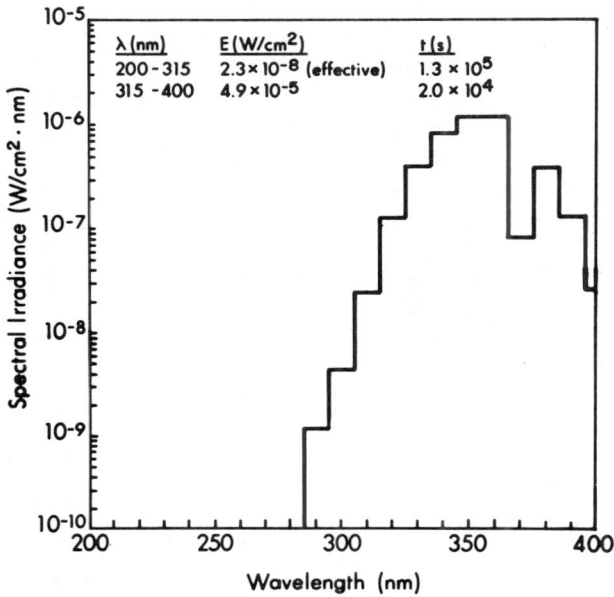

Figure 22-35. Lamp Spectrum. Absolute spectral irradiance of the Ultraviolet Products, Inc., mineral light longwave UVSL25.

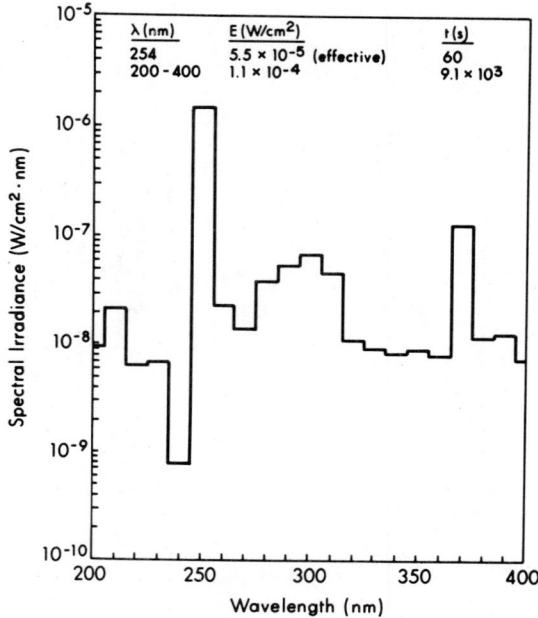

Figure 22-36. Lamp Spectrum. Absolute spectral irradiance of the Ultraviolet Products, Inc., mineral light shortwave UVSL25.

Black lights should be positioned in any application so that individuals are not normally exposed to UV irradiances exceeding 1 mW/cm². The eyes should not be chronically exposed to that level even though present standards make no such distinction between eye and skin exposure. Most readers have probably stared at a black light and surely noticed the fuzzy and annoying appearance of the lamp. This hazy appearance is due to two effects: to chromatic aberration in the cornea and lens of the eye at these wavelengths; and to lenticular fluorescence. The haze and annoyance can be easily eliminated by special plastic goggles which filter out UV-A radiation. These glare reduction goggles are available from several ultraviolet specialty companies, (e.g., UV Products Inc., San Gabriel, California).

22.5.4 Ultraviolet Curing Equipment

In the past few years there has been a substantial increase in the industrial use of ultraviolet radiation sources in UV curing applications. These UV sources are generally partially or totally enclosed and are used to "dry" (photochemically cure) ink in high-speed printing presses, to cure special paints, or to cure special orthopedic plastic cast materials. In the latter application a bank of UV-A fluorescent lamps are used. UV curing of dental filling resins makes use of special, portable UV

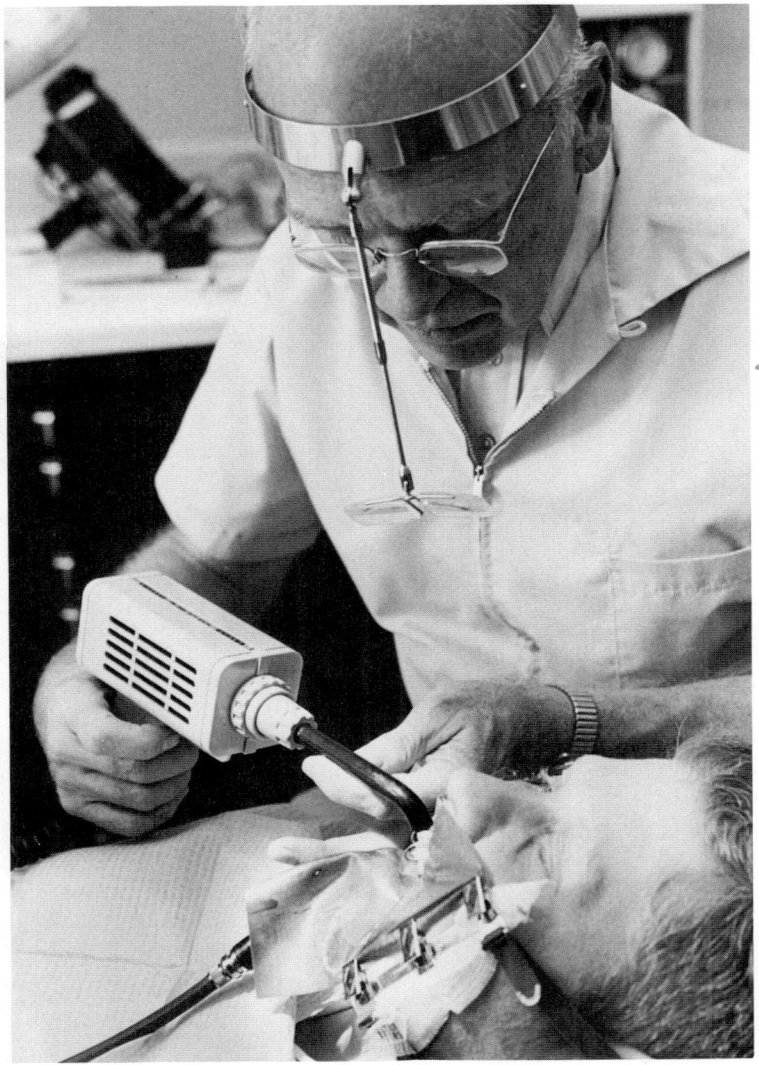

Figure 22-37. UV-A Dental Curing Device. This dental treatment "gun" permits the concentration of high intensities of UV-A radiation upon a UV-curable dental preparation inside the mouth. Although concern was expressed about UV leakage through side louvers in early models of this device, the problem was corrected and present models are safe when used in accordance with the dentist's instructions. Obviously the quartz rod beam director should not be placed next to the eye. (Photograph courtesy of U.S. Department of Commerce, National Bureau of Standards).

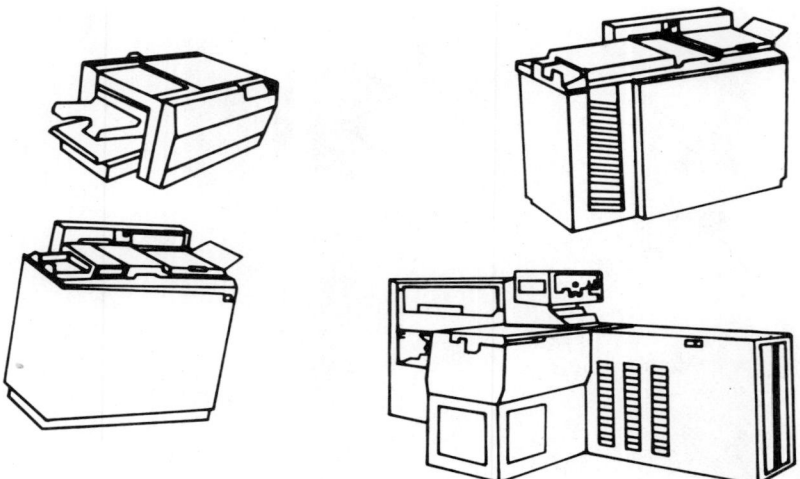

Figure 22-38. Office Copying Machines. Copying machines generally employ tungsten lamps, fluorescent lamps or xenon flashtubes and may be either a desk-top unit (upper left) or a console unit.

lamp guns (see Fig. 22-37). The enclosed systems, when properly designed, have interlocked enclosures and do not emit ultraviolet radiation into any part of the work space that can be occupied. Obviously, warning labels should exist at access panels to such equipment, and maintenance instructions should be adequate to protect the personnel from being exposed to hazardous levels. Carbon, xenon and mercury-arc lamps are often employed for high irradiance applications. Therefore, it is well to keep in mind that lamps used in these devices may emit radiation outside of the UV-A band.

22.5.5 Office Copying Machines and Graphic Arts Lighting

A wide variety of electrophotographic copying machines exist today. These machines may be small desk-top units or high-speed duplicating units found in printing shops (Figure 22-38). Except for units which have a feed-through feature and an enclosed light source, the light sources used in this equipment can produce glare. Glass platens upon which the document is exposed will always eliminate UV-B or UV-C leakage from the lamp. Tungsten or fluorescent CW lamps are generally used (Envall and Shangold, 1978). Xenon flashlamps have been used in high speed equipment. Some incandescent sources and most flashlamps can produce a *theoretical*

Lamps and Lighting Systems 745

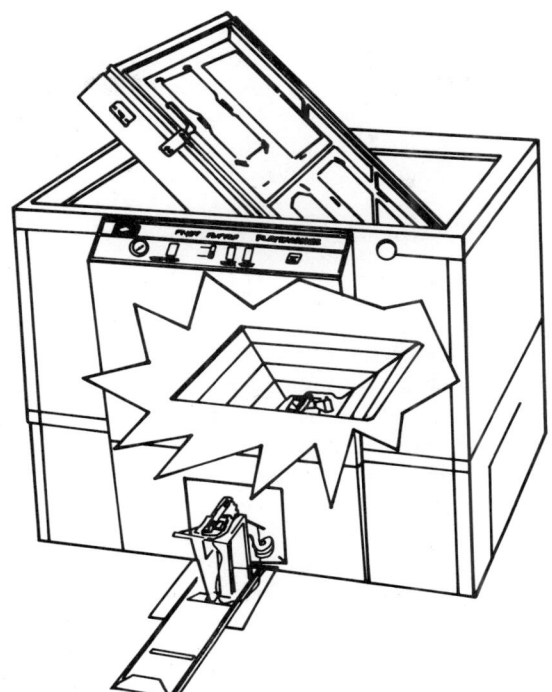

Figure 22-39. Printing-Plate Exposure Cabinet. This "flip-top" platemaker is commonly found in many printing plants. Hazardous UV radiation may leak through the seam between the top and the console. The cutaway shows the location of the tungsten-halide or arc lamp. Adapted from a drawing in Catalog G101 of the nuArc Co., Inc., of Chicago, IL.

blue-light hazard if one assumes an operator may run the machine almost constantly for a full day with the document cover removed. Some fluorescent lamps have unusually high luminance values since the fluorescent material is not coated around the entire tube and one can view the fluorescence off the inside of the tube. Manufacturers of machines with xenon flashlamps have either interlocked the document cover or diffused the light source. Operators should be cautioned not to stare into the light source and to always use the document cover when feasible.

In printing plants, and other graphic arts facilities, arc lamps and tungsten halogen lamps are used to expose copy for making negatives and photo-offset press plates. Large camera units should be located away from major work and traffic areas or screened. Employees should be cautioned to avoid staring at exposed lamps. Good exhaust ventilation for carbon arcs and xenon-arc lamps is also important. Although printing plate exposure cabinets (e.g., the nuArc Flip-Top Platemaker) reduce glare and eliminate most safety concerns, the operators should be warned against standing over the open slit that sometimes exists on the top of these types of units. If xenon-arc or carbon-arc sources are used in these cabinets (Figure 22-39), potentially hazardous UV levels will be present along this top slit. Most light sources used in this industry must emit intense UV-A and blue light to match the spectral response of graphic arts films and plates. Employees may therefore find it advisable to wear shortwave filtration glasses (e.g., "Noviol" lenses). Appendix F contains some source emission data and hazard analysis of copying machines.

22.5.6 CRT Displays and Control Measures for Glare from Visible Sources

Flashblindness, discomfort glare, and veiling glare have been previously discussed in Sections 4.10, 4.11 and 4.12. All these conditions contribute to the feeling of unease in a worker. Much of the attitude that optical sources are "dangerous" arises from the uncomfortable sensations associated with poor lighting conditions of the industrial environment. One of the most common causes of poor lighting is glare. The halo of glare associated with well-defined bright light sources has been discussed previously in Section 4.11 and 4.12. Similar problems are encountered with much lower intensity light sources which extend over the entire field of vision. This is a form of veiling glare in which every bright spot within the visual field is surrounded by a halo of scattered light. The halo is contributed by the forward scatter in the optical system of the eye or by some intervening optical elements such as a dirty window or dirty telescope objective. If the glare source is uniform over the entire field, then overall contrast is diminished which degrades acuity as well as other visual functions.

In order to assure proper performance under glare conditions, the observer's eye should contribute as little scattering as possible to the task (see Wolbarsht, 1977, for review). In any case, with all large visible light sources, an important part of the control measure procedure should be not only the elimination of the actual hazards but an attempt to present the light in an acceptable fashion from the standpoint of comfort.

Perhaps the best example of a glare problem relates to the use of cathode-ray-tube (CRT) visual display units (VDU's) which are now common in the computer, data processing, and printing industries. When first introduced a few years ago, many employees complained of headaches, eye fatigue, and other ailments they attributed to their VDU. Some suggested that the source of the problem must be some radiation not detectable by one's senses (e.g., UV, IR, or RF radiation). Measurements of such radiations have always clearly demonstrated that no *hazardous* conditions could exist (see, for example, Peterson et al., 1979). The phosphor luminance of most units are less than 0.05 cd/cm^2. Glare from windows or overhead lighting can reflect from the surface of the VDU screen or screen window. These reflections can be especially annoying if either of those surfaces are specular. In this instance, the eye may attempt to accommodate (focus) on the image of the glare source (several meters away) and then on the display (perhaps 50 cm). In practically no other occupation does one find such a visual environment with two competing object planes upon which to accommodate. The cures for such problems are obvious: diffuse all viewing surfaces and locate the screen such that a glare source is not seen

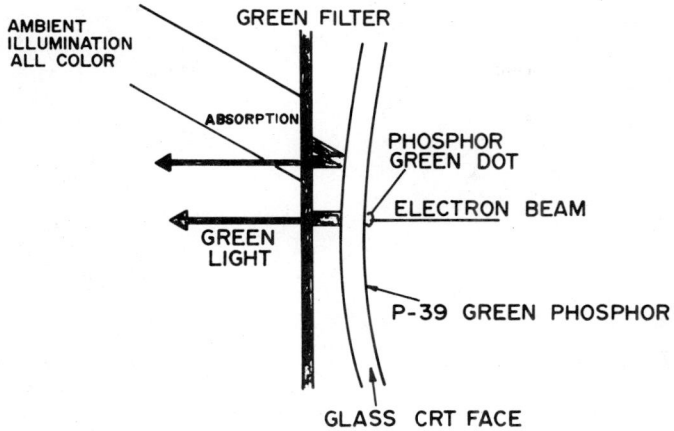

Figure 22-40. Cathode-Ray Tube (CRT) Visual Display. Although CRT displays pose no health hazards, eye fatigue and headaches are common for viewers working in a poorly desinged installation. Diffused screens, color-shield filters and proper location are used to reduce glare. (Wolbarsht et al., 1980.)

when looking at the screen. Figure 22-40 also illustrates how colored filters may be used to reduce glare.

22.5.7 Hospital Light Sources

Two categories of light sources found in medical and dental facilities are worthy of mention: operating-room (OR) lights and phototherapy lamps.

Operating-room light designers have expended a considerable effort to reduce the infrared heat load on a patient. Dichroic mirrors are used to reflect visible and transmit IR to the rear of the OR spotlight (Beck and Heimburger, 1973). The often recommended level of illumination on the operating table in a surgical suite is 27,000 lux (Health Care Facilities Subcommittee of the IES, 1978). These high illumination levels require projection optics (Figure 22-41) which are also diffused to reduce the projected luminance. Projection optics are reviewed in Chapter 23. The glass filters over the surgical spotlights are more than adequate to filter out UV-B and UV-C radiation.

Another use of visible light in hospitals is phototherapy of newborn infants who have excessive bilirubin in their blood (hyperbilirubenemia). Intense blue light is most effective in breaking down the bilirubin and special blue lights are used for this purpose (Figure 22-42). This application is probably a unique situation of an actual blue-light hazard. For this reason the eyes of the infant undergoing treatment

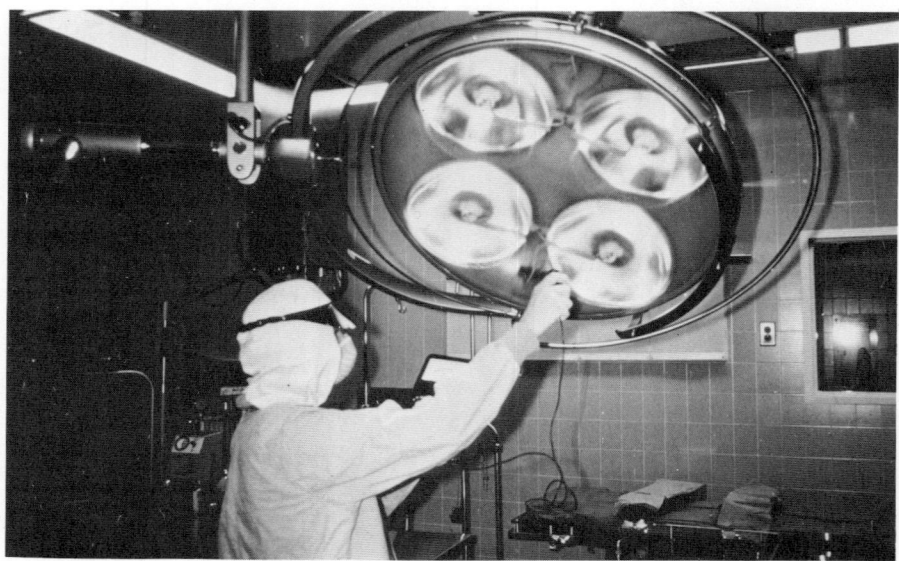

Figure 22-41. Operating-Room Spotlight. A technician checks the light output and UV-A output in an operating-room spotlight.

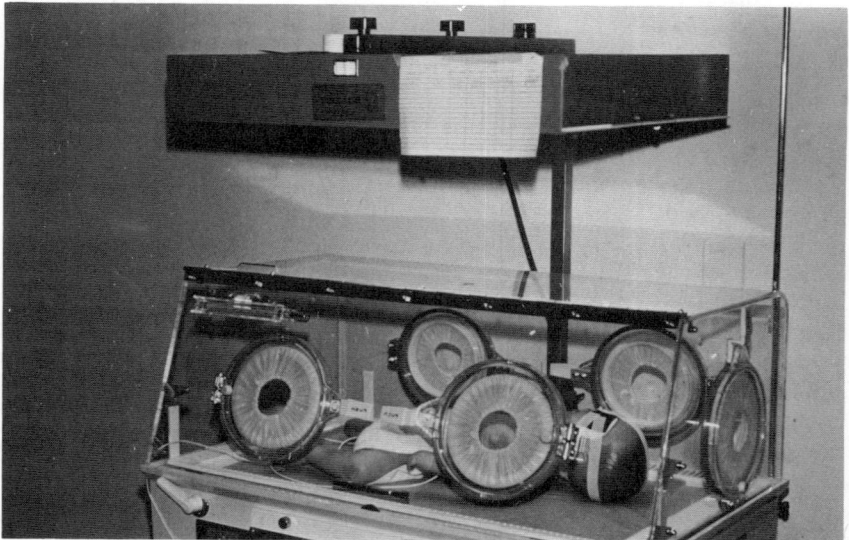

Figure 22-42. Neonatal Phototherapy. A rack of fluorescent lamps are used to illuminate a premature infant with hyperbilirubenemia. Note that the infant wears dark eye patches to protect the retina from blue-light exposure.

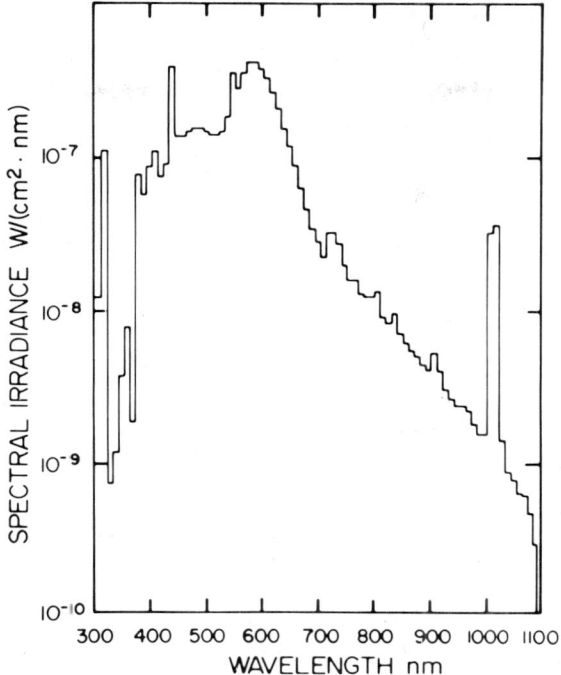

Figure 22-43. Cool White Fluorescent Lamp Spectrum. The spectral irradiance of most 20-W and 40-W fluorescent lamps are somewhat similar except for the change in phosphor and slight change in glass envelope. The spectral irradiance plot shown above is for a representative 20-W General Electric Cool White lamp at 80 cm. The illuminance at the point of measurement 0.082 lm/cm^2; E_{eff} was 0.14 μW/cm^2. Note the strong line at 313 nm.

must be protected. Black, opaque eye patches are generally used. Nurses are not at risk since the lamps are generally not visible to a standing individual and would not be stared at in any case. It is important that a clear plastic or glass filter be placed between the infant and the lamps to eliminate any UV-B radiation from the fluorescent lamps used for neonatal phototherapy as shown in Fig. 14-3 on p. 445. Although blue fluorescent lamps are used in many hospitals, white fluorescent lamps (e.g., Figs. 22-43 and 22-44) are also used extensively.

22.5.8 Photographic Flashbulbs

The only hazard control for the bright visible flash from flashbulbs and electronic flashlamps is to maintain an adequate exposure distance. Most of these lamps at unrealistically close viewing distances exceed present hazard criteria.

A commonly used flashcube provides a good example of a noncoherent,

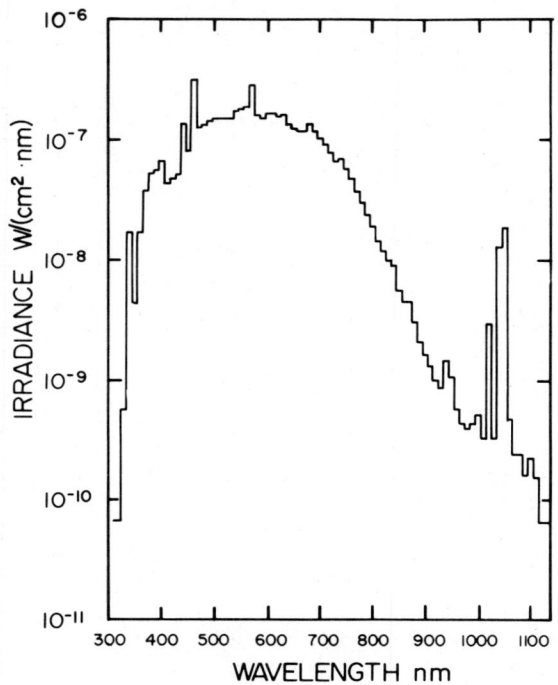

Figure 22-44. Vitalite Fluorescent Lamp Spectrum. The Duro Test Vitalite fluorescent lamp is designed to more closely simulate a solar spectrum. The glass envelope is sufficient to reduce UV-B levels below many other types of fluorescent lamps. Note the reduction of the 313-nm line. The illuminance at the point of measurement was 0.043 lm/cm² and E_{eff} was 0.02 μW/cm²

pulsed, extended source. A photograph of the radiance pattern is shown in Figure 22-45. The effective emitting area is about half of the reflector area. The flashcube has a reflector diameter (D_L) of about 2.5 cm and an effective pulse duration t of about 10 ms. The pulsed luminance Lp was determined to be approximately 450 cd·s/(cm²·sr). Assuming the flashcube's spectrum to be a fair approximation of the sun in the visible region, (Figure 22-46) one can estimate K to be about 120 lm/W. So $I_e \sim 3.8$ J/(cm²·sr) for the spectral region of 250-1400 nm. A further measurement with a broad-band thermal detector resulted in a total radiance of 5.4 J/(cm²·sr) showing a substantial infrared contribution. The tentative ACGIH pulsed-source criteria of Eqn. 10-3 (page 340) can be expressed as:

$$L \text{ (Haz)} = \sqrt{t}/\alpha t \quad W/(cm^2 \cdot sr), \tag{22-15}$$

or by converting α to D_L/r, an equivalent expression is:

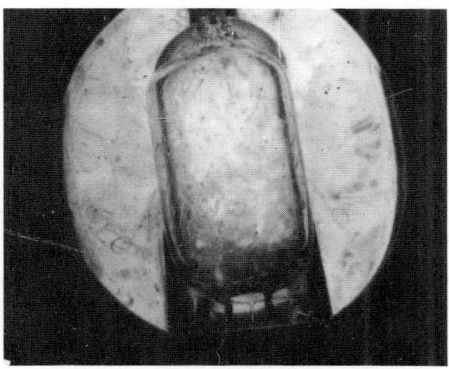

Figure 22-45. Flashcube. An intrabeam photograph of a flashcube was necessary to establish the radiating source size. It was assumed that the effective area of the source was half of the circular area defined by the 2.5-cm diameter reflector.

$$r\,(\text{Haz}) = L \cdot D_L \cdot \sqrt{t} \qquad (22\text{-}16)$$

if the angle α is less than 0.1 rad. To compute the hazard distance from this source the radiance L must be converted to integrated radiance L_p:

$$L_p = L \cdot t \qquad (22\text{-}17)$$

Combining equations (22-16) and (22-17) results in:

$$r\,(\text{Haz}) = L_p \cdot D_L \cdot \sqrt{t}/t \qquad (22\text{-}18)$$

Then, for the flashcube in this example, where the R factor (ACGIH) would be about 1.0 the:

$$\begin{aligned} r\,(\text{Haz}) &= (3.8)\,(2.5)\,(0.1)/(0.01) \\ &= 95 \text{ cm} \end{aligned}$$

At normal photographic distances the flashcube is perfectly safe. But this result also strongly suggests that flashcubes should not be fired at point-blank range at a person with dilated pupils. It also illustrates that the tentative ACGIH criteria are somewhat overly conservative for short exposure durations. Hochheimer and Caulkins (1977) measured similar flashcubes, Hi Power Flashcubes and M-3B and M-5 flashbulbs to obtain a range of values for L_p of 2.4 to 6.9 J/(cm²·sr) which agree well with our measurements of a variety of such sources.

The integrated radiances of xenon electronic photographic flashlamps are generally of the order of 1 J/(cm²·sr) with pulse durations of 2 to 4 ms. Their

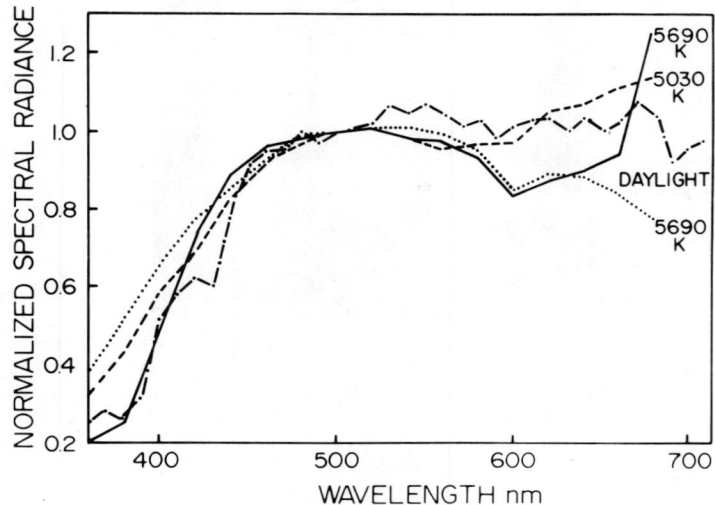

Figure 22-46. Relative Spectra of Three Photographic Flashbulbs. Most present-day photographic flash bulbs are designed for color film and must therefore mimic the spectrum of "daylight." The spectral radiance is normalized at 500 nm (after Henderson and Marsden, 1972).

source sizes D_L are normally larger than those of flashcubes. Specialized microsecond duration flashlamps have been used in technical applications (Edgerton and Barstow, 1959). The principal safety precautions applicable to all of these flash sources is to either diffuse them (increase D_L) or to maintain a safe separation distance of at least 1 m from human subjects.

22.5.9 HID Lamps

High-intensity-discharge (HID) lamps—specifically those containing mercury—have two envelopes: quartz, inner discharge tube and an outer glass jacket. In gymnasiums, high-bay industrial areas, and public buildings these lamps are often not enclosed in a protective fixture. The outer jacket can be broken in some instances by flying projectiles without damaging the inner discharge tube (Figure 22-47). If the lamp does not extinguish, substantial levels of actinic UV radiation will be emitted. Effective UV irradiances as high as 0.384 mW/cm² have been measured at a distance of 2 meters from 400-W mercury lamps (Piltingsrud and Fong, 1978). In 1979 the U.S. Department of Health, Education and Welfare, Food and Drug Administration (FDA), Bureau of Radiological Health (BRH), published new regulations

Lamps and Lighting Systems

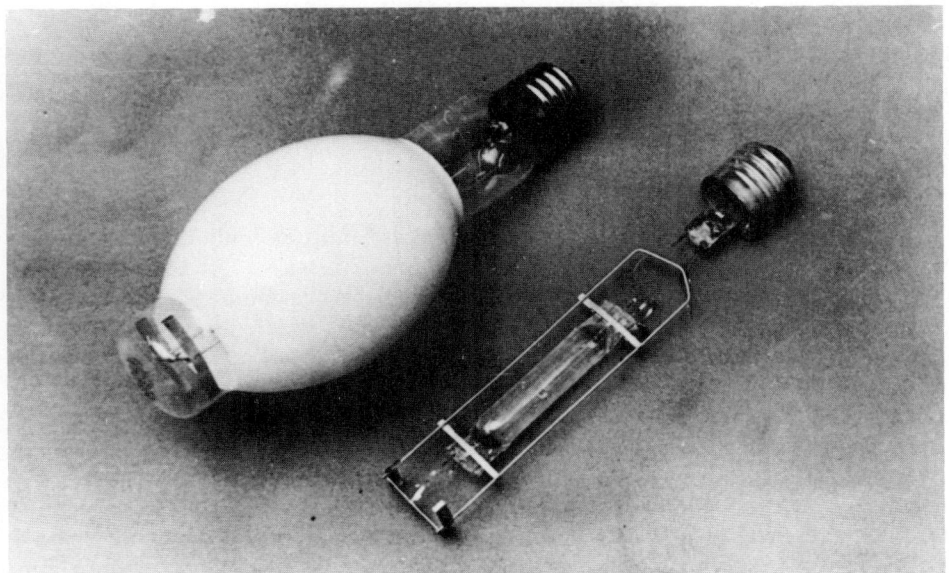

Figure 22-47. HID Lamp Damage. The outer jacket of a Mercury-HID lamp (left) can be broken such that the inner discharge tube can still function (courtesy of Bureau of Radiological Health).

(USDHEW-FDA, 1979) requiring manufacturers to install a self-extinguishing feature on all lamps not intended for use in enclosed protective fixtures as in street lights. The lamp would have to extinguish within 15 min of substantial breakage or removal of the outer envelope. More stringent rules would apply after September 1981. For lamps not having this feature, the advertisements for the lamps and packaging must bear the following warning:

WARNING: This lamp can cause serious skin burn and eye inflammation from shortwave ultraviolet radiation if outer envelope of the lamp is broken or punctured. Do not use where people will remain for more than a few minutes unless adequate shielding or other safety precautions are used. Lamps that will automatically extinguish when the outer envelope is broken or punctured are commercially available.

22.5.10 Infrared and Light-Emitting Diodes

LED displays do not emit luminance or radiance levels of concern. The red

LED displays in calculators are less than 0.02 cd/cm². Only with infrared GaAlAs (830 to 860 nm) and GaAs (900 to 970 nm) diode emitters is there ever a concern. The Siemens Corp. in Germany has argued in their sales literature that their infrared emitters were safe based upon retinal thermal injury studies. Siemens reported that a nearly linear relationship existed between the infrared emitted power Φ_e and the length of the emitter d_s (in mm):

$$\Phi_e \simeq k_s \cdot d_s \quad \text{for } d_s < 2 \text{ mm} \tag{22-19}$$

where k_s = 250 mW/mm. It was argued that these emitters could never be imaged on the retina to cause a hazardous retinal irradiance. This may well be true when one considers that bringing such an emitter closer than the near point of the eye (15 to 25 cm) can result in no greater concentration of infrared radiation since the image area would increase with closer viewing distance.

A useful example of a GaAs emitter would be one used in an arcade shooting-gallery rifle or a toy gun. A diffused-source GaAs, 940-nm diode with a peak-intensity rating I of 180 mW/sr has a beam spread of 15° (0.054 sr). Therefore the radiant power is 9.7 mW. The projected source size determined through intrabeam infrared photography was 1.3 mm in diameter (i.e., A_s was 0.013 cm²). For an average adult, the closest point of approach to the eye where the emitter would be sharply imaged on the retina is 25 cm (i.e., the near point). For a child's eye one may wish to consider a conservatively short near-point distance of 10 cm. At this distance the angular subtense of the source α is (0.13 cm)/(10 cm) or 0.013 rad. The source radiance is:

$$\begin{aligned} L &= I/A_s \\ &= (0.18 \text{ W/sr}) / (0.013 \text{ cm}^2) \\ &= 13.6 \text{ W/(cm}^2 \cdot \text{sr}) \end{aligned} \tag{22-20}$$

The ACGIH non-laser infrared source criteria requires that the radiance in W/(cm²·sr) not exceed L(Haz) (Eqn. 10-9, page 341). Hence, at a viewing distance r of 10 cm, where α is 0.013 rad:

$$\begin{aligned} L \text{ (Haz)} &= [0.6/\alpha] \text{ W/(cm}^2 \cdot \text{sr}) \\ &= [0.6/0.013] \text{ W/(cm}^2 \cdot \text{sr}) \\ &= 46 \text{ W/(cm}^2 \cdot \text{sr}) \end{aligned} \tag{22-21}$$

Therefore the diode can be operated CW or, as would be more likely, as a train of pulses with the same peak intensity. Obviously, if the diode is safe to view for the CW case, it is certainly safe if some of the total energy emitted each second were removed from the beam. For example, if the pulses were 30 μs in duration and the PRF were 240 Hz. then the duty cycle would be only (240) 3 × 10⁻⁵), or 0.007, and the average power output would be reduced from 9.7 mW to 0.07 mW. One should not compare the L (Haz) value to the *average* radiance value of a repetitively pulsed infrared emitter. In the absence of criteria for such repetitively pulsed, non-laser IR-A sources one could apply the laser safety criteria but would always

Lamps and Lighting Systems

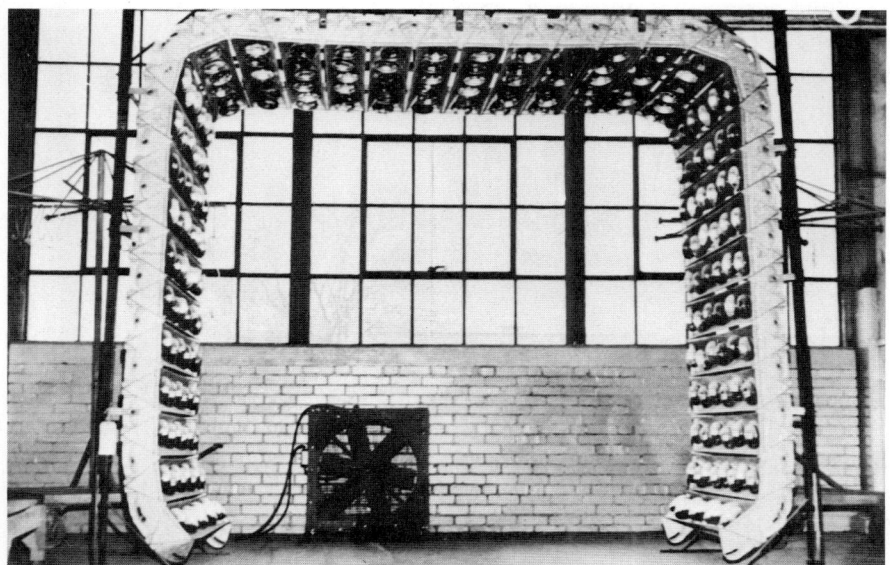

Figure 22-48. Infrared Lamp Array for Paint Drying. Arrays of type R40 infrared lamps (typically 250-W to 500-W each) are used in baking enamel paints. This array would be used for paint drying of automotive vehicles.

obtain an overestimate of the hazard. The previously illustrated procedure of comparing L (Haz) to the peak radiance of the diode also overstates the hazard. Fortunately, in the case of the example, the conservative approach resulted in a finding of no hazard.

22.5.11 Industrial and Home Baking Applications

There are many industrial infrared heating and drying applications which make use of arrays of infrared lamps. Paint-drying arrays as shown in Figure 22-48 are one of the most common. Irradiance levels within the baking facility are typically 0.1 to 0.8 W/cm^2 —well above levels for heat stress. Personnel should be limited to momentary exposure while in these areas. More intense infrared sources used in ovens represent potential skin burns and cataract hazards (Wolbarsht, 1978), and glass or metal doors with interlocks are desirable in these installations. Such enclosures are also very important for home appliance infrared ovens. In the past it was not uncommon to find less expensive infrared oven appliances without a front glass cover door. Warning labels are advisable for some such ovens. The infrared heating lamps used in commercial cooking establishments should be oriented in such a way the infrared beam is not directed at personnel. The infrared radiant intensity I of a Type R40/10, 250-W heat lamp is about 10 W/sr. Hence, at a distance r of 100 cm the irradiance E would be:

$$E = I/r^2 \qquad (22\text{-}22)$$
$$= 10/10^4$$
$$= 10^{-3} \text{ W/cm}^2.$$

22.5.12 Infrared Sources in Hospitals

In hospital neonatal-care facilities, infrared infant warmers may expose the infant to 10-30 mW/cm², a rather excessive level for the eyes. The use of eye patches and exposure timers are prudent in this application. High-intensity infrared lamps have often been used in the past in physical therapy facilities. Certainly, where these are used the eyes should be protected from the beam.

22.6 CONCEPT OF A LAMP SAFETY STANDARD FOR HIGH-INTENSITY SOURCES

Since lamp or arc sources may be hazardous from several aspects, it may be helpful to develop a hazard classification scheme similar to the one applied to laser products. The following scheme is only an attempt on the part of the authors to illustrate this concept and is not necessarily recommended as a final proposal for a standard. Both lamps and total lighting system could be included. The categories could be as follows:
• Group 1. *Safe Sources.* These lamps would be considered safe to view all day long. No warning label should be required. Example: a 60-W frosted tungsten filament lamp or a TV-display cathode-ray tube.
• Group 2. *Low-risk Sources.* These lamps would be safe for momentary 0.25-s, unintentional viewing. Examples: most spotlights and movie-projector lamp bulbs. A caution label should be required on the lamp socket base, and possibly on the projection system itself. No ultraviolet or infrared hazard would exist beyond 10 cm from the lamp or projected beam.
• Group 3. *Moderate-risk Sources.* These lamps would be unsafe to view at close range even momentarily. Presumably, skin injury could also occur from ultraviolet radiation as from germicidal lamps and sun lamps. A danger label clearly visible on the equipment using the lamp could be required. A common device which might fit into this category would be a home movie spot lamp with a 600-W to 1000-W tungsten-iodide bulb without a Fresnel lens. The emergent beam irradiance is far in excess of that required to ignite paper within a half meter of the source (Chapter 23). Obviously the basis for the determination of a hazard classification group would differ for each type of hazard criteria (i.e., retinal or skin) but each measurement for classification would be at a specified accessible approach distance using a standard aperture and solid angle of acceptance. The minimum approach distance could vary

Lamps and Lighting Systems 757

with application. Other examples in this category could include some very high-intensity, short-pulse, laser flash tubes, and 20 kW xenon-arc searchlights.
- Group 4. *High-risk Sources.* These sources would cause skin burns within a standard exposure duration (e.g., within 10 s) at a standard distance at which the effective UV irradiance would exceed 0.3 mW/cm^2, or the total irradiance across the entire spectrum would exceed 0.2 W/cm^2. Examples of such sources would be an open carbon-arc spotlight or an open 1-kW mercury lamp.

At the time of publication of this book, Committee Z-311 of the American National Standards Institute (ANSI) was attempting to develop a safety standard for "Lamps and Lighting Systems." Mr. I. Matelsky of the General Electric Co., Cleveland, Ohio, was chairman.

22.7 REVIEW QUESTIONS

1. How does the ACGIH proposed retinal-thermal-hazard threshold limit value vary with retinal image size? How does the old Sliney/Freasier criteria, as demonstrated in Table 22-3, vary with image size?

2. The effective UV-B irradiance measured at a distance of 7 m from a carbon arc searchlight is 10 μW/cm^2. What is the permissible exposure duration at this location?

3. What is the approximate radiance of a tungsten filament at 3200° K? What is the retinal hazard factor R (Sliney and Freasier) and retinal thermal hazard factor $\overline{R}$ (ACGIH)?

4. A tungsten filament operating at 2900° with an emissivity of 0.4 in the near infrared region is employed as a heat lamp. It uses an IR pass-band filter which cuts on at 750 nm and cuts off at 2000 nm. Estimate the radiance of this source if the filter has a transmission of 0.7 within its pass band. The use of the graph given in Figure 22-19 may be helpful.

5. A 4-ft fluorescent lamp is measured at 50 cm using two instruments. An illuminance meter provides a result of 2 lm/cm^2. By contrast, the calculated illuminance from the spectral irradiance measured by a spectroradiometer is 0.9 lm/cm^2. What are the likely reasons for this 100% discrepancy?

6. A quartz-tangsten-halogen lamp operates at 3000° K. The emitting surface area is 0.4 cm^2. The source is nearly Lambertian. Estimate the effective UV irradiance at 30 cm from the source.

7. Explain the significance of the following fluorescent lamp marking: T12F40CW.

8. A mercury vapor lamp is measured at a distance of 32 cm. The spectral irradiance of the continuum is unmeasurable at wavelengths below 325 nm with an

instrument having a sensitivity of 0.01 $\mu W/(cm^2 \cdot nm)$. The line irradiance at 297 nm, 303 nm, and 313 nm are 0.2 $\mu W/cm^2$, 4 $\mu W/cm^2$, and 12 $\mu W/cm^2$ respectively. What would be the maximum permissible exposure duration at 32 cm from the lamp?

9. Express the empirical equations of the Army/ACGIH broad-band source limits (Eqns. 10-4 through 10-9) in the preferable SI units (i.e., W/m^2, J/m^2, etc.).

10. A GaAs infrared-emitting diode emits 20 mW at 940 nm in a 0.4-sr beam from an active emitter area of 0.6 mm × 0.6 mm. Calculate the radiant intensity, radiance, radiant existance and estimate whether this source can be a hazard.

22.8 REFERENCES

Anonymous, 1956, The lamp makers' story, (Survey Issue) *Illum. Eng.* **51**(1):1–144.
Ash, G.S., 1979, Vital contrast for the display industry, *Opt. Spec.* **13**(9):44–47.
Baum, W.A., and Dunkelman, L., 1950, Ultraviolet radiation of the high pressure xenon arc, *J. Opt. Soc. Am.* **40**(11):782–786.
Beck, W.C., and Heimburger, R.F., 1973, Illumination hazard in the operating room, *Arch. Surg.* **107**:560–562.
Bickford, E.D., Clark, G.W., and Spears, G.R., 1974, Measurement of ultraviolet irradiance from illuminants in terms of proposed public health standards, *J. Illum. Eng. Soc.* **4**(1):43–48 and **5**(4):234–236.
Bresler, R.R., 1949, Cutaneous burns due to fluorescent light, *J. Am. Med. Assn.* **140**(17):1334–1336.
Bridges, J.M., and Ott, W.R., 1977, Vacuum ultraviolet radiometry. 3: The argon mini-arc as a new secondary standard of special radiance, *Appl. Opt.* **16**:367–376.
Briffa, D.V., and Warin, A.P., 1979, Photochemotherapy in psoriasis: a review, *J. Royal Soc. Med.* **72**:440–446.
Campbell, J.H., and Kershaw, D.C., 1956, Flashing characteristics of fluorescent lamps, *Illum. Eng.* **51**(11):755–760.
Committee on Light Sources of the IES, 1963, Effect of temperature on fluorescent lamps, *Illum. Eng.* **58**(2):101–105.
Committee on Photobiology, 1979, Risks associated with use of UV-A irradiators being used in treating psoriasis and other conditions, *Photochem. and Photobio.* **30**:199–202.
Council on Physical Medicine, 1946, Eye discomfort caused by improperly shielded black light ultraviolet lamps, *J. Am. Med. Assn.* **131**(4):287.
Dickinson, A.B., 1979, Remember operator needs when selecting CRT displays, *Instr. Control Sys.* **52**(3):37–41.
Eby, J., 1970, A computer based spectroradiometer system, *Appl. Opt.* **9**:888–894.
Edgerton, H.E., and Barstow, F.E., 1959, Multiflash photography, *Photogr. Sci. Eng.* **3**(6):288–290.
Elenbaas, W., 1972, "Light Sources," Crane, Russak and Company, Inc., New York.
Envall, K.R., and Shangold, E.J., 1978, "Survey of Photocopier and Related Products," HEW Pub. (FDA) 78-8060, U.S. Dept. of Health, Education, and Welfare, Food and Drug Adminis., Bureau of Radiological Health, Rockville, MD.
Forbes, P.D., Davies, R.E., D'Aloisio, L.C., and Cole, C., 1976, Emission spectrum differences in fluorescent blacklight lamps, *Photochem. and Photobiol.* **24**:613.
Geeraets, W.J., and Clarke, A.M., 1976, Phototherapy of the cornea: some aspects to be considered, *Ophthalmologica* **172**:449–455.

General Electric Company, 1969, "Product Heating with Infrared Lamps," pamphlet TP-116-R, Large Lamp Dept., General Electric, Nela Park, Cleveland, OH.

General Electric Company, 1969, "High Intensity Discharge Lamps," pamphlet TP-109, Large Lamp Dept., General Electric, Nela Park, Cleveland, OH.

Glauser, S.C., 1971, "Action Spectrum for the Photodestruction of Bilirubin," *Proc. Soc. Exper. Biol. Med.* **136**:518.

Goncz, J.H., and Newell, P.B., 1966, Spectra of pulsed and continuous xenon discharges, *J. Opt. Soc. Am.* **56**(1):87–92.

Guth, S.K., 1970, Lighting for visual performance and visual comfort, *J. Am. Optom. Assn.* **41**(1):63–71.

Hattenburg, A.T., 1967, Spectral radiance of a low current graphite arc, *Appl. Opt.* **6**(1):95.

Health Care Facilities Subcommittee, 1978, "Lighting for Health Care Facilities," Publication No. CP-29, Illumination Engineering Society, New York.

Henderson, S.T., and Marsden, A.M., 1972, "Lamps and Lighting," Crane, Russak and Co., New York.

Hochheimer, B.F., and Calkins, J.L., 1977, The integrated radiance of flashbulbs, *Opt. Eng.* **16**(2):212–213.

Holladay, L.L., 1928, Proportion of energy radiated by incandescent solids in various spectral regions, *J. Opt. Soc. Am.* **17**(5):329–342.

Illuminating Engineering Society, 1958, IES guide for photometric testing of searchlights, *Illum. Eng.* **53**(3):155–162.

Ivey, H.F., 1972, Color and efficiency of fluorescent and fluorescent-mercury lamps, *J. Opt. Soc. Am.* **62**(6):814–822.

Ivey, H.F., 1960, Problems and progress in electroluminescent lamps, *Illum. Eng.* **55**(1):13–20.

Jackson, D.A., 1976, Pressure shifts and broadenings in the arc spectrum of xenon, *J. Opt. Soc. Am.* **66**(10):1014–1018.

Johnson, J., 1962, Zero-length searchlight photometry system, *Illum. Eng.* **57**(3):187–194.

Kaufman, J.E., and Christensen, (eds.), 1972, "IES Lighting Handbook," 5th Ed., The Illuminattion Engineering Society, New York.

Klein, M.V., 1970, "Optics," John Wiley and Sons, New York (see especially Chap. 4).

Krizek, D.T., and Koch, E.J., 1979, Use of regression analysis to estimate UV spectral irradiance from broad band radiometer readings under FS-40 fluorescent sunlamps filtered with cellulose acetate, *Photochem. and Photobiol.* **30**:483–489.

Leighton, L.G., 1962, Characteristics of ribbon filament lamps, *Illum. Eng.* **57**(3):121–126.

Levin, R.E., Clark, G.W., Spears, G.R., and Bickford, E.D., 1977, Ultraviolet radiation—considerations in interior lighting design—part 1, *J. Illum. Eng. Soc.* **7**(1):80–89.

Liberman, I., and Zollweg, R.J., 1973, Air operable alumina envelope arc lamps, *Appl. Opt.* **12**(8):1740–1741.

Lienhard, O.E., and McInally, J.A., 1962, New compact-arc lamps of high power and high brightness, *Illum. Eng.* **57**(3):172-176.

Lienhard, O.E., 1965, Xenon compact-arc lamps with liquid-cooled electrodes, *Illum. Eng.* **55**(5):348–352.

Lucey, J.F., 1970, Phototherapy of jaundice 1969, *Birth Defects: Orig. Article Series*, **6**(2):63–70.

Maas, J.B., Jayson, J.K., and Kleiber, D.A., 1974, Effects of spectral differences in illumination on fatigue, *J. Appl. Psy.* **59**(4):524–526.

Martt, E.C., Smialek, L.J., and Green, A.C., 1964, Iodides in mercury arcs—for improved color and efficiency, *Illum. Eng.* **59**(1):34–39.

McKinlay, A.F., Harlen, F., and Clark, I.M., 1978, "A Limited Survey and Evaluation of Ultraviolet Radiation Hazards in University Laboratories," NRPB-R72, National Radiological Protection Board, Harwell, Didcot, Oxon.

Morris, R.W., 1947, Considerations affecting the design of flashing signal filament lamps, *Illum. Eng.* **42**(6):625–630.

National Industrial Pollution Control Council, 1972, "Fluorescent Lamps, The Environmental Compatibility of Fluorescent and Other Mercury-Containing Lamps." National Industrial Pollution Control Council, U.S. Dept. of Commerce, Washington, D.C.

National Radiological Protection Board, 1978, "Protection Against Ultraviolet Radiation in the Workplace," (ISBN O 85951 063 8), National Radiological Protection Board, Harwell, Didcot, Oxon, UK.

Nicodemus, F.E., 1976, "Self-Study Manual on Optical Radiation Measurements," NBS Technical Note 910-1, National Bureau of Standards, Optical Physics Div., U.S. Government-Printing Office, Washington, D.C.

Null, M.R., and Lozier, W.W., 1962, Carbon arc as a radiation standard, *J. Opt. Soc. Am.* 52(10): 1156–1160.

Ohta, N., and Wyszecki, G., 1975, Colorimetric significance of mercury-emission lines in fluorescent lamps, *J. Opt. Soc. Am.* 65(11):1354-1358.

Owens, D.A., 1979, The Mandelbaum effect: evidence for an accommodative bias toward intermediate viewing distances, *J. Opt. Soc. Am.* 69(5):646–652.

Parrish, J.A., Fitzpatrick, T.B., Tanebaum, L., and Pathak, M.A., 1974, Photochemotherapy of psoriasis with oral methoxsalen and longwave ultraviolet light, *New England J. Med.* 291: 1207–1222.

Parrish, J.A., Pathak, M.A., and Fitzpatrick, T.B., 1971, Protection of skin from germicidal ultraviolet radiation in the operating room by topical chemicals, *New England J. Med.* 284(22): 1257–1258.

Piltingsrud,H.V., Odland, L.T., and Fong, C.W., 1976, An evaluation of fluorescent light sources for use in phototherapy of neonatal jaundice, *Am. Indus. Hyg. Assn. J.* 437–444 (July 1976).

Piltingsrud, H. V., and Fong, C.W., 1978, An evaluation of ultraviolet radiation personnel hazards from selected.400-Watt high intensity discharge lamps, *Am. Indus. Hyg. Assn. J.*, 39(5): 406–413 (May 1978).

Potter, W.M., and Reid, K.M., 1959, Incandescent lamp design life for residential lighting, *Illum. Eng.* 54(12):751–757.

Sanders, C.L., and Jerome, C.W., 1973, Interlaboratory comparison of measurements of the spectral irradiance from fluorescent and incandescent lamps: a report, *Appl. Opt.* 12(9):2088–2098.

Segal, S.M., 1955, A study of high intensity light sources, *Illum. Eng.* 50(5):259–262.

Sisson, T.R.C., 1972, Phototherapy of jaundice in the newborn infant. Effect of various light intensities, *J. Pediatrics*, 81:35–40.

Sliney, D.H., 1978, "Nonionizing Radiation Protection Special Study No. 25-42-0388-79, Ultraviolet Radiation Sources Used in Dermatology, September-December 1978," (NTIS No. ADA 067251), U. S. Army Environmental Hygiene Agency, Aberdeen Proving Ground, MD.

Sliney, D.H., and Freasier, B.C., 1973, The evaluation of optical radiation hazards, *Appl. Opt.* 12(1):1-23.

Song, P.S., and Tapley, K.J., Jr., 1979, Photochemistry and Photobiology of Psoralens, *Photochem. Photobiol.* 29:1177-1197.

Spears, G.R., 1974, Radiant flux measurements of ultraviolet emitting light sources, *J. Illum. Eng. Soc.* (October 1974).

Staley, K.A., 1960, "Fundamentals of Light and Lighting," Bulletin LD-2, General Electric Large Lamp Department, Nela Park, Cleveland, OH.

Thorington, L., Cunningham, L., and Parascandola, J., 1971, The illuminant in the prevention and phototherapy of hyperbilirubinemia, *Illum. Eng.* 66(4):240–250.

Thouret, W.E., and Strauss, H.S., 1962, New designs demonstrate versatility of xenon high-pressure lamps, *Illum. Eng.* 57(3):150–158.

Thouret, W.E., Strauss, H.S., Cortorillo, S.F., and Kee, H., 1965, High-brightness xenon lamps with liquid-cooled electrodes, using standard lamp manufacturing techniques, *Illum. Eng.* 339-347 (May 1965).

U.S. Department of Health, Education and Welfare, Food and Drug Administration, 1979, Mercury vapor lamps; radiation safety performance standards, 21CFR1040.30, *Fed. Reg.* 44(175):52191–52196.

U.S. Department of Health, Education and Welfare, Food and Drug Administration, 1977, Sunlamp products, *Fed. Reg.* **42**(251):65189–65193.

Walsh, J.W.T., 1965, "Photometry," Dover Press, New York.

Waymouth, J.F., Gungle, W.C., Harris, J.M., and Koury, F., 1965, A new metal halide arc lamp, *Illum. Eng.* **60**(2):85–88.

Weiss, M.M., and Petersen, R.C., 1979, Electromagnetic radiation emitted from video computer terminals, *Am. Ind. Hyg. Assoc. J.* **40**:300–309.

Wolbarsht, M.L., 1977, Tests for glare sensitivity and peripheral vision in driver applicants, *J. Safety Res.* **9**(3):128–139.

Wolbarsht, M. L., 1978, The effects of optical radiation on the anterior structures of the eye, *in* "Current Concepts in Ergophthalmology," pp. 29–46, Societas Ergophthalmologica Internationalis, Stockholm, Sweden.

Wolbarsht, M. L., O'Foghludha, F. A., Sliney, D. H., Smith, A. A., Jr., and Johsnon, G. A., 1980, Electromagnetic emission from visual display units: A non-hazard, *in* "On the Ocular Effects of Non-ionizing Radiation" (M. L. Wolbarsht and D. H. Sliney, eds.), *Proc. Soc. Photo-Opt. Instrum. Eng.* (SPIE), Vol. 229, Bellingham, WA, pp. 187–193.

Chapter 23
Projection Systems

23.1 INTRODUCTION

As a general rule, broad-band sources which employ projection optics are the most difficult to evaluate. In addition to the problems encountered in evaluating exposed lamps, one must characterize the projected beam and projected source size. When one views a collimated light source from within the beam (other than a laser) he will see a magnified view of the actual source. The source is generally a high-brightness lamp. The brighter the lamp, the greater the maximal irradiance in the projected beam. This is a consequence of the Law of Conservation of Brightness (Radiance) as will be explained later in this chapter. Some lamps that are normally safe to view become hazardous to view through projection optics, despite the fact that the lamp cannot be made brighter by optics. This increase in hazard is an outcome of the dependence of retinal injury upon image size. Besides the obvious projection sources—such as spotlights, searchlights, slide projectors, and movie projectors—solar concentrators and other non-imaging light collectors may also require hazard evaluation. In this chapter we shall examine how the *Law of Conservation of Radiance* permits one to evaluate the retinal hazards from projector systems. As a further aid to understanding, several specific systems will be evaluated by example.

23.2 PROJECTION OPTICS

Collimating optics may consist of refracting elements (lenses), reflecting elements (curved mirrors) or both. Figure 23-1 illustrates simple refracting and reflecting collimation systems. A source is positioned at the focal point of the system. The smaller the source, the greater the degree of collimation that may be achieved. And the shorter the focal length of the lens, the greater the fraction of light that can be collected. Obviously an extremely short-focal-length lens could not

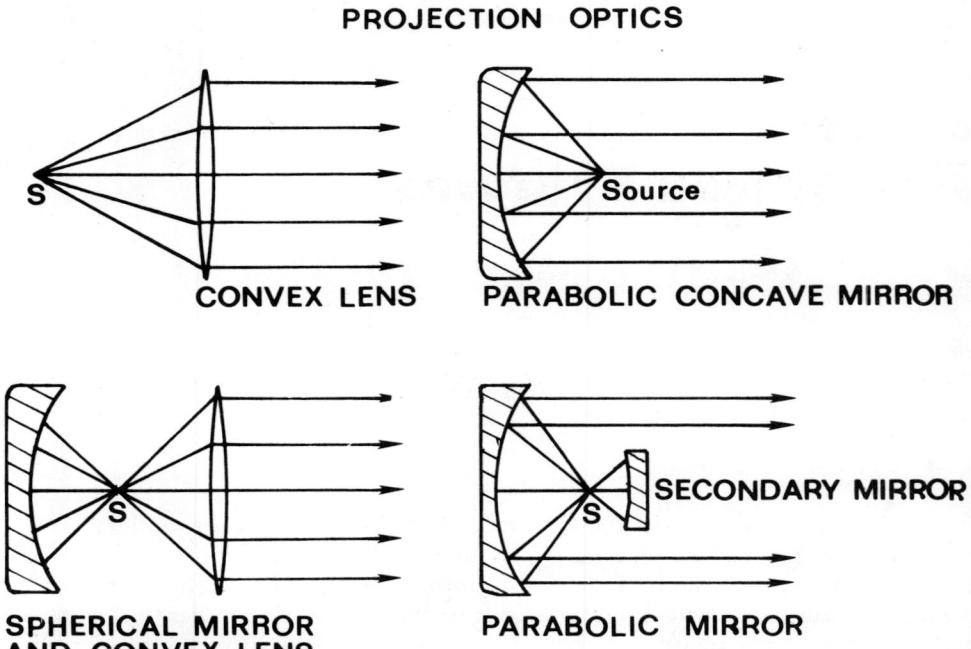

Figure 23-1. The simplest projection system is a single positive lens (top left) or parabolic mirror (top right) with a brilliant source at its focal point. Slightly more sophisticated systems (bottom) employ a spherical reflector to supplement the primary projection element.

even collect the radiation radiated into one hemisphere. To redirect some of the light lost to the other hemisphere, spherical reflecting elements are sometimes used. In fact many projector lamps have the reflector built into the lamp itself.

Since a short-focal-length lens will be very thick at its center, the French physicist Auguste Fresnel developed a segmented lens which has the same refracting surfaces but is thinner and of lighter weight by virtue of the fact that some of the glass has been "removed." The *Fresnel lens*, as it is called, is more effective as a collimator but cannot be used to form whole images. Figure 23-2 illustrates the principal of the Fresnel lens. Such lenses are used in automobile headlights, railway beacons, traffic lights, and lighthouses. But the Fresnel lens cannot be used in the imaging projection optics of movie and slide projectors. Modern plastic molding techniques have permitted the development of thin, fine-element plastic Fresnel lenses which permit higher quality collimation and even some degree of imaging.

Projection Systems

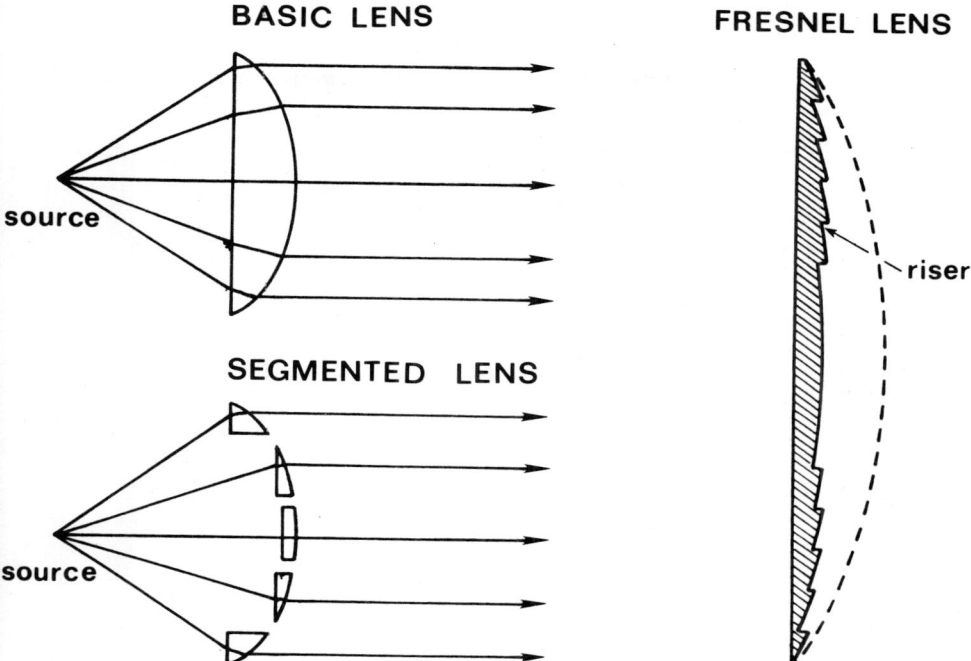

Figure 23-2. The Fresnel Lens. Fresnel lenses are used in many non-imaging projection optics. The basic concept is to replace a heavy, thick lens (top left) by segments of a lens (bottom left) to form a cut or molded segmented lens (right).

The projected beam irradiance of an ideal searchlight, or other collimating system, will remain nearly constant within a region known as the *near-field*. Then at a distance termed the *flash distance* r_f the irradiance will begin to decrease inversely as the square of the distance r from the searchlight. This would only be true for a perfect system with a small diffused, spherical Lambertian source at the focus. Nevertheless, as can be seen in Figure 23-3, there is clearly a near-field and a far-field. The flash distance r_f can be estimated if the reflector focal length (or lens focal length) f, the diameters of the source, and the reflector aperture diameter a, are known:

$$r_f \simeq a \cdot f / s \qquad (23\text{-}1)$$

In actual practice the proper value of the aperture a is normally 50% to 70% the full reflector diameter. For an example, a searchlight has an arc lamp with a source spot size of 2 mm, and a 50-cm diameter, 15-cm focal-length reflector. The flash distance would be:

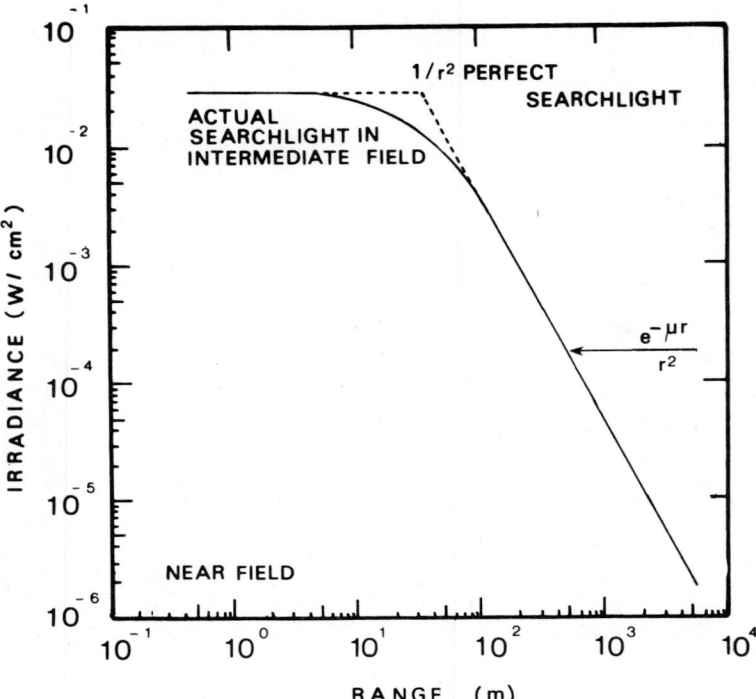

Figure 23-3. Searchlight Beam Irradiance vs Range. The beam irradiance of a 2.2 kW xenon-arc searchlight is nearly constant in the near-field to a distance of 23 m. The flash distance is 23 m. At greater distances, the far field, the irradiance decreases inversely as the square of the distance — or more rapidly due to atmospheric attenuation.

$$r_f \simeq (50 \text{ cm})(15 \text{ cm}) / (0.2 \text{ cm})$$
$$\simeq 3250 \text{ cm}$$
$$\simeq 32.5 \text{ m}$$

The divergence ϕ, or *beam spread*, of a searchlight is approximately:

$$\phi \simeq s/f \qquad (23\text{-}2)$$

Hence, to continue the example, the divergence of this searchlight would be:

$$\phi \simeq (0.2 \text{ cm}) / (15 \text{ cm})$$
$$\simeq 0.013 \text{ rad}$$
$$\simeq 13 \text{ mrad}$$
$$\simeq 0.76°$$

For searchlights it is characteristic to specify the source size and beam spread at 1/10 th-peak intensity points. The one photometric specification that is typically available for a searchlight, headlight, or beacon is the *luminous intensity* I (or *candlepower*). The candlepower I is estimated by:

$$I \simeq \rho \cdot \tau \cdot L \cdot A_s \qquad (23\text{-}3)$$

where ρ is the reflectance of any reflecting element, τ is the total transmittance of glass or plastic lenses, windows or filters in the beam, L is the source luminance or radiance, and A_s is the projected area of the souce at the flash distance. For example, if the arc lamp has a luminance L_v of 10^5 cd/cm², the reflectors' reflectance is 0.90, the glass cover's transmittance is 0.92 and A_s is the area of the 50-cm diameter reflector less a 10-cm-diameter central lamp occluder (i.e., 1963 cm² less 76 cm², or 1885 cm²) then:

$$\begin{aligned} I_v &\simeq (0.9)(0.92)(10^5)(1885) \\ &\simeq 1.56 \times 10^8 \text{ cd} \\ &\simeq 156 \text{ Mcd} \end{aligned}$$

As a comparison, Table 23-1 lists the peak candlepower of several representative searchlights, beacons, and spotlights. The principal value of specifying luminous intensity is that the illuminance E_v at a range r *in the far field* can be calculated very simply by:

$$E_v = I_v/r^2 \qquad (23\text{-}4)$$

Formula 23-4 applies equally to irradiance E_e and radiant intensity I_e. As an example, one can calculate the irradiance at 120 m (12,000 cm) from a spotlight with a radiant intensity of 1.5×10^5 W/sr:

$$\begin{aligned} E_e &= I_e/r^2 \\ &= 1.5 \times 10^5 / (1.2 \times 10^4)^2 \\ &= 1.0 \times 10^{-3} \text{ W/cm}^2 \\ &= 1.0 \text{ mW/cm}^2 \end{aligned}$$

It must be emphasized that Eqn. 23-4 applies only in the far field and that luminous and radiant intensity must be *measured* in the far field. If one knows K (in lm/W) one can convert from the radiometric system to the photometric system. For example, if a 100 lm/W xenon lamp were used in this particular searchlight, E_v would be 0.1 lm/cm². This illuminance would be only an estimate, however, since the spectrum will change with r due to stronger scattering of blue light and K will also change.

23.3 PROJECTED RADIANCE

If an individual were to stand in the center of a searchlight beam, he would

TABLE 23-1. Some Representative Beacons and Searchlights*

Type and Application	Light Source	Electrical Power (kW)	I (cd) × 10⁶	Beam Divergence (degrees) Horiz.	Vert.	Approx. Hazard Distance (m)
48-cm diam. Sea Search Airborne Searchlight	Carbon-arc	8.4	75	3.5	4	175†
150-cm diam. WWII Anti-aircraft Searchlight	Carbon-arc	12	500	1.25	1.5	450†
60-cm diam. Ship's Navigation Spotlight	Incandescent Lamp	55	2	4.25	3.5	36†
60-cm diam. Airfield Beacon	Incandescent Lamp	3	3	3.75	3.75	40†
90-cm diam. Airfield Beacon	Incandescent Lamp	1	3	4.5	4.5	40†
90-cm diam. Air Navigation Beacon	Hg-Xe Short-arc Lamp	2.5	100	1	1.25	200†
60-cm diam. Navigation Beacon	Hg-Xe Short-arc Lamp	2.5	40	2	2	130†
20-cm diam. Signaling Beacon	PAR-64 Xe Lamp	0.15	0.2	4	6	10†
58-cm × 41-cm Battlefield Tank Searchlight	Xe Short-arc	2.2	140	2	0.8	200
76-cm diam. Battlefield Searchlight	Xe Short-arc Lamp	20	800	1.75	1.75	600

* Source of Photometric Data: Kaufman and Christensen, 1972.
† Estimated.

see a magnified view of the source (Figure 23-4). At close range-within the near-field the magnified image will subtend an angle smaller than the angle subtended by the reflector aperture (Figure 23-5). When he is located at the flash distance r_f, (or minimum-inverse-square distance) he sees the reflector fully filled, i.e., "flashed." Beyond the flash distance he may see a slightly brighter, central element of the source if his eye is located on the searchlight axis; if so, it may be stated that he is in the "intermediate field." At still greater distances atmospheric attenuation and aberrations in the projection optics would actually decrease the projected radiance. If the individual stands off-axis (Figure 23-6) he will see the projected source to one side of center when he is in the near field. An excellent discussion of this subject may be found in Klein (1970). To demonstrate these principles, one may look into a high quality flashlight or projection lantern at different locations from withiin a beam. To comfortably view the flashlight, a shade 4 or 5 welding filter may be used.

One interesting result of the flashing of a searchlight relates to retinal image size. The retinal image size during intrabeam viewing does not vary with viewing distance within the near field! As a consequence of the Law of Conservation of

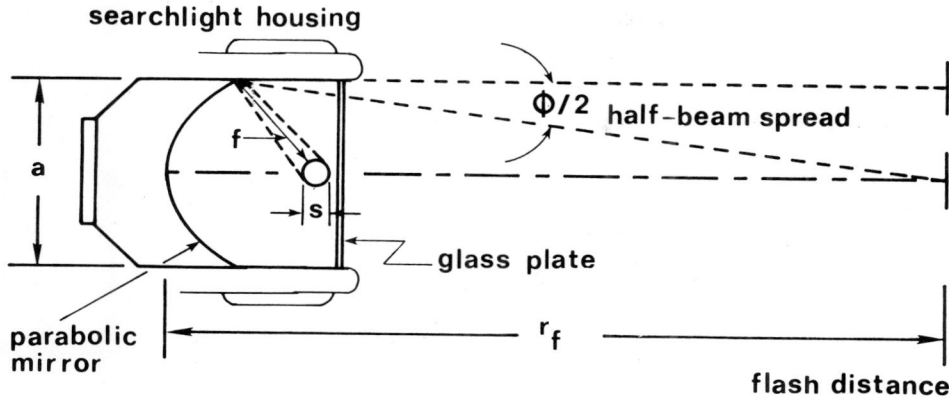

Figure 23-4. Searchlight Beam. The searchlight beam spread (divergence) is determined by the source size s and the reflector focal length f. The flash distance r_f is also determined by these two parameters plus the reflector diameter a.

Radiance, the projected solid angle of the source Ω_s must remain constant regardless of viewing distance if the irradiance is to remain constant in the near field. Figure 23-7 shows how the beam irradiance stays nearly constant in the near field. Figure 15-6 (p. 490) illustrated how Ω changed for an uncollimated light source when the irradiance decreased inversely as the square of the distance. This would also be the situation when viewing a searchlight beyond the flash distance.

The Law of Conservation of Radiance states that the radiance of a source cannot be *increased* by an optical system (Klein, 1970, and Nicodemus, 1976). It may be *decreased* by attenuating media (lenses, glass plates, poor reflectors and the atmosphere) and by field stops (the searchlight aperture or the aperture in viewing optics). Except for close viewing distances the pupil of the eye or the objective of a viewing telescope will not affect the radiance or projected source size. Nevertheless, when taking intrabeam photographs of a searchlight it is always wise to place a 7-mm limiting aperture in front of the camera objective. The transmission, reflection and collection loses of a projection system are often grouped together in a general term known as the *projector efficiency* ϵ. This concept is generally used only by optical designers and is generally not too helpful in specific calculations for hazard evaluation.

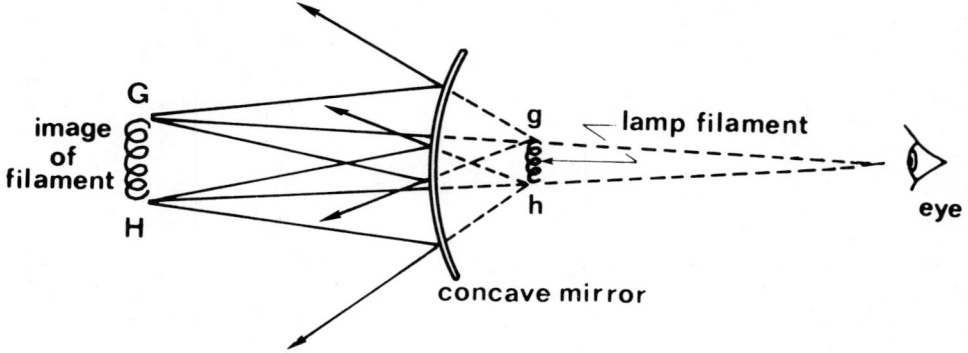

Figure 23-5. Magnification of the Source in a Searchlight. This ray diagram shows how the projected size of a tungsten filament at the focal point of a convex mirror is magnified as seen by the observer.

23.4 EVALUATING A PROJECTION SYSTEM

The principle of Conservation of Brightness, or Conservation of Radiance, permits a very practical technique for estimating the maximum radiance of a projector system such as a searchlight motion picture projector. The introduction of any optical system to collimate a source may provide a greater illuminance or irradiance at the cornea. However it cannot increase the retinal irradiance since the apparent source size will change proportionately. Of course the retinal irradiance can be decreased by transmission losses in optical elements or by stops in either the viewing system (for example binoculars or telescopes) or in the projector. Therefore only the source radiance and spectrum are required for preliminary hazard analysis of an optical projection system. If the effect of radiance of the source is below 1 W/(cm² · sr) there is no potential for a chorioretinal burn hazard. Therefore actual measurements of the projected radiance and effective source area as a function of intrabeam viewing distance for the device are not required for retinal thermal injury studies. However if the source has a luminance exceeding 1 cd/cm² which may correspond to a radiance as low as 10^{-3} W/(cm² · sr) then the source spectrum should still be weighted against the B_λ function for the consideration of long-term retinal injury hazards. Since source radiance L_s, projected radiance L_p, projector efficiency

Projection Systems

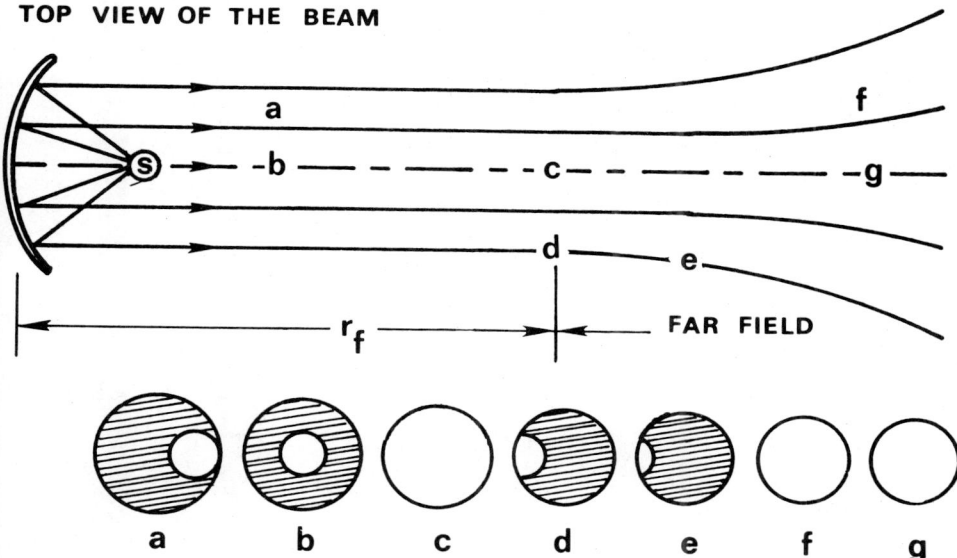

Figure 23-6. Projected Image of the Source by Searchlight Optics. The top panel shows the intrabeam viewing locations A through G of an observer. The bottom panel shows the appearance of the magnified image of the uniform disc source. In reality, the source is never so uniform but the effects shown in this figure nevertheless are obvious to an intrabeam observer.

ϵ, source area A_s, projected source area A_P, beam irradiance E, and beam solid angle Ω_P, are all interrelated by the law of conservation of brightness, the required radiometric measurements can be limited or can be confirmed by calculations using other parameters.

When irradiance is known as a function of range from the source (often the simplest measurement) and the radiance of the source is known, the effective projected source area at range r is:

$$A_p(r) = [E(r) \cdot r^2] / L \qquad (23-5)$$

In the foregoing we have generally considered the source area as uniform or we have been concerned only with maximum radiance. In practice a relatively uniform source is seldom encountered and an *effective* area, *effective* beam solid angle, and *effective* radiance, usually defined as one-half of peak, or 1/e of peak may be used. The uncertainties in the biological data upon which the hazard criteria are based, and the use of safety factors, make a more sophisticated approach unnecessary if not impossible with the present state of knowledge. If the source radiance is not known one may assume the worst case, that is, a practical "point" source.

If radiometric parameters of the source are known—often the case with short arc lamps—other parameters may be estimated. For a projector system one may calculate a lower limit for the projected area of the source. We will call this Ap

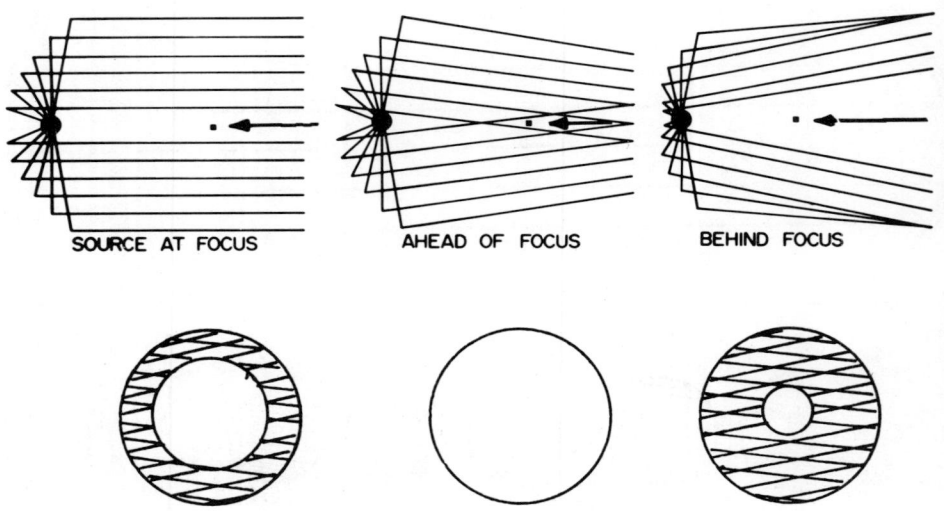

Figure 23-7. Adjustable Beam Spread. Some searchlights and theater spotlights have an adjustable beam spread. This feature is accomplished in some projectors by moving the source along the axis of the reflector in and out of focus (top). To satisfy the Law of Conservation of Radiance, the projected source size (bottom) must increase and decrease with the beam irradiance at a given point.

(min).

$$A_p \text{ (min)} = (4\pi / \Omega) A_s \qquad (23\text{-}6)$$

For purposes of hazard analysis where an irradiance E is known at viewing distance r, the worst-case condition for intrabeam viewing of a projected source exists for the smallest effective image area, hence projected source area. The designer of an optical projection system may use Eq. 23-6 to determine the minimum projector area for a safe radiance. The designer may be required to make a safe device that must also deliver an irradiance E at a given distance within a beam solid angle Ω. In the use of Eq. 23-6 one must realize that an accurate value of A_s is required, and such a value is often difficult to obtain. If the radiance is known accurately one could underestimate the hazard at a given viewing distance by underestimating the actual source size or projected source size. Using the relation of projected source area A_p, the irradiance E at distance r, and the solid angle Ω_p subtended by A_p at a distance r, one may determine the projected radiance and image size using the relation:

$$L = E/\Omega_p \qquad (23\text{-}7)$$

Formulae 23-6 and 23-7 are particularly useful when evaluating focused-beam systems. As shown in Figure 23-7, the projected source size is greatest when viewed from within the beam focal area. The projected source size is reduced when the beam is diverged. In all cases, to satisfy the Law of Conservation of Radiance, Eqn. 23-7 must hold. With an increased irradiance near the beam focus, the source size must be larger.

Several cross checks of calculations and measurements are normally desirable to provide the confidence for the ultimate test: the evaluator should be willing to expose himself to the worst-case conditions that he considers permissible.

One of the most useful cross checks of hazard calculations and measurements is to make use of photometric as well as radiometric data. If the luminous efficacy of radiation K is known, then it is possible to convert from one system to another. Then, simple measurements with inexpensive luminance and illuminance meters become useful to corroborate the measurements made with more sophisticated radiometers. It is very difficult to impart the experience necessary to evaluate such sources in a mere book chapter. There are many pitfalls in radiometric measurements, many opportunities to make a calculation error. For this reason, Table 23-1 provides the approximate characteristics of several typical optical projection systems and Tables 22-1 and 22-2 provide typical lamp source characteristics as useful checks against measured values. Additionally, the next section of this chapter shall consider several examples of optical sources and projection systems. These illustrate the application of both the simplified Threshold Limit Value criteria as well as the more comprehensive technique of plotting retinal irradiance as calculated at a variety of distances with the hazard criteria expressed in terms of retinal irradiance for a given image size.

Table 22-3 provides maximum permissible absorbed retinal irradiances recommended by Sliney and Freasier as a function of retinal image size. Of particular note is the fact that the limit varies little with the shorter dimension of the elongated image, but varies principally only with the longer dimension. This is based upon numerous unpublished retinal thermal injury calculations performed by Freasier. The results of this table also form the basis for the certain requirements for applying the tentative ACGIH Threshold Limit Values for light sources. The proposed TLV is expressed in terms of radiance where the limiting angle α is always the *greatest* angular subtense of the source if the source is not circularly symmetric. (Section 10.5.2).

23.5 EXAMPLES OF SPECIFIC PROJECTORS

23.5.1 Example 1: Tungsten-Halogen Lamp Spotlight

A typical tungsten-halogen spotlight has a 500-W doubly coiled tungsten lamp (3100 K) mounted in a 6-cm-diameter reflector. The spotlight is sold for use with home movie cameras. Tungsten has an approximate emissivity of 0.4 for this color temperature. From Figs. 22-20, 22-22, and 22-23 the total radiance L of the filament is approximately 150 W/(cm^2·sr), and the product L·R = 20 W/(cm^2·sr), and the absorbed chorioretinal dose rate is 0.4 W/cm^2 for a 3-mm pupil and 2.2 W/cm^2 for a 7-mm pupil. Assume that there is no loss in brightness when the filament image is projected. Since the radiance is much greater than 1 W/cm^2·sr),

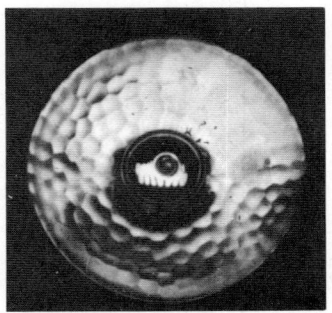

Figure 23-8. Intrabeam Photograph of Movie Light. The photograph shows both the filament and the reflected, but somewhat diffused image of the filament. Such a photograph, taken with a very dark neutral-density filter, is necessary to ascertain the projected source size as seen at a given viewing distance.

radiometric measurements are required to ascertain if a hazard exists. Fig. 23-8 shows a photograph of the source, indicating a projected area of 1.0 cm × 0.4 cm for the filament and approximately 3 cm × 4 cm for the brightest area on the reflector (approximately one-half the luminance of the filament). The measured, projected radiance of the filament was only slightly less than predicted. Using Eqn. (4-1) on page 121, the retinal image size of the filament would be 700 μm × 300 μm at a viewing distance of 25 cm and the reflected image would be 2000 μm × 3000 μm. From Table 22-3, the Sliney-Freasier hazard criterion is 2.6 W/cm² for the filament. Hence, the filament should not be viewed even momentarily at distances less than 25 cm. Using Fig. 22-21, we note that the luminance is approximately 300 cd/cm², three orders of magnitude above levels considered as comfortable to view.

The application of the Army/ACGIH criteria requires an estimate of the radiance weighted against B_λ and R_λ. From Fig. 22-24 the blue-light radiance is about 1.4 W/cm²·sr), and from Fig. 22-22 the ACGIH weighting factor $\overline{R}$ is 0.57. Hence the radiance weighted against the thermal retinal hazard function (i.e., $\overline{R} \cdot L$) is about 85 W/cm²·sr). Applying Eqn. 10-3 (page 340) results in a maximum permissible angular subtense α of 2.3 radians for a momentary 0.25-s viewing duration. This large angle could in practice not be achieved. Hence only a blue-light retinal hazard exists in reality. The maximum viewing duration t_{max} (Eqn. 10-8, page 340) is 71 s.

The emergent beam irradiance of ~20 W/cm² also presents a fire hazard. A fire hazard exists to a distance of 60 cm where the beam irradiance falls below 0.5 W/cm². Fig. 23-9 shows one of the authors demonstrating the fire hazard of this movie spotlight.

In short, the spotlight would not present a short-term retinal injury problem at distances at which the spotlight could be viewed; however, we have the interesting situation where the cornea and skin could be burned, but not the retina. Subjects should not be allowed to stare into the source for periods greater than a minute.

Projection Systems

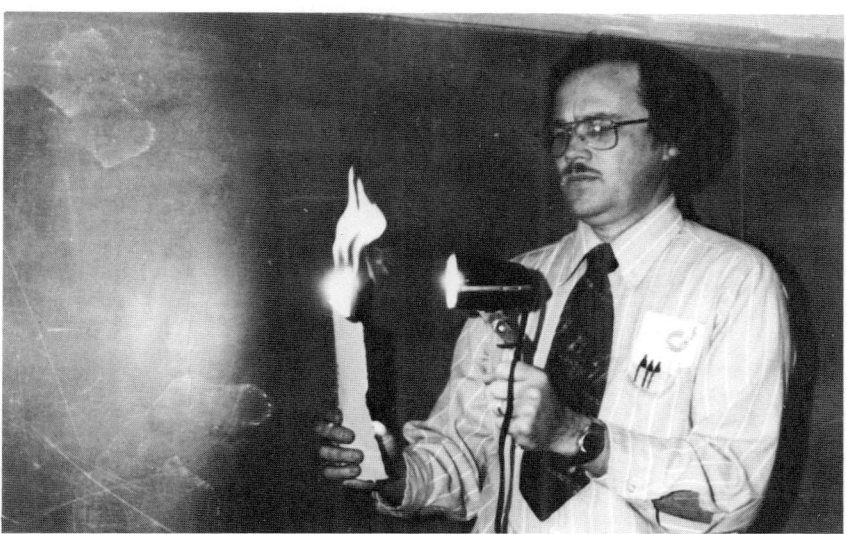

Figure 23-9. Fire Hazard. A small tungsten-halogen, home movie spotlight can quickly ignite paper and other flammable materials within 60 cm. One of the authors ignites a piece of paper in less than 10 seconds.

Fortunately, the dazzle should limit any such attempts. It might be noted that placing a diffuser or Fresnel lens over the reflector would reduce both the radiance and the potential for injury.

23.5.2 Example 2: Xenon-Short-Arc Searchlight

For a searchlight having a uniform source, one would expect the projected radiance to remain constant with a variation of viewing distance and the irradiance in the near field to remain constant, and then at a point known as the *flash distance,* or *minimum inverse square distance,* begin to decrease inversely as the square of the viewing distance. The flash distance is found when the reflector is flashed, i.e., where the image of the source (the arc) completely fills the reflector or projector lens (Sec. 23-4). This theoretical treatment assumes a perfect reflector and a uniform radiance across the arc. Actual arcs, however, do not provide such a convenient radiance distribution. Actual radiance measurements of searchlights often show a significant increase in projected radiance along the beam axis with increase in viewing distance, since the brighter, central region of the arc is being imaged at the axis. Fig. 23-10 shows the retinal irradiance calculated for an individual located near the beam axis of a 2.2-kW xenon, short-arc searchlight having an arc size of 4 mm ×

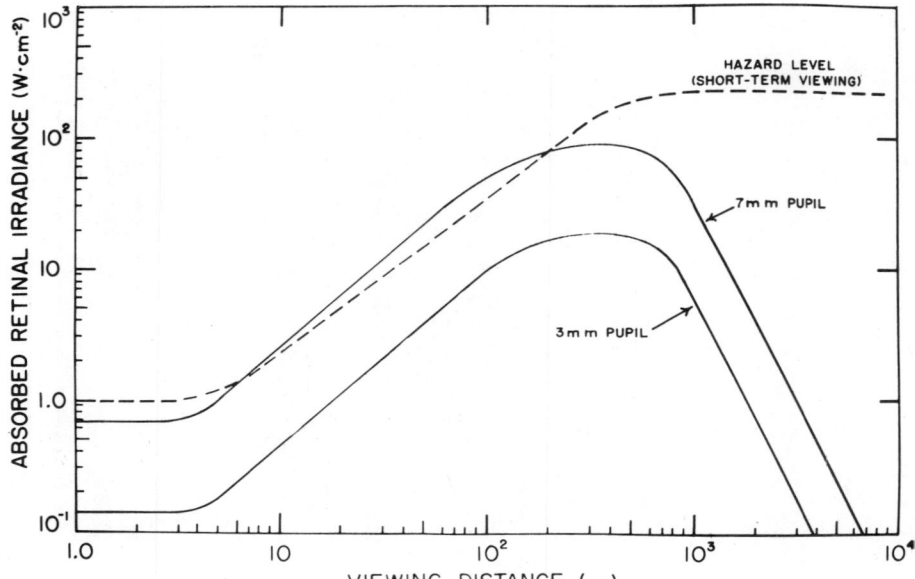

Figure 23.10. Hazard Analysis of a 2.2-kW Xenon-Arc Searchlight. The retinal irradiance from the searchlight is plotted as a function of viewing distance. The hazard level (Sliney-Freasier method) for short-term viewing increases with decreasing image size, indicating a hazardous viewing distance of 220 m for a 7-mm pupil. The "caution distance," as defined by Sliney and Freasier, was defined as the distance where the absorbed retinal irradiance fell below 0.1 W/cm^2. This level occurred at 4000 m for a 3 mm pupil and 7000 m for a 7-mm pupil (Sliney and Freasier, 1973).

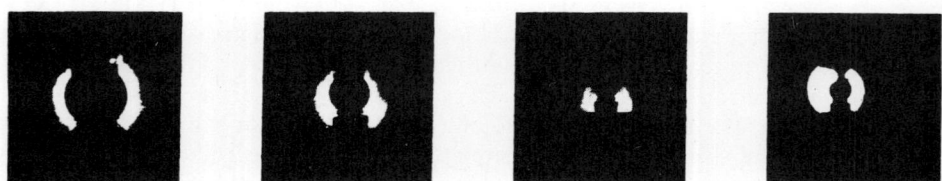

Figure 23-11. Intrabeam Photographs of a 2.2-kW Searchlight. The photographs show how the fraction of the reflector that is "flashed" increases with distance. The reflector is flashed in the right-hand photograph. The center of the source is occluded by the lamp chimney (from Sliney and Freasier, 1973).

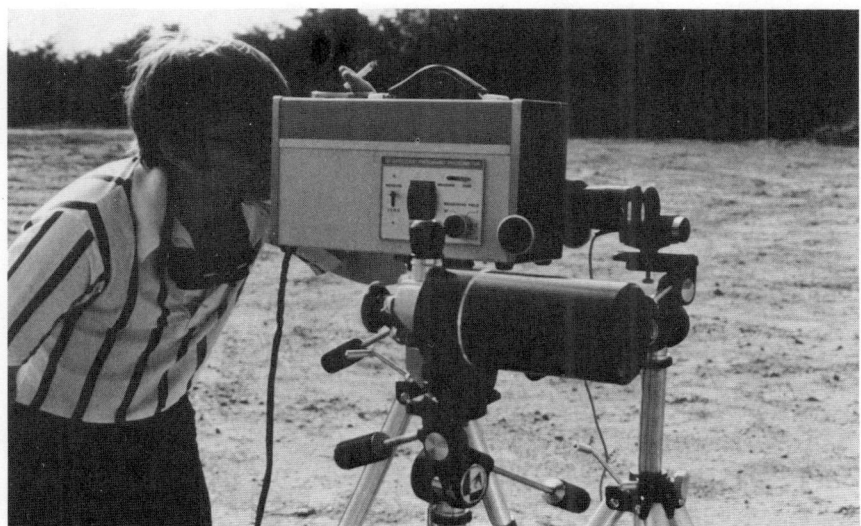

Figure 23-12. Intrabeam Radiometry and Photometry. A variety of instruments, including a thin-film-thermopile irradiance meter, an illuminance meter, a spectroradiometer, a camera, and a high resolution spot photometer are used to measure the searchlight at several distances downrange from the searchlight.

2.5 mm measured at half-peak radiance points, a 0.3° × 0.5° beam spread, a 43 cm × 57.5 cm reflector, and a total luminous flux of 8×10^4 lm. To obtain the values in Fig. 23-10, irradiance measurements and photographs of the projected source (Fig. 23-11) were used in addition to photometric brightness measurements. It was determined that the luminous efficacy of radiation from the searchlight was approximately 130 lm/W. Because the brightest portion of the arc filled the reflector only at a distance of approximately 200 m, the peak radiance values occurred only within that range. Instruments such as shown in Fig. 23-12 were used to measure and photograph the source at 1 m, 5 m, 10 m, 20 m, 40 m, 80 m, 160 m, 300 m, 600 m, and 1000 m downrange. So many intrabeam measurements were necessitated by the changing radiance characteristics with range. Despite an increase in projected radiance within the central spot, the searchlights' beam irradiance closely followed the theoretical prediction of Fig. 23-3.

Applying the ACGIH/Army criteria is also complicated by the searchlights' change in average radiance and in image size with increasing viewing distance. The highest projected radiance was about 1500 W/(cm² · sr). The $\overline{R}$ factor was 1.6 and the blue-light radiance was 170 W/(cm² · sr). The $\overline{R}$ factor is a weighted R_λ, term, i.e.,

$$\sum_{400}^{1400} L_\lambda \cdot R_\lambda \cdot \Delta\lambda = L \cdot \overline{R} \qquad (23\text{-}8)$$

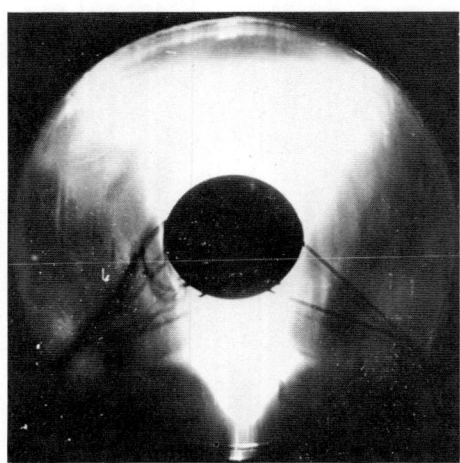 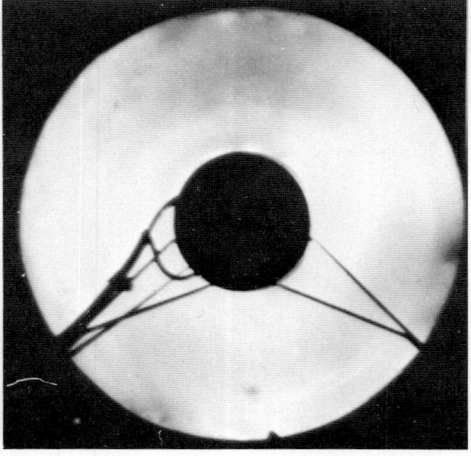

Figure 23-13. Intrabeam Photograph of an Axially-mounted Arc Searchlight. The illuminance and radiance distribution in this type of projector is much more uniform than the searchlight in Fig. 23-11. The left-hand photograph was taken in the near field.

The maximum safe angular subtense for viewing the source, from rearranging Eqn. (10-3) and employing Eqn. (23-8) is:

$$\alpha_{max} = (\sqrt{t}) / (t \cdot L \cdot \overline{R}) \qquad (23\text{-}9)$$

For momentary viewing Eqn. (23-9) gives:

$$\alpha_{max} = (\sqrt{0.25}) / (0.25)(1500)(1.6)$$
$$= 0.0008 \text{ rad}$$

which is less than the angle (1.3 mrad) which corresponds to the minimal effective retinal image size (0.022 mm). When α is 1.3 mrad L (Haz) is 1540 W/(cm² · sr) for a 0.25-s exposure. This radiance corresponds to an *irradiance* E (Haz) of:

$$E\,(Haz) = (2.0 \text{ mW/cm}^2) / \overline{R} \qquad (23\text{-}10)$$

or, for this searchlight:

$$E\,(Haz) = 1.3 \text{ mW/cm}^2.$$

Interestingly enough, this criterion is actually more conservative than the 2.5-mW/cm² criterion for momentary, intrabeam visible laser exposure. From

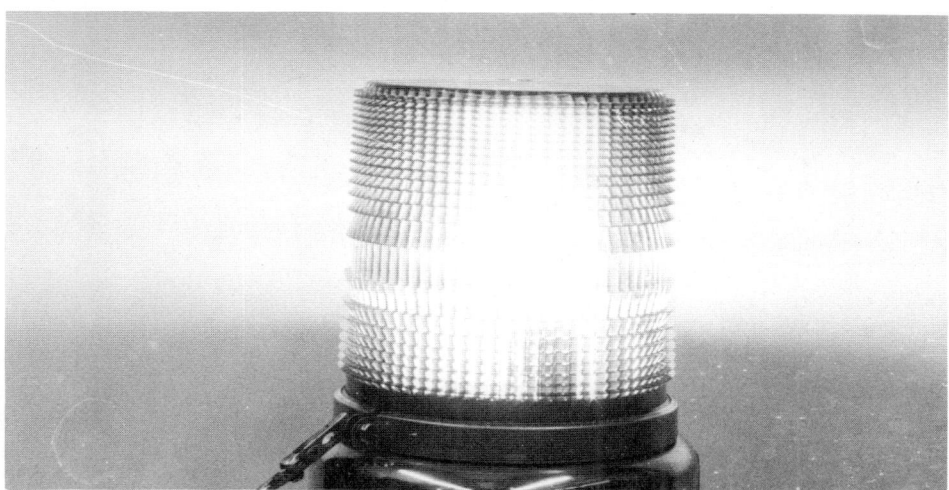

Figure 23-14. Emergency Vehicle Light. The photograph shows an intrabeam photograph of a xenon-flash warning light and the irradiance pattern on a wall immediately behind the light. Note how the Fresnel lens collimates the light into a beam with a wide-angle (360°) horizontal beam spread and a relatively tight, 10° vertical beam spread.

Fig. 23-3, this irradiance occurs at a distance of 180 m. Since the blue-light radiance was 170 W/cm²·sr), corresponding t_{max} (from Eqn. 10-4) was 0.59 s, which was less conservative than the thermal hazard criterion and was therefore not applied. Eqn. (10-6) on page 340 would be applied if the searchlight were to be stared into for an extended period. In conclusion, the application of the Sliney-Freasier method and the ACGIH method resulted in approximately the same hazard distance for momentary viewing. Sec. 23.6 will consider the safety precautions that are applicable to searchlights.

23.5.3 Example 3: Emergency-Vehicle Lights

As was demonstrated in the first example (Sec. 23.5.1) tungsten lamps are not normally a retinal hazard. Such lamps, mounted with rotating reflectors and placed in a clear-lens or Fresnel-lens dome, are used extensively in emergency vehicles (fire trucks, tow trucks, police cars, and ambulances). Aside from an annoyance factor at night, these are not hazards. Howell, Kelly and Pierce (1978) have provided an excellent review of the state-of-the-art in these lights. More recent types of emergency vehicle lights have employed xenon flash lamps. Fig. 23-14 shows an intrabeam photograph of such a source, which had the following measured parameters:

- Candlepower: 2,000,000 cd
- Beam spread: 10° vertical; 360° vertical
- Dome color: Aviation Blue (Police)
- Pulse Duration: 0.1 ms
- Pulse Repetition: two pulses placed 0.17 s apart every 0.9 s.
- Projected Source Size: 8 cm (horiz.) by 14 cm (vert.)
- Luminous Efficacy of Radiation K: 123 lm/W
- Average Projected Radiance: 0.28 W/(cm² · sr)
- Average Projected Blue-Light Radiance: 0.024 W/(cm² · sr)
- Retinal Hazard Factor (Sl-Fr) R: 0.43
- Retinal Hazard Factor (ACGIH) $\overline{R}$: 1.48
- Projected Pulsed Radiance L_p: 0.098 J/(cm² · sr) in central 2-cm² area

The blue-light hazard criteria should be applied for lengthy staring into the source; t_{max} from Eqn. 10-8 would be 4,170 s, or 1.2 hours. From a practical standpoint it is unrealistic to assume that anyone could stare into the source for that time period. Applying a maximum value for α of 0.1 rad (Sec. 10.5.2, page 340) leads to a value of L (Haz) of 0.1 J/(cm² · sr) for a single 0.1 ms pulse. Since the 0.1-ms pulse duration is less than the recommended range of applicable pulse durations for the ACGIH criteria, this limit will be overly conservative. The laser safety criterion for viewing an extended 0.1-ms extended source is 0.46 J/(cm² · sr). Hence, even with a repetitive pulse correction (from Fig. 8-11, page 290) the strobe is safe to view.

A secondary safety problem should always be considered for any flashing light—flicker sickness. Photo-induced seizures in susceptible epileptics represent the only documented health hazard from exposure to low-frequency intermittent light. The critical frequency for this effect is from 8 to 16 Hz; and this is well above the PRF of this strobe. Within the frequency of 8 to 16 Hz, most people will experience some slight feeling of disorientation, but only in pitch darkness.

23.5.4 Example 4: Slide Projector

Movie projectors and slide projectors generally use tungsten filament lamps operating at approximately 3200 K. Xenon-arc lamps and carbon arcs are often used in large theaters.

A typical 35-mm slide projector generally uses a 250-W to 500-W projection lamp. Fig. 23-15 shows an intrabeam photograph of the projected luminance profile of a 300-W singly coiled tungsten lamp as seen through the 6-cm diameter lens of a 35-mm slide projector. An illuminance of 0.2 lm/cm² and an irradiance (350 nm to 1400 nm) of 2.3 mW/cm² were measured at a distance of 3 m from the lens. Since the intrabeam photograph at 3 m and at several other intermediate distances showed approximately half the area of the 6-cm diameter (28-cm² area) lens filled, an area of 14 cm² was used for A_s. Then the projected luminance L_v and radiance L_e at a distance r of 300 cm would be:

$$L_v = (E \cdot r^2) / A_s \qquad (23\text{-}11)$$
$$= (0.2 \text{ lm/cm}^2)(300 \text{ cm})^2 / (14 \text{ cm}^2)$$
$$= 1300 \text{ cd/cm}^2$$

Projection Systems

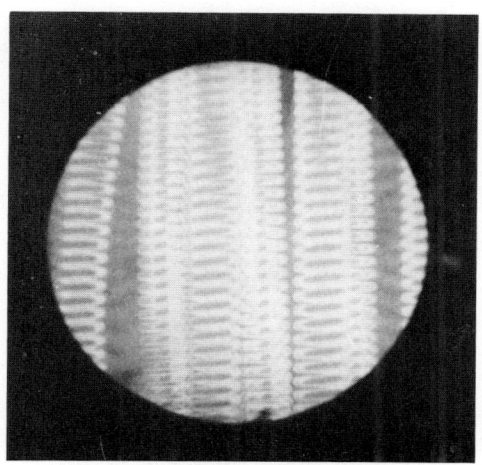

Figure 23-15. Intrabeam Photograph of a Slide Projector. Typical slide projectors use small coiled coil tungsten halogen lamps, or a larger, more conventional singly coiled tungsten lamp. The photograph shows the array of filaments of a single coiled lamp viewed through the 6-cm diameter projection lens at 3-m from the projector.

and similarly:

$$L_e = 1.5 \text{ W}/(\text{cm}^2 \cdot \text{sr})$$

Since $\bar{R}$ for such a tungsten source is approximately 1.0 for a similar tungsten lamp in Table 22-2, the maximum safe angular subtense for viewing α_{max} (Eqn. 23-9) is 1.3 rad for momentary, 0.25-s exposures. As this angle is far greater than 0.1 rad, one may conclude that no thermal injury exists. Even for a 10-s exposure, Eqn. (23-9) leads to an angle of 0.21 rad.

The luminance for the source is far too great to comfortably view, and afterimages would result from staring into the projector. The projected blue-light radiance extrapolated from the measured radiance and the radiance of a filament in Table 22-2 would be 0.02 W/(cm² · sr). From Eqn. (10-8) on page 340 the maximum stare-time would be 5000 s or 1.4 hours. Hence, one may conclude that there is not a realistic hazard from such a source, although slide-show lecturers should be cautioned not to needlessly stare into the source.

23.5.5 Example 5: Infrared Heat Gun

A variety of appliances make use of a focused beam of IR-A radiation from a tungsten lamp or arc source. Fig. 23-16 shows an infrared heat gun which employed a 500-W tungsten-halogen source filtered by a visible blocking filter. Following eye complaints by a user, Sensintaffar, Sliney and Parr (1978) evaluated this infrared, non-contact soldering tool. Using the more recent ACGIH criteria (Sec. 10.5.4, page 341) for estimating the IR-A retinal hazard, one may update this evaluation.

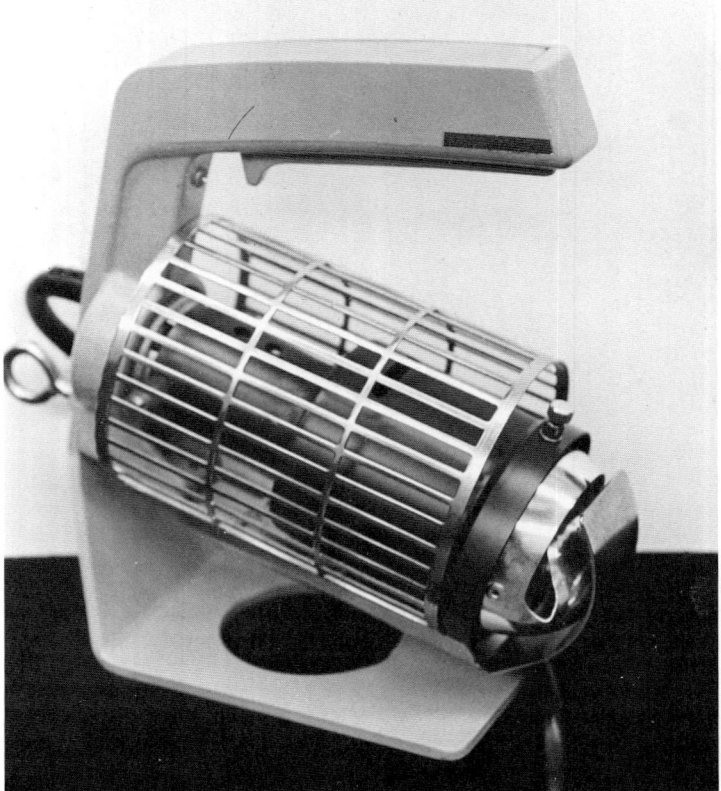
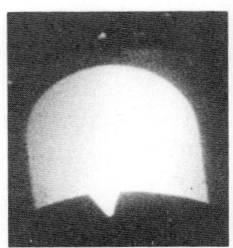

Figure 23-16. Infrared Heat Gun. This infrared handtool was designed for soldering and for heating heat-shrinkable plastic sleeves and fitting. The item to be heated is placed into the holding pot on the lower right. An intrabeam infrared photograph of the source [inset] was taken with the shield opened.

The operator would normally use his hands to hold the wires to be connected or covered but his hands would not be away from the focal-spot heating zone within the nose cone. However, on the unit examined, a beam of infrared radiation did escape from the nose cone and this was measured. Fig. 23-17 shows the spectrum of the source, illustrating that most of the emitted power was at wavelengths beyond 750 nm. The total irradiance was measured as a function of distance from the heating zone as plotted in Fig. 23-18. The source area (inset in Fig. 23-16) subtended a solid angle of 1 msr at 50 cm, where the beam irradiance was 12 mW/cm^2. This leads to a projected radiance of 12 W/(cm^2·sr). Applying Eqn. (10-9) on page 341

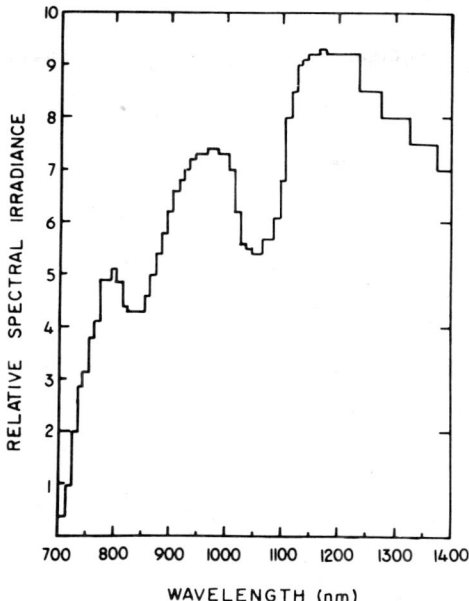

Figure 23-17. Relative Spectral Irradiance of IR Handtool. The irregular increase in spectral irradiance from 700 nm to 1200 nm resulted from the nature of the interference filter used to block out visible radiation.

leads to a maximum safe viewing angular subtense α_{max} of 0.05 rad. Since the greatest dimension of the source D_L was 1.8 cm, the hazardous viewing distance r (Haz) was:

$$\begin{aligned}\text{r (Haz)} &= D_L / \alpha_{max} \\ &= (1.8 \text{ cm}) / (0.05 \text{ rad}) \\ &= 36 \text{ cm}\end{aligned} \quad (23\text{-}12)$$

The typical viewing distance would normally exceed 36 cm, but not in all cases. The employee who complained of eye irritation viewed the workpiece (which occluded some of the source) at 20 cm. Since the source was operated intermittently, there was probably no serious retinal hazard. However, the total beam irradiance exceeded 0.1 W/cm² at viewing distances less than 17 cm. This irradiance would certainly dry the cornea and cause eye irritation following prolonged exposure. Shortly after concern was expressed about the complete safety of this tool, the manufacturer modified the design to include a dark, heat-absorbing filter shield over the source. This completely eliminated any potential hazard.

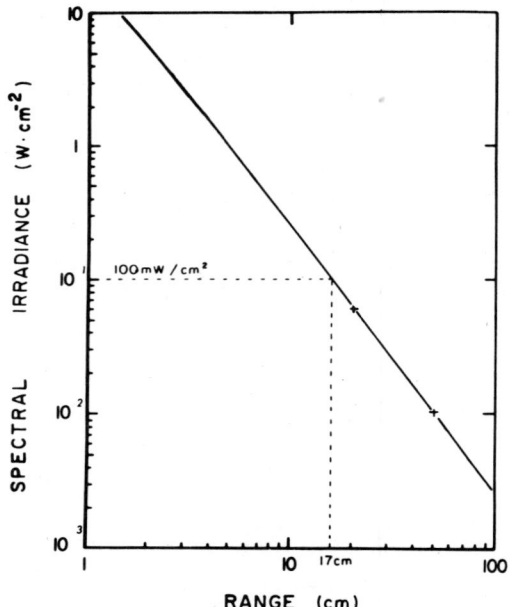

Figure 23-18. Irradiance from an IR Handtool. The total irradiance measured with a thin-film-thermopile radiometer followed the inverse square law at distances greater than 5 to 10 cm. A skin irradiance of 100 mW/cm² is considered maximal for localized exposure (as from a laser).

23.5.6 Example 6: Eye Movement Recorder

A variety of scientific instruments—oculometers—have been designed to monitor and record eye movements (Young and Sheena, 1975). One of the types of oculometer methods uses an infrared emitting diode or a filtered tungsten source to produce a corneal reflex which is then monitored through different electro-optical techniques. Infrared radiation is used to avoid interfering with the subject's performance of a visual task under study.

The potential ocular hazards of a Honeywell Remote Oculometer described by Merchant and Morrissette (1974) were evaluated as follows. A 150-W tungsten halogen lamp (type FCS) is used with projection optics which include IR-A passband filters to limit the spectrum to the region between 750 nm and 1100 nm (Fig. 23-19). An intrabeam photograph of the projected source showed the filament (somewhat similar to Fig. 23-15), which completely filled the 2.5-cm diameter projection lens at distances greater than 35 cm from this lens. Thus, the projected

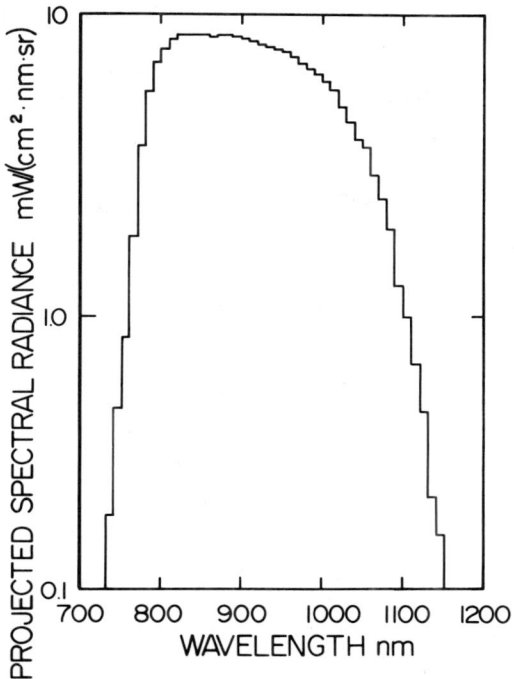

Figure 23-19. Spectral Radiance of Honeywell Remote Oculometer. Special filters are used to limit the IR-A radiation to the band between 750 nm and 1100 nm. (Courtesy of Dr. John Merchant, Honeywell, Inc.)

source area was 4.9 cm². The total projected radiance of the source was 4.5 W/(cm²·sr). For continuous viewing of an IR-A source Eqn. (10-9) is applied. This provides an angle α_{max} of 0.13 rad, which is greater than the practical limit of 0.1 rad applicable to Eqn. 10-9. The angle of 0.13 rad, if inserted into Eqn. (23-12), leads to a viewing distance of (2.5 cm) / (0.13 rad) or 19 cm. This distance is much less than the useful range of the instrument. The subject normally is located at approximately 100 cm from the last projection lens of the oculometer. Hence one may conclude that this oculometer does not pose a retinal hazard. The ACGIH IR-A criteria also recommends against chronic exposure of the anterior of the eye to an irradiance exceeding 10 mW/cm². This irradiance occurs at 50 cm and at the subject's eye, the irradiance is only 2.5 mW/cm². Since the machine will not function at viewing distances much less than 90 to 100 cm, there is no practical hazard. Nevertheless, the instruction manual should probably include a caution not to stare at the source within 50 cm.

Another device, the Stanford Research Institute (SRI) Eyetracker, uses a GaAs infrared-emitting diode (930 nm). In this system the corneal irradiance is up to

4 mW/cm², but the projected angle α of the source is 7.5° (0.13 rad) and the average projected radiance is 0.3 W/(cm² · sr). Using Eqn. (10-9) on page 341, the IR-A L (Haz) for an α of 0.13 rad is 4.6 W/(cm² · sr). Hence there is no hazard with this device either.

23.6 SEARCHLIGHT SAFETY MEASURES

The searchlight is one of the few types of high intensity light sources to which the public is potentially exposed. Open carbon-arc searchlights emit hazardous levels of actinic ultraviolet radiation. These searchlights should have a glass plate or Fresnel lens (Fig. 23-2) in front of the arc to filter out the actinic ultraviolet radiation, but some searchlights do not, particularly the older units left over as surplus equipment from World War II. This older type of equipment is most often found in carnivals and with similar groups where an understanding of the ultraviolet radiation hazard is very limited. Fortunately most searchlight units are used simply to direct a beam straight up into the sky, and scattered ultraviolet radiation incident upon people near the searchlight unit is minimal. To prevent both retinal injury and possible ultraviolet injury to the skin and eye, operators should be trained in safety measures. Operators should obviously be instructed never to point carbon-arc searchlights at personnel. Warning labels should be placed on the searchlight units to indicate this hazard.

Searchlight maintenance workers should have welding goggles available if they should have to look directly at the arc. Alignment of the carbon arc or the xenon arc to the center of the parabolic mirror focal point is accomplished in a variety of different ways. The least desirable method is visually positioning the arc point. The most acceptable method is to direct the beam on a fixed grid some distance away. It is normally desirable to place this target grid well above head level if the ceiling in the test facility is high enough.

23.7 OPHTHALMIC INSTRUMENTS

The exposure limits developed for both laser and non-laser are based upon certain assumptions that do not always apply during ophthalmic procedures. Exposure limits for pulsed exposure generally assume a 7-mm pupil, but limits for exposure durations exceeding a few seconds assume some minimal eye movement and in the case of visible light, a constricted 3-mm pupil. For some ophthalmic diagnostic or surgical procedures, the pupil may be dilated and the eye immobilized. As little is known of the effects of drugs and anesthesia upon retinal susceptibility to photochemical injury, caution should be used when the hazards of these types of instruments are evaluated with standard exposure limits.

23.7.1 Diagnostic Instruments

The most commonly used ophthalmic instruments which use potentially hazardous light sources are the *ophthalmoscope*, the *slit lamp* and *fundus camera*. All of these instruments use tungsten filament lamps. Almost all do not have an IR-A absorbing filter. Radiometric measurements of a wide variety of these instruments show that the total retinal irradiance never exceeds 0.5 W/cm^2, well below the retinal thermal injury level. The fundus camera flash lamp needs a separate evaluation (Wolbarsht et al., 1976).

Such light sources are sometimes directed at the retina in Maxwellian view (Westheimer, 1966) where the beam of light entering the eye is focused at the plane of the pupil. Although this technique delivers the greatest total power to the retina, it cannot in theory increase the retinal irradiance over that which would occur for the same pupil size when the source is imaged on the retina.

The radiance of a 3200 K tungsten filament is approximately 60 W/(cm$^2 \cdot$sr) and the blue-light radiance, 1 W/(cm$^2 \cdot$sr). Using Eqn. 4-4 on page 123, the maximal retinal irradiance for a filament imaged on the retina, with an 8-mm pupil, is less than 4 W/cm^2 (or an absorbed irradiance of 2.5 W/cm^2). The corresponding blue light retinal irradiance is less than 0.07 W/(cm$^2 \cdot$sr). The attenuation of projecting optics would always lower these values. In practice then, the concern would be for thermally enhanced photochemical injury. The lowest reported blue-light lesion threshold is approximately 30 J/cm^2 at the retina (Ham, Mueller, and Sliney, 1975). Therefore, a blue-light hazard would exist within a time period of (30 J/cm^2) / (0.07 W/cm^2), or 430 s (7 minutes). Indeed, Kuwabara and Gorn (1968), using an indirect-ophthalmoscope, were able to cause a visible retinal injury in the eye of a rhesus monkey with an irradiance of 0.27 W/cm^2 for 15 minutes.

Calkins and Hochheimer (1979) reported their measurements of a variety of slit lamps and ophthalmoscopes and compared these with laser exposure limits. Using a slit-lamp to produce a retinal irradiance of 0.3 W/cm^2 for 40 minutes, they detected sub-visible retinal injury through the use of fluorescein angiography.

In actual practice the retina is not illuminated by these diagnostic instruments under these worst-case conditions for such extensive periods. The illumination pattern moves across the retina and the instrument is not usually turned to its maximum setting. The retinal irradiance for the lower settings of slit lamps and indirect ophthalmoscopes may typically be a factor of two or three lower than for the higher setting. The potential risks could nevertheless be reduced considerably. The thermal load to the lens could be greatly reduced by the insertion of IR-A blocking filters in the projection optics of the instrument. The blue-light hazard could be reduced by further filtering of some of the shorter wavelength radiation. The development of flying-spot retinal scanners and other image conversion techniques will also lead to reduced retinal irradiances during diagnostic procedures.

23.7.2 Operating Room Instruments

The operation microscope can deliver the greatest retinal irradiance for the greatest duration, and changes in operating-room procedures could have the greatest impact upon reducing this potential hazard (Calkins and Hochheimer, 1979). The operation microscope light (tungsten source) if moved from about 15 cm from the eye to only 0.5 to 1.0 cm could be greatly reduced in radiance and thereby lower

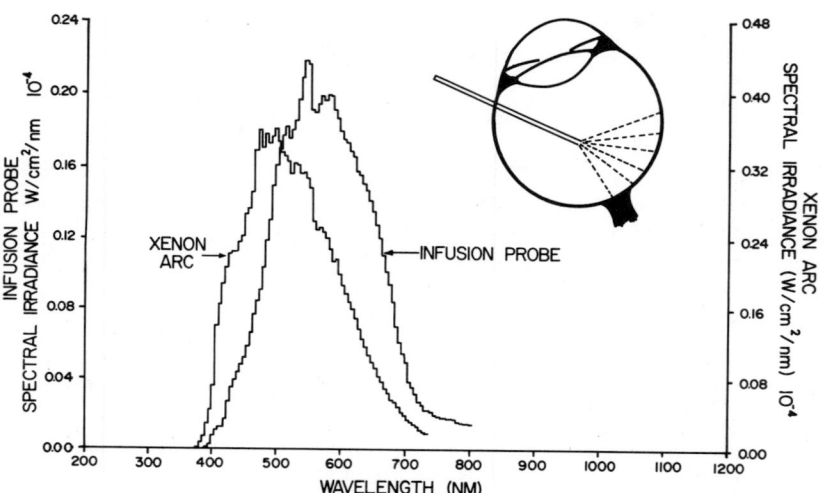

Figure 23-20. Spectral Irradiance of two Different Fiber Optic Bundles Used in Vitrectomy for Illumination. These probes are introduced in the eye as shown in the inset through the *pars plana*. The one described as the "original" is the same one described by Fuller *et al.* (1978), and its other characteristics are given in Table 23-2. The xenon-arc source-probe combination is that denoted "straight" in the xenon-arc illuminator section of Table 23-2.

the retinal irradiance considerably. Calkins and Hochheimer also recommended the use of a gel foam to diffuse the light source during suturing. Since the light dries the cornea, the surgeon generally tries to avoid excessive light levels.

Optical fiber probes are now being used in medicine, particularly in surgery, to deliver high intensity (in many cases infrared-free) illumination for both diagnostic and therapeutic purposes. By and large these uses are without hazard. However, one in particular needs some caution, that is, a new surgical technique, vitrectomy, especially the *pars plana* approach as developed by Machemer (Machemer and Aaberg, 1979). This operation uses the optical fibers to introduce light inside of the eye (Parel *et al.*, 1974, and Fuller *et al.*, 1978). The optical setup for this procedure is shown in the inset of Fig. 23-20. The spectral irradiance of two kinds of fibers with two different sources are shown in the main part of Fig. 23-20. The total output of these two fibers (and two others) are shown in Table 23-2. The blue-light hazard has been calculated on the basis of the spectral irradiance assuming the fiber optics bundle to be about 2 mm from the retina, at which distance the light would cover an approximate 3-mm to 5-mm diameter circular area. The xenon-arc source, with its output heavily weighted toward the blue, has a shorter safe exposure duration by a factor of 10 or more as compared with a tungsten-halogen source, even though its total output is greater by less than 4. Obviously, this hazard can be decreased by lowering the output in the blue end of the spectrum. How much reduction in the blue can be tolerated is still a subject of investigation, particularly

TABLE 23-2. Intraocular Optical Fiber Probes

	Tungsten Halogen Lamp		Xenon-Arc Lamp Zeiss NAG XBO 75 W	
	Original*	High Output, Designs for Vision	Straight	Hook
Output: UV, Visible IR-A (mW)	14.7	29	75	75
Output: UV, Visible All IR (mW)	22	33	95	95
Blue-Light Radiance [mW/(cm$^2 \cdot$sr)] at probe tip †	0.19	0.18	1.8	1.8
Safe Exposure Duration (min) 2 mm from retina	55	35	2.5	2.5

* The measurements of the "original" probe are to be compared with those made by Fuller *et al.* (1978). All the fibers and light sources were furnished through the courtesy of Dr. Robert Machemer, Chairman, Department of Ophthalmology, Duke University.

† The blue-light hazard evaluation is based on the 1978 proposed ACGIH standards for TLV broadband exposures.

when the surgeon's ability to recognize his landmarks and to accomplish the object of his surgery are considered. Thus, a benefit *vs.* risk analysis will be required to consider reducing the level of blue light for surgery, or to shorten the surgical exposure if more blue light is essential.

23.8 SOLAR SIMULATORS

23.8.1 Solar Simulator in Dermatology

Small arc-lamp projectors are sometimes used in dermatology to perform photosensitization tests of the skin. A useful chart (Fig. 23-21) developed by Berger is useful for comparing levels of UV and IR upon the skin that may be tolerated for limited periods.

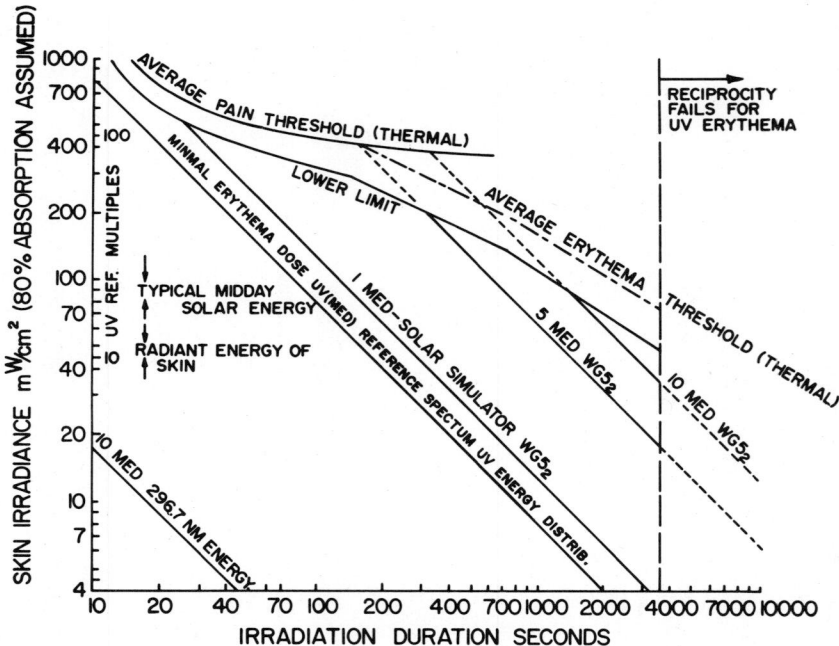

Figure 23-21. Dermatological Solar Simulator Chart. This chart, prepared by Daniel Berger (1969) of the Skin and Cancer Hospital, Temple University, shows the exposure limitations required to prevent thermal injury of the skin while still achieving a UV-induced effect.

23.8.2 Aerospace Solar Simulators

Solar simulators are used throughout the facilities of the National Aeronautics and Space Administration (NASA), in university laboratories, and in the aerospace industry. Most simulators use high-power xenon-arc lamps, although other arc sources have been used. Generally, these sources are completely enclosed within an opaque test chamber such as the one shown in Fig. 23-22. Questions of eye safety arise regarding safe handling of the high-pressure lamps during installation and maintenance as well as safe filters for windows in the test chamber. Polycarbonate plastic lamp covers or metal covers should always be used during installation of the lamps. A shade 12 to shade 14 welding filter glass should be used to view the arc. Normally the windows are not located such that a magnified image of the arc(s) can be viewed and, therefore, only the blue-light retinal injury is of particular concern.

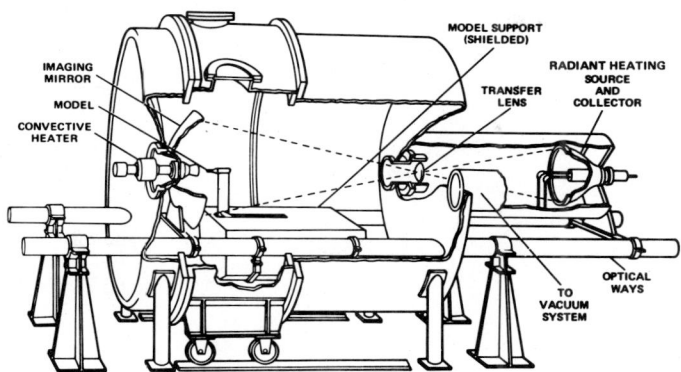

Figure 23-22. Solar Simulator for Aerospace Research. Solar simulators used for testing materials to be exposed to extraterrestrial sunlight are often evacuated and almost always completely enclosed. Shade 12 to 14 welding filters are used in viewing ports. (Drawing courtesy of NASA Ames Research Center, Moffett Field, CA)

23.9 HAZARDS FROM SOLAR FURNACES AND SOLAR POWER FACILITIES

As supplies of conventional fossil fuels have become diminished, there has been an increased interest in the use of the energy of solar radiation to supplement or even, to a large extent, replace other sources. Most small-scale applications such as solar heaters in individual houses or solar cell arrays do not present any unusual hazards, but large-size solar collectors could pose serious problems. Large solar furnaces are not new and are to be found at research laboratories in deserts, in the French Alps, and elsewhere throughout the world. These have been used for many years to produce very high radiant flux densities to study thermal effects in material. Still larger solar power facilities are envisioned for the future (Hildebrandt and Vant-Hull, 1977). Fig. 23-23 shows an artist's conception of a large-scale solar power facility to be located in the southwestern United States. It consists of a tall (possibly 200 m) central tower which collects reflected solar power from an array of heliostat mirrors. As the sun moves through the sky throughout the day, the heliostats move to keep the sun's rays on the solar collector at the top of the tower. In this collector, enormous temperatures are produced for the generation of electrical energy. Presumably this area at the top of the tower would be inaccessible to personnel during normal operation. However, the question must be asked as to the hazard that would result if a heliostat were misdirected toward an occupied area.

The field of heliostats would normally be arranged in a circular pattern around the central tower. Each heliostat might typically have an area between 5 and 40 m². Although the heliostat mirrors could be parabolic, spherical, or flat-surfaced, production ease and space utilization will probably demand a square shape. Any

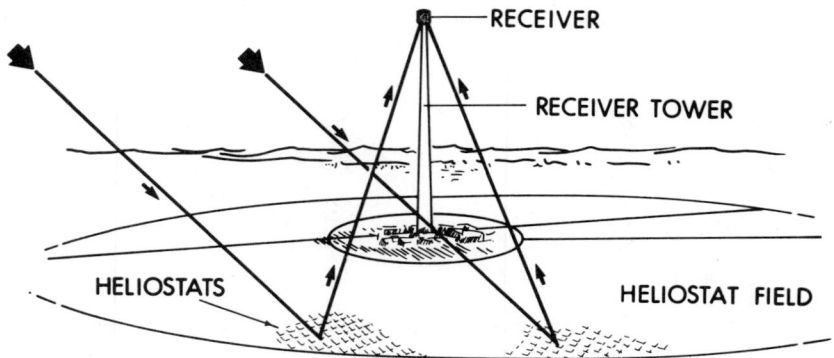

Figure 23-23. Solar Thermal Power Facility. One concept for a centralized solar power facility calls for a central receiver tower surrounded by heliostat mirrors. The heliostats move with the sun to maintain the reflected sunlight on the receiver. (After Ham and Sliney, 1978)

curved mirrors will have a focal length of the order of 100 m appropriate to the distance between the heliostat and the collector. Very large heliostats could be multifaceted with a common focal point. The reflectance of most polished mirrors ranges roughly from 0.85 to 0.95. For a solar reflector the upper value would be the theoretical limit, but it might be met with new mirror technology.

The total terrestrial irradiance from the sun does not vary a great deal from 0.1 W/cm^2 for solar elevation angles above 30°, but as the solar irradiance varies so would the irradiance of the heliostat's reflected beam. For a person standing on the ground looking at a heliostat which might be directed at him as a result of accidental misalignment or as a result of an alignment procedure, the maximal corneal irradiance would probably occur with the sun's zenith angle between 50° and 75°, since the off-axis aberrations would be least for those angles.

In theory, because of the Law of Conservation of Radiance, in an aberration-free specular system, neither the irradiance in the focal plane of the mirror, nor the projected radiance (hence retinal irradiance) of the sun, will vary much for zenith angles between 0° and 70°. For a preliminary hazard analysis, a theoretically aberration-free system and a maximal retinal image size can be assumed. The greatest effect of changing zenith angle will be the change from a nearly square retinal image for a square mirror at near normal angles of incidence to a foreshortened rectangular image for off-normal incidence angles. That is, both small and large zenith angles would have the smallest images for a person on the ground looking up at the heliostat. The irradiance in the reflected beam would vary with the mirrored area of the heliostat. Naturally the beam irradiance would increase as one goes farther from the heliostat and moves toward the focal spot. The Law of Conservation of Radiance thus indicates that the focal irradiance will vary little with zenith angles, and that only the image area will change with off-axis incidence of the sun's rays.

Projection Systems

The maximal beam irradiance E_f (at the receiving tower) in the focal spot is related to the total radiant power P (in Watts) in the beam and the focal spot area (A_f in cm²) as follows:

$$E_f = P/A_f \qquad (23\text{-}13)$$

The focal beam area (A_f) of a square reflector can be estimated for normal incidence as:

$$A_f = f^2 \cdot \phi^2 \qquad (23\text{-}14)$$

where f is the focal length of the heliostat in cm, ϕ is the source divergence angle in radians. The width of the spot is $f\phi$ since the diffraction effects from the mirror edges are minor. The sun subtends an angle of 9.3×10^{-3} rad which determines the divergence ϕ of the sun's rays. These calculations can be based upon geometrical optics, since the calculated Airy disc for these heliostats is considerably smaller than the geometrically determined image size. For a short (e.g., 75-m) focal length reflector, the focal spot diameter (D_f in cm) is:

$$\begin{aligned} D_f &= f\phi \\ &= 7500 \text{ cm} \times 9.3 \times 10^{-3} \text{ rad or } 70 \text{ cm} \end{aligned} \qquad (23\text{-}15)$$

which leads to a focal spot area of 0.49 m². The focal irradiance E_f in W/cm² by Eqn. (23-13) and Eqn. (23-14) is:

$$\begin{aligned} E_f &= (0.1 \text{ W/cm}^2)(0.88)(40 \text{ m}^2) / (0.49 \text{ m}^2) \\ &= 7.8 \text{ W/cm}^2 \end{aligned}$$

where the total power P in the beam is 39 kW as the product of the reflectance of the heliostat mirror (0.88), the solar irradiance (0.1 W/cm²), and the area of reflectance in cm² by Eqn. (23-15). The beam irradiance in the focal spot of the largest heliostat that could be located at the outer radius of the field, e.g., on the 1000-m radius, with an appropriate focal length is calculated in the same way using Eqn. (23-16). E_f is only 45 mW/cm² at this distance since the focal area at that distance is 86.5 m². Obviously a flat mirror is superior at the greater distances.

Our own experience in working with searchlights indicates that skin and corneal irradiances of only 20 to 30 mW/cm² added to a direct solar irradiance of 100 mW/cm² would be very uncomfortable at an ambient temperature of 20° C. An additional irradiance of 7.8 W/cm² added to a whole-body irradiance of 0.1 W/cm² would produce temperature elevations in the skin to the threshold of pain within one second of exposure. As shown in Figs. (4-26) on page 148 and (5-1) on page 163, an irradiance of 5-20 W/cm² would be expected to result in skin and corneal burns for an exposure duration of the order of one second, although the blink reflex would probably protect the cornea. An individual would probably take evasive action within one to three seconds, although there is little laboratory data to support that time period—only common experience.

The analysis of the hazards to the retina is more complicated. It is simple enough to calculate the retinal irradiance E_r anywhere in the beam. From Eqn. 4-4 on page 123 it is simply:

$$E_r = 0{,}27\, \rho L_s\, \tau \cdot d_e^2 \qquad (23\text{-}16)$$

where d_e is the pupil diameter in cm², ρ the heliostat reflectance, L_s the projected radiance from the heliostat in W/(cm²·sr) and τ the transmittance of the ocular medium. The total radiance of the sun as viewed near zenith from sea level is approximately 1600 W/(cm²·sr), or 1000 W/(cm²·sr) between 400 nm and 1400 nm. The average transmittance of the ocular media for the solar spectrum is taken to be 0.74 and the pupil diameter when looking directly at the sun is 0.2 cm or less in the normal individual. Eccles and Flynn (1944) determined the pupil size in the human during direct staring at the sun to be 1.6 mm on the average. The retinal irradiance when looking at the heliostat (where the solar radiance has been reduced by the factor of $\rho-0.85$) is then 11 W/cm². The eye's natural aversion response to bright light, of the order of 0.13 to 0.2 s, is adequate to protect against direct viewing of the sun when the image is 158 µm. Moreover, the actual threshold of injury for a 0.13-s, 158-µm exposure in the human has been shown to be more than 10 times the value of 8 W/cm².

A retinal hazard analysis need only be concerned with the focal irradiance for a single heliostat, since the projected radiance for all of the heliostats is the same in theory. The only variable is the retinal image size which is crucial (see Fig. 6-14 on page 208). Of course the reflected beam irradiance varies outside of the focal spot. An individual standing in the focal area of a heliostat and looking back at the sun's projection would see the reflector "flashed" in at least one dimension. That is to say, he would see a reflector having a radiance of ρL_s. The image of the sun would fill the full reflector area at normal angles of incidence. At intermediate distances the sun's image would have a radiance of ρL_s but the image would not fill the reflector's area. The product of the projected radiance of the sun and the solid angle of the source Ω_s in steradians would be the beam irradiance at that point. If two heliostats were oriented so that an individual would be in the focal spot of both, the irradiance at his cornea would be the sum of the two focal irradiances, but he would see two separate images, each having a radiance of ρL_s. The Law of Conservation of Radiance prohibits overlap of the images on the retina. This is just the same as viewing the sun through magnifying optics (e.g., a binocular). The retina cannot be exposed to a greater irradiance viewing the sun through optics than with the unaided eye. Collecting optics only increase the retinal image size and reduce the retinal irradiance by the loss factor of the optical system, in this case a reduction of at least 5%.

As discussed in Section 4.5.6 (page 130), studies of thermal injury to the retina have shown that the threshold of injury decreases approximately as the inverse of the retinal image size, and this is reflected in Eqn. (10-3) on page 399. This dependence is clearly valid for exposure durations of 0.1 s to 10 s. Therefore, to estimate the same degree of risk for a magnified view of the solar disk as a view of the solar disc as a view of the sun unaided by optics, one can express the maximal safe retinal irradiance E_r by the following formula:

$$E_r \text{ (safe)} = (1.7 \text{ mm}/d_r) \text{ W/cm}^2 \qquad (23\text{-}17)$$

where d_r must be expressed in millimeters. Hence, the comparable risk level for a 1-mm image is 1.34 W/cm². This formula provides an irradiance ten times below that found to cause injury within the normal aversion response (blink reflex) time of 0.13 to 0.2 s. The largest heliostat retinal image size can be calculated by the following formula which could be derived either by simple trigonometry or by the Law of Conservation of Radiance. At the focal spot:

$$\begin{aligned} d_r &= f_e \cdot D_h/f & (23\text{-}18) \\ &= f_e \cdot D_h \cdot \phi/D_f \\ &= (17 \text{ mm}) (9.3 \times 10^{-3} \text{ rad}) D_h/D_f \\ &= (0.16 \text{ mm}) D_h/D_f \end{aligned}$$

where f_e is the focal length of the eye (1.7 cm), f the focal length of the heliostat, D_f the width of focal spot, and D_h the width of heliostat. For the heliostat with the shorter focal length (75 m), D_f was 70 cm and the width of the square (40-m² area) reflector was 6.3; therefore, from Eqn. (23-15) the largest retinal image size would be:

$$\begin{aligned} D_f &= (0.16 \text{ mm}) (630 \text{ cm}) (70 \text{ cm}) \\ &= 1.4 \text{ mm} \end{aligned}$$

By Eqn. (23-18) a safe retinal irradiance is 0.76 W/cm², or 10% of the normal, unaided viewing irradiance. The darkest shade of sunglasses reduces the luminance of a white-light source by this amount. Thus, commercially available dark sunglasses would protect an individual in the heliostat beam on the same footing as any unprotected person standing outside in daylight unless his pupils are dilated when shaded by the sunglasses. Even if the pupils are not constricted to 2 mm (usual in daylight) a very significant safety factor below retinal injury thresholds is present for momentary viewing. However, the most serious hazard clearly exists if one is within the focal length of several heliostats.

If the ACGIH criterion of Eqn. (10-3) is applied to a 0.25-s exposure, L (Haz) for the shorter focal-length reflector would be 24 W/(cm² · sr), since α would be (6.3)/(75) or 0.084 rad. By this criterion, filter lenses with a maximal transmittance of 2.4%, should be worn, i.e., a shade 5 welding filter.

During normal operation, personnel on the ground would not be in the reflective beam of a heliostat. It is impossible to determine theoretically what would be the radiance of the diffuse reflection coming from the heliostats for an individual standing near the array. This would have to be measured. Nevertheless, this type of viewing situation should not present a hazardous condition. Scattered ultraviolet radiation could be of concern in the vicinity of the heliostats or tower; but again, measurements would be required to assess these potential problems.

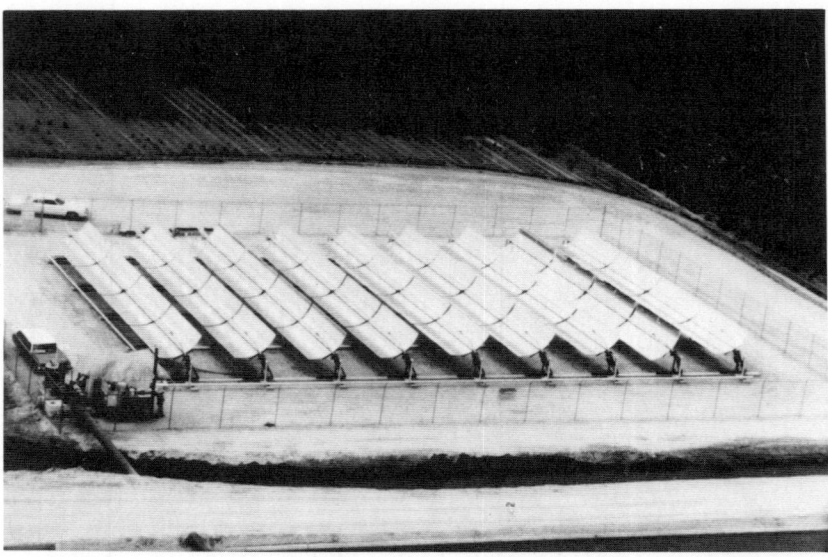

Figure 23-24. Cylindical-Mirror Solar Collector Array. These solar collectors are part of Northwestern Life Insurance Company's solar powered irrigation pump system which Battelle Memorial Institute helped develop. Note that a fence prevents entry of unauthorized personnel. No potential hazard could exist outside of the fence (Photograph courtesy of Battelle Memorial Institute).

During testing and alignment one might expect that the focal spot of the reflector could be on the ground, but even in this situation the normal aversion response of the eye would normally preclude a serious hazardous condition, unless many heliostats were directed toward the same location. A large-area, short-focal-length heliostat could produce sufficient irradiance to cause skin burns within 3 s. Only at the top of the central tower would a very serious personnel hazard exist, and this area should be declared a denied occupancy "Off Limits" area for personnel.

Personnel in aircraft could not simultaneously be in the center of focus of several heliostats, or even near a focal point without having other problems. In any case, since the aircraft would be moving, the duration of any exposure would be hazardous.

The hazards of a worst-case event for aircraft can be quickly calculated, if it is assumed that several adjacent heliostats were misdirected and aimed at a point in space beyond the central tower. The Law of Conservation of Radiance may be applied to estimate the radiance and image size of the sources seen by an observer in an aircraft passing through the beams. Our experience with projection systems indicates that the radiance of the sources would remain at approximately 1 kW/(cm^2·sr) wherever an observer is in the beam. Farther from the focal point, the image size will decrease. In other words, at the beam focal points, the images of adjacent heliostats would practically blend into one large image (if the heliostats themselves were practically touching), but the image areas would decrease in direct proportion to the decreased beam irradiance. By geometrical optics, it is easily argued that the beam irradiances due to a single heliostat at one focal distance beyond the tower on the opposite side must be less than "one sun" (0.1 W/cm^2). Also, the angular subtense of the source at this distance from the heliostat would be slightly less than the sun itself (9.3 mrad). The angular subtense α_H of the heliostat itself would be:

$$\alpha_H = D_h/2 \cdot f \qquad (23\text{-}19)$$
$$= 2 \text{ m}/200 \text{ m}$$
$$= 10 \text{ mrad}$$

for the smaller mirrors (5-m^2 area) and 28 mrad for the larger heliostats. Hence, one may conclude that for the smaller mirrors, that the retinal images from adjacent heliostats would almost be touching at two focal lengths from the heliostats. Using the same approach for a viewing distance of three or four focal lengths, it can also be concluded that the images at those viewing distances would be close to one another. On the other hand, the image of nine adjacent heliostats would have a total angular subtense of only three suns, which has been shown to be marginally hazardous for a 0.2-s exposure. For an aircraft observer, the viewing duration would not be so lengthy. The probability that so many heliostats could be misdirected to the same point in space seems sufficiently remote to discount such a hazardous event.

The risk of accidental injury to the skin and eye can be reduced if the areas of the shorter focal-length heliostats near the tower are limited to a few square meters. This would limit the focal beam irradiance for any heliostat to a level where the aversion responses to bright light and to skin temperature elevations would offer sufficient protection.

A completely different type of solar heating or solar thermal power system utilizes cylindrical-mirror collectors (Figs. 23-24 and 23-25). A cylindrical mirror has a focal line, not a focal point. The absorber (a pipe) is placed along this line. An observer viewing from in or near the focal line would see a bright vertical line extending nearly from the top to the bottom of the mirror. The angular width of the line would be the angular subtense of the sun (9.3 mrad). The retinal image would be 158 μm wide and perhaps several mm long. This would be an extremely hazardous viewing condition, because of the strong dependence of injury threshold on image length (see Table 22-3, page 726). Fortunately, most such reflector systems are mounted above eye level and are of relatively short focal length. Hence, the eye hazard is limited to a very small area. Maintenance workers would have to be cautioned to avoid the focal zone whenever the mirror is aimed at the sun.

23.10 REVIEW QUESTIONS

1. State the Principle of Conservation of Radiance. Why is it useful in evaluating projector systems?

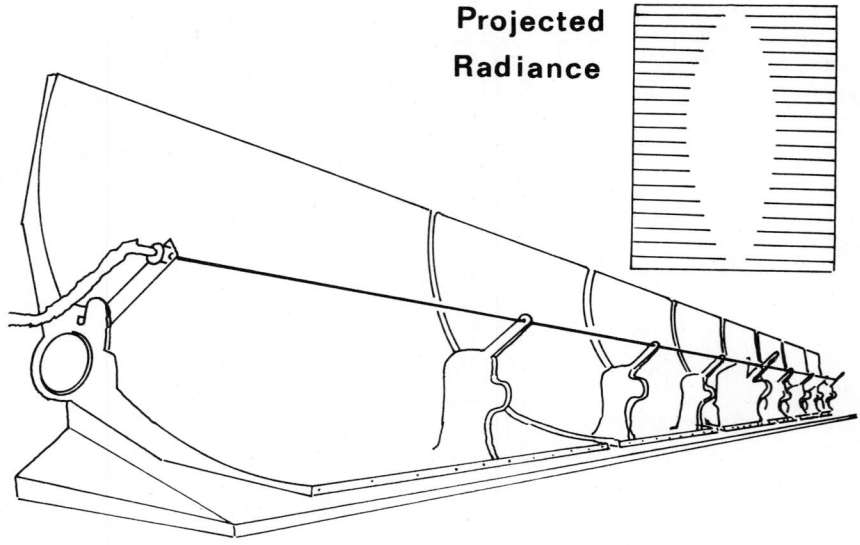

Figure 23-25. Projected Radiance of a Cylindrical Solar Collector. The projected reflected radiance of the sun would appear as a brilliant, narrow vertical strip to an observer near the mirror axis only, as shown in the upper right inset.

2. A searchlight has a beam luminous intensity of 40,000,000 cd and a luminous efficacy of radiation of 110 lm/W. What is the beam illuminance and irradiance at 135 m from the searchlight? What is the beam radiant intensity?

3. A xenon-arc searchlight uses a 1000-W Xenon-arc lamp with an arc spot of 2 mm. The searchlight reflector has a focal length of 20 cm and a clear aperture of 30 cm. What is the flash distance? What is the beam spread? If the land radiance is 1.2 kW/(cm² · sr), what is the irradiance in the near field?

4. A 10-cm diameter magnifying glass with a focal length of 25 cm focuses the rays of the noon-day summer sun on a person's forearm. What is the focal spot diameter and the focal spot irradiance?

5. What is meant by *Maxwellian view*?

6. What is the maximal *absorbed* retinal irradiance for a 3200-K tungsten-filament slit lamp if the slit is imaged on the retina through a 6-mm pupil and the optical

transmission of the slit-lamp projection optics is 0.62?

7. The zenith angle of the sun is normally large when the sun is directly viewed (Chapter 6) and man has adapted to these conditions. What are the implications of this adaptation for solar energy collection systems?

8. The corneal irradiance from an infrared diode (930 nm) used in an eye tracker is 12 mW/cm^2 and the retinal image size is 2.1 mm. Does this device pose an eye hazard?

9. A 50-cm diameter searchlight at 110 m (in the far-field) has an axial beam irradiance of 3.8 mW/cm^2. What is the radiance of the searchlight? If $\bar{R}$ is 1.6, what is the hazardous momentary (0.25-s) viewing distance?

10. Write a general expression for L (Haz) for a momentary (0.25-s) viewing condition for the ACGIH retinal thermal hazard criteria.

23.11 REFERENCES

Beck, W.C., and Heimburger, R. F., 1973, Illumination in the operating room, *Arch. Surg.* **107** (10):560–562.

Berger, D. S., 1969, Specification and design of solar ultravoilet solar simulators, *J. Invest. Dermatol.* **53**:192–199.

Born, M., and Wolf, E., 1970, "Principles of Optics," 4th ed., Pergamon Press, New York (especially pp. 188–190).

Calkins, J. L., and Hochheimer, B. F., 1980, Retinal light exposure from ophthalmoscopes, slit lamps, and overhead surgical lamps: an analysis of potential hazards, to be published in *Invest. Ophthalmol. Vis. Sci.*, **19**(9): 1009–1015.

Calkins, J. L., and Hochheimer, B. F., 1979, Retinal light exposure from operation microscopes, *Arch. Ophthalmol.*, **91**(12), 2363-2367.

Eccles, J.C., and Flynn, A.J., 1944, Experimental photo-retinitis, *Med. J. Australia* **1**:339–342.

Fuller, D., Machemer, R., and Knighton, R.W., 1978, Retinal damage produced by intraocular fiber optic light. *Am. J. Ophthalmol.*, **85**:519–537.

Haith, M., 1969, Infrared television recording and measurement of ocular behavior in the human infant, *Am. Psychologist*, **24**:279–283.

Ham, W.T., Jr., and Sliney, D.H., 1978, "Physiological Effects of Redirected Solar Radiation," Report ER-651, Research Project 955-1, Prepared with Black and Veatch Consulting Engineers for the Electrical Power Research Institute, Palo Alto, CA. (August, 1978).

Hildebrandt, A.F., and Vant-Hull, L.L., 1977, Power with heliostats, *Science*, **197** (4309): 1139–1146.

Hochheimer, B. F., D'Anna, S. and Calkins, J. 1979, Retinal damage from light, *Am. J. Ophthalmol.*, **88**(6), 1039-1044.

Howett, G. L. , Kelly, K.L. and Pierce, E.T., 1978, "Emergency Vehicle Warning Lights," NBS Special Publication 480-16, U.S. Department of Commerce, National Bureau of Standards, Washington, D.C., (September, 1978).

Howett, G.L., 1979, "Some Psychophysical Tests of the Conspicuities of Emergency Vehicle Warning Lights," NBC Special Publication 480-36, U.S. Department of Commerce, National Bureau of Standards, Washington, D.C.,(September, 1978).

Illuminating Engineering Society, 1958, I.E.S. Guide for photometric testing of searchlights, *Illum. Eng.*, **53**(3):155–162.

Johnson, J., 1962, Zero-length searchlight photometry system, *Illum. Eng.*, **57**(3):187–194.
Kaufman, J.E., and Christensen (eds.), 1972, "IES Lighting Handbook," 5th edition, Illuminating Engineering Society, New York.
Klein, M.V., 1970, "Optics," John Wiley and Sons, New York (especially pp. 135–139).
Machemer, R. and Aaberg, T.M., 1979, "Vitrectomy," Grune and Stratton, New York.
Merchant, J., and Morrisette, R., 1974, Remote measurement of eye direction allowing subject motion over one cubic foot of space, *IEEE Trans. Biomed. Eng.*, **BME-21**:309–317.
Parel, J.M., Machemer, R., and Aumaye, W., 1974, A new concept for vitreous surgery, IV. Improvements in instrumentation and illumination, *Am. J. Ophthalmol.*, 77(1):6–12.
Projector, T.H., 1953, Versatile goniometer for projection photometry, *Illum. Eng.*, 53(4)192–198.
Sensintaffar, E.L., Sliney, D.H., and Parr, W.H., 1978, An analysis of a reported occupational exposure to infrared radiation, *Am. Industr. Hyg. Assn. J.*, 32:415–431.
Sigmund, M., 1977, Plastic optical systems for electronics, *Electro-Opt. Syst. Des.*, 9(8):36–39.
Sliney, D. H., Bason, F.C., and Freasier, B.C., 1971, Instrumentation and measurement of ultraviolet, visible and infrared radiation, *Am. Industr. Hyg. Assn. J.*, 32:415–431.
Sliney, D. H., and Freasier, B.C., 1973, Evaluation of optical radiation hazards, *Appl. Opt.*, **12**(1):1–24.
Waldram, J.M., 1952, The photometry of projected light, *Illum. Eng.*, 47(3):397–401.
Walsh, J.W.T., 1965, "Photometry," 3rd ed., Dover Publications, New York.
Welford, W.T., and Winston, R., 1978, "The Optics of Nonimaging Concentrators, Light and Solar Energy," Academic Press, New York.
Wolbarsht, M.L., Landers, M. B., III, Wadsworth, J.A.C., Anderson, W. B., Jr., 1976, "Retinitis Pigmentosa: Clinical management based on current concepts, *in* Retinitis Pigmentosa: Clinical Implications of Current Research, M. B. Landers, III, M. L. Wolbarsht, J. E. Dowling and A. M. Laties, eds., Plenum Press, New York, pp. 181-196.

Chapter 24
Welding Arcs

24.1 INTRODUCTION

Surely the greatest population of personnel exposed to intense sources of optical radiation would be welders and welders' helpers. The American Welding Society (AWS) estimates that there may be as many as 500,000 welders in the USA (Emmett and Horstman, 1976). There are two broad categories of welding equipment—gas (acetylene) welding equipment and electric-arc welding equipment. A gas welding or cutting torch has a luminance not much greater than a candle flame, typically ranging from 1 to 20 cd/cm^2, and the ultraviolet emission is quite small. The optical radiation hazards of such torches are virtually nonexistent. Welding filter goggles used with such torches are to reduce glare, and generally are little more darker than very dark sunglasses having a shade number of the order of 3 to 5 (visual transmittance of 5 to 15 percent). On the other hand electric welding arcs may be 1,000 times brighter than gas torches and emit ultraviolet radiation at proportionately greater levels. This chapter is devoted to the hazards and the protective measures associated with working with welding and cutting electric arcs and other open-arc processes such as plasma arc spraying and plasma torches. All of this equipment is used in heavy industry, principally for working with heavy plate steel and aluminum.

Few are the welders specializing in using arc welding equipment who have not, at least once in their life, experienced "welder's flash," the familiar term for *ultraviolet photokeratitis*, and the accompanying ultraviolet erythema or "skin burn." Yet retinal injury from staring at the arc, which has been shown in a few instances, is quite rare—probably due to the natural aversion response from viewing the dazzling arc.

The detailed measurements of welding arcs and other open-arc processes made it possible to corroborate the value of the ultraviolet envelope exposure limit for ultraviolet radiation which was discussed previously in Section 10. Where people received threshold photokeratitis or skin erythema it was sometimes possible to measure the exposure dose that they received and to compare these levels with the duration required to exceed the threshold limit value for ultraviolet radiation.

Protective shields, curtains, and screens for bystanders as well as welding goggles for the welder are the standard protective equipment used in welding. Protective procedures and protective equipment for the welder have been developed empirically over the last three quarters of a century. Only very recently have detailed measurements of the radiometric output of welding arcs been available. When these measurements were carefully compared with exposure limits being developed for protection against bright light sources, it was shown that the empirically-developed protective equipment standards are in fact well founded. This chapter will review the hazards and give a case history of one retinal injury from a welding arc; summarize the knowledge of the output characteristics of different types of welding arcs; and consider the protective procedures and protective clothing recommended for arc welding and related open-arc processes.

24.2 WELDING ARC CHARACTERISTICS

The most common high-intensity arc is probably the welding arc. These arcs vary in brightness and in ultraviolet radiation content, primarily as a function of arc current, shielding gas, and the metals being welded.

24.2.1 Types of Welding Arcs Processes

There are a variety of different welding arc processes and cutting processes which vary in their ultraviolet and visible light output. Table 24-1 summarizes the principal techniques and the standard nomenclature used by the American Welding Society (AWS). Although arc currents vary from approximately 50 amperes up to nearly 1,000 amperes for different processes, there is no one process that covers this entire range of currents. For instance Gas Tungsten Arc Welding (GTAW) on soft metals such as aluminum may use only 50 amperes; however a very high-powered plasma cutting (PAC) torch may exceed 1,000 amperes.

Arc welding requires a large current, generally of a relatively low voltage after the arc has been struck. The arc is struck between an *electrode* and the workpiece—the *base metal*. The electrode may have either a largely non-consumable metallic tip or it may be a consumable rod of carbon or a consumable metal rod or wire. In some processes, a separate wire or rod—a *welding rod**—may be used to supply *filler metal*. Welding does not necessarily require the addition of filler metal from a consumable electrode or welding rod. Fusion of two metal surfaces can be produced with only the high temperature of the arc. Some welding processes may employ automatic wire feed systems and be totally automated. In other semi-automatic operations, the welder must advance the welding arc along the workpiece, but the wire is fed automatically.

---

*The term "welding rod," as used by the AWS, applies to a rod of filler material that is not an electrode. It must not be confused with rod-shaped electrodes used in Shielded Metal Arc Welding.

Welding Arcs

TABLE 24-1. Arc Welding Processes

Welding Process	AWS Designation	Electrode	Shielding Gases	Remarks
Carbon Arc Welding	CAW	Carbon electrode	None	Earliest Process. No longer commonly employed in industry.
Shielded Metal Arc Welding (also known as "stick" welding)	SMAW	Consumable stick electrode	Some shielding. Gas produced from welding rod.	Common in the field and in small shops. Produces excessive fumes.
Gas Tungsten Arc Welding	GTAW	Noncomsumable tungsten electrode	Argon most common gas. Helium used for penetrating welds.	Relatively clean process
Gas Metal Arc Welding	GMAW	Consumable wire electrode	Argon, CO_2 and CO_2/Ar are typical	Metal flows across arc from electrode to workpiece
Flux Core Arc Welding	FCAW	Consumable wire electrode with flux core	External (e.g., CO_2) or flux generated gas	Variation of GMAW
Plasma Arc Welding	PAW	Nonconsumable tungsten electrode	Argon and others	Three principal modes: melt-in, keyhole, and needle arc

Many electric arc welding processes make use of a direct current (dc) rather than alternating current. In any direct-current arc the specifications of polarity can be very important. If the electrode is a cathode and is negative (dcen), the AWS refers to this as *direct current straight polarity*, or DCSP. If the welding electrode is an anode, or electrode positive (dcep), this is referred to as *direct current reverse polarity* (DCRP). In the normal DCSP condition the base metal being bombarded by the electrons is hotter than the electrode and a deep, "penetrating" weld is produced. In contrast, DCRP produces a wider, shallower weld and the electrode is hotter than the base metal. An ac arc will produce intermediate characteristics of DCRP and DCSP welds since the arc polarity reverses every half cycle. The advantages and disadvantages of all of these different modes is the subject of welding texts (e.g., Weisman, 1976) and will not be discussed here.

24.2.1.1 The Carbon-Arc

Carbon-arc welding (CAW) and carbon-arc cutting (CAC) were the first arc welding and cutting processes. They were developed near the close of the nineteenth century. These processes, although uncommon today, are still employed in some special applications. A carbon electrode is typically the cathode and the base metal is the anode. The intense heat of the arc melts the surfaces of the base metal to be joined. Often a separate filler rod (the "welding rod") is also used. In air-carbon-arc cutting (AAC) a high pressure stream of air at about 550 kPa blows away the molten metal through the kerf. The *kerf* is the slot cut in a metal plate. The carbon electrodes are generally coated with copper to increase current capacity. AAC is one of the more common arc cutting and gouging processes.

24.2.1.2 The Shielded Metal Arc

Shielded-Metal-Arc Welding (SMAW) evolved from CAW when it was realized that the carbon electrode could be replaced by a consumable electrode—eliminating any need for a welding rod. To reduce oxidation, the electrode wire is coated with materials such as fluorides, oxides, carbonates, metal alloys, and binders to stabilize the arc, to produce gases to shield the weld from oxygen and atmospheric contaminants, and to introduce metals to alloy the weld (Weisman, 1976). SMAW is used principally with nickel and ferrous base metals. The electrodes are typically 2 to 6 mm (3/32 to ¼ inch) in diameter and are controlled by the welder in a clamp-type *electrode holder*. Because of the rod shape of the electrode, SMAW is sometimes referred to as *stick welding*.

The arc is struck by the welder when he briefly touches the electrode to the work piece and withdraws it to an optimum gap. A very experienced welder can advance the rod and maintain an optimum arc gap that produces a reasonably stable optical emission for short periods of time. But the optical radiation emitted from this type of arc when the stick is held by most welders will fluctuate substantially with time. Figure 24-1 illustrates the time course of optical emissions from a SMAW arc and other arcs.

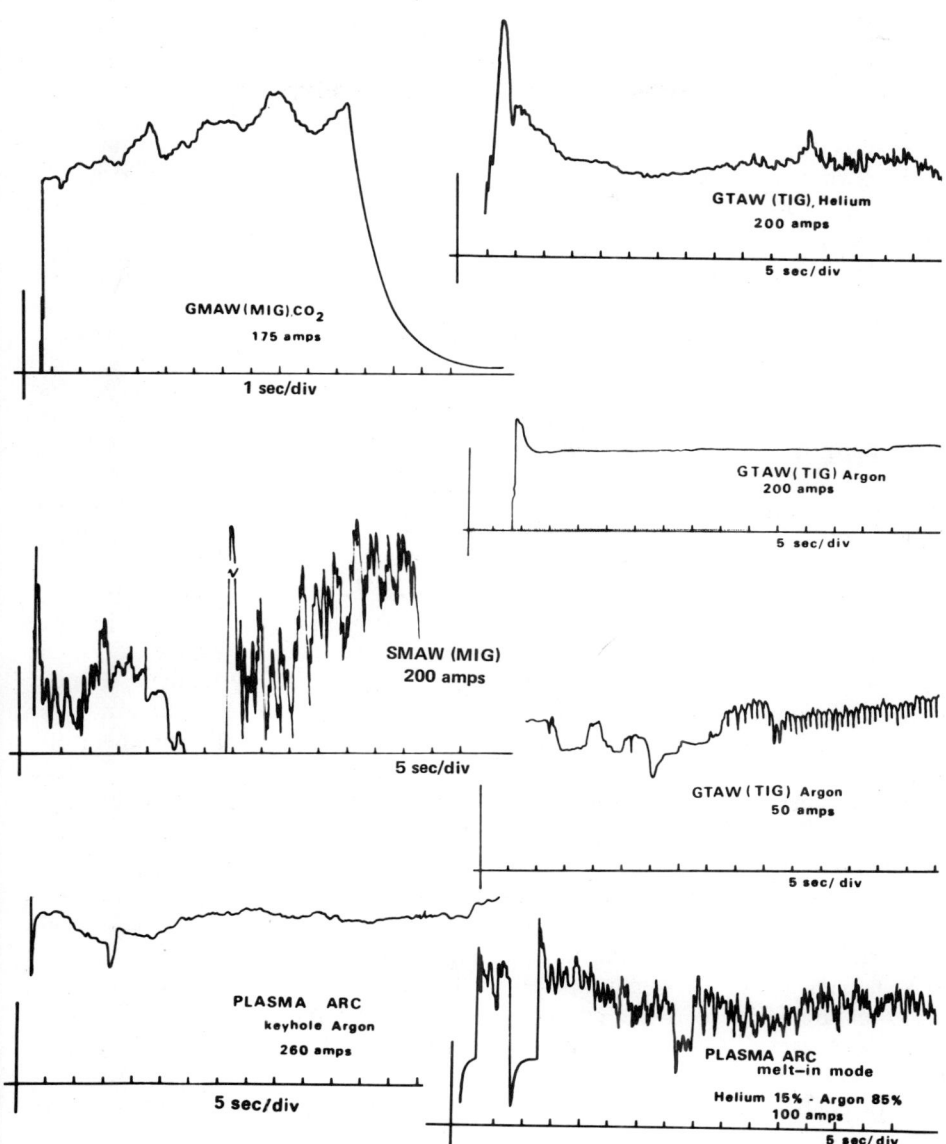

Figure 24-1. Arc Light Output Histories. The light output histories of a variety of arcs studied by Marshall *et al.* (1977) are shown. Because of the nature of the measurement study a great effort was made to minimize excursions in light output of these arcs. Note that hand-held SMAW (stick welding) shows the greatest arc instability. Note the wide fluctuation in SMAW compared to GTAW.

The principal advantage of SMAW is its cost and simplicity. Most arc welding machines found in home and garage use are SMAW machines. Such units often sell for less than $200, although portable, industrial units sell for more than $1,000. The size of the power supplies and cost make SMAW machines the favored units used in pipeline construction, heavy construction and shipbuilding. Most small power supplies operate between 30 A and 250 A, although some heavy units may have capabilities of 600 A. A shielded metal arc may also be used for cutting at higher currents and slower speeds to permit melt-though. It is then referred to as *shielded metal arc cutting* (SMAC). This is not a standard cutting process.

24.2.1.3 The Gas Tungsten Arc

During World War II a dramatically different types of welding process—originally called *heliarc* welding or *tungsten-inert-gas* (TIG) welding—was developed. Now properly termed *gas-tungsten-arc welding* (GTAW), this process was developed in the aircraft industry to permit effective welding of aluminum and magnesium alloys. GTAW employs a *nonconsumable* tungsten electrode and often a separate welding rod of filler metal. The lack of any flux meant that *slag* did not have to be removed from the weld as is required in SMAW.

An inert gas shield is provided through a concentric gas nozzle surrounding the electrode. Figure 24.2 (left panel) illustrates the process. Because of the requirements for compressed gas, a specialized welding gun, and more sophisticated current regulation equipment, this process is found most often in heavy industry. Helium was used predominantly at first (hence the term "heliarc"), whereas argon is now far more common as the inert gas. Helium, because of its higher ionization temperature, produces a hotter arc and is still preferred (despite its high cost) for specialized applications where a deeper penetrating arc is desired. Regardless of the shielding gas used, GTAW is generally regarded as the process which produces the highest quality conventional weld.

GTAW machines have more sophisticated constant current power supplies. A high frequency starting current is often used to strike the arc so that the electrode is not required to initially touch the base metal. High frequency is also employed with ac GTAW where it is superimposed on the 60-Hz ac current (ACHF condition) to maintain arc ignition. Power supplies used for GTAW range from moderate units with a 200-A capacity which may draw as much as 8 kW, to 500-A units which can require 30-kW service.

Gas tungsten arc cutting (GTAC) would probably use the same arc producing equipment as GTAW, but is run to permit burn-through of the base metal. As in other arc cutting (AC) procedures, the arc is largely burried in the base metal and the optical radiation emitted is thereby greatly reduced. GTAC is not a commonly used AC process.

24.2.1.4 Gas Metal Arc Welding

Gas-metal-arc welding (GMAW) is one form of *metal-inert-gas* (MIG) welding.

Welding Arcs

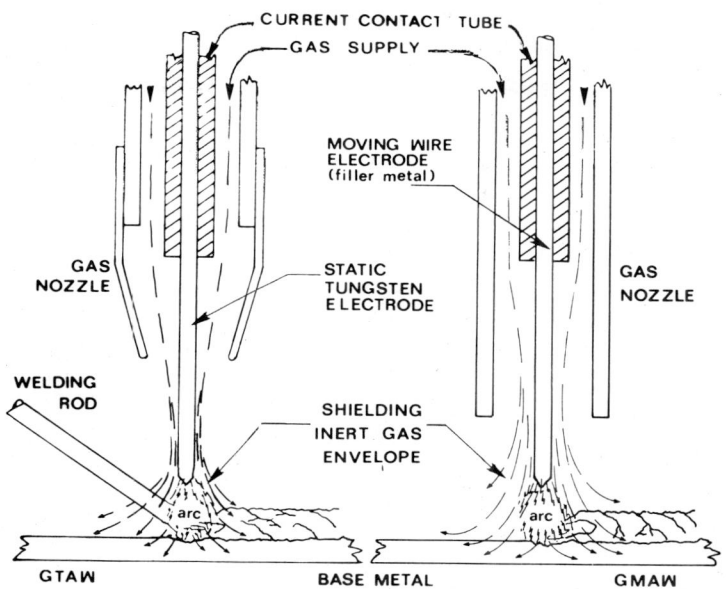

Figure 24-2. Geometry of Inert Gas Welding Heads. The GTAW process (left) and the GMAW process (right) differ in that a consumable electrode is used in GMAW. The inert gas shield (e.g., Ar or He) helps stabilize the arc and eliminates atmospheric contamination at the weld (after Wooding, 1953).

GMAW was an outgrowth of the development of GTAW. As in the GTAW process, an inert shielding gas such as argon, helium or CO_2 enshrouds the arc, but the GMAW electrode is consumable wire (right-hand panel of Figure 24-2). GMAW is a much faster process than GTAW.

Since metal is being transferred from the electrode and deposited in the weld, the nature of this transfer can greatly affect the arc characteristics and resultant weld. Specialized GMAW current modes are used to achieve specific forms of metal transfer. *Spray transfer* GMAW with an argon-shielded, high-current, DCRP arc produces a fine "spray" of metal droplets at rates of hundreds per second. In spray transfer there is little apparent "sputtering" of the arc because of the smooth transfer of metal. This results in a rather stable emission of optical radiation. In the *pulsed arc* (GMAW-P) the spray of droplets is produced primarily during high-current pulses, although a steady arc sustaining current exists between pulses. In the *buried arc* process, CO_2-rich gas mixtures are used to inhibit spray transfer and create globular metal transfer (with resulting spatter); the arc is often "buried" in its own crater in the steel with less optical radiation emitted. The *short-circuiting arc* (GMAW-S) process for welding thin sections also produces a train of high-current pulses resulting from a controlled short circuit at least every 20 ms.

The various GMAW variations probably account for the largest volume of industrial welding. This is surely true if one includes the sister process, FCAW. These two type of MIG welding are considered the most effective of filler-type welding methods (Weisman, 1976).

Gas metal arc cutting (GMAC) uses the GMAW welding machine to achieve burn-through, but this is not a common AC process.

24.2.1.5 Flux Cored Arc Welding

Flux-cored-arc welding (FCAW) is a variation of metal-inert-gas (MIG) welding where the electrode wire is replaced by cored wire—a fine electrode tubing filled with flux. The flux may produce the shielding gas *(self shielding)*; however, external gas shielding (often CO_2), as in the GMAW arrangement (Figure 24-2) is frequently used. The power supplies, guns, and electrode feel rolls are essentially the same as those used in GMAW. Cored electrodes are most commonly 1.6 mm (1/16 inch) in diameter, although electrode diameters of 2.4 mm (3/32 inch) are also used.

24.2.1.6 The Plasma Arc

A more recently developed welding process—*plasma arc welding* (PAW)—resulted from progress in plasma physics during the 1950's and 1960's. Although requiring more sophisticated and more costly equipment, PAW features a more stable, more concentrated arc which permits faster welds of higher quality than most competing processes. A pilot arc of argon introduced through an orfice inside a nozzle assembly reaches very high temperatures and ionizes a blanket of shielding gases to produce a second, larger plasma. The larger plasma forms the tight, "transferred" welding arc which exists between a tungsten electrode and the base metal. Welding rod is sometimes used as in the GTAW process.

PAW techniques are generally of three variations: the *melt-in-mode*, the *keyhole mode* for a very penetrating arc, and the *needle arc* for low currents. The PAW arc, although rich in ultraviolet emission because of its high temperature, does not always emit high levels of optical radiation since it is often buried to a considerable extent in the base metal.

Plasma arc cutting (PAC) is a common AC process. At high currents of 600 to 1000 A, PAC is used to cut very thick plate steel in excess of 2 cm in thickness. The elongated, high-velocity jet arc that can be achieved in specialized plasma arc cutting nozzles makes this possible. The high-velocity jet forces molten metal through the kerf. Water injection is used to cool the workpiece. Sometimes UV absorbing dyes are added to this water. The high noise levels created by the plasma arc have led to the development of a water muffler which is a shield of flowing water which enshrouds the arc. The PAC power supply can be quite expensive due to the high open-circuit voltages required to maintain a high arc voltage. Gas mixtures for PAC generally make use of argon with hydrogen or hydrogen with nitrogen. As in other AC processes the arc is largely occluded from view by the base metal.

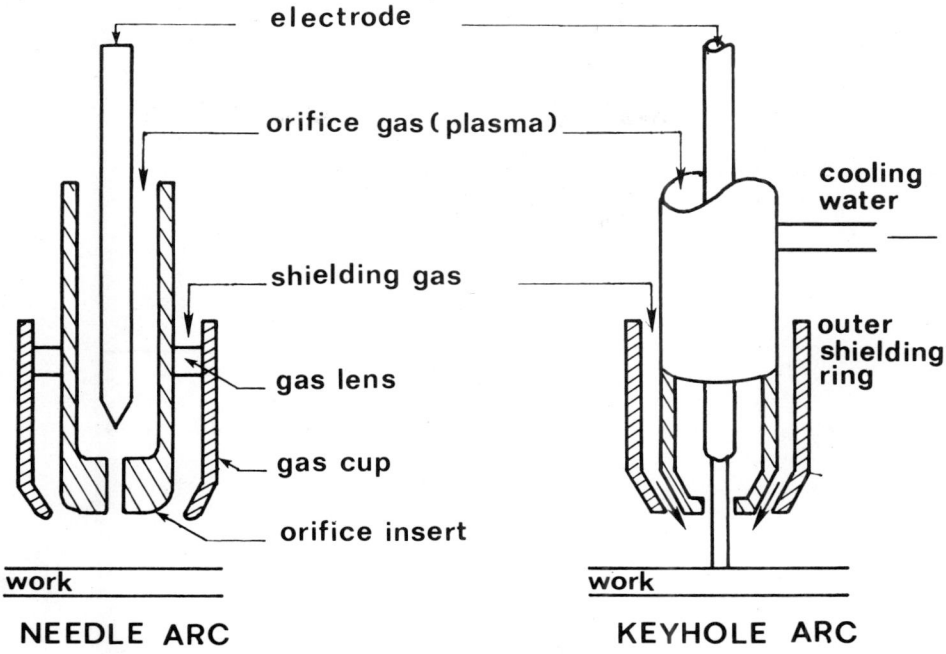

Figure 24-3. Plasma Arc Welding Torch. Argon flowing from the orfice forms the pilot-arc plasma. Shielding gas (e.g., Ar and He) is introduced through the encircling outer nozzle cup assembly. Adapted from catalogs of the Linde Division of Union Carbide Corporation.

Plasma arc spraying (PSP)—a surface treatment process—is one process where the intense plasma arc may be completely exposed. This results in exceedingly high levels of ultraviolet and visible radiation in the vicinity of this equipment.

24.2.2 Arc Size and Temperature Profile

The heated gas in the welding and cutting arcs may range from 5,000 to 30,000 K (and even 50,000 K). Glickstein (1976) studied welding arc temperatures in GTAW arcs as part of a careful study of GTAW plasma physics. For a 100-A arc with a 2-mm arc gap and a water-cooled copper anode, he found that the temperature ranged from approximately 8,000 K near the anode to 11,000 K near the cathode. For increasing currents the average, mid-plane arc temperature increased gradually from about 8000 K at 50 A to 11000 at 200 A for a 2-mm gap. Depending upon the temperature of the plasma, different spectroscopic lines will appear in the spectrum. The temperature can therefore be measured by looking for the presence or absence of certain lines. In fact, through the use of a rapid-scan spectroradiometer one can see the presence of some lines in ac welding arcs only during certain peak current periods. The increasing temperature with increasing current also predicts

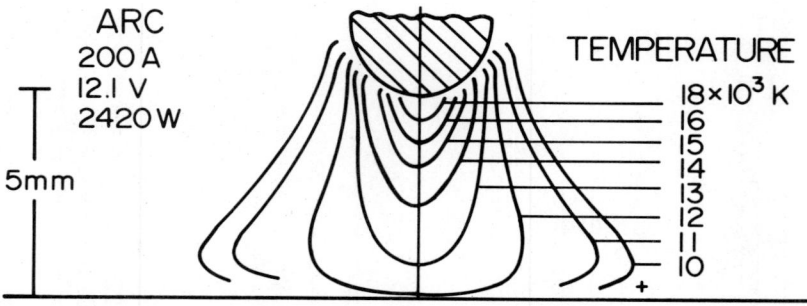

Figure 24-4. Welding Arc Isothermal Profile. The lines of equal temperature are for a 200-A, 5-mm argon tungsten arc (from Weisman, 1976, AWS Welding Handbook, with permission).

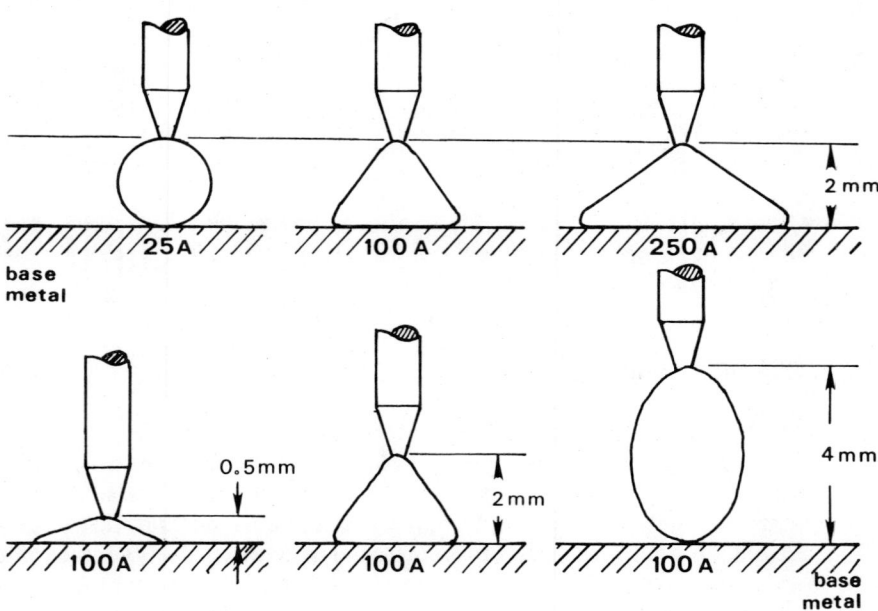

Figure 24-5. Welding Arc Shapes. The influence of current is shown in the top three simplified arc profiles and the influence of arc gap is shown in the bottom three profiles. The profiles are based on photographs taken of argon tungsten arcs by Glickstein (1976).

that the size of the plasma will increase. The arc width increased approximately as the current raised to the ¾-power in the Glickstein study. The arc temperatures for both a cooled anode and a stationary molten anode were found to be the same.

The AWS *Welding Handbook* (Weisman, 1976) shows a somewhat higher average temperature for a 5-mm arc gap for an argon tungsten arc (Figure 24-4). The arc profile of Figure 24-4 is similar in shape to those profiles (Figure 24-5) found by Glickstein (1976). The arc becomes elongated with increasing electrode gap and spreads out for both decreasing gap size and higher currents. Figure 24-6 shows iso-density traces of several arcs photographed by Marshall *et al.* (1977). Using such iso-density traces it is possible to develop the iso-luminance and iso-radiance distributions necessary for retinal hazard analysis. Note that the source size as defined at half-peak-luminance points or $1/e$-peak-luminance points is always smaller than the arc gap. Hence the central arc will amost always be a "point source" for all but the welder himself.

24.2.3 Optical Radiation Emitted from Welding Arcs

A large number of measurements of the spectra and radiance of welding arcs were performed by Lyon, Marshall, Sliney and their associates at USAEHA in conjunction with the American Welding Society (AWS) during 1975–1978 (Lyon *et al.*, 1976; Marshall *et al.*, 1977; Hinrichs, 1978). These measurements of more than 100 different arcs revealed that there are several fundamental relationships between arc current and type of welding arc. These relationships put a scientifically sound basis under the recommendations for limiting exposure duration for unprotected ancillary personnel and visitors as well as the recommendations for eye protection and skin protection for welders. The principal difficulty in performing reliable spectroradiometric, radiometric and photometric measurements of open arc processes relate to attaining a stable arc and eliminating electromagnetic interference from the arc. To reduce erroneous measurements from RF radiation generated by the various arcs, the instruments were either operated from internal batteries or from a constant voltage isolation transformer. Detector cables were shielded with coaxial braid and carefully grounded to the detector and readout chassis. These shielding techniques were periodically checked by placing a nonmetallic opaque shield over each detector aperture during operation of the arc. This assured that no instrument readings occured when optical radiation was blocked from a detector. Four spectroradiometers, two illuminance meters, a spot luminance meter, three ultraviolet irradiance meters and two irradiance meters were employed simultaneously to measure the arc characteristics and to permit direct intercomparisons. Figure 24-7 shows a photograph of the controlled experimental arrangement used for GTAW and GMAW measurements. Cold, degreased, rolled steel and aluminum was rotated under the arc gun to achieve a stable arc and constant arc gap. Such comprehensive measurements under the controlled conditions of welding engineering laboratories were made possible through the AWS Radiation Committee, the Union Carbide Corporation's Linde Division and other industrial concerns.

Figures 24-8 through 24-11 provide some characteristic spectra of welding arcs to indicate the range of values that may be expected. Of particular interest is the

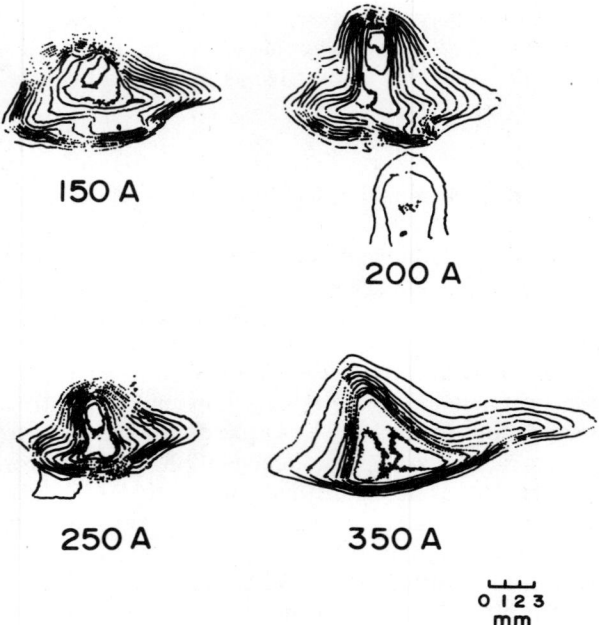

Figure 24-6. Welding Arc Iso-density Curves. These microdensitometer scans of welding arcs are iso-luminance traces. The contour intervals (CI) were typically about 0.16 density units. Hence, as one moves from the edge of the arc to the center each contour is 45% higher in luminance that the previous contour. The reflected arc luminance from the horizontal workpiece is sometimes evident.

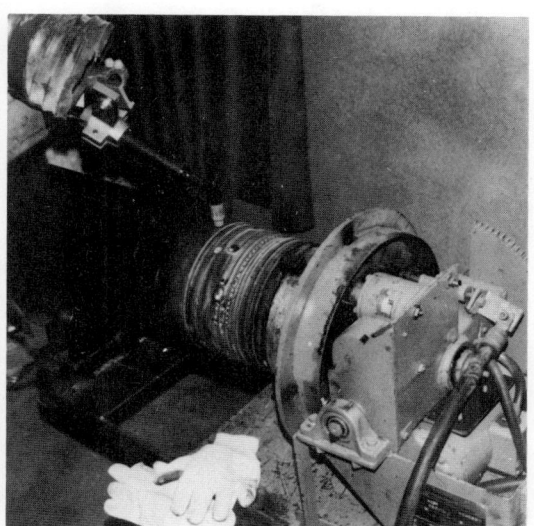 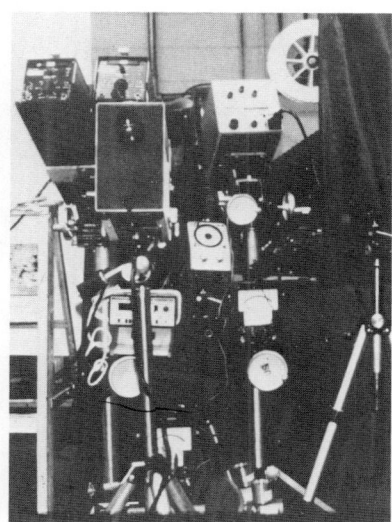

Figure 24-7. Welding Arc Measurements. A variable speed rotating pipe fixture (left) permits a stable arc with a constant arc gap. Radiometric and photometric detectors were placed one meter from the arc at an angle of maximum irradiance (right). Local exhaust ventilation removed as much of the welding fumes and vapors as possible.

fact that, although there is much structure in each spectrum due to the metals being involved and to the shielding gases, the average spectral irradiance does not vary greatly from the UV to the near-infrared and may be typically of the order of 1 μW/(cm^2·nm) at a distance of 1 m. There have been many attempts to measure the spectra and some attempts to measure the luminance of welding arcs; these are given in the reference list at the close of this chapter. Most of the measurements have been made for only a few typical arc currents.

Measuring a welding-arc spectrum achieves two primary goals. Absolute spectral irradiance values in the UV-B and UV-C when weighted against S_λ (the UV-Hazard Function; see section 10.3.4) provide the effective UV irradiance E_{eff} as shown in Figure 14.4, page 444. The permissible exposure duration for unprotected personnel (T_{max}) can then be calculated for that point where the measurement was made:

$$T_{max} = (0.003 \text{ J/cm}^2) / E_{eff} \qquad (24\text{-}1)$$

Measurements with UV-hazard meters are often less reliable (Section 14.8). The second use of the spectrum is to determine the relative fractions of visible and infrared, the luminous efficacy of the arc and to weight the visible spectrum against the

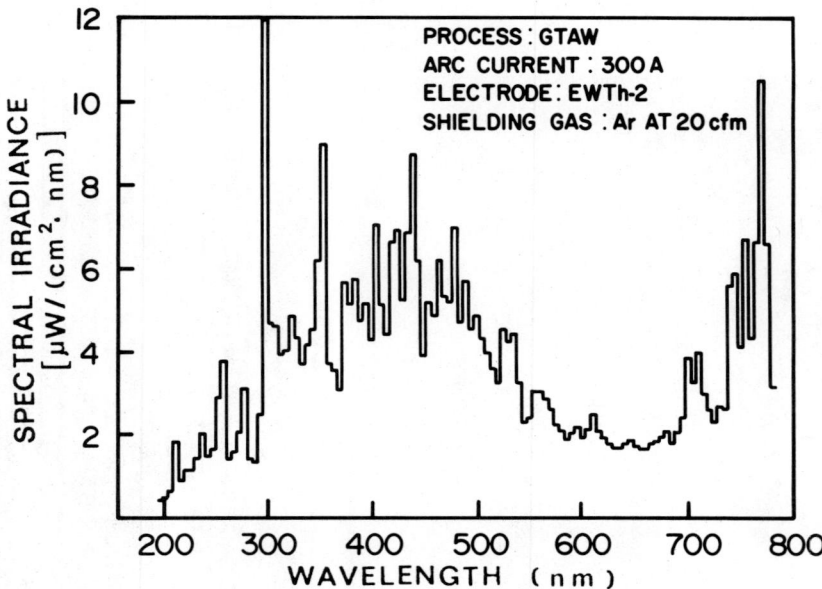

Figure 24-8. Gas Tungsten Arc Welding Spectrum for Argon Shielding Gas. Measurements were made at 100 cm from 1/16-inch arc on mild steel with 1/8-inch diameter electrode.

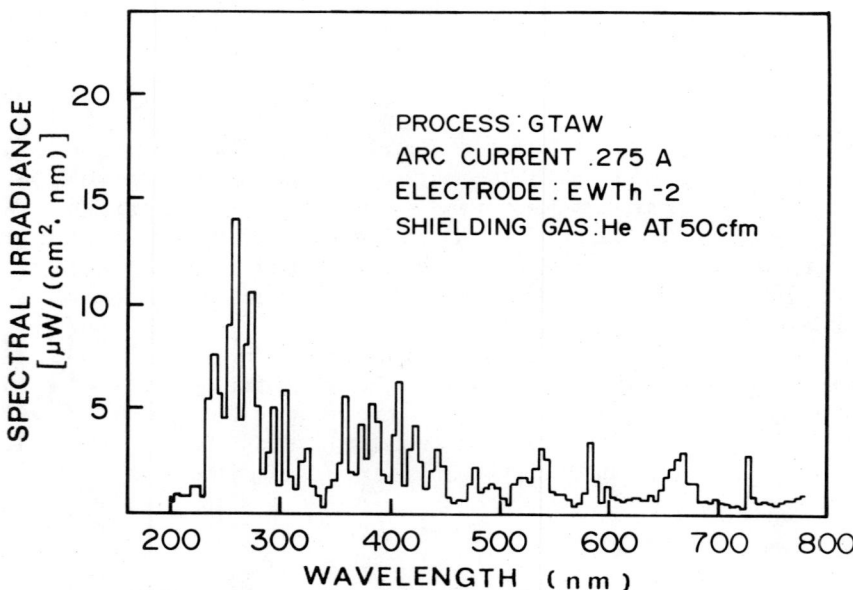

Figure 24-9. Gas Tungsten Arc Welding Spectrum for Helium Shielding Gas. Compare this spectrum with Figure 24-8 to show the influence of the shielding gas upon the spectral distribution. The measurement distance, arc gap, and electrode diameter were the same.

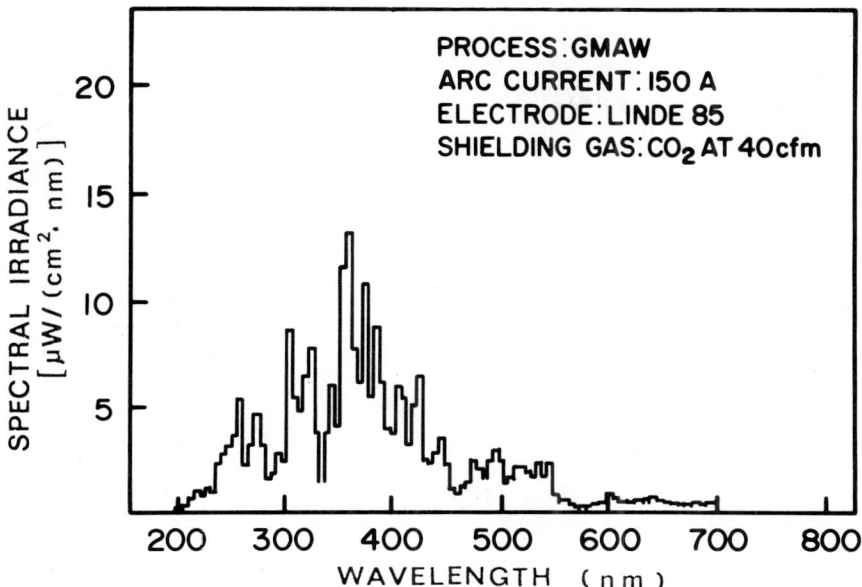

Figure 24-10. Gas Metal Arc Welding Spectrum for Carbon-Dioxide Shielding Gas. Measurements were made at 100 cm from arc on mild steel for 0.035-inch diameter electrode. Note the strong emission in the ultraviolet portion of the spectrum.

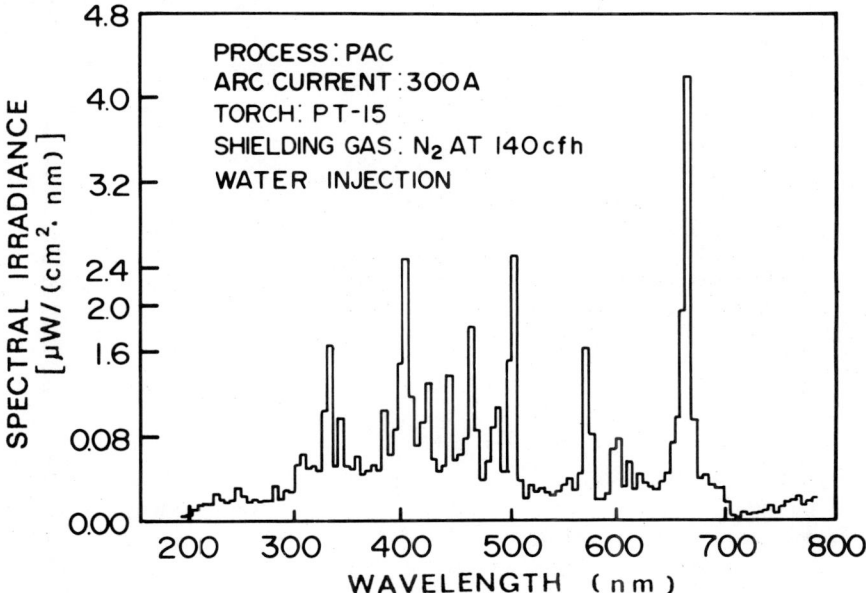

Figure 24-11. Plasma Arc Cutting Spectrum for Nitrogen Shielding Gas. Measurements were made at 190 cm from 1/4-inch arc on 5/8-inch thick mild steel with 0.156-inch diameter nozzle.

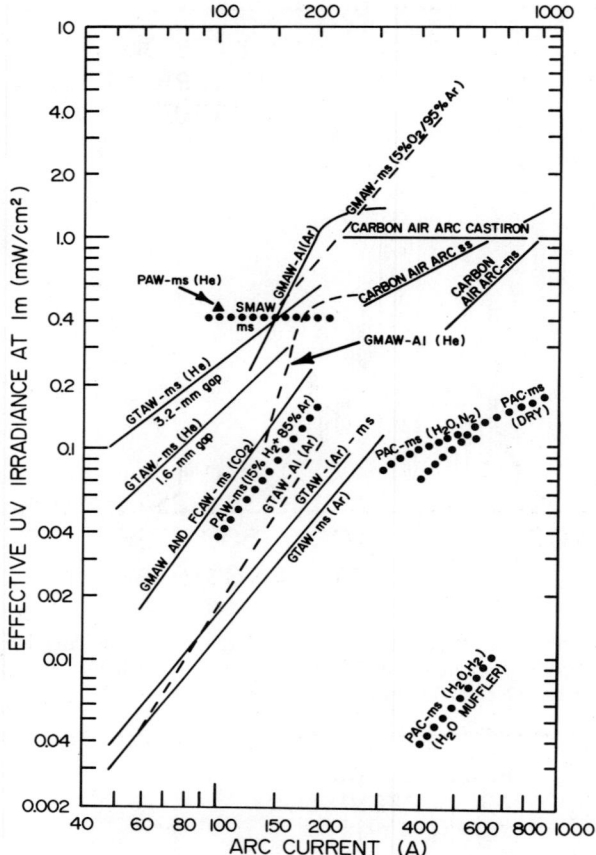

Figure 24-12. Effective UV Irradiance of Welding Arcs. The effective UV irradiances at one meter from a variety of welding and cutting arcs are shown as a function of arc current. The heavy dotted lines are values extrapolated from measurements made at approximately 2 m. Note the general trend of E_{eff} increasing as the square of the arc current. Departures from this approximate rule occur when the resistance across the arc changes appreciably or, as in the case of SMAW, when fume generation greatly reduces the UV flux density. The data shown are primarily from Lyon *et al.* (1976).

Blue-light Hazard Function, B_λ, which in conjunction with measurements of luminance and source size A_s (Figure 24-6) permits a determination using Eqs. 10-4 and 10-5 (or a corroboration) of the blue-light-weighted radiance L_B and the maximum time T_{max} for fixating upon the arc at close range:

$$T_{max} = [\ 100\ J/(cm^2 \cdot sr)\ ] / L_B \qquad (24\text{-}2)$$

Table 24-2 provides a summary of the principal measured and calculated characteristics of a large variety of arcs studied by USAEHA. Some of the arc currents and arc gaps listed in the Table would never be used in actual welding, but were chosen to obtain the data points required to understand the influence of different variables upon ultraviolet emission and luminance.

One of the primary motivations for the AWS/USAEHA studies was to characterize the ultraviolet radiation hazards of open arc processes. The effective UV irradiance was obtained from the spectral measurements and corroborated by several portable UV meters.

Figure 24-12 shows how the effective ultraviolet irradiance for most arcs varies approximately as the square of the arc current (Lyon et al., 1976). In no cases did this effective irradiance exceed:

$$E_{eff} \leqslant k_1 I_a^2 / r^2 \qquad (24\text{-}3)$$

where k_1 is 4×10^{-4} W/A² when E_{eff} is in W/cm², I_a is the current in A and r is the distance from the arc in cm. Note that exposed welding arcs produced the highest UV irradiances whereas AC processes and penetrating welding arcs emit less radiation for the same current. The large quantities of fumes produced by SMAW clearly reduced the UV emissions for the increased arc currents. The explanations for other departures from the current-squared relationship are not so clear. Obviously the optical radiant power available from the arc is limited by the electrical input power $I_a^2 \cdot R_a$, where R_a is the resistance across the arc. Hence, strong variations in the resistance across the gap should result in changes in arc emissions. The amount of radiated power is not available for heating the base metal and successful attempts to increase the efficiency of the arc in heating welding rods, base metals and consumable electrodes may be reflected in a reduction of optical radiation.

The primary contributor to excessive ultraviolet radiation from an arc is the combination of the specific shielding gas and the base metal used in the process. For instance, argon gas used in gas-metal-arc welding apparently is responsible for the very strong ultraviolet emission that is characteristic of that process. Note that GMAW of aluminum with Ar produces at least twice the UV as with He. GMAW and FCAW of mild steel with CO_2 produces the least UV for these processes. Remember that in GMAW there is metal transfer and metal is flowing through the arc. The use of helium as a shielding gas greatly increases the ultraviolet emission in PAW and GTAW of mild steel (ms). On the other hand, there is no difference in UV emissions from GTAW of aluminum with either He or Ar shielding gas. It is somewhat puzzling that the choice of shielding gas makes such an enormous difference in the ultraviolet emission from GTAW arcs when working with mild steel. Yet for GTAW of aluminum there is no difference in the ultraviolet radiation levels between He and Ar shielding. From an optical radiation hazard standpoint, the most hazardous processes for both skin erythema and photokeratitis at any given arc current appear to be argon-shielded GMAW for ferrous alloys and aluminum, and GTAW of ferrous alloys with He.

The size of the arc gap plays a role in UV emissions for GTAW arcs. This is quite evident for GTAW of mild steel with He and less dramatic with Ar as seen in

TABLE 24-2. Summary of Radiometric Measurements of the Welding Arcs.

Process	Base Metal	Current I (A)	Shield Gas	Arc Gap mm (in)	Luminance L_V (cd/cm^2)	Blue Light Radiance [W/(cm$^2 \cdot$sr)]	Radiance [W/(cm$^2 \cdot$sr)]	Arc Area (mm^2)	Effective † UV Irradiance (µW/cm^2)
GTAW	Steel	50	Ar	1.6 (1/16)	2.1 × 10^3	—	—	—	3.0
,,	,,	100	,,	,,	3.9 × 10^3	9.26	94.6	3.5	18
,,	,,	150	,,	,,	4.5 × 10^3	12	76.6	6.2	24
,,	,,	200	,,	,,	6.4 × 10^3	22.5	474	4.3	38
,,	,,	250	,,	,,	9.0 × 10^3	60.7	353	4.3	71
,,	,,	300	,,	,,	1.0 × 10^4	135	738	2.9	100
,,	,,	200	,,	,,	7.5 × 10^3	—	—	—	38
,,	,,	50	,,	3.2 (1/8)	2.5 × 10^3	8.65	60.4	2.3	2.7
,,	,,	100	,,	,,	4.2 × 10^3	—	*110	5.2	—
,,	,,	188	,,	,,	7.5 × 10^3	—	*160	9.5	—
,,	,,	300	,,	,,	6.3 × 10^3	45.2	345	8.3	120
,,	,,	250	He	,,	4.8 × 10^3	24.8	281	6.4	450
,,	,,	200	,,	,,	2.7 × 10^3	—	* 60	10	300
,,	,,	100	,,	,,	4.5 × 10^2	—	* 39	6.1	230
,,	,,	50	,,	,,	4.5 × 10^2	1.41	28.4	6.9	80
,,	,,	50	,,	1.6 (1/16)	2.4 × 10^2	4.38	75.3	1.9	40
,,	,,	100	,,	,,	1.5 × 10^2	—	* 15.9	8.8	150
,,	,,	200	,,	,,	3.6 × 10^2	5.22	* 81.4	4.3	290
,,	,,	275	,,	,,	3.3 × 10^2	28.9	47.2	25	270
,,	,,	300	Ar	4.8 (3/16)	9.0 × 10^3	—	183	19	110
,,	,,	200	,,	,,	7.5 × 10^3	—	—	—	60
,,	,,	100	,,	,,	4.6 × 10^3	9.63	54.2	9.9	18
,,	,,	200	,,	3.1 (1/8)	6.6 × 10^3	—	—	—	41
,,	Al	50	,,	,,	4.2 × 10^3	3.26	29.8	8.1	2.8
,,	,,	100	,,	,,	4.5 × 10^3	—	* 25.1	3.5	11
,,	,,	200	,,	,,	5.2 × 10^3	9.3	57.7	17	27
,,	,,	265	,,	,,	2.8 × 10^3	—	—	—	60
,,	,,	250	,,	,,	1.5 × 10^3	—	158	19	60
,,	,,	250	,,	4.8 (3/16)	1.5 × 10^3	—	* 37.6	82.4	86
,,	,,	250	,,	6.4 (1/4)	5.0 × 10^3	—	*112	40.3	—
,,	,,	200	,,	4.8 (3/16)	5.3 × 10^3	—	*102	26.5	42

Welding Arcs

Process	Material	Current	Gas	Electrode	Col6	Col7	Col8	Col9	Col10
"	"	100	"	"	2.5 × 10³	—	—	—	20
"	"	50	"	"	7.0 × 10³	—	—	—	3
"	"	50	He	"	4.4 × 10³	—	—	2.6	2.5
"	"	65	"	3.2 (1/8)	—	—	—	1.9	5
"	"	100	"	"	—	—	—	7.1	11
"	"	200	"	"	1.2 × 10³	—	—	—	90
"	"	200	"	4.8 (3/16)	—	—	—	—	90
"	"	150	"	N/A	—	—	—	—	16
GMAW	Steel	90	CO_2	"	8.3 × 10³	17.5	*19	1.2	49
"	"	150	"	"	—	53.7	*245	3.5	130
"	"	150	O_2 + Ar	"	—	—	*56	17.3	—
"	"	190	"	9.5 (3/8)	1.9 × 10⁴	—	131	13.9	650
"	"	200	"	6.4 (1/4)	2.4 × 10⁴	—	379	10.4	780
"	"	250	"	9.5 (3/8)	2.3 × 10⁴	64.5	*173	17.3	1300
"	"	260	"	6.4 (1/4)	1.9 × 10⁴	—	*321	9.5	1300
"	"	350	"	9.5 (3/8)	3.0 × 10⁴	—	709	3.5	1700
"	"	350	"	6.4 (1/4)	9.0 × 10⁴	—	*116	2.2	2300
"	"	350	CO_2	9.5 (3/8)	2.1 × 10⁴	—	*737	5.2	100
FCAW	"	250	"	N/A	1.0 × 10⁴	—	*2890	2.6	170
"	"	350	"	"	2.0 × 10⁴	—	*909	9.2	300
"	"	250	"	"	3.0 × 10⁴	—	*385	6.9	20
"	"	175	"	"	2.6 × 10⁴	—	*1540	19	21
GMAW	Al	300	Ar	6.4 (1/4)	1.6 × 10⁴	—	*489	34	1250
"	"	300	"	9.5 (3/8)	1.7 × 10⁴	—	*362	26.3	1150
"	"	300	He	6.4 (1/4)	1.1 × 10⁴	—	*289	21.8	500
"	"	200	"	"	5.4 × 10³	—	*131	27.5	500
"	"	200	Ar	"	3.9 × 10³	—	*114	19.4	1050
"	"	130	"	"	8.1 × 10³	—	*68.8	2.01	200
"	"	125	He	"	3.0 × 10³	—	*101	—	50
PAC/W	Steel	300	N_2	6.4 (1/4)	2.4 × 10³	—	*64.4	—	11
"	"	300	"	9.5 (3/8)	3.6 × 10³	—	*299	—	17
"	"	300	"	12.7 (1/2)	3.0 × 10³	—	*80.6	22	18
"	"	400	"	6.4 (1/4)	3.3 × 10³	—	—	—	15
"	"	400	"	9.5 (3/8)	1.5 × 10³	—	—	—	40
"	"	400	"	12.7 (1/2)	4.2 × 10³	—	82.4	36	11
"	"	500	"	9.5 (3/8)	4.5 × 10³	—	—	—	30
"	"	500	"	12.7 (1/2)	4.5 × 10³	—	—	—	13

TABLE 24-2. Summary of Radiometric Measurements of the Welding Arcs – (Continued)

Process	Base Metal	Current $I(A)$	Shield Gas	Arc Gap mm (in)	Luminance L_V [cd/cm^2]	Blue Light Radiance [W/(cm^2·sr)]	Radiance [W/(cm^2·sr)]	Arc Area (mm^2)	Effective † UV Irradiance (µW/cm^2)
PAC/W	Steel	600	N$_2$	9.5 (3/8)	6.9 × 10^3	—	—	—	27
,,	,,	600	,,	12.7 (1/2)	8.1 × 10^3	—	*224	54	32
,,	,,	750	,,	12.7 (1/2)	8.4 × 10^3	—	*978	15	42
,,	,,	1000	,,	12.7 (1/2)	4.5 × 10^3	—	—	—	55
,,	,,	1000	,,	19.0 (3/4)	4.8 × 10^3	—	—	—	70
PAC/W & Muffler	,,	400	N$_2$	6.4 (1/4)	1.4 × 10^2	—	—	—	0.5
,,	,,	400	,,	9.5 (3/8)	1.8 × 10^2	0.16	1.4	430	1.0
,,	,,	400	,,	12.7 (1/2)	2.1 × 10^2	—	* 2.8	142	1.1
,,	,,	600	,,	9.5 (3/8)	4.5 × 10^2	0.74	7.2	160	2.0
,,	,,	600	,,	12.7 (1/2)	1.1 × 10^3	—	* 8.5	142	2.7
PAW	,,	260	Ar	4.8 (3/16)	1.8 × 10^3	—	—	10	20
,,	,,	260	15% H 85% Ar	,,	1.2 × 10^4	—	—	8.3	30
,,	,,	240	,,	,,	9.9 × 10^3	—	—	—	9
,,	,,	275	,,	,,	1.1 × 10^4	—	*571	1.75	10
,,	,,	100	,,	,,	4.8 × 10^3	—	—	—	7
,,	,,	200	,,	,,	3.0 × 10^3	—	—	—	40
,,	,,	200	Ar	,,	3.0 × 10^3	—	*113	11.3	20
,,	,,	100	15% H 85% Ar	,,	6.9 × 10^3	—	—	—	9
,,	,,	100	He	,,	1.6 × 10^3	—	*333	1.92	110
,,	,,	200	,,	,,	6.9 × 10^3	—	—	—	—
SMAW	,,	100	None	3.2 (1/8)	1.5 × 10^3	8.94	68.4	30.9	60
,,	,,	100	,,	,,	—	2.17	45.3	23.2	10
,,	,,	100	,,	,,	1.3 × 10^4	—	* 26.8	44.7	110
,,	,,	200	,,	,,	2.7 × 10^4	—	*145	55.1	110
,,	,,	200	,,	,,	2.3 × 10^4	—	*111	71.9	25
,,	,,	200	,,	,,	4.1 × 10^4	—	* 85.5	46.8	50
AAC	,,	300	N/A	6.4 (1/4)	2.0 × 10^3	—	290	—	559

	Material	Current	Electrode	Irradiance				
"		500	N/A	9.5 (3/8)	4.6 × 10³	14	280	32	430
"		800	"	3.1 (1/8)	7.0 × 10³	3.2	81	100	750
"		600	"	6.4 (1/4)	6.0 × 10³	18	270	49	610
"		600	"	4.8 (3/16)	6.0 × 10³	1.8	150	85	280
"	Cast Iron	600	"	8.0 (5/16)	9.0 × 10³	11	—	150	990
"		800	"	6.4 (1/4)	5.0 × 10³	22	420	41	920
"		350	"	3.1 (1/8)	8.0 × 10⁴	—	—	160	740
"		350	"	3.1 (1/8)	1.1 × 10³	7.8	120	110	860
"		230	"	—	8.0 × 10⁴	4.2	140	71	910
"	Stainless	600	"	4.8 (3/16)	3.5 × 10⁴	2.6	310	49	640
"		800	"	4.8 (3/16)	7.8 × 10³	0.7	260	80	1100
"		300	"	3.1 (1/8)	1.0 × 10⁵	—	—	140	560
"	Al	220	"	3.1 (1/8)	—	—	—	—	100
"		400	"	—	2.0 × 10³	—	—	—	120
"		400	"	—	1.0 × 10⁴	—	—	—	200
"		600	"	—	6.0 × 10³	—	—	—	72
"	Steel	400	"	3.1 (1/8)	10 × 10³	—	—	—	600
"		400	"	4.8 (3/16)	1.0 × 10⁴	—	—	—	760
"		400	"	6.4 (1/4)	8.6 × 10³	—	—	—	1060

† The irradiance measurements for PAC, PAW and SMAW were at 200 cm; all others were at 100 cm.

Figure 24-12. In other processes the arc gap played no significant role and the curves in Figure 24-12 reflect data for differing arc gaps. In some cases a large nozzle will occlude much of the radiation from an arc where the gap is small.

In another study it was shown that even small quantities of magnesium (Mg) greatly increase UV emissions near 280 nm. In this study by Bartley, McKinnery and Wiegand (to be published), the spectral irradiance between 274 nm and 289 nm was carefully monitored as a function of arc gap and alloy being welded. This 15-nm wavelength interval was chosen because it includes the strong Mg ion emission lines near 280 nm. For aluminum alloys being welded by GTAW the UV emissions were 10 times greater for small arc gaps (1 mm) on Al with 1% to 2.5% Mg than for Al alloys with no Mg. GMAW of Al alloys showed the same effect. Al welding with 5% Mg wire produced 10 times the UV in the 15-nm spectral band than did Mg-free wire.

In the USAEHA/AWS studies repeated spectroradiometer scans were made for each arc condition to obtain the highest spectral line emissions. Some repeated scans showed lower spectral irradiance values because of accumulation of airborne contaminants. This was particularly apparent with SMAW. Table 24-3 shows that SMAW produces much more airborne contaminants than GTAW or GMAW. Devore (1973) reported that ultraviolet emissions increase when the arc was passed over a previously welded seam. This could have been a geometrically introduced effect or a result of increased filler metal at the arc pool.

Field measurements of ultraviolet radiation taken at different angles around welding stations in welding shops and production lines have revealed that joint geometry is a major factor that influences whether people in the vicinity receive hazardous levels of ultraviolet radiation. A bead-on-plate welding geometry where the arc is exposed and above the weld plane of the metal surface results in a maximum ultraviolet irradiance. On the other hand there are cases—a particularly good example being a plasma arc cutting torch—where the arc is actually buried in the metal plate, and very little ultraviolet radiation actually escapes from the area of the arc. One welding process—*submerged arc welding* (SAW)—where the arc is buried in granular flux—results in no measurable ultraviolet radiation in the vicinity of the arc. Thus, in practice the joint geometry in a given pass greatly influences the portion of the arc exposed to a viewer (Figure 24-13) and also the ultraviolet radiation emitted in the direction of the viewer. The radiation emitted in the directions where the arc is clearly exposed to view is normally at least one order of magnitude greater than that emitted in any other direction. For instance, if the arc is partially occluded within the gap between the two horizontal plates being welded, the greatest radiant intensity is in a plane running along the groove perpendicular to the plate surfaces; and within this plane it is the direction of the movement of the welding electrode as shown in Figure 24-13. This direction corresponds to the direction from which one can obtain a full view of the arc. In the direction above the seam, but away from the direction of the arc movement, a clear view of the arc is obstructed by the weld puddle.

The luminance of an arc does not appear to generally follow any simple rules since the size of the arc density may actually increase with increasing current to some degree (Marshall *et al.*, 1977). It has been suggested that this occurs because of the strong magnetic field created by the enormous current. Eventually the field

TABLE 24-3. Approximate Fume Generation Rates For Some Welding Processes and Electrodes*

Process	Electrode	Shielding Gas	Approx. Current Amps	Polarity	Approx. Fume Generation Rate g/min
		MILD STEEL TEST PLATE			
GTAW	EWTh-2	Ar	50–300	DCSP	less than 0.2
GTAW	EWTh-2	He	50–275	DCSP	less than 0.2
GMAW	E70S-4	CO_2	90–350	DCRP	0.2 – 0.4
GMAW	E70S-4	95% Ar, 5% O_2	150–350	DCRP	0.2 – 0.4
FCAW	E70T-1	CO_2	175–350	DCRP	0.9 – 1.3
SMAW	E6013	none	100–200	DCRP	0.9 – 1.2
SMAW	E7018	none	100–200	DCRP	0.5 – 0.7
SMAW	E7024	none	100–200	DCRP	0.3 – 0.5
		ALUMINUM TEST PLATE			
GTAW	EWTh-2	Ar	50–265	AC-HF	less than 0.2
GTAW	EWTh-2	He	50–200	AC-HR	less than 0.2
GMAW	E5356	Ar	150–300	DCRP	less than 0.2
GMAW	E5356	He	125–300	DCRP	less than 0.2

* Source: AWS Committee on Safety and Health, as reported in Marshall et al. (1977).

becomes so great (typically at 50 to 100 A) that it actually tends to confine the size of the arc. This more confined arc also provides a smoother welding process as there is a steady flow of metal globules in the welding site rather than the characteristic sputtering which is typical of lower current welding arcs. Figure 24-14 illustrates how the luminance of some GTAW arcs begin to increase—perhaps as this magnetic confinement of the arc takes place. The measured luminance of the other arcs seldom was as great as the GTAW of Al with Ar. The luminance values L_v (cd/cm^2) for all of the processes remained below a maximum value L_v (max) of:

$$L_v \text{ (max)} = k_2 \, I_a^2 \tag{24-4}$$

where k_2 was 2.0 cd/(cm$^2 \cdot$ W^2) if the arc current I_a was expressed in A.

The radiance of the arc varies in a fashion similar to the luminance although not as rapidly. The higher current arcs are hotter and are therefore richer in visible light. The luminous efficacy is greater for the hotter arcs. Figure 24-15 illustrates the high radiance of the GMAW-ms (CO_2) and PAW-ms (Ar) processes—two processes which did not have strong UV emissions. These arcs are sufficiently bright that a retinal thermal burn hazard could in theory exist if the source sizes were much larger. Indeed, if one were to observe such an arc without eye protection at close

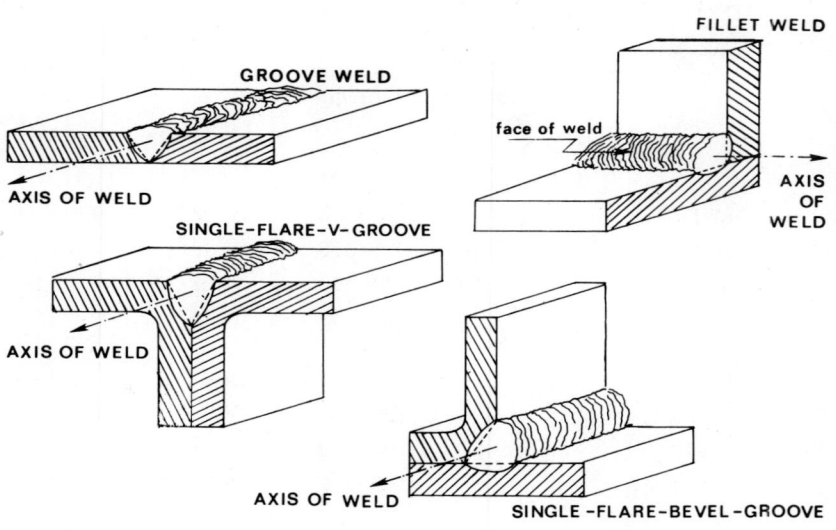

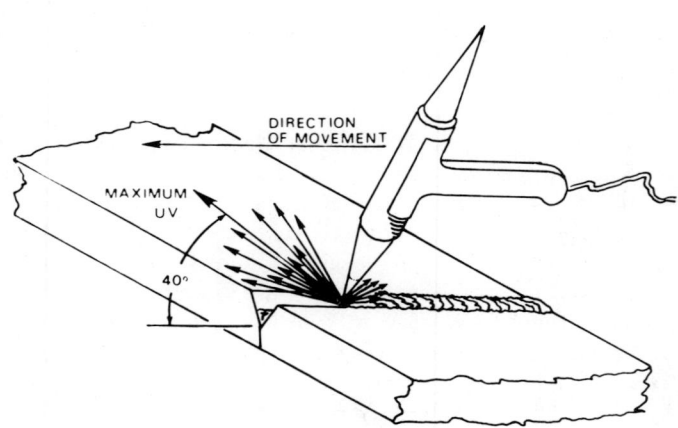

Figure 24-13. Weld Geometry. The type of weld—groove weld or fillet weld (top)— does not significantly effect the total UV emission unless the arc is obscured by the torch nozzle or the edge of a deep groove (bottom). The angle of maximum emission to the side of a seam occurs at about 40° from the plate surface. The maximum in the plane of the weld is in the direction of arc movement at an angle of 20° to 40° from the plane of the plate.

Welding Arcs

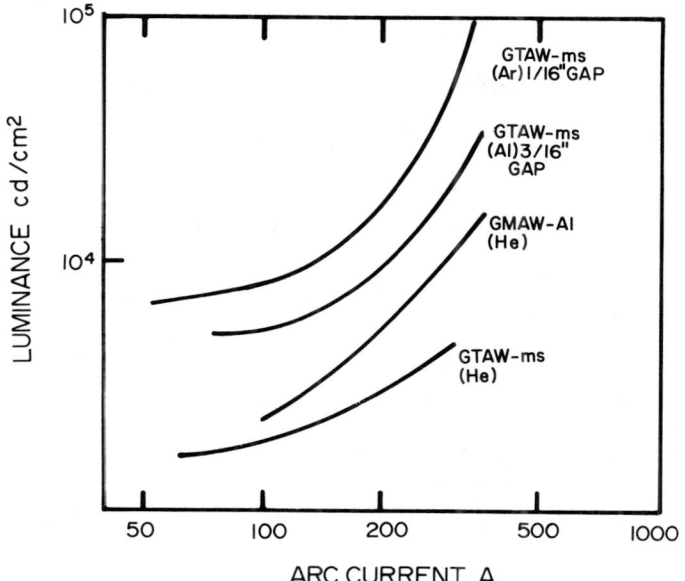

Figure 24-14. Luminance of GTAW Arcs. The peak luminance GTAW arcs on mild steel when shielded with argon increase rapidly at current between 100 A and 200 A. Increasing the arc gap from 1.6 mm to 4.8 mm (from .1/16 inch to 3/16 inch) forces an increase in arc size and a corresponding decrease in luminance. In actual welding operations the arc gap would normally be increased with increasing current and the increase in arc luminance would not be so marked. Two other luminance plots are provided for comparison (data from Marshall *et al.*, 1977).

range with high-powered magnifying optics, a retinal thermal injury might occur. Presumably no person would ever attempt such a foolish act.

For a realistic retinal hazard analysis it is far more important to examine the blue-light hazard. As noted above, the thermal injury hazard is essentially non-existent in practice. At close viewing distances the blue-light radiance (Section 10.5.3, page 340) must be calculated. This value will then be used in determining the minimal acceptable shade for eye protection. Blue-light radiances are listed in Table 24.2. A plot of the maximum measured values of Marshall *et al.* (1977) is provided in Figure 24-16.

For most arc viewing distances beyond the welder, the arc is effectively a "point source" for the purpose of hazard analysis. To calculate the potential retinal hazard to distant viewers and to determine the maximal "stare time" T_{max}, the blue-light irradiance must be known. Figure 24-17 provides the blue-light irradiance values at one meter from most of the arc processes studied. Note that the blue-light irradiance generally follows an I^2 trend since the total power and not the size of the arc plays the critical role in determining this quantity.

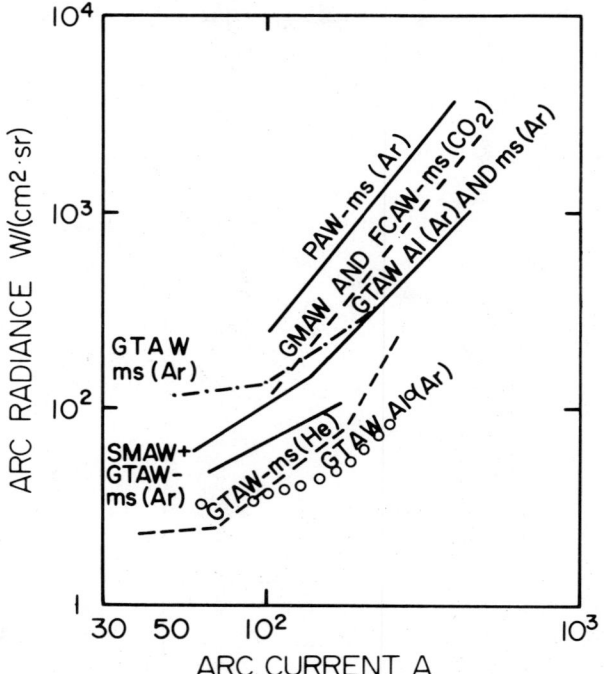

Figure 24-15. Radiance of Welding Arcs. The peak (center spot) radiance of a variety of welding arcs are plotted for comparison. Note that although PAW with Ar shielding and GMAW with CO_2 shielding on mild steel produced only moderate levels of UV, these two processes produce the highest radiances (data from Marshall et al., 1977).

Infrared radiation (principally IR-A) has sometimes erroneously been attributed to be a potential retinal hazard (e.g., Clark, 1968). Of course, the understanding of blue-light retinal injury is quite recent, and therefore only now can one argue effectively that the IR-A irradiance is not a significant retinal hazard. In most processes the IR-A and IR-B from the arc and heated base metal is insufficient to be considered a hazard to the anterior structures of the eye. Normally, less than half of the arc's irradiance may be found in the IR. Sutter et al. (1972) measured the infrared spectral irradiance of several welding arcs. Three representative spectra from their study are provided in Figure 24-18. Note that welding of Al with Ar produces considerable line structure in the IR-A. The spectral irradiance values in the IR-A are generally about the same as in the visible. Except for AAC, Sliney and his associates did not measure significant infrared irradiances in the arc processes they studied. Some infrared attenuation of welding filters is still probably advisable. But based upon present knowledge, the infrared radiation and light of wavelengths greater than 550 nm play virtually no hazardous role and levels of these radiations are below EL's at distances greater than 1 m.

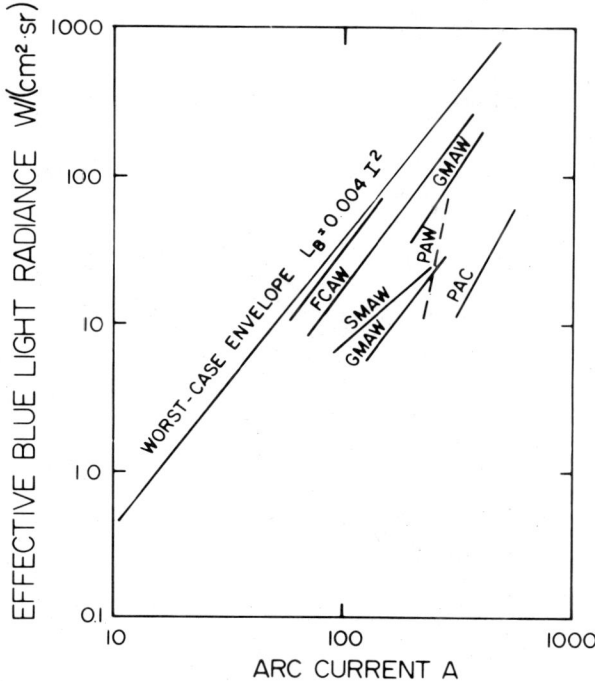

Figure 24-16. Blue-Light Radiances of Welding Arcs. The maximal values of blue-light radiance L_B are plotted for the processes given in Table 24-2. Many arcs have values of L_B for the given current that are well below these values.

24.3 HAZARDS TO THE SKIN

The optical radiation hazards to the skin from welding and cutting arcs are limited to ultraviolet erythema. Most arc welders wear face masks, heavy clothing, leather gloves, and sometimes leather or metal-shielded aprons to protect them from the ultraviolet rays. By comparison, a worker using an acetylene torch does not require such heavy clothing or face protection and his goggles normally cover only his eyes because of the very low UV emissions (Moss *et al.*, 1979). The skin hazards from welding are not of course limited to ultraviolet radiation. Hazards also exist from red-hot flying particles of metal. Sometimes welders, who limit their work to spot welding and tacking, or occasional use of arc welding equipment in conjunction with other machine shop work, are seen without complete skin covering although they do not develop erythema. They may develop a resistant tan and reduced skin sensitivity to the ultraviolet radiation. One could argue that welders exposed chronically to ultraviolet radiation could develop skin cancer. However, perhaps because of the usual practice to cover up, there has been no obvious increase in the incidence

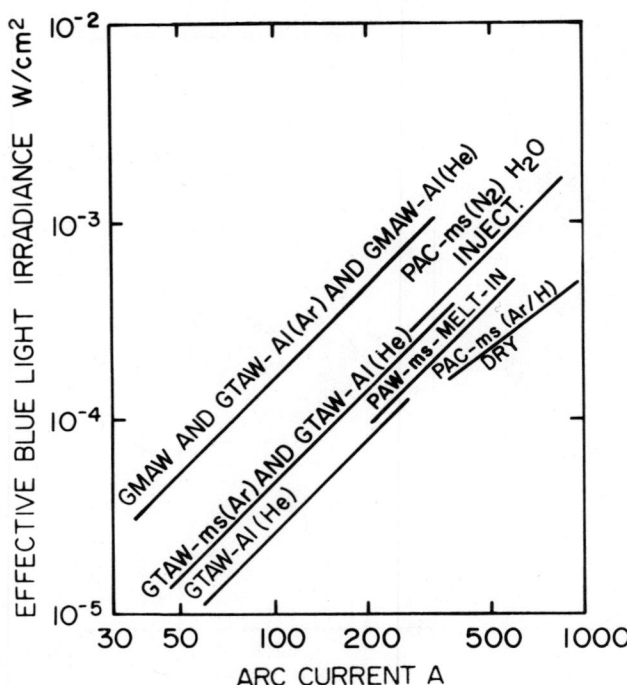

Figure 24-17. Blue-Light Irradiances of Welding Arcs. The relative blue-light hazards of different arc processes is far better illustrated by plotting blue-light irradiance than blue-light radiance. The values in this graph for a 1-m distance may be used for calculating arc stare times as a function of viewing distance and arc current (data from Marshall *et al.*, 1977).

of skin cancer in the welding population. Generally, when an experienced welder receives a skin burn it is due to an unexpected reflection. For example, when the welder is within a steel tank or large pipe there is a good chance that ultraviolet radiation will be reflected from the other side of the pipe or container and strike unprotected or poorly protected back and neck areas. Other injuries to the skin occur during very hot weather when welders take chances by compromising between exposing much of their skin area to decrease their discomfort due to heat, yet covering to attempt to shield themselves from the UV.

24.4 EYE HAZARDS

24.4.1 Corneal Injuries

Unlike the small protective goggles for use with acetylene welding equipment,

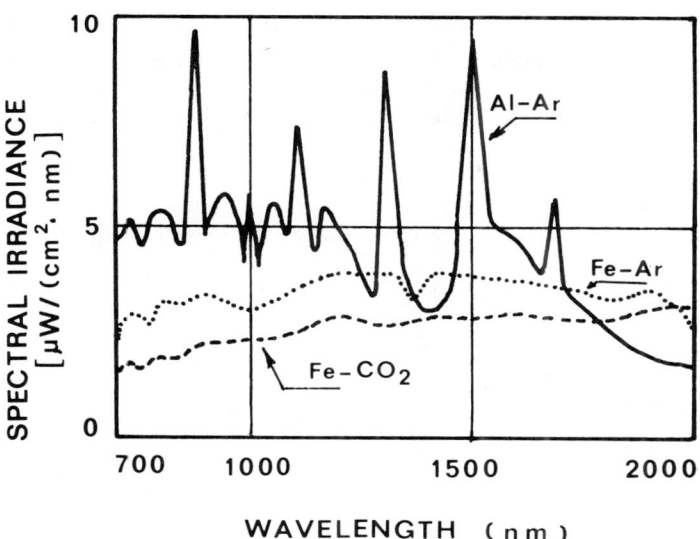

Figure 24-18. Infrared Spectral Irradiances for Three Types of Arcs. The three plots show that the spectral irradiance values for most arcs are generally no greater in the IR-A than in the visible. These plots show the line spectra only for Ar. Arc currents were 280 A (Fe) and 200 A (Al). Measurements were made at 50 cm; from Hübner et al. (1970).

arc welding requires a welding helmet. Cases of welder's flash are often reported in areas where helmets are difficult to use and where the welders' helpers or ancillary personnel are in the proximity of exposed arcs. For example, in steel fabrication in large shipyards, cases of welder's flash are not uncommon in riveters and other specialists who do not wear eye protection, yet are incidently exposed to open welding arcs, albeit sometimes at considerable distances. Sometimes beginning welders feel that they must show their "manhood" by refusing to wear welding face protection. This practice is quickly corrected after one or two experiences with arc flash because of the severe pain accompanying photokeratitis. Ultraviolet effects upon the eye are well documented, as discussed in Chapter 4.

Normally the improperly protected welder does not experience any pain or tearing during the welding operation if simple safety goggles or sunglasses are worn; but the ultraviolet radiation transmitted by such spectacles—or reflected through the sides of such spectacles—is often sufficient to cause the delayed photokeratitis. The full symptoms of photokeratitis are normally not experienced until the worker has left the job site. The duration between the time of exposure and the onset of symptoms varies depending upon the severity of exposure. For severe overexposures the sensation of sand in the eyes, blepharospasm, etc. may have an onset only two or three hours following the excessive exposure. At near-threshold conditions the effect may not even be noted until after the individual has retired for the evening, and suddenly awakes with a painful sensation of sand in the eyes late at night. Indeed the industrial physician and industrial nurse are always careful to inquire further of an employee who claims to have suffered welding flash if the symptoms first appear in the morning on the job site. It is not unheard of that a welder, desiring an excuse to leave the job site early, may claim eye irritation due to the welding. Such an immediate effect suggests that the photokeratitis may in fact be due to a chemical agent or an organic disease state, and not due to the ultraviolet radiation. If there is a lack of visible symptoms, the complaint may be due to "goldbricking" (malingering).

24.4.2 Retinal Injuries from Welding Arcs

As noted before, retinal injuries from staring at welding arcs are extremely rare. In no cases are welding arcs so brilliant that retinal injury can occur within the period of the blink reflex. Retinal thermal injury is virtually impossible because of the small retinal image size even at close range. One of the most authoritative texts in the field of opthalmology (Duke-Elder and McFaul, 1972) states that permanent retinal injury from viewing welding arcs is exceptional, and that the open welding arc "can usually be fixed for several minutes without any damage being done to the retina beyond temporary functional impairment and derangement of vision." Nevertheless retinal injury has been reported from short circuit-arcs of electric current of the same magnitude used in welding. Today, many electric power companies provide their maintenance workers with ultraviolet-absorbing safety glasses to protect against ultraviolet photokeratitis from short-circuit arcs, but there has been generally little concern for retinal injury. Minton (1949) referred to two cases of foveal lesions which developed in arc welders who failed to wear appropriate eye protection when striking their arcs. During the construction of the Paris subway at the turn of the century, numerous cases of eye injury, including retinal injury from viewing welding arcs, were reported (Terrien, 1904). This is not surprising, since the ambient illumination in these subway tunnels was very poor, pupils were dilated, and protective filters had not really been developed at that time. Even the Crookes glass (dark filter glass) was yet to be proposed in the literature. In most of the cases reported of retinal injury the observer was typically 2 m from the arc and for one reason or another, perhaps somewhat hypnotized, stared at the arc for some length of time.

24.4.3 A Case Report

It is useful to note the course of events and development of an eye injury from a welding arc that was recently documented (Naidoff and Sliney, 1974). An 18-year-old arc welding student (Caucasian) reported to a hospital emergency room with swollen eyelids, decreased vision in the right eye and complained of pain. The symptoms began a few hours after he had stared at an GTAW arc on aluminum for approximately 5 to 10 minutes without any form of protective lens. Figure 24-19

Welding Arcs

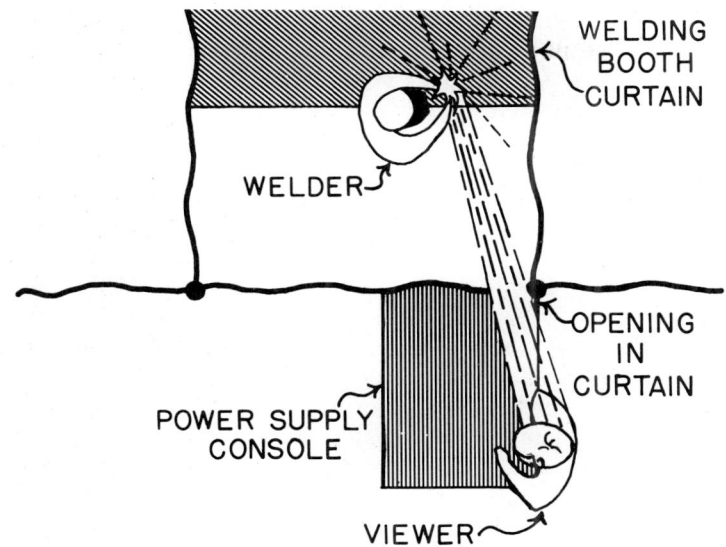

Figure 24-19. A Welding Accident. A student in a welding class leaned against a power supply adjacent to a welding booth and stared at an arc through a break in the curtain using only his right eye.

shows his location as he leaned against a power supply console with only the right side of his face and his right eye fully exposed to the rays of the arc. For this reason his left eye was not affected. He claimed that he had been drowsy, was dazzled by the arc and continued to stare at it. The ocular pain and eyelid edema were most severe the evening following the incident. The eyelid edema that evening was sufficient to totally close the eyelids. The eyelid swelling gradually decreased and after two days, when he was able to reopen his right eyelid he realized the loss of vision and visited an ophthalmologist.

A few months prior to the incident he had received a routine physical examination and his visual acuity was recorded as 20/20 in both eyes at that time. There had been no past history of ocular disease or of visual problems. On examination, the visual acuity in the right eye was 3/200 with eccentric fixation, and was 20/20 in the left eye. The left eye and left facial area were normal and the subsequent discussion pertains to the right eye only. There was periorbital edema (2+), and erythema (2+) that extended to the frontal and maxillary areas. A moderate blepharotosis covered at least half of the pupil. The bulbar conjunctiva showed 2+ injection; however, the cornea at that time was normal and did not stain with fluorescein. The right pupil was slightly larger than the left and its consensual reaction to light was greater than its direct reaction. The left pupil behaved in the opposite manner. Motility and tensions were normal. Field examination on the tangent screen using both the 9/1000 and the 2/1000 white test objects revealed a dense, approximately

4° central scotoma, and peripheral constriction to 20 to 25°. Ophthalmoscopic and contact lens examination of the fundus revealed a bright yellow foveal lesion situated deep in the retina of 0.25 to 0.2 disc diameter in size, surrounded by a pale yellow macular edema. The entire retinal lesion was approximately 0.75 disc diameters in size. The remaining retina including the disc, appeared normal.

On the fifth day after the accident the acuity was essentially unchanged and only a minimal eyelid edema and trace conjunctival injection remained. When seen on the ninth day, visual acuity was still only 5/200. The pupils at that time reacted normally and pigment granules were seen for the first time surrounding the oval yellow unpigmented foveal lesion that measured approximately 250 × 500 μm. The pigment granules were located in the formerly pale yellow edematous parafoveal area. By the twelfth day following exposure the visual acuity had improved to 20/30, and the pigment granules had increased in number surrounding the fovea. By four weeks after the incident the visual acuity was essentially 20/20 minus a small central scotoma which remained, and was still observed, 16 months after the incident. There was a generalized increase in pigment in the macula particularly along the foveal border 16 months following the exposure.

The arc that the student had stared at with one eye was an 80-ampere, gas-tungsten arc (GTAW, or TIG), and the exposure distance was approximately 200 cm from the arc. Reconstructing the exposure, it was revealed that the total irradiance was only 1 mW/cm^2 (0.4 mW/cm^2 within the retinal hazard region). The illuminance was 0.035 lm/cm^2 and the arc size was approximately 2 mm. Hence the total source radiance was approximately 1000 W/(cm^2·sr) and the corresponding luminance 35,000 cd/cm^2. The ultraviolet irradiance weighted against the envelope TLV for ultraviolet radiation indeed suggested an exposure duration of at least five minutes to corroborate the student's story. A 2-mm arc viewed at 200 cm would subtend a viewing angle of 1 mrad; hence the geometrical retinal image size would be only 17 μm. Of course, from our knowledge of eye movements it is certain that the site in the retina would not be continuously exposed; this would explain the larger retinal lesion size. The student's pupil was probably approximately 3 mm in diameter.

It should be emphasized that this case history is an extreme, but it does point out that although severe temporary injury to the cornea existed, it cleared completely. The retinal damage from blue light also subsided, leaving behind only a very minimal loss of vision, a small central scotoma, which would not generally be considered incapacitating by any stretch of the imagination. Therefore we could generally argue, based upon our present biomedical knowledge, that the ocular hazards due to optical radiation from welding are largely acute in nature (Naidoff and Sliney, 1974).

24.5 EPIDEMIOLOGICAL STUDIES

From epidemiological studies it should be possible to show whether there is a true risk associated with exposure to ultraviolet radiation and bright light sources over long periods of time—many years. Some studies, such as that performed by

Emmett and others (1979) at one large industrial firm showed that there was no significant increase in skin cancer among welders, nor were there any obvious ocular changes. On the other hand Gupta and Singh (1968) have shown that in a population of welders in India there was an increased incidence of defects in color vision which they attributed to the bright welding arcs. It could be argued that the protective measures followed in that country may not be equivalent to the protective measures followed in the USA; and that therefore, such changes would not necessarily be expected in the population of U.S. welders. Nevertheless, the possibility that welders as a general population may have a slight reduction in night vision, or some changes in color vision thresholds, or altered dark adaptation curves relative to the normal population cannot be completely ruled out. However, such a study awaits a future investigator. If such changes really do exist they would have to be quite subtle since any substantial or obvious difference between welders and the normal population would have been detected long ago due to the large numbers of arc welders in any population. Indeed, the lack of any obvious visual changes lends some credence to the arguments against excessively conservative safety levels for CW lasers and other optical sources where the exposure is only casual.

24.6 FIRST AID

For severe and extensive cases of welder's flash and ultraviolet erythema, medical care is essential, particularly in the case of ultraviolet photokeratitis. The injured site should not be exposed to further ultraviolet irradiation, including solar radiation, until healing is complete. Because of the extreme pain accompanying photokeratitis, the use of pressure compresses (often cold) to the eye is common. As the discomfort is from the eyelids irritating the deepithelialized cornea, the main therapy is to immobilize the lids by pressure until the epithelium is regenerated. Topical anesthetics may actually delay the regeneration, as well as inhibiting the pain. Thus the value of anesthetics or other medicines to relieve the pain is debatable. It is not uncommon for the experienced welder to have a bottle of eye drops (local anesthetic) in his tool kit, probably obtained from an ophthalmologist for his first case of welder's flash, but these are probably useless from age, or possibly harmful. Customarily the patient wears dark shaded glasses for additional relief from discomfort (photophobia) until the healing has been completed. Normally, because of the rapid turnover of the corneal epithelium, healing is complete, except in the severest cases, within a period of 48 hours following the exposure.

For mild exposure of the skin, cold creams or similar oils or greases including salad oil or shortening will relieve pain. The best of these "folk" remedies seems to be a hair-setting gel, Dippity-Do® (Gillete Co.), which has been extensively tested on sunburn. Medicated creams, butter, or oleomargine should *not* be applied.

Of course, optical radiation does not present the only occupational hazard to the welder. Fumes and gases generated in arc welding (Table 24-3) present substantial potential hazards. Because of the potential for severe electrical shock when working with electric arc welding equipment, cardiopulmonary resuscitation should be available, and personnel should be trained in the proper procedures (see Section 28.7).

24.7 EVALUATING WELDING OPERATIONS

Of particular concern in a welding shop are the potential exposures of passersby in aisles, or supervisors behind standup desks in the work area. The greatest hazard exists when the light of the direct arc can be seen as incident on any individual. Besides being uncomfortably bright, exposed arcs may very well be exposing ancillary personnel to hazardous radiation levels. In evaluating a production line already in progress the best way to determine whether there is really a hazard is to ask the individuals if they have encountered injuries. It is very difficult to assess adequately the total duration of welding in a day and the cumulative daily exposure of people walking around in the vicinity of the welding processes. It is even more foolish to argue with experienced personnel actually working in the area of the welding arc by claiming that they should be getting injured when in fact they are not. Table 24-4 provides a sample of exposure durations at a reference distance of 2 m for a variety of commonly-encountered welding processes where the arc is exposed. If the joint geometry is such that part of the arc is occluded or not directly observed, then of course these levels of ultraviolet radiation would be greatly reduced, and therefore, the permissible exposure durations at the distance stated would be greatly increased. The ultraviolet irradiation from the direct arc is not noticeably increased in joint geometries such as fillet welding where ultraviolet radiation would reflect from the adjacent metal.

Although reflected radiation can contribute to exposure in some conditions, in comparison to the direct radiation from a completely exposed arc, it is insignificant. The problem of reflected ultraviolet radiation only arises when an individual is shielded from the direct arc and receives reflected radiation for extensive time periods. One general observation is that if one is at least 30 m (100 ft) from any common welding arc within a range of current of 50 to 350 amperes there is essentially no chance of receiving ultraviolet erythema or photokeratitis in any daily exposure.

24.8 WELDING HAZARD INDEX

At the US Army Environmental Hygiene Agency a welding hazard index (WHI) was developed for different conditions, which permits the calculation of a maximal safe duration for bystanders at a given distance from the arc when shields are not feasible (as occasionally occurs in some industrial production lines). This index, however, is not necessary in most operations where the welder is located in a booth. The ultraviolet radiation emitted by an open welding arc normally appears to increase approximately as the square of the arc current. Figure 24-12 showed an example of measured ultraviolet radiation as a function of arc current for several types of welding processes. It was this type of data that permitted the development of a welding hazard index (WHI) for estimating the maximum permissible exposure duration t_{max} (in s) at a distance r (in cm) for an arc current I_a (in A):

$$t_{max} = (1000)(r^2) / (WHI)(I_a^2) \qquad (24\text{-}5)$$

TABLE 24-4
Representative Maximum Exposure Durations Welding Arcs Viewed at a Distance of 2 m*

Process (AWS Abbrev.)	Current (A)	Base Metal	t_{max} (UV) (S)	t_{max} (Blue Light) (S)
GTAW (He)	100	ms††	50	120
"	250	"	30	28
GTAW (Ar)	100	"	700	60
"	250	"	110	12
"	50	Al	4000	110
"	100	"	1000	33
GMAW (Ar)	150	"	26	13
"	300	"	12	5
GMAW (CO_2)	90	ms	300	50
"	150	"	100	20
"	350	"	16	4
GMAW (Ar/O_2)	150	"	30	10
"	250	"	10	5
"	350	"	5	3
SMAW	100	"	24	18
"	200	"	60	8
PAW (Ar)	200	"	120 †	22
"	260	"	80 †	7

* t_{max} is the total integrated on time for an exposed arc with good local exhaust ventilation. In actual situations most welding arcs are partially occluded with greater t_{max} Values reported by Lyon et al. (1976) and Marshall et al. (1977).
† Occluded arc.
†† Mild steel.

The welding hazard indexes given in Table 24-5 permit the estimation of the total permissible exposure duration in any daily work period for exposure to ultraviolet radiation. When establishing a plant layout, such a table is particularly time (and money) saving in this stage of arranging welding stations, determining whether welding booths are necessary, and locating aisle ways for heavy traffic and supervisory stations. Obviously, if it can be predicted that a particular location of a supervisor's desk would give exposures to the permissible ultraviolet level in less than two hours, the need for rearranging welding sites, or possibly installing a protective shield between the desk and the nearest welding site, can be anticipated.

The serious shortcoming of the welding hazard index, WHI, is that it predicts worst-case conditions. The WHI applies to arcs which are completely exposed, where there is excellent fume extraction. In reality these conditions are rarely achieved. Hence the WHI has limited applications. If the arc is not significantly exposed, the calculated value of t_{max} may be multiplied by a factor of at least ten. It must be remembered, however, that the use of the WHI is useful only for planning new layouts, or for ruling out any concern where even the worst-case calculations indicate a safe condition.

TABLE 24-5. Welding Hazard Index (WHI)*

Process	Shielding Gas	Base Metal	WHI (UV)
GTAW	He	ms	85
,,	Ar	,,	6.3
,,	Ar	Al	3.3
,,	He	,,	6.7
GMAW	CO_2	ms	15
FCAW	CO_2	,,	6
GMAW	Ar	,,	60
,,	Ar	Al	70
,,	He	,,	40
SMAW°	N/A	ms	130
PAW†	He	,,	140
,,	Ar, H	,,	50

* Representative values based upon actual measurements with good local exhaust ventilation.
† Arc is not exposed, but largely occluded by the base metal.
° Varies greatly with welding rod. An extreme case is given.

EXAMPLE: Find t_{max} for a gas-tungsten arc (GTAW) operating at 150 A on aluminum (Argon shielding gas) as viewed at 60 feet. From Table 24-5 the WHI is 3.3. The distance, 60 feet (0.3048 m/ft), is 18.3 m or 1830 cm. Hence by equation 24-5:

$$t_{max} = (1000)(1830)^2 / (3.3)(150)^2$$
$$= 4.5 \times 10^4 \text{ s}$$
$$= 750 \text{ minutes}$$
$$= 12.5 \text{ hours}$$

Obviously there is no UV hazard at this point, but a separate calculation would be required to show **if** lengthy staring at the arc could be safe. Fortunately one can consider the blue light hazard as academic since the natural aversion response of the eye limits one from staring at the arc.

24.9 ENGINEERING PROTECTIVE MEASURES

As in the control of other health and safety hazards, the primary protective measure should be the engineering controls. That is, welding stations should be designed to reduce greatly the exposure to intense optical radiation. Figure 24-20 shows an ideal welding booth with adequate ventilation to protect the welder against any potentially hazardous fumes, vapors and gases which may be released during welding and cutting operations. Such a booth might be particularly desirable in

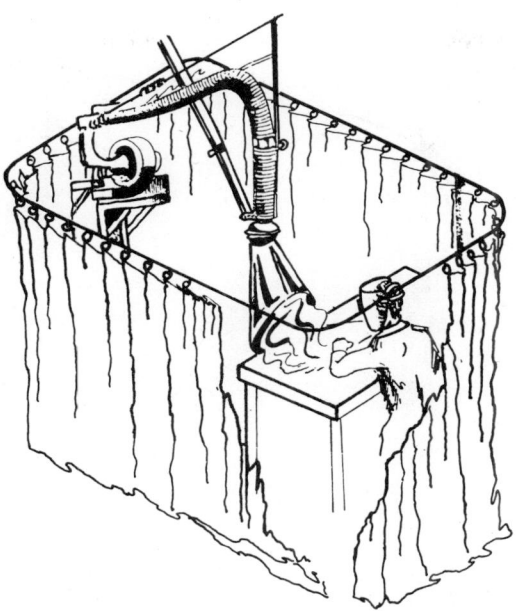

Figure 24-20. An Ideal Welding Booth. The use of local exhaust ventilation is very important when a booth is used to shield adjacent workers from actinic radiations. However, the more efficient that extraction becomes, the more ultraviolet radiation is transmitted through the fume cloud. Adapted from NIOSH.

certain types of plasma-arc and SMAW applications where the ultraviolet levels can be quite excessive. Obviously booths such as shown in Figure 24-20 are not possible in rapidly moving production lines, for example, in automobile assembly lines. In these cases the maximum use of baffles and personnel protective equipment may be necessary.

Locating the welding stations at a certain distance from occupied areas obviously is desirable, as distance is a very effective protective measure. Some materials may be particularly reflective in the ultraviolet, but as can be seen in Figures 15-13 to 15-18 (pp. 500-503) few materials reflect much in the UV-B and C. It is generally known that paints containing small quantities of titanium oxide or zinc oxide tend to have especially low reflectance in the ultraviolet. These types of paints are often recommended for painting cabinets and other structures in the vicinity of welding stations. Carbon-particle paints offer no more UV reduction and increase glare, hence they are not recommended. Light, diffused (perhaps even fluorescent) paints can reduce glare and improve lighting conditions within the

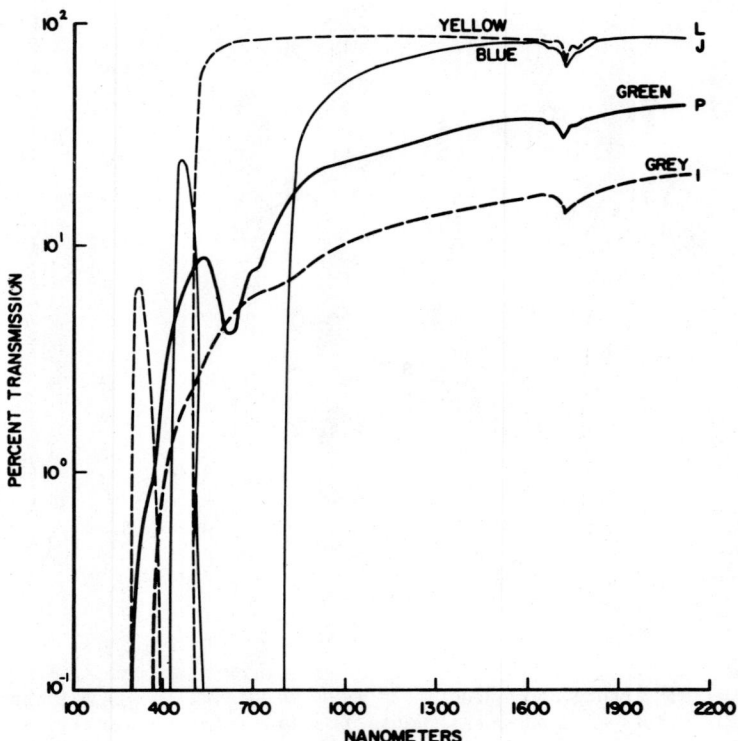

Figure 24-21. Transparent Welding Curtains. The spectral transmittance curves of several commercially available plastic welding curtains are shown for comparison. All provide adequate UV protection (adapted from Moss and Gawenda, 1978).

booth. Figures 15-13 to 15-18 provide some spectral reflectance curves of polished metals and typical paints. Oxidized or painted metal surfaces have lower reflectances than clean metal surfaces. Flaked metal paints should be avoided.

Welding curtains are often used to create a temporary booth. In the past most such curtains have been made of a heavy canvas material, which is very effective in attenuating ultraviolet radiation. However, semi-transparent welding curtains made of ultraviolet-absorbing plastic materials are becoming increasingly popular. Unfortunately some vendors have substituted cheaper, non-ultraviolet-absorbing curtains, generally out of ignorance of the different properties of seemingly similar plastic curtain materials. Normally the plastic curtains are yellow, green or orange to reduce the dazzle of the arc. The arc may appear visibly more dazzling through the yellow curtains; although it may actually be safer, due to the greater attenuation of the blue light which is the greater retinal hazard. Figure 24-21 provides some spectral transmission data of welding curtains examined by Mr. Eugene Moss and associates at NIOSH. Although the visual transmittance may seem to be excessively high, the transmission curve is somewhat misleading as most curtains, either because they become dirty quickly, or because of manufacturing techniques, are somewhat translucent and diffusing rather than truly transparent. For this reason the image of the arc is blurred and the effective luminance and blue light radiance is reduced. Such curtains are probably quite adequate where protection to passers-by is to be afforded. The reason such curtains have become quite popular is that supervisors can more readily determine when a welder is working than with the older opaque welding curtains. Also, an injured welder can be more readily seen and help can be summoned sooner. One study (Entwistle, 1964) indicated that there are more fall injuries and burns than arc flash incidents. Although many curtains are self-extinguishing, they will burn and holes do form where hot objects touch the plastic. For this reason, curtains should be periodically inspected, and patched or replaced if the holes are located at points where full attenuation is required. The arc should normally be kept at least 100 cm from the arc.

One particularly innovative curtain, developed by Miller and Stephens of the Jet Propulsion Laboratory, incorporates phosphorescent dyes which absorb UV and re-emit visible light which enhances the diffused illumination at the work place, thus reducing glare for the welder. These curtains were also designed with a fade-resistant orange dye that is particularly effective in filtering out harmful blue light. Furthermore, the curtain surface has been fabricated to diffuse the image of the arc, reducing its luminance while still permitting the observation of the welder. This type of orange curtain is marketed as Spectra® by the Wilson Sales Company of Rosemead, California. Mr. David F. Wilson, president of that company originated the transparent plastic welding curtain in the late 1960's.

The German Standardization Institute, DIN, issued a standard on welding curtains (DIN 32 504) in 1978. It recommended that transparent welding curtains be graded with shade numbers and that a curtain meet the same basic UV, VIS, and IR transmission specifications that apply to filter plates in eye protectors. This recommendation cannot be met by present curtains and it would be difficult to completely satisfy in any case. In particular, the organic dyes that have been used in plastic curtains do not absorb IR-A radiation. Indeed, fade-resistant IR-A absorbing dyes are unusual and expensive. The appropriate question to ask is: How much IR-A attenuation is really necessary for curtain applications?

The role of the welding curtain is clearly different from the role of the helmet filter plate. The minimum arc-viewing distance is about 100 cm for the curtain and 30 cm for the filter plate. The filter plate must be transparent; the curtain may be translucent. The filter plate must be designed to protect the welder's retina for extended time periods while the welder stares at the arc. By contrast, the curtain must protect passers-by and onlookers while still permitting some visibility of the welder as well as his arc. At a viewing distance of 30 cm the irradiance in all spectral bands is about ten-times the value at just 1 m and 40-times the value at 2 m. Since plastic curtains cannot be brought close to the arc, a highly conservative (close) viewing distance for an onlooker would be 1 m—and 2 m would be a typical viewing distance. Arc currents greater than 400-500 A would necessitate placing the curtain

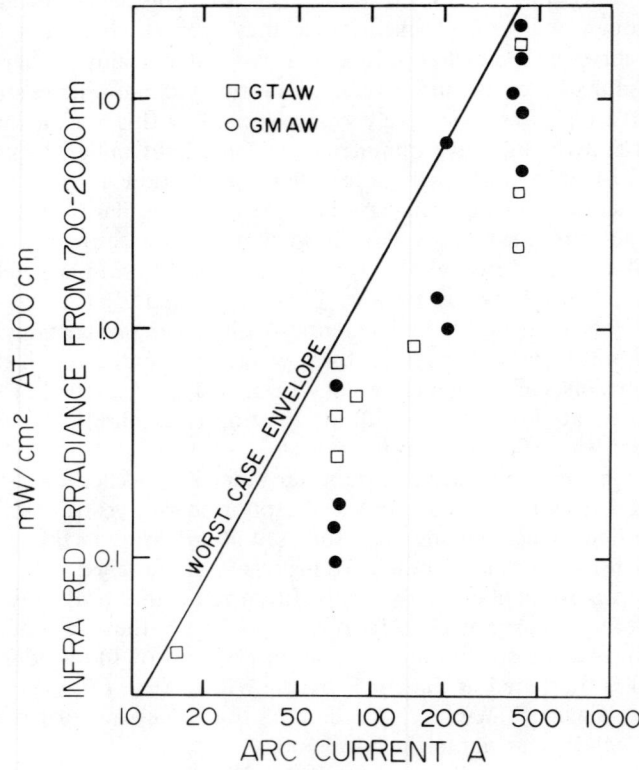

Figure 24-22. Infrared Irradiances of Welding Arcs. A worst-case curve is drawn through the measured values of Sutter *et al.* (1972) for infrared irradiance (750–2,000 nm). The curve and representative data points were adjusted for a reference distance of 100 cm although the measurements were made at 50 cm.

at still greater distances. The minimum curtain filtration requirements can therefore be determined for a worst-case, exposed arc at 500 A. At this current, equation 24-3 predicts a UV irradiance of 10 mW/cm² at 1 m. The corresponding blue-light irradiance would be 2 mW/cm² at 1 m (from Figure 24-17). The 8-hour exposure limit for actinic UV is 10^{-7} W/cm², for UV-A is 1 mW/cm², and for blue light (worst-case, non-diffused arc spot) is 10^{-6} W/cm². Many of the present plastic curtains (e.g., Spectra®) have transmittance values in these spectral bands which are easily sufficient to reduce the UV and VIS radiation well below these limits. The presently recommended limit for infrared radiation is 10 mW/cm² if there is no retinal hazard to be concerned with. Indeed if blue light and UV-A are filtered out, the lens could in theory be exposed to much higher IR-A levels. For this reason very little attention was paid to IR-A and IR-B measurements during the USAEHA/AWS arc measurement program. Only during AAC were hazardous IR-A levels measured. A far more complete study of arc emissions in this spectral range was performed in Germany.

Measurements by Sutter *et al.* (1972) at the Physikalisch-Technische Bundesanstalt (PTB, the equivalent in the U.S. of the National Bureau of Standards) in Braunschweig, West Germany, provide the best available IR and VIS spectral data for a wide variety of arcs. The spectra of three arcs in the spectral region of interest are shown in Figure 24-18. Sutter and his associates tabulated their irradiance data within several spectral bands. By plotting the irradiance values for the spectral range of 750 nm—2,000 nm (IR-A plus part of the IR-B band), it was possible to obtain a general relation which would predict the *maximum* near-infrared thermal load on the anterior structures of the eye. As was shown for the UV-weighted and blue-light irradiances, this irradiance E (750—2,000 nm) did not increase more rapidly than the square of the arc current I_a (Figure 24-22). The IR-A and IR-B would also decrease inversely as the square of the viewing distance r (in cm) for distances greater than 30-50 cm. The effective infrared source size is greater than the arc size—particularly in AC operations—because of the incandescence of the metallic workpiece. This worst-case formulation for currents between 40 A and 200 A is:

$$E (750-2,000 \text{ nm}) = k_3 \, I_a^2 / r^2 \qquad (24\text{-}6)$$

where $k_3 = 9 \times 10^{-4}$ W/A². If we calculate E (750—2,000 nm) at 100 cm for a current I_a of 200 A, we obtain 7 mW/cm². The highest irradiance value in the 2,000-nm band obtained by Sutter was 833 W/m² (long arc on stainless steel) for 420 A at 50 cm. This would correspond to 20.8 mW/cm² at 100 cm. Since this irradiance is only a factor of two above the long-term exposure limit, it should not be of great concern for incidental viewing. In actual practice, the soot that quickly covers a curtain plus the geometrical occlusion that is characteristic of all welding and cutting processes would reduce the time-averaged infrared irradiance to 10 mW/cm² behind a curtain 100 cm from an arc. Lest one too quickly dismisses any concern for IR-A hazards, one should remember that the welder, whose face plate is located only 30 cm from the arc—can receive ocular irradiances exceeding 100 mW/cm² at currents above 150 A. Heat-stress considerations would also dictate that infrared attenuation factors be greater than the minimum factor necessary to reduce the irradiance at the eye to 10 mW/cm². Our conclusion, then, based upon health and safety considerations, is that no substantial IR-A attenuation is necessary for curtains, but attenuation is required for helmet face plates. Specific recommendations for filter specifications will be presented in Section 24-12.

24.10 WELDING EYE AND FACE PROTECTION

Few people make use of welding goggles for arc welding because of the need to protect the face as well as the eye. Instead, a welding helmet or shield is used as shown in Figure 24-23. As noted previously (Section 16.11, page 542) the specifications for welding filters have been developed empirically and the values have been substantiated recently by the detailed measurement of a large variety of welding arcs. Table 24-6 provides the present American National Standard limits which were developed largely by Stair and associates at the National Bureau of Standards during

TABLE 24-6. Transmittances and Tolerances in Transmittance of Various Shade of Filter Lenses (ANSI Z87.1, 1968)

Shade Number	Optical Density			Luminous Transmittance			Maximum Infrared Transmittance	Maximum Spectral Transmittance in the Ultraviolet and Violet			
	Maximum	Standard	Minimum	Maximum	Standard	Minimum		313 nm	334 nm	365 nm	405 nm
				Percent	Percent	Percent	Percent	Percent	Percent	Percent	Percent
1.5	0.26	0.214	0.17	67	61.5	55	25	0.2	0.8	25	65
1.7	0.36	0.300	0.26	55	50.1	43	20	0.2	0.7	20	50
2.0	0.54	0.429	0.36	43	37.3	29	15	0.2	0.5	14	35
2.5	0.75	0.643	0.54	29	22.8	18.0	12	0.2	0.3	5	15
3.0	1.07	0.857	0.75	18.0	13.9	8.50	9.0	0.2	0.2	0.5	6
4.0	1.50	1.286	1.07	8.50	5.18	3.16	5.0	0.2	0.2	0.5	1.0
5.0	1.93	1.714	1.50	3.16	1.93	1.18	2.5	0.2	0.2	0.2	0.5
6.0	2.36	2.143	1.93	1.18	0.72	0.44	1.5	0.1	0.1	0.1	0.5
7.0	2.79	2.571	2.36	0.44	0.27	0.164	1.3	0.1	0.1	0.1	0.5
8.0	3.21	3.000	2.79	0.164	0.100	0.061	1.0	0.1	0.1	0.1	0.5
9.0	3.64	3.429	3.21	0.061	0.037	0.023	0.8	0.1	0.1	0.1	0.5
10.0	4.07	3.857	3.64	0.023	0.0139	0.0085	0.6	0.1	0.1	0.1	0.1
11.0	4.50	4.286	4.07	0.0085	0.0052	0.0032	0.5	0.05	0.05	0.05	0.1
12.0	4.93	4.714	4.50	0.0032	0.0019	0.0012	0.5	0.05	0.05	0.05	0.1
13.0	5.36	5.143	4.93	0.0012	0.00072	0.00044	0.4	0.05	0.05	0.05	0.1
14.0	5.79	5.571	5.36	0.00044	0.00027	0.00016	0.3	0.05	0.05	0.05	0.1

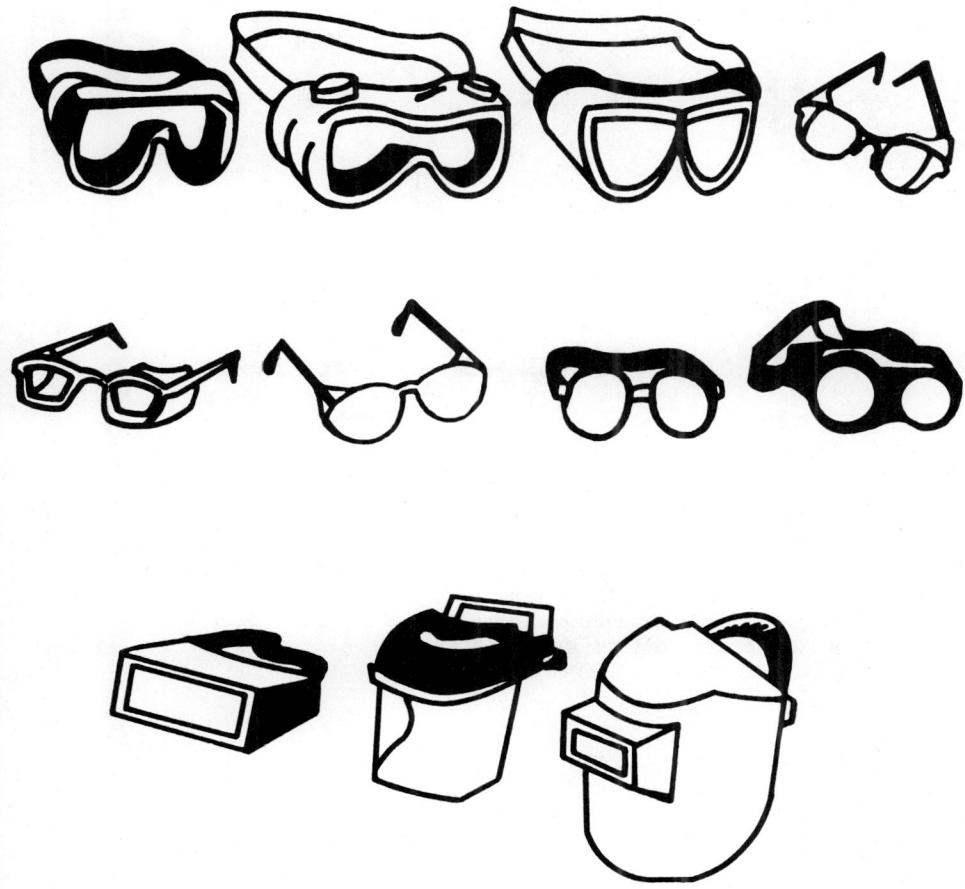

Figure 24-23. Eye Protection for Welders. A variety of eye protectors are available for welders. Face masks are required for arc welding; whereas, simple goggles are adequate for gas welding and cutting.

the 1940's (Stair, 1948). The specified transmission values are given at wavelengths of the mercury lamp. Now that the need for protection against blue light is understood, the specification should be extended to at least the 436-nm line of the mercury spectrum.

Eye protection is specified in terms of shade number which is a logarithmic notation of visual transmission. As noted in Section 16.11, the shade number S# of eye protection is:

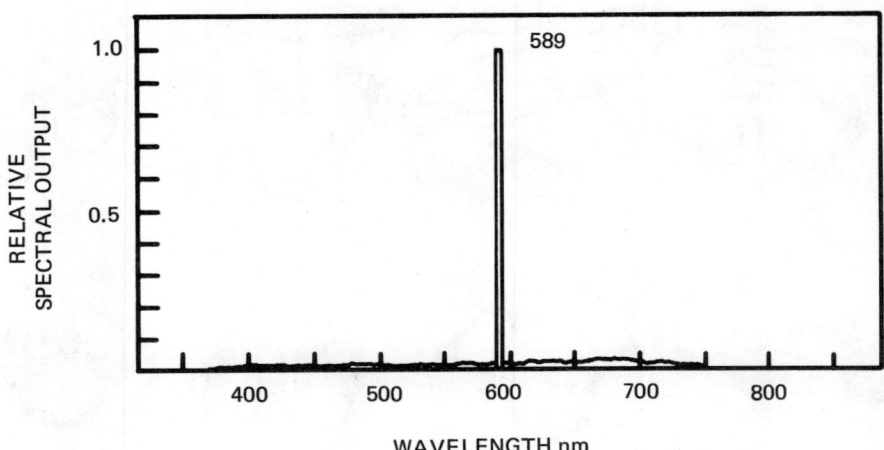

Figure 24-24. Relative Spectrum of a Low-Pressure Sodium Arc Lamp. Since most of the radiant power emitted by this type of lamp is centered in a doublet at 589 nm and 589.6 nm, a special spike-transmission filter which transmits this yellow doublet but heavily attenuates the rest of the spectrum can provide adequate eye protection while still accepting the visible light from overhead lamps. In theory, a multi-spike filter designed to transmit the lines of the mercury or mercury-hallide spectra could perform a similar role with better color rendering of the workpiece being welded.

$$S\# = (7/3)D + 1 \qquad (24\text{-}4)$$

where D is the optical density in the visible spectrum. For example, if the filter density is 3, the attenuation factor is 10^3 or 1000, and the shade number stamped on the filter should be 8. For gas welding a shade number stamped on the filter would be 4 to 8 depending upon the work. For arc welding a shade of 10 to 13 is typical, with shade 10 being the most widely selling shade. The welder chooses the shade which permits comfortable viewing of his workpiece. We have found that this "comfortable" shade typically reduces the luminance of the arc to approximately 1 to 4 cd/cm² (1 to 4 × 10^4 cd/m²).

One technique, which has not been used in the USA but has found favor in Sweden, is to use welding filters with a spike transmission at 589 nm which corresponds to the peak emission of low-pressure sodium vapor lamps (Figure 24-24). If these filters are used in conjunction with low-pressure sodium vapor lamps to illuminate the workpiece, the welder can view his work comfortably with reduced glare from the arc, provided that the arc does not have a strong sodium flare itself. A note of caution to prospective users of this technique is, however, in order. Such filters would be of little use with the high-pressure sodium arc lamps now commonly found in use in this country, since the high-pressure lamp actually has very little radiant output at 589 nm due to self-absorption by the arc. In any case, the ANSI specifications for ultraviolet and infrared transmission decrease with increasing shade number (Table 24-6). Because of the difficulty of testing welding filters and the enormous difficulty of measuring such high optical densities, manufacturers often do not have the capability to determine if their goggles or filter plates really meet these specifications completely. Most goggles marketed in the United States for welding protection that have a given shade stamped on them do adequately meet the recommended range of transmission values. Fortunately, the attenuation factors in the ultraviolet region are generally far in excess of that specified. A recent NIOSH study by Campbell (1976) did reveal, however that a surprisingly high percentage of commercial filters did not fully meet all of the requirements of the ANSI Z87.1 (1968) standard. For example, some plastic filter plates were darker than the specified shade. This may have been due to aging and to possible ultraviolet exposure. Other filters exceeded the 405-nm (violet) transmission limit. This latter failure is of greater concern since short-wavelength light emitted by the arc is the principal retinal hazard. The more common failures found by Campbell related to improper dimensions, or other aspects such as haze, impact resistance, or filter marking, which do not relate to filtration of optical radiation. The filters tested by Campbell were all advertised to meet the requirements of the ANSI Z87.1(1968) standard. Some filter plates are not even advertised to meet the standard. However, in industry, OSHA regulations (specifically 29 CFR 1926.102) require employers to assure that all filters used in the workplace meet the ANSI Z87.1(1968) standard for eye and face protection.

In recent years, several dynamic filter devices have been placed on the market. There is at present no standard for acceptance of such filters. The techniques for achieving rapid closure, or darkening, of the filter range from foot-switch and optically triggered filter shutters (mechanical closure) to photochromic, liquid crystal, and PLZT (electro-optic) filters. The PLZT filters can close within 0.1 ms. A commercially available liquid crystal filter mounted in a helmet closes within 150 ms (Harsch and Fergason, 1978). Unfortunately, most of these devices probably transmit too much blue light during repeated striking of the arc prior to full filter closure. One problem that has been noted with liquid crystal filters has been the loss of density when they were overheated. In theory, a good dynamic filter system would have a yellow filter with excellent ultraviolet and blue-light attenuation when in the "open" (clear) position.

For a long time there has been a debate over the adequacy of infrared attenuation by welding filters. The authors feel that the present Z87.1(1968) requirements are more than adequate. However, except for more stringent infrared filtration requirements, an ISO draft standard for welding filter plates that was circulating for review in 1978 differed only slightly from the ANSI standard values.

Filter requirements in the visible part of the spectrum have normally not been under much debate. Only in the case of SMAW welding arc processes was it found in the recent measurements of Marshall and colleagues (1977) that the recommended

TABLE 24-7. Guide for Selection of Shade Numbers

Operation	Electrode Size mm (32nd")	Arc Current (A)	Minimum Protective Shade	ANSI Z49.1* Suggested Shade No. (Comfort)
SMAW	< 2.5 (< 3)	< 60	7	–
	2.5-4 (3-5)	60–160	8	10
	4-6.4 (5-8)	160–250	10	12
	> 6.4 (> 8)	> 250	11	14
GMAW and		< 60	7	–
FCAW		60–160	10	11
		160–250	10	†12
		> 250	11	–
GTAW		< 50	8	10
		50–150	8	12
		> 150	10	14
AAC (light)		< 500	10	12
(heavy)††		> 500	11	14
PAW		< 20	6	6 to 8
		20–100	8	10
		100–400	10	12
		> 400	11	14
PAC (light)**		< 300	8	9
(medium)		300–400	9	12
(heavy)		> 400	10	14

* Where ANSI Z49.1 did not specify shades varying with current, these values were inserted based upon experience for comfortable viewing.
** These limits apply where the actual arc is clearly seen; and experience has shown that lighter filters may be used when the arc is occluded by the workpiece.
† The ANSI Standard distinguished only between ferrous and non-ferrous welding, not between current levels.
†† Only in AAC is there substantial IR.

shade numbers (Table 24-7) for specific welding processes were not totally adequate to reduce transmitted luminances to a comfortable level of 1 to 4 cd/cm^2, but in all cases, the recommended shades were considered safe for continuous, day-long viewing of short-wavelength light emitted by the welding arc.

24.11 PROTECTIVE CLOTHING FOR WELDERS

Most welders learn from early experience which fabrics attenuate ultraviolet radiation and which do not. Leather gloves and leather aprons and jackets are generally considered the most desirable. Woven fabrics vary greatly in their attenuation properties. Obviously, loosely woven fabrics through which one can readily see light when held up to a lamp will not be as effective as tighter woven materials. Cotton fabrics generally have UV-B diffuse transmission ranging from 5% to 30%, rayon and rayon blends transmit somewhat less (10 to 15%), and heavy wool and flannel materials may transmit 1% or less. Poplin is reported to have very low transmittance. Nylon is very ineffective and may typically transmit 20% to 40%. Attenuation is greatly enhanced by layered clothing.

The choice of clothing obviously rests with the welder. His experience with his own skin's UV sensitivity and his work environment (contribution of reflections, arc geometry, arc current, etc.) will provide the greatest assurance that any acute or delayed skin effects from welding arc radiation will be minimized.

24.12 RECOMMENDATIONS FOR FUTURE PROTECTIVE FILTER/CURTAIN REQUIREMENTS

24.12.1 Welding Filter Plates

The extensive measurements of Marshall *et al.* (1977) and Lyon, *et al.* (1976) revealed that the present Z87.1 method of specifying shade numbers was lacking in two areas and could be improved. Table 24-7 summarizes the minimum requirements found necessary from these studies and compares these values with the presently recommended shade numbers. As standards for recommended shade numbers have been incorporated into regulations, the proviso that the shade numbers be considered "typical" but not minumum has sometimes been dropped. However, the minimum shade values in Table 24-7 could be used for regulations designed to preclude retinal injury. The ANSI Z49.1 (1973) standard worded the consensus opinion on acceptable (comfort) shades as follows:

"The choice of a filter shade may be made on the basis of visual acuity and may, therefore, vary widely from one individual to another, particularly under different current densities, materials, and welding processes. However, the degree of protection from radiant energy afforded by the filter plate or lens when chosen to allow visual acuity will still remain in excess of the needs of eye filter protection. Filter plate shades as low as shade 8 have proven suitably radiation-absorbent for protection from the arc welding processes."

Although this ANSI statement is largely true, it requires that the specification of UV and blue-light transmission values for filter plates be revised. Table 24-8 provides a recommendation by the authors in this regard.

The specification for filtration of actinic ultraviolet radation as developed in the 1930's was limited to measurements at 313nm. There was no requirement for additional filtration at shorter wavelengths. This simplistic specification may well be

TABLE 24-8. Recommendations of the Authors
For Revision to Standards for Welding Filters

S#	Maximum Transmission Values (percent)			
	Ultraviolet Radiation*		Blue Light†	Infrared††
	(200-305 nm)	(313 nm)	(400-500 nm)	(760-3,000 nm)
2	0.1	0.2	1.0	80
3	0.07	0.2	0.7	40
4	0.04	0.2	0.4	20
5	0.02	0.2	0.2	10
6	0.01	0.1	0.1	5
7	0.007	0.1	0.07	3
8	0.004	0.1	0.04	2
9	0.002	0.1	0.02	1.5
10	0.001	0.1	0.01	1
11	0.0007	0.05	0.007	0.7
12	0.0004	0.05	0.004	0.4
13	0.0002	0.05	0.002	0.2
14	0.0001	0.05	0.001	0.1

* The spectral transmission (percent) between 200 nm and 305 nm should not exceed this value in the 200-305 nm column. The line transmission at 313 nm is the same as previously recommended.

† The spectral transmission (percent) should not exceed the value given between 400 and 500 nm. The old 405-nm values should be deleted, and the 436-nm line of mercury could be used as a check.

†† These recommended infrared transmission values (percent) should be sufficient to reduce the ocular exposure in the IR-A below 1 mW/cm^2.

adequate, for if the transmission at 313 nm is limited to perhaps 0.1%, it is assumed that the attenuation at shorter wavelengths will be far greater. Indeed, glass materials which attenuate strongly at 313 nm attenuate even more strongly at shorter wavelengths. However, with the advent of plastic welding filters, this assumption may possibly break down.

If new types of welding filters are developed incorporating crystalline substrates and dichroic coating, a mere check at 313 nm may not be sufficient, since the main objective of the 313-nm test is to assure attenuation *below* 313 nm of an optical density (OD) of 5.0 to 6.0 for arc welding. This region is often termed the actinic ultraviolet region. The requirement of a maximal transmittance for all UV below 313 nm would be a superior specification for future welding filters.

At the time the visible filtration requirements were developed, the blue light hazard was unknown. Hence, there was no limitation on the filter transmittance from 400 to 500 nm. In theory at least, a blue filter plate could be designed with a low visual transmittance overall and at 405 nm, yet with high transmittance between

410 and 500 nm. Even the transmittance limits at 405 nm were very lenient. It is therefore recommended that some filtration between 400 and 500 nm, or at least at 436 nm (another line of the mercury lamp spectrum), be specified. Table 24-8 lists these recommendations for modification of the filtration requirements.

The arc measurements performed under the USAEHA/AWS program suggested that the present IR requirements for filter attenuation are probably more than sufficient. At shade 4, the lowest shade typically used in gas welding and cutting, the ANSI recommendation (Table 24-6) for maximal IR transmittance is 0.05 (i.e., 5%). This transmittance specification would therefore limit irradiances to 200 mW/cm^2 on the front surface of the plate since the eye would receive the permissible exposure limit of 10 mW/cm^2 in that case. An irradiance of 200 mW/cm^2 may be encountered in some foundry operations, but not from gas welding sources. Moss and Murray (1979) measured a maximum near-IR (700-1100 nm) irradiance of 0.58 mW/cm^2 at 1 m from gas welding operations. At 30 cm from the torch, the corresponding level would be 6.4 mW/cm^2. From this, the total IR-A plus IR-B (760-3000 nm) irradiance at 30 cm can be estimated as about 30 mW/cm^2. This necessitates a maximal filter transmittance in that region of 0.33, which indicates that the Z87.1 IR-transmittance recommendations are quite conservative.

For arc welding shades (10 to 13), the Z87.1 standard recommends maximal IR transmittances of 0.004 (shade 13) to 0.006 (shade 10). The measurements of Sutter, *et al.* (1972) as shown in Figure 24-22 (page 840) suggest that a maximal IR transmittance of 0.25 at 200-A arc current and 0.015 at 1000 A would be required for a 30-cm viewing distance to reduce the corneal irradiance to 10 mW/cm^2.

The discussion above suggests that the IR transmittance specifications of ANSI Z87.1 may be overly restrictive. However, before the filter-plate specifications are relaxed, prototype filters with high IR transmission should be tried by welders to see if thermal comfort is adversely affected. After all, there may have been an empirical basis for the strong infrared absorption requirements. As a preliminary, cautious approach, the recommended infrared transmission values in Table 24.8 were derived on the basis that the IR-A irradiance should be reduced to 1.0 mW/cm^2 rather than 10 mW/cm^2.

24.12.2 Welding Filter Curtains

Shifting our attention to "see-through" welding curtains, it would appear that there should be no concern whatsoever regarding a lack of attenuation in the infrared for this type of product. IR-A and IR-B irradiances exceeding 10 mW/cm^2 beyond 1 m only occur at currents above 250 A. Since "see-through" curtains are not intended for continuous viewing, there is no serious hazard if the curtains do transmit 50% or even 90% in the 700-2000-nm wavelength range. See Figure 24-21. Since welding curtains are not meant for high-resolution seeing, no one would be expected to stare at the arc for long periods of time. There is probably not much merit in having more than one or two shades. Most present-day curtains have a shade ranging from 1 to 4 if one measures *diffuse* rather than *direct transmission*. The *effective* shade number for reducing the small-spot luminance of the arc may be 4

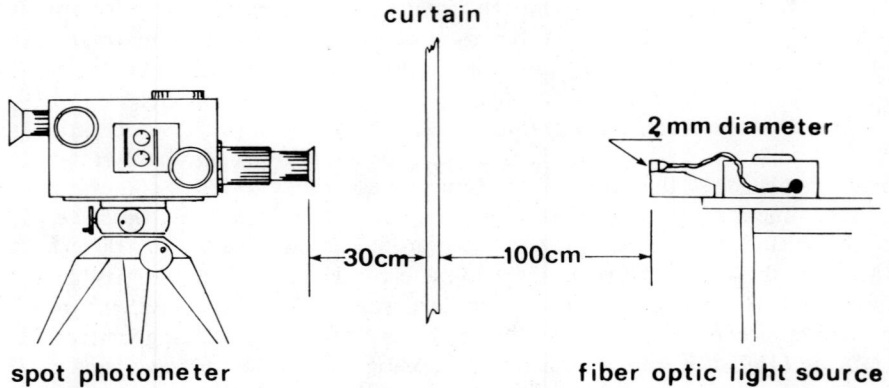

Figure 24-25. Prototype Filter-Curtain Test Set-up. A spot photometer having a 0.1-degree (1.7 mrad) field-of-view is placed 30 cm from a curtain being tested. A 2-mm diameter diffuse light source, such as a fiber optic source, is placed 100 cm behind the curtain. The luminance reduction factor with the curtain in place determines the *effective shade number* using the luminous transmission values in table 24-6.

to 10. Hence, it would be desirable to establish a testing procedure which would indicate the arc luminance reduction factor. For example, a spot photometer that just subtends a diffuse, 2-mm diameter light source placed 100 cm behind a curtain could be used to measure this fact. The spot photometer with a field-of-view of 0.1-degree would be placed at a reasonable viewing distance of 30 cm from the curtain, as shown in Figure 24-25. The same test, modified to measure blue-light radiance reduction (e.g., by using a scotopic filter) should be the basis of maximal blue light transmittance. The authors feel that this blue light reduction factor should be at least 10,000, and the luminance reduction factor at least 10. The actinic UV reduction factor should be 100,000, since viewing is not a factor in creating a skin or eye hazard to an adjacent bystander.

In conclusion, the recommendations for a standard for welding curtains should be: OD 5 between 200 nm and 315 nm, an effective OD for blue light radiance reduction (400-500 nm) of OD 4 and a luminance reduction of 10. These attenuation factors are readily achievable and are already met by some commercially available plastic curtains.

24.13 FLAMES AND MOLTEN METAL

24.13.1 Potential Hazards

The potential hazards from prolonged viewing of flames, gas torches, acetylene torches, and the pools of motlen metal and incandescent metal bars in industry

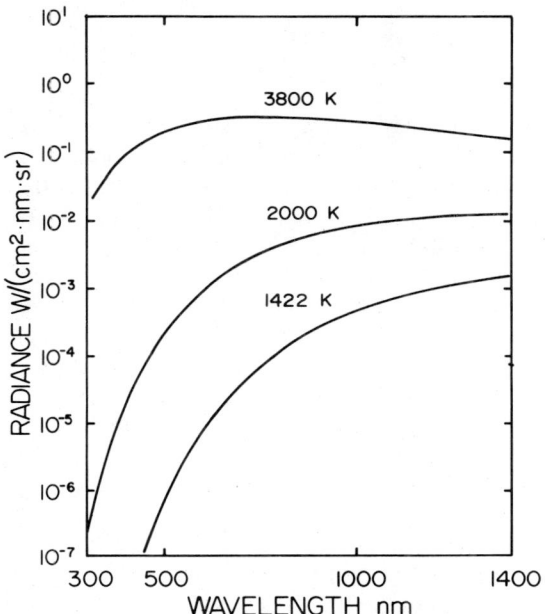

Figure 24-26. Blackbody Spectral Radiance Curves. These three spectral radiance curves across the retinal hazard region are useful in evaluating eye hazards in foundry operations. The lower two curves correspond to the temperatures of low-melting-point and high-melting-point metals in melting furnaces and the uppermost curve (3800 K) corresponds approximately to an open carbon arc which may often be found in electric furnaces.

must often be evaluated. These are encountered in foundries, steel mills, and many heavy industrial operations. A complete summary of the IR sources encountered in industrial operations, with the luminance and total irradiance at given distances would be difficult to compile. The optical radiation from these sources does not pose a retinal hazard problem, but rather a problem of total-body infrared heat stress. Possibly infrared effects upon the anterior of the eye also can be of concern. Open-arc processes such as welding and carbon arcs, and the electric arc furnaces used for melt-down of scrap metal, are often considered in the same category. Obviously, the open-arc processes are also of concern in the visible and ultraviolet. The ultraviolet emitted by blackbody emitters below 2000 K is not a problem in heavy industry. Figure 22-19 (on page 725) provides plots of values from blackbody tables which can be used to estimate the radiant exitance of a molten or incandescent metal surface in different spectral regions. The Stefan-Boltzmann Law makes it possible to calculate readily the total radiant exitance from a blackbody of known temperature, and with emissivity, of a graybody (Section 22.4.5). Figure 22-19 can also be used to determine what fraction of that total radiance or radiant exitance lies within a given wavelength region. For example, one can calculate the radiance of an incandescent source at the melting point of soft iron (1800 K), within the wavelength region between 400 and 1400 nm. Eqn. 2-25 (page 38) is used to calculate a total blackbody radiance value of 19 W/(cm^2·sr), by knowing the Stefan-Boltzmann constant which is 5.7 pW/(cm^2·K^4). Figure 22-19 is used by multiplying the first wavelength, 0.4 μm, by 1800 K to give KT = 720 for the value on the horizontal scale. The first curve shows that there is less than 1 % at wavelengths below 0.4 μm. Multiplying 1.4 μm by 1800 K gives a value for KT of 2520. Again from the right-hand curve in Figure 22-19, one finds that 82% of the radiation is found to be at wavelengths beyond 1400 nm. Hence the total radiance between 400 nm and 1400 nm is 18% of the total for all wavelengths, or (0.18)(19) = 3.4 W/(cm^2·sr). This radiance can then be used to estimate retinal hazards, which in this case do not exist. If there were a real concern for retinal hazards, one could go directly to Figures 22-23 and 22-24 which provide such information. These curves are based upon theoretical blackbody calculations of radiance and then calculations of retinal irradiance, where the transmission of the ocular media and the absorption in the retina have already been considered through the use of Equation (22-11) on page 727 (Sliney and Freasier, 1973). The radiance of a blackbody can also be used to estimate the irradiance at a distance from a pool of molten iron or other metal using Equation (22-12) on page 731. In this regard, it would be useful for the reader to review Section 22.4.5., which begins on page 728. Figure 24-26 provides three particularly useful blackbody radiance curves which correspond to the absolute melting-point temperatures of a high-temperature alloy and of soft iron, along with a very rough approximation of the blackbody equivalent temperature of a carbon arc.

Conventional methods of evaluating heat stress (Section 10.8, page 342) are appropriate for evaluating the thermal hazards to workers in foundries and steel mills, and will not be further discussed here. Of greater interest in this section are eye protective filters and infrared shields. Figure 16-19 (page 558) showed the infrared transmittance characteristics of infrared-reflective coatings used for heat control. Around heavy foundry operations such as the one shown in Figure 24-27, workers will typically wear dark glasses with high attenuation in the infrared region.

24.13.2 Infrared Protection Measures for Heavy Industry

In steel mills and other industrial facilities where infrared levels exceed 10 mW/cm^2, infrared- ("heat-") absorbing glasses are used for shielding. All types of glass absorb heavily at wavelengths beyond 4 μm, but only special "heat-absorbing" formulations absorb strongly in the 1 to 2 μm spectral region. Table 24-9 compares the infrared and visible transmission of a variety of commercial filters.

To avoid excessive temperature rises in the glass, an electrically conductive (EC) coating is often placed on the front surface of the glass to reflect as much of the incident infrared radiation as possible. This combination is sometimes referred to

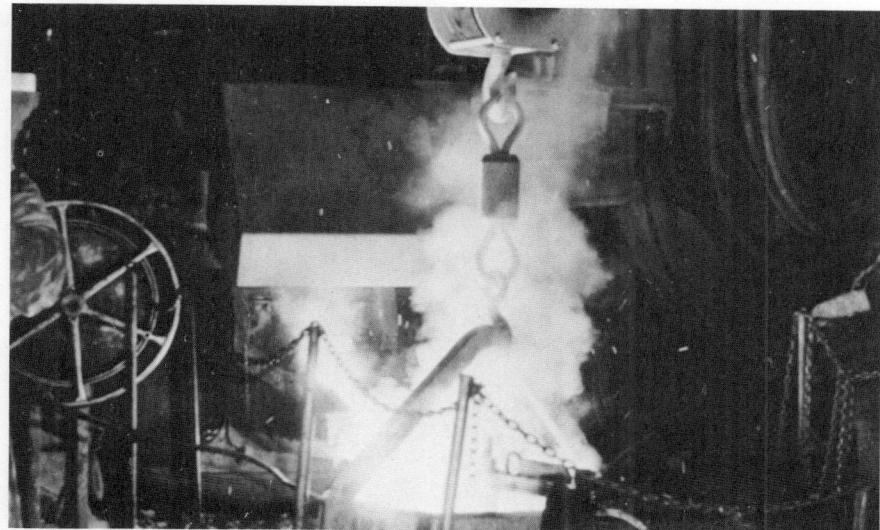

Figure 24-27. Steel Melting Furnace. The high levels of IR-B radiant energy from large vats of molten metal can produce conditions of heat stress and also require the use of dark spectacles or goggles with good infrared attenuating properties.

as a "hot mirror." The use of EC films on solar cells and spacecraft has stimulated a sophisticated technology for their fabrication (Hass *et al.*, 1979). Although, as discussed above, ultraviolet radiation from molten metal is not a problem, the carbon arcs often found in steel foundry furnaces may be hazardous to view directly.

When cobalt-blue glass lenses are used to check the temperature of the melt in electric furnaces, certain precautions shoud be exercised. Such glasses do not attenuate the hazardous blue light from the electric arc, hence the user should be cautioned to look only at the melt only for short periods and to avoid direct viewing of the arc. Fortunately, many furnaces are designed so that the arc itself is not seen at the normal viewing angles. Some IR-A radiation is also transmitted by cobalt blue glass, and this added to the short-wavelength light is not advisable for chronic exposure of the lens of the eye.

Figure 24-26 compares the spectra of blackbodies approximating incandescent and molten steel with an approximation of a carbon-arc spectrum. The molten steel has a low luminance, but more than 90% of its emission is beyond 1400 nm. This poses a severe whole-body thermal load. Section 16.19.3 discusses the aluminized protective clothing available for these environments. Also, the possibility that this long-wavelength radiation might facilitate cataractogenesis should be kept in mind (See Section 4.6).

TABLE 24-9. IR Transmission and Visual Transmission of Various Commercial Eye-Protective Filters†

Filter	Infrared Transmission (Percent)	Visible Transmission (Percent)
American Optical		
Clear	53	91
Cruxite	60	82
Didymium	46	48
MD Calobar	15	52
True Color	21	21
Cobalt Blue	32	0.74
Dark Calobar	9.4	37
Noviol	69	88
Plastic	22	94
Extra Dark Calobar	0.56	6.2
Filterweld	2.4	20
AO 584 Laser Goggle	6.3	36
Polysnap	29	92
Schott		
KG 3, 1 mm	7.1	86
BG-18, 3 mm	12	32
KG 3, 6.5 mm	<0.5	56
3M EC Coatings		
A33	12	32
A18	4.8	16
Eastern Safety*		
Visitors' Goggles	22	91
Safety Visor	22	91
Glendale Optical		
Glenweld Shade 1.3	20	67

† The infrared transmission values were measured using a thermopile against a lamp having a blackbody curve associated with a temperature of 1250 K. The visual transmission values were measured using the sun as a source and a photopic-filter detector to simulate the response of the eye. Some of the common filters are available in darker or lighter shades. Measurements were performed by W. J. Marshall and D. Crews, USAEHA.

* Characteristic of almost all clear plastic safety eyewear.

24.14 REVIEW QUESTIONS

1. Is it possible to receive a retinal injury from a welding arc?

2. Is there a first aid for welder's flash?

3. What is the recommended shade number for acetylene welding? What is the accepted shade number for shielded metal arc welding (SMAW) at 280 amps using ¼" wire?

4. What is the ANSI maximum ultraviolet transmittance at 313 nm for a shade 13 safety filter? How does this transmittance vary from the specifications for a shade 10 welding filter?

5. What is the typical range of luminance values for an open-arc welding arc?

6. For which welding geometries would hazardous reflected ultraviolet radiation be expected?

7. Give an example of a type of welding operation where shields and curtains are not practical.

8. A welder reports to an occupational health clinic complaining of welder's flash. He had been welding one hour just before he reported to the clinic. What would be a likely diagnosis?

9. An operator of a submerged arc-welding machine develops cataracts and claims it is due to the working with his submerged arc welding machine. Do you think this is possible?

10. What is the WHI for 250-A GMAW (Ar) on steel? What is the permissible exposure duration for UV exposure at 6 m from this arc?

24.15 REFERENCES

AMA Department of Environmental, Public and Occupational Health, 1972, Eye protection against indirect exposure to arc welding, *J. Am. Med. Assn.* **221**:1171.

American Conference of Governmental Industrial Hygienists, 1979, "Threshold Limit Values for Chemical Substances and Physical Agents in the Workroom Environment with Intended Changes for 1979," ACGIH, Cincinnati, OH.

American National Standards Institute (ANSI), 1973, "Safety in Welding and Cutting," Standard No. Z49.1-1973, ANSI, New York.

American Society for Testing and Materials (ASTM), 1961, "Standard Test for Haze and Luminous Transmittance of Transparent Plastics," ASTM Designation D 1003-61, ASTM, 1916 Race St., Philadelphia, PA.

American National Standards Institute (ANSI), 1968, "Standard Practice for Occupational and Educational Eye and Face Protection," Standard No. Z87.1-1968, New York.

Anonymous, 1969, Plasma jet cutting technique—the need to conform to safety rules, *Bedrijf en Teckniek - A*, **24**(618):450–452.

Bartley, D.L., McKinnery, W.N., and Wiegand, K.R., (to be published), "Ultraviolet Emissions from the Arc Welding of Aluminum-Magnesium Alloys," NIOSH, Cincinnati, OH.

Bates, C.C., 1952, The effects on the human eye of the radiant energy given off by various welding processes, *Sheet Metal Industr.*, **29**:349–357.

Bennett, A.P., Farmery, C., and Harlen, F., 1979, "Safety Aspects of Ultraviolet Emission from Welding Arcs," Report R/M/N1063, Central Electricity Generating Board, Research Division, Marchwood Engineering Laboratories, United Kingdom.

Campbell, D.L., 1976, "Welding Filter Plates," HEW Publication No. (NIOSH) 76-18, U.S. Department of Health, Education and Welfare, Washington, DC.

Carter, T.J, 1939, Electric welding, *U.S. Nav. Med. Bull.* **37**(1):138–142.

Chou, T.S., and Pfender, E., 1973, Spot formation at the anode of high intensity arcs, *Warme und Stoff*, **6**:69–77.

Clark, B.A.J., 1969, "Special-transmissive Requirements for Welding Filters," International Institute of Welding, London, Document VII pp.365–369.

Clark, B.A.J., 1968, Welding filters and thermal damage to the retina, *Austral. J. Optom.*, **51**(4): 91–98.

Coblentz, W.W., and Stair, R., 1930, Correlation of the shade numbers and densities of eye-protective glasses, *J. Opt. Soc. Am.*, **20**(11):624–629.

Dahlberg, J.A., 1971, The intensity and spectral distribution for ultraviolet emission from welding arcs in relation to the photodecomposition of gases, *Ann. Occup. Hyg.*, **14**:259–267.

Devore, R.K., 1973, "The Effective Spectral Irradiance of Ultraviolet Radiations from Inert-Gas-Shielded Welding Processes in Relation to the Arc Current Density," A Thesis submitted to the Texas A&M University (December 1973).

Dreessen, W.C., Brinton, H.P., Keenan, R.G., Thomas, T.R., Place, E.H., and Fuller, J.E., 1947, "Health of Arc Welders in Steel Ship Construction," U.S. Public Health Bulletin No. 298, Federal Security Agency, Washington, DC (185 pages)

Drinker, P., 1944, The measurement and prevention of eye flash, *Welding J.*, **23**(6):505–506.

Duke-Elder, S., and MacFaul, P.A., 1972, "Injuries, Non-Mechanical Injuries," in "System of Ophthalmology," (S. Duke-Elder, ed.) Vol. 14, part 2, C.V. Mosby, St. Louis.

Edebrooke, C.M., and Edwards, 1967, Industrial radiation cataract: the hazards and the protective measures, *Ann. Occ. Health*, **10**:293–304.

Emmett, E.A., and Horstman, S.W., 1976, Factors influencing the output of ultraviolet radiation during welding, *J. Occ. Med.*, **18**(1):41–44.

Emmett, E. A., Buncher, C. R., Suskind, R. R., and Rowe, K., 1980, A pilot study of skin and eye abnormalities among welders, in press.

English, P.E., 1973, Temperature and steel, *Iron Steel*, **46**(2):125–129.

English, W.P., 1973, Eye protection for welders, *ASSE J.*, **18**(7):39–43.

Entwistle, H., 1964, A case book of welding accidents, *Ann. Occup. Hyg.*, **7**:207–221.

Ferry, J.J., 1954, Ultraviolet emission during inert-arc welding, *Am. Industr. Hyg. Quart.*, **15**(1): 73–77.

Frant, R., 1968, Radiation problems associated with welding, *Z. Schweisstechnik - J. Soudure*, **58**(9):285–289.

Geeraets, W.J., and Berry, E.R., 1968, Ocular spectral characteristics as related to hazards from lasers and other light sources, *Am. J. Ophthal.*, **66**:15–20.

Glickstein, S.S., 1976, Temperature measurements in a free-burning arc, *Welding J. Pes. Suppl.*, **55**(8)222s–227s.

Gupta, M.N., and Singh, H., 1968, "Ocular Effects and Visual Performance in Welder," Report No. 27 of the Central Labour Institute, Ministry of Labour, Government of India, Sion-Bombay.

Hass, G., Heaney, J., and Toft, A., 1979, Transparent electrically conducting thin films for spacecraft temperature control applications, *Appl. Opt.*, **18**(10):1488–1489.

Heins, A.P (ed.), 1975, Occupational safety and health effects associated with reduced levels of illumination, USDHEW Publication (NIOSH) (75)142, National Institute of Occupational Health and Safety, Cincinnati, OH.

Hicken, G.K., and Jackson, C.E., 1966, The effects of applied magnetic fields on welding arcs, *Welding J.*, **45**(11):515s–525s.

Hinricks, J.F., 1978, Project committee on radiation-summary report, *Welding J.,* **57**(1):62,65.
Hogan, J., 1978, "The Use of Dye as Ultraviolet Inhibitor in Plasma Cutting Applications," Tech. Bulletin 3/10/78, Hypertherm, Inc., Hanover, NH.
Hogger, D., 1944, Die Gesundheitsgefathdungen im Berufe des Schweissers, *Gesundh. u. Wohlf.,* **24**:549–566.
Hornell, A., and Wulcan, J., 1972, "Spektralfordelningen hos Svetsljusbagar i Vaglangdsomradet 200-1200 nm," Thesis for the School of Electrical Engineering, Chalmers University of Technology, Goteborg, Sweden.
Horstman, S.W., Emmett, E.A., and Kneidielt, 1976, Field study of potential ultraviolet exposure from arc welding, *Welding Research,* **55**(5):121s–126s.
Horstman, S.W., and Ingram, J.W., 1979, A critical evaluation of the protection provided by common safety glasses from ultraviolet emissions in welding operations, *Am. Ind. Hyg. Assoc. J.,* **40**(3):770–780.
Hoyaux, M.F., 1968, "Arc Physics," Springer-Verlag, New York.
Hübner, H.J., Krause, E., Ruge, J., and Sutter, E., 1972, Strahlungsmessungen beim Lichtbogenschweissen nach verschiedenen Verfahren (einschliesslich Plasmaschneiden)–Beitrag zur Uberarbeitung von DIN 4647 Blatt 1, "Verwendung von Sichtscheiben for Augenschutzgerate, Schweisserschutz-filter," *Schweissen and Schneiden (Welding and Cutting)* **24**:290
Hübner, H.J., Sutter, E., and Wicke, K., 1970, Messung der Strahlungsleistung beim Schweissen und Folgerungen fur den Schutz der Augen gegan Infrarotstrahlung, *Optik,* **31**(5):462–476 (Available in English translation as National Research Council of Canada translation TT 1463).
Ingram, J.W., and Horst, J.W., 1977, A field study of near ultraviolet welding irradiance, *Am. Ind. Hyg. Assoc. J.* , **38**:456–461.
Jackson, C.E., 1960, The science of arc welding, *Welding J,* **39**(4-6):129s–140s, 177s–190s, and 225s–230s.
Kinsey, V.E., Cogan, D.G., and Drinker, P., 1943, Measuring eye flash from welding, *J. Am. Med. Assn.,* **123**(7):403–404.
Kleinfeld, M., Giel, C., and Tabershaw, J.R., 1957, Health hazards assocated with inert-gas-shielded metal-arc welding, *AMA Arch. Industr. Health,* **15**(11):27–31.
La Marre, D.A., 1977, Development of criteria and test methods for eye and face protective devices, Publication DHEW(NIOSH) 78-110, National Institute of Occupational Health and Safety, Cincinnati, OH.
Lesnewich, A., 1958, Control of melting rate and metal transfer in gas-shielded metal-arc welding, *Welding J.,* **37**(8-9):1–19s.
Levin, M., Ostberg, O., Knave, B., and Ottosson, A., 1976, Matning av Optisk Stralning–Arbetshygienisk Bedomning av Ljusbagen i plasmakaannarc (Measurements and criteria of optical radiations of the plasma torch), Underokingsrapport AMMF 103/76, Arbetarskddsstyrelsen.
Ludwig, H.C., 1968, Current density at anode spot size in the gas tungsten arc, *Welding J.,* **47**: 234s–240s.
Lyon, T.L., Sliney, D.H., Marshall, W.J., Krial, N.P., and DelValle, P.F., 1976, "Evaluation of the Potential Hazards from Actinic Ultraviolet Radiation Generated by Electric Welding and Cutting Arcs," Report No. 42-0053-77, USA Environmental Hygiene Agency, Aberdeen Proving Ground, Maryland (Available from NTIS, Springfield, VA, as ADA 033768).
Madden, R.P., 1975, Ultraviolet transfer standard detection and evaluation and calibration of NIOSH UV hazard monitor, HEW Publication NIOSH 75-131.
Malek, B., 1970, The problems with health protection plasma torch welding, *Zvaranie,* **19**(2): 46–52.
Malek, B., Novotna, J., and Trnka, J., 1973, "The Hygienic Significance of Radiation in the Wavelength Range from 200 nm to Visible Length in Electric Arc Welding," Document VIII-531-73, International Institute of Welding, Bratislava.
Marshall, W.J., Sliney, D.H., Lyon, T.L., Krial, N.P., and DelValle, P.F., 1977, "Evaluation of Potential Retinal Hazards from Optical Radiation Generated from Electric Welding and Cutting Arc," Report No. 42-0326-77, USA Environmental Hygiene Agency, Aberdeen Proving Ground, MD (Available from NTIS, Springfield, VA as ADA 043023).

Marshall, W.J., Sliney, D.H., Hoikkala, M., and Moss, C.E., 1979, "Optical Radiation Levels Produced by Air-Carbon-Arc Cutting Processes," U.S. Dept. of Health, Education, and Welfare, National Institute of Occupational Safety and Health, Cincinnati, OH (November 1979)

Maurelli, C., 1948, Vetri di protezione per i saldatori nelle nuove norme della B.S.I., *Securitas,* 33:32–36.

Mechev, V.S., and Eroshenko, L.E., 1972, Research into the spectrum of radiation by the argon-shielded arc close to the electrodes, *Automatic Weld.,* 25(8):57–61.

Mechev, V.S., and Eroshenko, L.E., 1970, Determining the temperature of the plasma in a arc discharge in argon, *Avt. Svarka,* 8:1–6.

Migai, K.V., 1969, Special clothing and footwear for electric welders, *Automatic Welding,* 22(10):63–67.

Minton, J., 1949, Occupational diseases of the lens and retina, *Brit. Med. J.,* 1:392–395.

Moss, C.E., and Gawenda, M.C., 1978, Optical radiation transmission levels through transparent welding curtains, NIOSH Research Report 78-176.

Moss, C.E., and Murray, W.E., 1979, Optical radiation levels produced in gas welding, torch brazing and oxygen cutting, *Welding J.,* 58(9):37–46.

Naidoff, M.A., and Sliney, D.H., 1974, Retinal injury from a welding arc, *Am. J. Opthal.,* 77(5):663–668.

National Institute of Occupational Safety and Health (NIOSH), 1978, "Safety and Health in Arc Welding and Gas Welding and Cutting," DHEW (NIOSH) Publication No. 78-138, National Institute of Occupational Safety and Health, Cincinnati, OH.

Nestor, O.H., 1962, High intensity current distributions at the anode of high current, inert gas arcs, *J. Appl. Phys.,* 33:1638–1648.

Olsen, H.N., 1962, Determination of properties of an optically thin argon plasma, in "Temperature, Its Measurement and Control in Science and Industry," (C.M. Herzfeld, ed.) Vol. III, Part 1, pp. 593–606, Reinhold Publishing Co., N.Y.

Pattee, H.E., Myers, L.B., Evans, R.M., and Monroe, R.E., 1973, Effects of arc radiation and heat on welders, *Welding J. Res.,* 52(5):297–308.

Powell, C.H., Goldman, L., and Key, M.M., 1968, Investigative studies of plasma torch hazards, *Am. Industr. Hyg. Assn. J.,* 29(4):381–385.

Rauh, F., 1927, Ein eigenartiger Fall von Veranderung der Netzhautmitte, *Z. f. Augenheilik.,* 63:48–64.

Rieke, F.E., 1943, Arc flash conjunctivitis: antinic conjunctivitis from electric welding arcs, *J. Am. Med. Assn.,* 122:734–736.

Rosskopf, T., 1953, Relation between welding current and appropriate transmission of filter glasses, *Welding J.,* 32(8):689–691.

Ruprecht, K.W., 1976, Foveo-maculopathy resulting from arc welding, *Zentralblat Arbeitsmed.,* 26:200–203.

Russ, D.S., 1973, The short-term effects on health of manual arc welding, *J. Soc. Occup. Med.,* 23(3):92–95.

Rutgers, G.A.W., 1950, Protective glasses for welding, *Doc. Opthalomogica,* 4:320–333.

Shaw, C.B., 1975, Diagnostic studies of the GTAW arc, *Welding J.,* 54:33s, 81s.

Sliney, D.H., and Freasier, B.C., 1973, Evaluation of optical radiation hazards, *Appl. Optics,* 12(1):1–24.

Stair, R., 1948, "Spectral-Transmissive Properties and Use of Eye-Protective Glasses," National Bureau of Standards Circular 471, U.S. Department of Commerce, National Bureau of Standards, Washington, DC.

Stutz, G.F.A., 1925, Observations of spectro-photometric measurements of paint vehicles and pigments in the ultraviolet, *J. Franklin Inst.,* 220:87–102.

Sutter, E., Hübner, H.J., Krause, E., and Ruge, J., 1972, "Strahlungsmessungen an Verschiedenen Lichtbogen-Schweissverfahren," Report No. Optik 2/72 of the Physikalish-Technische Bundesanstalt, Braunschweig, W. Germany.

Sutter, E., and Zander, K., 1973, Anforderungen an den IR- und UV-Transmissionsgrad von Augenschutzfiltern, *Zentralb. Arbeitsmed. Arbeitsschutz,* 23(9):275-279 (September 1973).

Szafran, L., 1965, Znetnienia soczewki o cichach zacmy hutniczej u spawacza, (A lens opacity with the morphological features of smelting cataract in a welder), *Med. Pracy.*, **16**(3):246–284.
Tengroth, B., 1976, Safety glasses in welding, *Env. Res.*, **11**(:283–284.
Terrien, F., 1902, Des trouble visual provoque por l'electricete, *Arch. Ophthalomol.*, **22**:692–696.
Tseng, C.F., and Savage, W.F., 1971, Effect of arc oscillation, *Welding J.*, **50**(11):777–786.
Van Someren, E., and Rollason, E.C., 1948, Radiation from the welding arc, *Welding J. Res. Suppl.*, **27**(9):448–452s and **28**:566.
Weisman, C., (ed.), 1976, "Welding Handbook, Fundamentals of Welding," Vol. 1, 7th Edn., American Welding Society, Miami, FL.
Wheater, R.H., 1976, Eye damage from repeated exposure to welding arcs, *JAMA*, **236**:2224.
Wickstrom, 1972, Welding health hazards, *Ehkaise Tapaturmia–Forebygg Olycksfall*, **2**:4–9.
Wolbarsht, M.L., 1978, The effects of optical radiation on the anterior structures of the eye, *in* "Current Concept in Ergophthalmogy," (Tengroth, *et al*, eds.) pp. 29–46, Societas Ergophthalmological Internationalis, Karolinske Institute, Stockholm, Sweden.
Wolfe, W.L., and Zissis, G.J., 1978, "The Infrared Handbook," Office of Naval Research, Washington, DC.
Wurdemann, H.V., 1936, The formation of a hole in the macula, light burn from exposure to electric welding, *Am. J. Ophthalmol.*, **19**:457–4.

Chapter 25
Safety Programs and Formal Training
By James Smith, IBM

25.1 INTRODUCTION

It should be evident from previous chapters that the use of lasers may present potential hazards if not properly used. In addition, there are several legislative and voluntary standards that have been promulgated or issued that require specific controls over the usage of lasers. As a result, it is necessary to establish a laser safety program that assures the safe use of lasers and compliance with all applicable standards.

Although this chapter is devoted primarily to laser safety and training programs, the same philosophy may be used to establish programs for use with other types of radiation.

Several of the "user" standards require user knowledge of laser safety, or more simply stated, some form of training. In addition to direct requirements for training programs, experience has shown that a good laser safety program contains training, or education as a major ingredient. The training program may in turn contain major ingredients for sound safety program management. Controls for laser safety may be of an engineering type, or of an administrative nature. A properly devised training program may be structured to contain many of the desired administrative type controls.

25.2 LASER SAFETY PROGRAM

In each company or organization, management should establish a laser safety program. The type and structure of the program should be chosen to best satisfy the needs of each organization. The program should provide for the designation of a specific individual assigned the authority and responsibility for maintaining and enforcing the laser safety program. It should be pointed out that this individual may not be devoting all his time to this task. The American National Standards Institute Z-136.1 Standard for the Safe Use of Lasers (1976), as well as several other standards and organizations, refers to this individual as the Laser Safety Officer, or LSO.

The LSO, whether full or part time, may be designated from among such personnel as a radiation protection officer, industrial hygienist, safety engineer, or perhaps even a user. He should have the authority for supervising the control of laser hazards. He or she may also provide consultative services on hazard evaluation, establish regulations for the control of the program with authority to suspend or restrict laser activity if hazard controls are not adequate, maintain laser inventory records, approve all protective equipment such as laser eyewear prior to use, investigate all known or suspected accidents from laser activity, assure that adequate warning systems and signs are installed in appropriate locations, and assure that adequate training in laser safety is provided for all employees using lasers. The training aspects will be covered in depth later.

Where the LSO job is full time, and the organizational requirements are large, the LSO may require additional assistance, which is recognized by ANSI Z-136.1 as the Deputy Laser Safety Officer.

The laser safety program should clearly delegate responsibilities to others in addition to the LSO. Some consideration should be given to define clearly the responsibilities as they relate to laser safety to Supervisors, employees working with lasers, and others where required. One company's internal standard (Charschan *et al.*, 1972) contains sections on specific responsibilities for the Local Safety Organization, Supervisor, Engineering and R & D Organizations, Installer and Operator, Medical, and Purchasing Organization. The Purchasing Organization responsibilities are a strong checkpoint to assist the LSO in assuring that lasers, laser systems and laser safety equipment will not be purchased unless previously approved by the LSO.

25.3 TRAINING OBJECTIVES/CONSIDERATIONS

There are many things to consider when establishing training objectives. The first two questions that may be asked are "who" and "why." Trainees may be individuals who will work with the laser on an every day basis. They may be individuals who will have little or no requirement to work on, or with, the laser directly, but may be assigned to routinely work in the general vicinity where lasers are in use. The trainee may be a manager, or supervisor of individuals working with lasers. A trainee may also be a Laser Safety Officer.

The "who" will in turn influence the "why." The one common denominator in the "why" is to assure the safe use of lasers. Some of the considerations to be evaluated are: the class of laser; engineering controls that are in use; frequency of use; the specific job the trainee has with respect to the laser; and the amount of previous training.

Should the individual receive training only to the extent that he may push the proper button at the proper time safely, or should he receive additional training on the basic concepts of lasers and laser hazards? To what extent should training present the substance and nature of applicable standards to the trainee? Will the trainee be responsible for protecting others, such as bystanders and passers-by?

Is the laser application confined to a fixed indoor location, or is it mobile or outdoors? What is the probability that the trainee will be directed to become involved with lasers other than the ones he is initially being trained for? Is the application a single laser used for a single purpose, or are there many lasers used for multiple applications?

It should be obvious by now that with all these considerations, it is impossible to set down a set of training objectives that would satisfy the needs of all. Because of this, some generalized training programs have been developed based on the classification of the laser(s) involved and the type of worker.

25.4 TRAINING

25.4.1 Area Workers Training

For purposes of developing training requirements, we shall define an "area worker" as one who does not have a job assignment requiring work on lasers, but is required to be in the vicinity of lasers. Examples of area workers would be construction workers in the vicinity of laser surveying equipment, production workers engaged in assembly or inspection tasks in the vicinity of a laser tool (laser welder for example), operating room staff assisting a surgeon performing surgery with a laser, etc.

Because an area worker's potential for exposure to hazard is generally less than for one who works directly with a laser, it would seem reasonable not to require as much training, or maybe none at all. Before that is determined, the class of laser(s) that the area worker will be in the vicinity of must be ascertained. If the laser is Class 1 without any enclosure, then there would be no potential hazard to anyone. However, if the laser is normally Class 1 by virtue of enclosures, and the laser within the enclosure is greater than Class 1, then consider the maintenance/service procedures. If any servicing will be done with the enclosure removed and the laser on, even though there will be strict procedures followed by the service personnel to protect area workers, it would be reasonable to provide some minimum training to area workers for at least an awareness of laser safety. This awareness training need not take the form of a classroom session, but may be only the required reading of a pamphlet on the subject, such as the LIA Laser Safety Guide (LIA, 1977). Too often the area worker is overlooked when considering laser safety, particularly when the laser is Class 1 only under normal operating conditions. Maintenance and service situations must always be considered when evaluating the need for area worker training.

If there are many area workers and laser workers involved with other than Class 1 lasers, it may be beneficial to give all area workers a minimum of at least an awareness of laser safety. This makes it easier to change area workers' job assignments, particularly if it requires working in the vicinity of a higher classification of laser.

25.4.2 Laser Workers Training

"Laser workers" are defined as any individuals whose work assignment causes them to work directly with lasers. This includes operators of lasers, technicians, maintenance personnel (including those who may spend only a small portion of their time on lasers), applications personnel, engineers, scientists, and the laser surveying transit operator, etc.

As with area workers, the class of laser the worker will be associated with must first be determined. It is important at this time to remember to look at the potential that the laser worker may work with a higher class laser at a later date. If a reasonable potential exists, then the training objectives should be established on the assumption that he will work with the higher class laser. This will reduce the need for additional training later, and not leave to chance that this will be overlooked just because the worker has been "trained" for the lower class laser.

Again, if the laser is Class 1, not enclosed, there is no potential hazard. If it is Class 1 by enclosure, then we must determine if the operator will be present during covers off servicing. If it is not a normal part of the operator's job to be present during maintenance, it must be asked if it would be probable that he assist for purposes of clarifying a defect condition, or the correction of one, as an aid to maintenance. Maintenance personnel's training needs are based on the worst case temporary classification of a laser with enclosures removed.

It can readily be seen that determination of training needs for laser workers is based on far more than classification of the laser system in normal use. It is based on the worst possible set of conditions. Extent of training for laser workers, depending on worst case potential classification, could range from a simple audio tape/slide presentation or lecture to a full 30-40 hrs. of instruction. Table 25-1 describes possible training choices for various classifications.

25.4.3 Management Training

One of the more difficult tasks in a laser safety program is to assure that the first line manager or supervisor has the proper awareness of laser safety. Often the manager is responsible for some paper work portion of the laser safety program, and he is not aware of it until one of his workers is involved in a violation. It is therefore desirable to provide the manager or supervisor of each area/laser worker with at least an awareness of laser safety. This may be in the form of a simple guideline pamphlet (LIA, 1977), or it may be the same level training as his workers.

Once a decision is made to include management and supervisory personnel in the training program, it is only one additional step to include some specific material for management only. If included, this additional material may be an effective means of assuring the Laser Safety Officer that management is fully aware of their role in the laser safety program. Topics that may be covered in management training are: inventory forms and procedures, workers' responsibilities in the program, the role of the Laser Safety Officer, requirements for training area/laser workers, accident reporting procedures, legal requirements, etc. Several industrial firms now require

TABLE 25-1. Training Requirements as a Function of Laser Classification and Type Worker

	Type of Worker	Highest Laser Classification			
		2	3a	3b	4
Safety Guide*	Area Worker	NR	R	SR	SR
	Laser Worker	R	SR	SR	SR
	Laser Safety Officer	SR	SR	SR	SR
Audio Tape/Slides†	Area Worker	NR	NR	R	SR
	Laser Worker	NR	R	SR	SR
	Laser Safety Officer	SR	SR	SR	SR
Text, Articles	Area Worker	NR	NR	NR	R
	Laser Worker	NR	NR	R	SR
	Laser Safety Officer	R	SR	SR	SR
Standards Review	Area Worker	NR	NR	NR	NR
	Laser Worker	NR	NR	NR	NR
	Laser Safety Officer	SR	SR	SR	SR
30-40 Hour Course††	Area Worker	NR	NR	NR	NR
	Laser Worker	NR	NR	NR	R
	Laser Safety Officer	R	SR	SR	SR

NR—not required; R—recommended; SR—strongly recommended.

*Such as LIA Laser Safety Guide (LIA, 1977)
†Such as Item 3, Table 25-2
††See Table 25-2, Short Courses

managers to take the laser safety training before the workers are permitted to use lasers.

The management training becomes even more effective if a certification program exists in which both laser workers and their management must be trained before the worker can be certified. This places more incentive on management to take the training. It also provides the Laser Safety Officer with a vehicle in which he can be sure that management receives the details necessary for him to administer his part of the laser safety program. One example of a training program incorporating mandatory training of management is given by Smith et al. (1977) and described in part in one of the example programs outlined later in this chapter (Sect. 25.5.3).

25.4.4 Laser Safety Officer Training

If the Laser Safety Officer (LSO) is to be the focal point of a laser safety program, then proper training becomes a necessity. Again, the level of training required will be somewhat dependent on the extent and classification of the lasers in use, but not to the same level as for area and laser workers. The LSO should be trained to at least one class higher than the laser worker. In large industrial and research organizations where new lasers and laser applications may arise on short notice, the LSO must be knowledgeable and able to make an assessment of potential hazards, and recommend appropriate controls. In this type of environment, the LSO must be skilled in the basics of laser safety hazard evaluation for those instances when the classification of the laser is not known, or when a system or the environment is modified. He must also be highly knowledgeable in the various control measures required for any class of laser under his jurisdiction. In addition to the topics described above, the LSO should be familiar with all applicable standards. This may include Federal, State, and voluntary standards.

Suitable training is not generally available within the employer's organization, and often outside courses are required to provide the necessary background for the LSO. Courses ranging from one day to one week in duration are periodically offered in laser safety by organizations such as the Laser Institute of America, and Rockwell Associates Seminar Management. Many of the shorter courses are offered in conjunction with conferences and symposium relating to lasers and associated technologies.

Some specific topics to be included in the LSO's training are: basic laser principles, bio-effects of lasers on eye and skin, non-radiation hazards such as electrical and chemical, classification of lasers, control measures, laser terminology, basic radiometry, laser parameter measurements, and laser standards. Most of the week duration courses cover these topics to varying degrees. They may also include workshop sessions on hazard analysis (including calculations) and measurements. Some courses also include a workshop or lab on the basic operation of a laser.

The LSO is often assumed to be a full time job, but this is not always the case. The LSO may have other responsibilities, and in fact, may even be a laser worker. Regardless of other duties, the LSO must still be trained to be the key individual responsible for effecting and enforcing the laser safety program.

25.5 EXAMPLE PROGRAMS

Training programs may be as varied as the many organizations requiring them. In cases where only one or two workers need be trained, it is often easier and more economical to send the individuals outside the company to a laser safety course. When many (sometimes hundreds or more) require the laser safety training, it becomes more necessary to establish training programs within the company.

If it has been determined that the training will be done in-company, it must be decided what type of training will best suit the needs of the company. This should be based on the objectives and the number of area and laser workers to be trained. Projected future training needs based on turnover of personnel and growth of technology should also be considered before selecting a particular type of training program. What resources are available for potential instructors? If the number of potential instructors is low, will they be available on a long term basis for future needs?

Three specific examples of training programs will be given. These are actual programs that have been used in a large industrial complex (Smith et al., 1977) to satisfy that particular facility. The content of the programs is intended as a guideline to present concepts and methods for training laser workers in industry. It is no way implied that these programs as described are required by legislative standards of any local, state, or federal agency.

25.5.1 Comprehensive Expandable Classroom Program

This is an early type of program developed with flexibility to allow removal of material and shortening of sessions for personnel who would be working only with low risk equipment. The session content to be described is for the high risk situation, and represents the longest course. The first three sessions were on the order of two hours each in duration. Since the fourth session dealt with specific equipment, the length varied with the complexity of the equipment. An additional challenge was imposed for this program by the decision that the same program would be used for manufacturing operators, maintenance personnel, engineers, technicians, and any others requiring laser safety training. This meant that the students in any given class would have a considerable spread in educational backgrounds. They would range from less than a high school diploma to advanced college degrees. The materials used had to be understood by the high school grad, yet not bore the college graduate. Therefore, most of the material was of low technical key, with only a small amount of higher level material thrown in for the benefit of the more advanced student.

The first classroom session, entitled "Introduction," comprised an oral presentation supported with well illustrated slides that described the basic Ruby laser and its principle of operation. The presentation covered briefly the more common types of various lasers, their wavelengths, modes of operation, and power/energy. The basic types of laser emission were discussed, such as conventional burst, long pulse, continuous wave (CW), Q-switched, etc. The session gave the student a basic overall picture of the laser, and provided information to make the later sessions more meaningful. The slides used as illustrations contained no mathematics, complicated relationships, or terms to confuse the less advanced student. In this session, it was fully realized that not every student would understand all the material presented, but each student would leave the class with much more knowledge about lasers than at the start.

The second classroom session, entitled "Safety." was the prime session of the course. Originally, the session was a slide illustrated lecture. The session described in very basic terms the bio-effects mechanisms for laser induced damage on human organs. Where possible, practical illustrations of damage were used. For example, in a class for students being trained in operation of CO_2 lasers, hot dogs, or chicken wings were irradiated with a CO_2 laser (Figure 25-1). The visible effect on the meat was far more impressive to the class than a statement such as, "An incident beam of X Watts/cm^2 on the skin will induce biological damage." Eyewear was covered in detail and examples of the use of improper laser safety goggles were shown, such as a quartz (used for CO_2 laser protection) with a piece of carbon paper taped behind the plate and a ruby laser fired *through* the plate, thereby blasting the carbon paper. This example illustrated that protective filter materials used for CO_2 lasers were not adequate for use with ruby lasers (Figure 25-2). The session also included a review of the company and facility laser safety requirements.

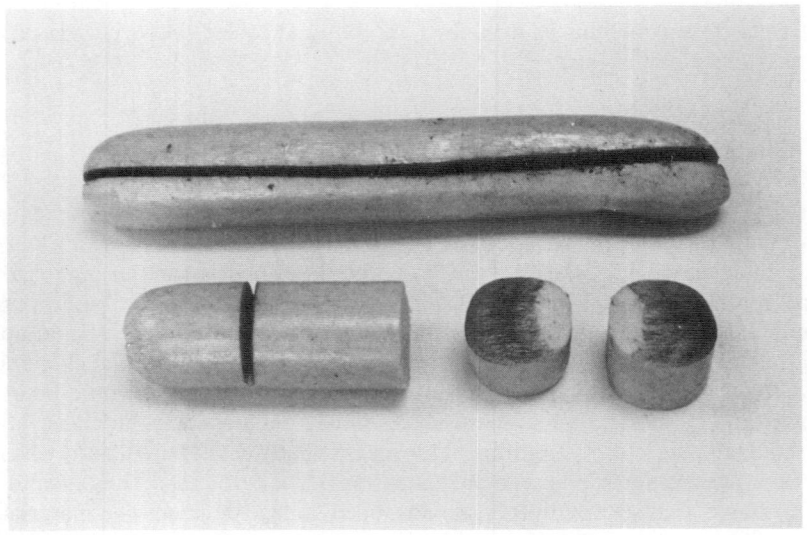

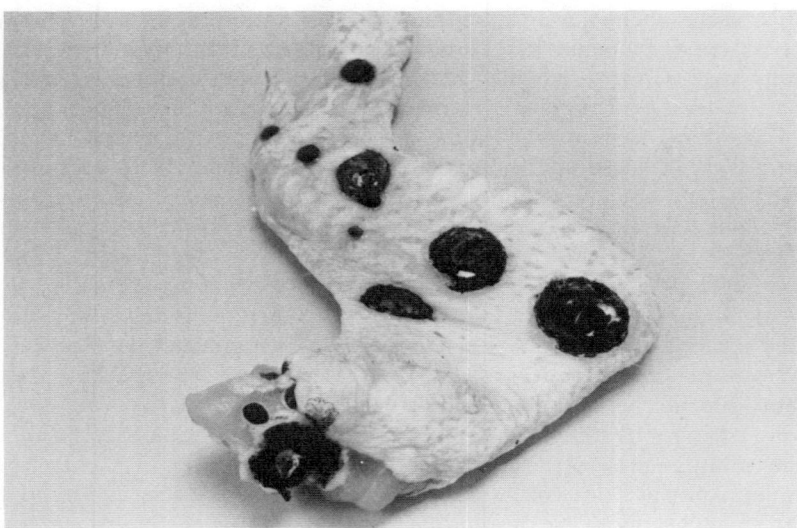

Figure 25-1. Laser Hazard Demonstration. A hot dog (top) and a chicken wing (bottom) irradiated by a focused CO_2 laser beam can aid in the demonstration of laser skin burn hazards.

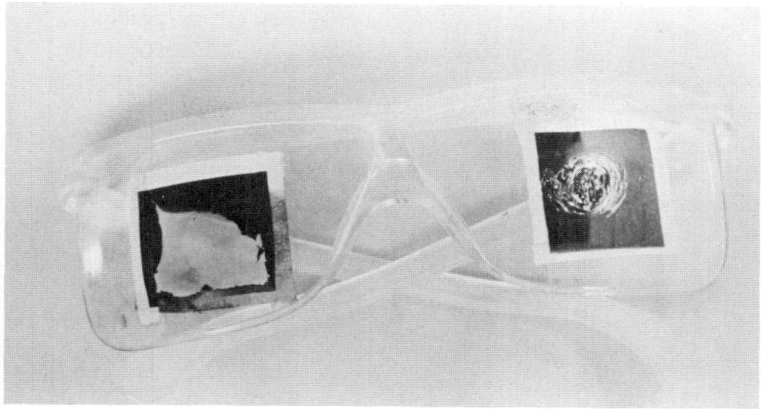

Figure 25-2. Carbon Paper Backed Clear Eyewear. Left side irradiated by Ruby laser and right side irradiated by CO_2 laser.

The third classroom session, entitled "Materials Processing with Lasers," was designed to acquaint students with the variety of laser applications within the company and industry in general, and to stimulate the imagination on the potential of lasers. Some 60-80 slides were utilized in this session illustrating the advantages, such as wavelength, power/energy, mode of operation, etc., of various types of lasers for specific applications.

The fourth and final classroom session, entitled "Systems Operations," dealt with the specific laser equipment of the students themselves. This session presented slides of the system, with and without covers removed, exposing all controls, adjustments, panels, work area, etc. The method of operation and operational procedures were covered in detail, using the slides to point out the switches, knobs, dials, etc., as they were discussed in the procedures. This classroom session eliminated the need for detailed introductory information to be repeated for each small group during the Practical Experience phase. If the total class numbers less than four students, this session can be eliminated, and the material covered in the Practical Experience phase.

The "Practical Experience," or On-Job-Training, was conducted as long as was necessary for the student to become sufficiently skilled in his job to meet all qualifications for certification in his specific category (operator, manufacturing technician, etc.). For complex systems, it was found desirable to bring in personnel from the laser manufacturer.

The course just described had several advantages. It taught the industrial users the potential hazards of lasers. The course superficially addressed basic "how-it-works" theory and applications. The sessions were flexible in content and duration because they were instructor controlled. Courses for complex high energy systems would use most of the materials. Applications utilizing low power helium-neon lasers could have the sessions condensed so that all classroom topics could be covered in a single two hour session. Because the classes had an instructor, there was excellent opportunity for discussion.

The classroom approach with instructors has its disadvantages. Some of the instructors come from line groups and had other responsibilities, making it difficult to schedule courses that would satisfy both student and instructors. If more than one instructor was used, the content varied from course to course. Also, with more than one instructor, it was not uncommon to have differences of opinion about the emphasis to be placed on the various aspects of laser safety. Finally, it was not practical to run a course for only a few students. If a course was scheduled only when sufficient students were available, there would be a long delay before any given student would be certified. Classes often contained a mix of employees in all categories requiring certification. Their education ranged from less than high school to advanced degrees in Engineering or Science. This factor was accentuated because the program was developed by a local facility rather than at the corporate level and other locations within the company developed similar but uncoordinated programs.

25.5.2 Movie-Tape/Slide Program

As time went on, the need for large classes diminished. It was difficult to obtain instructors for small groups, and the frequency of requests for one and two students to be trained in a short period of time increased. This situation clearly indicated the need for a program that could be scheduled on short notice for any number of students that would not require a trained instructor. The solution was to develop a Movie-Tape/Slide Program.

A one-hour program entitled "Laser Safety" was developed. Because safety was of primary importance, emphasis was placed on obtaining the visual aspects of the safety material. A film entitled "Laser Safety," (see Table 25-2) was chosen as the nucleus of the session. The film covered the basic bio-effects of laser beams on skin and eyes, and protective measures. The illustrations in the film were primarily of development and laboratory type laser installations. It was therefore necessary to supplement the movie heavily with slides that would illustrate industrial uses and environment more clearly. The slide program was developed in two sections: Hazards; and Control Measures.

The "hazards" section reemphasized some of the material in the movie. Slides of the effects of lasers on chicken wings, etc., were added. Associated hazards, particularly electrical, were covered in detail. Chemical hazards, including toxic vapor plumes, were also illustrated. The "control measures" section delt with the elimination or reduction of potential hazards with controls in three categories: engineering; personal protection; and administrative.

When the slide package was complete, the text for the slides was recorded and put onto standard "C" series cassettes. Some of the cassettes were produced with a 1KC "beep" to be used with automatic advancing slide projectors. The slide-tape package both supplemented and complemented the film. The program was then

TABLE 25-2. Sources of Laser Safety Training Media

1. Film		"Laser Safety," a 16 mm color film with sound, available from University of California, Extension Media Center, 2223 Fulton Street, Berkeley, California 94720.
2. Film		"Fundamentals of Lasers," a 16 mm color film with sound available from the Upjohn Company, Professional Communications, 700 Portage Road, Kalamazoo, Michigan 49001.
3. Slides		"Laser Safety Training Package," (80 slide set with audio tape cassette on industrial laser safety), available from Laser Institute of America, 4400 Executive Park Drive, Cincinnati, Ohio 45241.
4. Short Courses		Short Course on Laser Safety, conducted on a periodic basis by Laser Institute of America, 4100 Executive Park Drive, Cincinnati, Ohio 45241.
5. Short Courses		Rockwell Associates Seminar Management, 6282 Coachlite Way, Cincinnati, Ohio 45243.
6. Training Manuals		Technical Education Research Center, 4201 Lake Shore Drive, Suite 111, Waco, Texas 76710.

complete except for some means to introduce the basic fundamentals of lasers.

It was determined that laser fundamentals must be a part of the program if students were to fully understand the potential hazards related to the coherent nature of laser beams. A five-minute film entitled "The Fundamentals of Lasers" (see Table 25-2) was selected as the introduction. This film is an excerpt from the Upjohn *Vanguard of Medicine* series "Clinical Applications of Lasers." The film describes, in animated fashion, the laser and how it works; the contrast between ordinary white light and laser light in terms understandable to the non-engineer; how atoms in a uniform substance, such as a ruby crystal, are "excited;" why these atoms release photons; and how a chain reaction causes these photons to combine into a beam of very high intensity. Although the running time of the film is short, it does an excellent job of providing an adequate introduction for the primary topic of laser safety.

The final package consisted of: the introductory film; the film on laser safety, and the 80 slide-tape presentation, divided equally between hazards and control measures. This program did not have built in, on-the-job training (OJT) material. This was added by supplier representatives, engineers, previously certified personnel, etc. The primary advantage of this instruction package was the standardization of the material presented, which eliminated the need for an instructor in the classroom. The disadvantage was the lack of a question-and-answer opportunity. This could have been corrected by providing a monitor, but this would have eliminated one of the major advantages of the program however. Also, this program did not have any provision for testing the student.

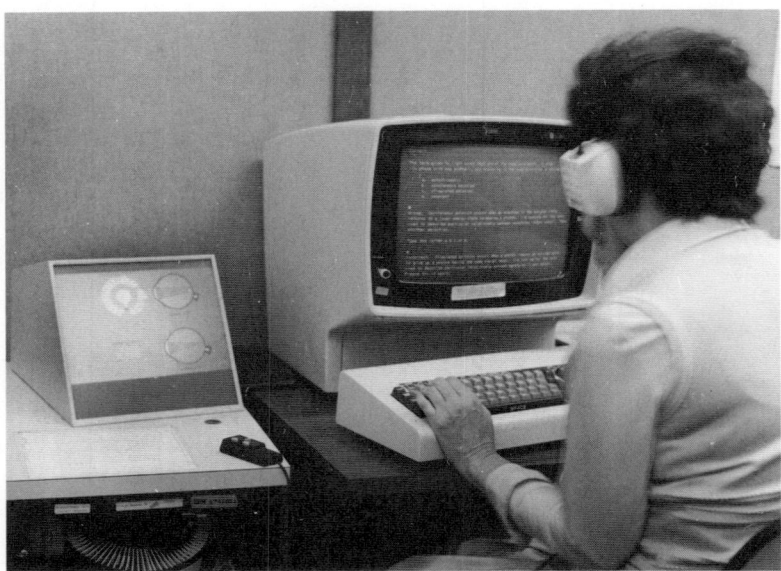

Figure 25-3. Student at CAI Terminal with Slide Set on Visual Monitor and Review Questions on Display.

25.5.3 Computer-Assisted Instruction (CAI)

In order to expedite the laser safety training program for individual requests (i.e., one or two at a time), a CAI course was developed. It was based on the existing movies/tape-slide presentation materials previously discussed. In addition, a special section was incorporated into the course which describes specific manager responsibilities.

The course was developed using a computer course writer language. Each student progresses through the course following directions and answering questions presented to him on a display terminal which consists of a CRT display tube and a keyboard (Fig. 25-3). Adjacent to the terminal is an audio/visual unit containing a cassette recorder and 35 mm slide projector. Each student progresses through the course at his own pace. The course structure is shown in Fig. 25-4. After the student "signs on" the course, he is presented the format of the course and asked if he is a manager. A list of specific course objectives is presented, along with additional objectives if he is a manager. Knowledge of these objectives is tested at the end of the course. All questions must be correctly answered in order to satisfactorily complete the course. Any questions missed on the quiz necessitates additional remedial material coupled with another similar question.

The student, after being given the course objectives, has the option of:

Safety Programs and Formal Training

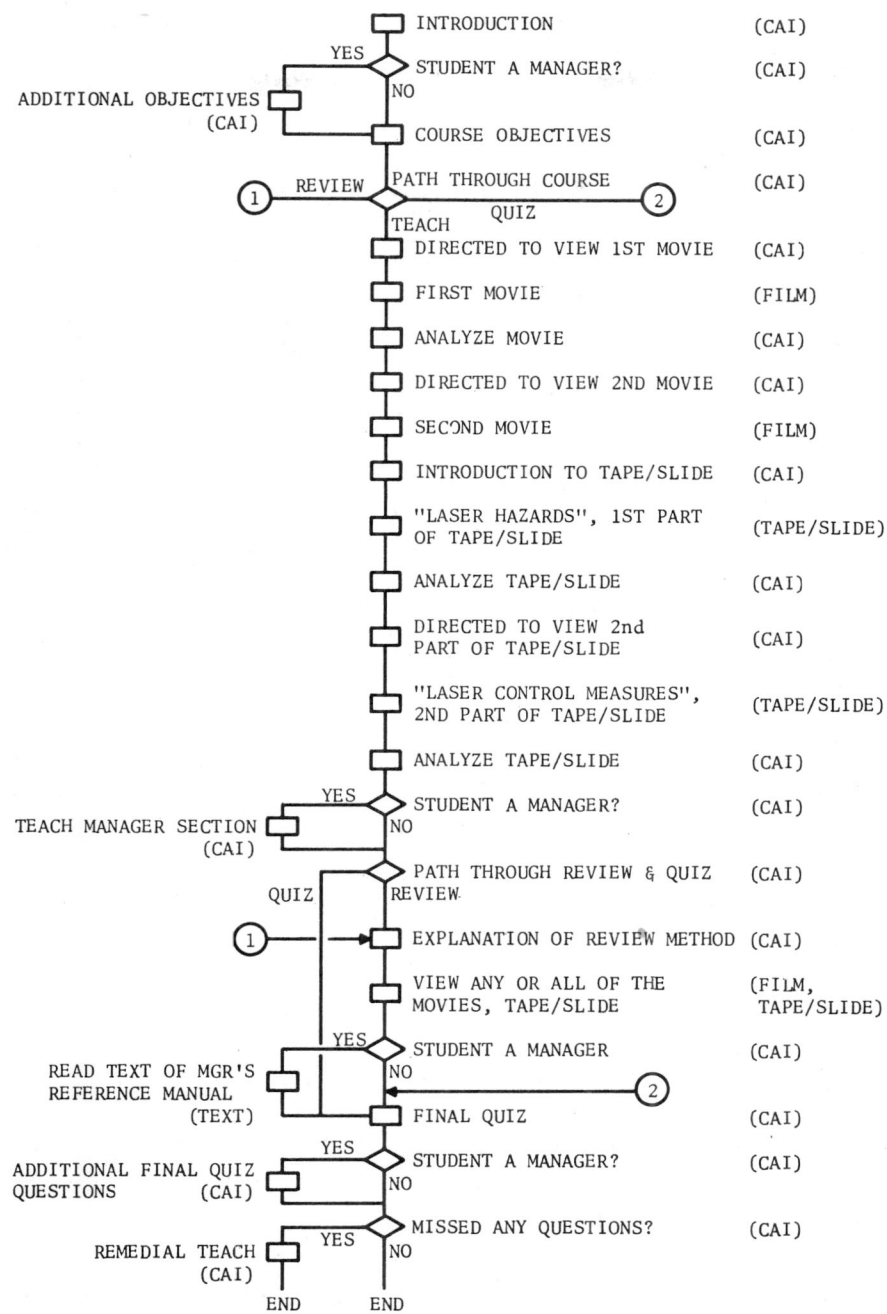

Figure 25-4. CAI Laser Safety Course Flow

1. Taking the quiz without going through the teach or review sequence.

2. Going directly to a review, and then the quiz.

3. Going through the complete teach and review sequence followed by the quiz.

During the teach sequence, the student is directed to view the first movie, entitled "The Fundamentals of Lasers." Upon completion of the film, he is asked questions, via the terminal, on its context. He is then directed to view the second movie entitled "Laser Safety." After the movie is finished, the student is directed to view the first section of the tape/slide presentation (the section on Hazards). Upon completion, he is again asked questions on the content of this section. The student is then directed to view the second section of the tape/slide presentation (the section on Control Measures). Upon completion, he is questioned on the information just viewed.

If the student is a manager, he receives additional information concerning his responsibilities in the laser field. A handout called the "Manager's Reference Manual" is also given to each manager taking the course.

Below is a sample question which a student would receive during the teach sequence, and the response given via the terminal to the student's answer:

Question presented to the student on the terminal screen.	*The most correct definition of laser light is:* a. A light source of single frequency, random direction and in phase. b. A light source of one wavelength, in phase and traveling in the same direction. c. A non-coherent light source. d. The light emitted by a fluorescent lamp. e. The photons that are released by spontaneous emission.
Student's answer *Terminal's response*	a *Wrong. Laser does not travel in a random direction. Try again.*
Student's answer *Terminal's response*	c *Incorrect. Laser is a coherent light source. Try it again.*
Student's answer *Terminal's response*	d *No. A fluorescent lamp certainly doesn't emit laser light. Look at the list and make another selection.*
Student's answer	e

Terminal's response	*You are pretty close. It takes more than spontaneous emission to produce the laser. The spontaneous emission is necessary to induce the stimulated emission. Together they produce the laser. Try again.*
Student's answer	b
Terminal's response	*Correct. Laser is a monochromatic coherent light.*

In the preceding example, the student is presented a multiple choice question at the top of the screen. He first enters the letter "a" on the terminal. Since "a" is incorrect, a remedial response is displayed on the screen directly below his answer. He is also told to try again. He then enters the letter "c." Since "a" is incorrect, a remedial response is displayed on the screen directly below his answer. He is also told to try again. He then enters the letter "c." Since this answer is incorrect, he is presented another remedial response. Finally, the student enters the letter "b" on the terminal. He is then told that he answered the question correctly.

The review sequence of the course consists of viewing the two films and the tape/slide presentation if the student feels he requires them. If the student is a manager, he will also be directed to read the summary portion of the "Managers Reference Manual." This document is issued to each manager when he takes the CAI Laser Safety Course. The course is a requirement for all managers of personnel involved with the use of lasers. The document is a culmination of many years of collaboration between safety management, safety engineers, and laser engineers. The need for the document became very evident from the questions asked by managers in regard to how they were to comply with the requirements put upon them by the company and outside standards. It also clarified managerial responsibilities pertaining to lasers beyond the area of personnel safety.

The advantage of the Laser Safety Manager's Manual is that it compiles the notification requirements, inventory data, employee training requirement, medical examinations, eye protection procedures, environment approval plan, and the certification requirements into one document. Samples of all the relevant forms, labels, signs, and a reproduction of the certification card are attached as reference figures. Furthermore, it isolates the management information for lasers from the comprehensive, more complex, and voluminous Manager's Manual. The laser manual is included as a handout for the manager when he takes the CAI course. The CAI quiz assures that the manager understands his role with records, forms, etc.

The advantages of the CAI course over a conventional classroom presentation are listed below:

a. Ideal for small numbers of students. There is no need to delay training due to an insufficient number of students.

b. The student progresses through the course at his own pace. Some students require more time to learn the material. The CAI method tends to reduce the pressure on the slower student. Individual students do not have to keep up as they would in a conventional class.

c. The instructional material is uniform. The student is not exposed to different instruction techniques.
d. Test administration via CAI is consistent. The test reinforces the material presented. Student education records are easily updated.
e. By administering the class via CAI, instructors are made available for other assignments. CAI also eliminates the preparation time required for a new instructor.

In CAI, a monitor is on duty to help students. However, the monitor is not knowledgeable of the content of all courses offered on CAI. The development author took steps to compensate for the possible lack of monitor expertise on the subject of lasers. He accomplished this by writing many questions to test the student periodically. When the student answers incorrectly, he is given a hint as to the correct answer, or an explanation of why his answer was wrong. Additional student feedback to the author, via a special command allowing the student to enter comments on the terminal, has led to the clarification of several points in the course. This feedback assists in constant improvement of the course. A quiz answer, data collection routine has been built into the course which will be used to evaluate and improve the test portion.

25.6 AUDIO/VISUAL SOURCES

Probably the greatest problem in initially setting up a training program such as the ones just described is obtaining audio/visual aids. This is not so much a problem as it is time consuming. A large portion of the slides may be obtained by writing to the authors (and/or their employers) of technical presentations, publications, technical articles in trade journals, etc., and requesting slide copies of some of their illustrations and figures. Of course, there will not be a 100% positive response, but it is surprising how many will respond positively, particularly if it has been made clear in the request that it is for use in a training program.

Another source of training material is film libraries. Today there are many films on lasers that may be borrowed, rented, or purchased. On the topic of laser safety, professional organizations may be of great help. For instance the Laser Institute of America has available an 80-slide program with audio cassette narration that closely resembles the tape/slide package used in the programs described earlier (from LIA). Other sources of technical material and training for laser safety instructors are seminars and courses on laser safety and related topics such as the week long courses on laser safety given by the Laser Institute of America and Rockwell Seminar Management (see Table 25-2). There are often one or two day courses in conjunction with trade shows or professional society conferences. Modular written test material on many aspects of lasers, including Laser Safety, has been prepared by organizations specializing in special text materials (Sources 5 and 6 in Table 25-2).

25.7 SUMMARY

Good industrial laser safety program management will combine standards, administrative controls and education to suit specific needs. Education is a key ingredient, and should be made a part of the administrative controls. The laser, like electricity, is not to be feared, but rather respected and used properly. A well planned industrial laser safety management program will assure this.

25.8 REFERENCES

American National Standards Institute, 1976, ANSI Z-136.1 Standard for the Safe Use of Lasers, 1430 Broadway, New York 10018.

Charschan, S. S. (ed.), 1972, Bell System Standard for the Safe Use of Lasers, Western Electric Company, Inc., Princeton, New Jersey 08540.

Laser Institute of America, 1977, LIA Laser Safety Guide, LIA, 4100 Executive Park Drive, Cincinnati, Ohio 45241.

Smith, J. F., Murphy, J. J., and Eberle, W. J., 1977, Industrial Laser Safety Program Management, IBM Corporation, System Products Division, Poughkeepsie, New York 12602.

Chapter 26
Medical Surveillance

26.1 INTRODUCTION

The term medical surveillance, as used in the field of occupational health refers to specific examinations of individuals working in a potentially hazardous environment. Such specific medical examinations normally serve one or more of three general purposes: (a) biological monitoring of specific occupational exposures, (b) to determine if an individual meets job standards, or (c) to ascertain if the developments of adverse physiological effects can be detected in an individual which may result from occupational (usually chronic) exposure to a chemical or a physical agent in time to be arrested or reversed. A fourth purpose (d), medical-legal does not have any significant or immediate value to the employee.

26.1.1 Monitoring Related to Occupation

Specific clinical laboratory tests may be used for biological monitoring to determine if certain chemical agents are present in the blood; for example, lead in the blood of lead workers. The primary use of such an examination is obvious. These tests perform a parallel service to industrial hygiene monitoring, and are required to determine the adverse effects of the worker's environment during actual exposure to that environment. For example, monitoring of internal body temperature is performed occasionally on individuals who are working in unusually hot environments. If the internal body temperature begins to approach a certain critical temperature then the employee is removed immediately from the environment. Although this is a more involved procedure than simply measuring the ambient temperature, it may be the only approach to assess adequately the adverse effect of the environment on the worker. If a functional impairment develops, or if factors leading to occupational disease are present, then the worker can be removed from the hazardous environment, or protective clothing and engineering controls employed to reduce or eliminate this risk. Biological monitoring is superior to industrial hygiene monitoring in that it accounts for variability in exposure, absorption, metabolism, etc.

26.1.2 Personnel Evaluation

The second justification for a medical examination is to ascertain if there is any functional impairment which could adversely affect job safety. For example, crane operators and airplane pilots are tested to ensure that they maintain sufficient visual capabilities and general medical fitness to perform their jobs, since such impairment could place themselves and many others at risk.

26.1.3 Health Evaluation

The third purpose is met by these tests suitable for biological monitoring of any anticipated effects of the potential hazard, even as audiograms of workers in a high noise area could be used to some extent as a biological monitor for temporary threshold shifts. Hopefully each monitoring will prevent any permanent loss of function. Examples of these tests in the current situation would be corneal epithelium examinations following UV-A exposure, lens examination with UV-B exposures, etc. The proper tests for monitoring should be versions of those discussed in detail in Section 26.4 for accident victims as modified for mass screening.

26.1.4 Medical-Legal

The fourth purpose for occupational medical surveillance, medical-legal, is strictly to protect the employer from false claims or to assist the employee in obtaining the proper compensation for a job related injury. It has no significant health value to the employee. This statement best applied to workers exposed to laser radiation. However, injuries to both the skin and the eyes, but most importantly to the eye, can occur from sources other than laser radiation. Some employers have required employees to undergo a pre-employment examination for the purpose of establishing a base line. Although this examination would serve no purpose if an injury developed from a non-laser source after the base-line examination, the examination would tend to screen out those few cases wherein a retinal or lens change had developed or was developing prior to the initial employment of the individual in a potentially hazardous laser examination. (An example of another type of occupational examination which is primarily required for a baseline is the pulmonary function test of workers exposed to hydrochloric acid, where the risk is from acute exposure. Following such an exposure such an exam shows the change from normal for that individual.) In recent years, however, the cost effectiveness of the base-line examination has come into serious question. In most states, in order for an individual to collect employment compensation for a job related injury, he must first be able to prove that functional impairment has taken place. The mere presence of a visible lesion without a significant affect on visual function would be unlikely to provide sufficient grounds for compensation.

26.2 RATIONALE OF MEDICAL EXAMINATIONS FOR LASER WORKERS

In the past decade many employees who worked routinely with lasers have been subjected to pre-placement, periodic, and end-of-job eye examinations. For instance, the original ANSI standard (1973) required annual eye examinations for all "high risk" workers. In a few, extremely rare instances, examinations of the skin were also conducted. These examinations originated when there was little knowledge of the adverse effects of laser radiation on man. As early as 1961 when the potential of the ruby laser to cause severe eye injury was recognized, it was considered wise to initiate a routine eye examination program for laser researchers. It was felt that these examinations would reveal any unexpected effects upon the eye which occurred at levels lower than had been predicted. In most large organizations, both governmental and industrial, even as late as 1970 one of the principal purposes of such periodic examinations was epidemiological. That is, the purpose was to show whether, in a large population of workers possibly exposed to lasers, unexpected or delayed effects were or were not developing. By 1976, the results of at least one large number of examinations had been negative. This indicates that the risks of laser exposure had been correctly assessed, and the protective procedures had been sufficient to prevent any ocular effects except in very rare circumstances. The only injuries have resulted from acute over-exposures which in themselves were sufficiently traumatic to alert the individuals to their loss of visual capability. All this has resulted in a changed rationale and a proposal has been made to change the requirements for medical surveillance in the current ANSI Z-136 Standard (1976). These proposals are given in Section 26.5. The data and an extensive discussion of the rationale behind this proposed medical surveillance of laser workers has been given by Hathaway *et al.* (1977). The proposed standard is similar to that already adopted by WHO(Suess, 1981).

The current question then is whether there is really any need for periodic examinations. The proposal suggests that indeed, the only eye examinations which clearly appear to have merit is the examination immediately after a suspected overexposure to laser radiation and the periodic subsequent re-examinations to provide documentation. This series would detail that any lesion produced followed a course consistent with an over-exposure to laser radiation, and would serve as a basis for proving or disproving a future claim for employee compensation. It could also assist in an understanding of the mechanism of the laser injury.

26.3 TYPES OF ROUTINE EYE EXAMINATION PROTOCOLS

26.3.1 Fundus

The fundus examinations with direct and indirect ophthalmoscopes have

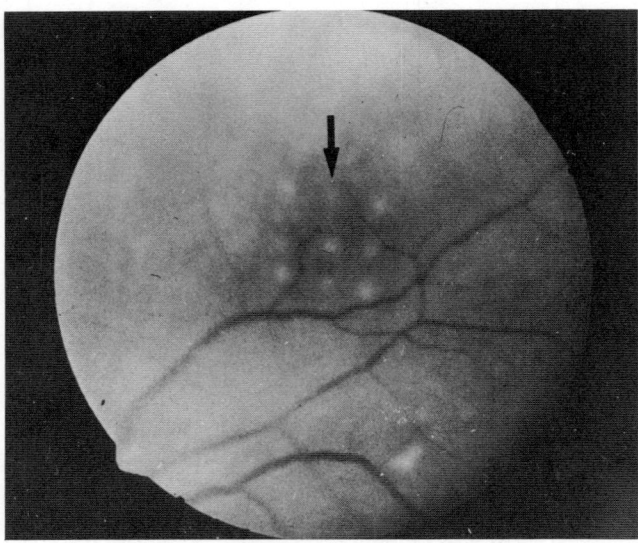

Figure 26-1. Laser Lesions in a Human Fundus. The grid pattern consists of a series of exposures at different power levels. The arrow indicates a threshold type lesion.

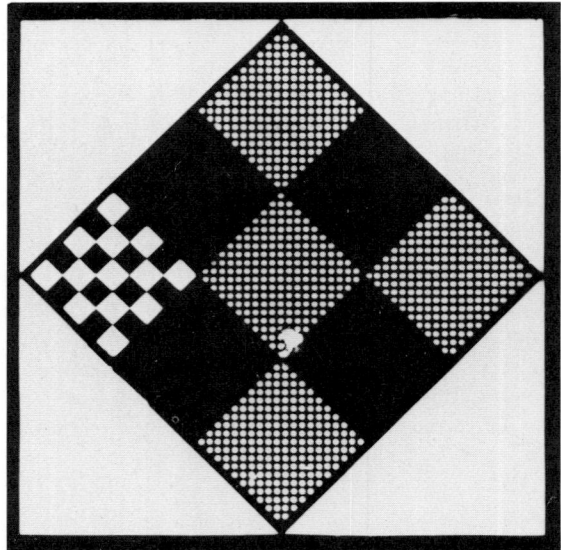

Figure 26-2. One Type of Visual Acuity Chart. The position of the large checker board must be selected. The visual acuity is given by the smallest correct selection from a series of patterns which progressingly decrease in size (visual angle).

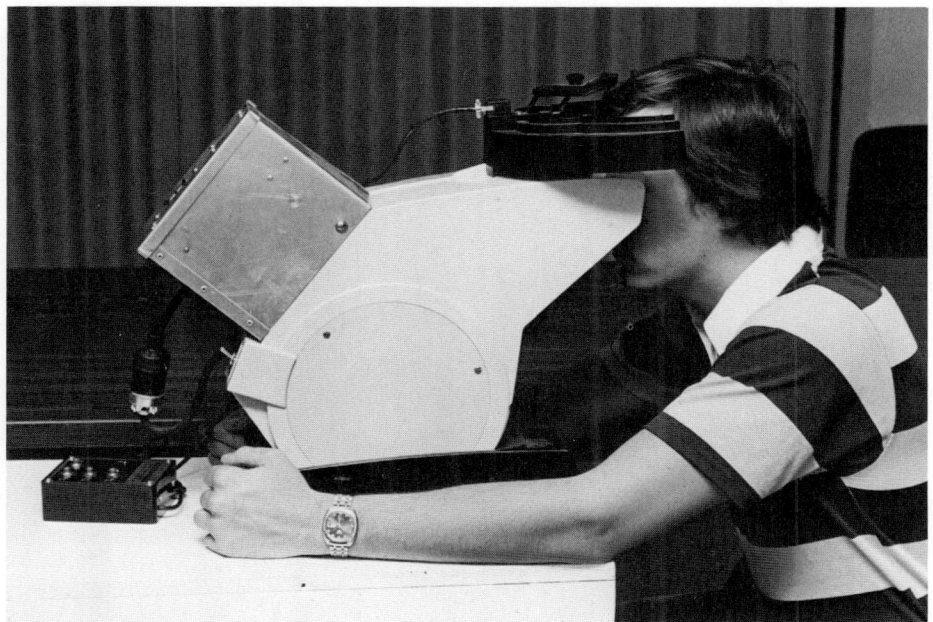

Figure 26-3. Test Machine for Visual Acuity with a Titmus Vision Tester. Patterns similar to those shown in Figure 26-1 are illuminated evenly and reproducibly, and can be easily changed.

been included in almost every protocol to date. Occasionally the protocol has even been restricted to a detailed retinal examination. However, these ophthalmoscopic examinations have severe limitations. Research studies on both animals and human volunteers have indicated that near-threshold retinal lesions (Figure 21-1) are not normally seen by an ophthalmoscopic examination, especially if delayed a few hours or a day. Whether such lesions would be accompanied by functional loss would depend upon their location. Only the lesions in or near the fovea could be detected and they would appear as a scotoma (or "blind spot") in the region of highest acuity. On the other hand, any marked suprathreshold laser exposure resulting in a significant visual defect would almost certainly become immediately apparent, and could then be found in an adequate eye examination.

26.3.2 Functional Examinations and Documentation

The routine and periodic eye examinations have also included visual acuity (Figures 26-2 and 26-3), visual fields and fundus photography (Figure 26-4) to document the presence or absence of abnormalities. When the limited information provided by these routine surveillance examinations is considered, along with the

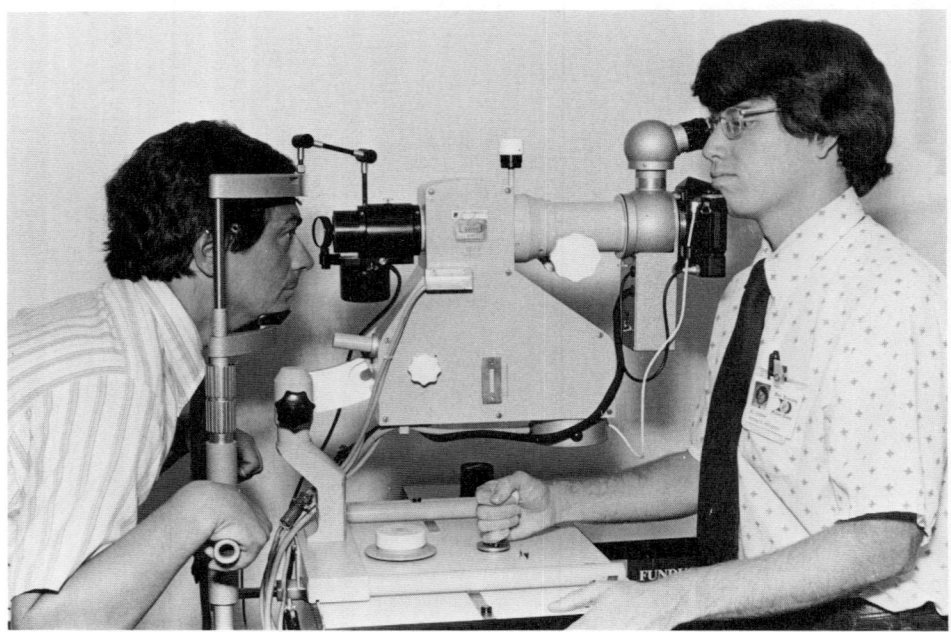

Figure 26-4. Fundus Photography with a Zeiss Instrument.

time spent by highly qualified (and expensive) medical personnel, it is obvious that detailed eye examinations need only be carried out as part of a general occupational health program. However, after any alleged injury resulting from an exposure to laser radiation, an adequate eye examination by a qualified expert clearly must be performed as soon as possible (and certainly within 24 hours). The current consensus [WHO (Suess, 1981)] is that a visual acuity test provides the most important information and should be performed in an expanded version. Many types of instruments have been devised to give more easily comparable results, one is shown in Figure 26-3. It is clearly the least expensive way if base-line examinations are deemed advisable by an employer. The visual acuity test reveals the only type of retinal dysfunction presently felt to result from acute laser exposure. Furthermore, it is possible that chronic exposures higher than the permissible exposure levels would cause a myriad of small nondetectable lesions which eventually would degrade the retinal mosaic to such a point that a functional loss of acuity would be revealed. At this time an ophthalmoscopic examination would certainly also begin to show some general retinal changes.

Other functional tests are more limited in their usefulness. For example, dark adaptation studies may be helpful in an initial, general examination, but will

Medical Surveillance

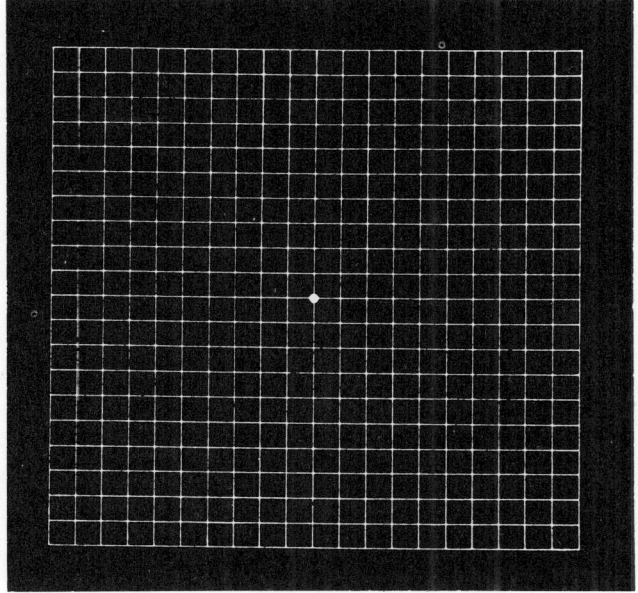

Figure 26-5. An Amsler Grid. The eye is fixed on the black spot. Any abnormalities (non-straight lines) are drawn by the patient with reference to the fixation spot.

rarely be of assistance in routine, periodic followups. Visual fields give similar information. Other than revealing the possible development of glaucoma they will also be of marginal assistance. Even scotomas resulting from laser injuries would only be found if in the macula. Peripheral lesions can only be found by searching in the visual space corresponding to the already known retinal abnormality or lesion.

The Amsler grid, Figure 26-5, resembles a piece of graph paper, and shows disturbances in the retina by distortions in the grid as described seen by the patient. The first documented use of a test similar to the Amsler grid was a musical staff. The retinal shrinkage around a lesion causes straight lines on the edge of the scotoma to bulge out. This was first noticed by an amateur astronomer, Reid (1819) who after a retinal burn resulting from viewing the sun through a telescope described the scotoma and the distortions of the musical scale in the neighborhood of the scotoma.

However, the functional test of visual acuity would probably indicate that some retinal pathology existed as early as could be revealed by an ophthalmoscopic examination. Since this test of visual acuity can be administered rapidly and with a minimum of time lost from work by the laser personnel, the rationale for choosing more extensive tests is not clear. Moreover, when the discomfort endured by the person during a complete ophthalmoscopic examination including fundus photography is considered along with the cost of such an examination, a simple visual acuity test alone certainly is preferred.

26.3.3 Anterior Portion of the Eye

The effects of chronic exposure on the parts of the eye anterior to the retina must also be considered. Exposure to near-infrared or ultraviolet laser radiation above the permissible exposure limits could in theory cause lens damage or cataracts. At present, visual screening procedures to detect the evolution of lenticular or corneal opacities by their adverse effect on glare sensitivity are being developed (Wolbarsht, 1977). In the future, therefore, examinations which are as simple to conduct as the visual acuity test may also be available to document the evolution of any changes in the anterior portion of the eye.

26.4 GUIDELINES FOR THE EXAMINATION OF LASER ACCIDENT VICTIMS

The assessment of an accident victim can be divided into two parts:
(1) to ascertain exactly what anatomical, physiological or functional conditions are present as compared with the pre-exposure state;
(2) to determine that the changes, (if any) are appropriate to the type of laser exposure.

26.4.1 External Examination—Lids, Brows, Cheek and Nose

Both ultraviolet and infrared C exposure can produce changes in the skin. Ultraviolet should produce characteristics of sunburn, pigment migration, with tenderness and blistering. Infrared radiation will produce erythema or a serious injury characteristic of a thermal burn. The burn should be present about the same time the cornea and conjunctiva become inflamed, but only if the beam was large enough to affect both the conjunctiva and surrounding skin. Threshold UV-exposures will produce pain, but only of a latent period of several hours.

26.4.2 Corneal Involvement (only following either an ultraviolet or infrared C laser exposure)

A. The sensitive region should be limited to the portion of the cornea and conjunctiva visible when the lids are open. The underside of the lid and unexposed portions of the conjunctiva should not be involved or irritated. Pain should appear only after a latent period of several hours for UV exposures.
B. Slit lamp or biomicroscope examination should show characteristics of ultraviolet exposure or thermal burn from infrared (laser) exposure, such as epithelial haze, granulation, etc.
C. The damage area should not be larger than the laser beam when a minimal exposure from a single short pulse is given. For example, the irritated region may be limited to one eye and even to a localized region on that eye.

26.4.3 Lens

Slit lamp examination may show vacuolation from intense, focused infrared. Ultraviolet exposures can produce lens problems, but only at or around the threshold for corneal involvement also. Usually, short pulse high intensity exposures from ultraviolet would affect both the lens and cornea. Unless the focal point of the laser beam can be accurately located by calculations to be in the anterior or posterior part of the lens, the reaction of the lens may not assist in reconstructing the optics of the exposure.

Ultraviolet exposures should affect the part of the lens in the pupil, whereas an infrared short pulse could give an opacity immediately behind the iris with spotting of the pupillary area. Only for longer IR exposures (at low power levels) would the portion of the lens shaded by the iris be spared, and the pupillary region alone involved (Wolbarsht et al., 1976, 1977).

26.4.4 Iris

Only very high intensity infrared and visible would be expected to affect the iris. In the ultraviolet the threshold for corneal damage would be far below that for iris damage. In any part of the spectrum focal illumination is almost required for damage of the iris without markedly affecting the cornea. High level, focal visible or IR exposure of the iris could cause irritation, leading to iritis, or it might go so far as to burn a hole, with hemorrhage if blood vessels are involved.

26.4.5 Vitreous

It is unlikely that any damage could be found in the vitreous other than that following changes in some other part of the eye, particularly the retina. Usually this results from a vascular involvement of the retina leading to hemorrhage into the vitreous. After a rather long latent period (months or years), large hemorrhages into the vitreous may lead to vitreous retraction and retinal detachment.

26.4.6 Retina

Examination of the retina with an indirect or direct ophthalmoscope, or even a biomicroscope with a Goldmann 3 mirror lens would be necessary to show sufficient detail of the supposed injury. After a threshold laser exposure, the lesion appears as a whitened area in the retina which quickly fades or will remain depending upon the exposure level. After a long period (months), the exposed area will appear hyperpigmented, even though it may have been almost depigmented immediately after the exposure. A single exposure from a small beam, short pulse laser could only produce damage in one eye unless unusual optical conditions are present. A large beam may affect both eyes, but the lesion(s) should be appropriate to the type of injury. A small lesion in the paramacular region should not change visual acuity in the other eye, whether exposed or unexposed. A macular lesion from a blue or green (Argon) laser should appear raised above a lesion formed in other parts of the retina. This results from a secondary lesion site around the macular pigment (Wolbarsht and Landers, 1975).

Functional tests for a scotoma when a lesion is seen may define the injury site more precisely. Occasionally a scotoma will extend into regions where no lesion is visible. Usually, however, such a scotoma disappears with time. The lesion itself will shrink after a period of a few months, and this should be evident in the distortion of the Amsler grid. Reports of pain accompanying a retinal injury should be weighed carefully. A near threshold lesion from a visible laser should be painless. Only high level suprathreshold exposures will occasionally produce a sensation of pain apparently in the cornea. This dislocation probably results from the anatomical anomaly that there are no pain fibers in the retina and those in the choroid are only fibers of passage that go to the cornea. This pain is transient, persistant pain would require considerable choroidal involvement.

26.5 CHANGES IN STANDARDS FOR MEDICAL SURVEILLANCE

At the time this was written a revised form of the medical surveillance section was under consideration by the National Committee for the ANSI Z-136 Standard. The proposed Medical Surveillance section is as follows:

6. MEDICAL SURVEILLANCE

<u>6.1 General.</u> The rationale for medical surveillance requirements for personnel working in a laser environment and specific information of value to examining or attending physicians are included in Appendix E. Medical surveillance requirements have been limited to those that are clearly indicated, based upon known risks of particular kinds of laser radiation. No medical surveillance is required for personnel using only Class 1 or Class 2 lasers and laser systems as defined in 3.3. Some employers may wish to provide their employees with additional examinations for medical-legal reasons, or to conform with established principles of what consititutes a thorough ophthalmologic or dermatologic examination or as part of a planned epidemiologic study. Further information is provided in Appendix E.

<u>6.2 Personnel Categories.</u> The category shall be determined by the Laser Safety Officer in charge of the installation involved. He should be responsible for having the appropriate examinations carried out. Those persons who should be under laser medical surveillance are defined in 6.2.1 and 6.2.2.

<u>6.2.1 Incidental Personnel.</u> Those whose work makes it possible but unlikely that they are exposed to laser energy sufficient to damage their eyes or skin; e.g., custodian, clerical, and supervisory personnel not working directly with laser devices.

<u>6.2.2 Laser Personnel.</u> Those who work routinely in laser environments. These individuals are ordinarily fully protected by engineering controls and/or administrative procedures.

6.3 General Procedures.

6.3.1 Incidental personnel shall have an eye examination for visual acuity (see Appendix E for further details).

6.3.2 Laser personnel shall be subject to the following:

(a) A medical history with emphasis on ocular and dermatologic systems and history of medication usage (particularly potentially photosensitizing drugs).

(b) Visual acuity determinations.

(c) Examination of various structures of the eye depending on wavelength of radiation produced by the lasers or laser systems that will be used (see paragraph 2.2, Appendix E, for details).

6.4 Frequency of Medical Examinations. For both incidental and laser personnel, required examinations shall be performed prior to participation in laser work. Following any suspected laser injury, the pertinent required examinations will be repeated in addition to whatever other examinations may be desired by the attending physician. Periodic examinations are not required.

Appendix E

E1. Purpose of Medical Surveillance. The basic reasons for performing medical surveillance of personnel working in a laser environment are the same as for other potential health hazards. Medical surveillance examinations may include assessment of physical fitness to safely perform assigned duties, biological monitoring of exposure to a specific agent, and early detection of biologic damage or effect.

Physical fitness assessments are used to determine whether an employee would be at increased or unusual risk in a particular environment. For workers using laser devices, the need for this type of assessment is most likely to be determined by factors other than laser radiation per se. Specific information on medical surveillance requirements that might exist because of other potential exposures such as toxic gases, noise, ionizing radiation, etc., are outside the scope of this Appendix.

Direct biological monitoring of laser radiation is impossible and practical indirect monitoring through the use of personal dosimeters is not available.

Early detection of biologic change or damage presupposes that chronic or subacute effects may result from exposure to a particular agent at levels below that required to produce acute injury. Active intervention must then be possible to arrest further biological damage or to allow recovery from biological effects. Although chronic injury from laser radiation in the ultraviolet, near-ultraviolet, blue portion of the visible, and near-infrared regions appears to be theoretically possible, risks to workers using laser devices are primarily from accidental acute injuries. Based upon risks involved with current uses of laser devices, medical surveillance requirements that should be incorporated into a formal standard appear to be minimal.

Other arguments in favor of performing extensive medical surveillance have been based on the fear that repeated accidents might occur and that workers would not report minimal acute injuries. The very small number of laser injuries that have been reported in the past 15 years and the excellent safety records with laser devices does not provide support to this argument.

E2. Medical Examinations.

E2.1 Rationale for Examinations.

E2.1.1 Preassignment Medical Examinations. Except for examination following suspected injury, these are the only examinations required by the standard. One purpose is to establish a baseline against which damage (primarily ocular) can be measured in event of an accidental injury. A second purpose is to identify certain workers who might be at special risk from chronic exposure to selected continuous wave lasers. For incidental workers only visual acuity measurement is required. For laser workers, medical histories, visual acuity measurement and selected examination protocols are required. The wavelength of laser radiation is the determinant of which specific protocols are required (see E2.2). Examinations should be performed by or under the supervision of an ophthalmologist or other qualified physician. Certain of the examination protocols may be performed by other qualified practitioners or technicians, under the supervision of a physician. Many ophthalmologists may prefer to perform more thorough eye examinations to assess total visual function as opposed to limiting examination to those areas that might be damaged by particular laser radiation. Some employers may find it advantageous to offer these more thorough examinations to their workers as a health benefit. For example, certain of the additional examinations such as tonometry, may be of value in detecting unknown disease conditions, in this case glaucoma. Even though this type of problem is unrelated to work with lasers, appropriate medical intervention will promote a healthier work force. Although chronic skin damage from laser radiation has not been reported, and indeed seems unlikely, this area has not been adequately studied. Limited skin examinations are suggested to serve as a baseline until future epidemiologic study indicates whether they are needed or not.

E2.1.2 Periodic Medical Examinations. Periodic examinations are not required by the Standard. At the present time no chronic health problems have been linked to work with laser radiation. Also, most uses of lasers do not result in chronic exposure of employees even to low levels of radiation. A large number of these examinations have been performed in the past and no indication of any detectable biologic change was noted. Employers may wish to offer their employees periodic eye examinations or other medical examinations as a health benefit; however, there does not appear to be any valid reason to require such examinations as part of a medical surveillance program.

E2.1.3 Termination Medical Examinations. The primary purpose of termination examinations is for the legal protection of the employer against unwarranted claims for damage that might occur after an employee leaves a particular job. The decision on whether to offer or require such examinations is left to individual employers.

E2.2 Examination Protocols.

E2.2.1 Medical History. Required for replacement examinations of all laser workers. The patient's past eye history and family eye history are reviewed. Any current complaints which he now has about his eyes are noted. Any history of skin problems is reviewed. Current and past medication use is reviewed. The patient's general health status should be inquired about with special emphasis upon diseases which can give ocular or skin problems. Certain medical conditions may cause the laser worker to be at increased risk if chronic exposure to ultraviolet or blue spectrum laser radiation is possible. Use of photosensitizing medications, such as phenothiazines and psoralens, lower the threshold for biologic effects in the cornea, lens, and retina of experimental animals. Aphakic individuals would be subject to additional retinal exposure from near-ultraviolet radiation. Unless chronic viewing of lower levels of laser radiation in these wavelengths is required, there should be no reasons to deny employment to these individuals. With current laser systems, chronic exposure even to low levels of blue laser radiation is very unusual.

E2.2.2 Visual Acuity. Required for preplacement examinations for all incidental and laser workers. Distance visual acuity should be tested both with and without corrective lenses to 20/15. Results should be recorded in Snellen figures. The visual acuity at near is tested at 35 cm and recorded in Jaeger-tested figures or Snellen figures with and without lenses, if any. Visual acuity screening instruments may be used.

E2.2.3 Manifest Refraction. Required for preplacement examinations of all laser workers when indicated. This is to measure the patient's refractive error, and the new visual acuity of the patient must be noted if the visual acuity is improved over that achieved with the patient's old lens prescription, or if he has no lenses at the time of the examination. This examination shall be carried out in all personnel whose best corrected distance visual acuity in either eye is less than 20/20.

E2.2.4 External Ocular Examination. Required for preplacement examinations for laser workers using laser systems producing radiation below 350 nm or above 1400 nm. This includes examination of brows, lids, lashes, conjunctiva, sclera, cornea, iris and pupillary size, equality, reactivity, and regularity.

E2.2.5 Examination by Slit Lamp. Required for preplacement examinations of laser workers using laser systems producing radiation below 420 nm or above 750 nm. The cornea, iris, and lens are examined with a biomicroscope and described.

E22.2.6 Examination of the Ocular Fundus with an Ophthalmoscope. Required for preplacement examinations of laser workers using laser systems producing radiation between 390 nm and 1400 nm and any aphakic worker. In the recording of this portion of the examination the points to be covered are: the presence or absence of opacities in the media: the sharpness of outline of the optic nerve; the size of the physiological cup, if present; the ratio of the size of the retinal veins to that of the retinal arteries; the presence or absence of a well-defined macula and the presence or absence of a foveolar reflex; and any retinal pathology that can be seen with a direct ophthalmoscope. Even small deviations from normal should be described and carefully localized.

E2.2.7 Skin Examination. Not required for preplacement examinations of laser workers; however, suggested for employees with history of photosensitivity or those working with ultraviolet lasers. Examination of the skin for presence of abnormal pigmentation or depigmentation, keratoses, malignancies, etc.

E2.2.8 Amsler Grid. Not required by the Standard. The Amsler grid sheet is presented to each eye separately and any distortion of the grid is noted by the patient and drawn by him. May be part of a thorough ophthalmologic examination.

E2.2.9 Tonometry. Not required by the Standard. This is the measurement of intraocular pressure. Should be part of a thorough ophthalmologic examination.

E2.2.10 Photograph of the Posterior Pole of the Fundus. Not required by the

Standard. This includes the area of the macula and head of the optic nerve and should be taken in color. May be obtained by the examining physician to more fully describe retinal abnormalities. Appropriate techniques to reduce the patient's exposure to optical radiation should be employed.

E2.2.11 Other Examinations. Further examinations should be done as deemed necessary by the examiner.

E3 Medical Referral Following Suspected or Known Laser Injury. Any employee with a suspected eye injury should be referred to an ophthalmologist. Persons with skin injuries should be seen by a physician.

E4 Epidemiologic Studies. In the past the use of laser systems has generally been stringently controlled, and the actual exposure to laser workers has been minimal or even nonexistent. It is not surprising that acute accidental injury has been rare and that the few reports of repeated eye examinations have not noted any chronic eye changes. For these reasons, the examination requirements of this standard are minimal. However, animal experiments with both laser and narrow-band radiation indicate the potential for chronic damage from both subacute or chronic exposure to certain wavelengths of radiation. Lens opacities have been produced by radiation in the 295–450 nm and the 750–1400 nm ranges.

Photochemical retinitis may be induced by exposure to 350–500 nm radiation. If chronic exposure is required of workers to even low levels of radiation in these wavelength regions, it is recommended that they be included in the long-term epidemiologic studies, with periodic examinations of the appropriate eye structures.

Epidemiologic studies of workers with chronic skin exposure to laser radiation (particularly ultraviolet) are suggested.

The most noticeable change proposed in 1979 is in the overall emphasis. It seems that the medical examination is now mostly for medical-legal reasons. The pre-placement eye examination will not aid in therapy or prevention of accidents, and annual (or other periodic) examinations are not required or even recommended. The most valuable examination for the worker is a careful one after any possible injury following exposure to a laser. The major part of ocular examination is a test of function, visual acuity. Other tests are specifically oriented towards the characteristics of the special laser involved or are otherwise useful in the assessment of general health. Record keeping is encouraged for epidemiological purposes.

A preliminary skin examination, is only considered if any UV radiation is associated with the laser, as then possible hypersensitivity of some individuals to ultraviolet may be detected. In addition, through the medical examination the worker can be alerted to changes in his UV sensitivity associated with drugs, diet, etc. However, except for any changes due to disease, there is no need for periodic examinations. Again the post-placement and terminal examinations are most useful for legal reasons.

The major portion of the proposed changes in the ANSI Z-136 Standard's Medical Surveillance section are actually part of the appendix. The appendix contains amplification of material in the body of the Standard, and is advisory in nature. The explicit call for epidemiological studies is possibly intended for the industrial organizations who may use the standard. Unfortunately such information, if gathered, will probably be a company secret unless release of information is required by the various state or Federal regulations. Even so, much of it might only be released by court action. It is debatable whether any changes due to chronic exposure could immediately be related to laser exposure. Possibly such data could only be gathered on a large scale basis by the National Institute of Occupational Safety and Health or some similar group. Only a prospective study type of program could establish a definite relation between chronic exposure and adverse physiological effects.

26.6 CASE HISTORIES

The case history of one individual who suffered corneal and retinal injuries from viewing a welding arc is presented in Section 24.4.3. Some examples of laser retinal injuries are presented in Section 15.8 (p. 508), and are referenced in Section 15.13. A review of these sections may be helpful to those interested in the subject of medical surveillance. One personal account of a laser accident by a scientist who viewed a reflected beam from a Class 4 neodymium laser is particularly instructive. This description, written by Dr. C. David Decker is reprinted below by permission of *Laser Focus* magazine which originally printed the account in its August 1977 issue. The account when read by laser research personnel often impresses them with the need for following appropriate laboratory laser safety measures. The account:

"The necessity for safety precautions with highpower lasers was forcibly brought home to me last January when I was partially blinded by a reflection from a relatively weak neodymium-yag laser beam. Retinal damage resulted from a 6-millijoule, 10-nanosecond pulse of invisible 1,064-nanometer radiation. I was not wearing protective goggles at the time, although they were available in the laboratory. As any experienced laser researcher knows, goggles not only cause tunnel vision and become fogged, they become very uncomfortable after several hours in the laboratory.

"When the beam struck my eye I heard a distinct popping sound, caused by a laser-induced explosion at the back of my eyeball. My vision was obscured almost immediately by streams of blood floating in the vitreous humor, and by what appeared to be particulate matter suspended in the vitreous humor. It was like viewing the world through a round fishbowl full of glycerol into which a quart of blood and a handful of black pepper have been partially mixed. There was local pain within a few minutes of the accident, but it did not become excruciating. The most immediate response after such an accident is horror. As a Vietnam War Veteran, I have seen several terrible scenes of human carnage, but none affected me more than viewing the world through my bloodified eyeball. In the aftermath of the accident, I went into shock, as is typical in personal injury accidents.

"As it turn out, my injury was severe but not nearly as bad as it might have been. I was not looking directly at the prism from which the beam had reflected, so the retinal damage is not in the fovea. The beam struck my retina between the fovea and the optic nerve, missing the optic nerve by about three millimeters. Had the

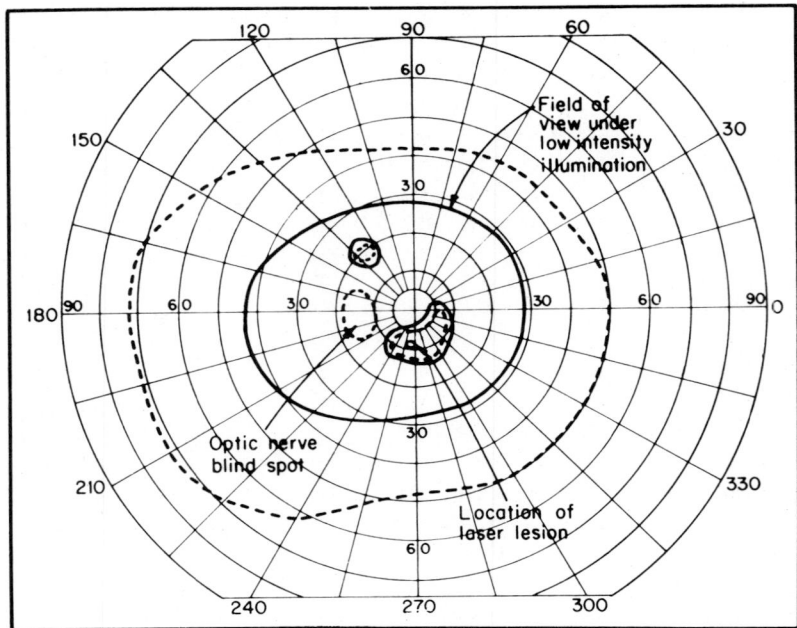

Figure 26-6. Accident Victim's Visual Field Chart. Eye damage caused by laser pulse is shown in this plot of field of view under high-intensity illumination (dotted lines) and under low-intensity illumination (solid lines). Outer circles show field of view; the two small regions inside the field of view are blind spots produced by laser damage. The blind spots are larger than the lesion and occupy a larger area under low illumination (from Decker, 1977, with permission of *Laser Focus*).

focused beam struck the fovea, I would have sustained a blind spot in the center of my field of vision. Had it struck the optic nerve, I probably would have lost the sight of that eye.

"The beam did strike so close to the optic nerve, however, that it severed nerve-fiber bundles radiating from the optic nerve. This has resulted in a crescent-shaped blind spot many times the size of the lesion. The diagram [Figure 26-6] is a Goldmann-Fields scan of the damaged eye, indicating the sightless portions of my field of view four months after the accident. The small blind spot at the top exists for no discernible reason; the lateral blind spot is the optic nerve blind spot. The effect of the large blind area is much like having a finger placed over one's field of vision. Also I still have numerous floating objects in the field of view of my damaged eye, although the blood streamers have disappeared. These "floaters" are more a daily hinderance than the blind areas, because the brain tries to integrate out the blind area when the undamaged eye is open. There is also recurrent pain in the eye, especially when I have been reading too long or when I get tired.

"The moral of all this is to be careful and to wear protective goggles when using highpower lasers. The temporary discomfort is far less than the permanent discomfort of eye damage. The type of reflected beam which injured me also is produced by the polarizers used in q switches, by intracavity diffraction gratings, and by all beamsplitters or polarizers used in optical chains."

26.7 CONCLUSIONS

It is appropriate to close this chapter with the concept that the proper exercise of current safety practices for workers in laser environments should eliminate any chance of acute exposure to damaging levels. However, eye injuries are still possible, although unlikely from chronic exposures to "low" levels. Therefore, efforts to prevent excessive chronic exposure should receive the most attention in any safety program. At present, even extensive (and costly) medical surveillance does not permit reliable detection of early changes from chronic exposure. Also, no treatment is presently known which could reverse any of the adverse retinal effects. Thus, previous medical surveillance seems to have served no useful purpose beyond furnishing a baseline for future changes resulting from accidents, and gathering data for epidemiological studies. Future medical surveillance can, therefore, be expected to be both minimal and more sophisticated. Table 21-1 provides a brief summary of points of interest in an examination as they relate to spectral bands.

26.8 REVIEW QUESTIONS

1. An ocular examination of an individual over-exposed to a ruby laser should emphasize:
   (a) the retina
   (b) the vitreous
   (c) the lens
   (d) the cornea

   Explain your choice.

2. An ocular examination of an individual over-exposed to a CO_2 laser should emphasize the anterior or posterior of the eye? Why?

3. What is an Amsler grid? What does it test?

4. An individual standing down range within a high-power, 1-meter-diameter ruby laser beam shows bilateral scotomas, each located one degree to the left of the visual axis. Are such scotomas likely to originate from viewing this laser source?

5. A scientist working with a sub-milliwatt CW neodymium YAG laser develops

Table 21-1. Examination Summary: Points of Interest

Effect	Possible Wavelength Region						
	UV-C	UV-B	UV-A	VIS	IR-A	IR-B	IR-C
1. Keratoconjuntivitis within Palpebral Fissure	√√	√√	√			√	√
2. Aqueous Flare					√		
3. Lenticular Changes			√√		√	†	
4. Retinal Lesions							
(a) Immediate Appearance				√	√		
(b) Delayed Appearance			†	√			
5. Retinal Hemmorhaging				√*	√*		

* Must be from a short-pulsed source √ likely
† Unlikely, but not impossible √√ most likely

lenticular opacities. Could this conceivably be related to laser exposure? From a He-Ne laser? From a CO_2 laser? From a pulsed N_2 laser?

6. A serviceman for a He-Ne laser scanner used in a supermarket checkout line complains of a burning sensation in both eyes, and has a pronounced photophobis. He blames his problems on an inadvertant over-exposure to the laser. Do you agree? Explain.

7. Would periodic examinations of the fundus have any value in the laser safety program of an industrial facility using CO_2 lasers? For one that uses only helium-neon lasers? Explain your answers.

8. Why do the proposed 1979 revisions for the ANSI Z-136 Standard suggest a detailed skin examination for other than medical-legal purposes?

9. A laboratory worker complains of pain in one eye after an alleged exposure by an argon laser. Fundus examination immediately after the alleged exposure shows a small, near-threshold lesion on the edge of the macula. The lesion is hyper-pigmented and a very small scotoma can be plotted on the visual field examination. The area around the lesion shows distortions in the Amsler grid with the lines bulging out around the lesion. The worker complains of persistent pain beginning at the time of the alleged exposure. The patient indicates that the pain is localized in the back of the eye "surrounding the part that looks at the scotoma." Are his symptoms consistent with the recent exposure? Explain your answer.

10. At present, visual acuity is considered the most valuable pre-placement test for screening laser workers. What is the rationale behind this test?

11. Based on present philosophy, would it be reasonable (advantageous) for a large organization in which many people are potentially exposed to low powered helium-neon lasers to have a physician on the staff specializing in eye examinations oriented toward the detection of minimal laser damage. Why?

26.9 REFERENCES

Alexander, R. W., Maida, A. S., Rufus, R. J., 1975, The validity of preemployment medical evaluation, *J. Occup. Med.* 17:687–692.
American National Standards Institute, New York, 1976, American National Standard for the Safe Use of Lasers, ANSI Z-136.1-1976, New York.
Brennan, D. H., 1973, Ocular examinations of laser workers and investigation of accidents, *Proc. Roy Soc. Med.* 66:844–845.
Decker, C. D., 1977, Accident victim's view, *Laser Focus* 13(8):6 (August 1977).
Dixon, E. M., 1973, Medical surveillance in industry, *J. Occup. Med.* 15:796–799.
Friedmann, A. I., 1978, The ophthalmic screening of laser workers, *Ann. Occup. Hyg.* 21:277–279.
Geeraets, W. J., and Nooney, T. W., 1973, Observations following high intensity white light exposure to the retina, *Am. J. Optom. & Arch. Am. Acad. Optom.* 50:405–412.
Hathaway, J. A., Stern N., Soles, E. M., and Leighton, E., 1977, Ocular medical surveillance on microwave and laser workers, *J. Occup. Med.* 19:683–688.
Hathaway, J. A., 1978, The needs for medical surveillance of laser and microwave workers, "Current Concepts in Ergophthalmology," pp. 139–160, Societas Ergophthalmologica Internationalis, Stockholm, Sweden.
Reid, T., 1819, "An Inquiry into the Human Mind on the Principles of Common Sense," Stirling, Slade, Ogle Allandice and Thompson, Edinburgh, Scotland.
Schilling, R. S. F., 1973, "Occupational Health Practices," Butterworth and Co., Ltd., London.
Suess, M. J. (Ed.), 1981, "Non-ionizing Radiation Protection," WHO Regional Publications Euro Series YVO.10, chapter on health aspects of optical radiation with particular reference to lasers. World Health Organization Regional Office for Europe, Copenhagen.
Tengroth, B., and Epstein, D. (Eds.), 1978, "Current Concepts in Ergophthalmology," Societas Ergophthalmologica Internationalis, Karolinska Institute, Stockholm, Sweden.
Wolbarsht, M. L., 1978, The effects of optical radiation on the anterior structures of the eye, *in* "Current Concepts in Ergophthalmology," pp. 29–46, Societas Ergophthalmologica Internationalis, Stockholm, Sweden.
Wolbarsht, M. L., 1977, Tests for glare sensitivity and peripheral vision in driver applicants, *J. Safety Res.* 9(3):128–139.
Wolbarsht, M. L., Orr, M. A., Yamanashi, B. S., Zigler, J. S., and Matheson, I. B. C., 1977, The origin of cataracts in the lens from infrared laser radiation, Duke Univ. Eye Center, Durham, N.C. (410455), Contract DAMD17-74-C-4133, Project 3E762772A813, U.S. Army Med. R&D Cmd., Washington, DC (October 1977).
Wolbarsht, M. L., and Landers, III, M. B., 1972, Laser exposures in the maculas of human volunteers, I. CW HeNe, CW Argon, Pulsed Ruby Laser Measurements, Technical report: ONR Contract N00014-67-A-0251-0011, 1-24 (December 1972).
Wolbarsht, M. L. and Landers, III, M. B., 1975, Laser exposures in the maculas of human volunteers, final report, ONR Contract N000 14-67-0251-0011, 1-41 (September 30, 1975).
World Health Organization, 1977, Manual on Non-ionizing Radiation Protection, Chapter on health aspects of optical radiation with particular reference to lasers.

World Health Organization, 1975, Early Detection of Health Impairment in Occupational Exposures to Health Hazards, Tech. Report Ser. No. 571, Geneva.

World Health Organization, 1973, Environmental and Health Monitoring in Occupational Health, Tech. Report Ser. No. 535, Geneva.

Zweng, H. C., and Rose, H. C., 1968, Eye examination standards and treatment, *in* "Laser Eye Effects," (H. G. Sperling, Ed.) pp. 87–89, Armed Forces-National Research Council Committee on Vision, Washington, DC.

Zweng, H. C., 1971, Lasers in ophthalmology, *in* "Laser Applications in Medicine and Biology," (M. L. Wolbarsht, Ed.) pp. 239–253, Plenum Press, New York.

Chapter 27
Ancillary Hazards

27.1 INTRODUCTION

The potential health hazards associated with high-powered laser systems (Class 4) are not limited to optical radiation hazards of the direct or reflected beam. In addition to the obvious hazards of optical radiation, many ancillary problems arise from the electrically energized power supplies, the often excessive noise from target interactions or from the laser itself, and from hazardous fumes, gases and vapors originating from the laser or target interactions. Indeed very high-power lasers which exceed 1 kW CW output power or 100 kW pulsed peak powers are often capable of producing all of these hazards (Sliney et al., 1975).

All of the present laser safety guidelines and standards, such as the BRH performance standard, the ANSI Z-136.1 standard, and the guide from the American Conference of Governmental Industrial Hygienists (ACGIH), classify CW lasers whose output power exceeds 0.5 W as "high power" because they are potentially both fire and skin hazards. As pointed out in Chapter 19, the optical hazards from reflections from a relatively low output Class 4 laser may actually be more severe than those from a very high power Class 4 laser since as a general rule the higher powered laser produces target damage, rather than seriously hazardous specular reflections. It is these very target reactions that are a major consideration of this chapter. Although an output power of 1 kW or more is an obvious fire and skin hazard, output powers in this range are used quite commonly in industrial applications.

The topics covered in this chapter will include the excessive noise levels above 85 db(A) that are sometimes present in the vicinity of TEA lasers, gas dynamic lasers and chemical lasers, X-radiation hazards and the many chemical laser constituents that incorporate toxic or chemically active materials which require special industrial hygiene attention. The potentially hazardous concentrations of combustion by-products from the exhaust of chemical and gas dynamic lasers will be covered as well as those contaminants produced at the target due to beam-target interaction. For this reason the exact type of laser in use as well as the general nature and extent of operator exposure must be considered, particularly if the laser system is located within an inadequately ventilated area. Another hazard of like nature is the ionizing radiation often produced by high-voltage electrical power supplies or electron-beam (E-beam) lasers. The hazards associated with high voltage electrical equipment, particularly high energy capacitors and power supplies will be considered separately in Chapter 28.

27.2 COMMON HIGH POWER LASERS AND THEIR APPLICATIONS

Although little has yet been published regarding the very high powered lasers being studied for military applications, many research laboratories and industrial facilities have been working with multikilowatt lasers in material processing application (see Chapter 19) and in an effort to produce laser-induced fusion. The earliest group of lasers capable of achieving the peak powers sufficiently high enough to be considered good candidates for such future applications as fusion are the infrared lasers, such a neodymium (1,064 μm), hydrogen-fluoride (2.6 to 3.3 μm) and deuterium-fluoride (3.5 to 4.2 μm), carbon-monoxide (approximately 5 μm), carbon-dioxide (10.6 μm) nitrous oxide (10.5–11 μm), and methanol (118.8 μm). Except for the neodymium laser, these lasers emit in the far-infrared and are not considered hazardous to the retina. In heavy welding and cutting applications only the CO_2 laser is commonly employed. There are other very high powered lasers which operate in the retinal-hazard and ultraviolet regions, e.g., the iodine laser (1,315 μm) and the hydrogen laser (UV) but they are uncommon.

27.3 AIRBORNE CONTAMINANTS

Many of the materials required for laser operation, as well as products produced by the laser during operation, or by beam interaction with target materials, are potentially hazardous to operating personnel. Laser fuels or exhaust products of chemical lasers can include carbon-monoxide, methane, sulfur dioxide, sulfur hexafluoride and other sulfur compounds, nitrogen, helium, fluorene, lithium, carbon-disulfide, hydrofluoric acid, hydrogen, carbon-dioxide, various fluorides, nitrogen oxides, and various refrigerants. Finally, beam interaction with metallic targets can produce airborne contaminants similar to those generated by arc welding on the same metals. The ACGIH suggests a single limit (TLV) for welding fumes (of not otherwise classified particulates) of 5 mg/m^3.

27.3.1 Contaminant Concentrations

Some allowable time-weighted exposure concentrations for probable, specific components of laser fuels, target byproducts, and the products of beam generation are listed in Table 27-1. The allowable time-weighted exposures are from the OSHA

Ancillary Hazards

Table 27-1. Representative Contaminants Associated with Laser Operation

Contaminants	Probable Source	OSHA Allowable Time Weighted Exposure**	OSHA Ceiling Value**
Asbestos	Target backstop	5 fibers/cc*	
Beryllium	Firebrick target	0.002 mg/m^3	
Cadmium oxide fume	Metal target	0.1 (0.04) mg/m^3	3 (0.2) mg/m^3
Carbon monoxide	Laser gas	50 (35) ppm	(200 ppm)
Carbon dioxide	Active laser medium	5,000 (10,000) ppm	50,000 ppm
Chromium	Metal targets	0.5 (0.025) mg/m^3	(0.05 mg/m^3)
Cobalt, metal fume, and dust	Metal targets	0.1 mg/m^3	
Copper fume	Metal targets	0.1 mg/m^3	
Fluorine	HF Chemical laser	0.1 ppm	
Hydrogen fluoride	Active medium of laser	3 (2.5) ppm	(5 ppm)
Iron oxide fume	Metal targets	10 (5†) mg/m^3	
Manganese	Metal targets		5 mg/m^3
Nickel	Metal targets	1 (0.015) mg/m^3	
Nitrogen dioxide	GDL discharge	5 ppm	(1 ppm)
Ozone	Target & Marx generators	0.1 ppm	
Sulfur Dioxide	Laser exhaust	5 (0.5) ppm	
Sulfur hexafluoride	Saturable absorber	1,000 ppm	
Uranium (soluble/insoluble)	Target	0.05/0.25 mg/m^3	
Vanadium fume (dust/fume)	Target		0.5/0.1 mg/m^3
Zinc oxide fume	Target	5 mg/m^3	

* > 5 μmeters in length.
**Values in parentheses denote changes recommended by NIOSH or ACGIH.
† Denotes change recommended by ACGIH.

Standards, Code of Federal Regulations sub-part G, Section 1910.1000 (U.S. Department of Labor, 1977). It is important to recognize that most of these values are for an eight-hour work day as part of a 40-hour work week, and that for some contaminants, occasional excursion above these values are permitted. General guidelines have been established to limit the magnitude of these excursions, and formulas for adding the permissible exposure limits (TLV's) of a combination of these airborne contaminants are also available, but definitive information is available only for a limited number. The formula most often used for calculating a threshold limit value (TLV) for a mixture of airborne contaminants that have similar toxicological effects is:

$$\frac{c_1}{T_1} + \frac{c_2}{T_2} + \frac{c_3}{T_3} + \cdots = 1 \qquad (27\text{-}1)$$

where c is the concentration in parts per million (ppm) and T is the TLV.

We do not wish to leave the reader with the deceptive notion that the measurements and calculations associated with the analysis of hazards from airborne contaminants are simple. These are not. Formula 27-1 is given only as an example and Table 27-1 is provided to give the reader a "feel" for TLV's. It lists OSHA permissible exposure limits. For those contaminants for which no excursion above a certain value is permitted, the values in Table 27-1 are termed "ceiling concentrations." This means that time-weighting is not permitted and that all exposure levels should fluctuate below the designated value. Those ceiling concentrations are analogous to exposure limits (MPE's) for pulsed laser exposures where no excursions above those limits are permitted. Values in parentheses are NIOSH or ACGIH recommendations for changes in the OSHA limits.

27.3.2 Removal by Ventilation

Exposure of operating personnel to the hazardous materials associated with laser operation should be kept below the established limits by local dilution ventilation, isolation, shielding, personnel protective devices, and other engineering or administrative controls.

Dilution ventilation is one of the most effective and frequently used control methods. For example, in an outdoor environment, over-exposure to airborne contaminants from vaporized target materials would not be expected because of ample dilution ventilation. For indoor operations local exhaust ventilation is probably the most effective control method. Airborne contaminants should be captured near the point of evolution even before they have a chance to be diluted in room air. In general, mechanical dilution (fan ventilation) is not an acceptable method for indoor control of the more toxic materials or where contaminants are generated from a point source. The more toxic materials in this regard are those with exposure limits below 100 ppm. For indoor operations, local exhaust (hood) ventilation is usually a more economical method of control than dilution ventilation since the required air volume flow rate is substantially less (Figure 27-1). Local exhaust systems should be designed to provide, at the point of contaminant evolution, a capture

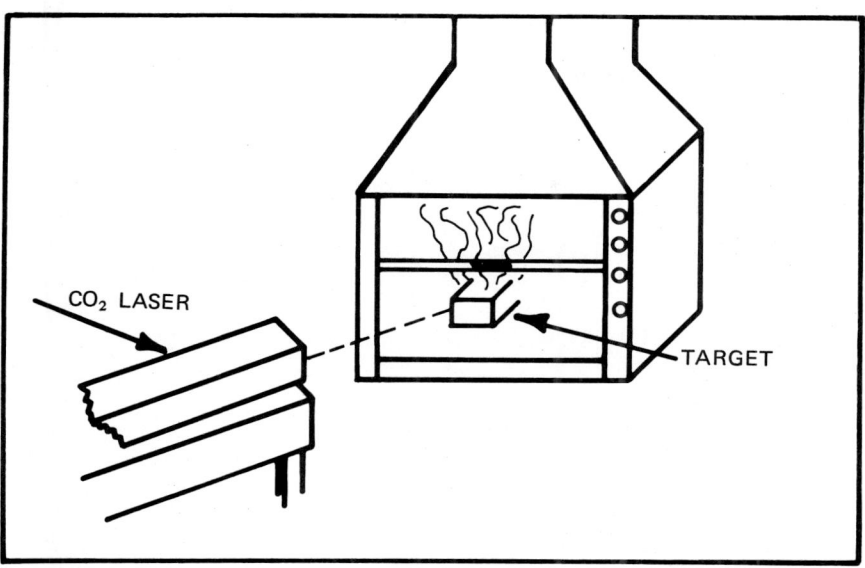

Figure 27-1. Fume Hood-Local Exhaust. A chemical fume hood is employed to exhaust hazardous fumes and vapors generated at the laser target.

velocity in the direction of the exhaust inlet of 100 to 150 linear-feet-per-minute. The exhaust inlet should be designed to minimize contaminant escape. For this purpose, total enclosure is optimal but not always obtainable. Thus, efforts should be made to enclose as much of the contaminant source as is practical. The location of the exhaust inlet should be selected to take advantage of the natural movement of the contaminant which, however, should not be allowed to pass through an individual's breathing zone en route. Disposal of chemical laser exhausts from large HF and DF lasers sometimes requires the use of self-contained laboratory scrubbing systems to remove SO_2 and HF vapors. Information particularly useful in the design of exhaust and dilution ventilation is extensively developed in the ACGIH industrial ventilation manual (1974) and the ANSI standard entitled "Fundamentals Governing the Design Operation of Local Exhaust Systems."

27.3.3 Contaminant Detection

Provisions should be made for contaminant detection around the larger laser systems, especially those where gas or liquid bulk storage facilities are maintained. It is important not only to maintain contaminant levels below allowable exposure limits, but also to provide early detection of system leaks. Since the presence of many of these contaminants, even in trace amounts, most often denotes leakage, detectors are generally located near the potential leakage sites and adjusted to respond to levels only slightly above ambient. These contaminant detection devices should be selected with great care; the sensitivity, accuracy, drift, maintenance requirements, and specificity should be considered as well as the operating environment (e.g., outdoors exposed to weather).

The fluorine lines which are used to feed HF and DF laser systems sometimes leak at welded joints. This is particularly common if one attempts to maintain a pressure of fluorine in the line above one atmosphere. Rupture of a fluorine line can result in a dangerous fire. In heavily occupied laboratory buildings, double-containment lines have been used. Leakage of fluorine into the interstitial space can be monitored by filling the jacket (interstitial space) with nitrogen and monitoring any change in nitrogen pressure.

27.3.4 Respiratory Protective Devices

In addition to detection equipment, respiratory protective devices for emergency use must also be provided in certain installations. Such safety equipment should be approved by the Bureau of Mines or the National Institute for Occupational Safety and Health (NIOSH) for use with many contaminant (s) likely to be encountered. Many of the contaminants associated with high power laser operations are described as simple asphyxiants; their principal action is the displacement of oxygen (e.g., nitrogen). Other materials are explosive (e.g., hydrogen) or toxic (e.g., ozone) or both. Some of the larger chemical and gas-dynamic laser systems include a large number of tanks or bulk storage facilities. Here a large leak or vessel rupture can result in the release of enormous quantities of hazardous material. Available emergency equipment should include approved, self-contained or air-supplied breathing devices, preferably of the pressure-demand type (Figure 27-2). All respiratory devices should be located in an area where they can be donned in a contaminant-free atmosphere and should be properly maintained and inspected as required by the OSHA standard in Section 1910.134 (U.S. Department of Labor, 1977).

In addition to the target site and the gas effluent from a flowing-gas laser, airborne contaminants are sometimes produced in unexpected locations. A common source of such airborne contaminants is beam interaction with optical elements in the laser system. For instance, infrared-transmitting optical materials (such as zinc-selenide, cadmium-telluride or selenium fluoride) occasionally degrade or vaporize under very high irradiances and decompose into toxic contaminants. Metal and plastic target materials may also produce airborne contaminants. Table 27-2 lists the thermal decomposition products of a variety of plastic materials that sometimes are heated to high temperature in laser operations.

27.3.5 Skin Hazards

Several liquid laser dyes and their common solvents are toxic but may not be

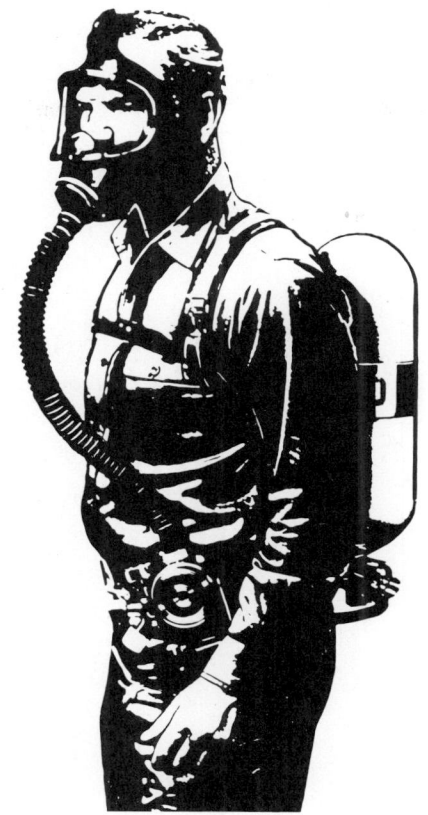

Figure 27-2. Respirator. Respirators are used only rarely in laser technology. This self-contained respirator could be employed in certain operations (courtesy MSA, Pittsburgh, PA).

properly labeled to indicate this. Also, for many dyes and solvents there is inadequate toxicity data. The manufacturer should normally be consulted on this question. The tests of one research group showed that the cyanine and carbosyanine (or polymethine) compounds were the most toxic of the 150 dyes used most extensively in the red and infrared portions of the spectrum. The cyanines are generally dissolved in dimethylsulfoxide (DMSO), a solvent that is by itself quite dangerous because of its ability to facilitate the transfer of molecules (which could be any airborne or splash contaminant) through biological membranes such as skin. The wisest approach in using any dye in a laser system is to wear rubber gloves, and in those rare instances where large quantities are used, accompany them with additional precautionary measures, such as the use of face masks, rubber aprons, and rubber sleeves. Many of the dye solvents are also highly flammable and fire protective controls should be included in the laboratory design.

Two types of materials used in electrical equipment have produced concern

Table 27-2. Pyrolysis Products from Polymers*†

Polymer	Decomposition Products
Alkyd Resin (oil modified)	methane(S), ethylene(S), ethane(S), propylene(S), propane (S), allyl alcohol(S), acetaldehyde(S), methacrolein(L).
Nitrocellulose	CO_2 and NO_X(L), CO(L), N(M), CH_4(M), C_2H_4(S), CH_3CHO(S), CH_3OH(S), C_2H_5OH(S).
Fluorocarbon Resins (Teflon, TFE, FEP)	CO_2(L), CF(M), COF(T), CF_2(M), CF_3(L), C_2F_2(T), OCF_3(T), C_3F_3(S), OC_2F_5(S), COF_2(L), CF_4(L).
Polyvinyl alcohol	carbon dioxide(M), carbon monoxide(L), methane(M), acetadehyde(M), ethyl alcohol(M), acetic acid(M).
Polyvinyl acetate	ethylene(S), ethane(S), acetic acid(L).
Polyacrylonitrile	Hydrogen Cyanide(S), methacrylonitrile(L), acetonitrile( ), propionitrile(I), alphamethyl-4-methyleneglutaronitrile(S), succinitrile(S), glutaronitrile(S).
Polystyrene	benzene(T), Toluene(S), alphamethylstyrene(S), 1,3-diphenylpropane(S), 1,3-diphenylbutene(M), allybenzene (S), styrene(L).
Polyvinyl chloride (copolymer with vinyl acetate)	methane(S), ethylene(S), ethane(S), propylene(S), propane(S), butene(S), butane(S), acetic acid(L), hydrochloric acid(M).
Phenol-formaldehyde resin	phenol(L), cresols(L), xylenols(S), formaldehyde(S).
Polyethylene	methane(S), ethylene(L), ethane(M), propane(S), propene (S), butane(M), butene(M), 1,-butadiene(S).
Polypropylene	propylene(L), butane(M), butene(M), pentane(S), 1,3-butadiene(S), methane(S), ethylene(S).
Styrene-butadiene	styrene(L), butadiene(S), vinylcyclohexene(S).
Polyester (saturated)	carbon monoxide(L), methane(S), carbon dioxide(L), ethylene(S), ethane(S), propylene(S), acetaldehyde(L).
Polyurethane	same as above, also isocyanic acid(S).

* Thermal degradation products listed in this table were obtained by heating the polymer to high temperatures under controlled conditions. Decomposition products from burning would be different.

Relative concentrations are denoted as follows: Large (L), Medium (M), Small (S), Trace (T).

† Source: Unknown.

in recent years: Polychlorinated biphenyls (PCB) are high viscocity liquid insulators used in electrical transformers because of their low vapor pressure. Related compounds, polybromenated biphenyls are used as fire retardants. Current control measures should be consulted if these substances are encountered.

27.3.6 Asbestos

The use of asbestos has raised many concerns in recent years because it is a lung carcinogen. The hazard is, however, limited to airborne asbestos fibers. Asbestos gloves, and asbestos backstops used in laser laboratories shoud not be considered hazardous. However, laboratory personnel and laser technicians should be warned not to attempt cutting or sawing asbestos sheeting because of the production of hazardous asbestos "dust." Recent recommendations of ACGIH (1979) would limit specific minerals which make up asbestos:

$$2 \text{ fibers longer than } 5 \ \mu\text{m per cc. for chrysotile}$$
$$0.2 \text{ fibers longer than } 5 \ \mu\text{m per cc. for crocidolite}$$
$$0.5 \text{ fibers longer than } 5 \ \mu\text{m per cc. for amosite}$$

There are clearly a large variety of potential industrial hygiene types of hazards associated with lasers. For this reason, it is generally wise to have an expert in the field of industrial hygiene review the design of any large laser system and to evaluate the layout of high powered laser research laboratories or industrial installations.

27.4 FIRE HAZARDS

As previously noted, solvents used in dye lasers are extremely flammable and, according to a report from Stanford Research Institute, have led to at least eight fires within a two year period in U.S. laboratories. Most of these fires were started by a high-voltage pulse through an alcohol solvent, although in one case a hot xenon arc lamp tube ignited the solvent. Probably the best control measure for this fire hazard is to restrict the operation of high-energy coaxial flash lamps to the average power levels recommended by the manufacturers and to use only non-volatile solvents. Another approach to the problem is, if possible, to replace the alcohol solvent with a water-alcohol mixture of more than 50% water. When alcohol must be used, the laser housing should enclose any exploding liquid (Grant and Hawley, 1975). If a fire occurs, dye pumps and laser pumps must be shut down quickly, which may be accomplished by the installation of a fluid-pressure or microphone-actuated switch.

It is common practice to increase the flashlamp voltage above the recommended operating level to compensate for the decrease output of aging lamps. This aging process results in an increase in the breakdown voltage of xenon-oxygen gas mixtures and is caused by the decomposition of the silicon dioxide in the glass or quartz envelope from repeated firing. The oxygen created by this decomposition increases the lamp threshold voltage. Therefore to prevent explosions, the threshold voltage can be monitored by placing a resistor in parallel with the lamp. One can choose the shunt resistance value at a power rating that will assure the burn-up of the resistor once the lamp breakdown voltage passes the maximal level.

The explosion hazard of dye laser solvents is shared by high-pressure xenon flash lamps (Figure 17-2). One model solid state pulsed laser manufactured between 1965 and 1970 was notorious for explosions, apparently because the flashlamp manufacturer's specifications were exceeded in the design of the high-voltage power supply. The enclosure around the flashlamp should always be sufficiently rugged to contain any explosion, although small pressure relief areas or holes should be provided.

High-power CW infrared lasers can produce substantial fire hazards from the direct beam. Unexpected specular reflections from metal surfaces can ignite flammable materials in the area of the laser operation. Fire resistant sheeting and other materials should be used to the maximum extent possible in the immediate vicinity of very high power laser operations. The fire fighting equipment required for laser operations can vary. Dry chemical fire extinguishers are often found in laboratories. However, laboratory personnel should be aware of the fact that such dry chemicals coat and etch optical surfaces, and may damage electronic components. Therefore, dry chemical extinguishers are less preferred than gas extinguishers, such as carbon dioxide or Freon® (Dupont). Other fire-fighting gas materials such as Halon 1301® (also a product of the Dupont Company) are quite effective in this regard. Water shares the disadvantages of dry chemical fire extinguishers in damaging some optical and electronic components and, in addition, may exacerbate an electrical fire, as well as presenting a shock hazard.

27.5 RADIATION HAZARDS

The high voltage power supplies used with some lasers often produce a limited quantity of low energy X radiation. This generally originates from the high-voltage vacuum tubes, such as rectifiers, thyratrons and crowbars used in laser power supplies. With the increased use of solid state electronics the X-ray potential is reduced or eliminated. Power supplies producing potentials greater than 15 kV with vacuum tubes may produce a sufficient quantity of X rays to present a significant health hazard. Normally such tubes have sufficient shielding to prevent the escape of hazardous levels. To measure such low energy X radiation it is important not to use a common geiger counter or similar instrument designed for very high energy ionizing radiation. A thin-window instrument, well shielded from the radio-frequency radiation often present in power supplies, should be used for this purpose.

In addition to the power supply itself, X rays are produced in large quantities from electron beam (E-beam) laser systems. However, the X-ray hazard from electron-beam machines is always anticipated in the design of such commercial equipment, and one should expect that adequate shielding has been placed around the system to preclude hazardous leakage levels. Safety personnel, however, should be on the lookout for modification, or poor maintenance practices, in an electron-beam system that could affect the efficiency of the shielding. If the operator of an

E-beam laser is not familiar with the X-radiation hazard, he might unknowingly remove a portion of the shielding, not realizing its value or purpose. An industrial X-ray facility which produces in excess of 100 mrad in any one hour is considered an "open protective" installation: some of the hazard control measures utilized for such X-ray installations can also be applied directly to an electron-beam laser system. Voltages of up to 500 kV may be generated by Marks-bank techniques and the X rays produced from such systems can present more serious control design problems since much heavier shielding materials must be used.

27.6 CRYOGENIC HAZARDS

Liquid nitrogen and other cryogenic fluids are utilized to cool some lasers and many high sensitivity photodetectors. Examples of cryogenically cooled lasers are CW solid state ruby lasers with continuous pumping by a high intensity lamp, or high-power gallium-arsenide laser arrays. Cryogenic cooling is most often encountered in infrared detectors such as the mercury-cadmium-telluride type. The signal-to-noise ratio of these detectors is greatly improved by the lower temperatures achieved with cryogenic cooling.

When cryogenic fluids evaporate they displace breatheable oxygen and thus should be used only in areas of good ventilation. Another safety hazard associated with the use of cryogenic fluids is the possibility of explosion from ice collecting in a valve or a connector. This explosive hazard is most common when the plumbing is not specifically designed to operate with cryogenic materials. The more hazardous cryogenic fluids such as liquid oxygen and liquid hydrogen are not typically used in laser research laboratories. Nevertheless, liquid oxygen, which is both a serious fire and explosive hazard, is often produced from room air. As the condensation temperature of oxygen is approximately 13° higher than the boiling point of liquid nitrogen, it may collect in open Dewar flasks of liquid nitrogen.

Both protective clothing and face shields should be used when handling large quantities of liquid nitrogen. Often protective gloves are not used in handling extremely small quantities of liquid nitrogen; in fact, the normal moisture and oil on the surface of the skin is sufficient to protect the hand from cold injury from a few small drops of liquid nitrogen. The small quantities of liquid nitrogen used to cool infrared sensitive detectors do not ordinarily present a serious health hazard.

There are a number of safety procedures required in the use of gas cannisters and cryogenic Dewar flasks to prevent serious accidents. It is now common practice to chain all gas cannisters to the wall or instrument system. This precludes a dangerous explosion should the cannister fall, and break the very vulnerable valve, with a resultant sudden release of the gas.

27.7 NOISE HAZARDS

Hearing conservation measures, including the use of protective devices, should be practiced when steady-state noise levels exceed 90 dB(A) for eight hours per day (by Federal regulation). However, an exposure of 115 dB(A) is permissible for a period of less than 15 minutes. For a pulsed laser impact that produces impulsive noise (i.e., less than 0.5), the maximum recommended exposure is 140 dB(A). The complete requirements for hearing conservation of the Occupational Health and Safety Administration (OSHA) are covered in sub-part G of Section 1910.95 (U.S. Department of Labor, 1977). Table 27-3 lists the ACGIH (1979) threshold limit values (TLV's) for noise.

As TEA lasers normally produce large impact noises, acoustical control measures are generally required. Often hazardous noise levels exist only in the immediate vicinity of the laser or target where other safety recommendations exclude personnel, thus obviating the need for control measures.

27.8 REVIEW QUESTIONS

1. What are the most likely causes of fires in a high-power laser facility?

2. What is the occupational limit for 2 hours exposure to loud noise according to ACGIH?

3. What is DMSO and why is it a potential hazard in some laser laboratories?

4. A safety officer notices the smell of ozone in a laser laboratory and recalls that an instructor once pointed out that "if you can smell it, the chances are it exceeds the permissible concentration." What should he do? Where should he look for the source of this ozone?

5. What is the permissible airborne concentration of carbon-monoxide? How much less hazardous is carbon-dioxide than carbon-monoxide?

6. Describe two types of hazards that are particularly of concern with high-powered pulsed dye lasers.

7. Calculate the permissible concentration for an atmosphere contaminated by both copper metal fumes and iron oxide fumes.

8. What is the maximum recommended exposure for an impact noise?

9. From what type of laser system might you expect to encounter such an impact noise?

10. A laser investigator comes to you and complains that the fire break that was installed as a backstop in his high-power laser research facility incandesces at such a bright level that he feels it is a potential eye hazard. He would prefer to replace these fire bricks with a softer fire brick that burns through and does not produce such an annoying glare during his experiment. What would you recommend?

Table 27-3a. Threshold Limit Values for Steady-State Noise

Duration per day Hours	Sound Level dBA*
16	80
8	85
4	90
2	95
1	100
1/2	105
1/4	110
1/8	115†

†No exposure to continuous or intermittent in excess of 115 dBA.

The sound level shall be determined by a sound level meter, conforming as a minimum to the requirements of the American National Standard Specification for Sound Level Meters, S1.4 (1971) Type S2A, and set to use the A-weighted network with slow meter response. Duration of exposure shall not exceed that shown in Table 27-3a.

These values apply to total duration of exposure per working day regardless of whether this is one continuous exposure or a number of short-term exposures but does not apply to impact or impulsive type of noise.

When the daily noise exposure is composed of two or more periods of noise exposure of different levels, their combined effect should be considered, rather than the individual effect of each. If the sum of the following fractions:

$$\frac{C_1}{T_1} + \frac{C_2}{T_2} + \cdots \frac{C_n}{T_n}$$

exceeds unity, then, the mixed exposure should be considered to exceed the threshold limit value, C_1 indicates the total duration of exposure at a specific noise level, and T_1 indicates the total duration of exposure permitted at that level. All on-the-job noise exposures of 80 dBA or greater shall be used in the above calculations.

Table 27-3b. Threshold Limit Values for Impulsive or Impact Noise

Peak Sound Pressure Level dB	Permitted Number of Impulses or Impacts per day
140	100
130	1,000
120	10,000

It is recommended that exposure to impulsive or impact noise shall not exceed the limits listed in Table 27-3b. No exposures in excess of 140 decibels peak sound pressure level are permitted. Impulsive or impact noise is considered to be those variations in noise levels that involve maxima at intervals of greater than one per second. Where the intervals are less than one second, it should be considered continuous.

It should be recognized that the application of the TLV for noise will not protect all workers from the adverse effects of noise exposure. A hearing conservation program with audiometric testing is necessary when workers are exposed to noise at or above the TLV levels.

27.9 REFERENCES

Adams, R. M., 1969, "Occupational Contact Dermatitis," 262 pages, Lippincott/Harper, New York.
American Conference of Governmental Industrial Hygienists, 1974, "Industrial Ventilation: A Manual of Recommended Practice," Cincinnati, OH.
American Conference of Governmental Industrial Hygienists, 1979, "Threshold Limit Values for Chemical Substances and Physical Agents in the Workroom Environment with Intended Changes for 1979," ACGIH, Cincinnati, OH.
American Industrial Hygiene Association, continually updated, "Hygienic Guide Series," Detroit.
American National Standards Institute, 1971, Fundamentals Governing the Design and Operation of Local Exhaust Systems, ANSI Z9.2, New York.
American National Standards Institute, 1971, Practices for Ventilation and Operation of Open-Surface Tanks, ANSI Z9.1–1971, New York.
ASPEN Systems Corporation Center for Compliance Information, 1978, "Toxic Substances Control Sourcebook," General Electric Co., Schenectady, New York.
Burns, W., 1973, "Noise and Man," 2nd ed., Lippincott/Harper, New York.
Clayton, G. D., and Clayton, F. E. (eds.), 1978, "Patty's Industrial Hygiene and Toxicology," 3rd rev. ed., Wiley-Interscience, New York.
Dezenburg, G. J., Roy, E. L., and McKnight, W. B., 1972, Performance of high voltage axially pulsed CO_2 lasers, *IEEE J. Quant. Elect.* **QE-8**(2):58.
Gafafer, W. M. (ed.), 1966, "Occupational Diseases–A Guide to their Recognition," U.S. Public Health Service Publication 1097, Washington, DC, Government Printing Office.
Grant, W. B., and Hawley, J. G., 1975, Prevention of fire damage due to exploding dye laser flashlamps, *Appl. Opt.* **14**(6):1257–1258.
Koller, L. R., 1965, "Ultraviolet Radiation," 2nd ed., John Wiley and Sons, New York.
Kues, H. A., and Lutty, G. A., 1975, Dyes can be deadly, *Laser Focus* **11**(5):58–60 (May 1975).
Mackison, F. W., Stricoff, R. S., and Partridge, L. J., 1978, "NIOSH/OSHA Pocket Guide to Chemical Hazards," DHEW(NIOSH) Publication No. 78-210, National Institute of Occupational Safety and Health, Cincinnati.
Marich, K. W., Orenberg, J. B., Treytl, W. J., and Glick, D., Health hazards in the use of the laser microprobe for toxic and infective samples, *Am. Ind. Hyg. Assn. J.* **33**(7):488–491.
National Bureau of Standards, 1963, "Handbook 93–Safety for Non-Medical X-ray and Sealed Gamma-ray Sources," ANSI Standard Z54.1-1963, Washington, DC.
National Fire Protection Association, 1977, "Fire Protection for Laboratories using Chemicals," NFPA 45, Boston, MA.
National Fire Protection Association, 1977, "Flammable and Combustable Liquids Code," NFPA 30, Boston, MA.
Patty, F. A. (ed.), 1958, "Industrial Hygiene and Toxicology," 2nd ed., Vol. I, Wiley-Interscience, New York.
Powell, C. H., and Hosey, A. D. (eds), 1973, "The Industrial Environment–Its Evaluation and Control," National Institute for Occupational Safety and Health, Government Printing Office, Washington, DC.
Proctor, N. H., and Hughes, J. P., 1978, "Chemical Hazards of the Workplace, 536 pages, Lippincott/Harper, New York.
Sliney, D. H., Vorpahl, K. W., and Winburn, D. C., 1975, Environmental health hazards from high-powered infrared laser devices, *Arch. Environ. Health* **30**(4):174–179.
Steere, N. V. (ed.), 1971, "Handbook of Laboratory Safety," 2nd ed., The Chemical Rubber Company, Cleveland.
U.S. Atomic Energy Commission Technical Bulletin 13, 1968, "Electrical Safety Guides for Research, Safety, and Fire Protection," Governmental Printing Office, Washington, DC.
U.S. Department of Labor, 1977, Title 29, Code of Federal Regulations 1910, Occupational Safety and Health Administration (OSHA) Standards, especially Section 1910.252(f)(3), Local Exhaust Hoods and Booths; Section 1910.1000, Air Contaminants; and Section 1910.1001, Asbestos; Section 1910.95 Noise.
Zabetakis, M. G., 1967, "Safety with Cryogenic Fluids," Plenum Press, New York.

Chapter 28
Electrical Hazards

28.1 INTRODUCTION

Ocular and skin hazards associated with laser radiation normally receive the greatest attention in any discussion of laser safety. However optical hazards in general are not potentially lethal, whereas electrocution is possible under certain circumstances. A few simple precautions can materially reduce the risks to personnel working with high-voltage power supplies used with many laser systems. An understanding of the physiologic basis of electrical shock and of cardiac arrest is important prior to discussing electrical safety. This chapter will not only consider the physiological basis of shock but will also attempt to provide guidelines for safe electrical design of laser equipment and safe test procedures to eliminate serious electrical safety problems.

28.2 ELECTRICAL ACCIDENTS

Most veterans of any laser research laboratory can recall at least one story of severe shock to a research worker from a high energy electrical power supply. Indeed an early survey conducted in the late 1960's to evaluate accidents associated with lasers revealed that electrical accidents occurred more frequently than injuries to the eye or skin from laser radiation. Although electrical safety precautions have long been standard practice in physics, electronics, and high-power laser laboratories, the large capacitor banks and very high voltage power supplies used in lasers require special attention. Accounts of some accidents and near-accidents are illustrative of what can happen when working with high voltage equipment (Franks and Sliney, 1975).

28.2.1 A Near Accident

A few years ago, a 25 kJ pulsed ruby laser power supply at one government research laboratory failed to discharge its capacitors when the power supply cabinet access panel was opened for a repair procedure. The operator tried to discharge the capacitors by means of an auxiliary grounding rod built into the supply. As a final safety check prior to touching the capacitor terminals he placed a portable voltmeter across the capacitors to assure that they were discharged. The voltmeter, set on the 300-volt range, was "pegged." The laser power supply employed two output terminals—a 3,000 J output used to power the oscillator stage flash lamps and a 25,000 J output which powered the amplifier stage flash lamps of the laser. The hazardous situation occurred when a faulty resistor (open circuit) in the charging circuit permitted a 10 kV capacitor to partially charge by arcing as shown in Figure 28-1. The capacitor would not completely discharge because of the open circuit, even when a dump switch was activated. An estimated 2-kV potential remained across the output terminals of the laser oscillator. Since no built-in meter was employed for this output (a meter monitored the voltage across the laser amplifier stage), there was no way of knowing that the capacitor was charged.

A grounding rod was supplied with the unit, but this, too, had become defective. It was dropped, causing a discontinuity (crack) in the rod. Despite the 2-kV potential existing across the capacitor, all reasonable precautions suggested that there was no charge on the capacitor. This high-voltage hazard was discovered by a cautious worker when he placed the portable voltmeter across the capacitor terminals. Fortunately, no injury occurred in this instance.

28.2.2 Severe Accidental Shocks

In another government laboratory an individual working on a laser system's high-voltage power supply accidentally placed his hands across a 30-kV terminal. Although he was thrown across the room and received skin burns at the points of contact with the high-voltage terminals, he did not suffer more than temporary disability.

In another case, a researcher was working with a Pockel cell electro-optic device which had been raised to a 32-kV potential. After switching off the power supply he touched the terminals gingerly with a shielded cable since there was a small capacitor in the circuit. A white spark traveled along the apparently dirty surface of the cable, and then continued across his hand and traveled along his sleeve to his elbow, thence to a metal cabinet. He jumped or perhaps was thrown across the room. He had no burns or scars from this incident but did have a sore arm for several days. A loud "crack" accompanied the discharge.

These cases are not unique. A technician at another government laboratory was momentarily shocked when his arm and head completed a circuit of 5-kV potential with a current of 70 mA. These accidents and reports of many similar nonfatal shocks from high voltage discharges lead to questions about possibly fatal electrical accidents with laser equipment.

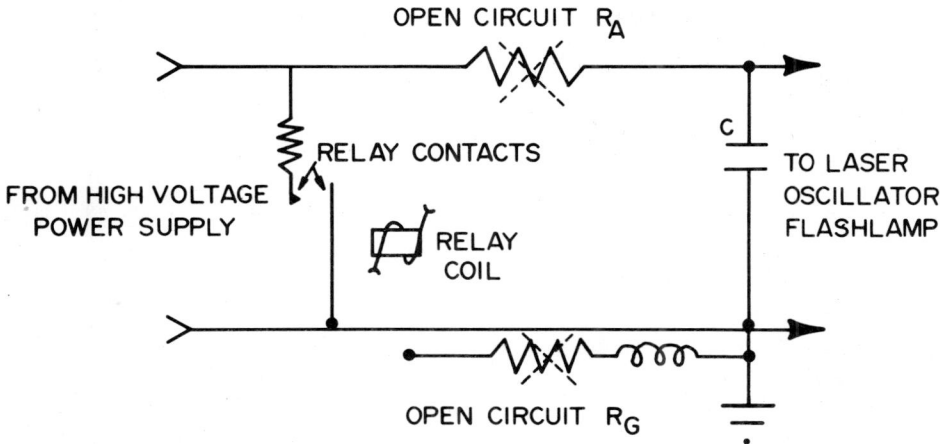

Figure 28-1. Laser Changing Circuit. R_A is open and permits capacitor C to partially charge by arcing. The capacitor is then isolated from the dumping circuit and will not discharge when the relay contacts are closed. The grounding rod R_g is touched to the capacitor terminals, but, since it is also open, prevents C from discharging.

28.2.3 Electrocutions

At least four individuals in the United States have been electrocuted while working with high voltage laser power supplies. An experienced technician at Space Rays, Inc., Burlington, Mass., lost his life in 1971 as a result of failing to reconnect a high-voltage transformer lead. He had previously cut this lead to reach some klystron tube circuit components. Later, when the power was restored, he reached into the power supply to trouble-shoot the apparent high-voltage failure. A doctoral candidate at the Massachusetts Institute of Technology, Cambridge, Massachusetts, was electrocuted in 1972 while working with a far-infrared gas laser with a floating end-plate potential of 4,000 V. MIT officials reported that safety covers were not in place on the power supply. A third person, a young man employed at a Massachusetts laser laboratory, was electrocuted in 1974 while working on a high-voltage power supply. He apparently did not take appropriate safety precautions. A fourth young man, another doctoral candidate, this time at Stanford University in Palo Alto, California, was electrocuted in 1976 when he touched current-carrying components of a high voltage power supply. The electrocution took place after midnight. The graduate student was overly fatigued. Clearly all of these accidents could have been avoided by strict adherence to long-established electrical safety guidelines.

Many people who work with electrical equipment also do not realize that it is possible literally to bring a person back from death after electrocution with fairly simple heart-lung resuscitative techniques.

A brief review of the physiology of electrical shock shall be presented here to give a better understanding of the appropriate resuscitative techniques. Later in this chapter, a typical chart will be shown that could be used in a laboratory where high-voltage electrical equipment is present.

28.3 PHYSIOLOGICAL EFFECTS OF ELECTRIC SHOCK

Most of the studies on electrical shock were performed during the 1930s and 1940s at the University of California at Berkeley and at Columbia University in New York. These pioneering research efforts are cited in references at the end of this chapter. In these studies it was determined that several factors established the severity of injury associated with electric shock. These factors are: the current path through the body; the frequency, if alternating current; the susceptibility of the heart in different phases of the cardiac cycle; the duration of the shock or discharge; repeated shocks in different phases of the heart cycle; the current magnitude (not voltage); skin resistance, and whether the voltage is sufficient to break down skin resistance (greater than 600 V). An in-depth discussion of the physiological effects of electric shock is beyond the scope of this presentation; however, some brief comments are helpful.

28.3.1 Current Magnitude

Current, not voltage, determines the physiological effect of electrical shock. It is useful to distinguish quantitatively between at least four levels of effects due to continuous electrical currents: (a) nonperceptible electrical currents; (b) perceptible (perhaps painful) currents below the so-called "let-go threshold;" (c) currents above the "let-go threshold;" and (d) currents which cause ventricular fibrillation (discoordinated heart action). For pulsed electrical discharges (as from a capacitor bank discharge), the distinction between categories (b) and (c) do not exist and the electrical energy (not current) determines the possibility of ventricular fibrillation. The currents passing through the human body which cause the various physiological responses are provided in Table 28-1. The thresholds of these effects are influenced by the current path through the body. The actual magnitude of current flow resulting from accidental contact of live electrical circuit components is determined by skin contact resistance. Current magnitude is determined by Ohm's law, that is:
$$I = V/R \qquad (28\text{-}1)$$
where I is the current through the body, V the applied voltage to the body contacts, and R the total resistance to current flow. Here R is the sum of two resistances in series: the contact resistance in the internal body resistance. The internal body

Table 28-1. Quantitative Effects of Electric Current On Man†

Physiologic Effect	Direct Current		Milliamperes Alternating Current			
			60-Hz		10,000 Hz	
	Men	Women	Men	Women	Men	Women
Slight sensation on hand	1	0.6	0.4	0.3	7	5
Perception threshold, median	5.2	3.5	1.1	0.7	12	8
Shock—not painful and muscular control not lost	9	6	1.8	1.2	17	11
Painful shock—muscular control lost by ½%	62	41	9	6	55	37
Painful shock—let-go threshold, median	76	51	16	10.5	75	50
Painful and severe shock—breathing difficult, muscular control lost by 99 ½%	90	60	23	15	94	63
Possible ventricular fibrillation						
Three-second shocks	500	500	675	675		
Short shocks (t in seconds)			$116/\sqrt{t}$	$116/\sqrt{t}$		
Capacitor discharges	50*	50*				

*Energy in Joules.
†Adapted from Dalziel (1943).

resistance is between 200 and 500 ohms, depending upon the particular current pathway, whereas contact resistance may vary between approximately 1,000 ohms and 100,000 ohms. High voltages (600 V cited in one reference) may cause breakdown of contact resistance resulting in negligible values. This is probably the only real significance of high voltage in regards to physiological effects of electrical currents.

Externally applied voltages which result in significant currents through the heart derange heart action, with ventricular fibrillation, but without damage to the cardiac tissues. Death results within a few minutes unless the fibrillation is arrested. A current through the body that results in a cardiac current just below the threshold for ventricular fibrillation is a maximum to which man may safely be subjected. Based upon numerous animal tests, this maximum current through a pathway between an arm and a leg is approximately 0.1 ampere for a duration of 1 s or greater; however, the threshold fibrillating current was affected by the species and size of the animal during these tests. The current pathway is a major variable also. For instance, the threshold current was nearly the same for paths from one arm to one leg, across the chest to an arm, and the head to one leg. A higher threshold current was required between the arms. From leg to leg the proportion of current reaching the region of the heart was so small that fibrillation did not take place even

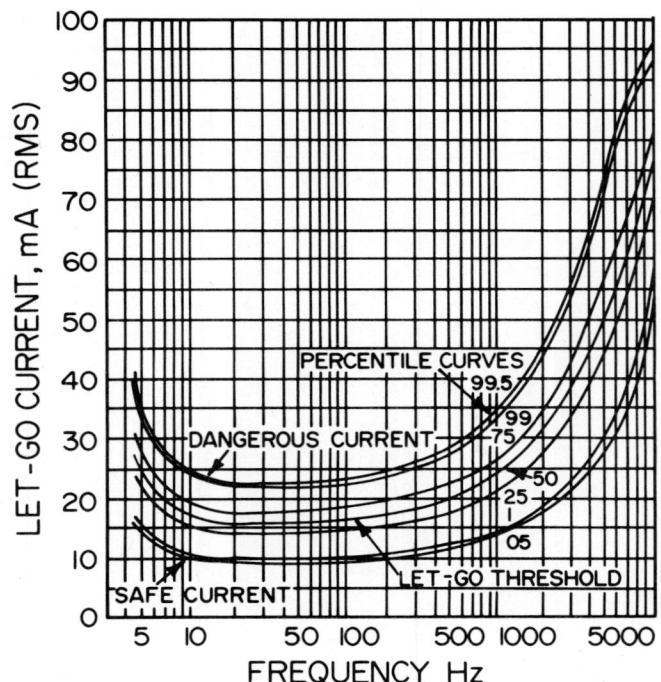

Figure 28-2. Effect of Frequency on Let-go Currents for Men. Values for women are approximately 66 percent of the current values shown on the curves. Current values become langercus progressively to an increasing number of persons as indicated by the percentile curves on the right hand side of the curves (redrawn from Dalziel, 1961).

at currents of 15 Amperes or greater, although such currents probably would burn the victim unless the contacts were very good and the shock was of short duration. There are many cases in the literature where an individual working with a high-voltage power supply suffered severe skin burns and was thrown across the room, but, as little of the current passed through the heart (hand to elbow, for example, there was no effect on the heart.

28.3.2 Frequency Effect

In addition to the current-path effect, the effect of frequency of an alternating current must be considered. The frequency affects shocks if the shocks are of 1 s or greater duration. The 25-Hz threshold current reported in the literature is approximately 25-percent higher than the 60-Hz threshold, and the DC current threshold is five times the threshold for the 60-Hz currents for shock durations of a fraction of a second. However, this relation probably does not hold for much greater shock durations since all thresholds were expected to approach one another. Figure 28-2 gives an indication of the frequency effect upon let-go current. The relative discomfort is greatest for frequencies between 10 and 200 Hz.

28.3.3 Ventricular Fibrillation

The phase relation of a short shock relative to the cardiac cycle is another major factor which influences the severity of shock. The time of the occurrence of short shocks in relationship to the cardiac cycle is considered important since the heart is only susceptible to fibrillation from shocks during the partial refractory phase—approximately 20-percent of the cycle (about 30 ms). This is simultaneous with the t-wave of the electrocardiogram. Hence, shocks of a duration of approximately 0.1 s or less do not produce ventricular fibrillation unless such shocks coincide in part, at least, with the sensitive, or partially refractory phase, of the cardiac cycle. The middle of the partially refractory phase is the most sensitive part. The threshold current varies inversely with shock duration, but not uniformly. It is more sensitive to change as the duration nears that of a complete heartbeat. The minimum threshold fibrillating current for shock durations of approximately 0.1 s or less can be more than 10 times that for 1 s or more. Shocks as long as one third or more of the heart cycle may cause ventricular fibrillation even though they would not extend into the sensitive phase. In those cases the heart continues its normal beat after a premature initiation which brings about prematurely a sensitive phase during the shock. Successive shocks do not have a cumulative effect on the susceptibility of the heart to fibrillation. Short shocks are more effective with currents up to several times the threshold, but then become ineffective with almost no fibrillation at currents around 25 amperes applied in the vicinity of the heart. At these current levels cardiac action ceases, and usually commences in a coordinated manner with the end of the electrical current. However, other serious accidents may be expected from such currents when brought about by accidental contact.

The literature on electrical shock is quite fascinating. A selected bibliography is presented at the end of this chapter. Some of the more interesting papers deal with individuals who have been struck by lightening and severely burned, yet recovered completely after several minutes without a heartbeat.

28.4 THE DANGEROUS ELECTRICAL SUPPLIES

Small lasers, such as those used in military laser rangefinders and small laser micromachining equipment that have output radiant energies ranging between 50–100 mJ, have typical electrical input energies of 10–20 J. A typical example is 1.6 kV at 10 μF. These electrical energies represent a potential shock hazard but would normally not be considered as a practical hazard except under unusual circumstances. A 1-mW helium-neon laser used in construction applications would typically have 10 W (2.5 mA at 4 kV) of electrical input power. Although power supplies used with helium-neon lasers used in construction and the high-powered infrared gas lasers used in cutting are capable of producing lethal voltages, operating personnel are normally protected by safe design. However, maintenance personnel can be exposed to hazardous conditions in the course of their repair work. The high-energy, Q-switched lasers often found in research laboratories may have electrical inputs of 1,000 J or more and associated voltages up to 100 kV. Some high-powered gas lasers also require input electrical voltages of 100 kV which can be achieved through the use of Marks Bank generators. Clearly research and maintenance personnel are those that are at high risk.

28.5 REGULATIONS, STANDARDS AND STANDARD OPERATING PROCEDURES (SOPs)

Most research laboratories that utilize high power lasers have SOPs that consider electrical hazards although many of these SOPs or regulations do not describe this hazard in depth. Neither do they provide detailed safety guidelines for working in the vicinity of such high voltage sources.

Among the many regulations and guide booklets in print on this subject, one of the most useful has been a publication of the old U.S. Atomic Energy Commission (later called the Energy Research and Development Administration or ERDA and now the Department of Energy); a booklet entitled "Electrical Safety Guides to Research," Safety and Fire Protection Technical Bulletin #13 was issued in December 1967 and is still widely used by safety professionals. Besides this document, one military standard (MIL Standard 454 C) which is used by many equipment manufacturers who specialize in military electronic equipment provides some information on the importance of grounding electrical chassis and dealing with safety in general. It however, does not go into detail on high voltage power supplies. The American National Standards Institute standard Z-136.1, 1976, The Safe Use of Lasers, does recommend that positive protection be afforded against contact with peak open circuit potentials over 42.5 V unless the current is limited to 0.5 mA. This standard also provides other specific guidelines for electrical safety.

Underwriters Laboratories (UL) in the USA has several equipment standards that relate to specific products which may use lasers. There is no general UV standard on all laser products. In Germany, an electrical standard specifically for laser equipment was promulgated by VDE in 1977 (VDE, 1977). It considers all laser equipment specialized environments and provides test procedures. There are no other standards known to the authors which are as complete or as rigorous as the German standard, although the International Electrotechnical Commission (IEC) Committee TC76 adopted many of the requirements for a proposed standard. The IEC draft standard was still in Committee in 1979.

28.6 SAFETY GUIDELINES TO PREVENT ELECTRICAL SHOCK

The following precautions should be followed by personnel working with hazardous electrical equipment (Franks and Sliney, 1975):

1. Avoid wearing rings, metallic watch bands, and other metallic apparel when working with electrical equipment or in the presence of strong induced fields.

2. Whenever possible, use only one hand for any manipulation of circuits or control devices.

3. Never handle electrical equipment when hands, feet, or body are wet, especially when perspiring or standing on a wet floor.

4. With high voltages, regard all floors as conductive and grounded for high voltages unless they are covered with well-maintained dry rubber matting of a type suitable for electrical work.

5. Be familiar with the following rescue procedures for application to apparent victims of electrocution:

    (a) kill the circuit

    (b) remove the victim with a non-conductor if he is still in contact with an energized circuit

    (c) initiate artificial mouth-to-mouth resuscitation immediately (or the technique of heart-lung resuscitation if known) and continue until relieved by a physician. The Chart on the next page can be copied and can be posted near hazardous equipment.

    (d) have someone call for emergency aid in all cases.

Extremely high energies and voltages are present in the power supplies for many lasers. High-energy pulsed lasers have capacitors charged to several kilovolts with associated energies of hundreds of joules. These high energies constitute potentially lethal shock hazards. Capacitors offer many potential hazards. The following engineering hazard control measures should be instituted in all laser laboratories where high energy pulsed and high power CW lasers are used:

1. Provide emergency shut-off switches. In some research laboratories these are incorporated in each laboratory bench outlet.

2. Provide enclosures—preferably a grounded metal enclosure—that is locked and/or interlocked and designed to prevent accidental contact with current-carrying conductors such as terminals and cables.

3. Automatically dump (crowbar) capacitors before opening any access door.

FIRST AID FOR SHOCK VICTIMS

1. If a person has stopped breathing or his heart has stopped beating, heart-lung resuscitation should be started at once. If the person is not breathing do the following: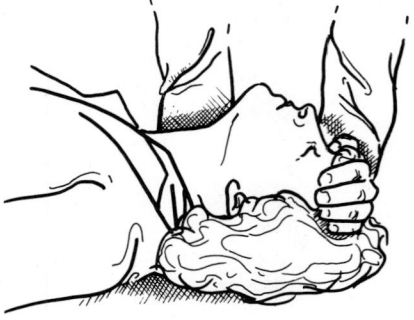
   (a) *Clear the throat.* Wipe out any matter in his mouth with your fingers or cloth wrapped around your fingers.
   (b) *Place the victim on his back.* Place him on a firm surface, such as the ground or floor, not on a bed or sofa.
   (c) *Tilt his head straight back (#1).* Extend the neck up as far as possible. This will automatically keep the tongue out of the airway.
   (d) *Open your mouth wide and place it tightly over the victim's mouth (#2).* At the same time pinch the victim's nostrils shut or close the nostrils with your cheek. Alternatively, close the victim's mouth and place your mouth over his nose. This latter method is preferable with babies and small children. Blow into the victim's mouth or nose with a smooth, steady action until the victim's chest seems to rise.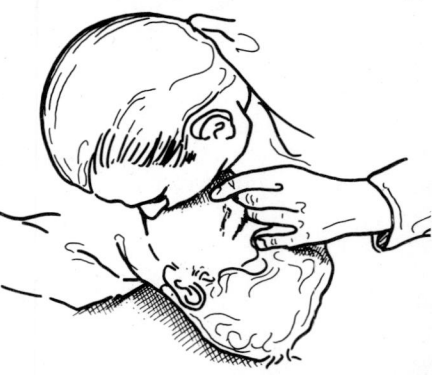
   (e) *Remove your mouth.* Listen for the return of air that indicates air exchange.
   (f) *Repeat.* Continue with relatively shallow breaths, appropriate for the victim's size, at the rate of one breath every five seconds. NOTE: If you are not getting air exchange quickly, recheck the position of his head, turn the victim on his side and give several sharp blows between the shoulder blades to jar foreign matter. After four or five breaths, stop and determine if his heart is beating by checking his pulse. If the heart is beating, return to mouth-to-mouth resuscitation and continue until breathing starts or until a physician tells you to stop.
2. If the heart has stopped, begin heart massage:
   (a) *Place the heel of one hand on the lower third of the breast bone,* the other hand on top of the first.
   (b) *Thrust downward from your shoulders* with enough force to depress the breast bone about 1½–2 inches.
   (c) *Relax at the end of each stroke* to permit natural expansion of the chest.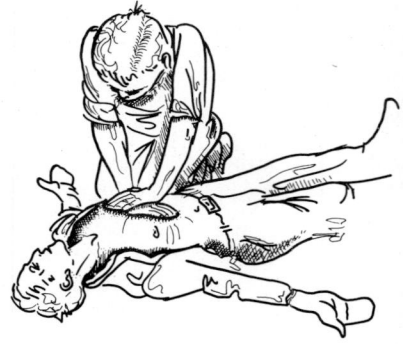
   (d) *Repeat* at the rate of about once each second. If you are alone with the victim you must alternate mouth-to-mouth breathing with heart massage at the ratio of about 2:15, that is, 2 breaths, then 15 heart compressions.
   (e) *If you have help,* use a ratio of 1:5; after five heart compressions, pause slightly to allow your partner to breathe once into the lungs of the victim.
3. *Call for help.* Continue one or both of the above while the victim is being transported to the hospital; until he revives; or until told to cease by a physician.

4. Where feasible, wait 24 hours before attempting any work on circuits involving very high energy capacitors.

5. Provide as short a discharge time constant as feasible in turn-off grounding system devices.

6. Check that each capacitor is discharged, shorted, and grounded prior to working in the area of the capacitors. Networks of gas discharge tubes (neon lamps) and resistors could be used to indicate simply the state of charge of the capacitors without affecting operation.

7. Install crowbars, grounding switches, cables, and other safety devices that can withstand the mechanical forces that often exist when fault or crowbar currents flow.

8. Provide suitable warning devices, such as signs and lights.

9. Place shorting straps on each capacitor during maintenance or storage.

10. Provide manual grounding equipment with a connecting cable visible for its entire length.

11. Provide a grounding stick that has a discharge resistor at its contact point and an insulated grounding cable (transparent insulation preferred) permanently attached to ground. Such a grounding stick should not be used to ground an entire large bank of capacitors as the time constant may be too long for the discharge. Large capacity shorting bars with resistors should be part of the stationary equipment. The use of resistors cut down on too rapid a discharge which might cause damage to capacitors and create large mechanical forces. Final assurance of discharge should be accomplished by using a solid conducting grounding rod. In one case on record the solid conducting grounding rod used for backup actually discharged a capacitor presumed to have been discharged by a resistive grounding rod. The explanation for this failure was a hairline crack in the ceramic resistor which had not been detected by the serviceman.

12. Encourage the use of shock preventive shields, power supply enclosures, and shielded leads even in all experimental, temporary, high-voltage circuits.

13. Provide safety devices, such as safety glasses, rubber gloves and insulating rubber floor mats.

14. Provide metering, control, and auxiliary circuits with protection from possibly high potentials, even during fault conditions.

15. Perform routine inspections for deformed or leaky capacitor-containers.

16. Prevent or contain fires by reducing combustible material in the vicinity of these capacitors. Avoide the use of PCB (polychlorinated biphenols) which have been used in the past in capacitors because of their high dielectric constants. PCB's produce extremely toxic vapors during fires.

17. Provide protection against projectiles that may be produced during faults by the use of suitable enclosures and barriers.

18. Consider live parts of circuits and components with peak open circuit potentials exceeding 42.5 V (and over 5 milliamperes) to be hazardous (American National Standard Z-136.1, "Safe Use of Lasers").

28.7 FIRST AID FOR SEVERE SHOCK VICTIMS

Not all laboratory and maintenance personnel are clearly familiar with first aid procedures for victims of severe shock. Only rarely does one find a poster that shows these first-aid procedures located near high-voltage power supplies. Some electrocution victims could have been saved if associates had realized the value of administering first-aid procedures as given in the Chart on the previous page, even if these first-aid procedures were administered after cessation of the heartbeat. Many cases of victims of lightening strikes being "brought back to life" by administering such first aid have been reported in the literature. The importance of continuing cardiopulmonary resuscitation in apparently "dead" victims of electric shock cannot be overemphasized. Cases have been recorded where complete recovery has been achieved even after many minutes of stopped or fibrillating heart action and after cessation of respiration.

An institution which has individuals working with hazardous electrical circuits should require these individuals and other coworkers to take a course (a lesson) in cardiopulmonary resuscitation. Although most health and safety specialists still agree to teaching mouth-to-mouth resuscitation, the teaching of closed-chest cardiac massage is controversial since the patient is possibly placed at risk if not properly performed. The argument for teaching this would be that a professional rescue team may not be sufficiently close to act in time. A further argument against the method in the chart is presented by Morley and Carter (1972) who argued that accident experience favored a different method: two blows on the chest followed by a manual method of artificial respiration. A manual method circulates blood whereas the mouth-to-mouth method does not. Franco (1969) emphasizes the "ABC's" of emergency respiration: A—Airway open; B—Breathe for the Patient; and C—Circulate his blood. He points out that external cardiac compression requires 80 to 120 pounds of pressure on the sternum to depress the patient's lower sternum 4 to 5 cm in the adult.

28.8 REVIEW QUESTIONS

1. High voltage alone is not in itself a major aspect of shock hazard. True or False? Why?

2. At what portion of the cardiac cycle is the heart most susceptible to the initiation of ventricular fibrillation by electrical shock?

3. What is the value of using a resistive grounding rod to discharge a high-voltage capacitor?

4. Why should a solid conductor grounding rod be used following the use of a resistive grounding rod?

5. Research laboratories should not have to follow any electrical safety standards since equipment is being put together, modified and dismantled, frequently on a daily basis. Do you agree?

6. Once an individual has been electrocuted, he cannot be revived. True or False?

7. What is ventricular fibrillation?

8. How could the charge of capacitors be monitored by neon lamps?

9. What would be the value of requiring a "buddy system" (i.e., a minimum of two must always be present) for activities where individuals are working with exposed electrical current-carrying conductors?

10. Why should electronics technicians working with high-current circuits be familiar with the techniques of cardiopulmonary resuscitation? What factors must be considered in any decision to teach such techniques?

28.9 REFERENCES

American Heart Association, 1967, "Cardiopulmonary Resuscitation, A Manual for Instructors," Committee on Cardiopulmonary Resuscitation, American Heart Association, New York.

Anonymous, 1971, 1972, 1974, Accident Reports, *Laser Focus* 7(4):8 (April 1971); 8(10):60 (April 1972); 10(9):4 (September 1974).

Castren, J. A., and Kytila, J., 1964, Eye symptoms caused by lightning, *Acta. Ophthal.* (Kobenhavn) 42:139–143.

Dalziel, C. F., 1960, Threshold 60-cycle fibrillating currents, *AIEE Trans. (Power apparatus and systems)* 50:667–673.

Dalziel, C. F., 1971, Deleterious effects of electric shock, "CRC Handbook of Laboratory Safety, (N. V. Steere, ed.) 2nd edn., pp. 521–527, Chemical Rubber Company, Cleveland, Ohio.

Dalziel, C. F., and Lee, W. R., 1969, Lethal electric currents, *IEEE Spectrum* 6(2):44–50.

Dalziel, C. F., 1961, Electricity—good and faithful servant, *Nat. Safety News* 84(3):28–29, 76, 78, 80, 82, 84.

Dalziel, C. F., 1956, The effects of electric shock on man, *IRE Trans. Med. Electr.* **PGME-5**.
Dalziel, C. F., 1946, Dangerous electric currents, *AIEE Trans. (Electrical Engineering)* **65**:8–9, 579–585.
Dalziel, C. F., 1943, Effect of wave form on let-go currents, *Electr. Eng.* **62**:739–744.
Dalziel, C. F., Lagen, J. B., and Thruston, J. L., 1941, Electric shock, *AIEE Trans. (Electrical Engineering)* **60**:1073.
Dalziel, C. F., and Lee, W. R., 1968, Reevaluation of lethal electric currents, *IEEE Trans. Ind. Gen. Appl.* **IGA-4**:467–476.
Dalziel, C. F., Ogden, E., Abbott, C. E., 1943, Effect of frequency on let-go currents, *AIEE Trans. (Electrical Engineering)* **62**(12):745–750.
Ehrenkranz, T. E., and Marsischky, G. W., 1971, Electrical equipment wiring and safety procedures, "CRC Handbook of Laboratory Safety," (N. V. Steere, ed.) 2nd edn., pp. 528–539, Chemical Rubber Co., Cleveland, Ohio.
Faraone, G., 1961, Five simultaneous cases of deaths caused by low-voltage and low-amperage electric currents, *Zacchia* **24**:359–368 (Italian).
Ferris, L. P., King, B. G., Spence, P. W., and Williams, H. B., 1936, Effect of electric shock on the heart, *Electr. Eng.* **55**:498–515.
Franco, S. C., 1969, Electric shock and cardiopulmonary resuscitation, *Arch. Environ. Health* **19**:261–264.
Fraunfelder, F. T., and Hanna, C., 1972, Electric cataracts, *Arch. Ophthal.* **87**(2):179–191 and **91**(6):469–473.
Hayworth, B., and Warrilow, D., 1978, Constant power changing supplies, *Electro-optical Syst. Des.* **10**(3):42–45 (March 1978).
Keesey, J. C., and Letcher, F. S., 1970, Human thresholds of electric shock at power transmission frequencies, *Arch. Environ. Health* **21**:547–551.
Kouwenhoven, W. B., Chestnut, R. W., Knickerbocker, G. G., Milnor, W. R., and Sass, D. J., 1959, AC shocks of varying parameters affecting the heart, *AIEE Trans. (Communications in electronics)* **78**:42, 163–169.
Kouwenhoven, W. B., 1956, Effect of capacitor discharges on the heart, *AIEE Trans. of Power Apparatus and Systems* **75**: (23 Part 3):12–15.
Kouwenhoven, W. B., Judd, J. R., and Knickerbocker, G. G., 1960, Closed chest cardiac massage, *J. Amer. Med. Assn.* **173**:1064–1067.
Lee, R. H., 1971, Electrical safety in industrial plants, *IEEE Trans. on Industry and General Applications IGA-7* **1**:10–16.
Levy, L. S., 1971, Physiological changes during electrical asphyxiation, *Brit. J. Industr. Med.* **28**:164–171.
Marriott, H. L., 1951, Lightning effects, "Medical Treatment–Principles and Their Application," (G. Evans, ed.) p. 300, Butterworth, London.
Mills, W., Switzer, W. E., and Moncrief, J. A., 1966, Electrical injuries, *J. Amer. Med. Assn.* **195**(10):852–854.
Milnor, W. R., Knickerbocker, G. G., and Kouwenhoven, W. B., 1958, Cardiac responses to transthoracic capacitor discharges in the dog, *Circulation Res.* **6**(1):60–65.
Morley, R., and Carter, A. O., 1972, First aid treatment of electric shock, *Arch. Environ. Health* **25**(4):276–285.
Murray, R., 1963, Hazards to health-electric shock, *New Engl. J. Med.* **268**(20):1127–1128.
NEPA, (updated), National Electrical Code, NFPA No. 70 (ANSI C1), National Fire Protection Association International, Boston.
Poehler, H. A., 1944, Effects of electric shock, *Electronics* **12**(7):140–142, 250–254.
Ravitch, M. M., Lane, R., Safar, P., Steichen, F. M., and Knowles, P., 1961, Lightning stroke, report of a case with recovery after cardiac massage and prolonged artificial respiration, *New Eng. J. Med.* **265**:36–38.
Taussig, H. G., 1969, Death from lightening and possibility of living again, *Amer. Sci.* **57**(3):306–316.
Thompson, G., 1933, Shock threshold fixes appliance insulation resistance, *Electr. World* **101**(24):793–795.

Underwriters Laboratories (UL), 1968, "Office Appliances and Business Equipment," UL467, and "Radio and Television Receiving Appliances," UL492, *Standards for Safety,* Underwriters Laboratories, Chicago.

U.S. Atomic Energy Commission, 1967, "Electrical Safety Guides for Research," Safety and Fire Protection Technical Bulletin No. 13, Division of Operational Safety, USAEC, Washington, DC (December 1967).

U.S. Department of the Air Force and the Army, 1975, "Prevention of Electrical Shock Hazards in Hospitals," AF Reg 160-3, TB Med 286, U.S. Department of the Air Force, Washington, DC (February 10, 1975).

U.S. Department of Defense, 1970, "Standard General Requirements for Electronic Equipment, MIL-STD-454 C, U.S. Department of Defence, Washington, DC (October 15, 1970).

VDE, 1977, "VDE Specification for the Electrical Safety of Laser Equipment and Installations," VDE 0836/2.77, DIN57836, VDE, Frankfurt (February 1977), in German.

Appendix A
Terms and Units of Measure - The International System of Units (SI)

The International System of Units, abbreviated SI, as defined in International Standard ISO 1000, is described in this appendix. International Standard ISO 1000 was approved by International Organization of Standards (ISO) Member Bodies from 30 countries including the United States.

The SI consists of the following:
1. Seven base units
2. All the derived units
3. Two supplementary units
4. The series of approved prefixes for multiples and submultiples of units.

The units which apply to optical safety, their definitions, their symbols, and the formation of multiple and submultiple units are presented in this appendix. Information related to style, use, and format is also provided.

A.1 THE THREE CLASSES OF UNITS IN THE SI

The units of the International System of Units are divided into three classes:
1. Base units
2. Derived units
3. Supplementary units.

Scientifically and technically this classification is partially arbitrary. The 10th General Conference of Weights and Measures (1954) adopted as base units of the SI the units of the quantities: length, mass, time, electric current, thermodynamic temperature, amount of substance, and luminous intensity which by convention are regarded as dimensionally independent. Associated with these quantities are seven well-defined units. This action was taken in the interest of achieving the advantages of having a single, practical, internationally accepted system for trade, education, science, and technology.

The derived units are the units of quantities that can be formed by combining base quantities and other derived quantities according to the rules of algebra. The units of these derived quantities are such that no numerical factors (factors of proportionality) are introduced into the fundamental equations defining these quantities. Thus the SI—composed of seven base units, a growing number of derived

TABLE A-1. SI Base and Supplementary Units

Quantity	Name	Symbol
SI base units:		
length	meter	m
mass*	kilogram	kg
time	second	s
electric current	ampere	A
thermodynamic temperature	kelvin	K
amount of substance	mole	mol
luminous intensity	candela	cd
SI supplementary units:		
plane angle	radian	rad
solid angle	steradian	sr

* "Weight" is the commonly used term for "mass."

units, and the supplementary units forms a coherent system of units. A coherent system of units is one in which all derived units can be expressed as products of ratios of the base units (and, in the SI, the supplementary units) without the introduction of numerical factors. Examples of derived quantities are speed, energy, and irradiance.

Two other units were adopted by the 11th General Conference of Weights and Measures (1960) as supplementary units primarily because it was not agreed that the two units were either base units or derived units. The quantities involved are plane angle and solid angle, and they may be regarded as base units or as derived units.

A.2 BASE UNITS OF THE SI

The SI is constructed from seven base units for independent quantities plus two supplementary units for plane angle and solid angle, listed in A-1.

Units for all other quantities are derived from these nine units. In Table A-2 are listed many SI derived units with special names which were derived from the base and supplementary units in a coherent manner, which means, in brief, that they are expressed as products and ratios of the nine base and supplementary units without numerical factors.

A.3 SUPPLEMENTARY UNITS

At present, there are only two units, both purely geometrical, in the SI which are classified as supplementary. They are presented before derived units because they may be used in derived units. Thus, for practical purposes these supplementary units

TABLE A-2. SI Derived Units with Special Names

Quantity	SI Unit Name	SI Unit Symbol	Expression in terms of other units
Area	square meter	m^2	m^2
Volume	cubic meter	m^3	m^3
Frequency	hertz	Hz	s^{-1}
Force	newton	N	$kg \cdot m/s^2$
Pressure, stress	pascal	Pa	N/m^2
Energy, work, quantity of heat	joule	J	$N \cdot m$
Power, radiant flux	watt	W	J/s
Quantity of electricity, electric charge	coulomb	C	$A \cdot s$
Electric potential, potential difference, electromotive force	volt	V	W/A
Capacitance	farad	F	C/V
Electric resistance	ohm	Ω	V/A
Conductance	siemens	S	A/V
Magnetic flux	weber	Wb	$V \cdot s$
Magnetic flux density	tesla	T	Wb/m^2
Inductance	henry	H	Wb/A
Luminous flux	lumen	lm	$cd \cdot sr$
Illuminance	lux	lx	lm/m^2
Celsius† temperature	degree Celsius	°C	K
Activity (of a radionuclide)†	becquerel	Bq	s^{-1}
Absorbed dose, specific energy imparted, kerma, absorbed dose index†	gray	Gy	J/kg
Wave number	1 per meter	$1/m$	$1/m$
Density, mass density	kilogram per cubic meter	kg/m^3	kg/m^3
Luminance	candela per square meter	cd/m^2	cd/m^2
Optical flux density, irradiance	watt per square meter	W/m^2	W/m^2
Energy density	joule per cubic meter	J/m^3	J/m^3
Radiant intensity	watt per steradian	W/sr	W/sr
Radiance	watt per square meter steradian	$W/(m^2 \cdot sr)$	$W/(m^2 \cdot sr)$

† In addition to the thermodynamic temperature (symbol T), expressed in kelvins (see Table A-1), use is also made of Celsius temperature (symbol t) defined by the equation:

$$t = T - T_e$$

where T_e 273.15 K by definition. The unit "degree Celsius" is equal to the unit "kelvin," but "degree Celsius" is a special name in place of "kelvin" for expressing Celsius temperature. A temperature interval or a Celsius temperature difference can be expressed in degrees, Celsius as well as in kelvins.

TABLE A-3. SI Units Used with the SI

Quantity	Name	Symbol	Expression in terms of other units	Expression In terms of SI units
Time	minute	min		60 s
Time	hour	h	60 min	3 600 s
Time	day	d	24 h	86 400 s
Plane angle	degree	°		$(\pi/180)$ rad
Plane angle	minute	′	$(1/60)°$	$(\pi/10\,800)$ rad
Plane angle	second	″	$(1/60)′$	$(\pi/648\,000)$ rad

The radian and steradian are defined in International Standard ISO 1000 as follows:
1. *radian.* The radian is the plane angle between two radii of a circle which cut off on the circumference an arc equal in length to the radius.
2. *steradian.* The steradian is the solid angle which, having its vertex in the center of a sphere, cuts off an area of the surface of the sphere equal to that of a square with sides of length equal to the radius of the sphere.

The use of degree (symbol°) and its decimal submultiples is permissible when use of the radian is not convenient. Solid angle always should be expressed in steradians.

TABLE A-4. SI Prefixes

Multiplication Factors	Prefix	SI Symbol
1 000 000 000 000 000 000 = 10^{18}	exa	E
1 000 000 000 000 000 = 10^{15}	peta	P
1 000 000 000 000 = 10^{12}	tera	T
1 000 000 000 = 10^{9}	giga	G
1 000 000 = 10^{6}	mega	M
1 000 = 10^{3}	kilo	k
100 = 10^{2}	hecto*	h
10 = 10^{1}	deka*	da
0.1 = 10^{-1}	deci*	d
0.01 = 10^{-2}	centi*	c
0.001 = 10^{-3}	milli	m
0.000 001 = 10^{-6}	micro	μ
0.000 000 001 = 10^{-9}	nano	n
0.000 000 000 001 = 10^{-12}	pico	p
0.000 000 000 000 001 = 10^{-15}	femto	f
0.000 000 000 000 000 001 = 10^{-18}	atto	a

* To be avoided where possible.

Table A-5. CIE Radiometric and Photometric Terms in Four Languages.

Symbol	English	French	German	Russian
Q_e	Radiant energy	énergie rayonnante	Strahlungsmenge	энергия излучения
Φ_e, P_e	Radiant Flux, or Radiant power	flux énergétique	Strahlungsfluss	поток излучения
E_e	Irradiance	éclairement énergétique	Bestrahlungsstärke	энергетическая освещенность
H_e	Radiant Exposure	exposition énergétique	Bestrahlung	энергетическая экспозиция
L_e	Radiance	luminance énergétique	Strahldichte	энергетическая яркость
I_e	Radiant Intensity	intensité énergétique	Strahlstärke	энергетическая сила света
Q_v	Quantity of Light	quantité de lumiere	Lichtmenge	световой поток
Φ_v, P_v	Luminous Flux	flux lumineux	Lichtstrom	световой энергия
E_v	Illuminance	éclairement lumineuse	Beleuchtungsstärke	освещенность
H_v	Light Exposure	exposition lumineuse	Belichtung	экспозиция
L_v	Luminance	luminance lumineuse	Leuchtdichte	яркость
I_v	Luminous Intensity	intensité lumineuse	Lichtstärke	сила света

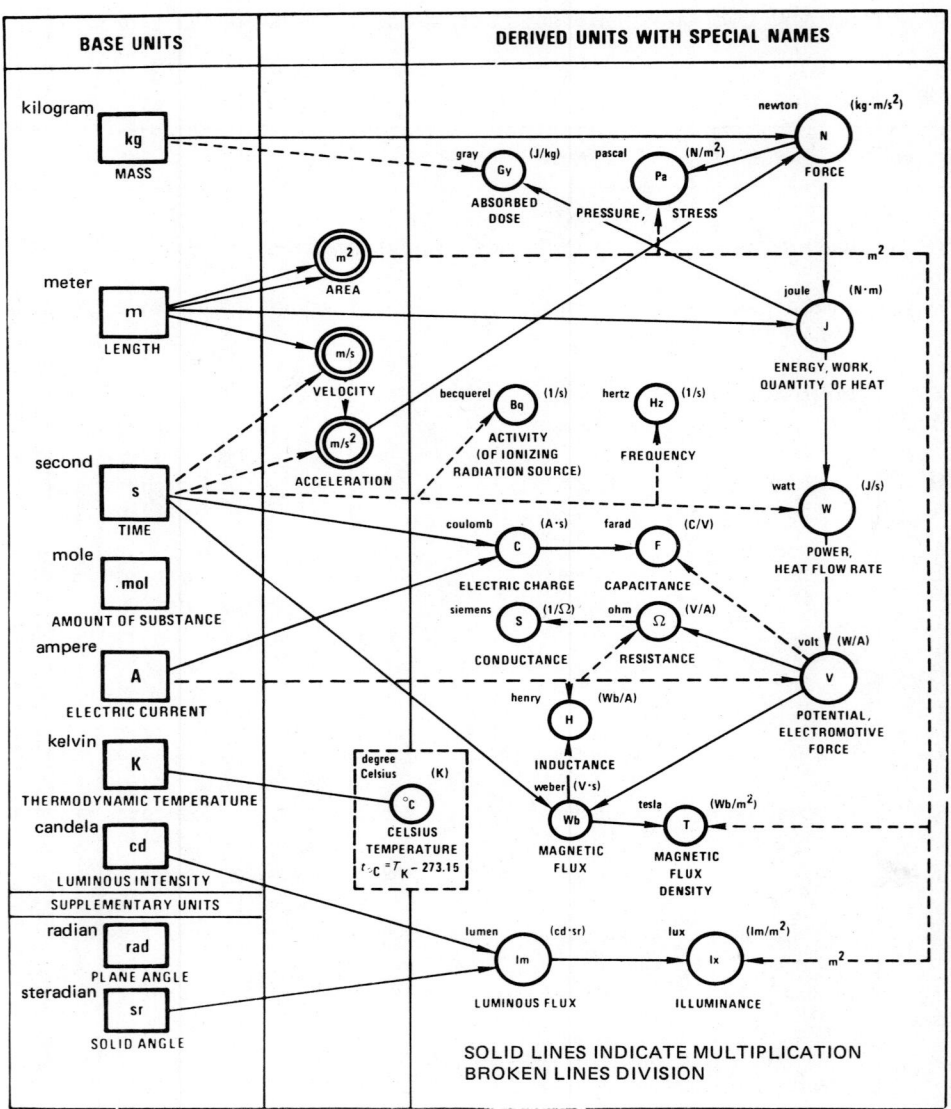

Figure A-1. Relationships of SI Units with Names. Diagram courtesy National Bureau of Standards.

A.4 CONVERSION FACTORS AND CONSTANTS

A.4.1 Useful Physical Constants

Acceleration due to gravity	g	$= 9.81$ m/s
Boltzmann constant	k	$= 1.381 \times 10^{-23}$ J/K
Charge of an electron	e	$= 1.602 \times 10^{-19}$ A·s
Impedance of free space	Z_0	$= \sqrt{\mu_0/\epsilon_0} = 376.7$ Ω
Maximum spectral luminous efficacy	K_m	$= 683$ lm/W
Permeability of free space	μ_0	$= 1.257 \times 10^{-6}$ V·s/A·m
Permittivity of free space	ϵ_0	$= 8.854 \times 10^{-12}$ A·s(V·m)
Planck constant	h	$= 6.626 \times 10^{-34}$ J·s
1st Radiation constant	c_1	$= 2\pi hc^2 = 3.741832 \times 10^{-16}$ W/m²
2nd Radiation constant	c_2	$= hc/k = 0.014388$ m·K
Stefan-Boltzmann constant	σ	$= 5.67032 \times 10^{-8}$ W·m²·K⁻⁴
Velocity of light in vacuum	c	$= 2.998 \times 10^8$ m/s

A.4.2 Useful Mathematical Constants

π	$= 3.14159$
π^2	$= 9.86960$
$\sqrt{\pi}$	$= 1.77245$
$1/\pi$	$= 0.31830$
$1/\sqrt{2\pi}$	$= 0.39894$
$1/2\pi$	$= 0.15915$
e	$= 2.71828$
e^2	$= 7.38905$
$\sqrt{e}$	$= 1.64872$
$1/e$	$= 0.36787$
$1/\sqrt{e}$	$= 0.60653$
$\log_e 10$	$= 2.30258$
$\log_{10} e$	$= 0.43429$

A.4.3 Useful Conversion Factors

Joule (J)	$= 10^7$ ergs $= 0.239$ cal
Electron volt (eV)	$= 1.602 \times 10^{-12}$ ergs $= 1.602 \times 10^{-19}$ J
Dyne	$= 1$ cm·g/s²
Erg	$= 1$ dyne cm
Watt (W)	$= 10^7$ erg/s¹
Newton (N)	$= 1$ mkg/s² $= 10^5$ dyne $= 1$ W·s/m
Calorie (cal)	$= 4.1868$ J
Torr	$= 133.32$ Pa
Pascal (Pa)	$= 0.0075$ torr

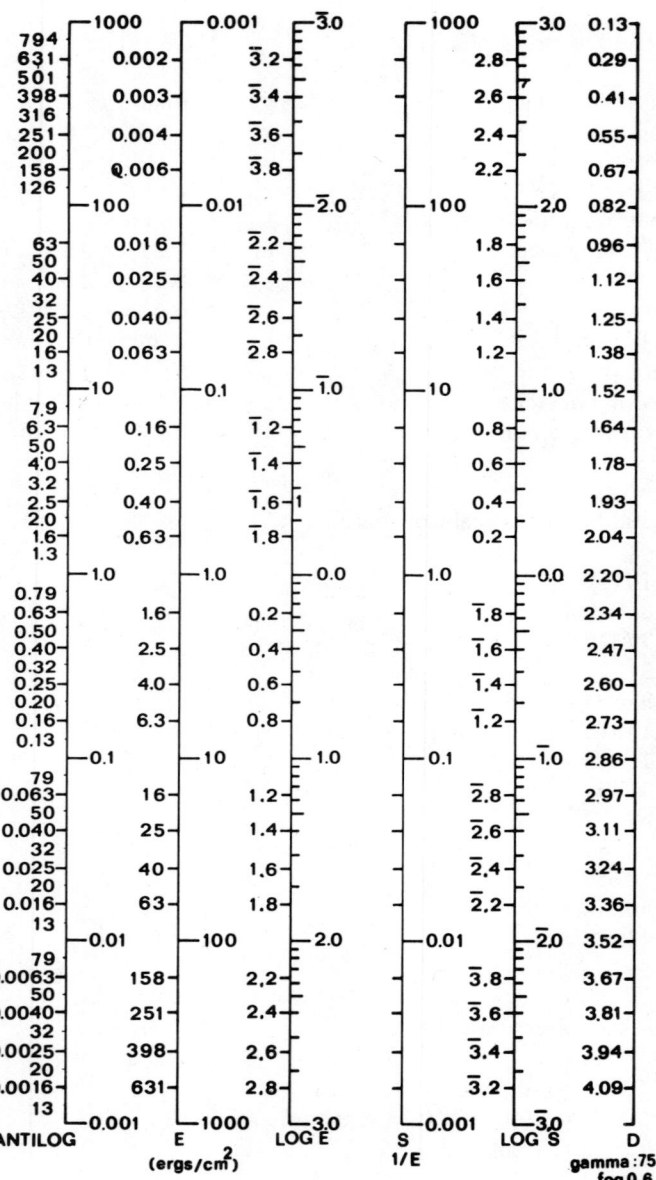

Figure A.2 Film Density versus Exposure Nomograph for Photographic Radiometry. A horizontal line links the exposure (E in ergs/cm^2) to the film sensitivity (S) and the actual density (D) of a film with a gamma of 0.75. This nomograph uses the USA convention for a sensitivity of 1 requiring an exposure of 1 erg/cm^2. This makes S equal to 1/E numerically. The left column (ANTILOG) is an expansion of the sensitivity (S).

TABLE A-6. Unitless Radiometric Definitions

UNITLESS RADIOMETRIC DEFINITIONS

Quantity	Symbol	Defining Equation	Unit
Absorptance •	a	$a = \dfrac{(*) \text{ absorbed}}{(*) \text{ incident}}$	(numeric)
Reflectance	ρ	$\rho = \dfrac{(*) \text{ reflected}}{(*) \text{ incident}}$	(numeric)
Transmittance	τ	$\tau = \dfrac{(*) \text{ transmitted}}{(*) \text{ incident}}$	(numeric)
Emissivity	ϵ	$\epsilon = \dfrac{(*) \text{ specimen}}{(*) \text{ blackbody at same temperature as specimen}}$	(numeric)

where (*) represents the appropriate quantity Q, Φ, M, E, I, or L.

• Radiant absorptance should not be confused with absorption coefficient.

TABLE A-7. Radiometric Conversion Factors

Radiant Exposure (exposure dose)

Multiply → To Obtain ↓ By ↘	erg/cm²	joule/cm²	W sec/cm²	µW sec/cm²
erg/cm²	1	10^{-7}	10^{-7}	0.1
joule/cm²	10^7	1	1	10^6
W sec/cm²	10^7	1	1	10^6
µW sec/cm²	10	10^{-6}	10^{-6}	1

Irradiance (exposure dose rate)

Multiply → To Obtain ↓ By ↘	erg/cm² · sec	joule/cm² · sec	W/cm²	µW/cm²
erg/cm² · sec	1	10^{-7}	10^{-7}	0.1
joule/cm² · sec	10^7	1	1	10^6
W/cm²	10^7	1	1	10^6
µW/cm²	10	10^{-6}	10^{-6}	1

TABLE A-8. Luminance Conversion Factors

Multiply Luminance in → To Obtain Luminance By in ↓	Footlambert	Nit	Millilambert	Candela/in^2
Footlambert (ftL)	1	0.2919	0.929	452
Nit (cd/m^2)	3.426	1	3.183	1,550
Millilambert (mL)	1.076	0.3142	1	487
Candela/in^2	0.00221	0.000645	0.00205	1
Candela/ft^2	0.3183	0.0929	0.2957	144
Stilb (cd/cm^2)	0.00034	0.0001	0.00032	0.155
Lambert	0.000108	0.000314	0.001	0.487

Multiply Luminance in → To Obtain Luminance By in ↓	Candela/ft^2	Stilb	Lambert	Apostilb (Blondel)
Footlambert (ftL)	3.142	2,919	929	0.0929
Nit (cd/m^2)	10.76	10,000	3,183	0.318
Millilambert (mL)	3.382	3,142	1,000	0.1
Candela/in^2	0.00694	6.45	2.05	0.0002
Candela/ft^2	1	929	295.7	0.0296
Stilb (cd/cm^2)	0.00108	1	0.318	0.000032
Lambert	0.00338	3.442	1	0.0001

TABLE A-9. Illumination Conversion Factors

Multiply Number of → To Obtain Number of ↓ By	Footcandles (ftcd)	Lux (lx)	Phot (lm/cm^2)	Milliphot (mlm/cm^2)
Footcandles (ftcd)	1	0.0929	929	0.929
Lux (lx)	10.76	1	10,000	10
Phot (lm/cm^2)	0.00108	0.0001	1	0.001
Milliphot (mlm/cm^2)	1.076	0.1	1,000	1

TABLE A-10. Energy of a Quantum of Optical Radiation

λ	Energy of quantum		
µm	erg	J	eV
0.2	$9.35 \cdot 10^{-12}$	$9.35 \cdot 10^{-19}$	$5.85 \cdot 10^0$
0.3	$6.23 \cdot 10^{-12}$	$6.23 \cdot 10^{-19}$	$3.90 \cdot 10^0$
0.4	$4.69 \cdot 10^{-12}$	$4.69 \cdot 10^{-19}$	$2.92 \cdot 10^0$
0.5	$3.74 \cdot 10^{-12}$	$3.74 \cdot 10^{-19}$	$2.34 \cdot 10^0$
0.6	$3.12 \cdot 10^{-12}$	$3.12 \cdot 10^{-19}$	$1.95 \cdot 10^0$
0.7	$2.67 \cdot 10^{-12}$	$2.67 \cdot 10^{-19}$	$1.67 \cdot 10^0$
0.8	$2.34 \cdot 10^{-12}$	$2.34 \cdot 10^{-19}$	$1.46 \cdot 10^0$
0.9	$2.08 \cdot 10^{-12}$	$2.08 \cdot 10^{-19}$	$1.30 \cdot 10^0$
1	$1.87 \cdot 10^{-12}$	$1.87 \cdot 10^{-19}$	$1.17 \cdot 10^0$
2	$9.35 \cdot 10^{-13}$	$9.35 \cdot 10^{-20}$	$5.85 \cdot 10^{-1}$
3	$6.23 \cdot 10^{-13}$	$6.23 \cdot 10^{-20}$	$3.90 \cdot 10^{-1}$
4	$4.69 \cdot 10^{-13}$	$4.69 \cdot 10^{-20}$	$2.92 \cdot 10^{-1}$
5	$3.74 \cdot 10^{-13}$	$3.74 \cdot 10^{-20}$	$2.34 \cdot 10^{-1}$
6	$3.12 \cdot 10^{-13}$	$3.12 \cdot 10^{-20}$	$1.95 \cdot 10^{-1}$
7	$2.67 \cdot 10^{-13}$	$2.67 \cdot 10^{-20}$	$1.67 \cdot 10^{-1}$
8	$2.34 \cdot 10^{-13}$	$2.34 \cdot 10^{-20}$	$1.46 \cdot 10^{-1}$
9	$2.08 \cdot 10^{-13}$	$2.08 \cdot 10^{-20}$	$1.30 \cdot 10^{-1}$
10	$1.87 \cdot 10^{-13}$	$1.87 \cdot 10^{-20}$	$1.17 \cdot 10^{-1}$
11	$1.70 \cdot 10^{-13}$	$1.70 \cdot 10^{-20}$	$1.06 \cdot 10^{-1}$
12	$1.56 \cdot 10^{-13}$	$1.56 \cdot 10^{-20}$	$9.85 \cdot 10^{-2}$
13	$1.44 \cdot 10^{-13}$	$1.44 \cdot 10^{-20}$	$9.00 \cdot 10^{-2}$
14	$1.33 \cdot 10^{-13}$	$1.33 \cdot 10^{-20}$	$8.35 \cdot 10^{-2}$

Note. $1 \text{ eV} = 1.59 \cdot 10^{-12} \text{ erg} = 1.59 \cdot 10^{-19} \text{ J}; \quad 1 \text{ J} = 6.29 \cdot 10^{20} \text{ eV}.$

TABLE A-11. Conversion Factors for Units of Length*

Multiply Number of → To Obtain Number of ↓ By ↘	Nano-meters (nm)	Micro-meters (μm)	Milli-meters (mm)	Centi-meters (cm)	Meters (m)	Kilo-meters (km)	Inches (in)	Feet (ft)
Nanometers (nm)	1	10^3	10^6	10^7	10^9	10^{12}	2.540×10^7	3.048×10^8
Micrometers (μm)	10^{-3}	1	10^3	10^4	10^6	10^9	2.540×10^4	3.048×10^5
Millimeters (mm)	10^{-6}	10^{-3}	1	10	10^3	10^6	2.540×10	3.048×10^2
Centimeters (cm)	10^{-7}	10^{-4}	10^{-1}	1	10^2	10^5	2.540	3.048×10
Meters (m)	10^{-9}	10^{-6}	10^{-3}	10^{-2}	1	10^3	2.540×10^{-2}	3.048×10^{-1}
Kilometers (km)	10^{-12}	10^{-9}	10^{-6}	10^{-5}	10^{-3}	1	3.048×10^{-5}	3.048×10^{-4}
Inches (in)	3.937×10^{-8}	3.937×10^{-5}	3.937×10^{-2}	3.937×10^{-1}	3.937×10	3.937×10^4	1	12
Feet (ft)	3.281×10^{-9}	3.281×10^{-6}	3.281×10^{-3}	3.281×10^{-2}	3.281	3.281×10^3	8.333×10^{-2}	1

*Obsolete Units of Length: 1 Angstrom (Å) = 0.1 nm
1 millimicron (mμ) = 1 nm
1 micron (μ) = 1 μm

To form a multiple of, for example, the metre, such that a unit 1000 times larger than the metre is formed, the prefix kilo is added forming kilometre (symbol km). The unit kilometre is 10^3 or 1000 times as large as the metre. The unit which is *smaller* than the second by a factor of 10^9 is the nanosecond (symbol ns), i.e., the nanosecond = 10^9 second.

REFERENCES

1. NBS 330, *The International System of Units (SI)*, Dept. of Commerce, National Bureau of Standards, April 1972.
2. International Organization for Standardization, *SI Units and Recommendations for the Use of Their Multiples and Certain Other Units*, International Standard ISO 1000, ISO, Switzerland, 1973.
3. American National Standards Institute, *Measuring Systems and Standards Organizations*, ANSI, NY n.d.
4. A. G. Chertove, *Units of Measurement of Physical Quantities*, translated by Scripta Technica, Inc., revised by Herbert J. Eagle, Hayden Book Company, Inc., NY, 1964.

5. American National Standards Institute, American Society for Testing and Materials, *Standards for Metric Practice*, ASTM E 380, ANSI NY, January 1976.
6. National Aeronautics and Space Administration, *The International System of Units: Physical Constants and Conversion Factors*, by E. A. Mechtly, rev. ed., NASA Office of Technology Utilization, Scientific and Technical Information Division, Washington, DC, 1969.
7. Commission International de l'Eclairage (International Commission on Illumination), 1970, International Lighting Vocabulary, Publication CIE No. 17 (E-1.1) Paris.

A.4.4 Speed

$$1 \text{ knot} = 1 \text{ nautical mile/hr}$$
$$1 \text{ mile/min} = 88 \text{ ft/sec} = 60 \text{ miles/hr}$$

A.4.5 Temperature Conversion Formulas

$$T_C = T_K - 273.16 = \frac{5}{9}(T_F - 32)$$
$$T_K = T_C + 273.16 = \frac{5}{9}(T_F + 459.69)$$
$$T_F = \frac{9}{5}T_C + 32 = \frac{9}{5}T_K - 459.69$$

A.4.6 Optical Units

$$\begin{aligned}
\text{Wave number} \quad & \eta(1/\text{cm}) \approx 10^4/\lambda(\mu m) \\
\text{Frequency} \quad & \nu(\text{Hz}) \approx 3 \times 10^{14}/\lambda(\mu m) \\
\text{Photon Energy} \quad & \mathscr{E}(\text{J}) \approx 1.987 \times 10^{-19}/\lambda(\mu m) \\
\text{Photon Energy} \quad & \mathscr{E}(\text{eV}) \approx 1.24/\lambda(\mu m)
\end{aligned}$$

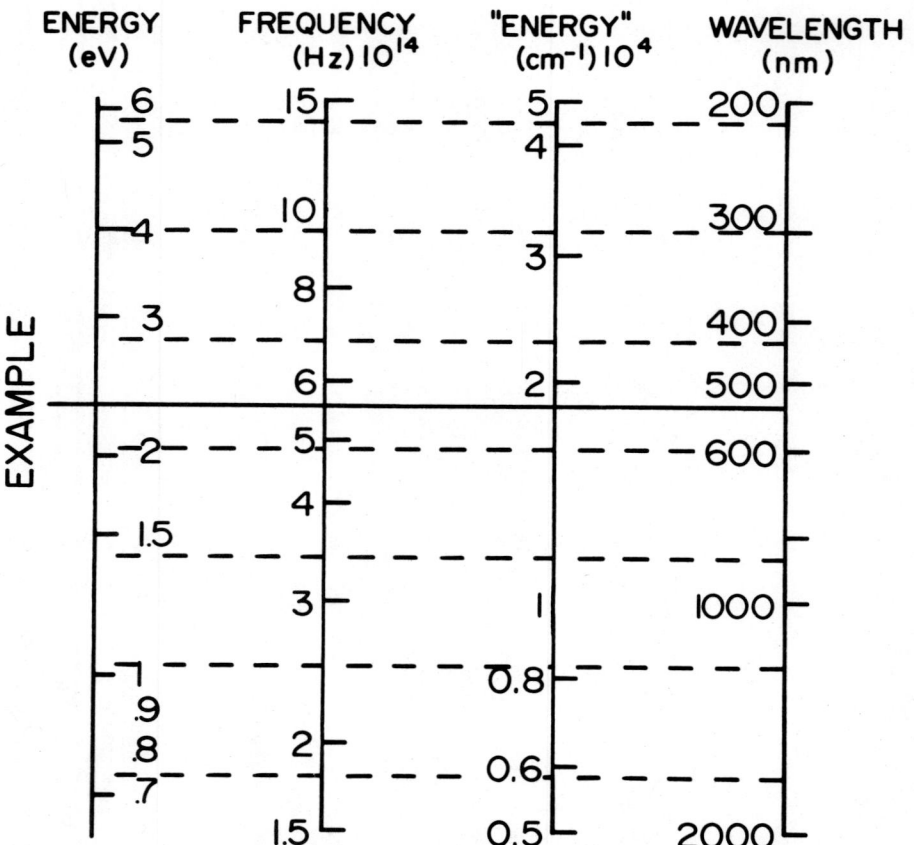

Figure A-3. Photon Energy Nomograph. Based on Photonetics Associates, Inc., Laser Focus, August, 1976.

TABLE A-12. Time

Multiply → To Obtain ↓ By ↘	yr	day	hr	min	SEC
1 year	1	365.2	8.766×10^3	5.259×10^5	3.156×10^7
1 day	2.738×10^{-3}	1	24	1440	8.640×10^4
1 hour	1.141×10^{-4}	4.167×10^{-2}	1	60	3600
1 minute	1.901×10^{-6}	6.944×10^{-4}	1.667×10^{-2}	1	60
1 SECOND	3.169×10^{-8}	1.157×10^{-5}	2.778×10^{-4}	1.667×10^{-2}	1

1 year = 365.24219879 days

TABLE A-13. Signs and Symbols
Greek Alphabet (Capital and Lower Case)

Capital	Lower Case	Greek Name
A	α	Alpha
B	β	Beta
Γ	γ	Gamma
Δ	δ	Delta
E	ϵ	Epsilon
Z	ζ	Zeta
H	η	Eta
Θ	θ	Theta
I	ι	Iota
K	κ	Kappa
Λ	λ	Lambda
M	μ	Mu
N	ν	Nu
Ξ	ξ	Xi
O	o	Omicron
Π	π	Pi
P	ρ	Rho
Σ	σ	Sigma
T	τ	Tau
Υ	υ	Upsilon
Φ	ϕ	Phi
X	χ	Chi
Ψ	ψ	Psi
Ω	ω	Omega

A.5 MATHEMATICAL SYMBOLS

a = Diameter of emergent laser beam (cm).

d_e = Diameter of the pupil of the eye (varies from approximately 0.2 to 0.7 cm).

D_{min} = Limiting object size of extended object (cm).

D_e = Diameter of the exit pupil of an optical system (cm).

D_L = Diameter of laser beam at range r (cm).

D_o = Diameter of objective of an optical system (cm).

e = Base of natural logarithms.

E, H = Radiant exposure (H) or irradiance (E) at range r, measured in $J \cdot cm^{-2}$ for pulsed laser and $W \cdot cm^{-2}$ for CW lasers.

E_o, H_o = Emergent beam radiant exposure (H_o) or irradiance (E_o) at zero range (units as for E, H).

f = Effective focal length of eye (1.7 cm).

F = Pulse repetition frequency (PRF, s^{-1} or Hz).

G = Ratio of retinal irradiance or radiant exposure received by optically aided eye to that received by unaided eyes.

L = Radiance of an extended source $[W/(cm^2 \cdot sr)]$.

L_p = Integrated radiance of an extended source $[J/(cm^2 \cdot sr)]$.

P = Magnifying power of an optical system.

Q = Total radiant energy output of a pulsed laser, measured in J.

r = Range from the laser to the viewer or to a diffuse target (cm).

r_1 = Range from the laser target to the viewer (cm).

$r_{1\,max}$ = Maximum range from the laser target to the viewer where extended source threshold limit value applies (cm).

R = Radius of curvature of a specular surface (cm).

S = Scan rate of a scanning laser (number of scans across eye per second).

T = Total exposure duration (in seconds) of a train of pulses.

T_i = Integrated "on-time" of a train of pulses.

T_{max} = Classification duration, i.e., a maximum duration of daily exposure inherent in the design of the laser device or maximum permissible exposure duration.

t	=	Duration of single pulse(s).
a	=	Viewing angle subtended by an extended source (in radians).
a_{min}	=	Minimum angle subtended by a source for which extended sources Threshold Limit Value applies (radians).
μ	=	Atmospheric attenuation coefficient (cm^{-1}) at a particular wavelength.
ϕ	=	Emergent beam divergence measured in radians.
Φ	=	Total radiant power (or radiant flux) output of a CW laser, or average radiant power of a repetitively pulsed laser, measured in watts.
ρ_λ	=	Spectral reflectance of a diffuse object at wavelength λ.
τ	=	Transmittance of a filter.
θ_s	=	Maximum angular sweep of a scanning beam (rad).
θ_v	=	Viewing angle.

A.6 NOMENCLATURE FOR RADIATION DOSIMETRY

The flow of energy or particles from the source to another location is specified in photochemistry and photobiology as either particle streams (electrons, neutrons, photons, etc.), or wave trains (electromagnetic radiation). Several different dosimetric schemes have evolved for each of these different specifications. However, for simplicity, if for no other reason, a simple dosimetric nomenclature should be available which is compatible with these other schemes. At the 1974 International Congress of Radiation, a working group proposed a set of terms as given in Table A-14. It should be noted that only particles (or wave trains) perpendicular to the area a are described. Therefore, "flosan" is not equivalent to the conventional "dose" except when the radiation comes from a single direction. "Dose" is rather the 4π steradian integral of "steric particle flosan". An equivalent analysis holds for the energy units.

TABLE A-14. Proposed Radiation Quantities

Quantities → Distributed with respect to ↓	Radiant energy Q [J]	Number of particles N [dimensionless]
time [s]	energy flux $P = \dfrac{dQ}{dt}$	particle flux $A = \dfrac{dN}{dt}$
area* [m²]	energy fluence $\Psi = \dfrac{dQ}{da}$	particle fluence $\gamma = \dfrac{dN}{da}$
volume [m³]	volumic energy $u = \dfrac{dQ}{dt}$	volumic number of particles $n = \dfrac{dN}{dt}$
area and time* [m² · s]	energy flosan $\psi = \dfrac{d^2 Q}{da\,dt}$	particle flosan $\Gamma = \dfrac{d^2 N}{da\,dt}$
solid angle and time [sr · s]	steric energy flux $I = \dfrac{d^2 Q}{dt\,d\Omega}$	steric particle flux $\dfrac{d^2 N}{dt\,d\Omega}$
area* solid angle and time [m² · sr · s]	energy radiance $L = \dfrac{d^3 Q}{dt\,da\,d\Omega}$	particle radiance $\dfrac{d^3 N}{dt\,da\,d\Omega}$

*The area da in this table is always taken perpendicular to the direction of propagation of an elementary radiation beam.

Note: Bracketed symbols represent abbreviations of units (in the International System, or SI) which should be used to express the corresponding quantity or variable: [J], joules; [s], seconds; [m], meter; [sr], steradian. The *energy fluence* for example, would be expressed in joules per square meter [J · m⁻²]; the *particle flux* in reciprocal seconds [s⁻¹], etc.

Appendix B
The Human Eye

B.1 THE STANDARD EYE

The optical constants of a "standard" eye — originally proposed by Gullstrand are presented in Figure B-1. The figure was adapted from a similar drawing in the US Department of Defense's Military Standardization Handbook No. 141, "Optical Design," 1962. The "standard" eye concept is used principally by the designers of optical instruments, but some of the "constants" may occasionally be useful as representative values for ocular hazard evaluation.

B.2 SPECTRAL WEIGHTING PROGRAM FOR EYE HAZARD COMPUTATIONS

W. J. Marshall, D. H. Sliney, and others at the US Army Environmental Hygiene Agency have developed a computer program to calculate weighted sums of the spectral irradiance or spectral radiance of a lamp or other broad-band source. As explained in Chapters 10, 14 and 22, the hazard analysis of such an optical source requires the weighted sum of several spectroradiometric parameters to estimate total retinal irradiance and biologically-weighted corneal and skin irradiance. Since it is just as easy to calculate the weighted sums of ten or twenty functions as it would be to calculate the weighted sum against S_λ and B_λ, a variety of other functions are also calculated. These other functions relate to earlier hazard functions and to functions used in scotopic, photopic and color vision studies. The functions are:

S_λ -- Ultraviolet Irradiance According to ACGIH Action Spectra (1973)
U_λ - Ultraviolet Irradiance According to CIE Action Spectra (1932)
A_λ - Ultraviolet Irradiance According to ANSI Action Spectra (Z136.1)
T -- Transmission of the Ocular Media x E_λ (Data of Ham)
T · A -- Transmission of the Ocular Media x Absorption of Retina x E_λ
R_λ -- Reciprocal of ANSI MPE Weighting Factor used in ACGIH TLV
V_λ -- Photopic Spectral Luminous Efficiency
V_λ' -- Scotopic Spectral Luminous Efficiency
B_λ -- Blue Light Hazard Function

$\bar{X}_\lambda$ – Spectral Tristimulus value (red)
$\bar{Y}_\lambda$ – Spectral Tristimulus value (green)
$\bar{Z}_\lambda$ – Spectral Tristimulua value (blue)
P_{445} – Dartnall Nomogram Absorption Coefficient for Blue
P_{535} – Dartnall Nomogram Absorption Coefficient for Green
P_{575} – Dartnall Nomobram Absorption Coefficient for Red

These functions are listed in Table B-1. The primary functions of importance are S_λ, $T \cdot A$, $1/C_A$, V_λ and B_λ. The photopic response of the eye V_λ is of value to check the spectral irradiance measurements and to extrapolate any of the weighted sums to points in space where illuminance or luminance values were taken, but where spectroradiometric measurements were not taken. Computations of total irradiance and radiance are also made by the program.

Figure B-2 provides a representation of the sequence of data cards. Figures B-3, B-4 and B-5 show flow diagrams of the computer program to aid any reader in designing his own computer program to achieve similar computations. Finally, Figure B-6 shows a cover data sheet developed by W. J. Marshall which illustrates the type of information necessary to record in order to complete the hazard analysis.

TABLE B-1. Relations Between Distances or Areas on the Retina and External Angle or Solid Angle

External Angle or Solid Angle		Distance or Area on the Retina
1 radian	≡	16.683 mm
0.05994 radian	≡	1 mm
1 degree	≡	0.2912 mm
3.434 degrees	≡	1 mm
1 minute	≡	4.853 μm
0.2061 minute	≡	1 μm
1 steradian	≡	278.3 mm^2
0.003593 steradian	≡	1 mm^2
1 square degree	≡	0.08478 mm^2
11.80 square degrees	≡	1 mm^2
1 square minute	≡	23.55 μm^2
0.04246 square minute	≡	1 μm^2

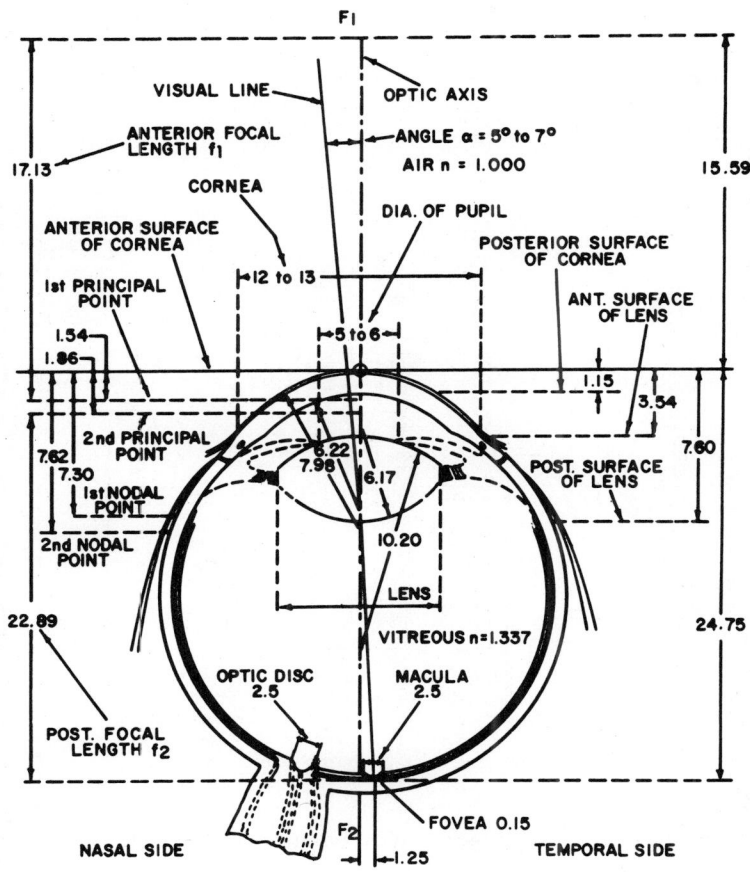

Figure B-1. Optical Constants For A "Standard Right Eye." Adapted from "Optical Design," MIL-HDBK-141, US Defense Department, 5 October 1962.

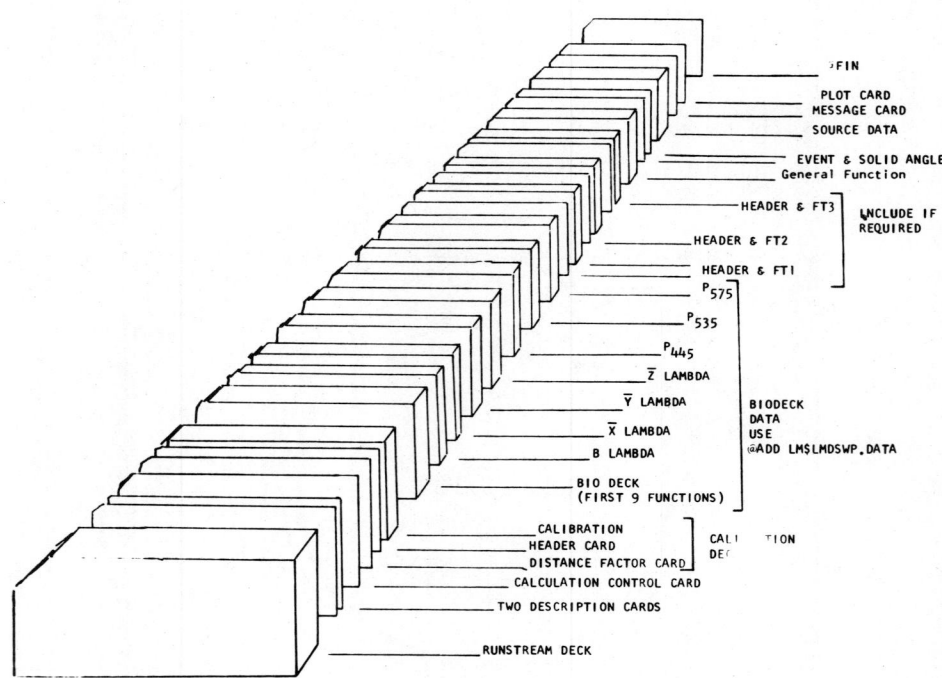

Figure B-2. Symbolic representation of spectral weighting program runstream.

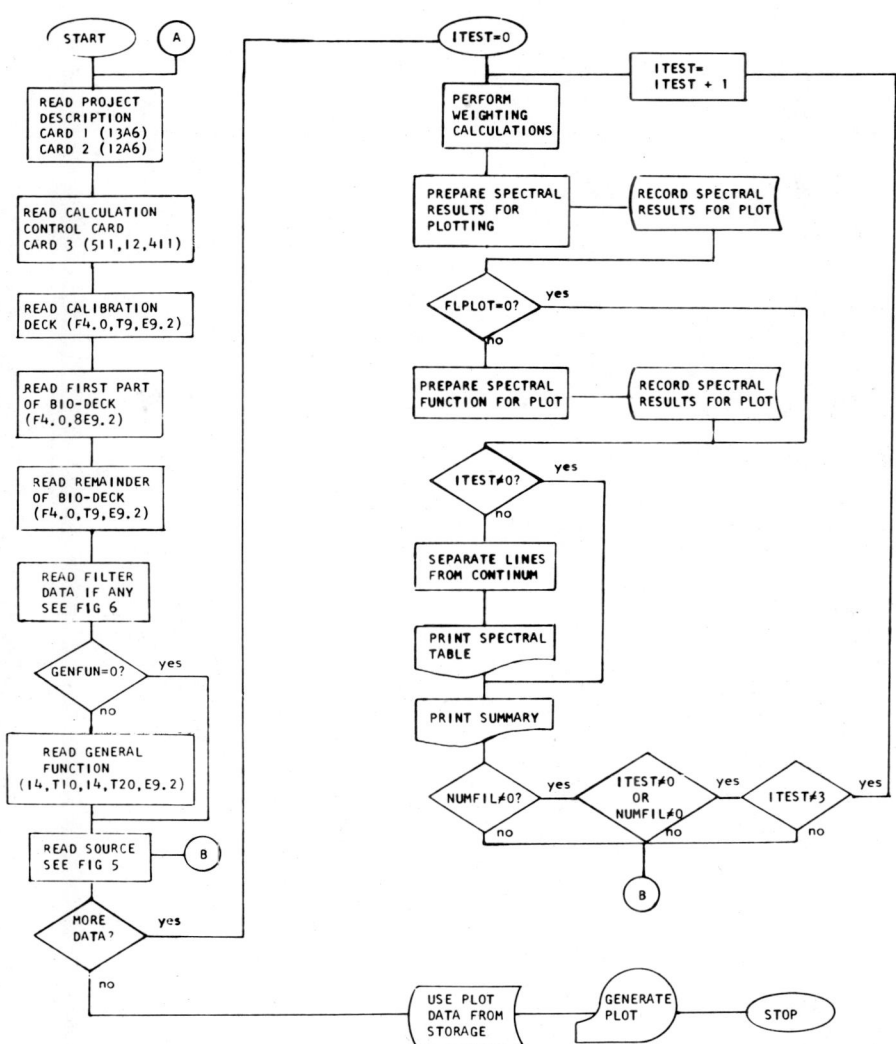

Figure B-3. General flowchart of SWP200 version of the spectral weighting program.

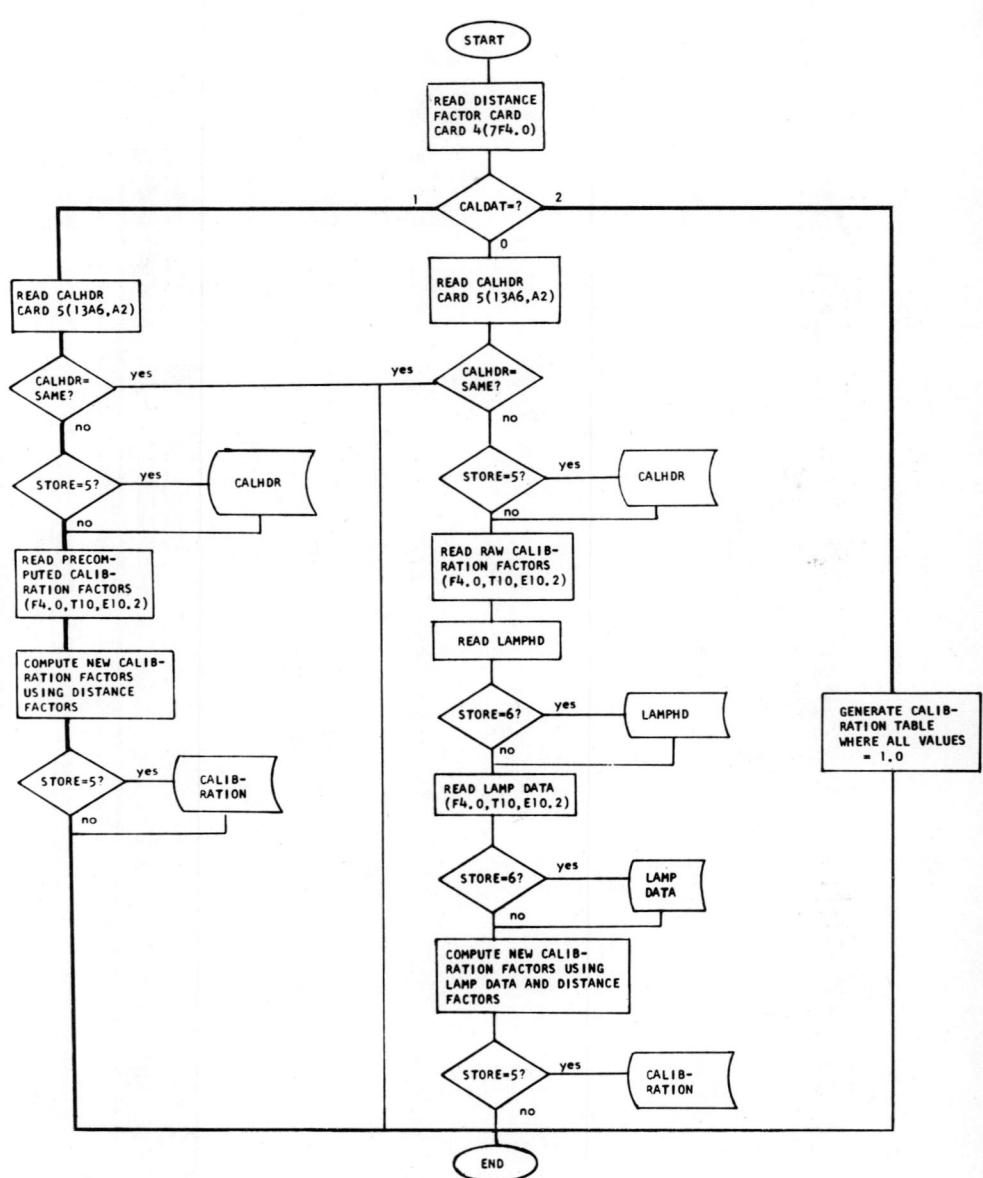

Figure B-4. Expanded flowchart for computing calibration factors.

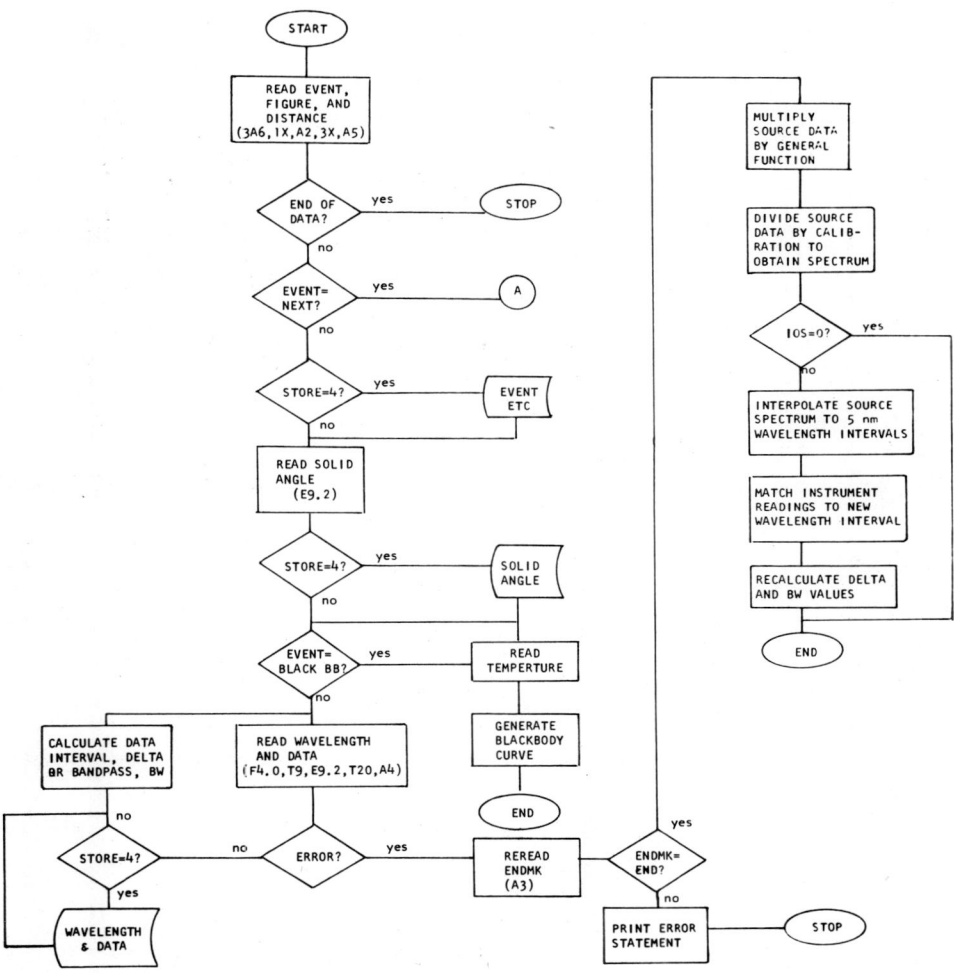

Figure B-5. Expanded flowchart for reading source data.

TABLE B-2 Spectral Weighting Functions for Eye Hazard Computations

λ nm	S_λ	U_λ	V_λ	V'_λ	T_λ	$T \cdot Ape_\lambda$	$1/C_A$	R_λ	λ nm	S_λ	U_λ	V_λ	V'_λ	T_λ	$T \cdot Ape_\lambda$	$1/C_A$	R_λ
200	3.0-02	0.0	0.0	0.0	0.0	0.0	0.0	1.0	266	8.6-01	2.3-01	0.0	0.0	0.0	0.0	0.0	1.0
201	3.3-02	0.0	0.0	0.0	0.0	0.0	0.0	1.0	267	8.8-01	2.1-01	0.0	0.0	0.0	0.0	0.0	1.0
202	4.0-02	0.0	0.0	0.0	0.0	0.0	0.0	1.0	268	9.4-01	1.8-01	0.0	0.0	0.0	0.0	0.0	1.0
203	4.4-02	0.0	0.0	0.0	0.0	0.0	0.0	1.0	269	9.7-01	1.6-01	0.0	0.0	0.0	0.0	0.0	1.0
204	5.0-02	0.0	0.0	0.0	0.0	0.0	0.0	1.0	270	1.0	1.4-01	0.0	0.0	0.0	0.0	0.0	1.0
205	5.3-02	0.0	0.0	0.0	0.0	0.0	0.0	1.0	271	1.0	1.3-01	0.0	0.0	0.0	0.0	0.0	1.0
206	5.9-02	0.0	0.0	0.0	0.0	0.0	0.0	1.0	272	1.0	1.1-01	0.0	0.0	0.0	0.0	0.0	1.0
207	6.3-02	0.0	0.0	0.0	0.0	0.0	0.0	1.0	273	9.7-01	1.0-01	0.0	0.0	0.0	0.0	0.0	1.0
208	6.8-02	0.0	0.0	0.0	0.0	0.0	0.0	1.0	274	9.7-01	9.0-02	0.0	0.0	0.0	0.0	0.0	1.0
209	7.1-02	0.0	0.0	0.0	0.0	0.0	0.0	1.0	275	9.5-01	7.4-02	0.0	0.0	0.0	0.0	0.0	1.0
210	7.5-02	0.0	0.0	0.0	0.0	0.0	0.0	1.0	276	9.4-01	6.8-02	0.0	0.0	0.0	0.0	0.0	1.0
211	8.1-02	0.0	0.0	0.0	0.0	0.0	0.0	1.0	277	9.2-01	6.4-02	0.0	0.0	0.0	0.0	0.0	1.0
212	8.6-02	0.0	0.0	0.0	0.0	0.0	0.0	1.0	278	9.1-01	6.2-02	0.0	0.0	0.0	0.0	0.0	1.0
213	9.0-02	0.0	0.0	0.0	0.0	0.0	0.0	1.0	279	9.1-01	6.1-02	0.0	0.0	0.0	0.0	0.0	1.0
214	9.2-02	0.0	0.0	0.0	0.0	0.0	0.0	1.0	280	9.0-01	6.0-02	0.0	0.0	0.0	0.0	0.0	1.0
215	9.7-02	0.0	0.0	0.0	0.0	0.0	0.0	1.0	281	8.8-01	6.1-02	0.0	0.0	0.0	0.0	0.0	1.0
216	1.0-01	0.0	0.0	0.0	0.0	0.0	0.0	1.0	282	8.6-01	6.2-02	0.0	0.0	0.0	0.0	0.0	1.0
217	1.1-01	0.0	0.0	0.0	0.0	0.0	0.0	1.0	283	8.4-01	6.6-02	0.0	0.0	0.0	0.0	0.0	1.0
218	1.1-01	0.0	0.0	0.0	0.0	0.0	0.0	1.0	284	8.2-01	7.6-02	0.0	0.0	0.0	0.0	0.0	1.0
219	1.1-01	0.0	0.0	0.0	0.0	0.0	0.0	1.0	285	8.1-01	9.0-02	0.0	0.0	0.0	0.0	0.0	1.0
220	1.2-01	0.0	0.0	0.0	0.0	0.0	0.0	1.0	286	7.8-01	1.1-01	0.0	0.0	0.0	0.0	0.0	1.0
221	1.2-01	0.0	0.0	0.0	0.0	0.0	0.0	1.0	287	7.5-01	1.3-01	0.0	0.0	0.0	0.0	0.0	1.0
222	1.3-01	0.0	0.0	0.0	0.0	0.0	0.0	1.0	288	7.1-01	1.7-01	0.0	0.0	0.0	0.0	0.0	1.0
223	1.4-01	0.0	0.0	0.0	0.0	0.0	0.0	1.0	289	7.0-01	2.2-01	0.0	0.0	0.0	0.0	0.0	1.0
224	1.4-01	0.0	0.0	0.0	0.0	0.0	0.0	1.0	290	6.5-01	3.1-01	0.0	0.0	0.0	0.0	0.0	1.0
225	1.5-01	0.0	0.0	0.0	0.0	0.0	0.0	1.0	291	6.3-01	4.6-01	0.0	0.0	0.0	0.0	0.0	1.0
226	1.5-01	0.0	0.0	0.0	0.0	0.0	0.0	1.0	292	5.9-01	6.4-01	0.0	0.0	0.0	0.0	0.0	1.0
227	1.6-01	0.0	0.0	0.0	0.0	0.0	0.0	1.0	293	5.7-01	8.0-01	0.0	0.0	0.0	0.0	0.0	1.0
228	1.7-01	0.0	0.0	0.0	0.0	0.0	0.0	1.0	294	5.4-01	9.2-01	0.0	0.0	0.0	0.0	0.0	1.0
229	1.7-01	0.0	0.0	0.0	0.0	0.0	0.0	1.0	295	5.0-01	9.8-01	0.0	0.0	0.0	0.0	0.0	1.0
230	1.8-01	0.0	0.0	0.0	0.0	0.0	0.0	1.0	296	4.7-01	9.9-01	0.0	0.0	0.0	0.0	0.0	1.0
231	1.9-01	0.0	0.0	0.0	0.0	0.0	0.0	1.0	297	4.3-01	1.0	0.0	0.0	0.0	0.0	0.0	1.0
232	2.0-01	0.0	0.0	0.0	0.0	0.0	0.0	1.0	298	3.8-01	9.8-01	0.0	0.0	0.0	0.0	0.0	1.0
233	2.1-01	0.0	0.0	0.0	0.0	0.0	0.0	1.0	299	3.3-01	9.0-01	0.0	0.0	0.0	0.0	0.0	1.0
234	2.1-01	0.0	0.0	0.0	0.0	0.0	0.0	1.0	300	3.0-01	8.3-01	0.0	0.0	0.0	0.0	0.0	1.0
235	2.2-01	0.0	0.0	0.0	0.0	0.0	0.0	1.0	301	2.7-01	7.2-01	0.0	0.0	0.0	0.0	0.0	1.0
236	2.3-01	0.0	0.0	0.0	0.0	0.0	0.0	1.0	302	2.0-01	6.0-01	0.0	0.0	0.0	0.0	0.0	1.0
237	2.4-01	0.0	0.0	0.0	0.0	0.0	0.0	1.0	303	1.1-01	5.2-01	0.0	0.0	0.0	0.0	0.0	7.5-01
238	2.5-01	0.0	0.0	0.0	0.0	0.0	0.0	1.0	304	7.6-02	4.4-01	0.0	0.0	0.0	0.0	0.0	5.0-01
239	2.6-01	0.0	0.0	0.0	0.0	0.0	0.0	1.0	305	6.0-02	3.3-01	0.0	0.0	0.0	0.0	0.0	3.0-01

TABLE B-2 Spectral Weighting Functions for Eye Hazard Computations (page 2)

λ nm	S_λ	U_λ	V_λ	V'_λ	T_λ	$T \cdot Ape_\lambda$	$1/C_A$	R_λ	λ nm	S_λ	U_λ	V_λ	V'_λ	T_λ	$T \cdot Ape_\lambda$	$1/C_A$	R_λ
240	2.7-01	5.6-01	0.0	0.0	0.0	0.0	0.0	1.0	306	5.0-02	3.0-01	0.0	0.0	0.0	0.0	0.0	1.9-01
241	2.9-01	5.6-01	0.0	0.0	0.0	0.0	0.0	1.0	307	3.3-02	2.5-01	0.0	0.0	0.0	0.0	0.0	1.2-01
242	3.0-01	5.6-01	0.0	0.0	0.0	0.0	0.0	1.0	308	2.5-02	2.0-01	0.0	0.0	0.0	0.0	0.0	7.5-02
243	3.2-01	5.7-01	0.0	0.0	0.0	0.0	0.0	1.0	309	1.9-02	1.5-01	0.0	0.0	0.0	0.0	0.0	4.8-02
244	3.3-01	5.7-01	0.0	0.0	0.0	0.0	0.0	1.0	310	1.3-02	1.1-01	0.0	0.0	0.0	0.0	0.0	3.0-02
245	3.5-01	5.8-01	0.0	0.0	0.0	0.0	0.0	1.0	311	1.0-02	8.2-02	0.0	0.0	0.0	0.0	0.0	1.9-02
246	3.6-01	5.8-01	0.0	0.0	0.0	0.0	0.0	1.0	312	7.5-03	5.8-02	0.0	0.0	0.0	0.0	0.0	1.2-02
247	3.8-01	5.8-01	0.0	0.0	0.0	0.0	0.0	1.0	313	6.0-03	5.0-02	0.0	0.0	0.0	0.0	0.0	8.0-03
248	3.9-01	5.8-01	0.0	0.0	0.0	0.0	0.0	1.0	314	4.3-03	2.9-02	0.0	0.0	0.0	0.0	0.0	5.0-03
249	4.1-01	5.8-01	0.0	0.0	0.0	0.0	0.0	1.0	315	3.0-03	1.0-02	0.0	0.0	0.0	0.0	0.0	3.0-03
250	4.3-01	5.7-01	0.0	0.0	0.0	0.0	0.0	1.0	316	0.0	9.1-03	0.0	0.0	0.0	0.0	0.0	0.0
251	4.4-01	5.6-01	0.0	0.0	0.0	0.0	0.0	1.0	317	0.0	8.0-03	0.0	0.0	0.0	0.0	0.0	0.0
252	4.5-01	5.6-01	0.0	0.0	0.0	0.0	0.0	1.0	318	0.0	6.8-03	0.0	0.0	0.0	0.0	0.0	0.0
253	4.7-01	5.5-01	0.0	0.0	0.0	0.0	0.0	1.0	319	0.0	5.6-03	0.0	0.0	0.0	0.0	0.0	0.0
254	5.0-01	5.4-01	0.0	0.0	0.0	0.0	0.0	1.0	320	0.0	5.0-03	0.0	0.0	0.0	0.0	0.0	0.0
255	5.2-01	5.3-01	0.0	0.0	0.0	0.0	0.0	1.0	321	0.0	4.2-03	0.0	0.0	0.0	0.0	0.0	0.0
256	5.5-01	5.2-01	0.0	0.0	0.0	0.0	0.0	1.0	322	0.0	3.6-03	0.0	0.0	0.0	0.0	0.0	0.0
257	5.8-01	5.0-01	0.0	0.0	0.0	0.0	0.0	1.0	325	0.0	3.0-03	0.0	0.0	0.0	0.0	0.0	0.0
258	6.0-01	4.8-01	0.0	0.0	0.0	0.0	0.0	1.0	330	0.0	0.0	0.0	0.0	0.0	0.0	0.0	0.0
259	6.3-01	4.5-01	0.0	0.0	0.0	0.0	0.0	1.0	335	0.0	0.0	0.0	0.0	0.0	0.0	0.0	0.0
260	6.5-01	4.2-01	0.0	0.0	0.0	0.0	0.0	1.0	340	0.0	0.0	0.0	0.0	0.0	0.0	0.0	0.0
261	6.8-01	4.0-01	0.0	0.0	0.0	0.0	0.0	1.0	345	0.0	0.0	0.0	0.0	0.0	0.0	0.0	0.0
262	7.1-01	3.6-01	0.0	0.0	0.0	0.0	0.0	1.0	350	0.0	0.0	0.0	0.0	0.0	0.0	0.0	0.0
263	7.5-01	3.2-01	0.0	0.0	0.0	0.0	0.0	1.0	355	0.0	0.0	0.0	0.0	0.0	0.0	0.0	0.0
264	7.9-01	2.9-01	0.0	0.0	0.0	0.0	0.0	1.0	360	0.0	0.0	0.0	0.0	0.0	0.0	0.0	0.0
265	8.1-01	2.6-01	0.0	0.0	0.0	0.0	0.0	1.0	365	0.0	0.0	0.0	0.0	0.0	0.0	0.0	0.0

See B.2 for explanation of headings.

TABLE B-2 Spectral Weighting Functions for Eye Hazard Computations (page 3)

λ nm	S_λ	U_λ	V_λ	V'_λ	T_λ	$T \cdot Ape_\lambda$	$1/C_A$	R_λ	B_λ	$\bar{X}_\lambda$	$\bar{Y}_\lambda$	$\bar{Z}_\lambda$
370	0.0	0.0	0.0	0.0	0.0	0.0	0.0	0.0				
375	0.0	0.0	0.0	0.0	0.0	0.0	0.0	0.0				
380	0.0	0.0	4.0-05	5.9-04	0.0	0.0	0.0	0.0		1.4-03		6.5-03
385	0.0	0.0	6.8-05	1.0-03	0.0	0.0	0.0	0.0		2.2-03		1.0-02
390	0.0	0.0	1.2-04	2.2-03	1.0-02	0.0	0.0	0.0		4.2-03	1.0-04	2.0-02
395	0.0	0.0	1.9-04	4.0-03	5.0-02	0.0	0.0	0.0		7.6-03	1.0-04	3.6-02
400	0.0	0.0	4.0-04	8.0-03	8.0-02	0.0	1.0	0.0	1.0-01	1.4-02	2.0-04	5.8-02
405	0.0	0.0	5.8-04	1.8-02	1.1-01	1.0-02	2.0	0.0	2.0-01	2.3-02	4.0-04	1.1-01
410	0.0	0.0	1.2-03	3.5-02	2.2-01	5.0-02	4.0	0.0	4.0-01	4.4-02	6.0-04	2.1-01
415	0.0	0.0	2.0-03	6.0-02	2.8-01	8.4-02	8.0	0.0	8.0-01	7.8-02	1.2-03	3.7-01
420	0.0	0.0	4.0-03	9.7-02	3.3-01	2.0-01	9.0	0.0	9.0-01	1.3-01	2.2-03	6.5-01
425	0.0	0.0	6.5-03	1.5-01	3.8-01	2.5-01	9.5	0.0	9.5-01	2.1-01	4.0-03	1.0
430	0.0	0.0	1.2-02	2.0-01	4.2-01	3.0-01	9.8	0.0	9.8-01	2.8-01	7.3-03	1.4
435	0.0	0.0	1.7-02	2.7-01	4.6-01	3.7-01	1.0+01	0.0	1.0	3.3-01	1.2-02	1.6
440	0.0	0.0	2.3-02	3.5-01	5.0-01	4.5-01	1.0+01	0.0	1.0	3.5-01	1.7-02	1.7
445	0.0	0.0	3.0-02	4.0-01	5.7-01	5.2-01	9.7	0.0	9.7-01	3.5-01	2.3-02	1.8
450	0.0	0.0	3.8-02	4.5-01	6.3-01	5.8-01	9.4	0.0	9.4-01	3.4-01	3.0-02	1.8
455	0.0	0.0	5.0-02	5.0-01	6.5-01	6.0-01	9.0	0.0	9.0-01	3.2-01	3.8-02	1.7
460	0.0	0.0	6.0-02	5.7-01	6.8-01	6.2-01	8.0	0.0	8.0-01	2.9-01	4.8-02	1.7
465	0.0	0.0	7.2-02	6.4-01	6.9-01	6.4-01	7.0	0.0	7.0-01	2.5-01	6.0-02	1.5
470	0.0	0.0	9.1-02	6.8-01	7.1-01	6.5-01	6.2	0.0	6.2-01	2.0-01	7.4-02	1.3
475	0.0	0.0	1.1-01	7.3-01	7.2-01	5.5-01	5.5	0.0	5.5-01	1.4-01	9.1-02	1.0
480	0.0	0.0	1.4-01	7.9-01	7.4-01	6.7-01	4.5	0.0	4.5-01	9.6-02	1.1-01	8.1-01
485	0.0	0.0	1.6-01	8.5-01	7.6-01	6.8-01	4.0	0.0	4.0-01	5.8-02	1.4-01	5.2-01
490	0.0	0.0	2.1-01	9.0-01	7.7-01	6.9-01	2.2	0.0	2.2-01	3.2-02	1.7-01	4.6-01
495	0.0	0.0	3.5-01	9.5-01	7.9-01	7.0-01	1.6	0.0	1.6-01	1.5-02	2.1-01	3.5-01
500	0.0	0.0	3.2-01	9.8-01	8.1-01	7.1-01	1.0	0.0	1.0-01	4.9-03	2.6-01	2.7-01
505	0.0	0.0	4.0-01	1.0	8.2-01	7.2-01	1.0	0.0	7.9-02	2.4-03	3.2-01	2.1-01
510	0.0	0.0	5.0-01	9.8-01	8.4-01	7.2-01	1.0	0.0	6.3-02	9.3-03	4.1-01	1.6-01
515	0.0	0.0	6.2-01	9.4-01	8.6-01	7.2-01	1.0	0.0	5.0-02	2.9-02	5.0-01	1.1-01
520	0.0	0.0	7.1-01	9.0-01	8.7-01	7.3-01	1.0	0.0	4.0-02	6.3-02	6.1-01	7.8-02
525	0.0	0.0	8.0-01	8.1-01	8.8-01	7.3-01	1.0	0.0	3.2-02	1.1-01	7.1-01	5.7-02
530	0.0	0.0	8.6-01	7.5-01	8.9-01	7.4-01	1.0	0.0	2.5-02	1.7-01	7.9-01	4.2-02
535	0.0	0.0	9.2-01	6.5-01	8.9-01	7.4-01	1.0	0.0	2.0-02	2.3-01	8.6-01	3.0-02
540	0.0	0.0	9.5-01	5.6-01	9.0-01	7.4-01	1.0	0.0	1.6-02	2.9-01	9.1-01	2.0-02
545	0.0	0.0	9.8-01	4.8-01	9.1-01	7.4-01	1.0	0.0	1.3-02	3.6-01	9.5-01	2.0-02
550	0.0	0.0	9.9-01	3.9-01	9.2-01	7.5-01	1.0	0.0	1.0-02	4.3-01	9.8-01	1.3-02
555	0.0	0.0	1.0	3.3-01	9.2-01	7.5-01	1.0	0.0	7.9-03	5.1-01	1.0	8.7-03
560	0.0	0.0	9.9-01	3.3-01	9.3-01	7.5-01	1.0	0.0	6.3-03	5.9-01	9.9-01	5.7-03
565	0.0	0.0	9.7-01	2.7-01	9.3-01	7.6-01	1.0	0.0	5.0-03	5.8-01	9.8-01	2.7-03

TABLE B-2 Spectral Weighting Functions for Eye Hazard Computations (page 4)

λ	S_λ	U_λ	V_λ	V'_λ	T_λ	$T \cdot Ape_\lambda$	$1/C_A$	R_λ	B_λ	$\bar{X}_\lambda$	$\bar{Y}_\lambda$	$\bar{Z}_\lambda$
570	0.0	0.0	9.5-01	2.1-01	9.4-01	7.6-01	1.0	0.0	4.0-03	7.6-01	9.5-01	2.1-03
575	0.0	0.0	9.1-01	1.7-01	9.4-01	7.5-01	1.0	0.0	3.2-03	8.4-01	9.1-01	1.8-03
580	0.0	0.0	8.7-01	1.2-01	9.5-01	7.5-01	1.0	0.0	2.5-03	9.2-01	8.7-01	1.7-03
585	0.0	0.0	8.1-01	1.0-01	9.5-01	7.4-01	1.0	0.0	2.0-03	9.8-01	8.2-01	1.4-03
590	0.0	0.0	7.6-01	6.5-02	9.5-01	7.4-01	1.0	0.0	1.6-03	1.0	7.6-01	1.1-03
595	0.0	0.0	7.1-01	5.3-02	9.6-01	7.3-01	1.0	0.0	1.3-03	1.1	7.0-01	1.0-03
600	0.0	0.0	6.3-01	3.3-02	9.6-01	7.3-01	1.0	0.0	1.0-03	1.1	6.3-01	8.0-04
605	0.0	0.0	5.8-01	2.3-02	9.6-01	7.2-01	1.0	0.0	1.0-03	1.0	5.7-01	6.0-04
610	0.0	0.0	5.0-01	1.6-02	9.6-01	7.2-01	1.0	0.0	1.0-03	1.0	5.0-01	3.0-04
615	0.0	0.0	4.5-01	1.1-02	9.6-01	7.1-01	1.0	0.0	1.0-03	9.4-01	4.4-01	2.0-04
620	0.0	0.0	3.6-01	7.4-03	9.6-01	7.0-01	1.0	0.0	1.0-03	8.5-01	3.8-01	2.0-04
625	0.0	0.0	3.2-01	4.3-03	9.6-01	6.9-01	1.0	0.0	1.0-03	7.5-01	3.2-01	1.0-04
630	0.0	0.0	2.7-01	3.3-03	9.6-01	6.8-01	1.0	0.0	1.0-03	6.4-01	2.7-01	
635	0.0	0.0	2.1-01	2.1-03	9.6-01	6.7-01	1.0	0.0	1.0-03	5.4-01	2.2-01	
640	0.0	0.0	1.8-01	1.5-03	9.6-01	6.6-01	1.0	0.0	1.0-03	4.5-01	1.8-01	
645	0.0	0.0	1.3-01	9.0-04	9.6-01	6.5-01	1.0	0.0	1.0-03	3.6-01	1.4-01	
650	0.0	0.0	1.1-01	6.8-04	9.6-01	6.5-01	1.0	0.0	1.0-03	2.8-01	1.1-01	
655	0.0	0.0	7.5-02	4.5-04	9.6-01	6.3-01	1.0	0.0	1.0-03	2.2-01	8.2-02	
660	0.0	0.0	6.1-02	3.1-04	9.6-01	6.2-01	1.0	0.0	1.0-03	1.6-01	6.1-02	
665	0.0	0.0	4.4-02	2.2-04	9.6-01	6.1-01	1.0	0.0	1.0-03	1.2-01	4.5-02	
670	0.0	0.0	3.2-02	1.5-04	9.6-01	6.0-01	1.0	0.0	1.0-01	9.7-02	3.2-02	
675	0.0	0.0	2.2-02	1.1-04	9.6-01	5.9-01	1.0	0.0	1.0-03	6.4-02	2.3-02	
680	0.0	0.0	1.7-02	7.1-05	9.6-01	5.9-01	1.0	0.0	1.0-03	4.7-02	1.7-02	
685	0.0	0.0	1.1-02	5.3-05	9.6-01	5.8-01	1.0	0.0	1.0-03	3.3-01	1.2-02	
690	0.0	0.0	8.2-03	3.5-05	9.6-01	5.7-01	1.0	0.0	1.0-03	2.3-02	8.2-03	
695	0.0	0.0	5.9-03	2.5-05	9.6-01	5.6-01	1.0	0.0	1.0-03	1.6-02	5.7-03	
700	0.0	0.0	4.1-03	1.8-05	9.6-01	5.5-01	1.0	0.0	1.0-03	1.1-02	4.1-03	
705	0.0	0.0	3.0-03	1.3-05	9.6-01	5.4-01	9.8-01	0.0	1.0-03	8.1-03	2.9-03	

See B.2 for explanation of headings.

LASER MICROWAVE DIVISION SPECTRAL WEIGHTING PROGRAM

COVER SHEET

A. Requestor's Name: _____

B. Source Description(DESCRP): _____

   (free format, two
   punched cards) _____

   _____

C. Calibration Deck Used: Deck Number _____

D. Calculation Control Card:

1	2	3	4	5	6	7	8	9	10	11

Box Number:

1. Number of Filters to be Processed(NUMFIL) -- Enter Number (max is 2).
2. Number of Columns for Filter 1(NOCOF1).
3. Number of Columns for Filter 2(NOCOF2).
4. Number of Columns for Filter 3(NOCOF3).
5. Form of Calibration Deck(CALDAT):
   a. Regular -- Enter "1".
   b. None Required -- Enter "2".
   c. Uncomputed -- Enter "0"(zero).
6-7. Specific Biological Function to be listed Spectrally(GENWEI). Enter Code:

   a. None -- 00   f. T·A -- 05   k. $\bar{x}_\lambda$ -- 10   p. P_{575} -- 15
   b. S_λ -- 01   g. R_λ -- 06   l. $\bar{y}_\lambda$ -- 11   q. FT1 -- 16
   c. U_λ -- 02   h. V_λ -- 07   m. $\bar{z}_\lambda$ -- 12   r. FT2 -- 17
   d. A_λ -- 03   i. V_λ' -- 08   n. P_{445} -- 13   s. FT3 or
   e. T_λ -- 04   j. B_λ -- 09   o. P_{535} -- 14   FT1*FT2 -- 18

8. General Function Used(GENFUN)? -- "1" is yes, zero or blank is no.
9. GENWEI Plotted(FLPLOT)? -- "1" is yes, zero or blank is no.
10. Input Deck to be Stored on File(STORE): a. None -- 0(zero)
    b. Filter one -- 1   d. Filter three -- 3   f. Calibration -- 5
    c. Filter two -- 2   e. Event -- 4   g. St. Lamp -- 6
11. Spectral Irradiance Interpolated(IOS)? -- "1" is yes, zero or blank is no.

E. Distance Factor Card -- Enter Correction Factors for Calibration Distance(DFU and DFV), Bandpass of measuring instruments(BANPAS), and Separating Wavelengths(BWAV1 and BWAV2). Default Values as Listed Below are used if Card is not filled in.

DFU	DFV	BANPAS(1)	BWAV1	BANPAS(2)	BWAV2	BANPAS(3)
(1.0)	(1.0)	(3.0)	(400)	(5.0)	(700)	(10.0)

1	2	3	4	5	6	7	8	9	10	11	12	13	14	15	16	17	18	19	20	21	22	23	24	25	26	27	28

F. Check List: ___ Source Description   ___ Instrument Readings
               ___ Calculation Control Card ___ Solid Angle
               ___ Calibration Deck   ___ End Cards
               ___ Header Cards   ___ Distance Factor Card

G. Number of Deck to be Stored: Deck Number _____

Figure B-6.   Cover sheet used for spectral weighting program.

B.3 TRANSMISSION THROUGH THE EYE

The absorption of the various parts of the eye have been discussed in 4.5.2.2. The spectral transmission of the rabbit and human eyes were shown in Figure 4-9 down to 1.4 μm. Figure B-7 shows measurements which extend down to 1.9 μm.

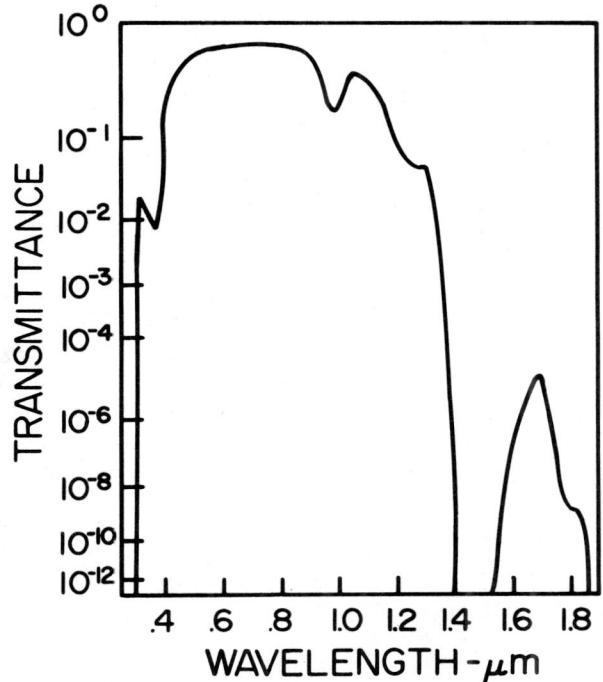

Figure B-7. Spectral transmittance through human eye. Between 0.3 and 1.3 μm, the curve is based on measurement of human ocular tissue. Beyond 1.3 μm, the transmittance is that of a 2.2 cm. layer of pure H_2O (adapted from D. J. Lund, G. H. Bresnick, M. B. Landers,III, J.D. Powell, J. E. Chester, and E. Carver. Ocular Hazards of the Q-Switched Erbium Laser. Invest. Ophthal. 9(6), 463-470, 1970).

Appendix C
Laser Wavelengths and Characteristics

TABLE C-1. Laser Wavelengths by Wavelength

Wavelength (nm)	Active Medium	Wavelength (nm)	Active Medium
172	Xenon	495.6	Xenon
173.6	Ruby (quad)	496.5	Argon, ionized, Ar^{2+}
193	Argon-fluoride excimer	497.5	Helium selenium
231.4	Ruby (trip)	499.5	Helium selenium
235.8	Neon, ionized, Ne^{3+}	500	Cadmium sulphide
248	Krypton-fluoride excimer	501.5	Argon, ionized, Ar^{2+}
266	Neodymium (quad)	501.7	Argon, ionized, Ar^{2+}
330	Zinc sulphide	506.8	Helium selenium
325	Helium cadmium vapor	514.5	Argon, ionized, Ar^{2+}
332.4	Neon, ionized, Ne^{2+}	517.5	Helium selenium
337.1	Argon-nitrogen	520.8	Krypton, ionized, Kr^{2+}
337.1	Nitrogen, molecular	522.7	Helium selenium
350	Xenon-fluoride excimer	525.3	Helium selenium
354.7	Neodymium (trip)	530	Neodymium, Nd/KDP
357.7	Argon nitrogen	530.5	Helium selenium
380.4	Argon nitrogen	530.9	Krypton, ionized, Kr^{2+}
441.6	Helium cadmium vapor	532	Neodymium, dobuled
457.7	Krypton, ionized, Kr^{2+}	539.5	Xenon
457.9	Argon, ionized, Ar^{2+}	540.1	Neon, ionized, Ne^{2+}
460.4	Helium selenium	552.3	Helium selenium
461.9	Krypton, ionized, Kr^{2+}	568.2	Krypton, ionized, Kr^{2+}
463.4	Krypton, ionized, Kr^{2+}	595.6	Xenon
464.8	Helium selenium	605.6	Helium selenium
465.8	Argon, ionized, Ar^{2+}	610	Europium, Eu^{3+}
468	Krypton, ionized, Kr^{2+}	632.8	Helium-neon
472.7	Argon, ionized, Ar^{2+}	644.4	Helium selenium
476.2	Krypton, ionized, Kr^{2+}	647.1	Krypton, ionized, Kr^{2+}
476.5	Argon, ionized, Ar^{2+}	649	Helium selenium
482.5	Krypton, ionized, Kr^{2+}	676.4	Krypton, ionized, Kr^{2+}
484.5	Helium selenium	687.1	Krypton, ionized, Kr^{2+}
484.6	Krypton, ionized, Kr^{2+}	690	Cadmium selenide
488	Argon, ionized, Ar^{2+}	692.9	Chromium

TABLE C-1. Laser Wavelengths by Wavelength (continued)

Wavelength (nm)	Active Medium	Wavelength (nm)	Active Medium
693.4	Chromium	2000-5000	Xenon
694.3 to 1000	Ruby	2046	Holmium
696.9	Samarium	2061	Xenon, atomic
708.2	Samarium	2360	Dysprosium
800	Cadmium telluride	2407	Uranium (SrF_2)
844.5	Argon-oxygen	2510	Uranium (CaF_2)
850	Er/y-Li fluoride	2556	Uranium (BaF_2)
850	Gallium arsenide	2600-3300 (15 lines)	HF
850	Gallium arsenide (77°K)	2613	Uranium (CaF_2)
850	Gallium aluminum arsenide	3200	Indium arsenide
900	Indium phosphide	3390	Helium-neon
905	Gallium arsenide	3392	Helium-neon
1037	Neodymium (SrF_2)	3500	Helium-xenon
1046.1	Neodymium (CaF_2)	3773	HC1
1046.8	Praseodymium ($CaWO_4$)	3800-4200 (25 lines)	DF
1047	Praseodymium ($SrMoO_4$)	4300	Lead sulphide
1060	Neodymium (BaF_2)	4800-8000 (50-70 lines)	CO
1060	Neodymium (glass)	5300	Indium antimonide
1064	Neodymium	6500	Lead telluride
1064.3	Neodymium ($CrMoO_4$)	7182.1	Cesium vapor
1064.5	Neodymium: YAG	8500	Lead selenide
1064.6	Neodymium ($CaWO_4$, pulsed)	9000-12000 (100 lines)	N_2O
1065	Neodymium ($CaWO_4$, CW)	10,000-20,000	HF
1123	Neodymium	10,600	CO_2
1152.3	Helium-neon	27,900	Water vapor
1153	Helium-neon	27,970	Water vapor
1315	Iodine (alkyl iodide)	33,700	Hydrocyanic acid, HCN
1318	Neodymium	47,700	Water vapor
1370	Neodymium	78,460	Water vapor
1454	Helium-carbon dioxide	95,800	Helium
1600	Gallium antimonide	118,000	Water vapor
1612	Erbium ($CaWO_4$)	118,400	Water vapor
1617	Erbium (CaF_2)	216.300	Helium
1910	Thulium (SrF_2)	311,000	HCN
1911	Thulium ($CaWO_4$)	337,000	HCN

TABLE C-2. LASER WAVELENGTHS BY MEDIUM

Part 1 — Chemical Lasers

Active Medium	Wavelength (nm)	Typical Operation
CO	50-70 lines from 4800 to 8000	CW
HF	15 lines from 2600 to 3300; 10,000 to 22,000	CW
DF	25 lines from 3800 to 4200	CW
H-CN	311,000 and 337,000	pulsed
H_2O (vapor)	27,970; 47,700; 78,460; 118,400	pulsed
N_2O	100 lines from 9000 to 12,000	
$LiNbO_3$	550 to 3500	
HCl	3773	

Part 2 — Crystal (Solid-State) Lasers

Active Medium	Wavelength (nm)	Typical Operation
Chromium, Cr^{3+} (Al_2O_3)	692.9	pulsed
" (77°K)	693.4	CW
Dysprosium, Dy_2^+ (CaF_2)	2360	pulsed, CW
Erbium, Er^{3+} ($CaWO_4$)	1612	pulsed
" (CaF_2)	1617	pulsed
Er/y-Li fluoride	850	pulsed
Europium, Eu^{3+}	610	pulsed
Holmium, glass	1950	pulsed
Holmium, Ho^{3+} ($CaWO_2$)	2046	pulsed
Neodymium, Nd^{3+}	1064, 1123, 1318, 1370	pulsed
" (quad)	266.0	pulsed
" (trip)	354.7	pulsed
" (doubled)	532.0	pulsed
" (SrF_2)	1037.0	pulsed
" (CaF_2)	1046.1	pulsed
Neodymium, glass	1060.0	pulsed
" (BaF_2)	1060.0	pulsed
" ($CrMoO_4$)	1064.3	pulsed
Neodymium: YAG	1064.5	pulsed, CW
" ($CaWO_4$)	1064.6	pulsed
" "	1065.0	CW
Nd/KOP	530.0	pulsed, CW
Praseodymium, Pr^{3+} ($CaWO_4$)	1046.8	pulsed
" ($SrMoO_4$)	1047.0	pulsed

Part 2 — Crystal (Solid-State) Lasers (continued)

Active Medium	Wavelength (nm)	Typical Operation
Ruby ($Al_2O_3Cr^{3+}$)	694.3 to 1100	pulsed
" (quad)	173.6	
" (trip)	231.4	
Samarium, Sm^{2+} (SrF_2)	696.9	pulsed
" (CaF_2)	708.2	pulsed
Thulium, Tm^{3+} (SrF_2)	1910.0	pulsed
" ($CaWO_4$)	1911.0	pulsed
Uranium, U^{3+} (SrF_2)	2407	pulsed
" (CaF_2)	2510, 2613	pulsed, CW
" (BaF_2)	2556	pulsed

Part 3 — Dye Lasers

Active Medium	Wavelength (nm)	Typical Operation
Organic dyes	560-640	CW argon laser excitation
Organic dyes	360-650	Pulsed N_2 excitation

Part 4 — Gas Lasers

Active Medium	Wavelength (nm)	Typical Operation
Argon, ionized, Ar^{2+}	457.9; 465.8; 472.7; 476.5; 488.0, 496.5, 501.5, 501.7, 514.5	CW
Argon-krypton, Ar/Kr	see Ar and Kr lines	
Argon-nitrogen, Ar/N_2	337.1, 357.7, 380.4	
Argon-oxygen, Ar/O_2	844.5	CW, pulsed
Cesium vapor, Cs	7182.1	CW
Carbon-dioxide, $CO_2 N_2$ He	10,600 (10.6 μm)	CW, pulsed
Helium, He	95,800; 216,300 (95.8, 216.3 μm)	CW
Helium cadmium vapor, HeCd	325.0, 441.6	CW
Helium carbon dioxide, $HeCO_2$	1454.0	CW, pulsed
Helium neon, HeNe	632.8, 1152.3, 1153.0, 3390.0, 3392.0	CW

Part 4 — Gas Lasers (continued)

Active Medium	Wavelength (nm)	Typical Operation
Helium selenide, HeSe	460.4, 464.8, 484.5, 497.5, 499.5, 506.8, 517.5, 522.7, 525.3, 530.5, 552.3, 605.6, 644.4, 649.0	CW
Helium-xenon, HeXe	3500 (3.5 μm)	CW
Hydrocyanic acid, HCN	33,700 (33.5 μm)	CW
Iodine (alkyl iodide)	1315.0	CW
Krypton, ionized, Kr^{2+}	457.7, 461.9, 463.4, 468.0, 476.2, 482.5, 484.6, 520.8, 530.9, 568.2, 647.1, 676.4, 687.1	CW
Neon, ionized, Ne^{3+}	235.8	pulsed
Neon, ionized, Ne^{2+}	332.4, 540.1	pulsed
Nitrogen, molecular, N_2	337.1	pulsed
Water vapor	27,900; 118,600 (27.9; 118.6 μm)	pulsed
Xenon, Xe	172.0, 495.6, 539.5, 595.6; 2000–5000 (2–5 μm)	CW, pulsed
Xenon, atomic, Xe	2061.0	pulsed

Part 5 — Semiconductor Lasers

Active Medium	Wavelength (nm)	Typical Operation
Cadmium selenide, CdSe	690	
Cadmium sulphide, CdS	500	
Cadmium telluride, CdTe	800	
Gallium antimonide, GaSb	1600	pulsed
Gallium arsenide, GaAs	850, 905	pulsed
Gallium arsenide, GaAs (77°K)	850	pulsed
Gallium aluminum arsenide, GaAlAs	850	pulsed
Indium antimonide, InSb	5300	
Indium arsenide, InAs	3200	
Indium phosphide, InP	900	
Lead selenide, PbSe	8500	
Lead sulphide, PbS	4300	
Lead telluride, PbTe	6500	
Zinc sulphide, ZnS	330	

Appendix D
List of Capital Letter Abbreviations

AC - Alternating Current

ACGIH - American Conference of Governmental Industrial Hygienists

ACGIH TLV Book - American Conference of Governmental Industrial Hygienists Threshold Limit Values

AEHA - Army Environmental Hygiene Agency (USA)

AEL - Acceptable Exposure Limits

ANSI - American National Standards Institute

ASL - Above Sea Level

AWS - American Welding Society

BG - Black Globe Temperature

BL - Blacklight Lamp (UV-A)

BRH - Bureau of Radiological Health (USA)

BSI - British Standards Institute

CAI - Computer Assisted Instruction

CBS - Columbia Broadcasting System

CCTV - Closed Circuit Television

CIE - Commission Internationle d'Eclairage (International Commission on Illumination)

CRC - Chemical Rubber Company

CRT - Cathode Ray Tube

CW - Continuous Wave

DB - Dry Bulb Temperature

DC - Direct Current

DF - Deuterium Fluoride

DIN - Deutsche Institut für Normung (German Standards Institute)

DMSO - Dimethylsulfoxide

DNA - Desoxyribose Nucleic Acid

DoD - Department of Defense (USA)

DT - Delayed Tanning

EC - Electrically Conductive Coating

ED_{50} dose - Effective Dose Level for 50% of Exposed Population

EG & G - Edgerton, Germeshausen, and Grier, Inc.

EIS - Environmental Impact Statements (USA)

EL - Exposure Limit (WHO)

EM - Electron Microscope

EPA - Environmental Protection Agency (USA)

ERDA - Energy Resources Development Agency (Now Department of Energy, USA)

ERG - Electroretinogram

FAA - Federal Aviation Administration (USA)

FDA - Food and Drug Administration (USA)

FO - Fiber Optic

Capital Abbreviations

FOV - Field of View (Acceptable Angle)

FS - Fluorescent Sunlight

GMAW - Gas Metal Arc Welding (Metal Ion Gas)

GTAW - Gas Tungsten Arc Welding (Tungsten Ion Gas)

GTE Sylvania - General Telephone and Electronics, Corp.

H-D - Hurter-Driffield (Photographic Film Exposure Density Wave)

HEW - Department of Health, Education and Welfare (USA)

HF - Hydrogen Fluoride

HID - High Intensity Discharge Mercury Fluorescent Lamp

IBM - International Business Machine, Corp.

IEC - International Electrotechnical Commission

IEC - TC 76 - International Electrotechnical Commission - Technical Committee 76 on Laser Safety

IES - Illuminating Engineers Society

I.P.D. - Immediate Pigment Darkening

IR-A - Near Infrared (760-1400 nm)

IR-B - Middle IR (1.4-3.0 μm)

IR-C - Far IR (3.0-1,000 μm)

IRPA - Internationale Radiation Protection Association

ISO - International Standards Organization

ITT - International Telephone and Telegraph, Inc.

LED - Light Emitting Diode

LIA - Laser Industries Association

LIDAR - Light Detection and Ranging

LRF - Laser Range Finder

LRSF - Laser Range Safety Fan

LRSO - Laser Range Safety Officer

LSO - Laser Safety Officer

MED - Minimal Erythemal Dose

MIL spec. - Military Specification (USA)

MPE - Maximum Permissible Exposure

MRD - Minimum Reactive Dose

MSA - Mine Safety Appliance

MTF - Modulation Transfer Function

NA - Numerical Aperture

NASA - National Aeronautics and Space Agency (USA)

NBS - National Bureau of Standards (USA)

NEI - National Eye Institute (USA), or Noise Equivalent Irradiance

NEP - Noise Equivalent Power

NIOSH - National Institute of Occupational Safety and Health (USA)

NOHD - Nominal Ocular Hazard Distance

NRC - National Research Council (USA)

OD - Optical Density

OJT - On the Job Training

OR - Operating Room (Surgical)

OSHA - Occupational Safety and Health Administration (USA)

PABA - Para-Amino-Benzoic-Acid

PCB - Polychlorinated Biphenyls

PLZT Filter - Polarized Light Zero Transmission Filter

POS - Point of Sale

PPM - Parts per Million, or Pulse Position Modulation

P.R.F. - Pulse Repetition Frequency

PRM - Pulse Rate Modulation

PWM - Pulse Width Modulation

RCA - Radio Corporation of America

R & D - Research and Development

R.F. - Radio Frequency

RFI - Radio Frequency Interference

RPE - Retinal Pigmented Epithelium

SHG - Second Harmonic Generation

SI - System Internationale

SOP - Standard Operating Procedure

SRI - Stanford Research Institute

T.C. 76 - See IEC - TC 76

TEA Laser - Tranverse Ecitation Atmospheric Laser

TEM - Transverse Electromagnetic Wave

TLV - Threshold Limit Value

TOTP - Total ON Time Pulse

UL - Underwriters Laboratory, Inc.

USAEHA - See AEHA

USAF - United States Air Force (USA)

USBRH - See BRH

USDHEW - See HEW

UV - Ultraviolet

UV-A - Near UV (315-400 nm)

UV-B - Far UV (280-315 nm)

UV-C - Extreme UV (100-280 nm)

VDU - Visual Display Unit

VER - Visual Evoked Response

VIS - Visible Radiation Range

WB - Wet Bulb Temperature

WBGT Index - Wet Bulb Globe Temperature Index

WHO - World Health Organization

Appendix E
Hazard Classification of Some Representative, Pre-1976 Lasers

Initially we ambitiously planned to list most of the lasers made prior to August 1976, the date when BRH Regulations required manufacturers to include the hazard classification on the label. The delayed completion of this text made such a list much less important. We give, therefore, a greatly abbreviated list containing only the more commonly encountered lasers whose hazard classification is not given on their labels. A far more complete listing is available in the NIOSH Technical Information Laser Hazard Classification Guide [HEW Publication No. (NIOSH) 76-183] from which this information has been extracted.

TABLE E-1
LASER HAZARD CLASSIFICATION GUIDE

MANUFACTURER/ MODEL ACTIVE MEDIUM	HAZARD CLASS (OSHA)	WAVE-LENGTH (NM)	DIA-METER (CM)	DIVER-GENCE (MRAD)	BEAM SHAPE	OUTPUT POWER/ENERGY	PULSE REP-RATE	PULSE WIDTH	BEAM IRRADIANCE/ RADIANT EXPOSURE ($W\,cm^{-2}$ or $J\,cm^{-2}$)	APPLICATION/ COMMENTS
AMERICAN OPTICAL AO-5Q NEODYMIUM GLASS	IV	1060	0.400	1.50	CIRC	0.100 J	1.00 P/M	0.040 μs	259 $mJ\,cm^{-2}$	RESEARCH & OEM
AMERICAN OPTICAL AO-11Q NEODYMIUM GLASS	IV	1060	0.600	1.50 2.50	CIRC	1.50 J	4.00 P/M	0.030 μs	3.89 $J\,cm^{-2}$	RESEARCH & OEM
AMERICAN OPTICAL 3100 HELIUM NEON (HeNe)	IIIb	632.8	0.200	0.300	CIRC	2.00 mW TEM_{00}	N/A		5.18 $mW\,cm^{-2}$	EDUCATION
AMERICAN OPTICAL 5000 NEODYMIUM GLASS	IV	1060		15.0		5000 J	12.0 P/H	3.00 ms	13.0 $kJ\,cm^{-2}$	RESEARCH & OEM
APOLLO LASERS 26200 NEODYMIUM GLASS	IV	1060	3.18	1.00	CIRC	5.00 GW PEAK	0.250 P/M	15.0 ns 25.0	31.4 $J\,cm^{-2}$	RESEARCH & OEM
AVCO EVERETT C-950-A NITROGEN (N_2)	IIIb	337.1	0.320 5.10	2.00 30.0	RECT	100 kW PEAK 100 mW AVER	2.00 TO 200 P/S	3.00 ns	184 $\mu J\,cm^{-2}$ 61.3 $mJ\,cm^{-2}$ 306 $\mu J\,cm^{-2}$	RESEARCH & OEM
BAUSCH & LOMB 41-17-03-05 HELIUM NEON (HeNe)	IIIb	632.8	0.015	7.00	CIRC	3.00 mW TEM_{00}	N/A		7.78 $mW\,cm^{-2}$	EDUCATION
BENDIX TL-1 HELIUM NEON (HeNe)	IIIb	632.8	0.200	0.400	CIRC	1.50 mW TEM_{00}	N/A		3.89 $mW\,cm^{-2}$	RESEARCH & OEM
CARSON LABS 202 ARGON/KRYPTON (Ar/Kr)	IV	476.5 TO 676.4	0.140	1.00	CIRC	1.00 W TEM_{00}	N/A		2.59 $W\,cm^{-2}$	RESEARCH & OEM
CHROMATIX CMX-4 UV OPTION DYE	IV	265.0 TO 350.0	0.300	1.00	CIRC	1.00 kW PEAK 1.00 kW AVER	5.00 P/S 30.0		28.2 $kW\,cm^{-2}$	SCIENTIFIC INSTR. PROVISIONAL-OSHA-CLASSIFICATION

Hazard Classification

TABLE E-1
LASER HAZARD CLASSIFICATION GUIDE (cont.)

MANUFACTURER/ MODEL ACTIVE MEDIUM	HAZARD CLASS (OSHA)	WAVE-LENGTH (NM)	DIA-METER (CM)	DIVER-GENCE (MRAD)	BEAM SHAPE	OUTPUT POWER/ENERGY	PULSE REP-RATE	PULSE WIDTH	BEAM IRRADIANCE/ RADIANT EXPOSURE ($W\,cm^{-2}$ or $J\,cm^{-2}$)	APPLICATION/ COMMENTS
COHERENT RADIATION COHERENT EYE SCANN HELIUM NEON (HeNe)	IIIb ENCL	632.8	(.1)	154	CIRC	1.20 mW AVER			3.11 mW cm^{-2}	RESEARCH & OEM CLASS I AS ENCLOSED PROVISIONAL -OSHA-CLASSIFICATION
COHERENT RADIATION CR - 8 ARGON (Ar)	IV	351.1 TO 528.7	0.140	0.500	CIRC	8.00 W TEM_{00}	N/A		1.02 kW cm^{-2}	RESEARCH & OEM
COHERENT RADIATION CR - 12 ARGON (Ar)	IV	351.1 TO 528.7	0.140 0.160	0.500 0.600	CIRC CIRC	1.50 W AVER 12.0			149 W cm^{-2} 1.19 kW cm^{-2}	RESEARCH & OEM PROVISIONAL -OSHA-CLASSIFICATION
COHERENT RADIATION 42 CARBON DIOXIDE (CO_2)	IV	10600	0.220		CIRC	50.0 W AVER	100 P/S	0.500 μs	26.2 J cm^{-2}	RESEARCH & OEM
COHERENT RADIATION 52A ARGON (Ar)	IV	457.9 488.0 514.5	0.140	0.800	CIRC	2.00 W TEM_{00}	N/A		5.18 W cm^{-2}	RESEARCH & OEM
COHERENT RADIATION 53 ARGON/KRYPTON (Ar/Kr) ARGON OR KRYPTON	IV	488.0 514.5 647.1 468.0	0.150	0.600	CIRC	6.00 W TEM_{00} 1.00	N/A		15.6 W cm^{-2} 2.59	RESEARCH & OEM
COHERENT RADIATION 54A ARGON (Ar)	IIIb	457.9 TO 514.4	0.078	0.900	CIRC	500 mW AVER			1.30 W cm^{-2}	RESEARCH & OEM PROVISIONAL -OSHA-CLASSIFICATION
COHERENT RADIATION CR - 084 HELIUM NEON (HeNe)	IIIb	632.8	0.050	1.20	CIRC	2.00 mW TEM_{00}	N/A		5.18 mW cm^{-2}	RESEARCH & OEM
COHERENT RADIATION CR490 RHODAMINE 6G		525.0 TO 700.0		1.00						RESEARCH & OEM INSUFFICIENT INFORMATION
COHERENT RADIATION 800 ARGON (Ar)	IV	514.5 488.0	0.140	0.800	CIRC	1.00 W	N/A		2.59 W cm^{-2}	MEDICAL

TABLE E-1
LASER HAZARD CLASSIFICATION GUIDE (cont.)

MANUFACTURER/ MODEL ACTIVE MEDIUM	HAZARD CLASS (OSHA)	WAVE- LENGTH (NM)	DIA- METER (CM)	DIVER- GENCE (MRAD)	BEAM SHAPE	OUTPUT POWER/ENERGY	PULSE REP-RATE	PULSE WIDTH	BEAM IRRADIANCE/ RADIANT EXPOSURE (W cm^{-2} or J cm^{-2})	APPLICATION/ COMMENTS
COHERENT RADIATION GRADOMAT I/II/III AND IV He Ne Ar or Kr	IIIb	632.8	0.700		CIRC	1.90 mW MAX	N/A		4.92 mW cm^{-2}	RESEARCH & OEM FOCUSED - 1.60 M AT 91 M
CONTROL LASER 904	IV	454.0 TO 647.1		0.600		4.00 W TEM$_{00}$ 5.00 W MULTI	N/A		10.4 W cm^{-2} 13.0	RESEARCH & OEM
CW RADIATION, INC. LS - 10 HELIUM NEON (HeNe)	IIIb	632.8				10.0 mW TEM$_{00}$	N/A		25.9 mW cm^{-2}	RESEARCH & OEM
EALING 25 - 7568 HELIUM NEON (HeNe)	IIIb	632.8	0.150	5.00	CIRC	1.50 mW TEM$_{00}$	N/A		3.89 mW cm^{-2}	EDUCATION
EDMUNDSCIENTIFIC 79005 HELIUM NEON (HeNe)	II	632.8	0.100	2.00	CIRC	.300 mW MULTI	N/A		778 μW cm^{-2}	RESEARCH & OEM
EOCOM CORP. 65R UV RANGE NO MEDIUM	IIIb	361.1 TO 363.8		0.110		400 mW	N/A		50.8 W cm^{-2}	MAT. PROCESSING THE "WRITE PART" OF LASERITE 65R
GENERAL PHOTONICS TWO - 12A NEODYMIUM YAG (Nd YAG)	IV	1064	0.071	1.00	CIRC	500 mW TEM$_{00}$ 1500 mW MULTI	N/A		1.30 W cm^{-2} 3.89	RESEARCH & OEM
GENERAL PHOTONICS TWO - 22 ND YAG DOUBLED	IV	532.0	0.071	1.00	CIRC	25.0 mW TEM$_{00}$			64.8 W cm^{-2}	RESEARCH & OEM PROVISIONAL-OSHA- CLASSIFICATION
GTE SYLVANIA 612 NEODYMIUM YAG (Nd YAG)	IV	1064	0.200	3.00	CIRC	10.0 W TEM$_{00}$ 200 W MULTI	N/A		25.9 mW cm^{-2} 518	RESEARCH & OEM
GTE SYLVANIA 941 - S CARBON DIOXIDE (CO$_2$)	IV	10600	0.400	4.00	CIRC	3.00 W TEM$_{00}$	N/A		47.6 W cm^{-2}	RESEARCH & OEM

TABLE E-1
LASER HAZARD CLASSIFICATION GUIDE (cont.)

MANUFACTURER/ MODEL ACTIVE MEDIUM	HAZARD CLASS (OSHA)	WAVE-LENGTH (NM)	DIA-METER (CM)	DIVER-GENCE (MRAD)	BEAM SHAPE	OUTPUT POWER/ENERGY	PULSE REP-RATE	PULSE WIDTH	BEAM IRRADIANCE/ RADIANT EXPOSURE ($W\,cm^{-2}$ or $J\,cm^{-2}$)	APPLICATION/ COMMENTS
HOLOBEAM INC. 250 - 2A NEODYMIUM YAG (Nd YAG)	IV	10600	0.300	35.0	CIRC	100 W	N/A		2.82 $kW\,cm^{-2}$	RESEARCH & OEM
HOLOBEAM INC. 256 - QG ND - YAG DOUBLED	IV	530.0	0.141	2.00	CIRC	3.0 kW PEAK 0.200 mJ	0.500 TO 24000 P/S	0.100 μs 0.250	1.94 $mJ\,cm^{-2}$ 518 $μJ\,cm^{-2}$	RESEARCH & OEM
HOLOBEAM INC. 500 - Q NEODYMIUM YAG (Nd YAG)	IV	1064	0.400	3.00	CIRC	100 mJ 8.00 MG PEAK	20.0 TO 50.0 P/S	12.0 ns	259 $mJ\,cm^{-2}$ 249	MAT. PROCESSING
HOLOBEAM INC. 910 SERIES ND - YAG Q SWITCHED	IIIb ENCL	1064	0.283	2.00	CIRC	3.00 kW PEAK	0.500 TO 24.0 kHz	15.0 μs 25.0	194 $mJ\,cm^{-2}$	MAT. PROCESSING CLASS I AS ENCLOSED
HOLOBEAM INC. LAZA - COM GA - AS	IV	905.0		1.00 300		8.00 W AVER	60.0 P/S	80.0 ns	346 $mJ\,cm^{-3}$	COMMUNICATOR
HONEYWELL 9000 CARBON DIOXIDE (CO_2)	IV	10600	0.600		CIRC	20.0 W TEM_{00}	N/A		141 $W\,cm^{-2}$	COMMUNICATOR
HUGHES AIRCRAFT 3035 - H HELIUM NEON (HeNe)	IIIb	632.8	0.130	0.100	CIRC	10.0 mW	N/A		25.9 $mW\,cm^{-2}$	RESEARCH & OEM
INTERNAT. LASER. SYS NC - 10/80 NEODYMIUM YAG (Nd YAG)	IV	1064	(.1)	5.00		1.00 MW PEAK 0.020 J	20.0 P/S	20.0 ns	51.8 $mJ\,cm^{-2}$	RESEARCH & OEM PROVISIONAL-OSHA-CLASSIFICATION
INTERNAT. LASER. SYS NT - 100P NEODYMIUM YAG (Nd YAG)	IV	1064		0.500		0.150 J	10.0 P/S	17.0 ns	389 $mJ\,cm^{-2}$	RESEARCH & OEM
JARRELL ASH MARK II MICROPROBE ND	IV	1060	0.005		CIRC	1.00 J		1.50 μs	2.59 $J\,cm^{-2}$	RESEARCH & OEM PROVISIONAL - OSHA-CLASSIFICATION

TABLE E-1
LASER HAZARD CLASSIFICATION GUIDE (cont.)

MANUFACTURER/ MODEL ACTIVE MEDIUM	HAZARD CLASS (OSHA)	WAVE-LENGTH (NM)	DIA-METER (CM)	DIVER-GENCE (MRAD)	BEAM SHAPE	OUTPUT POWER/ENERGY	PULSE REP-RATE	PULSE WIDTH	BEAM IRRADIANCE/ RADIANT EXPOSURE ($W\ cm^{-2}$ or $J\ cm^{-2}$)	APPLICATION/ COMMENTS
JODON HN-10 HELIUM NEON (HeNe)	IIIb	632.8	0.130	1.00	CIRC	15.0 mW TEM_{00}	N/A		38.9 mW cm^{-2}	RESEARCH & OEM
JODON HN-50 HELIUM NEON (HeNe)	IIIb	632.8 611.8	0.200	0.700	CIRC	50.0 mW AVER	N/A		3.17 W cm^{-2}	RESEARCH & OEM
KORAD KRT - MICROMACHINING NEODYMIUM YAG (Nd YAG)	IV	1064	(.1)			0.500 W AVER	800 TO 1200 P/S	25.0 ns	1.30 J cm^{-2}	MAT. PROCESSING PROVISIONAL - OSHA-CLASSIFICATION
KORAD K1QP RUBY	IV	694.3	0.800	10.0	CIRC	0.750 J MULTI 20.0 J TEM_{00}	1.00 P/M	20.0 ns	1.94 J cm^{-2} 51.8	SCIENTIFIC INSTR.
KORAD K1000QH RUBY	IV	694.3				4.00 J MULTI 200 mJ TEM_{00}	1.00 P/M	30.0 ns	10.4 J cm^{-2} 518 mJ cm^{-2}	HOLOGRAPHY
LASER DIODE LABS LSA-410 GA-AS	IIIb	905.0	(.1)	8.00		1.00 kW PEAK	1.00 TO 5.00 kHz	90.0 ns	233 $\mu J\ cm^{-2}$	RESEARCH & OEM PROVISIONAL - OSHA-CLASSIFICATION
LASER ENERGY INC N300 NITROGEN (N_2)	IIIb	337.1	0.317	2.00	CIRC	10.0 μJ 1.00 kW PEAK	4.00 TO 100 P/S		253 $\mu W\ cm^{-2}$	RESEARCH & OEM PROVISIONAL - OSHA-CLASSIFICATION
LEXEL 75-A ARGON (Ar)	IIIb	457.9 TO 582.7	0.090	1.50	CIRC	200 mW TEM_{00}	N/A		518 mW cm^{-2}	RESEARCH & OEM
LEXEL 96 ION LASER ARGON	IV	486.0 TO 514.5	0.013 0.018	0.600 1.50	CIRC CIRC	5.00 W TEM_{00}	N/A		13.0 W cm^{-2}	RESEARCH & OEM
LICONIX 405 HELIUM CADMIUM (HeCd)	IIIb	441.6 325.0	0.083	0.680	CIRC	40.0 mW TEM_{00} 15.0	N/A		5.08 W cm^{-2} 1.90	RESEARCH & OEM

TABLE E-1
LASER HAZARD CLASSIFICATION GUIDE (cont.)

MANUFACTURER/ MODEL ACTIVE MEDIUM	HAZARD CLASS (OSHA)	WAVE-LENGTH (NM)	DIA-METER (CM)	DIVER-GENCE (MRAD)	BEAM SHAPE	OUTPUT POWER/ENERGY	PULSE REP-RATE	PULSE WIDTH	BEAM IRRADIANCE/ RADIANT EXPOSURE ($W\ cm^{-2}$ or $J\ cm^{-2}$)	APPLICATION/ COMMENTS
LUMONICS TEA - 103 $CO_2 - N_2 - He$	IV	10600	3.81	2.10	CIRC	32.5 MW PEAK 9.75 J	1.00 P/S		$1.71\ W\ cm^{-2}$	RESEARCH & OEM PROVISIONAL -OSHA- CLASSIFICATION
METROLOGIC ML - 610 HELIUM NEON (HeNe)	IIIb	632.8	0.100	1.50	CIRC	1.00 mW	N/A		$2.59\ mW\ cm^{-2}$	RESEARCH & OEM
METROLOGIC ML - 680 HELIUM NEON (HeNe)	IIIb	632.8	0.100	1.00	CIRC	$1.50\ mW\ TEM_{00}$	N/A		$3.89\ mW\ cm^{-2}$	RESEARCH & OEM
METROLOGIC ML - 920 HELIUM NEON (HeNe)	IIIb	632.8	0.100	0.800	CIRC	$3.00\ mW\ TEM_{00}$	N/A		$7.78\ mW\ cm^{-2}$	RESEARCH & OEM
MOLECTRON SPECTROSCAN 10 DYE	IV	360.0 TO 740.0	0.030	1.50	CIRC	7.00 kW PEAK $35.0\ \mu J$	10.0 P/S 120	5.00 ns	$4.44\ mJ\ cm^{-2}$	RESEARCH & OEM
OPTICS TECHNOLOGY 170 HELIUM NEON (HeNe)	IIIb	632.8	0.100	1.00	CIRC	$3.00\ mW\ TEM_{00}$	N/A		$7.78\ mW\ cm^{-2}$	HOLOGRAPHY
ORIEL CORP. 6620 HELIUM NEON (HeNe)	IIIb	632.8		1.00	CIRC	$1.00\ mW\ TEM_{00}$	N/A		$2.59\ mW\ cm^{-2}$	RESEARCH & OEM
PERKIN ELMER 75 HELIUM NEON (HeNe)	IIIb	632.8	0.200	0.400	CIRC	1.00 mW	N/A		$2.59\ mW\ cm^{-2}$	RESEARCH & OEM
PHASE - R DL - 1000 DYE	IV	220.0 TO 950.0	1.00	3.00	CIRC	1.00 MW PEAK 0.500 J	0.100 P/S	$0.400\ \mu s$	$1.02\ J\ cm^{-2}$ 1.27	RESEARCH & OEM
PHOTON SOURCES 140 CARBON DIOXIDE (CO_2)	IV	10600	4.24	1.00	CIRC	250 W AVER	50.0 P/S	$10.0\ \mu s$ 100	$706\ nJ\ cm^{-2}$	RESEARCH & OEM NO LONGER MANU- FACTURED

TABLE E-1
LASER HAZARD CLASSIFICATION GUIDE (cont.)

MANUFACTURER/ MODEL ACTIVE MEDIUM	HAZARD CLASS (OSHA)	WAVE- LENGTH (NM)	DIA- METER (CM)	DIVER- GENCE (MRAD)	BEAM SHAPE	OUTPUT POWER/ENERGY	PULSE REP-RATE	PULSE WIDTH	BEAM IRRADIANCE/ RADIANT EXPOSURE ($W\,cm^{-2}$ or $J\,cm^{-2}$)	APPLICATION/ COMMENTS
QUANTRONIX 114-2 NEODYMIUM YAG (Nd YAG)	IV	1064	0.500	5.00	CIRC	9.00 W TEM_{00} 100 W MULTI	N/A		23.3 $W\,cm^{-2}$ 259	RESEARCH & OEM
RCA 40862 GAAS SINGLE DIODE	IIIb	905.0	(.1)	125		10.0 W PEAK	5.00 kHz	0.200 μs	5.18 $\mu J\,cm^{-2}$	RESEARCH & OEM PROVISIONAL-OSHA- CLASSIFICATION
RCA TA - 7763 GAAS SINGLE DIODE	IV	905.0	(.1)	125		2.00 kW PEAK	1000 P/S	0.200 μs	1.04 $mJ\,cm^{-2}$	RESEARCH & OEM
RCA TA - 7867 GAALAS	IIIb	855.0	(.1)	125		3.00 W PEAK	5.00 kHz	0.100 $\mu 2$	778 $nJ\,cm^{-2}$	RESEARCH & OEM PROVISIONAL-OSHA- CLASSIFICATION
SANTA BARBARA RC 32005 - TRANSMITTER GA - AS	I	904.0		5.00		2.00 W PEAK		100 ns	518 $nJ\,cm^{-2}$	COMMUNICATOR
SPECTRA PHYSICS 122 HELIUM NEON (HeNe)	IIIb	632.8				3.00 mW MULTI	N/A		7.78 $mW\,cm^{-2}$	RESEARCH & OEM
SPECTRA PHYSICS 123 HELIUM NEON (HeNe)	IIIb	632.8	0.900	1.30	CIRC	7.00 mW TEM_{00}	N/A		18.1 $mW\,cm^{-2}$	RESEARCH & OEM
SPECTRA PHYSICS 124 HELIUM NEON (HeNe)	IIIb	3390	0.110	1.00	CIRC	15.0 mW 30.0 mW MAX	N/A		1.90 $W\,cm^{-2}$ 3.81	RESEARCH & OEM
SPECTRA PHYSICS 125A HELIUM NEON (HeNe)	IIIb	632.8 3391 1152	0.700	7.00	CIRC	50.0 mW TEM_{00}	N/A		259 $mW\,cm^{-2}$	RESEARCH & OEM
SPECTRA PHYSICS 130 HELIUM NEON (HeNe)	IIIb	632.8	0.140	0.700	CIRC	2.00 mW TEM_{00} 0.100 mW TEM_{00}	N/A		5.18 $mW\,cm^{-2}$ 259 $\mu W\,cm^{-2}$	RESEARCH & OEM

TABLE E-1
LASER HAZARD CLASSIFICATION GUIDE (cont.)

MANUFACTURER/ MODEL ACTIVE MEDIUM	HAZARD CLASS (OSHA)	WAVE-LENGTH (NM)	DIA-METER (CM)	DIVER-GENCE (MRAD)	BEAM SHAPE	OUTPUT POWER/ENERGY	PULSE REP-RATE	PULSE WIDTH	BEAM IRRADIANCE/ RADIANT EXPOSURE (W cm^{-2} or J cm^{-2})	APPLICATION/ COMMENTS
SPECTRA PHYSICS 132 M HELIUM NEON (HeNe)	IIIb	632.8	0.100	5.00	CIRC	3.50 mW MULTI 6.00 mW MAX	N/A		9.07 mW cm^{-2} 15.6	RESEARCH & OEM
SPECTRA PHYSICS 133 HELIUM NEON (HeNe)	IIIb	632.8	0.090	1.00	CIRC	2.00 mW TEM$_{00}$ 4.00 mW MAX	N/A		5.18 mW cm^{-2} 10.4	RESEARCH & OEM
SPECTRA PHYSICS 133P HELIUM NEON (HeNe)	IIIb	632.8	0.070	1.20	CIRC	1.80 mW TEM$_{00}$ 4.00 mW MAX	N/A		4.67 mW cm^{-2} 10.4	RESEARCH & OEM
SPECTRA PHYSICS 141 ARGON (Ar)	IIIb	488.0 TO 514.5	0.160	0.700	CIRC	250 mW MULTI	N/A		648 mW cm^{-2}	RESEARCH & OEM
SPECTRA PHYSICS 165-00 ARGON (Ar)	IV	457.0 TO 514.5		0.500		2.00 W TEM$_{00}$ 6.00 mW MAX	N/A		5.18 W cm^{-2} 15.6	RESEARCH & OEM
SPECTRA PHYSICS 170-00 ARGON (Ar)	IIIb	351.1 TO 363.8	0.160	0.600	CIRC	140 mW TEM$_{00}$	N/A		13.9 W cm^{-2}	RESEARCH & OEM
SPECTRA PHYSICS 185 HELIUM CADMIUM (HeCd)	IIIb	441.6 TO 325.0	0.150	0.500	CIRC	50.0 mW TEM$_{00}$ 120 mW MAX	N/A		5.64 W cm^{-2} 13.5	RESEARCH & OEM
SPECTRA PHYSICS 833 TUNNEL LASER HELIUM NEON (HeNe)	IIIb	632.8				1.20 mW TEM$_{00}$ 2.20	N/A		3.11 mW cm^{-2} 5.70	LEVELING/ALIGNMENT
SPECTRA PHYSICS 944 LASER LEVEL SL HE NE	IIIb	632.8	0.660		CIRC	2.50 mW 3.00 mW MAX	N/A		6.48 mW cm^{-2} 7.78	LEVELING/ALIGNMENT
SYLVANIA 941 P & S CARBON DIOXIDE (CO$_2$)	IV	10600	0.500	5.00	CIRC	3.00 W TEM$_{00}$	N/A		30.5 W cm^{-2}	RESEARCH & OEM

TABLE E-1
LASER HAZARD CLASSIFICATION GUIDE (cont.)

MANUFACTURER/ MODEL ACTIVE MEDIUM	HAZARD CLASS (OSHA)	WAVE-LENGTH (NM)	DIA-METER (CM)	DIVER-GENCE (MRAD)	BEAM SHAPE	OUTPUT POWER/ENERGY	PULSE REP-RATE	PULSE WIDTH	BEAM IRRADIANCE/ RADIANT EXPOSURE ($W\,cm^{-2}$ or $J\,cm^{-2}$)	APPLICATION/ COMMENTS
SYLVANIA 948 CARBON DIOXIDE (CO_2)	IV	10600	0.600	5.00	CIRC	5.00 W TEM_{00} 10.0 W MULTI	N/A		35.3 W cm^{-2} 70.5	RESEARCH & OEM
TACHISTO TAC II-M215A CARBON DIOXIDE (CO_2)	IV	10600	0.600	3.00	CIRC	15.0 MW PEAK 2.00 J	0.200 TO 2.00 P/A	30.0 ns 50.0	5.29 J cm^{-2} 14.1	RESEARCH & OEM
TRICE V DEVELOPM. PLAN-O-LITE MOD.A HELIUM NEON (HeNe)	II	632.8	0.200 17.0	1.00 6280	RECT	3.50 mW	N/A		1.03 mW cm^{-2}	LEVELING/ALIGNMENT
UNITED AIRCRAFT J80 CARBON DIOXIDE (CO_2)	IV	10600		3.00		1.00 kW TEM_{00} 2.00 kW PEAK	N/A		127 kW cm^{-2}	RESEARCH & OEM
UNIVERSITY LABS 270 HELIUM NEON (HeNe)	IIIb	632.8	0.210	0.600	CIRC	10.0 mW TEM_{00}			25.9 mW cm^{-2}	RESEARCH & OEM
XEROX 200 He - Ne TELECOPIER	II ENCL	632.8	0.320		CIRC	0.850 mW	N/A		2.20 mW cm^{-2}	INT. ALARMS + COM. CLASS I AS ENCLOSED

Appendix F
Copy Machine Characteristics

TABLE F-1
SUMMARY OF RADIOMETRIC PARAMETERS
REPRESENTATIVE PRINTING AND GRAPHIC ARTS MACHINES

MANUFACTURERS MODEL NO.	LAMP TYPE	LAMP DIMENSIONS	APPROXIMATE LUMINANCE ($cd \cdot cm^{-2}$)	APPROXIMATE RADIANCE ($W \cdot cm^{-2} \cdot sr^{-1}$)	APPROXIMATE LUMINOUS EFFICACY (lm/W)	MAXIMUM IRRADIANCE AT GLASS PLATEN ($mW \cdot cm^{-2}$)	ENCLOSURE OR SHIELDING
Xerox 7000 (Console)	Xerox Type 122P209; Sylvania Type F23T8/WW/HO/35 Fluorescent	23" long 1" dia	1.3 (avg)	0.005	250	5.4	Rubber Matte Shield
Xerox 4000** (Console)	Xerox Type 122P316 (1 ea) Fluorescent	21" long 1.5" dia	3-4	0.01	250	1.4	Rubber Matte Shield
Xerox 3600-1 (Console)	Xerox Type 122P99*; GE Type F18T8/MG/XE Fluorescent, 12 ea	18" long 1" dia	1.3 (avg) 2.7 (max)	0.005 - 0.01	250	5.1	Rubber Matte Shield
Xerox 720 (Console)	Xerox Type 122P289 (2 ea)	18" long 1" dia	3	0.01	250	3	Rubber Matte Shield
Xerox 660-1 (desk copier)	Xerox Type 122P289 or 122P211 (2 ea) Fluorescent GE Type FP13/T5/GI6	13" long 0.62" dia	4	0.01	250	3	Metal Cabinet with Slot for Paper
Xerox 2400 CFP Computer Forms Printer	Xerox Type 122P118; F18T8/MG/XE GE Type F18T8/MG-XE Fluorescent	18" long " dia	3	0.01	250	NA	Shielded by Metal Cabinet
SCM Corp 111 (desk copier)	GE Type Q275T4/CL82 (2 ea) Tungsten Filament (300 W)	0.5" dia	750	10	75	10	Rubber Matte Shield
AB Dick 483-4600/ 625 (desk copier)	AB Dick Type 34442, Tungsten Filament 115 V, 600 W	11-1/2" long	1000	12	80	10	Metal Cover
Nu-Arc Platemaker Model FT-32 (Console)	Carbon Arc† 115 V, 17A 2kW	open arc	14,000	120	115	2.4	Shielded by Metal Cabinet

* Also used in Xerox Model 2400 Copying Machine
† Ultraviolet radiation hazard
** The Xerox 4500 has the same characteristics as the Xerox 4000

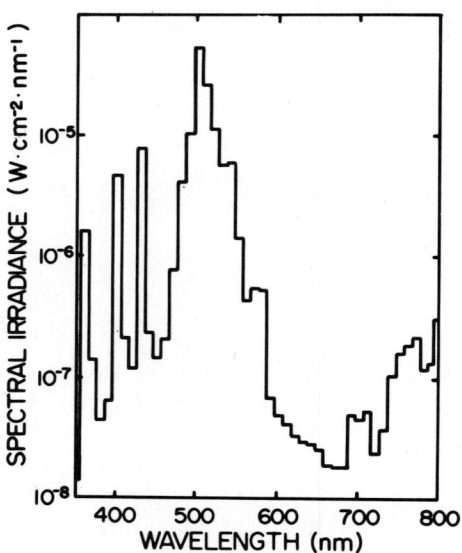

Figure F-1. Corneal Spectral Irradiance from Xerox Type 3600 Copier at Typical Viewing Height

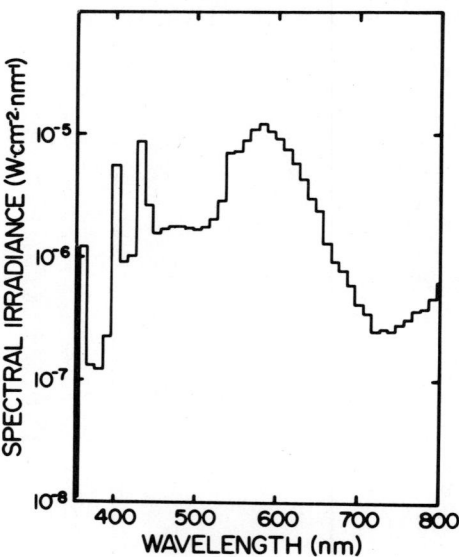

Figure F-2. Corneal Spectral Irradiance from Xerox Type 7000 Copier at Typical Viewing Height.

Copy Machine Characteristics

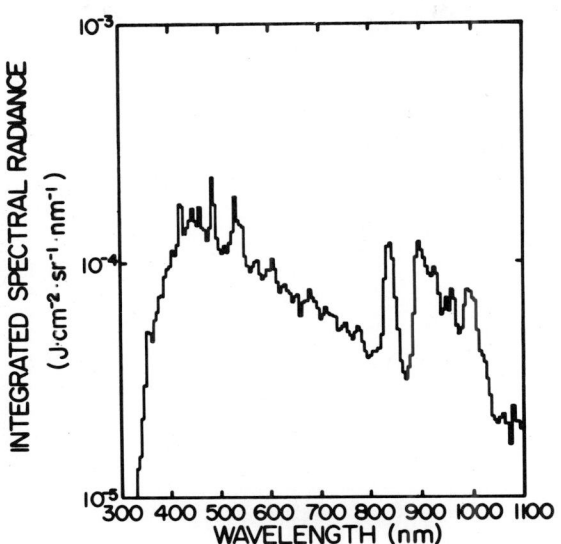

Figure F-3. Corneal Spectral Irradiance from Xerox Type 9200 Copier at Typical Viewing Height

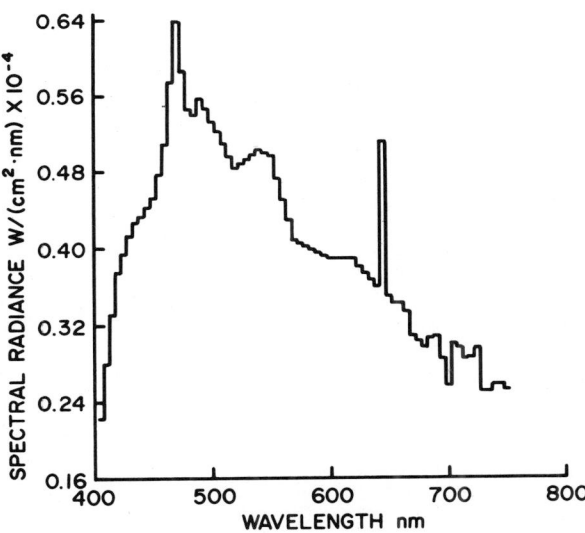

Figure F-4. Corneal Spectral Irradiance from Kodak Ektaprint 100 Copier at Typical Viewing Height.

TABLE F-2

LAMP RADIANCE CALCULATIONS FOR XEROX 3100

Wavelength λ (nm)	Spectral Radiance L_λ (W·cm^{-2}·sr^{-1}·nm^{-1})	Occ. Med. $T_\lambda \cdot A_\lambda$	Ret. Absorp. $L_\lambda \cdot T_\lambda \cdot A_\lambda$	Blue Haz. Factor R_λ	Blue Radiance $L_\lambda \cdot R_\lambda$ (W·cm^{-2}·sr^{-1}·nm^{-1})	Lum. Eff. V_λ	Photopic $L_\lambda \cdot V_\lambda$ (cd·cm^{-2}·nm^{-1}/680)
400	0.56	0.0	0	0.10	0.056	4 x 10^{-4}	----
405*	268	0.01	2.7	0.20	54	5.8 x 10^{-4}	0.16
410	0.46	0.05	0.02	0.40	0.18	1.2 x 10^{-3}	----
415	0.38	0.084	0.03	0.80	0.31	0.002	----
420	0.36	0.2	0.07	0.90	0.32	0.004	----
425	0.36	0.25	0.09	0.95	0.34	0.0065	----
430	0.53	0.30	0.16	0.98	0.52	0.012	----
435*	572	0.37	212	1.0	572	0.017	9.72
440	0.87	0.45	0.39	1.0	0.87	0.023	0.02
445	1.02	0.71	0.72	0.97	0.99	0.030	0.03
450	1.35	0.58	0.78	0.94	1.27	0.038	0.05
455	1.33	0.60	0.80	0.90	1.19	0.050	0.03
460	1.30	0.62	0.81	0.80	1.04	0.060	0.08
465	2.22	0.64	1.42	0.70	1.55	0.072	0.16
470	5.41	0.65	3.51	0.62	3.35	0.091	0.49
475	12.3	0.66	8.15	0.55	6.79	0.105	1.29
480	30.0	0.67	20.1	0.45	13.5	0.139	4.17
485	65.3	0.68	44.4	0.40	26.1	0.162	10.6
490	139	0.69	96.1	0.22	30.6	0.208	28.9
495	240	0.70	168	0.16	38.4	0.250	60.0
500	354	0.71	251	0.10	35.4	0.323	114
505	436	0.72	314	0.079	34.4	0.400	174
510	442	0.72	318	0.063	27.8	0.503	222
515	402	0.72	282	0.050	20.1	0.620	249
520	333	0.73	243	0.040	13.3	0.710	236
525	261	0.73	190	0.032	8.34	0.800	209
530	195	0.73	142	0.025	4.87	0.862	168
535	139	0.73	102	0.020	2.78	0.925	129
540	101	0.73	73.7	0.016	1.62	0.954	96
545*	424	0.74	314	0.013	5.5	0.980	416
550	47.2	0.74	34.9	0.010	0.47	0.995	46.8
555	32.8	0.75	24.6	0.008	0.26	1.0	32.8
560	22.4	0.75	16.8	0.006	0.13	0.995	22.2
565	15.0	0.75	11.2	0.005	0.075	0.97	14.5
570	10.4	0.76	7.87	0.004	0.041	0.95	9.8
575	7.40	0.76	5.62	0.0032	0.024	0.91	6.7
580*	95.4	0.74	70.6	0.0025	0.238	0.87	83.0
585	4.03	0.74	2.98	0.0020	0.008	0.81	3.3
590	3.39	0.73	2.48	0.0016	0.005	0.76	2.6
595	2.83	0.73	2.06	0.0013	0.004	0.71	2.0
600	2.93	0.73	2.14	0.001	0.003	0.63	1.85
605	2.32	0.72	1.67	0.001	0.002	0.58	1.34
610	0.8	0.72	0.59	0.001	<0.001	0.50	0.41
615 - 1005	----	---	----	----	-----	-----	<0.4
1010	.18	0.095	0.02	----	-----	0	----
1015	6.9	0.095	0.66	----	-----	0	----
1020	13.6	0.095	1.29	----	-----	0	----
1025	21.3	0.097	2.07	----	-----	0	----
1030	28.8	0.10	2.8	----	-----		----
1035	16.5	0.10	1.65	----	-----		----
1040	4.2	0.10	4.2	----	-----		----
1045 - 1125	----	---	----	----	-----	0	----
1130	5.6	0.13	0.73	----	-----	0	----
1135	9.7	0.12	1.17	----	-----	0	----
1140	7.5	0.12	0.90	----	-----		----
Summations	4680.74		2988.95		908.746		2356.4
Mult. by 5:	23403.7		14944.75		4543.82		11782

* Emission lines of Mercury

Data Summary: L = 23.4 mW·cm^{-2}·sr^{-1}; L(T·A) = 14.9 mW·cm^{-2}·sr^{-1}; L(blue) = 4.5 mW·cm^{-2}·sr^{-1}; L_v = 680(.01782) = 8.01 cd·cm^{-2}
Retinal Burn Hazard Factor R = 14.9/23.4 = 0.64
Luminous efficacy of radiation: K = 8.01 cd·cm^{-2} / 0.0234 W·cm^{-2}·sr^{-1} = 342 lm/W

Appendix G
Glossary of Terms Used in Welding and Biology

accommodation - the ability of the eye to adjust focus for various distances

aphakia - having no lens in the eye, e.g., after cataract removal

aqueous humor - fluid in the anterior chamber of the eye

base metal (material) - the metal (material) to be welded, brazed, soldered, or cut - see also substrate

blepharitis - inflammation of the eyelids

blepharospasm - spasm of eyelid muscles

blind spot - normal defect in visual field due to position at which optic nerve enters the eye

cataract - an opacity (cloudiness) of the lens

    incipient - any cataract in its early stages, or one which has sectors of opacity with clear spaces intervening

    congenital - one which originates before birth

    senile - a hard opacity of the lens occurring in the aged

    chorioretinitis - inflammation of the choroid and retina

choroid - vascular layer adjacent to the retina - its function is to nourish the retina

coalescence - the growing together or growth into one body of the materials being welded

cone, retinal - specialized visual cell in the retina; the cones are responsible for sharpness of vision and color vision

conjunctiva - the delicate membrane that lines the eyelids and covers the exposed surface of the eyeball

constricted arc (plasma arc welding and cutting) - a plasma arc column that is shaped by a constricting nozzle orifice

constricting nozzle (plasma arc welding and cutting) - a water cooled copper nozzle surrounding the electrode and containing the constricting orifice

constricting orifice (plasma arc welding and cutting) - the hole in the constricting nozzle through which the arc passes

contact tube - a device which transfers current to a continuous electrode

CO_2 welding - see preferred term gas metal arc welding

direct current electrode negative - the arrangement of direct current arc welding leads in which the work is the positive pole and the electrode is the negative pole of the welding arc - see also straight polarity

direct current electrode positive - the arrangement of direct current arc welding leads in which the work is the negative pole and the electrode is the positive pole of the welding arc - see also reverse polarity

direct current reverse polarity (DCRP) - see reverse polarity and direct current electrode positive

direct current straight polarity (DCSP) - see straight polarity and direct current electrode negative

electrode -

    arc welding electrode - a component of the welding circuit through which current is conducted between the electrode holder and the arc - see arc welding

    bare electrode - a filler metal electrode consisting of a single metal or alloy that has been produced into a wire, strip, or bar form and that has had no coating or covering applied to it other than that which was incidental to its manufacture or preservation

    covered electrode - a composite filler metal electrode consisting of a core of a bare electrode or metal cored electrode to which a covering sufficient to provide a slag layer on the weld metal has been applied - the covering may contain materials providing such functions as shielding from the atmosphere, deoxidation, and arc stabilization and can serve as a source of metallic additions to the weld

flux cored electrode - a composite filler metal electrode consisting of a metal tube or other hollow configuration containing ingredients to provide such functions as shielding atmosphere, deoxidation, arc stabilization and slag formation - alloying materials may be included in the core - external shielding may or may not be used

metal cored electrode - a composite filler metal electrode consisting of a metal tube or other hollow configuration containing alloying ingredients - minor amounts of ingredients providing such functions as arc stabilization and fluxing of oxides may be included - external shielding gas may or may not be used

tungsten electrode - a non-filler metal electrode used in arc welding or cutting, made principally of tungsten

electrode extension (gas metal arc welding, flux cored arc welding, submerged arc welding) - the length of unmelted electrode extending beyond the end of the contact tube during welding

electrode holder - a device used for mechanically holding the electrode while conducting current to it

electrode lead - the electrical conductor between the source of arc welding current and the electrode holder

electrode setback (plasma arc welding and cutting) - the distance the electrode is recessed behind the constricting orifice measured from the outer face of the nozzle

emmetropia - a state of perfect vision

etiology - the cause of a disease

flash blindness - temporary visual disturbance resulting from viewing an intense light source

flux cored arc welding (FCAW) - an arc welding process which produces coalescence of metals by heating them with an arc between a continuous filler metal (consumable) electrode and the work - shielding is provided by a flux contained within the tubular electrode - additional shielding may or may not be obtained from an externally supplied gas or gas mixture - see flux cored electrode

flux cored electrode - see electrode

fovea - a depression or pit in the center of the macula; it is the area of clearest vision

fundus - the interior surface of a hollow organ, as the retina of the eye

fusion - the melting together of filler metal and base metal (substrate), or of base metal only, which results in coalescence - see depth of fusion

fusion welding - any welding process or method which used fusion to complete the weld

gas metal arc welding (GMAW) - an arc welding process which produces coalescence of metals by heating them with an arc between a continuous filler metal (consumable) electrode and the work - shielding is obtained entirely from an externally supplied gas or gas mixture - some methods of this process are called MIG or CO_2 welding

gas tungsten arc welding (GTAW) - an arc welding process which produces coalescence of metals by heating them with an arc between a tungsten (nonconsumable) electrode and the work - shielding is obtained from a gas or gas mixture - pressure may or may not be used and filler metal may or may not be used (this process has sometimes been called TIG welding)

ground connection - an electrical connection of the welding machine frame to the earth for safety - see also work connection and work lead

ground lead - see preferred term work load

gun - arc welding gun - in semiautomatic, machine, and automatic welding, a manipulating device to transfer current and guide the electrode into the arc - it may include provisions for shielding and arc initiation

heat-affected zone - that portion of the base metal which has not been melted, but whose mechanical properties or microstructure have been altered by the heat of welding, brazing, soldering, or cutting

inert gas - a gas which does not normally combine chemically with the base metal or filler metal - see also protective atmosphere

inert- gas metal arc welding - see preferred term gas metal arc welding

inert-gas tungsten arc welding - see preferred term gas tungsten arc welding

infrared radiation - electromagnetic energy with wavelengths from 770 nm to 12000 nanometers

iritis - inflammation of the iris

irradiance - (E) - radiant flux (radiant power) per unit area incident upon a given surface [units of W/cm^2]

keratitis - inflammation of the cornea; usually characterized by loss of transparency and dullness

keyhole - a technique of welding in which a concentrated heat source penetrates completely through a workpiece forming a hole at the leading edge of the molten weld metal - as the heat source progresses, the molten metal fills in behind the hole to form the weld bead

lens, crystalline - lens of the eye: a transparent biconvex body situated between the anterior chamber (aqueous) and the posterior chamber (vitreous) through which the light rays are further focused on the retina - the cornea provides most of the refractive power of the eye

lenticular (adj) - pertaining to the lens of the eye

machine welding - welding with equipment which performs the welding operation under the constant observation and control of a welding operator - the equipment may or may not perform the loading and unloading of the work - see automatic welding

macula - an oval area in the center of the retina devoid of blood vessels; the area most responsible for color vision

manual welding - a welding operation performed and controlled completely by hand - see automatic welding, machine welding, and semiautomatic welding

MIG welding - see preferred terms gas metal arc welding, flux cored arc welding

miosis - reduction in the size of the pupil

molten weld pool - the liquid state of a weld prior to solidification as weld metal

nanometer - 10^{-9} meter, preferred unit for wavelength in the ultraviolet, visible and near-infrared spectral region

nontransferred arc (plasma arc welding and cutting, and thermal spraying) - an arc established between the electrode and the constricting nozzle - the workpiece is not in the electrical circuit - see transferred arc

nozzle - a device which directs shielding media

opacity - the condition of being nontransparent, a cataract

open-circuit voltage - the voltage between the output terminals of the welding machine when no current is flowing in the welding circuit

ophthalmologist - a medical practitioner specializing in the medical and surgical care of the eyes

ophthalmoscopy, direct - the observation of an upright mirrored image of the interior of the eye through the use of an ophthalmoscope

ophthalmoscopy, indirect - the observation of an inverted image of the interior of the eye

optic disc - the portion of the optic nerve within the eye which is formed by the meeting of all the retinal nerve fibers at the level of the retina

orbit - the cavity in the skull which contains the eyeball

orifice gas (plasma arc welding and cutting) - the gas that is directed into the torch to surround the electrode - it becomes ionized in the arc to form the plasma, and issues from the orifice in the torch nozzle as the plasma jet

orifice throat length (plasma arc welding and cutting) - the length of the constricting orifice

parent metal - see preferred term base metal

photophobia - abnormal sensitivity to and discomfort from light

pigment epithelium - a layer of cells in the retina containing pigment granules

pilot arc (plasma arc welding) - a low current continuous arc between the electrode and the constricting nozzle to ionize the gas and facilitate the start of the main welding arc

plasma - a gas that has been heated to an at least partially ionized condition, enabling it to conduct an electric current

plasma arc cutting (PAC) - an arc cutting process which severs metal by melting a localized area with a constricted arc and removing the molten material with a high velocity jet of hot, ionized gas issuing from the orifice

plasma arc welding (PAW) - an arc welding process which produces coalescence of metals by heating them with a constricted arc between an electrode and the workpiece (transferred arc) or the electrode and the constricting nozzle (nontransferred arc) - shielding is obtained from the hot, ionized gas issuing from the orifice which may be supplemented by an auxiliary source of shielding gas - shielding gas

Glossary 993

may be an inert gas or a mixture of gases - pressure may or may not be used, and filler metal may or may not be supplied

plenum (plasma arc welding and cutting, and thermal spraying) - the space between the inside wall of the constricting nozzle and the electrode

polarity - see direct current electrode negative, direct current electrode positive, straight polarity, and reverse polarity

pterygium - a growth of the conjunctiva considered to be due to a degenerative process caused by long continued irritation as from exposure to wind, dust, and possibly to ultraviolet radiation

puddle - see preferred term molten weld pool

pupil - the opening at the center of the iris of the eye for the transmission of light - the pupil size varies from 2 mm to 8 mm

radiance - ($\underline{L}$) - radiant flux (power) output per unit solid angle per unit area [units of $W/cm^2 \cdot sr$]

retina - the innermost coat of the posterior part of the eyeball, surrounding the vitreous body and responsible for vision

sclera - the tough, white, protective coat of the eye

scotoma - a blind or partially blind area in the visual field

semiautomatic arc welding - arc welding with equipment which controls only the filler metal feed - the advance of the welding is manually controlled

shielded metal arc welding (SMAW) - an arc welding process which produces coalescence of metals by heating them with an arc between a covered metal electrode and the work - shielding is obtained from decomposition of the electrode covering - pressure is not used and filler metal is obtained from the electrode

shielding gas - protective gas used to prevent atmospheric contamination

slit-lamp - an instrument producing a slender beam of light for illuminating any reasonably transparent structure, as the cornea, or lens

stick electrode - see electrode: covered electrode

stick electrode welding - see preferred term shielded metal arc welding

stickout - see preferred term electrode extension

strabismus - squint; failure of the two eyes simultaneously to direct their gaze at the same object because of muscle imbalance

straight polarity - the arrangement of direct current arc welding leads in which the work is the positive pole and the electrode is the negative pole of the welding arc - a synonym for direct current electrode negative

substrate - any base material to which a thermal sprayed coating or surfacing weld is applied

tear film - microscopically thin lipid film which constantly bathes cornea

torch - see preferred terms welding torch, cutting torch, spray torch

transferred arc (plasma arc welding) - a plasma arc established between the electrode and the workpiece

tungsten electrode - see electrode: tungsten electrode

vision, photopic - vision attributed to cone function characterized by the ability to discriminate colors and small detail; daylight vision

vision, scotopic - vision attributed to rod function characterized by the lack of ability to discriminate colors and small detail and effective primarily in the detection of movement and low luminous intensities - night vision

visual acuity - ability of the eye to sharply perceive the shape of objects in the direct line of vision

visual axis - the central line of gaze

visual cortex - final station of visual impulses in the brain; sensory area of brain responsible for vision

visual field - the area of physical space visible to an eye in a given position

vitreous or vitreous body - transparent, colorless mass of soft gelatinous material filling the posterior chamber of the eyeball (behind the lens)

weld - a localized coalescence of metals or nonmetals produced either by heating the materials to suitable temperatures, with or without the application of pressure, or by the application of pressure alone, and with or without the use of filler

welder - one who performs a manual or semiautomatic welding operation (sometimes erroneously used to denote a welding machine) welding - a materials joining process used in making welds (see the Master Chart of Welding and Allied Processes)

welding current - the current in the welding circuit during the making of a weld - in resistance welding, the current used during a preweld or postweld interval is excluded

welding electrode - see preferred term electrode

welding generator - a generator used for supplying current for welding

welding ground - see preferred term work connection

welding head - the part of a welding machine or automatic welding equipment in which a welding gun or torch is incorporated

welding leads - the work lead and electrode lead of an arc welding circuit

welding machine - equipment used to perform the welding operation - for example, spot welding machine, arc welding machine, seam welding machine, etc.

welding operator - one who operates machine or automatic welding equipment

welding procedure - the detailed methods and practices including all joint welding procedures involved in the production of a weldment - see joint welding procedure

welding processes - a materials joining process which produces coalescence of materials by heating them to suitable temperatures, with or without the application of pressure or by the application of pressure alone, and with or without the use of filler metal (see the Master Chart of Welding and Allied Processes)

welding rectifier - a device in a welding machine for converting alternating current to direct current

welding rod - a form of filler metal used for welding or brazing which does not conduct the electrical current

welding tip - a welding torch tip designed for welding

welding torch - a device used in oxyfuel gas welding or torch brazing for mixing and controlling the flow of gases

welding transformer - a transformer used for supplying current for welding - see also reactor (arc welding)

welding wire - see preferred terms electrode and welding rod

weld metal - that portion of a weld which has been melted during welding

weld metal area - the area of the weld metal as measured on the cross section of a weld

weldor - see preferred term welder

wire feed speed - the rate of speed in mm/s or in/min at which a filler metal is consumed in arc welding or thermal spraying

wire straightener - a device used for controlling the cast of coiled wire to enable it to be easily fed into the gun

work connection - the connection of the work lead to the work

work lead - the electric conductor between the source of arc welding current and the work

Appendix H
Sources of US Government Publications

Many publications of US Government Agencies are referenced in this text—in the US these are available at cost from NTIS, Springfield, Va.

NTIS has established a worldwide network of agents from whom NTIS documents can be obtained. If you are ordering from one of the eight countries specified below, you must order from the applicable NTIS agent; orders sent directly to NTIS will be returned. Prices of NTIS publications may vary with each agent. It is therefore recommended that you first contact your agent before ordering. If you are ordering from countries other than the eight specified, you may send your order to NTIS in the United States. Payment is required in US currency.

If you order from:

England Ireland Scotland Wales	Microinfo Ltd. The Post House High Street Alton, Hampshire GU34 1ES England
The Netherlands	NTIS Nederland Intermediair Postbus 3842 1000/AT Amsterdam The Netherlands
Japan	Mitsubishi Research Institute 8-1, Yuraku-Cho 1-Chome Chivoda-Ku Tokyo 100 Japan

Brazil	Nucleo de Informacoes Technologicas Barroslearn Producoef Didaticas Ltda Rua 24 de Maio, 62 Caixa Postal 6182 01000 Sao Paula - S.P. Brazil
Mexico	INFOTEC/CONACYT Division NTIS Aptdo. Postal 19-194 Mexico 12, D. F. Mexico-19, D. F.
All other countries	National Technical Information Service Springfield, Virginia 22161 U.S.A.

You may now use Visa or Master Charge for purchases from the Superintendent of Documents, Government Printing Office, Washington, DC 20402. Include your credit card number, Master Charge Interbank number and expiration date (month and year) with each order.

Appendix I
Hammer Safety

HAMMER SAFETY
By Richard C. Honey, Ph.D.

Reprinted from: Journal of Occupational Medicine, 10:245-246, May 1968, American Medical Occupational Association, 150 N. Wacker Drive, Chicago, Illinois 60606. With permission.

In developing codes of safe practice one often loses perspective of the relative magnitude of the hazard in question in relation to other hazards encountered in every day life. A number of articles have appeared in recent years to point out the problems when this perspective is lost. The best of those on Laser Safety was written by Dr. Richard Honey of Stanford Research Institute and is reprinted in part below. Dr. Honey was intimately concerned with the development of laser safety standards and from his experiences he distilled the following model code for the safe use of hammers. Although Dr. Honey's style is definitely "tongue-in-cheek", he nevertheless captures the exaggerated concern of some early laser standards formulators who felt that the only "safe" laser was one lacking emission.

I would like to describe today a series of experiments that we have conducted over the past two and one-half years on the hazards of the hammer. We have found that those instruments, so long a household item, have unsuspected dangers associated with their use. To wit, biologic tissue that has been struck with the hammer is subject to a rapid series of compression and decompression waves that are reflected and refracted through adjacent tissues in a manner that results in damage, and in extreme cases, to the destruction and death of the tissue. This sensitivity to damage has gone wholly undetected and even unsuspected for years.

In a series of experiments utilizing 2,571 mice, of which 1,321 were tested and 1,250 were controls, it was found that the destruction of tissue resulting from a hammer blow to the back of the cranial cavities of the experimental animals resulted in the deaths of 100% of the experimental animals, while 99.44% of the control mice survived. All of the experimental animals had identical portions of the epidermis on their cranial cavities exposed by careful shaving of all protective hair covering from the area.

Although the statistics resulting from the data reported above were quite startling, and quite convincing, nevertheless, it was felt that further investigation of the experimental results was necessary to determine, if possible, whether or not any uncontrolled variables had influenced the data. Therefore, autopsies were performed on all 2,571 mice. It was found that intracranial hemorrhages had occurred in all the tested animals; none had occurred in the controls. The deaths of the animals were attributed primarily to these hemorrhages. Upon careful examination, it was found that the seven deaths in the control group of 1,250 mice could be attributed to unrelated causes. Three deaths were the result of uncontrolled infections due to slight cuts in the cranial cavity. The other four deaths were from undetermined causes—although it was surmised that they may have been due to old age since the experiment extended over a much greater period of time than originally estimated. A check of the birth records of all mice involved indicated that these four mice were among the oldest in the entire group of control mice.

Therefore, it must be concluded that the hammer has some serious hazards associated with its use that have not been fully appreciated in the past—hazards that may limit the further extension of its use in the construction industry. However, realizing that the hammer has an enviable record and shows great promise as a means of expeditiously driving nails into wood, and that this is an essential element in the home construction industry, the following recommendations have been devised to insure the continued safe use of the hammer:

1. Never subject biologic tissue to a direct impact from a hammer.
2. All hammers should be contained within some suitable shield so that uninformed personnel who may be working or passing through an area cannot be injured by accidental exposures. Signs should be posted warning all persons that hazards exist within the room.
3. Some audible or visual signal should be used to indicate that a hammer is to be used. This warning should not call attention to the hammer, but rather away from it.
4. Flesh or biologic tissue should not be used as a detector for hammer blows. This is especially true since rebounds are difficult to predict and can make off-axis observation as dangerous as on-axis observation.
5. Operate the hammers whenever possible in well lighted rooms. This will keep the pupil of the eye small and, thus, provide more acute vision, and greater depth-of-field.
6. Look away or close the eyes during the count-down before the firing signal to avoid any possible rebound if the procedure dictates the use of an unshielded hammer.
7. If the hammer is to be used over distances greater than the length of an enclosed room, special precautions must be used to prevent accidental exposure to persons who may find themselves in the path. Hammers can do damage at distances up to several hundred feet depending on the conditions. A curious bystander can receive serious injury.
8. Any accident involving persistent pain should be reported immediately for medical attention.
9. The screens used for hammer demonstrations should be thick, soft and absorbent. Every precaution should be taken to prevent any type of rebound from hard, smooth surfaces during such a demonstration.
10. Protective mats (straight-jackets) should be provided for personnel protection. Some jackets protect against only certain types of hammers and must be

selected to match their design characteristics with the characteristics of the hammer. Some jackets may lose their protective ability after an initial exposure, and must be checked to assure that they retain adequate protective characteristics.

11. Keep left hand in pocket during countdown. If the experimental design does not permit this, fold left thumb out of point of impact.

Although it is realized that the experiments described above do not encompass all of the important cases, it is felt that these preliminary results were sufficiently alarming to warrant publication before the remaining data is accumulated.

Detailed recordings of typical pressure waves that propagate throughout the cranial cavity during the course of an experiment have been obtained. This was achieved using transducers implanted into the cranial cavity of the experimental animal prior to an experiment. The outputs of the transducers were recorded on high-frequency oscillographs, and it is felt that the records are accurate up to the precise moment when the hammer contacted each transducer during the course of each experiment.

Experiments in progress and planned for the future include:

1. *In situ measurements with mice:* Tests with mice from which no hair will be removed from the back of the cranial cavity, and no artificial constraints will be utilized to hold the mice in a fixed position. Some observers have felt that the holding devices may have killed the experimental animals. Unfortunately, the control mice in the reported experiment were not tested in the same holding device to test their survival rate. A special technician has been in training for the past four months, and has so refined the technique that he can strike a uniform hammer blow to the back of the cranial cavities of mice on the run with a 99.8% probability of success.

2. *In situ measurements with monkeys:* A similar series of experiments is planned using rhesus monkeys, since they have cranial cavities that more nearly resemble human cranial cavities. However, the training of a technician for this task has met with unexpected difficulties. Unless the rhesus monkeys have been suitably tranquilized, they can dodge any hammer blow administered even by the most agile technician tested to date. In fact, some of the slower technicians have been the victims of aggressive counter attacks by the rhesus monkey. All have survived to date, however. The careful training of one of the rhesus monkeys to perform this task is in progress.

3. *In situ measurements with humans:* Human volunteers have been solicited through the medical profession to contribute to this important project. Since these will be voluntary patients, it is not anticipated that any special holding devices will be required for them. Furthermore, the tests will begin immediately with unshaved specimens since it will more nearly approximate the hazard situation that exists in real life.

Author Index

Aaberg, T.M. [Machemer *et al.*] 788
Abbott, C. E. [Dalziel *et al.*] Chapter 28
Abel, L. A. Chapter 20
Adams, D. O. Chapter 4 [Adams *et al.*] 236
Adams, R. M. Chapter 27
Adhav, R. S. Chapter 15
Adler, F. H 72, 77
Agarwal, L. P. 202
Albrecht, R. [Noell and Albrecht] 134,
 [Noell and Albrecht] Chapter 6,
 [Noell and Albrecht] Chapter 7
Alcarez, E. C. [Livingston *et al.*] Chapter 13
Alcock, A. J. [Walker and Alcock] Chapter 11
Alexander, R. W. Chapter 26
Allen, L. Chapter 2
Allen R. E. [Bartoli *et al.*] Chapter 11
 [Kruer *et al.*] Chapter 11
Allen, R. G. [Gibbons and Allen] Chapter 4
 [Gibbons and Allen] 238 [Gibbons and Allen] 510
Altemeier, W. A. [Goldman *et al.*] Chapter 17
Altman, J. H. Chapter 12
Altobelli, K. K. [Hemstreet *et al.*] 245
Alvarado, J. A. [Hogan, Alvarado and Waddell] 71
AMA Council on Physical Medicine Chapter 10
American Conference of Governmental Industrial Hygienists Chapter 1, 170, Chapter 8, 221, Chapter 9, 337, 499, Chapter 19, Chapter 24, 900, 903, 907, 910
American Heart Association Chapter 28
American Industrial Hygiene Association Chapter 27
American Medical Association Department of Environmental Publicity and Occupational Health Chapter 24

American National Standards Institute 1, Chapter 8, Chapter 9, Chapter 10, 515, 542, 572, Chapter 18, Chapter 19, Chapter 20, 845, 847, 862, 879, 880, Chapter 27
American Society for Testing and Materials (ASTM) Chapter 24
Ames, A. E. [Bird *et al.*] Chapter 12
Andelin, J. P., Jr. [Title *et al.*] Chapter 11
Anderson, F. A. Chapter 7
Anderson, R. R. [Parrish *et al.*] 174
 [Parrish *et al.*] Chapter 10
Anderson, W. J. 549, 550
Andreou, D. Chapter 11
Andrews, J. R. [Lawton and Andrews] Chapter 11
Anglin, J. H., Jr. [Everett *et al.*] Chapter 5
Angstrom, A. K. 449
Arams, F. R. [Melchior *et al.*] Chapter 11
Armstrong, C. E. 509
Arnaud, J. A. Chapter 2, 369
Arndt, K. A. [Fitzpatrick *et al.*] Chapter 3
Arnold, G. P. [Greiner *et al.*] Chapter 11
Arnulf, A. 85
Asakura, T. [Yoshida and Asakura] 394
Ash, G. S. Chapter 22
Ashby, L. Chapter 10
ASPEN Systems Corporation Center for Compliance Information Chapter 27
Auth, D. C. [Gulacsik *et al.*] 577, Chapter 17
Avizonis, P. V. Chapter 12

Bachem, A. 113, Chapter 5
Badger, H. L. [McSparron *et al.*] Chapter 17
Bailey, N. A. Chapter 17
Baker, B. N. [Williams and Baker] 134
Baker, D. J. [Gardiner *et al.*] Chapter 12
Baker, D. W. [Harding and Baker] Chapter 17

Baker, H. J. Chapter 11
Ball, R. J. [Bartley and Ball] Chapter 4
Barnes, F. S. 132
Barstow, F. E. [Edgerton and Barstow] 752
Bartholomew, R. V. [Thursby et al.] 543
Bartley, D. L. 822
Bartley, S. H. Chapter 4
Bartoli, F. Chapter 11 [Kruer et al.] Chapter 11
Bason, F. C. [Sliney, Bason and Freasier] 353 [Sliney et al.] Chapter 11 [Sliney et al.] Chapter 14 [Sliney et al.] Chapter 19 [Sliney et al.] 776
Basov, N. G. Chapter 2
Bates, C. C. Chapter 24
Bates, C. E. [Wren et al.] 557 [Wren et al.] 558
Bauer, G. Chapter 11, Chapter 14, 538
Baum, W. A. Chapter 22
Baumann, C. A. [Rusch, Kline and Baumann] 175
Beatrice, E. S. [Frisch et al.] 102 [Frisch, Beatrice and Holst] 104 [Frisch, Beatrice and Holsen] 130, 132 [Zwick et al.] 137 [Adams et al.] Chapter 4, 233 [Adams et al.] 236 [Zwick and Beatrice] 237 [Beatrice and Frisch] 238 [Stuck et al.] 244 [Stuck et al.] 245 [Frisch et al.] Chapter 7 [Stuck et al.] Chapter 8, Chapter 13
Bebie, H. [van der Zypen et al.] 143
Beck, G. Chapter 11
Beck, W. C. 747, Chapter 23
Becklund [Williams and Becklund] Chapter 2
Becklund, O. A. [Williams and Becklund] Chapter 14
Bedell, R. B. [Adams et al.] Chapter 4 [Adams et al.] 236
Behrendt, T. [Clarke and Behrendt] 202 [Clarke and Behrendt] 203
Beiser, L. Chapter 20
Bekshaw, A. Ya. [Grimblatov et al.] Chapter 12
Bell, L. [Verhoeff, Bell and Walker] 117 [Verhoeff, Bell and Walker] 137 [Verhoeff, Bell and Walker] 147
Bell, W. E. [Sinclair and Bell] Chapter 2 [Sinclair and Bell] Chapter 12
Benary, V. [Riva et al.] 584
Benedek, G. B. 67
Bener, P. 193

Bennett, A. P. Chapter 24
Beran, M. Chapter 2, 425
Berger, D. 172, 330, 454, Chapter 23
Berggvist, T. Chapter 4
Bernstein, H. N. [Bernstein et al.] Chapter 4
Berry, C. Z. [Dahling et al.] Chapter 16
Berry, F. [Herreman et al.] Chapter 19
Berry, E. R. [Geeraets and Berry] 87 [Geeraets and Berry] 89 [Geeraets and Berry] 118 [Geeraets and Berry] 119 [Geeraets and Berry] 120 [Geeraets and Berry] 121 [Geeraets and Berry] Chapter 24
Berson, E. L. Chapter 6
Bettelheim, F. A. [Bettelheim and Kumbar] Chapter 3
Bickford, E. D. [Levin et al.] Chapter 22 Chapter 22
Bird, G. R. Chapter 12
Birky, M. M. Chapter 12
Birnbaum, G. Chapter 11
Birnbaum, M. Chapter 11
Birngruber, R. [Gabel et al.] 120 [Gabel, Birngruber and Hillenkamp] 127, Chapter 4 [Hillenkamp et al.] Chapter 4 [Wallow et al.] Chapter 7
Bitt, S. [Bitt et al.] Chapter 2
Bixler, H. A. [Spencer and Bixler] 538 [Spencer and Bixler] 543
Blabla, J. 594
Blackmon, W. Chapter 11
Blackwell, H. R. [Fry et al.] Chapter 4 [Bredemeyer et al.] 218
Blais, B. R. [Marlor et al.] Chapter 6
Blancard, P. 509
Blankenship, E. A. [Wick et al.] Chapter 12
Blevin, W. R. Chapter 11
Block, W. H. Chapter 11
Blonk, K. [Blancard et al.] 509
Bloom, A. L. Chapter 12
Blum, H. F. 172
Bode, H. G. Chapter 5
Boettner, E. A. 107, 118, 119 [Boettner and Wolter] 119, 121, Chapter 4, Chapter 7
Boivin, L. P. Chapter 11
Boogaard, J. [Munnik and Boogaard] 119 [Vos et al.] Chapter 4
Borish, I. M. 549, 550
Borkman, R. F. [Kurzel et al.] 115 [Lerman et al.] Chapter 4
Borland, R. B. [Borland et al.] 148

Author Index

Borland, R. G. 233, 235, 239
Born, M. Chapter 2, Chapter 23
Borwein, B. 106
Bostrom, R. G. 341
Bourzina, S. [Thoss and Bourzina] Chapter 3
Boyd, G. D. [Boyd and Gordon] Chapter 12
Boyden, D. G. [Marlor et al.] Chapter 6
 [Curtin and Boyden] Chapter 15, 486
 [Curtin and Boyden] 509
Boyne, H. S. 370
Boynton, R. M. Chapter 4
Bradley, D. J. 367
Bredemeier, H. [Campbell et al.] 148 [Stellar et al.] Chapter 17
Bredemeyer, A. [Bredemeyer et al.] 218
Bredemeyer, H. G. [Bredemeyer et al.] 218
Brennan, D. H. [Borland et al.] 148 [Borland et al.] 233 [Borland et al.] 235 [Borland et al.] 239, Chapter 26
Bresler, R. R. Chapter 22
Bresnick, G. H. Chapter 4 [Bresnick et al.] 219, 230, 231 [Lund et al.] 240
Bridger, J. M. [Saunders et al.] Chapter 14
Bridges, J. M. 733
Bridges, T. J. Chapter 11 Bridges,
Bridges, W. G. 407
Briffa, D. V. Chapter 22
Brinton, H P. [Dreessen et al.] Chapter 24
Bristow, M. P. F. Chapter 11
British Standards Institute Chapter 16, Chapter 18
Brooks, J. 162 [Schmidt et al.] Chapter 5 [Schmidt et al.] Chapter 6
Brown, D. J. [Randall, Brown and Sloan] 90
Brown, J. L. 139
Brownell, A. S. 168, 240
Bruce, W. R. [Skeen et al.] 219 [Skeen et al., b] 219 [Skeen et al., a and b] 244 [Hemstreet et al.] 245 [Skeen et al., a and b] 245 [Ward and Bruce] Chapter 7 [Skeen et al.] 280
Buck, A. L. Chapter 13
Bucker, H. Chapter 5
Buckler, M. J. 644
Buettner, K. 162, 165
Burch, D. E. Chapter 13
Burch, J. M. [Burch and Gates] Chapter 17
Bureau of Radiological Health (BRH) 1, 597
Burkes, W. T. [Mayyasi et al.] Chapter 4
Burkhart, J. [Geeraets et al.] Chapter 4 [Geeraets, Burkhart and Guerry] 237

Burnett, N. H. [Offerberger et al.] Chapter 11
Burnham, D. C. Chapter 12
Burnham, R. [Eden et al.] Chapter 2
Burns, W. Chapter 27
Burt, J. E. Chapter 14
Buser, R. G. Chapter 13
Butler, J. K. [Kressel and Butler] Chapter 11
Buzawa, M. J. [Hopkins and Buzawa] Chapter 20
Byer, R. L. [Roundy et al.] Chapter 11

Cain, C. P. Chapter 4
Calkins, J. L. [Hochheimer and Calkins] 751, 787, Chapter 23
Campbell, C. J. 148
Campbell, D. L. Chapter 24
Campbell, F. W. [Westheimer and Campbell] 85 [Campbell and Green] 85 [Campbell and Gubisch] 85 [Westheimer and Campbell] Chapter 4
Campbell, J. H. Chapter 22
Carlson, F. P. Chapter 2, 400
Carman, R. L. [Thomas et al.] Chapter 11
Carothers, M. L. [Sliney et al.] 335, [Sliney et al.] 369 [Sliney et al.] 445
Carpenter, J. A. 219
Carter, A. O. [Morley and Carter] 924
Carter, T. J. Chapter 24
Carver, C. [Lund et al.] 240
Case, W. E. [Geist et al.] Chapter 11
Castren, J. A. Chapter 28
Cavonius, D. R. Chapter 4, Chapter 7
Champagne, L. F. [Eden et al.] Chapter 2
Chan, G. [Geeraets et al.] 120
Chang, C. [Trosko and Chang] 227
Chang, H. [Vassiliadis et al.] Chapter 4
Chang, T. Y. [Bridges et al.] Chapter 11
Charbonneau, D. G. [Dobrowolski et al.] 556
Charlton, D. Chapter 20
Charschan, S. S. Chapter 2, Chapter 15, 609, 862
Chatterjee, A. 211
Cheng, S. S. [Runge and Cheng] Chapter 20
Cheo, P. K. [Bridges et al.] Chapter 11
Chernov, L. A. Chapter 13
Chester, J. E. [Lund et al.] 240
Chestnut, R. W. [Kourvenhoven et al.] Chapter 28
Chianta, M. A. [Stoll and Chianta] 557

Chick, E. W. [Hudnell and Chick] Chapter 4
Chin, S. L. [Girard et al.] Chapter 15
Ching, F. C. Chapter 6
Chisum, G. T. 139, 140
Choo, T. S. Chapter 24
Christensen [Kaufman and Christensen] 704
 [Kaufman and Christensen] 705
 [Kaufman and Christensen] 708
 [Kaufman and Christensen] 712
 [Kaufman and Christensen] 768
Churchkova, M. 450
Claesson, S. Chapter 5
Clark, A. M. [Moon et al.] 237 [Geeraets and Clarke] Chapter 22
Clark, B. A. H. 826
Clark, C. Chapter 5
Clark, G. W. [Levin et al.] Chapter 22
Clark, G. W. [Bickford et al.] Chapter 22
Clark, I. M. [McKinlay et al.] Chapter 22
Clark, J. H. Chapter 10
Clark, W. H. Jr. [Fitzpatrick et al.] Chapter 3
Clarke, A. M. [Ham et al.] 134 [Ham et al.] 135 [Ham et al.] 137 [Moon et al.] 137, 202, 203 [Ham et al.] 219 [Ham et al.] 237, 242 [Ham et al.] 594
Clayton, F. E. [Clayton and Clayton] Chapter 27
Clayton, G. D. Chapter 27
Cleary, S. F. 132 [Ham et al.] Chapter 4 [Ham et al.] 219 [Ham et al.] 237 [Ham et al.] 594
Clifford, S. F. Chapter 13
Cloud, T. M. Chapter 4
Coakley, J. M. [Bostrom and Coakley] 341 [Peterson et al.] Chapter 11, 445 [Envall et al.] 525 [Envall et al.] 528
Cobb, S. Chapter 4
Coblentz, W. W. 172, 330, 542, Chapter 24
Cochrane, A. L. [Wallace and colleagues] 147
Cogan, D. G. [Cogan and Kinsey] 110, 111, 112, 202 [Kinsey et al.] Chapter 24
Cole, C. [Forbes et al.] Chapter 22
Coleman, L. W. [Thomas et al.] Chapter 11
Collins, B. A. [MacNichol et al.] 137
Combs, G. F., Jr. 252
Commission International de l'Eclairage 19, 20, 55, 525, Chapter 20, 694
Committee on Photobiology 737
Committee on Light Sources of the IES Chapter 22

Connolly, J. S. [Zuclich and Connolly] 109 [Hemstreet et al.] 245
Considine, P. S. 128, Chapter 4
Coogan, P. S. 79, 120 [Lappin and Coogan] 134 [Lappin and Coogan] 219 [Lappin and Coogan] 236 [Lappin and Coogan] 238
Cook, R. B. 539, 543
Cooper, B. [Jacobson and co-workers] 146
Cope, F. W. Chapter 7
Cordes, F. D. 206
Cornsweet, T. N. Chapter 3
Cortorillo, S. F. [Thouret et al.] Chapter 22
Cotton, G. [Machta et al.] 191
Coulson, K. L. Chapter 6
Council on Physical Medicine Chapter 22
Cram, L. S. [Mullaney et al.] 584
Crawford, B. H. 69 [Stiles and Crawford] 92 [Stiles and Crawford] 93 [Stiles and Crawford] 118
Crescitelli, F. Chapter 21
Cripps, D. J. 172, 176
Crissman, H. A. [Mullaney et al.] 584
Crockett, S. [Lawwill et al.] 134 [Lawwill et al.] 136 [Lawwill et al.] 137 [Lawwill et al.] 238
Crookes, Sir William 542
Cuff, K. F. [Emmons et al.] Chapter 11
Cullen, A. P. [Pitts, Cullen and Hacker] 110 [Pitts and Cullen] 113 [Pitts, Cullen and Hacker] 114
Cumin, B. Chapter 11
Cunningham, L. [Thorington et al.] Chapter 22
Currier, G. [Lawwill et al.] 134 [Lawwill et al.] 136 [Lawwill et al.] 137 [Lawwill et al.] 238
Curtin, T. L. Chapter 15, 486, 509
Curtis, J. [Bernstein et al.] Chapter 4
Cushman, W. H. Chapter 4
Cutchen, J. T. [Harris and Cutchen] 543
Cylus, L. [Willis and Cylus] Chapter 5

Dabbert, W. F. 423, 429
D'Agati, A. P. [McClatehey and D'Agati] Chapter 13
Dahlberg, J. A. Chapter 24
Dahling, R. F. Chapter 16
Dall'Acqua, F. [Pathak et al.] Chapter 4
Dallas, A. G. [Bresnick et al.] Chapter 4 [Bresnick et al.] 219 [Bresnick et al.] 230 [Bresnick et al.] 231

Author Index

D'Aloisio, L. [Forbes et al.] Chapter 22
Dalziel, C. F. 917, 198, Chapter 28
Daniels, F., Jr. Chapter 5 [Johnson and Daniels] Chapter 5 [Johnson et al.] Chapter 5
Dankovic, D. [Boettner and Dankovic] Chapter 4 [Boettner and Dankovic] Chapter 7
D'Anna, S. [Hochheimer et al.] Chapter 23
Dannheim, F. 143
Daroff, R. B. [Abel et al.] Chapter 20
Daugherty, J. D. [Jacob et al.] Chapter 11
Davidoff, R. A. Chapter 4
Davidson, S. Chapter 4
Davies, J. M. 163, Chapter 6
Davies, J. R. Chapter 4
Davies, R. E. [Berger, Urbach and Davies] 172 [Berger et al.] 330 [Forbes et al.] Chapter 22
Davis, T. P. 164, 594
Davson, H. 98
Decker, C. D. Chapter 15, 893, 894
Dedrick, K. G. [Vassiliadis et al.] Chapter 4 [Vassiliadis et al.] Chapter 7 [Vassiliadis et al.] Chapter 10
DeGroot, A. J. [Smith et al.] 393
de Groot, S. G. 69, Chapter 4
Deitz, P. H. 423, 424 [Livingston et al.] Chapter 13
Delisle, C. [Girard et al.] Chapter 15
de la Claviere, B. [Arnaud et al.] 396
Dell'Osso, L. F. [Abel et al.] Chapter 20
Delmelle, M. Chapter 4
Del Valle, P. F. [Sliney et al.] Chapter 9 [Sliney et al.] Chapter 15 [Marshall et al.] 811 [Marshall et al.] 822 [Marshall et al.] 823 [Marshall et al.] 825 [Marshall et al.] 826 [Marshall et al.] 828 [Marshall et al.] 835 [Marshall et al.] 845 [Marshall et al,] 847 [Lyon et al.] 811 [Lyon et al.] 816 [Lyon et al.] 835 [Lyon et al.] 847
Denault, G. C. [Spencer et al.] Chapter 13
Dennis, J. E. [Smith and Dennis] 633
Department of the Air Force Chapter 1
Department of the Army Chapter 1
Derzko, Z. [Weseley and Derzko] 423
Devore, R. K. 822
Dewan, E. M. Chapter 4
Dewey, H. J. [Geist et al.] Chapter 11
Dezenburg, G. J. Chapter 27
Dickinson, A. B. Chapter 22

Dickson, L. D. 397
Diffey, B. L. 193
Dimitroff, J. M. [Jacquez et al.] 165
DIN Chapter 10
Ditchburn, R. W. Chapter 2, 79, 524
Dixon, E. M. Chapter 26
Djeu, N. [Eden et al.] Chapter 2
Dobrowolski, J. A. 556
Doda, D. D. [Garrisson et al.] 192
Donohue, D. [Eden et al.] Chapter 2
Doran, C. K. [Everett et al] Chapter 5
Doss, T. T. [Avizonis et al.] Chapter 12
Douglas, C. A. [McSparron et al.] Chapter 17
Dowdy, C. [Herreman et al.] Chapter 19
Doxey, B. C. 618, 619
Doyle, W. M. 357, 358, 359
Dratz, E. A. [Katz et al.] Chapter 4 [Stone et al.] Chapter 4
Dressen, W. C. Chapter 11
Dreffner, R. Chapter 19
Drinker, P. [Kinsey et al.] Chapter 24
Drummond, A. J. Chapter 11 [Angstrom and Drummond] 449
Dudley, W. W. 44
Duggar, B. C. [Williams and Duggar] 543
Duguay, M. A. Chapter 11
Duke-Elder, S. 68, 143, 146, 147, 830
Duley, W. W. Chapter 19
Dunkelman, L. [Baum and Dunkelman] Chapter 22
Dunn, K. L. 147
Dunsky, I. L. 219, 238 [Ebbers and Dunsky] 245 [Ebbers and Dunsky] Chapter 7, Chapter 21
Dunster, J. Chapter 10
Duntley, S. O. [Edwards et al.] Chapter 5
Dupuy, O. [Arnulf and Dupuy] 85

Eaglesfield, C. C. Chapter 2
Earl, F. L. [Bernstein et al.] Chapter 4
Ebbers, R. W. 114, 245, Chapter 7 [Thursby et al.] 543
Eberle, W. J. [Smith et al.] Chapter 25
Eberli, B. [Riva et al.] 584
Eby, J. Chapter 22
Eccles, J. C. 206, 794
Eckerle, K. L. Chapter 14
Edebrooke, C. M. Chapter 24
Eden, G. Chapter 2
Edgerton, H. E. 752
Edwards, E. Chapter 5
Edmunds, H. D. 644

Edwards, J. G. Chapter 11
Egbert, D. E. 79, 240, 254
Ehrenkranz, T. E. Chapter 28
Eisen, A. Z. [Fitzpatrick et al.] Chapter 3
Electronic Industries Association Chapter 9
Elenbaa, W. Chapter 14
Elgin, S. [Cavonius et al.] Chapter 4
　　[Cavonius et al.] Chapter 7
Ellenbass, W. 33, Chapter 22
Ellingson, O. L. Chapter 11
Elterman, L. Chapter 13
Elterman, P. B. Chapter 17
Emmett, E. A. 801, Chapter 24 [Horstman et al.] Chapter 24
Emmons, R. B. Chapter 11
Emsley, H. H. 98
Eng, J. [Dobrowolski et al.] 556
English, P. E. Chapter 24
English, W. P. Chapter 24
Engstrom R. W. Chapter 11, 418, 419
Enroth-Cugell, C. [Robson and Enroth-Cugell) Chapter 21
Entwhistle, H. 839
Envall, K. R. 525, 528, 744
Eppers, W. Chapter 13
Epstein, D. [Tengroth and Epstein] Chapter 26
Epstein, J. H. Chapter 5 [Willis et al.] Chapter 5
Ernest, 76
Eroshenko, L. E. [Machev and Eroshenko] Chapter 24
Esterowitz, L. [Bartoli et al.] Chapter 11 [Kruer et al.] Chapter 11
Evans, E. 162 [Schmidt et al.] Chapter 5 [Schmidt et al.] Chapter 6
Evans, R. M. [Pattee et al.] Chapter 24
Everett, H. D. [Everett et al.] Chapter 5
Everett, M. A. [Sayre, Olson and Everett] 172, 173, 174 [Olson et al.] Chapter 5 330
Ewald, R. A. 206
Eymers, J. G. [Fischer and co-workers] 146

Falconer, I. S. Chapter 11
Falkenstein, W. [Penzkofer and Falkenstein] Chapter 11
Fallon, J. P. Chapter 12
Fankhauser, F 233, Chapter 7
Faraone, G. Chapter 28
Farmery, C. [Bennett et al.] Chapter 24
Farrer, D. N. [Ham et al.] 237
Fears, T. R. [Scotto et al.] Chapter 6

Feke, G. T. [Riva et al.] 584
Fender, D. H. Chapter 3, Chapter 15, Chapter 18
Ferris, L. P. Chapter 28
Ferry, J. J. Chapter 24
Feyman, R. P. Chapter 2
Fidler, J. P. [Goldman et al.] Chapter 17
Fife, W. A. [Dunsky et al.] Chapter 21
Findlay, G. H. Chapter 5
Findley, G. B. [Green et al.] Chapter 5
Fine, B. S. [MacKeen et al.] Chapter 4 [Tso et al.] Chapter 4, 240
Fine, S. [MacKeen et al.] Chapter 4
Finkelstein, N. [Edwards et al.] Chapter 5
Finley, R. D. [Young and Finley] Chapter 6
Finney, D. J. 232
Firester, A. H. [Gorog et al.] 45, 396
Fischer, F. P. 146
Fisher, E. 175
Fisher, M. B. [Melchior et al.] Chapter 11
Fishlock, D. Chapter 2
Fite, K. V. Chapter 21
Fitzpatrick, T. B. Chapter 3 [Parrish et al.] Chapter 4 [Pathak et al.] Chapter 4 174, 177, 178, 179 [Parrish et al.] Chapter 5 [Pathak et al.] Chapter 5, Chapter 6, Chapter 15 [Parrish et al.] 553, Chapter 16 [Parrish et al.] Chapter 22
Flamant, F. 69
Fligsten, K. G. Chapter 11
Flocks, M. [Vassiliadis et al.] Chapter 4
Florian, H. J. Chapter 17
Flowers, W. 119, 120
Flynn, A. J. [Eccles and Flynn] 206 [Eccles and Flynn] 794
Flynn, J. A. F. 208
Fong, C. W. Chapter 10 [Piltingsrud and Fong] 752
Forbes, P. D. Chapter 22
Fordon, L. [MacDonald and Fordon] 137 [MacDonald and Fordon] 207
Foulks, G. N. Chapter 4
Fowles, G. R. Chapter 2
Fox, R. E. 543, Chapter 21
Fox, S. H. [Goldman et al.] Chapter 17
Franco, S. C. Chapter 28, 924
Francom, M. Chapter 2
Franke, E. A. [Arnaud et al.] 396
Franke, J. M. [Arnaud et al.] 396
Frankhauser, F. [van der Zypen et al.] 143
Franks, J. K. [Sliney et al.] 87, 88 [Sliney et al.] Chapter [Sliney et al.] Chapter 9 [Sliney et al.] Chapter 15

Frant, R. Chapter 24
Franzen, D. L. Chapter 11
Fraunfelder, F. T. 199, Chapter 28
Frazier, G. F. [Scherman and Frazier] Chapter 19
Freasier, B. C. [Sliney and Freasier] 122 [Sliney and Freasier] 124 [Sliney and Freasier] 125 [Sliney and Freasier] 126 [Sliney and Freasier] 171 [Sliney and Freasier] Chapter 6 [Sliney and Freasier] 330 [Sliney and Freasier] 335 [Sliney and Freasier] 336 [Sliney and Freasier] 337 [Sliney, Bason and Freasier] 353 [Sliney et al.] Chapter 11 [Sliney et al.] Chapter 14 [Sliney and Freasier] 542 [Sliney et al.] Chapter 19, 655 [Sliney and Freasier] 668 [Sliney and Freasier] 698 [Sliney and Freasier] 724 [Sliney and Freasier] 727 [Sliney and Freasier] 729 [Sliney and Freasier] 730 [Sliney and Freasier] 732 [Sliney et al.] 776, Chapter 23 [Sliney and Freasier] 852
Freeman, R. G. 172, 173, 330 [Berger et al.] 454
Fridovich, I. 252
Fried, D. L. Chapter 13
Friedmann, A. I. Chapter 26
Friend, J. [Foulks et al.] Chapter 4
Frisch, G. D. 102, 104, 130 [Bresnick et al.] Chapter 4 [Bresnick et al.] 219 [Bresnick et al.] 230 [Bresnick et al.] 231 [Beatrice and Frisch] 238, Chapter 7 [Beatrice and Frisch] Chapter 13
Fry, G. A. Chapter 4
Fuller, D. 788
Fuller, J. E. [Dressen et al.] Chapter 24

Gabel, V. P. 120, 127 [Birngruber et al.] Chapter 4 [Hillenkamp et al.] Chapter 4 [Wallow et al.] Chapter 7
Gaddy, O. L. [Block and Gaddy] Chapter 11
Gafafer, W. M. Chapter 27
Gamaleya, N. F. 577
Garbor, D. Chapter 20
Garbuny, M. Chapter 2, Chapter 14
Gardiner, H. A. B. Chapter 12
Gardner, C. S. Chapter 21
Garrisson, L. M. 192

Garza, C. G. [Skeen et al.] 219 [Skeen et al.] 219 [Skeen et al. a and b] 244 [Skeen et al. a and b] 245 [Skeen et al.] 280
Gates, D. M. 189
Gates, J. W. C. [Burch and Gates] Chapter 17
Gauer, O. [Hausser and Gauer] Chapter 5
Gawenda, M. C. [Moss and Gawenda] 838
Gebel, R. K. H. [Anderson and Gebel] 549 [Anderson and Gebel] 550, 551
Gebhard, J. W. [DeGroot and Gebhard] 69 [DeGroot and Gebhard] Chapter 4
Gebhardt, G. 426, 431, 432
Geeraets, W. J. 87, 89, 118, 119, 120 [Geeraets and Berry] 120, 121, 134 [Ham et al.] 135, Chapter 6 [Ham et al.] Chapter 6 [Ham et al.] 218 [Ham et al.] 219 [Geeraets, Burkhart and Guerry] 237 [Farrer, Ham et al.] 237 [Clarke et al.] 242, Chapter 7 [Ham et al.] 543 [Ham et al.] 549 [Ham et al.] 594, Chapter 22, Chapter 24, Chapter 26
Gehring, P. Chapter 10
Geist, [Doyle, McIntosh and Geist] 357 [Blevin and Geist] Chapter 11, Chapter 11
Geller, M. [Mooradian et al.] Chapter 13
General Electric Company Chapter 22
Ger, R. [Kaplan et al.] Chapter 17
Gerathewohl, S. J. Chapter 4, Chapter 6 [Gerathewohl and Strughold] 223
Giacomotti, L. [Hiller and colleagues] 211
Gibbons, M. G. Chapter 13
Gibbons, W. [Pitts and Gibbons] 110
Gibbons, W. D. Chapter 4, 238, 245, 510
Gibson, A. F. Chapter 11
Gibson, G. L. M. Chapter 7
Giel, C. [Kleinfeld et al.] Chapter 24
Gillham, E. J. Chapter 14
Gilmartin, T. J. Chapter 13
Ginsburg, B. L. Chapter 4
Girard, A. Chapter 15
Glaros, S. S. [Manes et al.] Chapter 11
Glaser, P. E. Chapter 14
Glauser, S. C. Chapter 22
Glick, D. [Marich et al.] Chapter 17 [Marich et al.] Chapter 27
Glickstein, S. S. 809, 810, 811
Goedertier, P. V. [Gorog et al.] 45
Goldberg, B. [Klein and Goldberg] 190

Goldman, A. I. 132, 133, Chapter 7
Goldman, H. 143, 145
Goldman, J. R. Chapter 17
Goldman, L. 101, 167, 168, [Rockwell and Goldman] 169, 169, Chapter 8, Chapter 15, 577, Chapter 20 [Powell et al.] Chapter 24
Goncz, J. H. Chapter 22
Goodeve, C. G. Chapter 3
Goodson, J. E. Chapter 20
Goody, R. M. Chapter 6
Gordon, J. P. [Boyd and Gordon] Chapter 12
Gori, G. B. [Scotto et al.] Chapter 6
Gorog, I. 45
Gould, J. C. [Makous and Gould] Chapter 20
Gracheva, M. E. Chapter 13
Grahm, E. S. [Farrer, Ham et al.] 237
Graham, C. H. 93
Graham, P. A. [Wallace and colleagues] 147
Grant, W. B. 907
Gray, D. E. Chapter 15
Graymore, C. N. Chapter 3
Green, A. C. [Martt et al.] Chapter 22
Green, A. E. S. Chapter 5 [Garrisson et al.] 192, Chapter 6 [Johnson et al.] Chapter 6, Chapter 15
Green, D. G. [Campbell and Green] 85, 584
Green, J. B. Chapter 4
Green, S. I. Chapter 11
Greenwood, R. A. [Scherr et al.] 521
Greiner, N. R. Chapter 11
Griffin, A. C. [Cloud et al.] Chapter 4
Grimblatov, V. M. Chapter 12
Grover, D. Chapter 4
Grum, F. [Altman et al.] Chapter 12
Gryvnak, D. A. [Burch et al.] Chapter 13
Gubisch, R. W. [Campbell and Gubisch] 85, 124, 125, 242, Chapter 7, 687
Guerry, D., III [Geeraets et al.] 120 [Ham et al.] 135 [Geeraets et al.] Chapter 4 [Geeraets, Burkhart and Guerry] 237
Gulacsik, C. 577
Gullberg, K. Chapter 7
Gungle, W. C. [Waymouth et al.] Chapter 22
Gunn, S. R. Chapter 11
Gupta, M. N. 138, 833
Gurvich, A. S. [Gracheva and Gurvich] Chapter 13
Guth, S. K. Chapter 22

Haas, R. A. [Manes et al.] Chapter 11
Hacker, P. D. [Pitts, Cullen and Hacker] 110 [Pitts, Cullen and Hacker] 113 [Pitts, Cullen and Hacker] 114
Hadland, R. 367
Hadley, M. E. Chapter 6
Haertling, G. H. Chapter 16
Haith, M. Chapter 23
Hakim, R. [Cloud et al.] Chapter 4
Hall, R. B. [Pond et al.] Chapter 11
Halliday, D. Chapter 2, 82
Ham, W. R. [Schmidt et al.] Chapter 5
Ham, W. T. Jr. 79 [Geeraets et al.] 120 [Goldman et al.] 133, 134, 135, 136, 137 [Moon et al.] 137 [Evans et al.] 162, 201, 206 [Schmidt et al.] Chapter 6, 218 [Ham et al.] 219 [Mueller and Ham] 236 [Moon et al.] 237 [Farrar, Ham et al.] 237, 238 [Mueller and Ham] 240 [Clarke et al.] 242 [Mueller and Ham] 254 [Goldman et al.] Chapter 7 [Ham, Mueller and Sliney] 336, 543, 549, 594, 792
Hamerski, W. 112
Hammer, W. 474, 475
Hammell, H. T. [Hardy and co-workers] 162 [Hardy and co-workers] 165
Hanna, C. [Fraunfelder and Hanna] 199 [Fraunfelder and Hanna] Chapter 28
Hansson, H. A. Chapter 4
Harber, L. C. [Fitzpatrick et al.] Chapter 3 [Fitzpatrick et al.] 174 [Fitzpatrick et al.] 177 [Fitzpatrick et al.] 178 [Fitzpatrick et al.] 179 [Fitzpatrick et al.] Chapter 15
Harding, D. C. Chapter 17
Hardy, J. D. Chapter 3, 162, 165 [Clark et al.] Chapter 5, Chapter 6
Harlen, F. [McKinlay et al.] Chapter 22 [Bennett et al.] Chapter 24
Harley, R. D. [Peckham and Harley] 136 [Peckham and Harley] 138 [Peckham and Harley] 210
Harosi, F. I. [MacNichol et al.] 137
Harrington, D. O. Chapter 3
Harris, J. M. [Waymouth et al.] Chapter 22
Harris, J. O., Jr. 543
Hartman, B. [Gullberg et al.] Chapter 7
Hartmann, B. [Berggvist et al.] Chapter 4
Harwerth, R. S. 134, 135, 137 [Sperling and Harwerth] 237
Hass, G. 853

Author Index

Hass, W. [Machta et al.] 191
Hasselbalch, K. A. Chapter 5
Hatch, T. F. Chapter 7
Hatfield, E. M. 137, Chapter 6
Hathaway, J. A. 881
Hattenburg, A. T. Chapter 22
Hausser, I. Chapter 5
Hausser, K. W. 171, 172, 188
Hawkins, S. R. [Emmons et al.] Chapter 11
Hawley, J. G. [Grant and Hawley] 907
Hayes, J. R. 120, 128, 132, 133 [Vassiliadis et al.] 138
Hayworth, B. Chapter 28
Hazzard, G. Chapter 10
Health Care Facilities Subcommittee Chapter 22
Heaney, J. [Hass et al.] 853
Heard, H. G. Chapter 11, Chapter 12
Hecht, J. Chapter 20
Hedblom, E. E. 549
Hedinger, R. A. [Green and Hedinger] Chapter 6
Heffner, D. K. Chapter 11
Heimburger, R. F. [Beck and Heimburger] 747 [Beck and Heimburger] Chapter 23
Heimlich, R. [Avizonis et al.] Chapter 12
Heins, A. P. Chapter 24
Heller, M. E. [Firester et al.] 396
Hemstreet, H. W. 245
Henderson, S. T. Chapter 6, 752
Henriques, F. C., Jr. 162 [Moritz and Henriques] Chapter 5
Henkes, H. E. 509
Henry, D. E. [Rentschler et al.] 456
Herreman, G. O. Chapter 19
Herzberger, M. Chapter 2
Hicken, G. K. Chapter 24
Hickey, J. 646
Hildebrandt, A. F. 791
Hill, J. H. [Chisum and Hill] Chapter 4
Hill, R. J. Chapter 13
Hillenkamp, F. [Gabel et al.] 120 [Gabel, Birngruber and Hillenkamp] 127 [Birngruber et al.] Chapter 4, Chapter 4 [Wallow et al.] Chapter 7, Chapter 17
Hiller, R. 211
Hinricks, J. F. 811, Chapter 24
Hirleman, E. D. Chapter 12
Hoag, A. A. Chapter 12
Hoag, E. 615

Hochheimer, G. 584 [Calkins and Hochheimer] 751, 787, Chapter 23
Hogan, J. Chapter 24
Hogan, M. J. 71
Hogger, D. Chapter 24
Hogue, J. M. [Coblentz, Stair and Hogue] 172
Hoikkala, M. [Marshall et al.] 811 [Marshall et al.] 822 [Marshall et al.] 823 [Marshall et al.] 825 [Marshall et al.] 826 [Marshall et al.] 828 [Marshall et al.] 835 [Marshall et al.] 845 [Marshall et al.] 847
Holladay, L. L. 141 [Luckiesh, Holladay and Taylor] 172, Chapter 22
Hollyfield, J. G. Chapter 3
Holm, D. M. [Mullaney et al.] 584
Holmberg, B. Chapter 7
Holsen, R. C. [Frisch et al.] 102 [Frisch Beatrice and Holsen] 130 [Frisch et al.] Chapter 7
Holst, G. C. [Bresnick et al.] 219 [Bresnick et al.] 230 [Bresnick et al.] 231 [Robbins et al.] Chapter 7, Chapter 16
Holst, G. E. [Frisch, Beatrice and Holst] 104 [Bresnick et al.] Chapter 4
Honey, R. C. [Vassiliadis et al.] Chapter 4
Hopkins, R. E. Chapter 20
Hora, H. [Schwarz and Hora] Chapter 19
Hori, Y. [Pathak et al.] Chapter 5
Hornby, P. [Goldman et al.] Chapter 15 [Goldman and Hornby] Chapter 17
Hornell, A. Chapter 24
Horst, J. W. [Ingram and Horst] Chapter 24
Horstman, S. W. 801, Chapter 24
Hortman, S. W. [Emmett and Hortman] Chapter 24
Hosey, A. D. Chapter 27
Howett, G. L. Chapter 23
Hoyaux, M. F. Chapter 24
Hoyle, R. C. [Riggle et al.] 577
Hubbard, W. M. [Arnaud et al.] 396
Hubner, H. J. [Bauer et al.] 538 [Sutter et al.] 826, 829 [Sutter et al.] 840 [Sutter et al.] 841 [Sutter et al.] 849 Chapter 24
Hudnell, A. B. Chapter 4
Hudson, H. T. [Freeman et al.] 172 [Freeman et al.] 173 [Owens et al.] Chapter 5 [Freeman et al.] 330
Hudson, R. D., Jr. 362, 420

Hudson, J. W. [Hudson and Hudson] Chapter 11
Hudson, R. J. Jr. Chapter 2
Hughes, J. P. [Proctor et al.] Chapter 27
Hughes, W. F. [Coogan et al.] 79 [Coogan et al.] 120
Hurvich, L. M. [Jameson and Hurvich] Chapter 3
Huss, J. [Jacquez et al.] 165
Hutzler, P. [Hillenkamp et al.] Chapter 17
Hysell, D. K. [Brownell et al.] 168

Iceland, W. F. Chapter 19
Illuminating Engineering Society Chapter 10, 702, Chapter 23
Ingelstam, E. Chapter 17
Ingram, J. W. Chapter 24
International Electrotechnical Commission Chapter 8, 310, Chapter 15
International Standards Organization Chapter 2
Iris, L. [Blancard et al.] 509
Ivey, H. F. Chapter 22

Jackson, C. E. [Hicken and Jackson] Chapter 24, Chapter 24
Jackson, D. A. Chapter 22
Jackson, J. K. [Stair et al.] Chapter 14
Jacob, J. H. Chapter 11
Jacobs, I [Hardy et al.] Chapter 6, Chapter 20
Jacobson, H. J. 509
Jacobson, J. H. 146
Jacquez, J. A. 165
Jaeger, T. [Mooradian et al.] Chapter 2
Jako, G. J. [Snow et al] 581
James, R. H. Chapter 11 [Peterson et al.] Chapter 11
Jameson, D. Chapter 3
Jander, S. Chapter 19
Jankow, R. [Cook and Jankow] 539 [Cook and Jankow] 543
Jaramillo, J. G. [Lytle et al.] Chapter 15
Jayson, J. K. [Maas et al.] Chapter 22
Jenkins, D. [Zwick and Jenkins] 128 [Zwick and Jenkins] 633
Jenkins, D. L. 583 Chapter 11
Jenkins, F. A. Chapter 2
Jerome, C. W. [Sanders and Jerome] Chapter 22
John, J. [Blabla and John] 594
Johnson, B. E. [Daniels et al.] Chapter 5 Chapter 5

Johnson, E. G. Chapter 12
Johnson, F. S. Chapter 6
Johnson, G. [Ullrich and Johnson] 501 [Ullrich and Johnson] 503
Johnson, J. Chapter 22, Chapter 23
Johnson, J. C. Chapter 11
Johnson, L. C. [Davidoff and Johnson] Chapter 4
Johnston, W. L. [Mayyasi et al.] Chapter 4
Johnson, W. T. [Dabbert and Johnson] 423
Jones, A. E. 239
Jones, D. G. C. [Allen and Jones] Chapter 2
Jones, O. C. Chapter 14
Jones, R. C. [Bird et al.] Chapter 12
Joseph, A. S. Chapter 11
Josephy, P. D. [Dobrowolski et al.] 556
Judd, J. R. [Kouwenhoven et al.] Chapter 28
Juhlin, L. [Claesson et al.] Chapter 5

Kahn, G. Chapter 16
Kalugin, V. V. [Grimblatov et al.] Chapter 12
Kamibayashi, T. Chapter 11
Kaplan, Z. Chapter 17
Kasha, M. Chapter 14
Kashuba, V. A. Chapter 19
Kaste, R. C. [Sliney et al.] 335 [Sliney et al.] 369 [Sliney et al.] 445
Katz, M. L. Chapter 4 [Stone et al.] Chapter 4
Kaufman, J. E. 704, 705, 708, 712, 768
Kee, H. [Thouret et al.] Chapter 22
Keenan, R. G. [Dressen et al.] Chapter 24
Keesey, J. C. Chapter 28
Keeton, W. T. [Kreithen and Keeton] 684
Kellen, P. F. [Fallon and Kellen] Chapter 12
Kelly, K. L. [Howett et al.] Chapter 23
Kerr, J. R. Chapter 13
Kershaw, D. C. [Campbell and Kershaw] Chapter 22
Ketcham, A. S. [Riggle et al.] 577
Key, M. M. [Powell et al.] Chapter 24
Khitun, V. A. Chapter 4
Kimmitt, M. F. [Gibson et al.] Chapter 11
Kholodilou, A. A. [Novikov and Kholodilnu] Chapter 16
Kiesling, G. A. Chapter 20
Kinder, J. [Hillenkamp et al.] Chapter 17
King, B. G. [Ferris et al.] Chapter 28
King, T. A. [Baker and King] Chapter 11

Kingslake, R. Chapter 2
Kinsey, V. E. [Cogan and Kinsey] 110 [Cogan and Kinsey] 111 [Cogan and Kinsey] 112, 118, Chapter 24
Klang, G. Chapter 4
Klauder, J. R. Chapter 2
Kleiber, D. A. [Maas et al.] Chapter 22
Klein, M. V. Chapter 22, 768, 769
Klein, R. M. 449
Klein, W. H. 190
Kleinfeld, M. Chapter 24
Kleman, B. [Berggvist et al.] Chapter 4
Klenk, K. F. [Green et al.] Chapter 5
Kletz, T. A. Chapter 10
Kligman, A. 174 [Willis et al.] Chapter 5
Kline, B. E. [Rusch, Kline and Baumann] 175
Kline, M. V. Chapter 2 [Kline and Ray] Chapter 2
Knave, B. [Levin et al.] Chapter 24
Kneidielt [Horstman et al.] Chapter 24
Knickerbocker, G. G. [Kouwenhoven et al.] Chapter 28
Knighton, R. W. [Fuller et al.] 788
Knowles, P. [Ravitch et al.] Chapter 28
Knox, J. D. [Gorog et al.] 45
Knox, J. M. [Freeman et al.] 172 [Freeman et al.] 173 [Ogura and Knox] Chapter 5 [Owens et al.] Chapter 5 [Freeman et al.] 330
Knudtzon Chapter 6
Koch, E. J. [Krizek and Koch] Chapter 22
Kock, E. [Gullberg et al.] Chapter 7
Koechner, W. Chapter 2
Kogelnick, H. 407, 409
Kohtiao, A. [Jacobson and co-workers] 146
Koller, L. R. Chapter 2, Chapter 14, Chapter 15, Chapter 27
Komhyr, W. [Machta et al.] 191
Konig, H. [Goldman et al.] Chapter 4, Chapter 4
Korff, D. [Poirier and Korff] Chapter 13
Korzun, P. A. [Khitun et al.] Chapter 4
Koury, F. [Waymouth et al.] Chapter 22
Kouwenhoven, W. B. Chapter 28
Kramer, D. M. [Pathak et al.] Chapter 4
Krasnov, M. M. Chapter 17
Krause, E. [Sutter et al.] 826 [Sutter et al.] 840 [Sutter et al.] 841 [Sutter et al.] 849 [Hubner et al.] Chapter 24
Krauskopf, J. 85
Krautwald, R. C. [Mooradian et al.] Chapter 13

Kreithen, M. L. 684
Kressel, H. Chapter 11
Krial, N. P. 101 [Sliney et al.] Chapter 9 [Sliney et al.] Chapter 15 [Marshall et al.] 811 [Lyon et al.] 811 [Marshall et al.] 822 [Lyon et al.] 816 [Marshall et al.] 823 [Marshall et al.] 825 [Marshall et al.] 826 [Marshall et al.] 828 [Lyon et al.] 835 [Marshall et al.] 835 [Marshall et al.] 845 [Lyon et al.] 847 [Marshall et al.] 847
Kripke, B. J. [Snow et al.] 581
Krizek, D. T. Chapter 22
Kruer, M. [Bartoli et al.] Chapter 11, Chapter 11
Kruse, P. W. Chapter 2
Kubo, U. [Nakatsuka and Kubo] Chapter 11
Kuck, J. [Lerman et al.] Chapter 4
Kues, H. A. Chapter 27
Kuhfeld, R. [Hickey and Kuhfeld] 646
Kukita, A. [Fitzpatrick et al.] Chapter 3 [Fitzpatrick et al.] 174 [Fitzpatrick et al.] 177 [Fitzpatrick et al.] 178 [Fitzpatrick et al.] 179 [Fitzpatrick et al.] Chapter 15
Kuizenga, D. J. [Roundy et al.] Chapter 11
Kumbar, M. [Bettelheim and Kumbar] Chapter 3
Kunz, Y. W. [MacNichol et al.] 137
Kuppenheim, H. F. [Jacquez et al.] 165
Kurchatova, C. [Churchkova and Kurchatova] 450
Kurtin, W. E. [Zuclich and Kurtin] 114
Kurzel, R. B. 113, 115, 207, 210
Kuwabara, T. 134 [Bernstein et al.] Chapter 4, Chapter 6
Kuzina, F. D. [Tkachuk and Kuzina] 372
Kytila, J. [Castren and Kytila] Chapter 28

Labo, J. A. Chapter 11
Ladany, I. [Gorog et al.] 45
Lagen, J. B. [Dalzul et al.] Chapter 28
Lam, U. T. Y. [Auth et al.] Chapter 17
LaMarre, D. A. Chapter 16, Chapter 24
Land, C. E. Chapter 16
Landers, M. B. III 105, 133 [Bresnick et al.] Chapter 4 [Bresnick et al.] 219 [Bresnick et al.] 230 [Bresnick et al.] 231 [Lund et al.] 240 [Wolbarsht and Landers] 581 [Wolbarsht and Landers] Chapter 26

Landry, R. J. 366, 374, [Envall et al.] 525 [Envall et al.] 528
Lane, R. [Ravitch et al.] Chapter 28
Langer, H. Chapter 3
Langley, R. K. 146
LaPiana, F. G. [Tso and LaPiana] Chapter [Tso and LaPiana] 202
Lappin, P. W. 134 [Dunsky and Lappin] 219, 219 [Lappin and Coogan] 236 [Dunsky and Lappin] 238, 238, 594
Laser Focus 296, 657
Laser Institute of America Chapter 1, Chapter 7, Chapter 15, 863, 864, 876
Laubereau, A. [Penzkofer et al.] Chapter 11
Laudieri, P. C. [Labo et al.] Chapter 11
Laures, P. Chapter 12
Lawrence, N. S. [Clifford et al.] Chapter 13
Lawrence, R. S. [Ochs and Lawrence] 425 Chapter 13
Lawton, R. A. [Young and Lawton] Chapter 11
Lawwill, T. 134, 136, 137, Chapter 6, 238
Lee, J. A. H. Chapter 7
Lee, R. H. Chapter 28
Lee, W. R. [Dalziel and Lee] Chapter 28
Leebeek, H. J. [Walraven and Leebeek] 88
LeGrand, I 84
LeGrand, Y 141
Lehmiller, D. J. [Carpenter et al.] 219
Lehmkuhle, S. W. [Fox et al.] Chapter 21
Leibowitz, H. M. 148
Leighton, E. [Hathaway et al.] 881
Leighton, L. G. Chapter 22
Leighton, R. B. [Feynman et al.] Chapter 2
Lengyel, B. A. Chapter 2
Lerman, S. 115, Chapter 4
Lesnewich, A. Chapter 24
L'Esperance, F. A. Chapter 4, Chapter 17
Levi, L. Chapter 2, Chapter 12
Levin, M. Chapter 24
Levine, J. S. [MacNichol et al.] 137
Levy, L. S. Chapter 28
Levin, R. E. Chapter 22
Li, T. [Kogelnick and Li] 409
Liberman, I Chapter 22
Lienhard, O. E. Chapter 22
Lind, M. A. [Geist et al.] Chapter 11, Chapter 11
Linfoot, E. H. Chapter 2
Liotet, S. A. [Blancard et al.] 509

Little, H. L. [Zweng et al.] Chapter 4
Little, V. I. Chapter 11
Livingston, P. C. 136, 138, 210
Livingston, P. M. Chapter 13
Livingston, S. [Marshall et al.] Chapter 4
Lobitz, W. [Montagna and Lobitz] Chapter 3
Locke, E. V. Chapter 19
Loewen, E. G. Chapter 12, 442
Logan, G. Chapter 5
Letcher, F. S. [Keesey and Letcher] Chapter 28
Longhurst, R. S. Chapter 2
Loomis, W. F. Chapter 5
Lotmar, W. [Fankhauser and Lotmar] 233
Lowenstein, E. V. Chapter 15 [Smith and Lowenstein] Chapter 15
Lozier, W. W. [Null and Lozier] Chapter 22
Lucas, N. S. Chapter 5
Lucey, J. F. Chapter 22
Luckiesh, M. 172
Ludvigh, E. 118
Ludwig, H. C. Chapter 24
Lund, D. J. [Beatrice and Lund] 132 [Beatrice et al.] 233, 240 [Stuck et al.] 244 [Stuck et al.] 245 [Wallow et al.] Chapter 7 [Stuck et al.] Chapter 8, Appendix B, p. 959.
Lurie, M. [Stone et al.] Chapter 4
Luther, F. M. [Burt and Luther] Chapter 14
Lutty, G. A. [Kues and Lutty] Chapter 27
Lyon, T. L. [Sliney et al.] Chapter 9 [Sliney et al.] Chapter 15 [Lyon et al.] 811 [Marshall et al.] 811 [Marshall et al.] 822 [Marshall et al.] 823 [Marshall et al.] 825 [Marshall et al.] 826 [Marshall et al.] 828 [Marshall et al.] 835 [Marshall et al.] 845 [Marshall et al.] 847 [Lyon et al.] 847
Lytle, J. D. Chapter 15

MacDonald, J. E. 137, 207
MacKeen, D. Chapter 4
MacNichol, E. F., Jr. 137
McAquistan, R. B. [Kruse et al.] Chapter 2
McCall, G. H. Chapter 11
McCarthy, E. F. [Ludvigh and McCarthy] 118
McCartney, A. J. [Jones and McCartney] 239
McCartney, E. J. Chapter 13
McClatchey, R. A. 421
McClure, J. D. [Nichols et al.] Chapter 11

McCulloch, C. [Langley, Mortimer and McCulloch] 146
McCullough, E. C. 193
McFaul, P. [Duke-Elder and McFaul] 143 [Duke-Elder and McFaul] 146, Chapter 8 [Duke-Elder and McFaul] 830
McGlauchlin, L. D. [Kruse et al.] Chapter 2
McGowan, J. W. [Borwein et al.] 106
McInally, J. A. [Lienhard and McInally] Chapter 22
McIntosh, B. C. [Doyle, McIntosh and Geist] 357 [Doyle and McIntosh] 358 [Doyle and McIntosh] 359
McKeenan, W. [Jacquez et al.] 165
McKinlay, A. F. Chapter 22
McKinnery, W. N. [Bartley et al.] 822
McKnight, W. B. [Dezenburg et al.] Chapter 27
McLeod, D. S. [Flowers et al.] 119 [Flowers et al.] 120
McLean, J. M. [Jacobson and McLean] 509
McNair, J. N. [Penner and McNair] 137 [Penner and McNair] 202
McSparron, D. A. Chapter 14, Chapter 17

Maas, J. B. Chapter 22
Machemer, R. [Fuller et al.] 788 [Parel et al.] 788
Machta, L. 191
Machtwey, D. S. [Rundel and Machtwey] Chapter 6
Mackison, F. W. Chapter 27
Macomber, J. D. [Rier and Macomber] Chapter 11
Madden, R. P. Chapter 14, Chapter 24
Mader, F. [Goldman et al.] Chapter 4
Maggs, P. N. D. [Gibson et al.] Chapter 11
Magnus, I. A. Chapter 3, 172 [Berger et al.] 454
Maher, E. F. [Egbert and Maher] 240 [Egbert and Maher] 254
Maida, A. S. [Alexander et al.] Chapter 26
Mainster, M. A. Chapter 4 [White et al.] Chapter 4, 207 [White et al.] 208, 687
Maksymonko, G. [Smathers and Maksymonko] Chapter 11
Makous, W. L. Chapter 20
Malek, B. Chapter 24
Malik, S. R. K. [Agarwal and Malik] 202
Malina, F. J. Chapter 20
Mandel, G. [Johnson et al.] Chapter 5

Mandeville, G. D. [Arnaud et al.] 396
Manes, K. R. Chapter 11
Marich, K. W. Chapter 17, Chapter 27
Marlor, R. L. Chapter 6
Marmor, M. F. [Stone et al.] Chapter 4
Marriott, H. L. Chapter 28
Marshall, C. [Marshall et al.] Chapter 4
Marshall, J. Chapter 4 [Borlund et al.] 233 [Borlund et al.] 235 [Borlund et al.] 239
Marsischky, G. W. [Ehrenkranz and Marsischky] Chapter 28
Marsden, A. M. [Henderson and Marsden] 752
Marshall, W. J. 244 [Sliney et al.] Chapter 9 [Sliney et al.] 335 [Sliney et al.] 369 [Sliney et al.] 445 [Sliney et al.] Chapter 15, 670, 805, 811, 822, 823 825, 826, 282, 835 [Lyon et al.] 835 845 [Lyon et al.] 847
Marsh, G. E. [Dobrowolski et al.] 556
Marston, D. R. [Labo et al.] Chapter 11
Martin, D. H. Chapter 14
Martin, G. 685
Martin-Marietta 502
Martt, E. C. Chapter 22
Massey, G. A. [Johnson et al.] Chapter 11
Matelsky, I. 107, Chapter 10
Matheson, I. B. C. [Wolbarsht et al.] 110 [Wolbarsht et al.] 145 [Wolbarsht et al.] 887
Mattick, A. T. [Duguay and Mattick] Chapter 11
Maurelli, C. Chapter 24
Mautner, W. J. [Davis and Mautner] 594
Maystre, D. [Loewen et al.] Chapter 12
Mayyasi, A. M. Chapter 4
Maney, M. N. Chapter 9
Mechev, V. S. Chapter 24
Medeiros, J. A. [Borwein et al.] 106
Medvedovskaya, T. P. 136
Meisner, M. D. [Hardy et al.] Chapter 6
Melchior, H. Chapter 11
Mellerio, J. Chapter 4
Menkin, M. F. [Dewan et al.] Chapter 4
Menzel, R. [Snyder and Menzel] Chapter 3
Merchant, J. 784
Merrill, J. J. [Gardiner et al.] Chapter 12
Meyer, M. R. [Snow et al.] 581
Meyer, R. [Goldman and Meyer] Chapter 17
Meyer-Arendt, J. R. Chapter 2
Meyer-Schwickerath, G. Chapter 4, 581
Michaelson, S. M. [Goldman et al.] Chapter 8

Middleton, W. E. K. 416
Miehe, J. A. [Cumin et al.] Chapter 11
Migai, K. V. Chapter 24
Miller, J. H. [Green et al.] Chapter 6
Miller, N. D. 139
Miller, W. C. [Hoag and Miller] Chapter 12
Miller, W. H. [Snyder and Miller] Chapter 21
Mills, W. Chapter 28
Milnor, W. R. [Kouwenhoven et al.] Chapter 28
Minnik 119
Minton, J. 830, Chapter 24
Miyakawa, T. Chapter 11
Mo, T. [Green et al.] Chapter 5 [Green et al.] Chapter 6 [Johnson et al.] Chapter 6
Mohan, K. [Peterson et al.] Chapter 11 [McSparron et al.] Chapter 14
Mohon, N. Chapter 17
Mohr, R. W. [Auth et al] Chapter 17
Mollsen, J. A. [Coogan et al.] 79 [Coogan et al.] 120
Moncrief, J. A. [Mills et al.] Chapter 28
Monroe, R. E. [Pattee et al.] Chapter 24
Montagna, W. [Montagna and Lobitz] Chapter 3 [Montagna and Parakkal] Chapter 3
Moon, M. E. [Ham et al.] 134 [Ham et al.] 137, 137, 237 [Ham et al.] Chapter 7
Mooradian, A. Chapter 2, Chapter 13
Morgan, R. L. [Lowenstein et al.] Chapter 15
Mortiz, A. R. [Henriques and associates] 162, Chapter 5
Morley, R. 924
Morris, R. W. Chapter 22
Morrisette, R. [Merchant and Morrisette] 787
Mortensen, R. L. Chapter 9
Mortimer, C. B. [Langley, Mortimer and McCulloch] 146
Morway, P. E. [Chisum and Morway] Chapter 4
Moser, H. O. Chapter 12
Moss, C. E. [Marshall et al.] 811 [Marshall et al.] 822 [Marshall et al.] 823 [Marshall et al.] 825 [Marshall et al.] 826, 827 [Marshall et al.] 828 [Marshall et al.] 835, 838 [Marshall et al.] 845 [Marshall et al.] 847, 849
Mueller, H. A. [Goldman et al.] 133 [Goldman et al.] 134 [Ham et al.] 134 [Ham et al.] 135 [Ham et al.] 136 [Ham et al.] 137 [Moon et al.] 137 [Ham and colleagues] 201 [Ham and colleagues] 206 [Ham et al.] 218 [Ham et al.] 219, 236 [Moon et al.] 237 [Farrer, Ham et al.] 237 [Ham et al.] 238, 240, 254 [Goldman et al.] Chapter 7 [Ham, Mueller and Sliney] 336 [Ham et al.] 543 [Ham et al.] 549 [Ham et al.] 594
Mullaney, P. F. 584
Munnik, A. A. [Vos et al.] Chapter 4
Murgatroyd, D. [Hardy and co-workers] 162 [Hardy and co-workers] 165
Murphy, J. J. [Smith et al.] 866
Murray, L. E. [Garrisson et al.] 192
Murray, R. Chapter 28
Murray, W. E. [Moss et al.] 827 [Moss and Murray] 849
Muzyka, D. F. [Pasachoff and Muzyka] 451
Myers, L. B. [Pattee et al.] Chapter 24

Naidoff, M. A. 219, 830, 832
Najac, H. W. [Jacobson and co-workers] 146
Nakatsuka, M. Chapter 11
National Academy of Sciences 195, 196, 197
National Bureau of Standards Chapter 27
National Fire Protection Association Chapter 27
National Industrial Pollution Control Council Chapter 22
National Radiological Protection Board Chapter 22
Nelson, C. N. [Altman et al.] Chapter 12
NEPA Chapter 28
Nestor, O. H. Chapter 24
Neviere, M. [Loewen et al.] Chapter 12
New, G. H. C. [Bradley and New] 367
Newell, P. B. [Goncz and Newell] Chapter 22
Newsome, D. A. Chapter 4
Nichols, D. B. Chapter 11 [Pond et al.] Chapter 11
Nicholson, A. N. [Borland et al.] 148 Chapter 21
Nicodemus, F. E. (ed.) Chapter 11, Chapter 14, 500, Chapter 22
Niland, R. A. [Falconer et al.] Chapter 11
NIOSH 328, Chapter 24
Noell, W. 134, Chapter 6, Chapter 7
Nooney, D. W. Chapter 6 [Geeraets and Nooney] Chapter 26

Author Index

Norris, B. [Gibson et al.] Chapter 11
North, J. C. Chapter 20
Northam, N. B. [Jacob et al.] Chapter 11
Novikov, N. P. Chapter 16
Novotna, J. Chapter 24
Null, M. R. Chapter 22

Obukhova, Ye. A. [Khitun et al.] Chapter 4
Occupational Safety and Health Administration (OSHA) 1
Ochs, G. R. 425 [Clifford et al.] Chapter 13, Chapter 13
Odland, L. T. Chapter 10 [Piltingsrud et al.] Chapter 22
Offerberger, A. A. Chapter 11
Ogden, E. [Dalziel et al.] Chapter 28
Ogilvie, J. C. Chapter 4
Ogura, R. M. Chapter 5
Ohta, N. Chapter 22
Olsen, H. N. Chapter 24
Olson, R. L. [Sayre, Olson and Everett] 172 [Everett et al.] 173, Chapter 5 [Everett et al.] 330
Orenberg, J. B. [Marich et al.] Chapter 17 [Marich et al.] Chapter 27
Orr, M. A. [Wolbarsht et al.] 110 [Wolbarsht et al.] 145 [Wolbarsht et al.] 887
Orszag, M. [Adhav and Orszag] Chapter 15
Ostberg, O. [Levin et al.] Chapter 24
O'Steen, W. K. Chapter 4
Ostertag, E. Chapter 11
Ott, W. R. [Saunders et al.] Chapter 14, 733
Ottosson, A. [Levin et al.] Chapter 24
Owens, D. A. Chapter 22
Owens, D. W. [Freeman et al.] 172 [Freeman et al.] 173, Chapter 5 [Freeman et al.] 330

Palmisano, W. A. [Sliney and Palmisano] 280 [Sliney and Palmisano] 221 [Sliney and Palmisano] Chapter 15
Parakkal, P. F. [Montagna and Parakkal] Chapter 3
Parascandola, J. [Thorington et al.] Chapter 22
Parel, J. M. 788
Parker, G. S. Chapter 20
Parker, L. [Abel et al.] Chapter 20
Parr, W. H. [Pitts and Cullen] 110 [Pitts and Cullen] 113, 163 [Brownell et al.] 168, 168 [Sonsinstaffar et al.] 781

Parrent, G., Jr. [Beran and Parrent] Chapter 2
Parrish, J. A. Chapter 3, Chapter 4 [Pathak et al.] Chapter 4, 174 [Ying et al.] Chapter 5, Chapter 10, 553 [Fitzpatrick et al.] Chapter 16, Chapter 22
Parry, G. Chapter 13
Partridge, L. J. [Mackison et al.] Chapter 27
Pasachoff, J. M. 451
Pathak, M. A. [Fitzpatrick et al.] Chapter 3 [Parrish et al.] Chapter 4, Chapter 4 [Fitzpatrick et al.] 174 [Fitzpatrick et al.] 177 [Fitzpatrick et al.] 178 [Fitzpatrick et al.] 179 [Parrish et al.] 174, Chapter 5 [Ying et al.] Chapter 5 [Fitzpatrick et al.] Chapter 15 [Parrish et al.] 553 [Fitzpatrick et al.] Chapter 16 [Parrish et al.] Chapter 22
Pattee, H. E. Chapter 24
Patty, F. A. Chapter 27
Peabody, R. R. [Vassiliadis et al.] Chapter 4 [Zweng et al.] Chapter 4, Chapter 7
Peacock, G. R. [Leibowitz and Peacock] 148
Pearson, J. E. 425
Pease, H. [Hoag et al.] 615
Peckham, R. H. 136, 138, 210
Pembrook, J. D. [Burch et al.] Chapter 13
Pendleton, W. R. [Gardiner et al.] Chapter 12
Pendorf, R. Chapter 13
Penner, R. 137, 202
Penning, F. M. Chapter 14
Penzkofer, A. Chapter 11
Peppers, N. A. [Vassiliadis et al.] Chapter 4 [Peabody et al.] Chapter 7
Pert, G. J. Chapter 15
Peters, G. A. Chapter 15
Petersen. R. C. [Weiss and Petersen] Chapter 22
Peterson, R. W. [Landry and Peterson] 366 [Landry and Peterson] 374 [James et al.] Chapter 11, Chapter 11 [Envall et al.] 525 [Envall et al.] 528 [Van Pelt et al.] 633
Pfender, E. [Chov and Pfender] Chapter 24
Phelan, R. J. [Smith and Phelan] Chapter 11
Phillion, D. W. [Roundy et al.] Chapter 11
Pierce, E. T. [Howett et al.] Chapter 23
Pierce, R. L. Chapter 11
Pierson, A. H. 443
Piltingsrud, H. V. Chapter 10, Chapter 14, 752

Pirie, A. 115, Chapter 6
Pitts, D. G. 109, 110, 111, 112, 113, 114, 118 [Parrish et al.] 174, 237, 330 [Parrish et al.] Chapter 10
Pitts, S. M. [Flowers et al.] 119 [Flowers et al.] 120
Place, E. H. [Dressen et al.] Chapter 24
Plass, G. M. Chapter 13
Plato 116
Poehler, H. A. Chapter 28
Pohl, R. W. Chapter 2
Poirier, J. L. Chapter 13
Polanyi, T. Chapter 2 [Stellar et al.] Chapter 17
Polis, B. D. [Cope et al.] Chapter 7
Polyak, S. 72, 79, 85
Pond, C. R. Chapter 11
Pope, T. P. [Tittle et al.] Chapter 11
Post, P. W. [Daniels et al.] Chapter 5
Potter, W. M. Chapter 22
Potts [Ernest and Potts] 76
Powell, C. H. Chapter 24, Chapter 27
Powell, J. O. [Tso et al.] 104 [Bresnick et al.] Chapter 4 [Bresnick et al.] 219 [Bresnick et al.] 230 [Bresnick et al.] 231 [Lund et al.] 240
Pressley, R. J. Chapter 2
Preston, F. R. [Marlor et al.] Chapter 6
Preston, J. S. [Jones and Preston] Chapter 14
Priebe, A. [Welch and Priebe] 128 [Welch and Priebe] 327
Prince, J. H. 684
Pritchard, B. S. [Fry et al.] Chapter 4
Proctor, N. H. Chapter 27
Projector, T. H. Chapter 4, Chapter 23
Pusey, P. N. Chapter 13

Rabson, T. A. [Bitt et al.] Chapter 2
Ragnarsson, S. I. [Ingelstam and Ragnarsson] Chapter 17
Ramsay, C. A. [Cripps, Ramsay and Ruch] 172 [Cripps et al.] 176
Ramsey, J. D. Chapter 10
Randall, H. G. [Randall, Brown and Sloan] 90
Randolph, D. I. [Davies and Randolph] Chapter 4 [Beatrice et al.] 233
Rapp, L. M. Chapter 4
Rassow, B. [Dannheim and Rassow] 143
Rathkey, A. S. 509
Rauh, F. Chapter 24
Ravitch, M. M. Chapter 28

Ray, I. W. [Kline and Ray] Chapter 2
Raybold, R. C. [McSparron et al.] Chapter 14
Rayborn, M. E. [Hollyfield and Rayborn] Chapter 3
RCA Corporation
Ready, J. F. Chapter 19
Reeves, P. 69, Chapter 4
Reid, K. M. [Potter and Reid] Chapter 22
Reid, T. 885
Reitz, P. R. [Charlton and Reitz] Chapter 20
Rentschler, H. C. 456
Rentzepis, P. M. Chapter 17
Resnick, R. [Halliday and Resnick] Chapter 2 [Halliday and Resnick] 82
Rice, D. K. Chapter 13
Rice, R. O. Chapter 11
Richey, E. O. [Thursby et al.] 543 [Dunsky et al.] Chapter 21
Richfield, D. [Goldman et al.] 169
Rieke, F. E. Chapter 24
Riggle, G. C. 577
Rinalducci, E. J. [Boynton et al.] Chapter 4
Ritchey, C. L. [Ewald and Ritchey] 206
Rittler, M. C. [Campbell et al.] 148
Riva, C. E. 584
Roach, T. 452
Robbins, D. O. [Cavonius et al.] Chapter 4 [Cavonius et al.] Chapter 7, Chapter 7
Roberts, A. M. [Van Pelt et al.] 633
Robinson, N. Chapter 6
Robson, J. G. Chapter 21
Rock, J. [Dewan et al.] Chapter 4
Rockwell, R. J., Jr. [Goldman and Rockwell] 101, 167, 168, 169 [Goldman et al.] 169 [Goldman et al.] Chapter 8, Chapter 11 [Goldman et al.] Chapter 15 [Goldman and Rockwell] 577 [Goldman et al.] Chapter 17, Chapter 19, 632
Rodemann, A. [Mohon and Rodemann] Chapter 17
Rodighiero, G. [Pathak et al.] Chapter 4
Roger, F. C. 199
Rohde, R. S. [Buser and Rohde] Chapter 13
Rollason, E. C. [Van Someren and Rollason] Chapter 24
Rosan, R. C. [Vassiliadis et al.] 138 [Vassiliadis et al.] 239
Rose, H. C. [Zweng and Rose] Chapter 26

Rose, H. W. [Vassiliadis et al.] Chapter 4 [Peabody et al.] Chapter 7
Rosen, A. N. 584
Rosenberg, G. V. Chapter 13
Ross, D. Chapter 2
Ross, M. Chapter 2
Rosskopf, T. Chapter 24
Rottier, P. B. [Rottier and van der Leun] 172 [Berger et al.] 454
Roundy, C. B. Chapter 11
Roy, E. L. [Dezenburg et al.] Chapter 27
Royston, D. D. Chapter 20
Rubin, C. E. [Auth et al.] Chapter 17
Ruch, D. M. [Cripps, Ramsay and Ruch] 172 [Cripps et al.] 176
Ruffin, R. S. [Ham et al.] 218
Ruffolo, J. J., Jr. 79 [Ham et al.] 134 [Ham et al.] 137 [Moon et al.] 137 [Moon et al.] 237 [Ham et al.] Chapter 7
Rufus, R. J. [Alexander et al.] Chapter 26
Ruge, J. [Sutter et al.] 826 [Sutter et al.] 840 [Sutter et al.] 841 [Sutter et al.] 849 [Hubner et al.] Chapter 24
Rugh, E. R. [Jacob et al.] Chapter 11
Rundel, R. D. Chapter 6
Runge, P. K. Chapter 20
Ruprecht, K. W. Chapter 24
Rusch, H. P. 175
Russ, D. S. Chapter 24
Rutgers, G. A. W. Chapter 24
Ryan, M. L. [Ogilvie and Ryan] Chapter 4
Ryan, L. 101

Safar, P. [Ravitch et al.] Chapter 28
Said, F. S. Chapter 3, Chapter 4
Sanders, C. L. Chapter 22
Sands, M. [Feynman et al.] Chapter 2
Sans, W. M., Jr. Chapter 5
Sanwal, M. [Borwein et al.] 106
Sass, D. J. [Kouwenhoven et al.] Chapter 28
Saunders, R. D. [McSparron et al.] Chapter 14, Chapter 14
Savage, W. F. [Tseng and Savage] Chapter 24
Saxman, A. C. [Wick et al.] Chapter 12
Sayre, R. M. 172 [Everett et al.] 173 [Everett et al.] 174 [Olson et al.] Chapter 5 [Everett et al.] 330 [Berger et al.] 454
Schaefer, A. R. Chapter 11
Schell, P. G. Chapter 12

Scherman, G. H. Chapter 19
Scherr, A. E. 521
Schierer, P. Chapter 11
Schilling, R. S. F. Chapter 26
Schlaer, R. Chapter 21
Schleusener, S. A. [White et al.] Chapter 13
Schmidt, F. H. [Geeraets et al.] 120 [Evans et al.] 162
Schmidt, K. Chapter 5, Chapter 10
Schmidt, L. B. [Geist et al.] Chapter 11 [West and Schmidt] Chapter 11
Schmidt, R. H. Chapter 5, Chapter 6
Schmitt, L. B. [Franzen and Schmitt] Chapter 11
Schneider, W. E. [Stair et al.] Chapter 14
Schott Glass Company 525
Schreibeis, W. J. 521
Schreiber, M. M. [Dahling et al.] Chapter 16
Schultz, F. V. Chapter 14
Schultz, J. [Zigman et al.] Chapter 4
Schulze, R. Chapter 6
Schwarz, H. J. Chapter 19
Scott, M. L. [Combs and Scott] 252
Scott, W. D. [Wren et al.] 557 [Wren et al.] 558
Scotto, J. Chapter 6
Sears, D. [Ebbers and Sears] 114
Segal, S. M. Chapter 22
Seidly, E. Chapter 5
Seiji, M. [Fitzpatrick et al.] Chapter 3 [Fitzpatrick et al.] 174 [Fitzpatrick et al.] 177 [Fitzpatrick et al.] 178 [Fitzpatrick et al.] 179 [Fitzpatrick et al.] Chapter 15
Seka, W. Chapter 12
Selby, J. E. A. [McClatchey and Selby] 421
Semmlow, J. Chapter 4
Sensinstaffar, E. L. 781
Sephens, D. H. [Mooradian et al.] Chapter 13
Sever, R. J. [Cope et al.] Chapter 7
Shangold, E. J. 744
Shapiro, S. I. [Dahling et al.] Chapter 16
Sharon, U. [Kaplan et al.] Chapter 17
Shaw, C. B. Chapter 24
Shaw, H. E. [Landers et al.] 105 [Landers et al.] 133
Sheng, P. [Firester et al.] 396
Sherashov, S. G. 110, Chapter 4
Shostak, V. I. [Khitun et al.] Chapter 4
Shumaker, J. B. [Saunders and Shumaker] Chapter 14
Siegman, A. E. Chapter 2

Sigmund, M. Chapter 23
Siler, V. E. [Goldman et al.] Chapter 17
Silverstein, F. E. [Gulacsik et al.] 577 [Auth et al.] Chapter 17
Sims, S. D. [Solon and Sims] Chapter 20
Sinclair, D. C. Chapter 2, Chapter 12
Singh, H. [Gupta and Singh] 138 [Gupta and Singh] 833
Sipp, B. [Cumin et al.] Chapter 11
Sisson, T. R. C. Chapter 22
Skeen, C. H. 219, 244, 245, 280
Sliney, D. H. 69, 83, 85, 87, 88, 101, 118, 122, 124, 125, 126, 129 [Wolbarsht and Sliney] 132 [Ham et al.] 136 [Ham et al.] 137, 137, 148, 171, 200 [Ham and colleagues] 201, 204, 205 [Ham and colleagues] 206, 209 [Sliney and Palmisano] 218 [Naidoff and Sliney] 219 [Wolbarsht and Sliney] 219 [Sliney and Palmisano] 221, 221 [Ham et al.] 238, 241, 242 [Wolbarsht and Sliney] 243 [Goldman et al.] Chapter 8, 322, 328, 330, 331, 335 [Ham, Mueller and Sliney] 336, 336, 337, 351, 353, 369, Chapter 11, 423, 425, 428, Chapter 445, 455, Chapter 15, 521, 522, 539, 542, Chapter 17, Chapter 18, Chapter 19, [Rockwell et al.] 632, 655, 668, 698, 724, 727, 729, 730, 732, 776, Chapter 23 [Sensinstaffar et al.] 781 [Ham and Sliney] 792 [Lyon et al.] 811 [Marshall et al.] 811 [Lyon et al.] 816 [Marshall et al.] 822 [Marshall et al.] 823 [Marshall et al.] 825 [Marshall et al.] 826 [Marshall et al.] 828 [Naidoff and Sliney] 830 [Naidoff and Sliney] 832 [Marshall et al.] 835 [Lyon et al.] 835 [Marshall et al.] 845 [Marshall et al.] 847 [Lyon et al.] 847, 852, 899
Sloan, L. L. [Randall, Brown and Sloan] 90
Smathers, S. E. Chapter 11
Smialek, L. J. [Martt et al.] Chapter 22
Smith, D. C. [Gebhardt and Smith] Chapter 13
Smith, D. L. [Manes et al.] Chapter 11
Smith, D. R. [Lowenstein et al.] Chapter 15, Chapter 15
Smith, F. G. Chapter 2
Smith, F. K. [Chisum et al.] Chapter 4
Smith, H. E. 136, 206, 210
Smith, J. F. [Rockwell et al.] 632, 866

Smith, K. C. 227, 228
Smith, K. O. [Rentschler et al.] 456
Smith, L. D. 633
Smith, M. G. [Skeen et al. a and b] 219 [Skeen et al. a and b] 244 [Skeen et al. a and b] 245 [Skeen et al.] 280
Smith, P. W. Chapter 2
Smith, R. A. Chapter 14
Smith, R. L. 379
Smith, T. C. [Boivin and Smith] Chapter 11
Smith, W. J. Chapter 2
Smith, W. L. 393
Smith, W. V. Chapter 2
Smy, P. R. [Offerberger et al.] Chapter 11
Snow, J. C. 581
Snyder, A. W. Chapter 3, Chapter 21
Snyder, D. S. Chapter 5
Soles, E. M. [Hathaway et al.] 881
Soloman, S. [Fisher and Soloman] 175
Solon, L. R. Chapter 17, Chapter 20
Sommerfeld, A. Chapter 2
Song, P. S. Chapter 22
Sorato, M. [Blancard et al.] 509
Soronkin, P. P. [Smith and Soronkin] Chapter 2
Spears, D. L. Chapter 11
Spears, G. R. Chapter 14, 723 [Bickford et al.] Chapter 22 [Levin et al.] Chapter 22, Chapter 22
Specht, W. A. 616
Spence, P. W. [Ferris et al.] Chapter 28
Spencer, D. J. Chapter 13, 538, 543
Sperling, H. G. [Harworth and Sperling] 134 [Harworth and Sperling] 135 [Harworth and Sperling] 137 [Harworth and Sperling] Chapter 6, 237
SPIE Chapter 14
Spitzmas, M. Chapter 4
Spracklen, H. R. [Thomas et al.] Chapter 11
Staal, J. [Hoag et al.] 615
Stair, R. [Coblentz, Stair and Hogue] 172 [Coblentz and Stair] 330, Chapter 14 [Coblentz and Stair] 542, 542, 843 [Coblentz and Stair] Chapter 24
Staley, K. A. Chapter 22
Stark, L. [Semmlow and Stark] Chapter 4
State of New York Chapter 15
Steere, N. V. Chapter 27
Steichen, F. M. [Ravitch et al.] Chapter 28
Steinkamp, J. A. [Mullaney et al.] 584
Stellar, S. Chapter 17
Stencil, J. A. [Piltingsrud and Stencil] Chapter 14

Stern, N. [Hathaway et al.] 881
Stern, W. K. Chapter 5
Sternhein, C. [Boynton et al.] Chapter 4
Stevens, C. C. [Hemstreet et al.] 245
Stevenson, W. H. [Hirleman and Stevenson] Chapter 12
Stewart, H. F. [Van Pelt et al.] 633
Stier, M. T. [Traub and Stier] Chapter 13
Stiles, W. S. 92, 93 [Wyszecki and Stiles] Chapter 3, 118
Stimson, A. Chapter 11
Stokinger, H. E. Chapter 7
Stokseth [Mooradian et al.] Chapter 2
Stoll, A. M. 557
Stone, W. L. [Katz et al.] Chapter 4, Chapter 4
Stotts, L. B. [Mooradian et al.] Chapter 13
Stratton, K. [Pathak and Stratton] Chapter 5
Straub, H. W. 521
Strauss, H. S. [Thouret et al.] Chapter 22
Stricoff, R. S. [Mackison et al.] Chapter 27
Strohbehn, J. W. Chapter 13
Stroke, G. W. Chapter 2, Chapter 20
Strong, J. Chapter 2
Strong, M. S. [Snow et al.] 581
Strughold, H. [Gerathewohl and Strughold] Chapter 4 [Gerathewohl and Strughold] Chapter 6 [Gerathewohl and Strughold] 223
Stuck, B. E. [Beatrice et al.] 233 [Brownell and Stuck] 240, 244, 245, Chapter 8
Stutz, G. F. A. Chapter 24
Sudashan, F. C. G. [Klauder and Sudashan] Chapter 2
Sutter, E. [Bauer et al.] 538, 826 [Hubner et al.] 829, 840, 841, 849 [Hubner et al.] Chapter 24, Chapter 24
Suzaki, Y. Chapter 12
Svelto, O. Chapter 2
Svetlik, J. 410
Svoboda, J. R. Chapter 6
Swope, C. H. 521, 530
Sweetnam, P. M. [Wallace and colleagues] 147
Switzer, W. E. [Mills et al.] Chapter 28
Szabo, G. [Pathak et al.] Chapter 5
Szafran, L. 146, Chapter 24

Tabershaw, J. R. [Kleinfeld et al.] Chapter 24
Taboada, J. [Zuclich and Taboada] 109

Takeda, Y. Chapter 20
Takimoto, H. H. [Spencer et al.] Chapter 13
Tanebaum, L. [Parrish et al.] Chapter 22
Tanenbaum, L. [Parrish et al.] Chapter 4
Tapaszto, I. 112, Chapter 4
Tapley, K. J., Jr. [Song and Tapley] Chapter 22
Tartarski, V. I. Chapter 13
Tavssig, H. G.
Taylor, A. H. [Luckiesh, Holladay and Taylor] 172
Taylor, S. L. 632
Tengroth, B. [Gullberg et al.] Chapter 7 [Goldman et al.] Chapter 8, Chapter 24, Chapter 26
Terrien, F. 830
Terus, W. S. [Blum and Terus] 172
Thacker, P. D. 369
Thebault, J. [Cumin et al.] Chapter 11
Thekakara, M. P. Chapter 6
Thoft, R. A. [Foulks et al.] Chapter 4
Thomas, S. W. Chapter 11
Thomas, T. R. [Dressen et al.] Chapter 24
Thomas, W., Jr., Chapter 12, 503
Thompson, G. Chapter 28
Thomson, J. H. [Smith and Thomson] Chapter 2
Thomson, M. L. Chapter 5
Thorington, L. Chapter 22
Thoss, F. Chapter 3
Thouret, W. E. Chapter 22
Thruston, J. L. [Dalziel et al.] Chapter 28
Thursby, W. R. 543
Tichibana, A. Chapter 12
Timberlake, G. T. [Riva et al.] 584
Timmerman, C. C. Chapter 20
Tips, J.H., Jr. [White et al.] Chapter 4 [White et al.] 208 [Skeen et al. a and b] 219 [Skeen et al. a and b] 244 [Skeen et al. a and b] 245 [Skeen et al.] 280 [Mainster et al.] 687
Title, A. M. Chapter 11
Tittel, F. K. [Bitt et al.] Chapter 2
Tkachuk, R. 372
Tobias, I. Chapter 2
Toft, A. [Hass et al.] 853
Townes, C. H. Chapter 2
Traub, W. A. Chapter 13
Treacy, E. B. Chapter 11
Treagar, R. T. Chapter 5
Tredici, T. J. [Pitts and Tredici] 109 [Pitts and Tredici] 110 [Carpenter et al.] 219 [Pitts and Tredici] 330

Treytl, W. J. [Marich et al.] Chapter 17 [Marich et al.] Chapter 27
Tricker, R. A. R. 419
Tripp, G. R. [Thomas et al.] Chapter 11
Trnka, J. [Malek et al.] Chapter 24
Troll, D. [Owens et al.] Chapter 5
Trosko, J. E. [Trosko and Chang] 227
Tseng, C. F. Chapter 24
Tso, M. O. M. 104, 136, 203
Tsunoda, Y. [Takeda and Tsunoda] Chapter 20
Tucker, R. J. [Scherr et al.] 521
Turk, M. I. [Falconer et al.] Chapter 11
Twersky, V. Chapter 4
Tyrar, G. [Schell and Tyrar] Chapter 12
Tyte, D. C. [Kimmitt et al.] Chapter 11

Ulett, G. A. 143
Ullrich, O. A. 501, 503
Underwriter's Laboratory Chapter 28
Urbach, R. Chapter 6, 165 [Berger, Urbach and Davies] 172 [Parrish et al.] 174, 175, 191, 194, 197, 198, 199 [Berger et al.] 330 [Parrish et al.] Chapter 10
US Atomic Energy Commission Chapter 27, Chapter 28
US Congress Chapter 9
US Department of the Air Force Chapter 7, 655, Chapter 28
US Department of the Army Chapter 7, Chapter 15, 655, Chapter 28
US Department of Commerce Chapter 7
US Department of Defense Chapter 28
US Department of Health, Education and Welfare 226, 247, 308, Chapter 9, Chapter 10, 576
US Department of Health, Education and Welfare (Bureau of Radiological Health 375, 379
US Department of Health, Education and Welfare (Food and Drug Administration) 334, Chapter 20, 752, 753
US Department of Labor 597, 902, 904, 910
US Department of the Navy Chapter 21
US Naval Research Laboratory Chapter 2

Vahle, W. [Hausser and Vahle] 171 [Hausser and Vahle] 172 [Hausser and Vahle] 188
Valley, S. L. 201, 420, 421
Valtonen, E. J. Chapter 5
Van de Hulst, H. C. Chapter 13

van de Hulst, H. W. Chapter 2
van den Brink 85
van der Leun [Rottier and van der Luen] 172, 174
van der Linde, D. [Penzkofer et al.] Chapter 11
van der Zypen, E. 143
van Meeteren, A. [Vos et al.] Chapter 3 [Vos et al.] Chapter 4
von Helmholtz, H. Chapter 3
van Norren, D. Chapter 4
Van Pelt, W. F. 633
Van Scott, E. J. [Fitzpatrick et al.] Chapter 3
Van Someren, E. Chapter 24
Vant-Holl, L. L. [Hildebrandt et al.] 791
Vass, Z. [Tapaszto and Vass] 112 [Tapaszto and Vass] Chapter 4
Vassiliadis, A. 132, 138, 148, 149, 219, 238, 239 [Peabody et al.] Chapter 7, Chapter 10
Vaughan, C. W. [Snow et al.] 581
Vaughn, J. H. [Fitzpatrick et al.] Chapter 3
Vaughan, T. [Zigman and Vaughan] Chapter 4
VDE 920
Vechet, B. Chapter 14
Verhoeff, F. 117, 137, 147
Vermuellen, D. [Fischer and co-workers] 146
Vinegar, R. [Clark et al.] Chapter 5
Viveash, J. D. [Borland et al.] 233 [Borland et al.] 235 [Borland et al.] 239
Vogt, A. 144
Vorpahl, K. W. [Sliney et al.] 899
Vos, J. J. Chapter 3 [van Norren and Vos] Chapter 4, Chapter 4

Waddell, J. E. [Hogan, Alvarado and Waddell] 71
Waldram, J. M. Chapter 23
Walkenbach, J. E. Chapter 7
Walker, A. C. Chapter 11
Walker, A. E. [Marshall et al.] Chapter 4
Walker, C. B. [Verhoeff, Bell and Walker] 117 [Verhoeff, Bell and Walker] 137 [Verhoeff, Bell and Walker] 147
Walker, R. F. [Glaser and Walker] Chapter 14
Wallace, J. 147
Wallace, R. A. [Campbell et al.] 148
Wallow, I. H. L. [Tso et al.] 104, Chapter 7

Walls, G. L. 684
Walraven, J. [Vos et al.] Chapter 3, 141, [Vos et al.] Chapter 4
Walraven, P. L. 88
Walsh, J. W. T. Chapter 2, 90, Chapter 11, Chapter 14, Chapter 22, Chapter 23
Waltermire, J. A. [Everett et al.] 173
Wangemann, R. T. [Sliney et al.] 87, 88 [Sliney et al.] Chapter 4
Ward, B. Chapter 7
Warin, A. P. [Briffa and Warin] Chapter 22
Warner, C. G. [Wallace and colleagues] 147
Warrilow, D. [Hayworth and Warrilow] Chapter 28
Warwick, R. Chapter 3
Watkins, W. R. [White et al.] Chapter 13
Watson, C. W. [Davidson and Watson] Chapter 4
Watt, B. E. Chapter 11
Waymouth, J. F. Chapter 22
Weale, R. A. [Said and Weale] Chapter 3 [Said and Weale] Chapter 4
Weaver, E. G. [Bitt et al.] Chapter 2
Weber, M. J. [Smith et al.] 393
Weiner, M. J. Chapter 19
Weisman, C. 804, 808, 810, 811
Weiss, M. M. Chapter 22
Welch, A. J. 128 [Cain and Welch] Chapter 4 [Welch and Priebe] 237
Welford, W. T. Chapter 2, Chapter 23
Wenzel, R. G. [Greiner et al.] Chapter 11
Weseley, M. L. 423
Wessels, S. R. [Fite and Wessels] Chapter 21
West, E. D. Chapter 11
Westendorf, D. H. [Fox et al.] Chapter 21
Westheimer, G. 85, Chapter 4
Wettermark, G. [Claesson et al.] Chapter 5
Wheater, R. H. Chapter 24
White, H. E. [Jenkins and White] Chapter 2
White, K. O. Chapter 13
White, T. H. 129
White, T. J. 128, 208 [Mainster et al.] 687
Whitman, A. M. 425
Wick, R. V. Chapter 12
Wicke, K. [Hubner et al.] 829
Wickstrom Chapter 24
Wiegard, K. R. [Bartley et al.] 822
Wiegmann, O. A. [Bredemeyer et al.] 218
Wilcox, G. [Kahn and Wilcox] Chapter 16
Wildavsky, A. Chapter 9
Wilhelm, D. L. [Logan and Wilhelm] Chapter 5
Wilkening, G. M. Chapter 17
Wilkerson, G. W. [Lytle et al.] Chapter 15
Williams, C. S. Chapter 2, Chapter 12, Chapter 14
Williams, D. R. Chapter 16
Williams, D. W. 543
Williams, H. B. [Ferris et al.] Chapter 28
Williams, R. C. [Geeraets et al.] 120 [Ham et al.] 135 [Evans et al.] 162 [Schmidt et al.] Chapter 5 [Ham et al.] Chapter 6 [Schmidt et al.] Chapter 6 [Ham et al.] 218 [Ham et al.] 219 [Farrer, Ham et al.] 237 [Ham et al.] 543 [Ham et al.] 549 [Ham et al.] 594
Williams, T. B. 134
Williams, T. P. [Rapp and Williams] Chapter 4
Willis, I. Chapter 5
Wilson, P. W. [White et al.] Chapter 4 [White et al.] 208 [Mainster et al.] 687
Wilson, R. M. Chapter 19
Wilson, W. M. [Green et al.] Chapter 5
Winburn, D. C. [Sliney et al.] Chapter 17, 899
Winell, M. [Holmberg and Winell] Chapter 7
Winer, I. M. Chapter 12
Winkelmann, R. K. [Epstein and Winkelmann] Chapter 5
Winston, R. [Welford and Winston] Chapter 23
Withrow, A. P. [Withrow and Withrow] 495 [Withrow and Withrow] Chapter 16
Withrow, R. B. 495, Chapter 16
Witte, E. [Bode and Witte] Chapter 5
Wittke, J. P. [Gorog et al.] 45
Wolbarsht, M. L. [Sliney et al.] 87, 88, Chapter 3 [Landers et al.] 105, 110 [Kurzel et al.] 113 [Kurzel et al.] 115 [Hayes and Wolbarsht] 120 [Hayes and Wolbarsht] 128, 132 [Hayes and Wolbarsht] 132 [Landers et al.] 133 [Hayes and Wolbarsht] 133, 145 [Sliney et al.] Chapter 4 [Kurzel et al.] 207, 207 [Kurzel et al.] 210 [Vassiliadis et al.] 219 219, 237, 243, Chapter 7 [Goldman et al.] Chapter 8 [Fligsten and Wolbarsht] Chapter 11, 581, 746, 755, Chapter 24, 886, 887

Wolf, E. [Born and Wolf] Chapter 2, Chapter 2, Chapter 12 [Born and Wolf] Chapter 23
Wolfe, W. L. Chapter 13, Chapter 24
Wolter, J. R. [Boettner and Wolter] 107 [Boettner and Wolter] 118 [Boettner and Wolter] 119 [Boettner and Wolter] 121
Wood, R. W. Chapter 2
Woodlief, T., Jr. Chapter 12
World Health Organization (WHO) 881, 884
Worst [Van Pelt et al.] 633
Wren, J. E. 557, 558
Wright, M. J. [Kimmitt et al.] Chapter 11
Wright, R. E. Chapter 6
Wrolstad, K. H. [Nichols et al.] Chapter 11
Wulcan, J. [Hornell and Wulcan] Chapter 24
Wurdemann, H. V. Chapter 24
Wurtman, R. J. 194
Wyszecki, G. Chapter 3 [Ohta and Wyszecki] Chapter 22

Yacovissi, R. 655
Yamanashi, B. S. [Wolbarsht et al.] 110 [Kurzel et al.] 113 [Kurzel et al.] 115 [Wolbarsht et al.] 145 [Kurzel et al.] 207 [Kurzel et al.] 210 [Wolbarsht et al.] 887
Yarbus, A. L. Chapter 3, Chapter 4
Yeargers, E. [Everett et al.] 174
Ying, C. Y. [Parrish et al.] 174, Chapter 5
Yonemochi, S. Chapter 11
Yoshida, A. 394
Young, J. D. H. Chapter 6
Young, M. Chapter 11
Young, R. W. Chapter 3, 104
Yuen, K. [Hiller and colleagues] 211
Yulo, T. [Zigman et al.] Chapter 4
Yura, H. T. 425

Zabetakis, M. G. Chapter 27
Zalewski, E. F. [Lind and Zalewski] Chapter 11 [McSparron et al.] Chapter 14
Zander, K. [Sutter and Zander] Chapter 24
Zar, J. [Hoag et al.] 615
Zigler, J. S. [Wolbarsht et al.] 110 [Wolbarsht et al.] 145 [Wolbarsht et al.] 887
Zigman, S. [Grover and Zigman] Chapter 4, Chapter 4
Zimmerer, R. W. Chapter 11
Zimmerman, L. E. [Tso et al.] 104 [Tso et al.] Chapter 4
Zimmermann, J. [Seka and Zimmermann] Chapter 12
Zinn, K. M. Chapter 3
Zissis, G. J. [Wolfe and Zissis] Chapter 24
Zissis, G. W. [Wolf and Zissis] Chapter 2
Zollweg, R. J. [Liberman and Zollweg] Chapter 22
Zuclich, J. A. [Zuclich and Connolly] 109 113, 114, 115
Zuidema, H. [Henkes and Zuidema] 509
Zweng, H. C. [Vassiliadis et al.] 138, Chapter 4 [Vassiliadis et al.] 239 [Peabody et al.] Chapter 7 [Vassiliadis et al.] Chapter 10, Chapter 15, 509, Chapter 17, Chapter 26
Zwick, H. 128, 137 [Beatrice et al.] 233 237 [Robbins et al.] Chapter 7, 633

Subject Index

Abbreviation - 967-972
Absorption - 26ff
Access - See Human Access
Accessible emission limits - 288-294
Accidents -
    electrical - 5, 915-919
    laser - 508-510, 893-895
    medical examination - 886-889, 892
    welding - 830-832
Accommodation (of the eye) - 78
Accuracy - 378-379
Actinic UV - See Ultraviolet radiation
Airborne contaminants - 618-620, 900-907
Airspace - 634-635, 662-664, 674-679, 682-683
Airy disc - 31-32, 81-85, 124-126
Alignment lasers - 585, 591-598, 605-606, 681-682
α min. - 272, 275-277
Alpha min. - See α min.
Ancillary hazards - 575-576, 899-910. See also Cryogenic, Electrical, Fire, Noise hazards
Animals, laser hazards to - 684-685
Aperture stop - 241, 317, 349, 429, 505
Aphakic eyes - 109. See also Erythropsin
Aqueous flare - 143, 146, 896
Aqueous humor - 66, 67, 107

Argon laser - 219, 320, 581-583
Asbestos - 574, 901, 907
Atomic fireballs - See Nuclear weapons
Atmosphere - 415ff, 987
    absorption - 421
    attenuation - 415-422, 666
    blue light - 609-612
    scattering - 415-420, 631
    scintillation - 422-430
    turbulence - 422-433
    ultraviolet effect - 187-194
Attenuation - 26-29, 526
Aversion response - 222-223, 326, 485-486, 585
Aviators - 138, 675-677

Backstops - 9, 43, 514-515, 568-577, 670-673
Beam attenuators - 297, 301, 571
Beam divergence - 349, 385-394, 649-650, 766
Beam profile - 47-51, 351, 385-413, 477-480
    circular beam - 387-388
    elliptical beam - 388
    "hot spots" - 51, 424-425, 428-429, 482-483
    measurement of - 392-413, 462-464
    rectangular beam - 388, 650
    single mode - 51, 391
Beam traps - See Backstops
Bilirubin lamps - 747-749
Binoculars - 206-207, 501-505, 669-670

Blackbody radiation - 18, 34, 37-38, 347, 695-702, 725-733, 851-855
"Black light" - 176, 333-334, 736, 739-742
Blepharospasm - 109
Blink reflex - 222. See Aversion response
Blue-light retinal hazard - 336, 947-958
  Retinal injury - 135-138, 201-207, 336ff, 643-644
    from sun - 201-207
    from lamps - 336ff, 723, 747, 789
    from welding arcs - 551-552, 816-825
Body heat - See Thermal load
Brightness - 2, 56-60
Broad-band sources - 325-343, 439-467
Brow ridge - 66, 197-198, 200
Bruch's Membrane - 76
Building materials (reflectance) - 503

Calibration - 368-375, 376
Calorimetry - 347, 353-359
Carbon arcs - 711-714, 804-809
Carbon dioxide lasers - 148-149, 163-170, 225, 278, 320, 421, 577-581, 609, 614-617, 868-869, 899-900, 908
Cataract - 112-115, 144-147, 210-211. See also Lens (of the eye)
Caution Range - 671-672, 797
Ceilometer - 683
Chemical hazards - 5-6
Choroid - 76
Chromatic aberration - 25, 78-80, 86, 87
Classification (of laser hazards and lasers) - 2, 6, 7, 10, 221-226, 320, 471-473, 596, 973-982
Classification duration - 483-485

Coherence - 51-54
  retinal effects - 635
  spatial - 51-53
  temporal - 54
Collateral radiation - 288, 296
Color temperature - 697-698
Communication lasers - 645-648, 682
Conservation of radiance - 490-491, 763, 769, 792
Construction lasers - 591-608
Controlled areas - 572-573
Control measures (airborne contaminants) - 902-907
Control measures (electrical) - 920-924
Control measures (cryogenics) - 5, 6, 576
Control measures (infrared radiation) - 556-558, 571
Control measures (laser) - 510-516
  for Class 1 - 8, 296-299, 475
  for Class 2 - 8, 296-299
  for Class 3 - 8-9, 296-299, 514-516, 600-604
  for Class 4 - 9, 296-299, 513-514, 563-588, 657-682
  enclosures - 477, 571-575
  interlocks - See Interlocks
  laboratory - 563-588
  switches - 476
Control measures (ultraviolet radiation) - 556-559, 564-565, 733-744
Control measures (hammer) - 999-1001
Construction lasers - 222, 591-598. See also Alignment lasers
Consumer product lasers - 625
Copy machines - 644-655, 744-745, 983-986
Cornea - 4, 67, 68, 104, 106, 109-112, 115, 145, 147-149, 187-188, 199-200, 211, 240-242, 253-254, 505, 886, 896

Subject Index

CRT displays – 746-747
Cryogenic hazards – 909
Cylindrical mirrors – 797-798

Dark adaptation – 91-92, 548
Daylight – 752. See also Sun
Demonstration lasers – 308, 309, 435, 626-641
Dermis # (corium) – 95, 163
Design (hazard avoidance) – 475
Designators target – 655-657
Detectivity – 363-366
Detectors – 353-368
    calibration – 368-372
    quantum – 359-361
    specifications – 361-368
    thermal – 353-359
    UV – 359, 368
    windows – 360
Diagnostic (medical) lasers – 583-585
Diffraction – 29-32
Diffuse reflection – See Reflection, diffuse
Diode arrays – 667-669
Dispersion – 25
Distance measurement laser systems – 598-600, 655
Dye lasers – 43, 313, 320
Dynamic eye protectors – 543, 845

ED – 50-102, 103, 219, 229-232, 245-246, 594. See also Probit analysis
Electrical hazards – 5, 300, 913-927
Electrocution – 5, 915-919
Electromagnetic spectrum – 14-15
Emergency vehicle lights – 779-780
Emission indicator – 297, 301
Emissivity – 34
Emittance – 34
Enclosures – 225, 296-300, 574-575, 612, 630-631
Endoscopy – 577-580
Environmental assessment (wildlife) 684-685

Epidemiological studies – 892, 881, 892-893
Epidermis – 95, 163
Epileptics – 143, 206
Erbium laser – 278
Erythema – 110, 170-176, 188, 328-329, 790, 827
Erythropsia – 137, 207
Eskimos – 200
Exit pupil – See Aperture stop
Explosion hazards – 565-566
Exposure duration – 485-486
Exposure limits (laser) – 217, 226-244, 261-288
Extended sources – 274-277, 477-479
Eye – See also Retina, Cornea, Iris, Aqueous, Lens, Cataract, Vitreous body
    anatomy – 65-76, 947-949
    laser therapy – See Photocoagulators
    optical characteristics – 76-84, 117-128, 145, 947-949, 959
    physiology – 74-93. See also Aqueous, Choroid, Cornea, Lens, Macula lutea, Retina and Vitreous
    refractive power – 76-78
Eye hazards – 1, 4, 101-159, 187-188, 508-510, 521, 583, 947-958. See also Ultraviolet effects of eye, determination of threshold values – 102-103, 217-255
Eye injuries – 886-888
    first aid – 833
    laser – 508-510
    welding – 830-832
Eye movement recorders – 784-786
Eye protectors –
    infrared – 852-854
    laser – 10, 207, 511-512, 521-557, 563, 580, 612, 677, 689, 869, 895
    welding – 841-850

Far field - 53, 385, 765-767, 775
Fiber optics - See Optical fibers
Field-of-view - 317, 373, 464
Filaments - 698-699
Filters - See also Eye protectors
  laser - 494-496, 523-541,
    556-557, 677
  welding - 841-850
Fire hazards - 6, 9, 514, 616,
  906-908
First aid -
  electrical shock - 920-922
  ultraviolet injury - See
    also Welding chap
Flashblindness - 138-140
Flashburns (of the skin) - 146,
  161-162, 167
Flashing lights - 142-143, 206,
  780
Flash distance - 765-771
Flashlamps - 564, 714-716, 749-
  752, 779-780
Flicker, Flicker sickness -
  143, 704, 780
Focussed beam - 406, 409-411
Foundries - 852-853
Fovea centralis - 79, 84, 90,
  103, 684. See also Retina
Frequency doubling - 481
Fresnel reflection - 660-666.
  See Reflection, specular
Fresnel lenses - 764-765, 775,
  779-780

GaAs lasers - 278-291, 314, 320,
  648-653, 667-669, 683
Gaussian beam - 47-51, 391-400,
  406-412
Germicidal lamps - 455, 733-736
Germanium detectors - 360, 364
Glare - 110, 141, 886
  discomfort glare - 141
  disability glare - 141
  sensitivity - 886
  veiling glare - 141
Flassblowers - 138, 144-148

Hazard analysis -
  lamps - 716-733, 772ff
  laser - 471-520, 564, 566-
    568, 652
  projector systems - 763-
    797
  welding arcs - See Welding
    arcs, hazard analysis
Hazard distance - See NOHD
  for lasers - See NOHD
  for searchlights - 768,
    770-786
Heliostats - 791-797
Heat lamps - 164, 702, 755-756,
  781-784
Heat stress - 169-170, 211
Helium-cadmium laser - 315, 320
Helium-neon lasers - 281, 320
High intensity discharge (HID)
  lamps - 705-709, 752-753
Holography - 584-585, 620-621,
  627-628
Hospital lamp sources - 747-749,
  756
Hot spots (laser beams) - 51
Human access - 288, 295, 310
Hyperopia - 78

Ice reflections - 663-665
Image converters - 543-548, 567
Incandescent sources - 38, 135,
  693-757
  general - 38
  lamps - 135, 693ff
  ovens - 755-756
Infrared - 20
  effects upon eye - 101,
    105-106, 144-149, 253-
    254, 341, 669, 755-756,
    850-852
  effects upon skin - 161-170,
    852
  eye movement recorder -
    784-789
  heat gun - 781-784
  IR cataract - 106, 144-147
  protective filters - 536-
    538, 854
  reflection - 491
  sources - 480-481, 685, 702,
    755, 852-853

Subject Index

Infrared radiant heating - 164, 702, 751-753, 755-756, 781-784
Integrating spheres - 371, 463
Interference - See Measurement, pitfalls
Interlocks - 297, 300, 476-511, 513, 572
Inverse-square law - 765-767, 775
Iris (of the eye) - 66-69, 143-144, 887. See also Pupil
Irradiance - 55-58, 422-426, 650-651, 929-934

Key Control - 297, 301, 511, 577

Labels - 303, 304
Lambert's Law - 286, 372, 374, 730
Lamps - 693-761. See also Heat lamps
    arc lamps - 709-711, 721
    fluorescent - 703-705, 718
    gas discharge - 35
    high intensity discharge (HID) - 341, 705-709
    incandescent - 38, 695-703, 718
    light emitting diodes (LED's) - 716
    mercury - 703, 718
    safety standards - 752, 756-757, 760, 761
    sodium, high-pressure - 707-708, 718
    sodium, low pressure - 703, 718
Lamp specifications - 694, 719-723
Laser cane for the blind - 648-653
Lasers - 39ff
    CW - 42
    dye laser - 42, 313, 320
    gas - 42
    hazard classification - See Classification
    modes - 46-49
    mode-locked - 46
    Q-switched - 43, 312
    scanning - See Scanning lasers
    solid-state - 42
    wavelengths - 46, 480-481, 605-606, 961-965
Laser safety officer - 670, 862-866
Lenses - 25, 763-765
Lens (of the eye) - 4, 70-71, 106, 112-117, 119-120, 145, 887, 896
LIDAR - 9, 514, 655, 681-683
Lifeguards - 138, 207
Light emitting diodes (LED's) - 718
Light shows (laser) - 628-640
Limiting apertures - See Aperture stop
Luminance - 58, 60, 123, 929-934
    defined - 56
    of lamps - 134
    of natural surroundings - 210
    of sun - 210
Luminous intensity - 56, 58, 929-934
Luminous efficacy - 56
    of laser wavelengths - 369

Macula lutea - 80, 84
Maintenance - 305, 677-679
Manufacturing lasers - 609-623
Material processing lasers - 101, 609-617
Maximum permissible exposures (MPE) - 226-244. See also Exposure limits
Measurement - See also Photography, Radiometry, Spectro-radiometry, Beam profile measurement
    Beam profile - 392-406
    Compliance - 295, 317
    Illuminance - 723

Irradiance - 296, 723
Luminance - 723
Photometric - 722-724
Pitfalls - 29ff, 375-377, 811
Radiance - 296, 723
Radiant energy - 347-379
Radiant power - 295
Radiometric - 722-724
Rationale - 347-348
Scanning beams - 296
Source size - 462-464
Medical lasers - 308, 576-585
Medical light sources - 747-749
Medical surveillance (medical examinations) - 2, 679, 879-898
    eye examinations - 881-886
        following accidents - 886-888
    medical-legal aspects - 880-881
    rationale - 879-881, 889-890
    standards - 888-893
Medical treatment - See First aid
Melanin - 95-96, 132-137, 143, 169
Mie scattering - 415-419, 421-422
Military lasers - 307
Minimum-inverse-square distance - See Flash distance
Mode locking - 46, 133, 366-368, 481-482
Modulation transfer function (MTF) - 84
Multiple wavelengths - 480-481
Myopia - 78

Near Field - 53, 385, 765-767, 775
Neodymium lasers - 219, 316, 319, 320, 577-579
NOHD (Nominal Ocular Hazard Distance) - 389-391, 430-431, 433, 440-441, 488-489, 657, 670-677, 682, 686-689

Noise equivalent power - 362-363
Noise hazards - 6, 618, 909-911
Non-destructive testing - 620
Non-linear optical effects - 133
Nuclear weapons -
    flashburns - 162
    retinal effects - 117, 140
Numerical aperture - 645-646

Office machines (laser) - 625, 644-645
Operating room light sources - 787-789
Optical fibers - 645-648, 787-789
Ophthalmoscopic examination - 102, 786-787, 881-884, 891
Ophthalmic light sources - 786-789
Optical density - 524-525
Optical viewing instruments - 501-505, 669-670
Optically aided viewing - 501-505, 596-597, 669-670

Paints (reflectance) - 501-502
Palpebral fissure - 109
Photochromic glass - 549-551. See also Welding filters
Photocoagulators - 581-583
Photographic flash lamps - 749-750
Photography - 351, 388-405
    camera - 398-399
    electronic flash - 715
    film characteristics - 402-405, 936
    film plane exposure - 123
    flash bulbs - 749-752
    for beam profile measurement - 369, 400-404
    movie lamps - 774
    streak camera - 367
Photokeratitis (photophthalmia) - 106-112, 200, 328-329, 801, 830-833. See also Ultraviolet, effects on the eye

Photometric terms - 54-60, 694-695, 929-934, 938
Photometry - 54-60, 366, 368, 439
Photons - 15, 17, 34-36
Photophobia - 109
Photopic vision - 54, 86, 90, 525, 533
Photosensitizers - 115-116, 177-179
Photosensitive epileptics - See Epilepsy
Photosensitivity (skin) - 176-179, 486
Phototherapy - 736-742, 748
Planck, Max - See Blackbody radiation
Plasma arcs - 802, 805, 808
Plastics - 556-557
Polarization - 17, 24, 542-543
Precision - 378-379
Premature babies - See Bilirubin lamps
Presbyopia - 70, 78
Printing Plants -
  lasers - 617
  lamps - 744-746
Probability of exposure - 488-489, 679-680
Probit analysis - 103, 227-235
Projection optics - 477-480, 685-689, 763-800
Protective eye wear - See Eye protectors
Protective garments - 521, 557-558, 563, 580, 847
Protective housing - 296, 477-480, 563
Pump lamps - 564-566
Pupil (of the eye) - 69, 117-118, 223, 501-508, 666
Purkinje shift - 86
Pyroelectric detectors - 355-359, 365

Quantum - See Photon

Radiometers - 352-373, 451-456
Radiometry - 54-60, 347-384, 439-469, 929-934
  interference - See Measurement, pitfalls
  irradiance - 17, 225, 349, 439-440, 659
  photographic - 123
  radiance - 57, 123, 427-429, 439-440
  radiant energy - 347-379
  radiant exposure - 57, 349-352, 659, 666-669
  radiant power - 57, 347-379
  terms - 54-60, 350
  See also Spectroradiometry
Radiometric units - 54-60, 292, 347-353, 694-695, 929-934, 937, 939, 942, 944-946
Radium light sources - 714
Raleigh scattering - 415-419
Reciprocity - 108, 110, 173
Rectangular images - 726
Reflection - 21-23, 486-503, 613-614
  diffuse - 21-52, 286, 487, 489-503, 568-571, 639ff, 661
  natural surfaces - 110, 112, 196-199, 661-666
  retroreflection - 492-494, 680
  spectral reflectance - 501-503
  specular (regular) - 21-23, 487-488, 491-498, 509-510, 514, 553, 581-583, 658-668
Refractive index - 23
  of glass -
  of plastics -
  of air - 23
Refraction - 23-25
Remote control connector - 297
Repetitively pulsed lasers - 244-245, 269-270, 273-274, 280, 645-648, 656
Respirators - 904-905
Responsivity - 361-362

Retina – See also Eye, blue light hazard
  anatomy – 71-76
  examination – 887, 894, 896
  fovea – 79, 84, 90, 103, 684, 893-894
  hazard function – 121, 242
  hazards – 3-4, 103-104, 108-109, 201-210, 430-431, 440, 583, 594-595, 642, 644, 668, 792-797
  physiology – 71-76
  retinal burns – 116, 236-242, 252-255, 830-832, 887, 893-895
  retinal image – 77-84, 121-127, 130-131, 203, 233, 241-242, 430, 489-491, 583, 585, 643ff, 666, 668-669, 763, 792-797
  spectral properties – 120-121, 241
  temperature elevation – 128-130
  UV effects – 108-109
Retinal hazard region – 103, 723-729. See also Eye, retinal hazard
Retroreflections – 491-494
Ruby Lasers – 277, 312, 320, 688-689

Safety meters, monitors – 368, 451-456
Safety precautions – See Control measures
Safety Programs – 861-877
Safety standards, laser – 1, 217ff, 261ff, 285ff
  ACGIH – 218, 261, 285, 899
  ANSI – 220-254, 261, 285-287, 473, 593-597, 625-641, 656, 861-862, 881, 888-892
  BRH – 217, 285-322, 473, 576-579, 597, 612, 625, 631-632, 677, 682, 899
  BSI – 218-220, 249, 285
  FDA – See BRH
  Foreign – 248-251, 261, 881
  IEC – 249, 251, 261, 285, 304
  OSHA – 217, 261, 309, 597-598, 612
  States and local – 246-247
  USDHEW – See BRH
  US Air Force – 219-220, 655
  US Army – 218-220, 655
Safety standards, non-laser – 325-345, 756-757
  ACGIH standards – 328-341, 754, 774, 777-779
  ANSI standards – 341, 757
  AMA standards – 328
  blue light – 338-339
  BRH standards – 341, 752-753
  German – 834
  Infrared – 339, 341-342
  Light – 334-341
  Lamps – 341
  NIOSH UV criteria – 328-334
  ultraviolet – 327-334, 752-753
  US Army – 335-338
Scanning lasers – 298, 299, 303, 506-508, 635-639, 641-644, 664-668
Scattering – 32-33
  Rayleigh scattering – 32, 415-420
  Mie scattering – 32, 415-420
  atmospheric – 415-420
Science exhibits – 626-627
Sclera – 76, 993
Scotopic vision – 86, 90-91, 525, 533. See also Dark adaptation
Scotoma – 92, 103, 203, 993
Searchlights – 763-773, 775-779, 786
Service – 305
Shade number, welding goggles – 542, 841-844, 846

Subject Index

Shielding - 555-557
Silicon detectors - 360, 364-366
Skin - 6, 93-97, 161
    anatomy - 93-96
    cancer - 169, 175-176, 192, 833
    erythema - 170-174, 188, 790
    first aid for sunburn - 833
    hazards - 4-6, 161-181, 188-199, 241, 827-828, 904-907
    optical properties - 164-166
    physiology - 94-97
    protection - 552-553
    sensitizing materials - 5, 176-179
    tanning - 174-176, 188, 192-199
    testing - 790
Slide projectors - 780-781
Snow blindness - 109-112, 187, 200, 207-209. See also Ultraviolet effects on the eye and Photokeratitis
Solar furnaces and Solar collectors - 791-798
Solar retinitis - See Sun
Solar simulators - 789-791
Solid angle - 55-59
Speckle - 54, 583-584, 635
Spectral lines - 441-443, 465
Spectral reflectance - See Reflection, spectral
Spectral transmission -
    eye (ocular media) - 89
    filter - 360, 449
    glass - 449, 495
    plastics - 496
    quartz - 360
Spectroradiometry - 369, 439-466
    standards - 369
Standard operating procedures - 573-574, 920
Standards - See Safety standards
Stiles-Crawford Effect - 92-93

Stratum corneum - 95, 162, 174
Stray light - 445-451, 457-462
Streak cameras - 367-368
Surgical lasers - 577-581
Survey forms - 585-588, 958
Surveying lasers - 308
Sun - 207-211. See also Sun simulators
    angular subtense - 202
    direct viewing - 1, 130, 188-207, 548-552, 791-798
    eye hazards - 1, 115-117, 130, 136-138, 187-188, 199-211, 548-553, 791-798
    heat stress - 211, 794
    indirect exposure - 138, 207-211
    skin hazards - 187-198, 552-553, 794-798
    solar (eclipse) retinitis - 188, 201
    solar spectrum - 201, 203-206, 456, 752
    viewing with binoculars - 206-207
Sunglasses - 548-552. See also Eye protective wear
Suntanning - 95, 174-176, 188-192, 199
Surgical light sources - 786-789
System safety - 473-483

Tanning - See Suntanning
Target designators - See Designators, target
Target Designators - 655-657, 681-682
TEA lasers - 278, 899, 910
Telescopes - 501-505, 669-670
Testing -
    eye protection - 538-541
Thermal load and regulation - 97, 793
Thermal injury -
    general - 162
    retina - 116, 128-130, 236-242, 252-255, 887, 893-

895
  rate process — 162
  skin — 162, 793
Thermopiles — 353–355, 365
Thresholds of injury —
  general — 102, 217–255
  eye — 217–255, 594–595
  skin — 161–176
Training — 861–898
  by computer — 872–877
  demonstrations — 867–870
  example program — 866–877
  for Laser Safety Officer —
    865–866
  for management — 864–865
  for operators — 863–864
  lasers for — 680–681
  objectives — 862
  requirements — 865
  source materials — 871
Transmission — 25–26
Tungsten, emissivity of — 33
Turbulons — 427–430

Ultraviolet curing equipment —
  742–744
Ultraviolet radiation —
  CIE bands — 108
  effects on the eye — 4,
    106–116, 187–188, 199–
    201, 210–211, 253–254,
    329, 801, 830–833. See
    also Photokeratitis
  effects on the skin — 110,
    170–180, 329
  exposure limits — 262–264,
    327–334
  from the sun — 188–201
  measurement — 451–461, 813
  reflection — 110, 112, 197–
    199, 501–503
  retinal injury — 108–110,
    947–958
  sources — 180, 188–201, 516,
    564–565, 731–733, 752–
    753, 813–822

Ventilation — 902–903
Ventricular fibrillation — 919

Video display terminals — 746–
  747
Viewing conditions — 494
Viewing optics — 298, 299, 302,
  611–612
Vision —
  dark adaptation — 91–92
  infrared — 87–88
  loss — 102, 134
  photopic (day) — 86–87, 90–
    91
  scotopic (night) — 86–87,
    90–91
  ultraviolet — 87
Visual acuity — 81
  loss — 102
Vitreous body or humor — 145,
  661, 887

Warning signs, labels — 735
Water reflections — 662–664
Water vapor lasers — 318, 320
WBGT Index — 169–170, 342
Welder's flash — See Photokeratitis
Welding arcs — 801–850
  arc shapes — 810, 812
  blue light — 816–821, 825–
    828
  corneal injury — See Photo-
    keratitis
  fumes — 823
  hazard analysis — 85
  infrared radiation — 826,
    829, 840
  luminance — 823–825, 822–
    925
  retinal injury — 830–832
  spectra — 814–815
  temperature profiles —
    809–811
  types of welding — 802–809
  ultraviolet radiation —
    816–822, 824
Welding arc measurements — 455,
  809–827
Welding curtains — 836–841, 849–
  850

Subject Index

Welding filters — 542, 838-850
Welding hazard index — 834-836
Welders — 138, 801
Welder's flash — See Photokeratitis
Whole body exposure — 169
Wildlife, laser hazards to — 684-685
Windows — 494, 496, 556-557, 838

X radiation — 15
    accessible emission limits — 292
    control measures — 909
    sources — 6, 625, 908-909
Xenon-arc flashlamps — 717

Yogurt — 211